Wolff's
HEADACHE
and other head pain

Wolff's
HEADACHE
and other head pain

Seventh Edition

Edited by

STEPHEN D. SILBERSTEIN, M.D., F.A.C.P

Director, Jefferson Headache Center
Professor of Neurology
Thomas Jefferson University School of Medicine
Philadelphia, Pennsylvania

RICHARD B. LIPTON, M.D.

Professor of Neurology, Epidemiology and Social Medicine
Albert Einstein College of Medicine
New York, New York
Chief Science Officer
Innovative Medical Research
Stamford, Connecticut

DONALD J. DALESSIO, M.D.

Consultant in Neurology
Scripps Clinic and Research Foundation
La Jolla, California

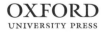

OXFORD
UNIVERSITY PRESS

OXFORD
UNIVERSITY PRESS

Oxford   New York
Athens   Auckland   Bangkok   Bogotá   Buenos Aires   Calcutta
Cape Town   Chennai   Dar es Salaam   Delhi   Florence   Hong Kong   Istanbul
Karachi   Kuala Lumpur   Madrid   Melbourne   Mexico City   Mumbai
Nairobi   Paris   São Paulo   Singapore   Taipei   Tokyo   Toronto   Warsaw

and associated companies in
Berlin   Ibadan

Published by Oxford University Press, Inc.
198 Madison Avenue, New York, New York 10016

Oxford is a registered trademark of Oxford University Press

Library of Congress Cataloging-in-Publication Data
Wolff's headache and other head pain.—7th ed. /
edited by Stephen D. Silberstein, Richard B. Lipton, Donald J. Dalessio.
p. ; cm.   Includes bibliographical references and index.
ISBN 0–19–513518–0
1. Headache.   I. Title: Headache and other head pain.   II. Wolff, Harold G. (Harold George), 1898–   .
III. Silberstein, Stephen D.   IV. Lipton, Richard B.   V. Dalessio, Donald J.
[DNLM: 1. Headache.   2. Headache Disorders.   WL 342 W856 2001]   RB128 .W68 2001
616.8′491—dc21   00–062428

The science of medicine is a rapidly changing field. As new research and clinical experience broaden our knowledge, changes in treatment and drug therapy do occur. The author and the publisher of this work have checked with sources believed to be reliable in their efforts to provide information that is accurate and complete, and in accordance with the standards accepted at the time of publication. However, in light of the possibility of human error or changes in the practice of medicine, neither the author, nor the publisher, nor any other party who has been involved in the preparation or publication of this work warrants that the information contained herein is in every respect accurate or complete. Readers are encouraged to confirm the information contained herein with other reliable sources, and are strongly advised to check the product information sheet provided by the pharmaceutical company for each drug they plan to administer.

1 2 3 4 5 6 7 8 9
Printed in the United States of America
on acid-free paper

To Marsha, Joshua, Aaron, and Irene Silberstein

To Gerald Lipton for his undying confidence that all of us can make a difference

For Leanne

Foreword

I take this opportunity to express my gratitude to Harold G. Wolff and the editors of this seventh edition, for providing the clinical neurological sciences with the "Headache Bible" that has prevailed since publication of the first edition in 1948. Wolff, both a clinician and a systematic investigator, introduced science to the study of headache.

In the Preface to the First Edition, Wolff, pithily capturing the essence of this almost universal symptom, wrote, "Headache may be equally intense, whether its implications are malignant or benign, and though there are few instances in human experience where so much pain may mean so little in terms of tissue injury, failure to separate the ominous from the trivial may cost life or create paralyzing fear." In addition, he stated presciently, "the major cerebral blood vessels are covered by a network of nerve fibers having to do with pain." Decades later, the currently prevailing neurovascular mechanism of migraine replaced Wolff's vasodilatation as the cause of migraine, but his hypothesis remains pragmatically and operationally sound in clinical practice. Although not necessarily mediated by his proposed mechanisms, vasodilating drugs cause headache and abort auras, while vasoconstrictors relieve migraine.

Wolff died in 1962, at the age of 64, shortly after completing the manuscript of the second edition. This edition was published in 1963, and it sparked my early interest in headaches as a neurology resident. Written entirely by Wolff, the second edition contained personal anecdotes that became lost in later editions. One that I remember was a footnote about circus performers standing on their heads to relieve migraine pain. The mechanism, according to Wolff, was the compensatory vasoconstriction required to prevent profound cephalic hyperemia. Indeed, while serving as a neurologist in the U.S. Army after my residency and caring for a patient population that followed orders and was in great physical shape, I often had soldiers with migraine doing head stands in the dispensaries and clinics. The headaches almost always aborted but, unfortunately, returned with great severity when the solders became upright. The Foreword to the Second Edition, written by E. Hugh Luckey, Professor and Chair of Medicine and former Dean at Cornell, described Wolff as convinced that "The pertinent problems in human biology are posed by the sick person." Wolff's motto was "Never a day without its question, its experiment, its observation of man in his environment." To Luckey, Wolff's approach was "holistic," when that term encompassed scholarship and experimentation rather than its contemporary trivialization by practitioners who reject evidence–based medicine.

Don Dalessio, a Wolff trainee at Cornell, took on the task of editing the third (1972) and subsequent editions. Steve Silberstein joined him for the sixth (1993), and Richard Lipton joined them both for this seventh edition.

The fourth edition (1980) was the first to be multiauthored, almost a necessity for a comprehensive text; the fifth (1986) expanded the contributing authors; and the sixth (1993) expanded the discussions of migraine pathophysiology and neuroimaging.

In the interval since the sixth edition, we have witnessed the introduction of the triptans, and enlarged our experience with neuroimaging, both of which are well covered in this edition. The number of contributors has doubled and includes the world's most authoritative experts. Six new chapters have been added, including "Headaches in Children and Adolescents" and "Communicating with the Patient."

Harold Wolff brought "headache" into the modern era, and this seventh edition, shepherded by Dalessio, Lipton, and Silberstein, is a just tribute to the Wolff legacy.

Robert B. Daroff, M.D.

Preface

With this seventh edition, *Wolff's Headache* spans five decades. We hope that this edition remains a vibrant and useful source of information for headache specialists and primary care doctors.

Since the sixth edition, there has been an explosion of new knowledge about headache. The mechanisms of cephalic pain and the genetics of headache are better understood. New treatments have emerged based on the mechanisms of headache. Numerous well designed clinical trials are available using the headache classification system of the International Headache Society.

This edition of *Wolff's Headache* is entirely new. There is a new senior editor (Silberstein) and a new junior editor (Lipton). Dr. Dalessio continues to be involved in the book he has shepherded since the second edition. Dr. Dalessio has added a personal remembrance of Dr. Harold Wolff, a much deserved tribute to the founding author of this work.

We have added new authors to the book and continued its international scope. There is a chapter on migraine genetics, which highlights new discoveries in the molecular genetics of familial hemiplegic migraine. Just as important is a new chapter on patient communication.

We have made a special effort to integrate new data with older, proven observations; still, much remains to be resolved and investigated. As Dr. Wolff observed in the preface to the first edition, "Here is the account as far as it has gone." We hope you will agree that it has gone far indeed.

Philadelphia	SDS
Bronx	RBL
La Jolla	DJD

Acknowledgments

We are indebted to the many individuals who participated in the creation of this volulme. A book, such as this, is the product of many minds and much hard work. We especially thank our contributors and their collaborators for their knowledge, insight, and clear writing as we worked toward a common goal.

Our thanks and appreciation to Lynne Kaiser for her editorial proficiency, to Linda Kelly for her organizational ability, and to them both for their dedication and commitment.

As always, our relationship with our publisher, Oxford University Press, has been outstanding and we are grateful to their excellent staff for their help and guidance.

Contents

IV. SPECIAL TOPICS

Contributors

JAMES U. ADELMAN, M.D.
Director, Headache Wellness Center
Greensboro, North Carolina

ROBERT D. AIKEN, M.D.
Assistant Professor of Neurology
Thomas Jefferson University Hospital
Philadelphia, Pennsylvania

MARIE GERMAINE BOUSSER, M.D.
Professor of Neurology
Lariboisiere Medical Faculty
Paris University
Paris, France

J. KEITH CAMPBELL, M.D.
Emeritus Professor of Neurology
Mayo Medical School and Mayo Clinic
Rochester, Minnesota

DAVID J. CAPOBIANCO, M.D.
Assistant Professor
Mayo Medical School
Mayo Clinic Jacksonville
Jacksonville, Florida

RICHARD J. CASELLI, M.D.
Chair, Department of Neurology
Mayo Clinic Scottsdale
Scottsdale, Arizona

JAMES J. CORBETT, M.D.
McCarty Professor and Chairman,
    Department of Neurology
Professor of Ophthalmology
University of Mississippi Medical Center
Jackson, Mississippi

F. MICHAEL CUTRER, M.D.
Director, The Headache Treatment and
    Research Center
Massachusetts General and Brigham and
    Women's Hospitals
Assistant Professor of Neurology
Harvard Medical School
Boston, Massachusetts

DONALD J. DALESSIO, M.D.
Consultant in Neurology
Scripps Clinic and Research Foundation
La Jolla, California

ROBERT B. DAROFF, M.D.
Professor of Neurology and Associate Dean
Case Western Reserve University School of
    Medicine
Cleveland, Ohio

DAVID W. DODICK, M.D.
Assistant Professor of Neurology
Director of Mayo Headache Center
Co-Director of Cerebrovascular Clinic
Mayo Clinic Scottsdale
Scottsdale Arizona

JOHN G. EDMEADS, M.D., F.R.C.P.C.,
    F.A.C.P.
Professor of Neurology
Sunnybrook and Women's Health Science
    Center
Toronto, Ontario, Canada

RANDOLPH W. EVANS, M.D.
Chief of Neurology
Park Plaza Hospital
Clinical Associate Professor
Department of Neurology
University of Texas at Houston Medical
    School
Houston, Texas

MICHEL D. FERRARI, M.D.
Associate Professor of Neurology
Leiden University Medical Centre
Leiden, The Netherlands

FREDERICK G. FREITAG, D.O.
Associate Director, Diamond Headache
    Clinic
Research and Educational Foundation
Clinical Assistant Professor of Family
    Medicine
Finch University Health Sciences/Chicago
    Medical School
North Chicago, Illinois

PETER J. GOADSBY, M.D., PH.D.
Professor of Clinical Neurology
Institute of Neurology
The National Hospital for Neurology and
    Neurosurgery
Queen Square
London, United Kingdom

JANINE GOOD, M.D.
Associate Professor of Neurology
University of Maryland Hospital
Baltimore, Maryland

STEVEN B. GRAFF-RADFORD, D.D.S.
Director, The Pain Center
Adjunct Associate Professor
UCLA School of Dentistry
Los Angeles, California

JOOST HAAN, M.D.
Professor of Neurology University Hospital
University of Leiden
Leiden, The Netherlands

SANDRA W. HAMELSKY, PH.D., M.P.H.
Medical Director
Bristol-Myers Squibb
Worldwide Consumer Medicines
Hillside, New Jersey

KENNETH A. HOLROYD, PH.D.
Professor of Clinical Health Psychology
Psychology Department
Ohio University
Athens, Ohio

GENE G. HUNDER, M.D.
Emeritus Professor of Medicine
Mayo Clinic
Rochester, Minnesota

STEVEN J. KITTNER, M.D.
Professor of Neurology
Department of Neurology and Department
    of Epidemiology and Preventive Medicine
University of Maryland at Baltimore
Geriatrics Research, Education, and
    Clinical Center
Baltimore Department of Veterans Affairs
    Medical Center
Baltimore, Maryland

GARY L. LIPCHIK, PH.D.
Co-Director, Pain Services
St. Vincent Rehabilitation and Pain Services
St. Vincent's Health Center
Erie, Pennsylvania

RICHARD B. LIPTON, M.D.
Professor of Neurology, Epidemiology and
    Social Medicine
Albert Einstein College of Medicine
New York, New York
Chief Science Officer
Innovative Medical Research
Stamford, Connecticut

TIMOTHY J. MARTIN, M.D.
Associate Professor of Ophthalmology
Wake Forest University School of Medicine
Winston-Salem, North Carolina

BAHRAM MOKRI, M.D.
Consultant in Neurology
Mayo Clinic
Professor of Neurology
Mayo Medical School
Rochester, Minnesota

LAWRENCE C. NEWMAN, M.D.
Assistant Professor of Neurology
Albert Einstein College of Medicine
Director of Headache Institute
St. Luke's Roosevelt Hospital
New York, New York

RUSSELL C. PACKARD, M.D.
Professor of Neuropsychiatry and Behavioral
    Science
Department of Neuropsychiatry
Director, Headache and Concussion Care
    Center
Texas Technical University
Health Sciences Center
Lubbock, Texas

DONALD B. PENZIEN, PH.D.
Associate Professor of Psychiatry and
    Human Behavior
Director, UMC Head Pain Center
University of Mississippi Medical Center
Jackson, Mississippi

NABIH RAMADAN, M.D.
Research Advisor, Eli Lilly & Co.
Adjunct Professor of Neurology
Indiana University School of Medicine
Indianapolis, Indiana

A. DAVID ROTHNER, M.D.
Director Emeritus, Section of Child
    Neurology
Director, Pediatric/Adolescent Headache
    Program
Cleveland Clinic Foundation
Cleveland, Ohio

TODD D. ROZEN, M.D.
Assistant Professor of Neurology
Thomas Jefferson University Hospital
Philadelphia, Pennsylvania

JOEL R. SAPER, M.D.
Director and Founder, Michigan Head Pain
    and Neurologic Institute
Ann Arbor, Michigan
Professor of Neurology
Michigan State University
Lansing, Michigan

AARON L. SHECHTER, B.A.
Jefferson Headache Center
Thomas Jefferson University Hospital
Philadelphia, Pennsylvania

FRED SHEFTELL, M.D.
Director, New England Center for
    Headache
Stamford, Connecticut
Clinical Assistant Professor of Psychiatry
New York Medical College
Valhalla, New York and
National President
American Council for Headache Education
    (ACHE)
Mt. Royal, New Jersey

STEPHEN D. SILBERSTEIN, M.D., F.A.C.P.
Director, Jefferson Headache Center
Professor of Neurology
Thomas Jefferson University School of
    Medicine
Philadelphia, Pennsylvania

SEYMOUR SOLOMON, M.D.
Professor of Neurology
Albert Einstein College of Medicine and
    Montefiore Medical Center
New York, New York

VALERIE SOUTH, R.N.
Chief Operating Officer, World Headache
    Alliance
Oakville, Ontario, Canada

WALTER F. STEWART, PH.D.
Adjunct Assistant Professor
Johns Hopkins University
School of Public Health
Department of Epidemiology
Baltimore, Maryland and
President, Innovative Medical Research
Towson, Maryland

MICHAEL WALL, M.D.
Professor, Ophthalmology and Medicine
Director of Neuro-ophthalmology
University of Iowa and Iowa City VA
    Hospital
Iowa City, Iowa

THOMAS O. WILLCOX, M.D.
Assistant Professor of Otolaryngology
Thomas Jefferson University
Philadelphia, Pennsylvania

PAUL WINNER, D.O.
Premiere Research at Palm Beach
    Headache Center
West Palm Beach, Florida

WILLIAM B. YOUNG, M.D.
Assistant Professor of Neurology
Thomas Jefferson University
Philadelphia, Pennsylvania

I

Introduction

Remembrances of
Dr. Harold G. Wolff

DONALD J. DALESSIO

Who was Harold G. Wolff, M.D., the man after whom this book is named? What sort of man was he? Where did he come from? What drove him? Why are we still quoting his work some 40 years after his death?

Harold Wolff was born in New York City in 1898. The son of an artist, he married an artist. He was educated at the Townsend Harris High School, City College, New York, and then at Harvard University, where he received his M.D. and later his M.A. degrees. At Harvard, he met his teacher and life-long friend, Stanley Cobb, a disciple of Walter B. Cannon. Cobb inspired in Wolff an intense interest in the motivation and purpose of living things and provided him with a solid knowledge of the nervous system. After clinical training at Roosevelt Hospital and the Cornell Clinic in New York City, Wolff returned to Harvard to pursue his research career in the laboratory of Dr. H.S. Forbes, working with Cobb, Lennox, Levine, Talbott, and others on the intricacies of cerebral circulation.

He early became interested in the question "How do the cerebral blood vessels, many of them covered with a network of nerve fibers, participate in migraine headache?" His pursuit of this query eventually led to his exhaustive and methodic study of headache. Wolff himself had occasional migraines; his relentless daily drive for accomplishment, permitting no resting points of satisfaction, epitomized the migraine personality he so vividly documented in hundreds of his patients.

When he was at Phipps Psychiatric Clinic, he collaborated with Horsley Gantt in the study of the conditioned reflex. (Their laboratory dog, Kompa, became famous.) Also while at Phipps, he published the classic study of delirium with Desmond Curran and formed his life-long friendship with Curt Richter. His work with Adolph Meyer, who had also influenced Stanley Cobb, contributed to development of Wolff's unified concept of the mind–body relationship.

He spent a year learning about the neurohumoral transmission of nerve impulses with Nobel Prize winner Otto Loewi in Graz, Austria; and for a briefer time, he enriched his understanding of the conditioned reflex in the laboratory of Ivan Pavlov in Leningrad. He had the tremendous inspiration of working with this great man at about the time of the big flood in the kennels, when Pavlov was forced to revamp his whole concept for the nature of conditioned reflexes to include the disruptive effects of such cataclysmic emotional events.

His study with Stewart Wolf of the famous Tom produced the classic *Human Gastric Function*. When Tom's face blanched, so did his stomach mucosa; and when Tom was hot under his collar and red-faced with anger, his stomach also flushed red. Such changes were no figment of the imagination. Students came, saw, and were convinced that a man's adaptive reactions are critical variables in gastric function.

When the New York Hospital–Cornell Medical Center opened in 1932, Wolff was appointed head of the Department of Neurology. Later, he succeeded to the chair of Foster Kennedy and took charge of the Cornell Neurology Service at Bellevue, as well as at the New York Hospital and Cornell Medical College, where he became Professor of Medicine in Neurology in the 1940s. In the 1950s, when one of his grateful patients created an endowed chair for him as part of her gift of $10 million to the center, he became the first Anne Parrish Titzell Professor of Medicine in Neurology at Cornell.

In the spring of 1933, Harold Wolff pioneered the formal, disciplined bedside teaching of neurology to second-year medical students. He insisted that the proper study of neurology began with a thorough mastering of the neurological examination, which could be learned only at the bedside.

Each year, the second-year class was given an outline of the neurological examination containing 101 questions, which fashioned what Wolff called the "irreducible minimum of information necessary for an understanding of the nervous system." What a daunting experience it was to receive that monograph! Yet those who persevered through it and learned the formal, structured method for writing down their observations knew how to do a neurological examination!

Harold Wolff's published papers numbered 539. His books and monographs written alone or in collaboration totaled 14, including several medical classics in addition to *Human Gastric Function, Stress and Disease, Headache and Other Head Pain, The Nose: Experimental Observations of Human Nasal Function*, and *Pain Sensations and Reactions*. Yet he did not neglect the arts or other activities of life. He was a mountain climber. He listened to music every day of his life and visited some art museum or picture gallery almost every week, usually taking some students and associates with him. Several have said that "the Boss" inspired them to start

their own collections. His daily squash game and, in the warm months, his daily swim in Riverdale, were well known. He ordered his schedule with strict attention to the clock so that he was always on time, always prepared.

For Harold Wolff, there was no day without its experiment. He spent long hours in his laboratories on the sixth floor, well known as the testing ground where pain might be induced, headache brought about, hypnotic suggestions used, anger aroused, or situations of frustration created for the sake of observation. The laboratories were themselves simple, not cluttered with the gear and impedimenta which characterize today's investigative units, for they were made to study people, not animals or molecules or other subunits but functioning human beings.

My introduction to headache and its problems occurred in 1956, when I came down from Yale Medical School in New Haven to intern in medicine at the New York Hospital. A part of that activity was a rotation on the neurology service, where I was first exposed to Dr. H.G. Wolff. To say that I was frightened at presenting cases to Dr. Wolff is to understate the matter. Despite John F. Fulton and the spirit of Harvey Cushing, in his later years, training in clinical neurology at Yale was none too explicit. Perhaps "diaphanous" might be descriptive of that training, or "ephemeral;" it was hardly substantive then.

Dr. Wolff, on the other hand, was at the top of his form, perhaps the most experienced clinical and experimental neurologist in the United States, editor of *Archives of Neurology*, president of the American Neurological Association, and trained by Ivan Pavlov, Otto Loewi, Adolph Meyer, and Stanley Cobb. He carried with him the aura of one who knows, and who knows that he knows. Asked once why he was not board-certified in neurology, he thought for a moment and said, "But who would test me?"

I survived my initial encounters with Dr. Wolff without obvious ego scars and went off to spend my time in the military service, as part of the NATO shield against the Ruskies, and was happily assigned to France and the American Hospital of Paris. Following this elegant European tour, I returned to New York Hospital in the summer of 1959. I began then under Dr. Wolff's service, and it is fair to say that his ratiocinative approach to his work shaped my thinking more than any other single influence. Not only did he direct the course of my work, but I came to know his family, particularly his wife, the noted artist Isabel Bishop, recently deceased. I find myself even now under his tutelage, almost 40 years after his death. During the last two decades, I have revised his book four times for Oxford University Press, established the Harold G. Wolff, M.D., Lecture Award for the American Association of Headache, now in its 33rd year, and given some lectures which he certainly would have given had he survived his 62nd year. For example, a symposium on pain was held in 1978 at the Association for Nervous and Mental Disease in New York; I gave the lecture on headache. Dr. Wolff organized a similar symposium for the Association in 1942 and gave the headache lecture. I found it a particularly poignant moment as I realized this, just before my lecture was to begin.

It was, in fact, on the squash court that I first came to know Dr. Wolff. The telephone would ring and a voice would say, "Dalessio, let's play at four today." There were squash courts at the top of New York Hospital, an eerie place on the 20th floor, where the wind would shriek about the stone battlements. We would meet there and play three rigorous games, and no more. It was during one of these early encounters that Wolff asked me to undertake some studies in migraine with him, and it was then that my interest in the subject and in neurology in general began.

My initial exposure to headache investigations came as the Wolff group was completing their studies on neurokinin, a bradykinin-like material implicated in neurogenic inflammation. I participated in the completion of these studies and then began to work on serotonin and its antagonists at about the time that the Sandoz group produced methysergide. Dr. Wolff seized on this new compound as a method for studying headache, serotonin, and serotonin antagonism; and as a result of these

studies, we became convinced that the drug acted both centrally and peripherally. The current interest in central pain and headache mechanisms was perhaps presaged by some of these investigations published in the early and mid-1960s.

Then, quite suddenly, in 1962 he was gone. He was attending a meeting at the National Institutes of Health when he failed to show up on time, a situation no one could remember happening before. His colleagues were filled with foreboding, went to his hotel, and found Dr. Wolff with a major hemispheric stroke. He was hospitalized but died shortly thereafter. I remember attending his funeral and the wake at his home. The latter was something of a party, as Dr. Wolff would have wanted it to be.

In closing, let me quote from Wolff's presidential address, read at the 86th meeting of the American Neurological Association, Atlantic City, NJ, on June 12, 1961.

It is unprofitable to establish a separate category of illness to be defined as psychosomatic. Rather, man's nervous system is implicated in all categories of disease.

In closing, let me indicate how such a formulation of the intimate involvement of the nervous system in disease may affect the growth and development of neurologic science, and, more particularly, neurologic medicine. It brings to human pathology a unifying concept which gives the teaching of neurologic medicine an even greater importance in the education of all who care for the sick. It could freshen the eye to see the major problems of medicine and challenge the best minds to new feats of exploration. It emphasizes that in pathological reactions in man, his goals, purposes, and aspirations are of the utmost importance. It offers a programmatic basis for the treatment of those aspects of disease that are uniquely human.

REFERENCES

Goodell, H. (1970). The influence on medicine and neurology of Harold G. Wolff, M.D. *Cornell Univ. Med. Coll. Q.* (Spring).

Wolff, H.G. (1961). Man's nervous system and disease. *Arch. Neurol.* 5:235–243, 1961.

2

Overview, Diagnosis, and Classification of Headache

STEPHEN D. SILBERSTEIN
RICHARD B. LIPTON
DONALD J. DALESSIO

Headache is one of the most common medical complaints of civilized humans, yet severe and chronic headaches are only infrequently caused by organic disease. In the United States, in 1 year, most of the population will have a headache and over 5% will seek medical aid; over 1% of physicians' office visits and emergency department visits are primarily for headache (Silberstein and Silberstein, 1990). Most recurrent headaches are symptoms of a chronic primary headache disorder, but ophthalmologic problems, sinusitis, dental disorders, infection, brain tumor, cerebral hemorrhage, and meningitis may all present with headache. Headache pain of benign origin may be intense; headache pain of malignant origin may be mild. Many patients fear that their headache is secondary to a serious medical problem and seek not only pain relief but also reassurance that they do not have a brain tumor or other life-threatening problem. For these reasons, every physician must be knowledgeable in the diagnosis and treatment of headache.

What makes headaches hurt? What are the underlying mechanisms of headache? How can headaches best be classified? These questions, basic to an understanding of headache, are discussed in detail throughout this book. The clinician who appreciates how and why headaches occur will proceed more directly to a specific diagnosis and an appropriate course of therapy.

The key to diagnosis is the history. If the physician thinks "analgesic" as soon as the patient describes headache, little will be accomplished. Pain and associated symptoms are subjective and must be described by the patient. Some patients are not good observers of their own complaints, even when those complaints are chronic. For individuals who have difficulty verbalizing their symptoms, clinicians will need time to take a precise history.

Remember, then, that the diagnosis of headache often depends upon patients' descriptions of their symptoms. It is helpful to discuss this dilemma directly with the patients and advise them that there are no precise clinical tests for many specific pain syndromes, including migraine headache, cluster headache, and the major neuralgias. Diagnostic tests help establish or exclude secondary disorders.

HEADACHE CLASSIFICATION AND THE INTERNATIONAL HEADACHE SOCIETY CRITERIA

Before 1988, the taxonomy of headache was not uniform and diagnostic criteria were rarely based on operational rules. In 1988, the International Headache Society (IHS) instituted a classification system for headache that has become the standard for headache diagnosis and clinical research (Headache Classification Committee of the International Headache Society, 1988). The IHS classification of headache provides operational definitions for all headache types. It divides headaches into two broad categories: the primary headache disorders (categories 1–4), which include migraine, tension-type headache, and cluster headache, and the secondary headache disorders (categories 5–12). We have summarized the new classification in Table 2–1 and the rules for classification in Table 2–2. Tables 2–3 through 2–6 describe migraine without aura, migraine with aura, tension-type headache, and cluster headache, respectively.

An attempt has been made throughout the book to use the IHS classification where it is applicable, although in some chapters the more traditional names for headache or both old and new names are used. In the chapter on chronic daily headache, new terminology is proposed.

How should the IHS classification be used? It is a formidable, 96-page document, albeit a useful one. The classification represents an enormous step forward in the codification of headache. The IHS criteria have been translated into many languages and have been the basis for clinical trials and epidemiologic research since 1990. The criteria are now being revised to make them more useful and inclusive. The IHS classification system diagnoses headache attacks, not disorders. If a patient has more than one type of headache, each type should be diagnosed separately. The IHS criteria were modeled after the DSM-III criteria of the American Psychiatric Association.

The IHS system uses both clinical features and laboratory tests to provide criteria of *inclusion* (features needed to establish a particular diagnosis) and *exclusion* (features that prevent assigning a particular diagnosis). For primary headaches, physical examination and laboratory investigations serve to exclude secondary disorders, or they may provide evidence to support the diagnosis of a secondary headache. Thus, the diagnosis of a primary headache disorder is based on the patient's report of symptoms of previous attacks, and accurate diagnosis requires explicit rules about the required symptom features. Each major category of primary headache has subtypes, which are differentiated based on the symptom profile (migraine with aura vs. migraine without aura), the temporal profile, or the attack frequency (episodic vs. chronic tension-type headache, episodic vs. chronic cluster headache). Details about subtyping are presented in the chapters about each major headache category.

The older classification system divided migraine headaches into two varieties, classic and common migraine. The nomenclature has been changed to reflect the presence or absence of the aura.

Common migraine (Table 2–3) is now called "migraine without aura" and is defined in terms of the duration and quality of the attack. To diagnose migraine without aura, the requirements under each lettered heading in Table 2–3 must be met. Some headings (e.g., Table 2–3A and B) have a single mandatory feature. Other headings include several alternative characteristics. For example, in Table 2–3C, only two of four pain features are required. No single pain feature under heading C is absolutely required for diagnosis. The exclusion criteria are provided under category E. They eliminate other headache disorders based on at least one of the history, physical, and neurologic examinations (E1) or laboratory tests (E2). Alternatively, a secondary headache disorder may be present if the onset of the primary and that of the secondary disorders are separated in time.

Migraine with aura (Table 2–4), formerly classic migraine, is also precisely defined, particularly with respect to the time of the onset and duration of the aura. Types of aura include (1) homonymous visual disturbance, (2) unilateral paresthesias and/or numbness, (3)

Table 2–1 International Headache Society classification system (Headache Classification Committee, 1988)

A. Primary headache disorders	7.5 Headache related to intrathecal injections
1. Migraine	7.6 Intracranial neoplasm
1.1 Migraine without aura	7.7 Headache associated with other
1.2 Migraine with aura	intracranial disorder
1.3 Ophthalmoplegic	8. Headache associated with substances or their
1.4 Retinal migraine	withdrawal
1.5 Childhood periodic syndromes that may	8.1 Headache induced by acute substance use
be precursors to or associated with	or exposure
migraine	8.2 Headache induced by chronic substance
1.6 Complications of migraine	use or exposure
1.7 Migrainous disorder not fulfilling above	8.3 Headache from substance withdrawal
criteria	(acute use)
2. Tension-type headache	8.4 Headache from substance withdrawal
2.1 Episodic	(chronic use)
2.2 Chronic	8.5 Headache associated with substances but
2.3 Headache not fulfilling above criteria	with uncertain mechanism
3. Cluster headache and chronic paroxysmal	9. Headache associated with noncephalic infection
hemicrania	9.1 Viral infection
3.1 Cluster headache	9.2 Bacterial infection
3.1.1 Periodicity undetermined	9.3 Headache related to other infection
3.1.2 Episodic	10. Headache associated with metabolic disorder
3.1.3 Chronic	10.1 Hypoxia
3.2 Chronic paroxysmal hemicrania	10.2 Hypercapnia
3.3 Cluster headache-like disorder not	10.3 Mixed hypoxia and hypercapnia
fulfilling above criteria	10.4 Hypoglycemia
4. Miscellaneous headaches unassociated with	10.5 Dialysis
structural lesion	10.6 Headache related to other metabolic
4.1 Idiopathic stabbing headache	abnormality
4.2 External compression headache	11. Headache or facial pain associated with
4.3 Cold stimulus headache	disorder of cranium, neck, eyes, ears, nose,
4.4 Benign cough headache	sinuses, teeth, mouth, or other facial or cranial
4.5 Benign exertional headache	structures
4.6 Headache associated with sexual activity	11.1 Cranial bone
B. Secondary headache disorders	11.2 Neck
5. Headache associated with head trauma	11.3 Eyes
5.1 Acute posttraumatic headache	11.4 Ears
5.2 Chronic posttraumatic headache	11.5 Nose and sinuses
6. Headache associated with vascular disorders	11.6 Teeth, jaws, and related structures
6.1 Acute ischemic cerebrovascular disease	11.7 Temporomandibular joint disease
6.2 Intracranial hematoma	12. Cranial neuralgias, nerve trunk pain, and
6.3 Subarachnoid hemorrhage	deafferentation pain
6.4 Unruptured vascular malformation	12.1 Persistent (in contrast to tic-like) pain of
6.5 Arteritis	cranial nerve origin
6.6 Carotid or vertebral artery pain	12.2 Trigeminal neuralgia
6.7 Venous thrombosis	12.2.1 Idiopathic trigeminal neuralgia
6.8 Arterial hypertension	12.2.2 Symptomatic trigeminal neuralgia
6.9 Headache associated with other vascular	12.3 Glossopharyngeal neuralgia
disorder	12.4 Nervus intermedius neuralgia
7. Headache associated with nonvascular	12.5 Superior laryngeal neuralgia
intracranial disorder	12.6 Occipital neuralgia
7.1 High cerebrospinal fluid pressure	12.7 Central causes of head and facial pain
7.2 Low cerebrospinal fluid pressure	other than tic douloureux
7.3 Intracranial infection	12.8 Facial pain not fulfilling criteria in groups
7.4 Intracranial sarcoidosis and other	11 or 12
noninfectious inflammatory diseases	13. Headache not classifiable

unilateral weakness, and (4) aphasia or unclassifiable speech difficulty. Most common is the visual aura.

Tension-type headache (Table 2–5) is the term now used to describe what was previously called "tension headache," "muscle contraction headache," "stress headache," or "ordinary headache." In earlier editions of this book, it was called "muscle contraction headache." The new IHS criteria distinguish

Table 2–2 General rules for classification

1. If the patient has more than one headache disorder, all should be diagnosed in the order of importance indicated by the patient.
2. To make a diagnosis, all letter headings of a set of diagnostic criteria must be fulfilled.
3. After each diagnosis, add estimated number of *headache days per year* in brackets.
4. Diagnostic criteria given at the one- or two-digit level must generally be met by the subforms, but exceptions and/or more specific criteria are listed under the subforms.
5. Patients who develop a particular form of headache for the first time in close temporal relation to the onset of one of the disorders listed in groups 5–11 are coded to these groups using the fourth digit to specify the type of headache. A causal relationship is not necessarily indicated however. Preexisting migraine, tension-type headache, or cluster headache aggravated in close temporal relation to one of the disorders listed in groups 5–11 are still coded as migraine, tension-type headache, or cluster headache (groups 1–3). If the number of headache days increases by 100% or more, the aggravating factor may be mentioned in parentheses, but it is not coded.
6. Code to the degree (number of digits) that suits your purpose.
7. If one headache type fits the diagnostic criteria for different categories of headache, code to the first headache category in the classification for which the criteria are fulfilled (1.7, 2.3, and 3.3 are not regarded as diagnoses if the headache also fulfills another diagnosis).
8. If a patient has a form of headache that fulfills one set of diagnostic criteria, similar episodes that do not quite satisfy the criteria also usually occur. This can be due to treatment, lack of ability to remember symptoms exactly, and other factors. Ask the patient to describe a typical untreated attack or an unsuccessfully treated attack, and ascertain that there have been enough of these attacks to establish the diagnosis. Then, estimate the days per year with this type of headache, adding treated attacks and less typical attacks.
9. A major obstacle to an exact diagnosis is reliance on the patient's history to determine whether criteria are met. In less clear cases, have the patient record the attack characteristics prospectively, using a headache diary, before the diagnosis is made.
10. If a fourth digit is to be used in association with a diagnosis at the two-digit level, insert 0 as the third digit.

Source: Headache Classification Committee of the International Headache Society (1988).

between patients with episodic tension-type headache and chronic tension-type headache. The major distinguishing feature is the frequency of the headache, i.e., fewer than 15 headache days per month for episodic tension-type headache or more than 15 headache days per month for chronic tension-type headache. A new chapter deals with the other varieties of chronic daily headache, with a proposed classification system for the following subtypes: chronic daily migraine, chronic tension-type headache, new daily persistent headache, and hemicrania continua.

Cluster headache (Table 2–6) is a disorder that affects predominantly men. Attacks are briefer and more frequent than migraine, are strictly unilateral, and usually occur in clusters that last for weeks (*episodic cluster*). Attacks that occur for more than 1 year without remission or with remissions that last less than 14 days define *chronic cluster*.

Group 4 of the classification (Table 2–1) deals with a variety of headache disorders that are not associated with a structural lesion. Some, like idiopathic stabbing headache, cold stimulus headache, and benign exertional headache, may be part of the migraine syndrome. The remainder of the headache disorders are secondary to, and considered symptomatic of, an organic disorder, although the clinical symptomology may be identical to one of the primary headache disorders. These will be discussed in their individual chapters. The cranial neural-

Table 2–3 Migraine without aura

1.1 Migraine without aura
Diagnostic criteria
A. At least 5 attacks fulfilling B–D
B. Headache lasting 4 to 72 hours (untreated or unsuccessfully treated)
C. Headache has at least two of the following characteristics:
1. Unilateral location
2. Pulsating quality
3. Moderate or severe intensity (inhibits or prohibits daily activities)
4. Aggravation by walking stairs or similar routine physical activity
D. During headache, at least one of the following:
1. Nausea and/or vomiting
2. Photophobia and phonophobia
E. No evidence of organic disease

Source: Headache Classification Committee of the International Headache Society (1988).

Table 2–4 Migraine with aura

1.2 Migraine with aura
Previously used terms: classic migraine; classical migraine; ophthalmic, hemiparesthetic, hemiplegic, or aphasic migraine
Diagnostic criteria
A. At least 2 attacks fulfilling B
B. At least 3 of the following 4 characteristics:
1. One or more fully reversible aura symptoms indicating focal cerebral cortical and/or brain stem dysfunction
2. At least one aura symptom develops gradually over more than 4 minutes or 2 or more symptoms occur in succession
3. No aura symptom lasts more than 60 minutes; if more than one aura symptom is present, accepted duration is proportionally increased
4. Headache follows aura with a free interval of less than 60 minutes (it may also begin before or simultaneously with the aura)
C. No evidence of organic disease

1.2.1 Migraine with typical aura
Diagnostic criteria
A. Fulfills criteria for 1.2, including all four criteria under B
B. One or more aura symptoms of the following types:
1. Homonymous visual disturbance
2. Unilateral paresthesias and/or numbness
3. Unilateral weakness
4. Aphasia or unclassifiable speech difficulty

Source: Headache Classification Committee of the International Headache Society (1988).

gias are considered by themselves in Chapter 23.

HEADACHE DIAGNOSIS

The first task in evaluating a headache patient is to identify or exclude secondary headache based on the history, the general medical examination, and the neurologic examination. If suspicious features are present, diagnostic testing may also be necessary. Once secondary headaches are excluded, the task is to then diagnose one (or more than one) specific primary headache disorder. In the initial eval-

Table 2–5 Tension-type headache

2.1 Episodic tension-type headache (ETTH)
Diagnostic criteria
A. At least 10 previous headache episodes fulfilling criteria B–D. Number of days with such headache <180/year (<15/month)
B. Headache lasting from 30 minutes to 7 days
C. At least 2 of the following pain characteristics:
1. Pressing/tightening (nonpulsating) quality
2. Mild or moderate intensity (may inhibit but does not prohibit activities)
3. Bilateral location
4. No aggravation by walking stairs or similar routine physical activity
D. Both of the following:
1. No nausea or vomiting (anorexia may occur)
2. Photophobia and phonophobia are absent, or one but not the other is present
E. No evidence of organic disease
2.1.1 ETTH associated with disorder of pericranial muscles
Diagnostic criteria
A. Fulfills criteria for ETTH
B. At least one of the following:
1. Increased tenderness of pericranial muscles demonstrated by manual palpation of pressure algometer
2. Increased EMG level of pericranial muscles at rest or during physiological tests

2.1.2 ETTH unassociated with disorder of pericranial muscles
Diagnostic criteria
A. Fulfills critria for ETTH
B. No increased tenderness of pericranial muscles; if studied, EMG of pericranial muscles shows normal levels of activity
2.1.3 Chronic tension-type headache
Diagnostic criteria
A. Average headache frequency 15 days/month (180 days/year) for 6 months, fulfilling criteria B–D
B. At least 2 of the following pain characteristics:
1. Pressing/tightening quality
2. Mild or moderate severity (may inhibit but does not prohibit activities)
3. Bilateral location
4. No aggravation by walking stairs or similar routine physical activity
C. Both of the following:
1. No vomiting
2. No more than one of the following: nausea, photophobia, or phonophobia
D. No evidence of organic disease
2.2.1 Chronic tension-type headache associated with disorder of pericranial muscles
2.2.2 Chronic tension-type headache unassociated with disorder of pericranial muscles

Source: Headache Classification Committee of the International Headache Society (1988).

Table 2–6 Cluster headache

3.1.1 Cluster headache
Diagnostic Criteria
A. At least 5 attacks fulfilling B–D
B. Severe unilateral orbital, supraorbital, and/or temporal pain lasting 15 to 180 minutes, untreated
C. Headache associated with at least one of the following signs, which have to be present on the pain side:
1. Conjunctival injection
2. Lacrimation
3. Nasal congestion
4. Rhinorrhea
5. Forehead and facial sweating
6. Miosis
7. Ptosis
8. Eyelid edema
D. Frequency of attacks: from 1 every other day to 8/day
E. No evidence of organic disease
3.1.2 Episodic cluster headache
Diagnostic criteria
A. Criteria on cluster
B. At least 2 periods of headaches (cluster periods) lasting (untreated patients) from 7 days to 1 year, separated by remissions of at least 14 days
3.1.3 Chronic cluster headache
Diagnostic criteria
A. Criteria on cluster
B. Absence of remission phases for 1 year or more with remissions lasting <14 days

Source: Headache Classification Committee of the International Headache Society (1988).

uation, the experienced physician looks for "headache alarms" that suggest the possibility of a secondary headache disorder.

Headache may arise in a number of metabolic disorders, particularly those that lead eventually to disordered cognitive states. These include, but are not limited to, hypernatremia, hyponatremia, acid-base abnormalities, and liver and kidney failure. Headache is usually a minor symptom in these conditions, which are marked by increasing irritability and weakness, confusion, disorientation, and eventually coma. As cerebral cortical functions deteriorate, headache is no longer a complaint. Exceptions to the rule are as follows:

1. *Hypercapnia*: Some individuals with chronic respiratory failure, primarily those with hypercapnia, will develop severe headache. Marked dilation of cerebral vasculature may occur, and at times papilledema may result.
2. *Acidosis*: Acidosis may be associated with headache. The cause is assumed to be the vasodilation that can occur as cerebral autoregulation is affected by the acidotic state.
3. *Hypoglycemia*: Hypoglycemia is associated with a headache that is usually holocranial and may be steady or throbbing.
4. *Thyroid disease*: Headache occurs particularly with hypothyroidism and generally disappears as the disturbance of metabolic function is corrected.
5. *Parathyroid disease*: A particularly intense form of chronic headache is seen in patients with hyperparathyroidism. Generally, the pain is bilateral, and muscular tenderness may be present. The headache generally improves as the disease is corrected (usually by surgery), but this may take as long as 6 months to accomplish.

HISTORY

Since most headache patients have normal neurologic and physical examinations, the most important tool for making a correct headache diagnosis is a detailed and relevant history (Silberstein, 1992). The headache history also provides an opportunity to establish a rapport that will serve as the basis for an ongoing relationship.

Patients often have more than one type of headache or a change in headache pattern over time. We begin with the headache that is the greatest concern to the patient, the one that motivated the person to seek care. We then explore any other headache patterns and their evolution.

The most common diagnoses are tension-type headache and migraine and associated variants. Headaches provoked by fever and hunger (missed meals) probably rank next in frequency, followed by those due to nasal and paranasal, ear, tooth, and eye disease. The headaches of meningitis, intracranial aneurysm, brain tumor, and brain abscess, though most important and singularly dramatic, are less common.

Age at Onset

Primary headaches often begin in childhood, adolescence, or the second or third decade of life. Headaches that begin after age 50 more frequently have an organic etiology, such as temporal arteritis, cerebrovascular disease, or tumor. Migraine often stops at menopause, but it occasionally starts at that time. Tension-type headaches can begin at any age. Hypnic headache often begins in the elderly.

Location

Is the headache bilateral or unilateral? Unilateral head pain that alternates sides suggests migraine. Cluster headache is almost always unilateral, with the pain centered around the eye, temple, or head.

The headache of migraine can occur anywhere in the head and face, with the most common site being the temple. The headache usually involves either the right or left side of the head, but it may be strictly unilateral or bilateral. The headache of tooth, sinus, or eye disease usually is frontal; but the pain may be referred to the back of the head and neck. Headaches associated with pituitary adenomas and parasellar tumors are often bitemporal.

Localized pain may occur in organic disease. The trigeminal nerve is the major source of innervation to the pain-producing structures in the supratentorial space. Infratentorial pain-producing structures receive innervation from the upper cervical, glossopharyngeal, and vagus nerves. For these reasons, supratentorial lesions often cause frontal headaches, and those situated infratentorially often produce pain in the occipital region, although overlap in the distribution of neurons projecting to the trigeminocervical complex leads to referral outside this strict pattern. When headache is strictly limited to the periorbital region, ocular pathology should be excluded. Trigeminal neuralgia may cause pain in any area of the face that is innervated by the trigeminal nerve.

The headaches of posterior fossa tumors, early in the development of the tumor and before the beginning of general brain displacement, are usually occipital. Headaches from supratentorial tumors, before serious brain displacement occurs, are usually frontal or vertex. If the tumor involves the dura or bone, the headache may be localized to the site of the lesion. Early in the course of the tumor or before general displacement of the brain has occurred, the headache commonly is on the side of the tumor.

Subdural hematoma may produce a headache of considerable intensity, usually localized over or near the site of the lesion, most commonly over the frontoparietal areas. The headache may be chronic, daily but intermittent, and characteristically continuous from the date of injury.

Although tension-type headache may be most intense in the neck, shoulders, and occiput, it can involve the frontal region. These headaches may be unilateral or bilateral.

Disease involving the dome of the diaphragm or the phrenic nerve causes pain high in the shoulder and neck. Myocardial ischemia can cause pain in the lower jaw and cervical occipital junction.

If headache is always on the same side, should one suspect an aneurysm? What does it mean to have a persistent focal headache? Should the patient be studied? Are angiograms indicated?

Focal headaches imply focal disease. The clinician should be alert for local infection, such as sinusitis or inflammation (cranial arteritis), or diseases of the facial organs, including the eyes and nose. He or she should also be concerned about endocrine and metabolic diseases, especially diabetes. However, if the headache is typically migrainous or suggests cluster headache, then it should be accepted as such. Aneurysms are, by and large, nonpainful entities. Angiomas do not often produce pain. Angiomas may rupture, bleed, clot, calcify, provoke seizures, and eventually inhibit learning; but they do not usually hurt.

Many patients with migraine always have their headache on the same side, and there is no requirement that the headache must shift from side to side. This first maxim, then, has produced many unnecessary studies and evoked much needless worry among clinicians. If focal disease is not present, the clinician should accept the persistent repetition of unilateral throbbing head pain as compatible with headache of several types, including migraine and cluster headaches.

Frequency

The frequency and pattern of headache may provide clues to the diagnosis. Cluster headache typically occurs in brief attacks, each lasting 30 to 90 minutes and recurring two to six times a day. Migraine may also occur at sporadic intervals and, thus, can mimic cluster headache. Episodic tension-type headaches occur fewer than 15 times a month; if they are more frequent, they are classified as chronic tension-type headache. Headache patterns may suggest useful preventive strategies. For example, menstrual migraines may respond to perimenstrual nonsteroidal antiinflammatory medications. Nocturnal cluster attacks may be prevented by administering ergotamine at bedtime. Organic headaches may be episodic or daily and continuous. Headaches that are organic in origin do not occur with any set pattern and may mimic the known primary headaches, but if the frequency of headache increases, diagnostic evaluation is needed.

Onset, Duration, Character, and Severity

The severity of the pain and the rapidity of onset and resolution are diagnostically important. We advise using a 1 to 10 scale, where 1 represents minimal discomfort and 10 the most excruciating pain the patient can imagine. While these numbers may not be comparable across patients, they are very useful for charting individual improvements. As most headaches vary in intensity during an attack and across different attacks, it is also useful to inquire about the range of pain experienced during a headache. The pain of cluster headache is described as deep and boring, as if a hot poker were being driven into the eye. The headaches of fever, migraine, hemangiomatous tumors, and arterial hypertension are characteristically throbbing or pulsating in quality. The headaches of

brain tumor and of meningitis, though occasionally pulsating, usually have a steady, aching quality. Tension-type headache is dull, nagging, and persistent and often described as feeling as though a band were wrapped around the head.

The most intense headaches are those associated with malignant hypertension and those due to meningitis, fever, migraine, and ruptured intracranial aneurysm. Beware of the acute-onset, "thunderclap" headache; it may be caused by a subarachnoid hemorrhage. Subarachnoid hemorrhage resulting from a ruptured intracranial aneurysm produces a headache that is sudden in onset, reaches great intensity in a very short time, and may be associated with unconsciousness or feelings of faintness. The onset of pain is soon followed by a stiff neck and blood in the lumbar spinal fluid. The intense headache of meningitis is accompanied by a stiff neck, which prevents passive flexion of the head on the chest, although the spasm of the neck muscles associated with migraine may also inhibit neck flexion.

Headaches associated with brain tumors, brain abscesses, sinus disease, tooth disease, and eye disease are usually only moderately severe. Hemorrhage into the parenchyma of the brain may not cause headache unless the hemorrhage breaks through into the ventricular or subarachnoid space or produces significant brain displacement; then, intense headache may result.

Course

Beware the headache that progressively worsens; it may have an organic cause. The longer the headache has existed in its present form, the more likely it is to be benign. Cluster headache occurs in bouts that last from 1 to 2 weeks or for as long as 4 to 5 months.

Chronologic Features

Migraine headaches typically last 4 to 72 hours but may be as brief as 20 or 30 minutes or last days or, rarely, weeks. The usual headache lasts less than 24 hours. A striking singular feature of migraine is the freedom from headache between prostrating attacks. The headaches of brain tumor are intermittent and vary in intensity but usually occur every day. Tension-type headache may persist for days, weeks, or even years.

Migraine headaches and headaches associated with hypertension frequently occur in the early morning hours, with the patient awakening in pain. Cluster headache commonly occurs after sleep onset. The headache of brain tumor may be more severe in the early part of the day, though not in the early hours of the morning, and may not have any diurnal pattern.

Migraine attacks are common during weekends, during the first period of vacation holidays, and immediately after vacation. Attacks are commonly triggered by menstruation. Migraineurs often have their headaches on specific days of the week.

Migraine headache occurs during periods of increased conflict, tension, or stress for the individual, for example, during early fall for the schoolteacher, during rush or holiday seasons for the merchant, or during very hot or humid weather for those who feel ineffective and prostrated during such climatic states. Headache associated with nasal and paranasal disease is usually more common during periods when upper respiratory infections prevail, namely, the darker months of the year. Exacerbations of tic douloureux are common in the spring and fall, notably March and October. The same may be true for cluster headaches.

Prodromes and Auras

Significant prodromes, such as mood changes or changes in appetite, can occur 1 to 2 days before a migraine headache. Auras such as scintillating scotoma or paresthesias precede and define classic migraine.

Associated Signs and Symptoms

Associated symptoms may occur prior to, concurrent with, or following the headache. Inquire about redness or tearing of the eyes, nasal congestion, nausea, vomiting, teeth grinding, and neck stiffness or tenderness.

Unilateral nasal congestion and tearing are associated with cluster headache. Nausea and vomiting are commonly associated with migraine. Teeth grinding and neck tenderness may be seen with tension-type headache.

Mucous Membrane Injection

Redness and swelling of the mucous membranes of the nose (with or without nosebleeds) and conjunctival injection may occur with migraine. The mucous membrane injection and engorgement may be conspicuous and give rise to headache in those with allergic sensitivities to inhalants and those in whom the nasal mucous membranes are involved during periods of major adaptive difficulties. With the exception of headache due to neoplastic invasion of paranasal structures and antral infection via the dental route, headache associated with disease of the nasal and paranasal sinuses does not occur without obvious congestion of the turbinates and nasal mucous membranes.

Gastrointestinal Disturbances

Anorexia, nausea, and vomiting, though most commonly associated with migraine, may occur with any headache; and the more intense the headache, the more likely these symptoms are to occur. Vomiting without nausea may occur with brain tumors, especially tumors of the posterior fossa. Nausea and vomiting with little or no headache may occur with migraine. Headache associated with sinus or eye disease is seldom associated with vomiting. Although constipation is commonly associated with migraine, diarrhea may also occur. Distention and flatulence are common in migraine and tension-type headaches but are seldom associated with other headaches.

Polyuria

Polyuria is commonly associated with migraine headache; it seldom occurs with other headaches. Tension states with headaches may be linked to urinary frequency.

Signs of Depression and Cognitive Dysfunction

Insomnia, early-morning awakening, fatigue, anorexia, change in libido, and malaise all are signs of depression, which is frequently associated with long-standing headache. Ask about changes in behavior and thinking; check with a family member.

Mood

The wish to retire from people and responsibilities and a dejected, depressed, irritable, or negativistic mental state bordering on prostration or stupor are dominant aspects of the migraine attack and may in some instances be more disturbing than the pain in the head. Apathy, listlessness, or even euphoria may be associated with brain-tumor headache.

Tension-type headache may occur in a tense, irritable person; but the patient is usually willing to accept attention, massage, or medication, in contrast to the patient with a migraine headache attack, who commonly expresses the wish to be left alone. Exaltation or feelings of especial well-being are rare sequels to the migraine headache attack. The suffering experienced with the headache of fever, meningitis, or ruptured aneurysm may be very great; but the mental state is that of reaction to severe pain.

Signs of Neurologic Dysfunction

Signs of neurologic dysfunction include weakness, paresthesia, aphasia, diplopia, visual loss, vertigo, and faintness, which suggest a space-occupying lesion or aneurysm; alternatively, they may be part of the neurologic symptoms of migraine.

Visual Disturbances

Both scintillating scotomata and visual field defects, such as unilateral or homonymous hemianopia, may occur with migraine headaches. Such visual defects may occur with brain-tumor headaches when the tumor is due to a lesion of the occipital lobes or is adjacent to the visual pathways. The visual disturbances of migraine, with the exception of blurred vision and diplopia, usually precede the headache. These phenomena usually last less than 1 hour. Enlarged pupils and lacrimation may cause faulty vision during a migraine headache, but when defects in visual acuity or the field of vision outlast the headache attack, it is likely that a cerebrovascular accident or brain tumor is the cause. Defects in color vision and colored rings around lights may occur with headache associated with glaucoma.

Vertigo and Other Sensory Disturbances

Vertigo may be a forerunner of a migraine headache attack. Vertigo is sometimes associated with the headaches of brain tumors, although feelings of unsteadiness are more common. Fleeting vertigo occurring with sudden movement or rotation of the head often accompanies post-traumatic headache and tension-type headache.

Ménière's (or labyrinthine) syndrome is occasionally associated with headache. Other sensory disturbances, such as paresthesias of the hands and face, may occur as a forerunner of the migraine headache. However, paresthesias that persist during the headache attack or outlast it are more common in patients with brain tumors or epilepsy.

Precipitating Factors

Identifying factors that precipitate or aggravate headache attacks is useful in establishing a diagnosis and implementing a treatment program. Recognizing triggers helps patients avoid precipitants. Alcohol, a newly prescribed drug, bright lights, fatigue, loss of sleep, hypoglycemia, stress, food additives, and certain drugs can provoke migraine. Migraine is often triggered by menstruation and relieved by pregnancy. Exercise or orgasm can trigger a migraine or result in the rupture of an aneurysm. Head trauma can both cause and trigger headache.

Relieving Factors

Identifying the factors that ameliorate the discomfort of the headache and the associated symptoms may provide useful diagnostic and therapeutic information. Migraineurs commonly volunteer that they must retire to a dark quiet room and lie motionless to obtain relief; many patients find that sleep will clear their attacks. Not infrequently, pressing on the superficial temporal artery brings relief but only during the period of compression. Hot or cold compresses are often applied. Cluster-headache patients note that sitting upright, rocking in a chair, pacing to and fro, or engaging in vigorous movement seems to lessen the pain. Tension-type headache may be alleviated by relaxation, rest, or sleep.

Effects of Position and Body Movement

In many instances, migraine is made worse by assuming a horizontal position and is relieved by an erect position. It is often made worse by ascending stairs, moving about rapidly, or lifting. Sitting quietly in an upright position often proves to be most comfortable. The recumbent position may at first intensify the headache associated with nasal and paranasal disease, but subsequently the headache subsides. A sudden change in position, usually from the sitting to the recumbent position, may intensify the headache of brain tumor. Unlike migraine headache, the headache of brain tumor is often worse when the patient is in the upright position. The head-down position aggravates most headaches, except those due to spinal drainage and occasionally those associated with brain tumor.

Straining at stool and coughing increase all but tension-type headache and headaches due to spinal drainage. Sharp flexion or extension of the head often reduces the intensity of post-lumbar puncture headache, whereas jugular compression increases the headache.

A major criterion that can be used in the diagnosis of cluster headache is the patient's behavior during the attack. Pacing, walking, sitting, and rocking are activities that are considered pathognomonic of this disorder. Frantic activity may occur. No other primary headache disorder is associated with such behavior.

Effect of Head Jolt

Headaches known to arise primarily from dilation of pain-sensitive intracranial vessels (i.e., histamine headache, hypoglycemic headache, and the headaches of fever, systemic infection, "hangover," post-lumbar puncture, and the early postconcussive state) or inflammation of pain-sensitive intracranial arteries and veins and their adjacent structures (the headache of meningitis) are particularly sensitive to head jolting. The threshold of jolt headache during these states may be depressed 2.0 to 3.0 g or more. Patients with intracranial masses (i.e., subdural hematoma or brain tumor) usually have a depressed threshold of jolt headache. The location of the headache induced by jolting may indicate the site of the lesion. The threshold of jolt headache may be lowered during a migraine headache.

Headaches not arising from involvement of intracranial structures of the head (i.e., tension-type headache, some migraine headaches, and the headache induced by the injection of hypertonic saline into the temporal muscle) are not significantly intensified by head jolting, and the threshold to jolt headache is not lowered.

Sleep

Migraine usually does not disrupt sleep. Brain tumor, sinus disease, and tension-type headache usually do not interfere with sleep. Complaints of long periods of sleep loss because of headache may be due to coexistent anxiety or depression. The headache of meningitis usually interrupts sleep. Migraine may also occur after periods of excessively prolonged or very deep sleep.

Cluster headache often occurs during rapid-eye-movement (REM) sleep.

Social History

Social factors may play a significant role in headache. The examiner should explore the patient's marital and family status, education, occupation, outside interests, and friendships. Has the patient recently had a major life change, such as marriage, divorce, separation, a new job, retirement, or death in the family? Is work satisfying or merely drudgery? Is there conflict in the workplace? What is the patient's employment? Exposure to drugs or toxins in the workplace may trigger headaches. Carbon monoxide exposure can occur in the workplace or the home due to poor ventilation. Inquire about other habits, such as the use of alcohol, tobacco, caffeine, or illicit drugs. A history of homosexual or bisexual activities should prompt a search for a potential infectious cause of the headache such as human immunodeficiency virus. Sleep habits may be significant. Sleep apnea is not uncommon in middle-aged obese men and may cause morning headache.

Family History

As some headache disorders are familial, it is useful to obtain a family history. Attempt to get a description of the headache and associated features, rather than accepting the patient's diagnosis of the relative's headache. Approximately 50% to 60% of migraineurs have a parent with the disorder, and as many as 80% have at least one first-degree relative with migraine. Cluster headaches rarely occur within the same family. Forty percent of patients with tension-type headaches have family members with similar headaches.

Familial headaches do not necessarily imply a genetic basis, although this seems to be the case in migraine sufferers. Shared environmental exposures may also cause familial headaches. For example, a leaky furnace may cause familial headaches induced by carbon monoxide.

Past Headache History

A history of prescribed medications and their dosages is useful for many reasons. First, treatment response may support a diagnosis. Second, a detailed history may help to explain past treatment failures. Unsuccessful treatment is often the result of incorrect dosing strategies or not allowing enough time to obtain a potential benefit.

The patient's current approach to headache treatment should be reviewed. Many headache sufferers overuse medications, willingly or unwittingly. Many over-the-counter pain relievers contain caffeine with acetaminophen (paracetamol) or aspirin. Excessive use of these agents, as well as narcotics, barbiturates, and ergots, can produce withdrawal or rebound headaches.

Multiplicity

It is not unusual for a patient to have different types of headache. The presence of preexisting migraine does not exclude other, perhaps more ominous, types of headache.

Impact of Headache

Consider the impact of the headache disorder on the patient's life. Patients who have severe disability may require a program of care to improve their lives. Ask patients how headaches affect their lives and what they were hoping for in seeking care. We recommend assessing headache disability using the Migraine Disability Assessment (MIDAS) questionnaire. This questionnaire measures the effect of headache on work or school, household work, and family, social, and leisure activities over the past three months. The 4-point grading system for the MIDAS questionnaire is as follows: Grade 1 (0–5 days) = little or no disability; Grade 2 (6–10 days) = mild disability; Grade 3 (11–20 days) = moderate disability; Grade 4 (21+ days) = severe disability. Grades 3 and 4 define a more disabled group of headache sufferers (Fig. 2–1).

Physical Examination

The physical examination can rule out systemic causes of headache. Include vital signs; examine the heart and lungs; auscultate the

Instructions: Please answer the following questions about ALL your headaches you have had over the past 3 months. Write your answer in the box next to each question. Write "0" if you did not do the activity in the past 3 months.

1. On how many days in the past 3 months did you miss work or school because of your headaches? _____ days
2. How many days in the past 3 months was your productivity at work or school reduced by half or more because of your headaches? (Do not include days you counted in question 1 when you missed work or school) _____ days
3. On how many days in the past 3 months did you not do household work because of your headaches? _____ days
4. How many days in the past 3 months was your productivity in household work reduced by half or more because of your headaches? (Do not include days you counted in question 3 when you missed work or school) _____ days
5. How many days in the past 3 months did you miss family social, or leisure activities because of your headaches? _____ days

MIDAS score   Total days _____

A. On how many days in the past 3 months did you have a headache? (If a headache lasted more than 1 day, count each day.) _____ days

B. On a scale of 0–10 how painful were these headaches? (Where 0 = no pain at all and 10 = pain as bad as it can be) _____

© Innovative Medical Research

Figure 2–1 Migraine Disability Assessment (MIDAS) questionnaire.

eyes, the carotids, and the vertebral arteries for bruits; perform funduscopy; and palpate the structures in and about the face and head (examine the temporomandibular joint for tenderness, decreased motility, asymmetry or clicking). A neurologic examination should be conducted, but the results may be normal even in the presence of intracranial disease. Include mental status (speak to a family member about changes in behavior), cranial nerves (including pupils and eye movements), reflexes, Babinski's sign, motor strength, and any evidence of meningeal irritation, such as neck stiffness or Kernig's or Brudzinski's sign (Edmeads, 1988).

Tenderness

Tenderness over the aching side of the head and of the nasal and paranasal sinuses, the teeth, and the ear may be conspicuous during migraine headache and for some hours there-after. Muscles may become tender to palpation with both migraine and tension-type headaches. Thus, brushing and combing the hair may be a painful experience during or after a migraine headache. Myositis and myalgia may be accompanied by tender areas in the muscles of the head and neck. Percussion of the head may cause pain over or near an underlying brain tumor or subdural hematoma.

Periostitis secondary to mastoiditis or frontal, ethmoid, or sphenoid sinus disease produces moderate to severe pain associated with focal tenderness. If the pain is sufficiently severe and continuous, it may become generalized. The tenderness, or hyperalgesia, associated with mastoid disease with periostitis is far greater than that associated with posterior fossa brain tumor.

Tenderness at the site of a head injury is often associated with a scar and may persist for years. Tender muscles or nodules often occur in parts of the head remote from the site of injury.

Pressure upon the temporal, frontal, supra-orbital, postauricular, occipital, and common carotid arteries often reduces the intensity of migraine headache and headache associated with arterial hypertension. Supporting the head makes any patient with headache feel more comfortable. The pain of tension-type headache may be intensified by firm manipulation of tender muscles or regions of tenderness; however, gentle massage and simple measures of physical therapy, including heat application, frequently will relieve this form of headache.

Ptosis of the eyelid may accompany the headache of brain tumor or a cerebral aneurysm of the circle of Willis, especially if there is a fixed and dilated pupil. Ptosis also occurs with ophthalmoplegic migraine, a symptom complex involving paresis of the muscles supplied by the third cranial nerve and occasionally those supplied by the fourth and sixth cranial nerves. It usually has its onset late in the headache attack, persists for days or weeks, and may be due to edema near or about the affected cranial nerves.

Horner's syndrome occurs with cluster headache. Photophobia, associated with any frontal or vertex headache, is commonly seen in patients with meningitis, migraine, nasal and paranasal disease, eye disease, brain tumor, and tension-type headache. Scleral and conjunctival injection may accompany the photophobia. If the intensity of the pain is very great, lacrimation and sweating of the homolateral forehead and side of the face may also occur.

When headache is associated with papilledema, it is in most instances a result of increased intracranial pressure due to an expanding intracranial mass. However, in patients with brain tumor, headache often occurs without papilledema and papilledema without headache. In the advanced phase of hypertensive encephalopathy, headache and papilledema occur. A subarachnoid hemorrhage from a ruptured aneurysm may cause intense headache without papilledema, but it is occasionally associated with a retinal hemorrhage. Meningitis does not affect the eye grounds except possibly to induce slight suffusion, unless there is increased intracranial pressure (and papilledema). There may be unilateral arterial and venous dilation in eye grounds during a migraine headache.

History After the Initial Visit

On occasion, a diagnosis may not be established on the first visit, or the initial assessment may be incorrect. It is useful to ask the patient to keep a headache diary for both diagnostic and treatment purposes. The frequency, severity, and duration of the headaches are logged, as are the medications and the possible headache triggers. On subsequent visits, reviewing the diary may uncover previously unrecognized patterns that can provide clues to diagnosis. The headache triggers that are identified may suggest behavioral interventions.

EMERGENCY PRESENTATION OF HEADACHE PATIENTS

Headache patients may present as an emergency for various reasons.

Acute Systemic Illness

The patient may have a new headache as the symptom of an acute systemic illness. Diagnosis in these cases is usually not difficult, and treatment is directed toward the underlying illness.

First or Worst Headache

The patient may have an attack of his "first or worst headache" (Edmeads, 1988), with or without a prior history of recurrent headache, or a progressively worsening headache. This presentation may be complicated by focal neurologic signs or symptoms of intractable nausea and vomiting.

"Last Straw" Syndrome

Finally, the headache may be part of a chronic headache disorder that either has failed to respond to the usual treatment or can no longer be tolerated (the "last straw" syndrome) (Edmeads, 1988). Most patients who present to the emergency department with the chief complaint of headache have a primary headache disorder or a systemic illness.

Causes for Concern

The physician should be especially concerned if the patient has any of the following (Silberstein, 1992; Edmeads, 1988): (1) a new-onset headache in a patient over the age of 50; (2) a sudden-onset headache; (3) a headache that is subacute in onset and gets progressively worse over days or weeks; (4) a headache associated with fever, nausea, and vomiting that cannot be explained by a systemic illness; (5) a headache associated with focal neurologic symptoms or signs, such as papilledema, changes in consciousness or cognition (such as difficulty in reading, writing, or thinking), or a stiff neck (other than the typical aura of migraine); (6) no obvious identifiable headache etiology; and (7) a new-onset headache in a patient with cancer or human immunodeficiency virus (Tables 2–7, 2–8).

If a cause for concern exists, neurologic consultation, neuroimaging studies (magnetic resonance imaging or computerized axial tomography), or lumbar puncture may be indicated.

CONCLUSION

Most patients who see a physician for a headache disorder have an acute exacerbation of a recurrent primary headache disorder or a headache associated with an acute febrile illness. However, all headaches should be taken seriously, and a diagnosis based on the new IHS criteria should be made, prior to instituting treatment if possible.

Successful treatment of a patient with headache often depends on the care and sympathy the physician gives. Cures should not be promised. Patience and perseverance on the part of both physician and patient may be necessary. The physician may find that his or her therapeutic suggestions have not achieved the desired result. It is important, then, not to become angry at the patient. Sometimes simple structuring of the environment will help the patient to modify some of his or her life goals. At times, the patient will demand a type of practical office psychotherapy, an informal program directed toward guidance and re-education of his or her emotional responses. With careful attention to the

Table 2–7 Diagnostic alarms in the evaluation of headache disorders

Headache alarm	Differential diagnosis	Possible work-up
Headache begins after age 50	Temporal arteritis, mass lesion	Erythrocyte sedimentation rate, neuroimaging
Sudden-onset headache	Subarachnoid hemorrhage, pituitary apoplexy, bleed into a mass or AVM, mass lesion (especially posterior fossa)	Neuroimaging, lumbar puncture
Accelerating pattern of headaches	Mass lesion, subdural hematoma, medication overuse	Neuroimaging, drug screen
New-onset headache in a patient with cancer or HIV	Meningitis (chronic or carcinomatous), brain abscess (including toxoplasmosis), metastasis	Neuroimaging, lumbar puncture
Headache with systemic illness (fever, stiff neck, rash)	Meningitis, encephalitis, Lyme disease, systemic infection, collagen, vascular disease	Neuroimaging, lumbar puncture, blood tests
Focal neurologic symptoms or signs of disease (other than typical aura)	Mass lesion, AVM, stroke, collagen vascular disease (including APL antibodies)	Neuroimaging, collagen vascular evaluation
Papilledema	Mass lesion, pseudotumor, meningitis	Neuroimaging, lumbar puncture

Key to abbreviations: AVM, arteriovenous malformation; APL, anterior pituitary-like; HIV, human immunodeficiency virus.

Table 2-8 Differential diagnosis of selected headache disorders

Headache type	Age at onset (years)	Location	Duration	Frequency/timing	Severity	Quality	Associated features
Migraine	10–40	Hemicranial	Several hours to 3 days	Variable	Moderate to severe	Throbbing, steady ache	Nausea, vomiting, photo/phono/ osmophobia, scotomata, neurologic deficits
Tension-type	20–50	Bilateral	30 min to 7 days +	Variable	Dull ache may wax/wane	Vise-like, band-like pressure	Generally none
Cluster	15–40	Unilateral peri/ retro-orbital	30–120 min	1–8×/day, nocturnal attacks	Excruciating	Boring, piercing	Ipsilateral conjunctival injection, lacrimation, nasal congestion, rhinorrhea, miosis, facial sweating
Mass lesion	Any	Any	Variable	Intermittent, nocturnal, upon arising	Moderate	Dull steady, throbbing	Vomiting, nuchal rigidity, neurologic deficits
Subarachnoid hemorrhage	Adult	Global, often occipitonuchal	Variable	N.A.	Excruciating	Explosive	Nausea, vomiting, nuchal rigidity, loss of consciousness, neurologic deficits
Trigeminal neuralgia	50–70	More common in 2nd & 3rd than 1st div. of trigeminal nerve	Seconds, occurs in volleys	Paroxysmal	Excruciating	Electric shock-like	Facial trigger points, spasm of facial muscles ipsilaterally (tic)
Giant cell arteritis	>55	Temporal, any region	Intermittent, then continuous	Constant, worse at night?	Variable	Variable	Tender scalp arteries, polymyalgia rheumatica, jaw claudication

whole patient, some resolution of the problem can be achieved in the majority of patients with headache complaints. If the physician suspects a serious thought disorder, psychiatric consultation is mandatory. Headache patients are generally easily treated. Many do not require medical assistance, and those who do usually respond to standard treatments. They are anxious to return to their endeavors and aggravated by the annoyance that headache invariably produces. Of course, there are exceptions, e.g., persons with migraine or cluster headache, or even tension-type headache, who need more careful management of their headache problems. Here again, most patients respond to appropriate therapies, and the vast majority can be helped by a knowledgeable physician.

THE DIFFICULT HEADACHE PATIENT

In 1978, James E. Groves published his now classic paper "Taking Care of the Hateful Patient." He described four classes of patients who might strike dread into a physician's heart but was careful to note that a single patient might encompass more than one of these attributes.

To these four stereotypes, we have added a fifth, called, for lack of a better term, the "day-ruiner." The day-ruiner usually arrives on the office doorstep, notes in hand, prepared to settle in for a prolonged period of intense discussion. Many of these patients appear to have found special comfort in prepaid organizations such as health maintenance organizations, which allow them to visit the physician's office frequently without the pain of paying for the interaction. They are characterized by striking adaptiveness and are capable of turning an ordinary 15-minute visit into an hour-long verbal wrestling match. Furthermore, they are often late but insist on being seen nonetheless, and they are frequently married to persons of similar personality. The day-ruiner is best described as demanding, manipulative, tangential, disorganized (or hyperorganized), frustrating, complaining, litigious, disputatious, and cantankerous. These stereotypes are familiar to most practicing physicians. Like other difficult patients, they sometimes engage in games with headache as the primary complaint, hence, the term "headache games."

A small group of difficult headache patients remains. This is the chronic group, characterized by persisting complaints and resistance to treatment; they are often very difficult to deal with professionally. It is this group that we have characterized and separated into the ten headache games that follow.

Headache Game 1

This is the "You're my last hope, doctor" game: "None of the other doctors I've seen have done me any good. Most of them shouldn't have licenses. All they're interested in is money. They order too many tests. But I know you'll be different, doctor."

Commentary

Do not fall into this trap. Often, this game is played by the person who accompanies the headache patient. Both parties (e.g., husband and wife or patient and child) may contribute. It is unlikely that all previous physicians seen by the patient have been greedy and incompetent. You can be sure that you are next on the list for this form of doctor-bashing.

Solution

Advise the patient that you are not a magician and no miracles are likely to occur. We tell patients that all physicians use the same medications. If you suspect your patient is litigious, be especially careful about criticizing your colleagues. Be helpful, assertive, and supportive; but maintain distance from these patients.

Headache Game 2

This is the "It's my diet" game: "I know it's some food I'm eating. Of course, I've given up most foods, and all I eat now are scallions and broccoli with garlic powder. I never touch sugar, and meat is so bad for you. But

I keep having headaches. Could I have some allergy tests?"

Commentary

We generally advise a healthy diet with regular meals and provide guidance regarding this matter. Although diet may be a provoking factor in migraine, it is important to point out that it is only one factor among many. Eating a rigidly restricted diet is unwise. It tends to reinforce obsessive habit patterns.

Solution

Send the patient for professional nutritional help, or have him or her purchase a cookbook for migraine patients. Alternatively, devise dietary guidelines of your own and instruct the patient in their use. Eating should be one of life's great pleasures. Emphasize that to your patient.

Headache Game 3

This is the "It's my sinuses" game: "I've had my nose fixed and two Caldwell-Lucs and turbinates removed, but I keep having sinus troubles. I can't breathe through my nose, and the pain at the bridge of my nose is awful. It radiates through my ears and down my back out my tailbone. If only I could get my nose and sinuses straightened out, everything would be fine."

Commentary

This is an example of obsessive preoccupation with a single organ system. Although chronic sinusitis can produce chronic headache, the diagnosis is usually readily evident. Given today's modern methods of investigation, there should be no real problem of establishing the diagnosis or excluding it. The pain pattern described here is also bizarre and does not fit anatomic guidelines.

Solution

Once a problem has been thoroughly investigated, one should move on to other etiolo-

gies. Discourage dwelling on a single organ system. Change the topic. Do not abet the situation by agreeing to another consultation, another study, or another operation.

Headache Game 4

This is the "It's my TMJ" game: "And my tongue burns, too. I've been to three dentists, had complete caps, my bite has been reworked, and I almost had both TM joints replaced; but at the last minute I decided against that procedure. My teeth and gums burn all the time, and my mouth is so sore I just can't stand it. Do you think it could be my dental fillings? Should I have another gum biopsy?"

Commentary

Unless you are doubly trained in dentistry, our advice is to deflect questions about temporomandibular joint (TMJ) disease to the dental profession. If patients come to us and say their problem is TMJ, we tell them immediately that they have been referred incorrectly and try to refer them appropriately.

Solution

Our test for TMJ disease is to have the patient open and close the mouth repeatedly. If there is no pain and the mouth capacity is adequate, we look elsewhere for a headache etiology. Magnetic resonance imaging of the TMJ may show degenerative changes, but that is true of almost every joint in the body as one ages. Conservative treatment of this problem is best. Try not to contribute to what may be an oral fixation, often a problem in these patients.

Headache Game 5

This is the "I need Demerol" game: "Now look, doctor, let's get one thing straight. I don't respond to anything but Demerol (or Percodan). I'm allergic to everything else or it doesn't work, so don't give me any nonsteroidal anti-inflammatory drugs, antidepressants, anxiolytics, etc.; and furthermore, I'm resistant to Demerol, so I need big doses, like 200 mg, and maybe repeated once or twice. And I'm not an addict, I know my body."

Commentary

This patient is seeking drugs. Requests for a specific narcotic, a specific dose, should always arouse suspicion. However, addiction implies daily use, with increasing doses to achieve the same effect. Appearing at an emergency room once every several months for an injection is not addiction.

Solution

Other drugs can be employed in this situation and are, in fact, more effective. Both sumatriptan and dihydroergotamine (DHE-45) can be used. If Demerol or another narcotic relieves your patient, it can be employed provided such use does not become a habit. You can always just say no.

Headache Game 6

This is the "Everything is wonderful in my life" game: "I have such terrible headaches and I don't know why. My husband/wife is so understanding, what a saint. My son is Phi Beta Kappa at Harvard, and my daughter just won three gold medals at the Olympics. We live in a beautiful house with plenty of money and I love my Jaguar convertible. And of course we travel constantly, always first class, staying at the best hotels, in season. Do you suppose if something was wrong I'd feel better?"

Commentary

This is the Pollyanna syndrome. Nobody has a perfect life, marriage, or relationship with a spouse and children. Patients like this need to learn that it is normal to have some problems that are difficult to resolve, and they do well in self-help group sessions where they can learn to vocalize deficiencies and gain support from group dynamics.

Solution

These patients are generally more easily managed than some of the other game players. A behavioral consultation may be helpful. Often, biofeedback is useful in this situation. Work with the patient with regular visits and reassurance.

Headache Game 7

This is the "I need alternative medicine" game: "All the doctors keep giving me are tranquilizers and pills. I know it's a hidden infection. I had food allergy testing and turned up positive to *Candida*. I'm on an anti-*Candida* diet, and it isn't easy but I'm sticking to it. I haven't seen any improvement yet, but I know I'm on the right track. I'd like your opinion, doctor, about *Candida*, and do you believe in homeopathy, chelation, and acupressure?"

Commentary

If patients wish to pursue alternatives to mainstream medicine, we do not raise objections. It is important, however, not to put your personal imprimatur on these projects, especially if they turn out to be expensive and unsuccessful. Be honest and give your opinion without becoming overbearing, angry, and dictatorial. Remember, you are not the patient's parent or caretaker, and you are not responsible for another's behavior.

Solution

Always guide your patient in the directions you believe are appropriate. Be specific in your recommendations, rather than providing alternatives and telling the patient "It's your choice." That is the essence of a professional opinion. Try not to become offended if your advice is not followed. A little humility is helpful. None of us has all the answers.

Headache Game 8

This is the "I'm allergic to everything" game: "I've been so weak and fatigued, and the headaches, my God, my head feels like it's splitting with water rushing out and my scalp is on fire and it hurts when I blink. But I found out I'm allergic to light, sound, smell, and touch; and so I'm moving to a colony in the high desert where there's no smog or odors or perfumes, where the air and water are clean and pure, and I'm going to grow everything organically and live like people are supposed to live. I'll show organized medicine. I'll make it all the way back, then I'm going to write a book and be on the Oprah show."

Commentary

Make sure that patients such as this are worked up to rule out endocrine disease, myasthenia, and the like. If that has been done, advise the patient that no disease has been found, and that allergy is not a cause of chronic fatigue. If the patient persists and begins to quote from those who lead the clinical ecology movement, advise that chronic fatigue has been a problem for every generation and was called "the vapors" or neurasthenia or effort syndrome in past years.

Solution

Treat the patient's opinion with courtesy and respect, but do not agree with him or her, especially if you believe that the proposed solution is not correct professionally. Suggest that the patient transfer to the care of another physician with a different outlook. Be honest but firm, and do not argue with the patient.

Headache Game 9

This is the "I need another test" game: "I'm sure there's something the matter, but the doctors can't find it. I've had three CAT scans, three MRIs, a TCI, an LP, and a bone scan, and it's all negative. Have you heard of the magnetoencephalograph? Should I have one of those? I'm going to keep going till I find an answer and I don't care how much it costs Medicare! They owe me. I worked hard for 40 years and always paid my taxes. By the way, do you accept assignment?"

Commentary

This patient is hypochondriacal and believes that a disease is present, despite overwhelming evidence to the contrary. If you follow the patient long enough, of course, the patient will be correct. We are all mortal, and sooner or later a discoverable disease will appear. Furthermore, if patients are covered by third-party insurance or by government funding, the cost of studies is not felt by them, which compounds the problem.

Solution

With newer tests of neurologic function, you may be able to convince these patients that no serious disease is present, particularly by going over the films with them. If this fails and further work-up is demanded, then stand your ground. Although there are no rewards for denying studies, it is still the honorable thing to do if you believe a study is not indicated.

Headache Game 10

This is the "impossible situation" game: "Hey, man, it's two o'clock in the morning and I'm having a terrible headache. I've been barfing since supper. I need a shot, but I don't have any medicine or syringes or needles. Could you call something in to a pharmacy? I don't want to go to an emergency room, either; it costs too much. And I don't know of any pharmacy that's open, and I don't have their telephone number either. I'd sure like some help. Do you have any suggestions? And by the way, before you order anything I need to remind you, in case you have forgotten, that I'm allergic to most medications. What if what you are going to give me doesn't work?"

Commentary

There are impossible situations in medicine, and this is one of them. The patient knows it full well. If, by some miracle, you could relieve all of these complaints, would the patient be happier? Probably not. It is especially disheartening when one hears the last sentence above because the patient, or an enabler, begins to question your plan of treatment before it is even undertaken. Negative thinking of this type is always counterproductive.

Solution

Deferred.

On Prescription Renewals

A final note on problem patients concerns prescription renewals. For the most part, prescriptions are renewed because the patient finds the medication useful and needs more. However, prescription renewals are a legal act and extend the physician–patient contract. Hence, you need to see your patient at reasonable intervals, depending on the drug ordered. This requires a good deal of record keeping, secretarial and clerical help, and overhead for telephone expenses, among others. It is surprising that so few physicians charge for this service. We have never done so.

Here is a partial list of reasons for prescription renewals that we have found either amusing or irritating. (1) My purse (wallet) was stolen, with my medicines. (2) I've lost the prescription. (3) I've switched pharmacies (×2, ×3, ×4). (4) I flushed the medicine down the toilet. (5) My medications all got wet in the rain. (6) My dog (cat, pig) ate the medications. (7) I'm on vacation and left my medications at home. (8) I couldn't reach my regular doctor during the week, so I'm calling you on the weekend (or at 2:00 A.M.). (9) My medications were in my pants, and I laundered them by mistake. (10) My grandmother has used all my medicines, and I didn't even know it. (11) My suppositories have melted. (12) The triplicate prescription has expired. (13) I didn't have your prescription filled when you wrote it, but now I need it.

Are there other guidelines to follow when dealing with difficult patients of these types? Four rules apply.

First, do not dump difficult patients on your colleagues under the guise of consulta-

tion. It is perfectly acceptable to ask for a second opinion, especially regarding management; but this should be done with the expectation that the patient will be returning to you. If you do transfer the patient to a colleague, it is appropriate to call and advise about your problems with the patient. At least then your colleague is forewarned.

Second, do not argue with difficult patients, especially about billing, insurance coverage, and disability status. When possible, pass them along to an ombudsman who is, preferably, not a physician. Many times an ombudsman skilled in interpersonal relationships can resolve issues with courtesy and dispatch and smooth over ruffled feelings, even if only temporarily.

Third, do not become involved physically. This also applies to any sort of sexual liaison. Patients assume physicians are trustworthy, and one simply cannot violate that trust. There is no excuse for placing hands on a patient in other than a professional manner for other than professional reasons.

Fourth, do not become disillusioned. Most patients are not in the above categories. Medicine remains a calling, a service profession, and a worthwhile life pursuit. With attention to courtesy and tactful use of some of the suggestions outlined above, even difficult headache patients can be managed successfully.

REFERENCES

Edmeads, J. (1988). Emergency management of headache. *Headache* 28:675–679.
Groves, I.E. (1978). Taking care of the hateful patient. *N. Eng. J. Med.* 298:883–887.
Headache Classification Committee of the International Headache Society. (1988). Classification and diagnostic criteria for headache disorders, cranial neuralgia, and facial pain. *Cephalalgia* 8:1–96.
Silberstein, S.D. (1992). Evaluation and emergency treatment of headache. *Headache* 32: 396–407.
Silberstein, S.D. and M.M. Silberstein. (1990). New concepts in the pathogenesis of headache. Part II. *Pain Manage.* 3:334–342.

3

Neuroimaging and Other Diagnostic Testing in Headache

RANDOLPH W. EVANS
TODD D. ROZEN
JAMES U. ADELMAN

Most headache disorders can be diagnosed without supplemental testing, utilizing the history and the physical and neurologic examinations. In some cases, however, diagnostic testing is necessary to distinguish primary headaches from those secondary headaches that have similar features. The differential diagnosis for headache is one of the longest in all of medicine, with more than 300 types. In this chapter, we discuss the rationale for performing diagnostic testing and review the use of neuroimaging, electroencephalography, lumbar puncture, and clinical laboratory studies. We also review diagnostic testing in adults and children with migraine who have a normal neurologic examination or who have their first or worst headache. We end the chapter with a review of diagnostic testing in individuals who are over 50 years of age.

REASONS FOR DIAGNOSTIC TESTING

Authorities differ over the indications for diagnostic testing. Saper et al. (1999) state: "In general, we believe that most patients with recurring, frequent headache will require some neurodiagnostic testing." Lance and Goadsby (1998) opine: "Only a small proportion of headache patients require investigation, other than a careful history and physical examination."

Although practice guidelines have been developed (Greenberg and Franklin, 1999), the indications for diagnostic testing vary and the neurologist must make decisions on a case-by-case basis. Clinical situations where neurologists consider diagnostic testing are listed in Table 3–1 (Frishberg, 1997; Silberstein et al., 1998).

There are many other reasons physicians recommend diagnostic testing: faulty cognitive reasoning; the medical decision rule that it is better to impute disease than to risk overlooking it; busy practice conditions, where tests are ordered as a shortcut; patient expectations; financial incentives; professional peer pressure, where recommendations for routine and esoteric tests are expected as a demonstration of competence; medicolegal reasons (Beresford, 1999; Woolf and Kamerow, 1990); and "our stubborn quest for diagnostic certainty" (Kassirer, 1989). The attitudes and demands of patients and families and the practice of defensive medicine are especially important reasons where headaches are concerned. In the era of managed care, equally

Table 3–1 Reasons to consider neuroimaging for headaches

Temporal profile and headache features
  1. The "first or worst" headache (ask about thunderclap headache)
  2. Subacute headache with increasing frequency or severity
  3. A progressive or new daily persistent headache
  4. Chronic daily headache
  5. Headache always on the same side
  6. Headache not responding to treatment
Demographics
  7. New-onset headache in patients who have cancer or who test positive for human immunodeficiency virus
  8. New-onset headache after age 50
  9. Patients with headache and seizures
Associated symptoms and signs
  10. Headache associated with symptoms and signs such as fever, stiff neck, nausea, and vomiting
  11. Headaches other than migraine with aura associated with focal neurologic symptoms or signs
  12. Headaches associated with papilledema, cognitive impairment, or personality change

Reproduced with permission from Evans, R.W. (1999). Headaches. In *Diagnostic Testing in Neurology* (R.W. Evans, ed.), p. 2. W.B. Saunders, Philadelphia.

compelling reasons for not ordering diagnostic studies include physician fears of deselection and at-risk capitation. Lack of funds and underinsurance continue to be barriers to appropriate diagnostic testing for many patients.

DIAGNOSTIC TESTING OPTIONS

Computed Tomography versus Magnetic Resonance Imaging

Computed tomography (CT) will detect most, but not all, abnormalities that can cause headache. It is generally preferable to magnetic resonance imaging (MRI) for the evaluation of acute subarachnoid hemorrhage (SAH), acute head trauma, and bony abnormalities. However, a number of disorders may be missed on routine CT of the head; these include vascular disease, neoplastic disease, cervicomedullary lesions, and infections (Table 3–2). The technique of MRI is more sensitive than CT for detecting posterior fossa and cervicomedullary lesions, ischemia, white

matter abnormalities (WMA), cerebral venous thrombosis, subdural and epidural hematomas, neoplasms (especially in the posterior fossa), meningeal disease [such as carcinomatosis, diffuse meningeal enhancement in low cerebrospinal fluid (CSF) pressure syndrome, and sarcoid], cerebritis, and brain abscess. Pituitary pathology is more likely to be detected on a routine MRI of the brain than on a routine CT.

Despite higher cost, MRI is generally preferred to CT for the evaluation of headaches. The yield of MRI may vary depending on the field strength of the magnet, the use of paramagnetic contrast, the selection of acquisition sequences, and the use of magnetic resonance angiography (as discussed later in this chapter) and venography. However, MRI may be contraindicated for some patients (e.g., those who have an aneurysm clip or pacemaker). In addition, about 8% of patients are claustrophobic, and about 2% are so claustrophobic that they cannot tolerate the study. Open MRI machines with improved image quality may help in this situation.

Table 3–2 Causes of headache that can be missed on routine computed tomographic scan of the head

Vascular disease
  Saccular aneurysms
  Arteriovenous malformations (especially posterior fossa)
  Subarachnoid hemorrhage
  Carotid or vertebral artery dissections
  Cerebral infarctions
  Cerebral venous thrombosis
  Vasculitis
  Subdural and epidural hematomas
Neoplastic disease
  Neoplasms (especially in the posterior fossa)
  Meningeal carcinomatosis
  Pituitary tumor and hemorrhage
Cervicomedullary lesions
  Chiari malformations
  Foramen magnum tumors
Infections
  Paranasal sinusitis
  Meningoencephalitis
  Cerebritis and brain abscess

Reproduced with permission from Evans, R.W. (1999). Headaches. In *Diagnostic Testing in Neurology* (R.W. Evans, ed.), p. 3. W.B. Saunders, Philadelphia.

Neuroimaging During Pregnancy

When there are appropriate indications, neuroimaging should be performed during pregnancy. A radiation dose of >15 rad is necessary to result in deformities that might justify pregnancy termination; however, with the use of lead shielding, a standard CT scan of the head exposes the fetus to <1 mrad. Magnetic resonance imaging is more sensitive for rare disorders that may occur during pregnancy, such as pituitary apoplexy, metastatic choriocarcinoma, and cerebral venous sinus thrombosis (in which case magnetic resonance venography should be added). It carries no known risk during pregnancy, but there is some disagreement about this because the magnets induce an electric field and slightly raise the core temperature (<1°C). Although there is no known risk of intravenous contrast for CT scan or gadolinium for MRI, contrast should be avoided if possible. The radiation dose for a typical cervical or intracranial arteriogram is <1 mrad.

Electroencephalography

In the pre-CT scan era, the electroencephalogram (EEG) was a standard test for evaluating headaches. Gronseth and Greenberg (1995) reviewed the literature that was published between 1941 and 1994 on the utility of EEG in the evaluation of patients with headache. Most of the articles had serious methodologic flaws, including referral bias, poor controls, nonblinded evaluations, and use of outdated criteria for normal EEG patterns. The only significant abnormality reported in studies with a relatively nonflawed design was prominent driving in response to photic stimulation (the "H response") in migraineurs, with a sensitivity ranging from 26% (Rowan, 1974) to 100% (Simon et al., 1982) and a specificity from 80% (Smyth and Winter, 1964) to 91% (Simon et al., 1982) (Fig. 3–1). This finding, while interesting, is not necessary for the clinical diagnosis of migraine. If the purpose of the EEG is to exclude an underlying structural lesion such as a neoplasm, CT or MRI is superior.

The report of the Quality Standards Subcommittee of the American Academy of Neurology (AAN) (1995) suggests the following practice parameter: "The electroencephalogram (EEG) is not useful in the routine evaluation of patients with headache. This does not exclude the use of EEG to evaluate head-

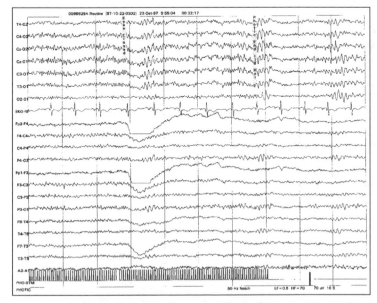

Figure 3–1 H response. (Reprinted from Silberstein, S.D., Lipton, R.B., and P.J. Goadsby (eds.) (1998). Diagnostic Testing and Ominous Causes of Headache. In *Headache in Clinical Practice* pp. 31–40. Isis Medical Media, Oxford.)

ache patients with associated symptoms suggesting a seizure disorder such as atypical migrainous aura or episodic loss of consciousness. Assuming head imaging capabilities are readily available, EEG is not recommended to exclude a structural cause for headache."

Lumbar Puncture

An MRI or CT scan is usually performed before a lumbar puncture, except when acute meningitis is suspected. Lumbar puncture can be diagnostic for meningitis or encephalitis, meningeal carcinomatosis or lymphomatosis, SAH, and high (i.e., pseudotumor cerebri) or low CSF pressure. When patients have blood dyscrasias, the platelet count should be 50,000 or greater before performing the lumbar puncture. The CSF opening pressure should always be measured when investigating headaches. The measurement should be taken while the patient is in a lateral decubitis position. When measuring the opening pressure, it is important for the patient to relax and at least partially extend the head and legs, to avoid recording a falsely elevated pressure.

A lumbar puncture is indicated when the headache is the first or worst of the patient's life, is accompanied by fever or other symptoms or signs that suggest an infectious cause, is subacute or progressive [in human immunodeficiency virus (HIV)-positive patient or a person with carcinoma], or is atypical.

There are numerous potential complications of lumbar puncture. The most common is a low CSF pressure headache or a postlumbar puncture headache, which occurs about 30% of the time when the conventional bevel-tipped or Quincke needle is used (Evans, 1998). The risk of headache can be dramatically reduced to about 5% by using an atraumatic needle, such as the Sprotte needle, and replacing the stylet before withdrawing the needle (Evans, 2000).

Clinical Laboratory Studies

Clinical laboratory studies are generally not helpful in diagnosing headaches. However, they are indicated at times, as in the following

instances: erythrocyte sedimentation rate or C-reactive protein to diagnose temporal arteritis; erythrocyte sedimentation rate, rheumatoid factor, and ANA in a patient with headaches and arthralgias to diagnose collagen vascular disease such as lupus (Amit et al., 1999); a mononucleosis spot in a teenager with headaches, sore throat, and cervical adenopathy; complete blood count (CBC), liver function tests, HIV test, or Lyme antibody in a patient with a suspected infection or a treatment-refractory chronic daily headache; an anticardiolipin antibody and lupus anticoagulant in a migraineur with extensive WMA on MRI or a prolonged aura (looking for an underlying coagulopathy); thyroid-stimulating hormone since headache may be a symptom in 14% of cases of hypothyroidism and hyperthyroidism is a contraindication for ergotamine therapy; a CBC since headache may be a symptom of anemia (headache typically occurs when the hemoglobin concentration is reduced by one-half or more); blood urea nitrogen and creatinine to exclude renal failure, which can cause headache; serum calcium since hypercalcemia can be associated with headaches; a CBC and platelet count because thrombotic thrombocytopenic purpura can cause headaches; and endocrine studies in a patient with headaches and a pituitary tumor.

Additionally, clinical laboratory studies may be indicated as a baseline and for monitoring certain medications, such as valproic acid for migraine prophylaxis, carbamazepine for trigeminal neuralgia, and lithium for chronic cluster headaches. Drug levels can also monitor patient compliance.

HEADACHES AND A NORMAL NEUROLOGIC EXAMINATION

Neuroimaging Studies in Adults

The yield of abnormal neuroimaging in studies of patients with headaches as the only neurologic symptom and normal neurologic examinations depends on a number of factors, including the duration of the headache, the study design (prospective vs. retrospective), who orders the scan, and the type of scan performed (Frishberg, 1994). The percentage of abnormal scans is higher when ordered by neurologists (Baker, 1983) or physicians at a tertiary care center (Laffey et al., 1978) than when ordered by primary care physicians. This represents case selection bias. In reported CT scan series, the yield varies depending on the generation of the scanner and whether iodinated contrast was used. The yield of MRI varies depending on the field strength of the magnet, the use of paramagnetic contrast, the selection of acquisition sequences, and the use of magnetic resonance angiography.

Frishberg (1994) reviewed eight CT scan studies of 1,825 patients with unspecified headache types and varying durations (Baker, 1983; Carrera et al., 1977; Laffey et al., 1978; Larson et al., 1980; Mitchell et al., 1993; Russell et al., 1978; Sargent et al., 1979; Weingarten et al., 1992). The summarized findings from these studies were combined with those from four additional studies of 1,566 CT scans in patients with headache and normal neurologic examinations (Akpek et al., 1995; Demaerel et al., 1996; Dumas et al., 1994; Sotaniemi et al., 1991) for a total of 3,389 scans. The overall percentages of various pathologies were as follows: brain tumors, 1%; arteriovenous malformations, 0.2%; hydrocephalus, 0.3%; aneurysm, 0.1%; subdural hematoma, 0.2%; and strokes (including chronic ischemic process), 1.1%. The studies cited did not give information about the detection of paranasal sinus disease, which may be the cause of some headaches.

Four studies of patients with chronic headaches and a normal neurologic examination have been done. In three of these studies combined, for a total of 1,282 patients, the only clinically significant pathology was one low-grade glioma and one saccular aneurysm (Akpek et al., 1995; Dumas et al., 1994; Weingarten et al., 1992). However, a fourth study, of 363 consecutive CT scans, found significant pathology in 11 (3%), including two intraventricular cysts, four meningiomas, and five malignant neoplasms (Demaerel et al., 1996).

Weingarten et al. (1992) extrapolated various data from a health maintenance organization of 100,800 adult patients. The estimated prevalence (in patients with chronic headache and a normal neurologic examination) of a CT scan demonstrating an abnormality requiring neurosurgical intervention may have been as low as 0.01%. It is not certain whether detecting additional pathology on MRI scan would change this percentage. For example, complaints of headache with a normal neurologic examination may be seen in patients with type I Arnold-Chiari malformation, which is easily detected on MRI, but not CT, scans (Khurana, 1991). Pituitary hemorrhage can produce a migraine-like acute headache (thunderclap headache) with a normal neurologic examination (Evans, 1997). Pituitary infarction, with severe headache, photophobia, and CSF pleocytosis, can initially be quite similar to aseptic meningitis or meningoencephalitis (Embil et al., 1997). Pituitary pathology is more likely to be detected on an MRI than a CT scan (Fig. 3–2).

Neuroimaging in Children

Five studies have investigated neuroimaging in children with headaches. Dooley et al. (1990) reported the retrospective findings on CT scans of 41 children who had headaches and normal neurologic examinations and were referred to a secondary or tertiary care facility. Only one scan was abnormal, demonstrating a choroid plexus papilloma. Chu and Shinnar (1992) obtained brain-imaging studies in 30 children 7 years of age or younger who had headaches and were referred to pediatric neurologists. The studies were normal (except for five that had incidental findings). Maytal et al. (1996) obtained MRI or CT scans or both for 78 children who were 3 to 18 years of age and had headaches. With the exception of six patients, the neurologic examinations were normal. The studies were normal except for incidental cerebral abnormalities in four children and mucoperiosteal thickening of the paranasal sinuses in seven.

Wöber-Bingöl and colleagues (1996) prospectively obtained MRI scans of 96 children, 5 to 18 years of age, who had headaches and normal neurologic examinations and were re-

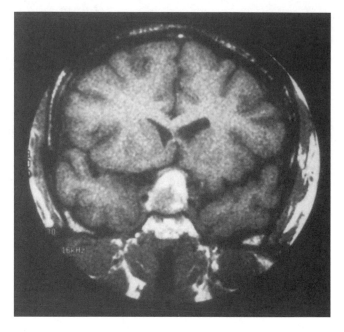

Figure 3–2 Magnetic resonance imaging pituitary apoplexy.

ferred to an outpatient headache clinic. The studies were normal except for 17 (17.7%) that revealed incidental findings. Finally, Medina et al. (1997) retrospectively reported MRI findings on 315 children who were 3 to 20 years of age (mean 11 years) and had headaches. Neurologic examinations were abnormal for 89 patients. Thirteen (4%) had surgical space-occupying lesions. After analyzing risk factors for these lesions as well as the prior literature, the authors suggested guidelines for neuroimaging in children with headache (Table 3–3).

Carlos et al. (2000), by retrospectively reviewing charts, identified all pediatric migraine patients who had had a CT or MRI to investigate their headaches. Ages ranged from 3 to 18 years. Of 194 charts reviewed, 93 patients (48%) had neuroimaging. Thirty-five patients had CT, 14 had MRI, and 9 had both. Reasons for imaging included age younger than 5 years, an atypical headache pattern, an abnormal neurologic examination, focal symptoms or signs during the headache, or parent/physician concerns of an intracranial mass lesion. Twenty-two patients had abnormalities on imaging (known previous abnormality, sinus disease, arachnoid cyst, asymmetry of ventricles, white matter lesions), but none was felt to be related to the

patients' headaches. The authors concluded that neuroimaging has limited value in evaluating pediatric patients with migraine.

American Academy of Neurology Practice Guideline

A report of the Quality Standards Subcommittee of the AAN entitled "The utility of neuroimaging in the evaluation of headache in patients with normal neurologic examina-

Table 3–3 Reasons to consider neuroimaging for children with headaches

1. Persistent headaches of less than 6 months duration that do not respond to medical treatment
2. Headaches associated with abnormal neurologic findings, especially if accompanied by papilledema, nystagmus, or gait or motor abnormalities
3. Persistent headaches associated with an absent family history of migraine
4. Persistent headaches associated with substantial episodes of confusion, disorientation, or emesis
5. Headaches that awaken a child repeatedly from sleep or occur immediately upon awakening
6. Family history or medical history of disorders that may predispose one to central nervous system lesions and clinical or laboratory findings suggestive of central nervous system involvement

Data from Medina, S., J.D. Pinter, D. Zurakowski et al. (1997). Children with headache: clinical predictors of surgical space-occupying lesions and the role of neuroimaging. *Radiology* 202: 819–824.

tions" (1994) stated that there is moderate clinical certainty to support the following statement: "At this time, there is insufficient evidence to define the role of CT and MRI in the evaluation of patients with headaches that are not consistent with migraine." Recommendations for future research included large prospective studies to define the clinical characteristics of chronic headaches which would help identify those patients at higher risk for intracranial disease and evaluating the role of repeated neuroimaging in patients with previously negative studies.

Risk/Benefit and Cost/Benefit of Neuroimaging

Table 3–4 summarizes the estimated risks and benefits of neuroimaging in patients with headaches and normal neurologic examinations. Although for many patients the scan helps to relieve anxiety, for others the scan may produce anxiety when nonspecific abnormalities, such as incidental anatomical variants or white matter lesions, are found.

NEUROIMAGING IN MIGRAINE

Incidence of Pathology

Frishberg (1994) reviewed four CT scan studies (Cala and Mastaglia, 1976; Cuetter and Aita, 1983; Hungerford et al., 1976; Masland et al., 1978), four MRI scan studies (Igarashi et al., 1991; Jacome and Leborgne, 1990; Osborn et al., 1991; Soges et al., 1988), and one combined MRI and CT scan study (Kuhn and Sheklar, 1990), for a total of 897 scans of patients with migraine. These findings were combined with more recent reports of one CT scan study of 284 patients (Dumas et al., 1994) and six studies of MRI scans of 444 patients (Cooney et al., 1996; de Benedittis et al., 1995; Fazekas et al., 1992; Pavese et al., 1994; Robbins and Friedman, 1992; Ziegler et al., 1991), for a total of 1,625 scans of patients with various types of migraine. Other than WMA, the studies showed no significant pathology except for four brain tumors (three of which were incidental findings) and one

arteriovenous malformation (in a patient with migraine and a seizure disorder).

White Matter Abnormalities

Twelve MRI studies have investigated WMA on scans of migraine patients. White matter abnormalities are foci of hyperintensity on both proton density and T2-weighted images in the deep and periventricular white matter, possibly due to interstitial edema, ischemia, perivascular demyelination, or gliosis. White matter abnormalities are easily detected on MRI but rarely seen on CT scan (Kuhn and Shekar, 1990) (Fig. 3–3).

The percentages of WMA for all types of migraine range from 12% (Osborn et al., 1991) to 46% (Soges et al., 1988). Such abnormalities have been reported as both more frequent (De Benedittis et al., 1995; Igarashi et al., 1991) and no more frequent (Pavese et al., 1994) in the frontal region of the centrum semiovale than in the white matter of the parietal, temporal, and occipital lobes. Five of the six studies that used controls found a higher incidence of WMA in migraineurs. The incidence of WMA in controls ranged from 2% (Pavese et al., 1994) to 14% (Fazekas et al., 1992). One small study reported a similar incidence of WMA in patients with tension-type headaches (34.3%) and those with migraine (32.1%), greater than the 7.4% in controls (De Benedittis et al., 1995).

Four studies comparing migraine with aura to migraine without aura (Cooney et al., 1996; De Benedittis et al., 1995; Pavese et al., 1994; Prager et al., 1991) found similar percentages of WMA, while two reported a higher percentage of WMA in migraine with aura (Fazekas et al., 1992; Igarashi et al., 1991). Three small studies found WMA in 17% of basilar migraine patients (Cooney et al., 1996; Jacome and Leborgne, 1990) and 38% (Fazekas et al., 1992). White matter abnormalities are variably reported as being more often present in adult migraineurs between the ages of 40 and 60 years (Cooney et al., 1996; Prager et al., 1991) and equally present (Fazekas et al., 1992) compared with those 40 years of age or younger. Cooney et al. (1996) found an increased frequency of WMA associated with age over 50 and with medical risk factors (hypertension, atherosclerotic heart disease, diabetic mellitus, autoimmune disorder, or demyelinating disease) but not with gender, migraine subtype, or duration of migraine symptoms.

Most migraineurs never develop changes on MRI. White matter lesions in migraineurs are preferentially located in the centrum semiovale and frontal subcortical white matter in individuals less than 40 years of age and involve the deep white matter at the level of the basal ganglia in migraineurs past the age of 40. The lesions correlate with increasing age but not with migraine subtype, headache frequency, or duration. The T2 lesions may not be specific or directly related to migraine. The same incidence of white matter lesions occurs in tension-type and migraine patients (De Benedittis et al., 1995).

While the cause of WMA in migraine is not certain, various hypotheses have been advanced, including increased platelet aggregability with microemboli, abnormal cerebrovascular regulation, and repeated attacks of hypoperfusion during the aura (De Benedittis et al., 1995; Igarashi et al., 1991; Pavese et al., 1994). Antiphospholipid antibodies might be another risk factor for WMA in migraine (Tietjen, 1992). The reported incidence of

antiphospholipid antibodies in migraine ranges from 0% (Hering et al., 1991) to 24% (Robbins, 1991). In one MRI study, however, the presence of WMA showed no correlation with the presence of anticardiolipin antibodies (Igarashi et al., 1991). The presence of anticardiolipin antibodies is not an additional risk factor for stroke in migraineurs (Daras et al., 1995). Tietjen et al. (1998) found that there was no increase in frequency of anticardiolipin positivity in adults under 60 years of age with transient focal neurologic events or in those with migraine with or without aura compared to control subjects.

A subgroup of migraineurs may have a genetic predisposition for white matter lesions on MRI scans. Cerebral autosomal dominant arteriopathy with subcortical infarcts and leukoencephalopathy (CADASIL) is a familial genetic disease with migraine as a common symptom and severe WMA on MRI as a consistent neuroimaging finding (Fig. 3–4). Chabriat et al. (1995) described several members of a family with an autosomal dominant illness manifested by migraine attacks and a significant leukoencephalopathy on MRI but without other specific manifestations of CADASIL. It is possible that there is a specific gene locus for migraine with white matter changes. Variable gene penetrance could

Table 3–4 Computed tomography (CT, with intravenous contrast) or magnetic resonance imaging (MRI, without contrast) in patients with headache and normal neurologic examinations

	CT	MRI	No test
Health outcomes			
Benefits			
Discovery of potentially treatable lesions			
Migraine	0.3%	0.4%	0
Any headache	2.4%	2.4%	0
Relief of anxiety	30%	30%	0
Harms			
Iodine reaction			
Mild	10%		
Moderate	1%		
Severe	0.01%		
Death	0.002%		
Claustrophobia			
Mild	5%	15%	0
Moderate (needs sedation)	1%	5–10%	
Severe (unable to comply)	1%–2%		
False-positive studies	No data	No data	
Cost (charges)	Varies widely depending on the payor		

Reproduced and modified with permission from Frishberg, B.M. (1994). The utility of neuroimaging in the evaluation of headache in patients with normal neurologic examinations. *Neurology* 44:1196.

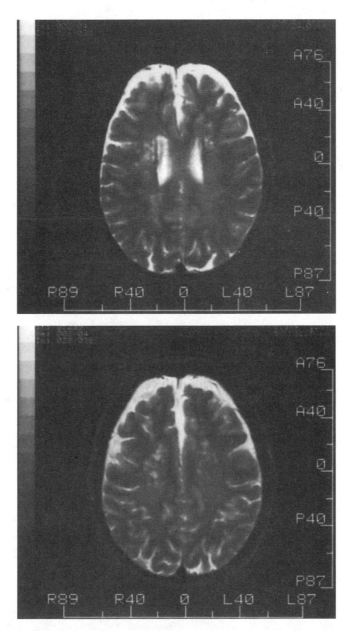

Figure 3–3 White matter abnormality on magnetic resonance imaging in migraine. (Reprinted with permission from Rozen, T.D., Silberstein, S.D., and D. Friedman (1999). Neuroimaging of Headache. In *Neuroimaging* (J.O. Greenberg, ed.) pp. 89–106. McGraw-Hill, New York.)

result in CADASIL at one extreme and individuals with tiny T2 hyperintense white
matter foci and migraine alone at the other
extreme.

Cerebral Atrophy

Diffuse cerebral atrophy with widening of the
lateral ventricles and cerebral sulci is equally
well detected by both MRI and CT scan
(Kuhn and Shekar, 1990). The incidence of
cerebral atrophy in migraineurs on CT and
MRI scan has been variably reported as 4%
(Cala and Mastaglia, 1976), 26% (Hungerford
et al., 1976), 28% (Prager et al., 1991), 35%
(Kuhn and Shekar, 1990), and 58% (du Boulay et al., 1983). The studies describe most
cases of atrophy as mild to moderate. The
cause of the atrophy, which can be a nonspecific finding based on often subjective criteria,

is not certain (Prager et al., 1991; Ziegler et
al., 1991). Two more recent studies have
found the incidence of atrophy in migraineurs
to be no greater than in controls (De Benedittis et al., 1995; Ziegler et al., 1991). The
high incidence of CT changes seen in migraineurs in early studies probably reflected
artifact and a failure to recognize the range
of normality on this new imaging technique.

Arteriovenous Malformations
and Migraine

The prevalence of arteriovenous malformations (AVMs) is about 0.5% in postmortem
studies (Brown et al., 1988). In contrast to
saccular aneurysms, up to 50% present with
symptoms or signs other than hemorrhage.
Headache without distinctive features (such
as frequency, duration, or severity) is the

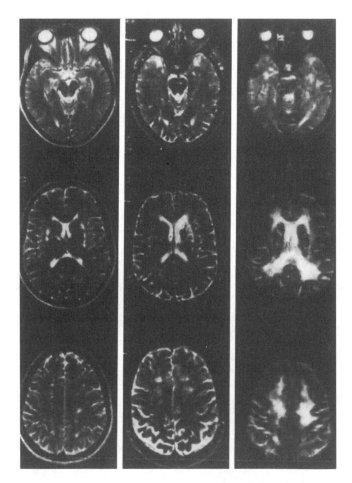

Figure 3–4 Cerebral autosomal
dominant arteriopathy with subcortical
infarcts and leukoencephalopathy
(CADASIL). (Reprinted with
permission from Rozen, T.D.,
Silberstein, S.D., and D. Friedman
(1999). Neuroimaging of Headache. In
Neuroimaging (J.O. Greenberg, ed.)
pp. 89–106, McGraw-Hill, New York.)

presenting symptom in up to 48% of cases (Arteriovenous Malformation Study Group, 1999) (Fig. 3–5).

Migraine-like headaches with and without visual symptoms can be associated with AVMs, especially in the occipital lobe, which is the predominant location of about 20% of parenchymal AVMs (Frishberg, 1997; Kupersmith et al., 1996). Although headaches always occurring on the same side (side-locked) are present in 95% of patients with AVMs (Bruyn, 1984), 17% of patients with migraine without aura and 15% of patients with migraine with aura have side-locked headaches (Leone et al., 1993). Migraine due to an AVM is usually atypical and rarely meets the International Headache Society criteria for migraine. Bruyn (1984) reported the following features in patients with migraine-like symptoms and AVMs: unusual associated signs (papilledema, field cut, cranial bruit); short duration of headache attacks (several hours); auras of short duration (5 to 10 minutes); auras always occurring on the same side; late age at onset of migraine with aura; absent family history for migraine; atypical sequence of aura, headache, and vomiting such that the headache would start before the aura; and the presence of seizures or coma.

American Academy of Neurology Practice Parameter and United States Headache Consortium Guideline

The report of the Quality Standards Subcommittee of the AAN (1994) suggests the following guideline for the use of neuroimaging in the evaluation of migraine: "In adult patients with recurrent headaches defined as migraine, including those with visual aura, with no recent change in headache pattern, no history of seizures, and no other focal neurologic signs or symptoms, the routine use of neuroimaging is not warranted. In patients with atypical headache patterns, a history of seizures, or focal neurologic signs or symptoms, CT or MRI may be indicated."

The U.S. Headache Consortium has concluded that neuroimaging is not usually warranted in migraine patients who have a normal neurologic examination; however, it should be considered when neuroimaging risk factors for intracranial pathology exist, such as when a patient with a nonacute headache lasting more than 4 weeks has an unexplained neurologic examination, an atypical headache or headache features, or an additional risk factor, such as immune deficiency (Frishberg et al., 2000). In the acute headache setting, which was outside of the original guidelines, risk factors for intracranial pathology include acute onset, occipitonuchal location, age >55 years, associated symptoms, and abnormal neurologic examination (Ramirez-Lassepas et al., 1997).

ACUTE, SEVERE, NEW-ONSET HEADACHES ("FIRST OR WORST")

Differential Diagnosis

Perhaps 1% of patients presenting to the emergency room have headache of acute onset as their chief complaint (Fodden et al., 1989). Table 3–5 lists the possible causes of acute, severe, new-onset headache (the "first or worst") (Dalessio, 1994; Silberstein, 1992). A prospective study of 148 patients with acute severe headaches seen by general practitioners in the Netherlands found SAH to be the cause in 25% of cases (Linn et al., 1994).

There are many causes of SAH (Table 3–6). About 80% are due to rupture of intracranial aneurysms (Wilterdink, 1994) and 5%, to rupture of intracranial AVMs. In about 15% of cases, an arteriogram does not demonstrate the cause of the bleeding. In about 50% of these arteriogram-negative cases, CT scan reveals blood confined to the cisterns around the midbrain, a perimesencephalic hemorrhage, which may be caused by a rupture of prepontine or interpeduncular cistern dilated veins or venous malformations. Other causes of arteriogram-negative SAH are listed in Table 3–6 (Khajavi and Chyatte, 2000).

In the United States, over 30,000 people per year are diagnosed with SAH from a ruptured saccular aneurysm, resulting in over 18,000 deaths (Raps et al., 1994). Based on a meta-analysis, the prevalence of saccular aneurysms in the general population is about

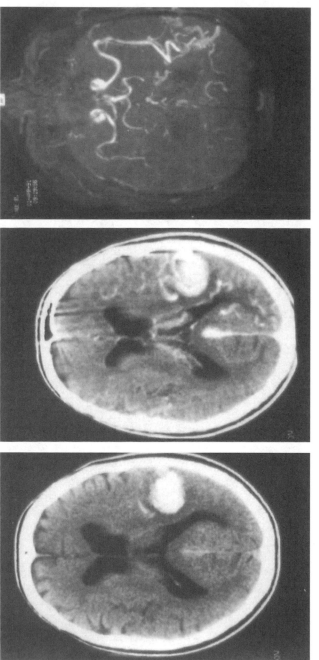

Figure 3–5 Arteriovenous malformation. (Reprinted with permission from Rozen, T.D., Silberstein, S.D., and D. Friedman (1999). Neuroimaging of Headache. In *Neuroimaging* (J.O. Greenberg, ed.) pp. 89–106, McGraw-Hill, New York.)

Table 3–5 Differential diagnosis of the acute, severe, new-onset headache ("First or Worst")

Crash migraine (Fisher, 1984)	Benign intracranial hypertension
Cluster	Post-lumbar puncture headache
Miscellaneous	Related to intrathecal injections
Benign exertional headache	Intracranial neoplasm
Benign orgasmic cephalgia	Pituitary apoplexy
Post-traumatic	Acute intoxications
Associated with vascular disorders	Associated with noncephalic infection
Acute ischemic cerebrovascular disease	Acute febrile illness
Subdural and epidural hematomas	Acute pyelonephritis
Parenchymal hemorrhage	Cephalic infection
Unruptured saccular aneurysm	Meningoencephalitis
Subarachnoid hemorrhage	Acute sinusitis
Systemic lupus erythematosus	Acute mountain sickness
Temporal arteritis	Disorders of eyes
Internal carotid and vertebral artery dissection	Acute optic neuritis
Cerebral venous thrombosis	Acute glaucoma
Acute hypertension	Cervicogenic
Pressor response	Greater occipital neuralgia (Pascual-Leone and
Pheochromocytoma	Pascual, 1992)
Pre-eclampsia	Cervical myositis
Associated with nonvascular intracranial disorders	Trigeminal neuralgia
Intermittent hydrocephalus	

Reproduced with permission from Evans, R.W. (1999). Headaches. In *Diagnostic Testing in Neurology* (R.W. Evans, ed.), p. 7. W.B. Saunders, Philadelphia.

2% (Rinkel et al., 1998). Perhaps 50% of SAHs will present with a Hunt and Hess grade I (no symptoms or minimal headache, slight nuchal rigidity) or grade II (moderate to severe headache, no neurologic deficit other than cranial nerve palsy). Although most patients with headache due to SAH will have the worst headache of their life with maximum intensity within 5 minutes but typically much faster (Linn et al., 1998), SAH can be easily overlooked (Johnston and Robinson, 1998). Ten percent of patients have no headache at onset and 8% describe a mild, gradually increasing headache (Walton, 1956; Weir, 1994). A stiff neck is absent in 36% of patients (Kassell et al., 1990). Physicians must be aware of the diverse presentations of SAH and should exclude aneurysmal SAH if a patient has the worst headache of his or her life or a dramatic, acute change in headache pattern.

Table 3–6 Causes of nontraumatic subarachnoid hemorrhage

80%	Intracranial saccular aneurysm	
5%	Intracranial arteriovenous malformation	
15%	Negative arteriogram	
	50%	Benign perimesencephalic hemorrhage
	50%	Other causes
		Occult aneurysm
		Mycotic aneurysm
		Vertebral or carotid artery dissection
		Dural arteriovenous malformation
		Spinal arteriovenous malformation
		Sickle cell anemia
		Coagulation disorders
		Drug abuse (cocaine and methamphetamine)
		Primary or metastatic intracranial tumors (e.g., pituitary, melanoma)
		Primary or metastatic cervical tumors
		Central nervous system infection (e.g., herpes encephalitis)
		Central nervous system vasculitis

Reproduced with permission from Evans, R.W. (1999). Headaches. In *Diagnostic Testing in Neurology* (R.W. Evans, ed.), p. 7. W.B. Saunders, Philadelphia.

Computed Tomography and Magnetic Resonance Imaging Scans and Aneurysmal Subarachnoid Hemorrhage

A CT scan without contrast is the neuroimaging study of choice for the detection of acute SAH (Table 3–7, Fig. 3–6). In a cooperative series of 3,521 patients, findings on the first CT scan after rupture of a saccular aneurysm were as follows: normal, 8.3%; decreased density, 1.1%; mass effect, 6.1%; aneurysm, 5%; hydrocephalus, 15.2%; intraventricular hematoma, 16.7%; intracerebral

Table 3–7 Approximate probability of recognizing an aneurysmal subarachnoid hemorrhage on computed tomographic scan after the initial event

Time	Probability (%)
Day 0	95 (Adams et al., 1983)
Day 3	74 (Adams et al., 1983)
1 week	50 (van Gijn and van Dongen, 1982)
2 weeks	30 (van Gijn and van Dongen, 1982)
3 weeks	Almost 0 (van Gijn and van Dongen, 1982)

Reproduced with permission from Evans, R.W. (1999). Headaches. In *Diagnostic Testing in Neurology* (R.W. Evans, ed.), p. 9. W.B. Saunders, Philadelphia.

hematoma, 17.4%; subdural hematoma, 1.3%; and SAH, 85.2% (Kassell et al., 1990). On day 0, CT scan detected aneurysmal SAH in 92% of patients, decreasing to 58% on day 5. On day 0, 3.3% of scans were normal; on day 1, this was 7.2%; and on day 5, this was 27.3%. False-positives can occur from mistaking calcification (e.g., of the falx cerebri) for blood or anoxic encephalopathy as diffuse SAH (Al-Yamany et al., 1999).

Van der Wee et al. (1995) studied a prospective series of 175 consecutive patients with sudden headache and a normal neurologic examination. The CT scans performed within the first 12 hours detected SAH in 117, for a detection rate of 98%. In the remaining 58 patients, lumbar puncture was performed 12 or more hours after the onset of the headache. Two of the 58 patients were found to have xanthochromic CSF by spectrophotometric analysis. Both of these patients had aneurysms.

Based on a prospective study of 100 patients, the probability of recognizing an aneurysmal hemorrhage on CT scan is 50% after 1 week, 30% after 2 weeks (mostly patients with hematomas), and almost nil after 3 weeks (van Gijn and van Dongen, 1982). The increased attenuation values in the basal cisterns and fissures usually disappear by day 5 to 9. Most hematomas resolve between days 14 and 22.

The pattern of hemorrhage in the absence of an intracerebral hematoma helps to locate

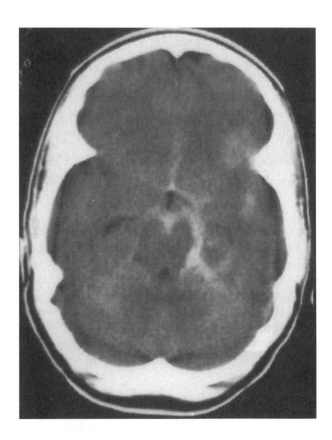

Figure 3–6 Subarachnoid bleed on computed tomography. (Reprinted with permission from Rozen, T.D., Silberstein, S.D., and D. Friedman (1999). Neuroimaging of Headache. In *Neuroimaging* (J.O. Greenberg, ed.) pp. 89–106, McGraw-Hill, New York.)

Table 3–8 Aneurysm sites suggested by the location of subarachnoid hemorrhage (SAH)

Site of aneurysm	Predominant location of SAH
Anterior communicating artery	Interhemispheric fissure and/or septum pellucidum
Middle cerebral artery	Sylvian fissure cistern
Posterior communicating artey	Suprasellar cistern
Infratentorial arteries	Posterior fossa cistern
Unknown origin	Diffuse, symmetrical cisterns

Reproduced with permission from Evans, R.W. (1999). Headaches. In *Diagnostic Testing in Neurology* (R.W. Evans, ed.), p. 9. W.B. Saunders, Philadelphia.

the ruptured saccular aneurysm (Table 3–8) (Ghoshhajra et al., 1979; Wang et al., 1995). Computed tomography is the most sensitive and specific test for diagnosing a ruptured anterior cerebral artery aneurysm or anterior communicating artery aneurysm (van der Jagt et al., 1999). Usually, SAH only in the prepontine cistern or interpeduncular fossa indicates a venous or capillary rupture (Rinkel et al., 1991b; Yuichi, 1981), although a basilar artery aneurysm is responsible about 5% of the time (Rinkel et al., 1991b).

In the acute setting, CT scan without contrast is preferred to MRI for the evaluation of possible SAH because of the wide availability of CT scans and their lower cost and faster scanning time. Ogawa et al. (1993) compared CT scan with MRI at 0.5 Tesla in the detection of aneurysmal SAH. Acute SAH was detected as an area of high signal intensity relative to that of normal CSF and the surrounding brain parenchyma on a moderately T2-weighted MRI sequence. For the detection of SAH, MRI was almost equal to CT scan in the first 24 hours and slightly superior in the acute stage up to 72 hours. From more than 3 to 14 days after the ictus, MRI was definitely superior to CT scan in the identification and delineation of SAH (Fig. 3–7).

Lumbar Puncture and Subarachnoid Hemorrhage

When a patient with a new-onset headache that is suspicious for SAH has a normal CT scan, a lumbar puncture should be performed. Since lumbar punctures can result in clinical deterioration and death after SAH, a CT scan should be performed first (Duffy, 1982; van Gijn, 1992).

Cerebrospinal Fluid Examination

Red blood cells (RBCs) are present in the CSF in virtually all cases of SAH. The RBCs clear in 6 to 30 days (Tourtellotte et al., 1964). When bloody CSF is obtained from the first lumbar puncture, the presence of a xanthochromic supernatant is the only certain way to distinguish SAH from a traumatic tap. Although a decrease in RBCs from the first to the third test tube can be seen after a traumatic tap (Fishman, 1992), a similar decrease can be seen after a previous bleed (Buruma et al., 1981). Conversely, after a traumatic tap, the number of RBCs may stay constant in all three tubes (Vermeulen et al., 1989). Since crenation occurs very soon after RBCs enter the CSF, the presence of crenated RBCs is not a reliable sign of SAH (Vermeulen and van Gijn, 1990).

When RBCs break down in the CSF, they release oxyhemoglobin, which is degraded to bilirubin by the third to fourth day by macrophages and other cells in the leptomeninges (Barrows et al., 1955). These two pigments are responsible for xanthochromia (which literally means "yellow color" but refers to a colored supernatant) after SAH. The CSF supernatant is pink or pink–orange due to oxyhemoglobin, yellow due to bilirubin, and an intermediate color if both are present. Methemoglobin, a reduction product of hemoglobin, is found in encapsulated subdural hematomas and in old loculated intracerebral hemorrhages (Fishman, 1992). Although oxyhemoglobin can be detected as early as 2 hours after entry of RBCs into the CSF, xanthochromia is not present in all cases until after 12 hours (Vermeulen et al., 1989). Therefore, to avoid confusing blood-stained CSF from a traumatic lumbar puncture with SAH, it has been suggested that lumbar puncture should be delayed until 12 hours after the ictus (Vermeulen and van Gijn, 1990). However, this is not always practical since pa-

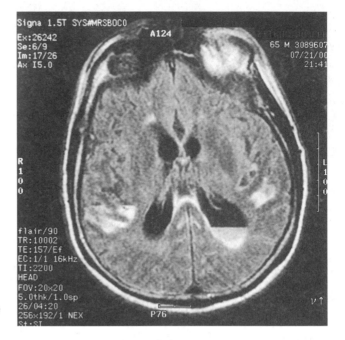

Figure 3–7 Subarachnoid hemorrhage on magnetic resonance imaging.

tients with severe headaches and a normal examination are frequently evaluated as outpatients or in the emergency room. If the initial lumbar puncture was negative but completed within 6 to 8 hours of the ictus, a second spinal tap looking for xanthochromia should be completed after the 12-hour mark if the physician believes the patient may have had SAH.

Xanthochromia is best detected by spectrophotometry since the naked eye can detect xanthochromia only about half of the time (Söderström, 1977; Vermeulin and van Gijn, 1990). *Absorption spectrophotometry*, which is a measurement of the light intensity in different regions of the visible spectrum (400–700 nm) after its transmission through an absorbing medium, can detect oxyhemoglobin and bilirubin by their characteristic maximum absorption bands of 415 and 455 nm, respectively (Vermeulen and van Gijn, 1990; Weir, 1994).

The probability of detecting xanthochromia by spectrophotometry at various times after SAH is shown in Table 3–9 (Vermeulen et al., 1989). Other causes of xanthochromia include the following: jaundice, usually with a total plasma bilirubin of 10 to 15 mg/dl; CSF protein >150 mg/dl; dietary hypercarotene-

mia; malignant melanomatosis; oral intake of rifampin; and traumatic lumbar punctures (Fishman, 1992). Because oxyhemoglobin can form in vivo, false-positives for SAH can occur from traumatic taps with even a small number of RBCs (Beetham et al., 1998; Morgenstern et al., 1998). Only bilirubin and methemoglobin can be formed in vitro.

Cerebral Arteriography, Magnetic Resonance Angiography, and Spiral Computed Tomographic Angiography

After SAH is diagnosed, a four-vessel cerebral arteriogram should be performed to locate

Table 3–9 Probability of detecting xanthochromia with spectrophotometry in cerebrospinal fluid at various times after a subarachnoid hemorrhage

Time	Probability (%)
12 hours	100
1 week	100
2 weeks	100
3 weeks	>70
4 weeks	>40

Data from Vermeulen, M., D. Hasan, B.G. Blijenberg, et al. (1989). Xanthochromia after subarachnoid hemorrhage needs no revisitation. *J. Neurol. Neurosurg. Psychiatry* 53:826–828.

the underlying aneurysm. About 20% of patients will have multiple aneurysms. Although saccular aneurysms are usually detected on the initial arteriogram, false-negatives can occur in 6% (Urbach et al., 1998) to 16% (Iwanaga et al., 1990) of patients, often missing an anterior communicating artery aneurysm. Potential reasons for false-negatives include vasospasm, aneurysmal thrombosis, observer error, and technical factors, such as inadequate oblique views (Iwanaga et al., 1990; Wolpert and Caplan, 1992). The arteriogram should be repeated after 2 weeks when vasospasm is found, the study is incomplete or inadequate, an aneurysmal pattern of blood is seen on the initial CT scan (Rinkel et al., 1991a), or a CT scan performed within 4 days after the SAH shows thin or thick subarachnoid blood, particularly in the basal frontal interhemispheric fissure (Iwanaga et al., 1990). Occasionally, a third arteriogram may be necessary to demonstrate an aneurysm (Mehdorn et al., 1992).

Cerebral arteriography occasionally causes neurologic complications. A prospective study of 1,000 consecutive cerebral arteriograms from the Barrow Neurological Institute reported a 1% overall incidence of neurologic deficit and a 0.5% incidence of persistent deficit (Heiserman et al., 1994). All of the complications occurred in patients with an average age of 73 years who were being evaluated for a history of stroke, transient ischemic event, or carotid bruit. Although there were no complications in the 137 cerebral arteriograms performed for SAH, complications associated with vasospasm can occur. A higher

incidence of complications may occur in departments that do a low volume of studies or when the studies are performed by inexperienced physicians (Gabrielsen, 1994).

Although magnetic resonance angiography (MRA) has not yet replaced cerebral arteriography, it is a useful screening procedure in some cases (i.e., when a patient declines an arteriogram or has a thunderclap headache with a normal CT scan and normal CSF examination) (Litt, 1994) (Fig. 3–8). Occasionally, MRA can detect a saccular aneurysm not seen on cerebral angiography (Rogg et al., 1999). Huston et al. (1994) compared aneurysms detected on cerebral arteriograms with time-of-flight and phase-contrast MRA and conventional MRI. The sensitivities of the sequences for detecting aneurysms ≥5 mm were as follows: T1-weighted, 37.5%; T2-weighted, 62.5%; phase-contrast, 75%; and time-of-flight, 87.5%. Retrospectively, aneurysms 3 mm or larger could be identified. In another MRA study of 51 patients with recent SAH, false-positives were reported in 2% and false-negatives in 5.9% of cases (Sankhla et al., 1996).

Spiral (helical) CT angiography can also be used to detect intracranial aneurysms (Fig. 3–9). Strayle-Batra et al. (1998) reported a series of 20 aneurysms found in 16 patients. With an examination time of 5 to 7 minutes, the sensitivity of spiral CT angiography compared to digital subtraction angiography was 85%, with detection of aneurysms ranging from 3 to 20 mm (mean 8.9 mm). There were no false-positives. The posterior communicat-

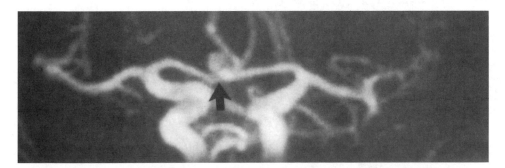

Figure 3–8 Aneurysm on magnetic resonance angiography. (Reprinted with permission from Rozen, T.D., Silberstein, S.D., and D. Friedman (1999). Neuroimaging of Headache. In *Neuroimaging* (J.O. Greenberg, ed.) pp. 89–106, McGraw-Hill, New York.)

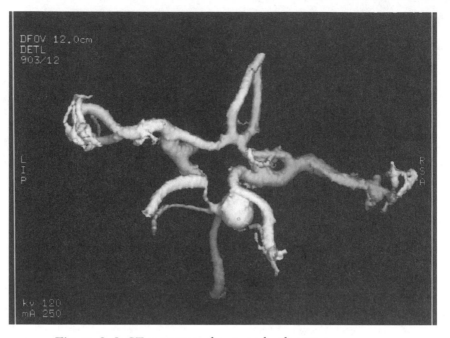

Figure 3–9 CT angiogram showing a basilar artery aneurysm.

ing artery was difficult to assess due to its close relationship to bony structures. Spiral CT offers an important addition as well as an alternative for those with contraindications to MRA, including pacemakers and claustrophobia.

NEW-ONSET HEADACHES IN PATIENTS OVER THE AGE OF 50

When new-onset headaches begin in patients over the age of 50, the physician should consider the various primary headache disorders as well as secondary headaches (Table 3–10). While new-onset tension-type headaches are rather common, it is unusual for migraine and cluster headaches to begin after age 50. Female cluster patients may have a second cluster incidence peak in the fifth or sixth decade (the first is in the second decade) (Rozen et al., 1999). Hypnic headaches (which occur only at night and awaken the patient from sleep at a consistent time) occur in those 40 years of age or older. The pain can be unilateral or bilateral, throbbing or nonthrobbing; it typically lasts 15 minutes to 6 hours (Dodick et al., 1998). The diagnosis of hypnic

headache is one of exclusion since many secondary headaches present as nocturnal syndromes. These include drug-withdrawal headaches, temporal arteritis, sleep apnea, oxygen desaturation, pheochromocytomas, primary and secondary neoplasms, communicating hydrocephalus, subdural hematomas, and vascular lesions (Gould and Silberstein, 1997). A good sleep history is necessary for all patients who have sleep-related headaches (i.e., they

Table 3–10 Common causes of headache beginning in the elderly

Secondary headache disorders
Mass lesions
Temporal arteritis
Medication-related headache
Trigeminal neuralgia
Postherpetic neuralgia
Systemic disease
Disease of the cranium, neck, eyes, ears, and nose
Cerebrovascular disease
Parkinson's disease
Primary headache disorders
Migraine
Tension-type headache
Cluster headache
Hypnic headache

Reproduced with permission from Lipton, R.B., D. Pfeffer, L.C. Newman et al. (1993). Headaches in the elderly. *J. Pain Symptom Manage.* 8:88.

awaken each morning with a headache or headaches awaken them from sleep). The sleep history should include questions about snoring, restless legs, nocturnal seizures, and rapid eye movement–related sleep problems. If a patient has treatment-refractory sleep-related headaches, a sleep study should be ordered to see if he or she has an underlying sleep disturbance.

The common causes of secondary headache disorders beginning in later life include mass lesions, such as subdural hematomas and neoplasms; temporal arteritis; medication-related headaches, including headaches caused by specific medications (e.g., nitrates) as well as medication-rebound or medication-withdrawal headaches; trigeminal neuralgia; postherpetic neuralgia; systemic disease, such as infection, acute hypertension, hypoxia, or hypercarbia, and other metabolic abnormalities, such as hypercalcemia or severe anemia; headaches associated with disorders of the cranium, neck, eyes, ears, and nose, including cervicogenic headache, glaucoma, otitis, sinusitis, and dental infections; cerebrovascular disease; and the one-third of patients with Parkinson's disease who report headaches (Edmeads, 1997; Lipton et al., 1993).

Pascual and Berciano (1994) performed a study of 193 patients 65 years of age and over seen by their neurology service over a 15-year period with de novo headache as their initial and main symptom. The most frequent diagnoses were tension-type headaches (in 43% of patients) and trigeminal neuralgia (in 19%). Only one patient met migraine criteria. Fifteen percent of patients had a secondary headache disorder due to conditions such as stroke, temporal arteritis, or intracranial neoplasm. Although the incidence of patients with de novo headaches attending a general hospital decreased with age, the risk of headache due to serious conditions increased ten times after age 65.

REFERENCES

Akpek, S., M. Arac, S. Atilla et al. (1995). Cost effectiveness of computed tomography in the evaluation of patients with headache. *Headache* 35:228–230.

Al-Yamany, M., J. Deck, and M. Bernstein. (1999). Pseudo-subarachnoid hemorrhage: A rare neuroimaging pitfall. *Can. J. Neurol. Sci.* 26:57–59.

American Academy of Neurology. (1994). The utility of neuroimaging in the evaluation of headache in patients with normal neurologic examinations. *Neurology* 44:1353–1354.

American Academy of Neurology. (1995). Practice parameter: The electroencephalogram in the evaluation of headache. *Neurology* 45:1411–1413.

Amit, M., Y. Molad, O. Levy et al. (1999). Headache and systemic lupus erythematosis and its relation to other disease manifestations. *Clin. Exp. Rheumatol.* 17:467–470.

Arteriovenous Malformation Study Group. (1999). Arteriovenous malformations of the brain in adults. *N. Engl. J. Med.* 340:1812–1818.

Baker, H. (1983). Cranial CT in the investigation of headache: Cost effectiveness for brain tumors. *J. Neuroradiol.* 10:112–116.

Barrows, L.J., F.T. Hunter, and B.Q. Banker. (1955). The nature and clinical significance of pigments in the cerebrospinal fluid. *Brain* 78:59–80.

Beetham, R., M.N. Fahie-Wilson, and D. Park. (1998). What is the role of spectrophotometry in the diagnosis of subarachnoid haemorrhage? *Ann. Clin. Biochem.* 35:1–4.

Beresford, H.R. (1999). Medicolegal aspects. In *Diagnostic Testing in Neurology* (R.W. Evans, ed.), pp. 479–488. W.B. Saunders, Philadelphia.

Brown, R.D., D.O. Wiebers, G. Forbes et al. (1988). The natural history of unruptured intracranial arteriovenous malformations. *J. Neurosurg.* 68:352–357

Bruyn, G.W. (1984). Intracranial arteriovenous malformation and migraine. *Cephalalgia* 4:191–207.

Buruma, O.J.S., H.L.F. Janson, F.A.J.T.M. Den Bergh et al. (1981). Blood-stained cerebrospinal fluid: Traumatic puncture or haemorrhage? *J. Neurol. Neurosurg. Psychiatry* 44:144–147.

Cala, L. and F. Mastaglia. (1976). Computerized axial tomography findings in a group of patients with migrainous headaches. *Proc. Aust. Acad. Neurol.* 13:35–41.

Carlos, R.A., C.S. Santos, S. Kumar et al. (2000). Neuroimaging studies in pediatric migraine headaches. *Headache* 40:404.

Carrera, G., D. Gerson, J. Schnur et al. (1977). Computerized tomography of the brain in patients with headache or temporal lobe epilepsy: Findings and cost effectiveness. *J. Comput. Assist. Tomogr.* 1:200–203.

Chabriat, H., E. Tournier-Lasserve, K. Vahedi et al. (1995). Autosomal dominant migraine with MRI white matter abnormalities mapping to the CADASIL locus. *Neurology* 45:1086–1091.

Chu, M.L. and S. Shinnar. (1992). Headaches in children younger than 7 years of age. *Arch Neurol* 49:79–82.

Cooney, B.S., R.I. Grossman, R.E. Farber et al. (1996). Frequency of magnetic resonance imaging abnormalities in patients with migraine. *Headache* 36:616–621.

Cuetter, A. and J. Aita. (1983). CT scanning in classic migraine [letter]. *Headache* 23:195.

Dalessio, D.J. (1994). Diagnosing the severe headache. *Neurology* 44(Suppl. 3):S6–S12.

Daras, M., B. Koppel, M. Leyfermann et al. (1995). Anticardiolipin antibodies in migraine patients: An additional risk factor for stroke? *Neurology* 45(Suppl. 4):A367–A368.

De Benedittis, G., A. Lorenzetti, C. Sina et al. (1995). Magnetic resonance imaging in migraine and tension-type headache. *Headache* 35:264–268.

Demaerel, P., I. Boelaert, G. Wilms et al. (1996). The role of cranial computed tomography in the diagnostic work-up of headache. *Headache* 36:347–348.

Dodick, D.W., A.C. Mosek, and J.K. Campbell. (1998). The hypnic ("alarm clock") headache syndrome. *Cephalalgia* 18:152–156.

Dooley, J.M., P.R. Camfield, M. O'Neill et al. (1990). The value of CT scans for children with headaches. *Can. J. Neurol. Sci.* 17:309–310.

du Boulay, G.H. and J.S. Ruiz. (1983). CT changes associated with migraine. *Am. J. Neuroradiol.* 4:472–473.

Duffy, G.P. (1982). Lumbar puncture in spontaneous subarachnoid haemorrhage. *BMJ* 285:1163–1164.

Dumas, M.D., W. Pexman, and J.H. Kreeft. (1994). Computed tomography evaluation of patients with chronic headache. *Can. Med. Assoc. J.* 151:1447–1452.

Edmeads, J. (1997). Headaches in older people. How are they different in this age-group? *Postgrad. Med.* 101:91–100.

Embil, J.M., M. Kramer, S. Kinnear et al. (1997). A blinding headache. *Lancet* 349:182.

Evans, R.W. (1997). Migraine-like headaches in pituitary apoplexy. *Headache* 37:455–456.

Evans, R.W. (1998). Complications of lumbar puncture. *Neurol. Clin.* 16:83–105.

Evans, R.W. (1999). Headaches. In *Diagnostic Testing in Neurology* (R.W. Evans, ed.), pp. 1–19. W.B. Saunders, Philadelphia.

Evans, R.W., C. Armon, E.M. Frohman et al. (2000). Assessment: Prevention of post-lumbar puncture headaches. *Neurology* 55:909–914.

Fazekas, F., M. Koch, R. Schmidt et al. (1992). The prevalence of cerebral damage varies with migraine type: A MRI study. *Headache* 32:287–291.

Fisher, C.M. (1984). Painful states: A neurological commentary. *Clin. Neurosurg.* 31:32–53.

Fishman, R.A. (1992). Examination of the cerebrospinal fluid: Techniques and complications. In *Cerebrospinal Fluid in Diseases of the Nervous System*, pp. 183–252. W.B. Saunders, Philadelphia.

Fodden, D.I., R.C. Peatfield, and P.L. Milsom. (1989). Beware the patient with a headache in the accident and emergency department. *Arch. Emerg. Med.* 6:7–12.

Frishberg, B.M. (1994). The utility of neuroimaging in the evaluation of headache in patients with normal neurologic examination. *Neurology* 44:1191–1197.

Frishberg, B.M. (1997). Neuroimaging in presumed primary headache disorders. *Semin. Neurol.* 17:373–382.

Frishberg, B., J.H. Rosenberg, D.B. Matchar et al. (2000). Evidence-based guidelines in the primary care setting: neuroimaging in patients with nonacute headache. This reference is only available on *www.aan.com*.

Gabrielsen, T.O. (1994). Neurologic complications of cerebral angiography. *AJNR Am. J. Neuroradiol.* 15:1408–1411.

Ghoshhajra, K., L. Scotti, J. Marasco et al. (1979). CT detection of intracranial aneurysm in subarachnoid hemorrhage. *AJR Am. J. Roentgenol.* 132:613–616.

Gould, J.D. and S.D. Silberstein. (1997). Unilateral hypnic headache: A case study. *Neurology* 49:1749–1751.

Greenberg, M.K. and G.M. Franklin. (1999). Practice parameters. In *Diagnostic Testing in Neurology* (R.W. Evans, ed.), pp. 485–488. W.B. Saunders, Philadelphia.

Gronseth, G.S. and M.K. Greenberg. (1995). The utility of electroencephalogram in the evaluation of patients presenting with headache: A review of the literature. *Neurology* 45:1263–1267.

Heiserman, J.E., B.L. Dean, J.A. Hodak et al. (1994). Neurologic complications of cerebral angiography. *AJNR Am. J. Neuroradiol.* 15:1401–1407.

Hering, R., E.G.M. Couturier, T.J. Steiner et al. (1991). Anticardiolipin antibodies in migraine. *Cephalalgia* 11:19–21.

Hungerford, G., G. du Boulay, and K. Zilkha. (1976). Computerized axial tomography in patients with severe migraine: A preliminary report. *J. Neurol. Neurosurg. Psychiatry* 39:990–994.

Huston, J., D.A. Nichols, P.H. Luetmer et al. (1994). Blinded prospective evaluation of sensitivity of MR angiography to known intracranial aneurysms: Importance of aneurysm size. *AJNR Am J. Neuroradiol.* 15:1607–1614.

Igarashi, H., F. Sakai, S. Kan et al. (1991). Magnetic resonance imaging of the brain in patients with migraine. *Cephalalgia* 11:69–74.

Iwanaga, H., S. Wakai, C. Ochiai et al. (1990). Ruptured cerebral aneurysms missed by initial angiographic study. *Neurosurgery* 27:45–51.

Jacome, D.E. and J. Leborgne. (1990). MRI studies in basilar artery migraine. *Headache* 30:88–90.

Johnston, S.D. and T.J. Robinson. (1998). Subarachnoid haemorrhage: Difficulties in diagnosis and treatment. *Postgrad. Med.* 74:743–748.

Kassell, N.F., J.C. Torner, E.C. Haley et al. (1990). The international cooperative study on the timing of aneurysm surgery. Part I: Overall management results. *J. Neurosurg.* 73:18–36.

Kassirer, J.P. (1989). Our stubborn quest for diagnostic certainty. A cause of excessive testing. *N. Engl. J. Med.* 320:1489–1491.

Khajavi, K. and D. Chyatte. (2000). Subarachnoid hemorrhage. In *Neurobase* (S. Gilman, ed.), Arbor Publishing, San Diego.

Khurana, R.K. (1991). Headache spectrum in Arnold-Chiari malformation. *Headache* 31:151–155.

Kuhn, M.J. and P.C. Shekar. (1990). A comparative study of magnetic resonance imaging and computed tomography in the evaluation of migraine. *Comput. Med. Imaging Graph.* 14:149–152.

Kupersmith, M.J., M.E. Vargas, A. Yashar et al. (1996). Occipital arteriovenous malformations: Visual disturbances and presentation. *Neurology* 46:953–957.

Laffey, P., W. Oaks, R. Sawmi et al. (1978). *Computerized Tomography in Clinical Medicine: Data Supplement.* Medical Directions, Philadelphia.

Lance. J.W. and P.J. Goadsby. (1998). *Mechanism and Management of Headache*, 6th ed. Butterworth Heinemann, Oxford.

Larson, E., G. Omenn, and H. Lewis. (1980). Diagnostic evaluation of headache: Impact of computerized tomography and cost effectiveness. *JAMA* 243:359–362.

Leone, M., D. D'Amico, F. Frediani et al. (1993). Clinical considerations on side-locked unilaterality in long lasting primary headaches. *Headache* 33:381–384.

Linn, F.H.H., G.J.E. Rinkel, A. Algra et al. (1998). Headache characteristics in subarachnoid haemorrhage and benign thunderclap headache. *J. Neurol. Neurosurg. Psychiatry* 65:791–793.

Linn, F.H.H., E.F.M. Wijdicks, Y. van der Graaf et al. (1994). Prospective study of sentinel headache in aneurysmal subarachnoid haemorrhage. *Lancet* 344:590–593.

Lipton, R.B., D. Pfeffer, L.C. Newman et al. (1993). Headaches in the elderly. *J. Pain Symptom Manage.* 8:87–97.

Litt, A.W. (1994). MR Angiography of intracranial aneurysms: Proceed, but with caution. *AJNR Am. J. Neuroradiol.* 15:1615–1616.

Masland, W., A. Friedman, and H. Buchsbaum. (1978). Computerized axial tomography of migraine. *Res. Clin. Stud. Headache* 6:136–140.

Maytal, J., R.S. Bienkowski, M. Patel et al. (1996). The value of brain imaging in children with headaches. *Pediatrics* 96:413–416.

Medina, S., J.D. Pinter, D. Zurakowski et al. (1997). Children with headache: Clinical predictors of surgical space-occupying lesions and the role of neuroimaging. *Radiology* 202:819–824.

Mehdorn, H.M., V. Dietrich, R. Kalff et al. (1992). Subarachnoid hemorrhage of unknown etiology: Long-term prognosis. *Neurosurg. Rev.* 15:27–31.

Mitchell, C., R. Osborn, and S. Grosskreutz. (1993). Computerized tomography in the headache patient: Is routine evaluation really necessary? *Headache* 33:82–86.

Mokri, B. (1997). Headache in spontaneous carotid and vertebral artery dissections. In *Headache* (P.J. Goadsby and S.D. Silberstein, eds.), pp. 327–353. Butterworth-Heinemann, Boston.

Morgenstern, L.B., H. Luna-Gonzales, J.C. Huber et al. (1998). Worst headache and subarachnoid hemorrhage: Prospective, modern computed tomography and spinal fluid analysis. *Ann. Emerg. Med.* 32:297–304.

Ogawa, T., A. Inugami, E. Shimosegawa et al. (1993). Subarachnoid hemorrhage: Evaluation with MR imaging. *Radiology* 186:345–351.

Osborn, R.E., D.C. Alder, and C.S. Mitchell. (1991). MR imaging of the brain in patients with migraine headaches. *AJNR Am. J. Neuroradiol.* 12:521–524.

Pascual, J. and J. Berciano. (1994). Experience in the diagnosis of headaches that start in elderly people. *J. Neurol. Neurosurg. Psychiatry* 57:1255–1257.

Pascual-Leone, A. and A.P.L. Pascual. (1992). Occipital neuralgia: Another benign cause of "thunderclap headache." *J. Neurol. Neurosurg. Psychiatry* 55:411.

Pavese, N., R. Canapicchi, A. Nuti et al. (1994). White matter MRI hyperintensities in a hundred and twenty-nine consecutive migraine patients. *Cephalalgia* 14:342–345.

Prager, J.M., J. Rosenblum, D.J. Mijulis et al. (1991). Evaluation of headache patients by MRI. *Headache Q* 2:192–196.

Ramirez-Lassepas, M., C.E. Espinosa, J.J. Cicero et al. (1997). Predictors of intracranial pathologic findings in patients who seek emergency care because of headache. *Arch. Neurol.* 54:1506–1509.

Raps, E.C., S.L. Galetta, J. Rogers et al. (1994). Unruptured aneurysms and headache. *Arch. Neurol.* 51:447–448.

Rinkel, G.J.E., M. Djibuti, A. Algra et al. (1998). Prevalence and risk of rupture of intracranial aneurysms. A systematic review. *Stroke* 29:251–256.

Rinkel, G.J.E., E.F.M. Wijdicks, D. Hasan et al. (1991a). Outcome in patients with subarachnoid haemorrhage and negative angiography according to pattern of haemorrhage on computed tomography. *Lancet* 338:964–968.

Rinkel, G.J.E., E.F.M. Wijdicks, M. Vermeulen et al. (1991b). Nonaneurysmal perimesencephalic subarachnoid hemorrhage: CT and MR patterns that differ from aneurysmal rupture. *Am. J. Neuroradiol.* 12:829–834.

Robbins, L. (1991). Migraine and anticardiolipin antibodies—case reports of 13 patients and the prevalence of antiphospholipid antibodies in migraineurs. *Headache* 31:537–539.

Robbins, L. and H. Friedman. (1992). MRI in migraineurs. *Headache* 32:507–508.

Rogg, J.M., S. Smeaton, C. Doberstein et al. (1999). Assessment of the value of MR imaging for examining patients with angiographically negative subarachnoid hemorrhage. *AJR Am. J. Roentgenol.* 172:201–206.

Rowan, A.J. (1974). The electroencephalographic characteristics of migraine. *Arch. Neurol.* 37: 95–99.

Rozen, T.D., R. Niknam, A.L. Shechter et al. (1999). Gender differences in clinical characteristics and treatment response in cluster headache patients. *Cephalalgia* 19:323.

Russell, D., P. Nakstad, and O. Sjaastad. (1978). Cluster headache: Pneumoencephalographic and cerebral computerized axial tomographic findings. *Headache* 18:272–273.

Sankhla, S.K., W.J. Gunawardena, C.M.A. Coutinho et al. (1996). Magnetic resonance angiography in the management of aneurysmal subarachnoid haemorrhage: A study of 51 cases. *Neuroradiology* 38:724–729.

Saper, J.R., S. Silberstein, C.D. Gordon et al. (1999). *Handbook of Headache Management*, 2nd ed. p. 20. Lippincott, Williams and Wilkins, Philadelphia.

Sargent, J., C. Lawson, P. Solbach et al. (1979). Use of CT scans in an outpatient headache population: An evaluation. *Headache* 19:388–390.

Silberstein, S.D. (1992). Evaluation and emergency treatment of headache. *Headache* 32: 396–407.

Silberstein, S.D., R.B. Lipton, and P.J. Goadsby. (1998). *Headache in Clinical Practice*. Isis Medical Media, Oxford.

Simon, R.H., A.W. Zimmerman, A. Tasman et al. (1982). Spectral analysis of photic stimulation in migraine. *Electroencephalogr. Clin. Neurophysiol.* 53:270–276.

Smyth, V.O.G. and A.L. Winter. (1964). The EEG in migraine. *Electroencephalogr. Clin. Neurophysiol.* 16:194.

Söderström, C.E. (1977). Diagnostic significance of CSF spectrophotometry and computer tomography in cerebrovascular disease. A comparative study in 231 cases. *Stroke* 5:606–612.

Soges, L.J., E.D. Cacayorin, G.R. Petro et al. (1988). Migraine: Evaluation by MR. *AJNR Am. J. Neuradiol.* 9:425–429.

Sotaniemi, K.A., M. Rantala, J. Pyhtinen et al. (1991). Clinical and CT correlates in the diagnosis of intracranial tumours. *J. Neurol. Neurosurg. Psychiatry* 54:645–647.

Strayle-Batra, M., M. Skalej, A.K. Wakhloo et al. (1998). Three-dimensional spiral CT angiography in the detection of cerebral aneurysm. *Acta Radiol.* 39:233–238.

Tietjen, G.E. (1992). Migraine and antiphospholipid antibodies. *Cephalalgia* 12:69–74.

Tietjen, G.E., M. Day, L. Norris et al. (1998). Role of anticardiolipin antibodies in young persons with migraine and transient focal neurologic events. A prospective study. *Neurology* 50: 1433–1440.

Tourtellotte, W.W., L.N. Metz, E.R. Bryan et al. (1964). Spontaneous subarachnoid hemorrhage. Factors affecting the rate of clearing of the cerebrospinal fluid. *Neurology* 14:301–306.

Urbach, H., J. Zentner, and L. Solymosi. (1998). The need for repeat angiography in subarachnoid haemorrhage. *Neuroradiology* 40:6–10.

van der Jagt, M., D. Hasan, H.W. Bijvoet et al. (1999). Validity of prediction of the site of ruptured intracranial aneurysms with CT. *Neurology* 52:34–39.

van der Wee, N., G.J.E. Rinkel, D. Hasan D et al. (1995). Detection of subarachnoid haemorrhage on early CT: Is lumbar puncture still needed after a negative scan? *J. Neurol. Neurosurg. Psychiatry* 58:357–359.

van Gijn, J. (1992). Subarachnoid hemorrhage. *Lancet* 339:653–655.

van Gijn, J. and K.J. van Dongen. (1982). The time course of aneurysmal haemorrhage on computed tomograms. *Neuroradiology* 23:153–156.

Vermeulen, M., D. Hasan, B.G. Blijenberg et al. (1989). Xanthochromia after subarachnoid haemorrhage needs no revisitation. *J. Neurol. Neurosurg. Psychiatry* 52:826–828.

Vermeulen, M. and J. van Gijn. (1990). The diagnosis of subarachnoid haemorrhage. *J. Neurol. Neurosurg. Psychiatry* 53:365–372.

Walton, J.N. (1956). *Subarachnoid Hemorrhage*. Edinburgh, E. & S. Livingstone.

Wang, A.M., J.H. Bisese, and C.T.L. Jackson. (1995). Computed tomography of cerebrovascular disease. In *Cerebrovascular Disease. Imaging and Interventional Treatment Options* (C.L. Rumbaugh, A.M. Wang, and F.Y. Tsai, eds.), pp. 153–187. Igaku-Shoin, New York.

Weingarten, S., M. Kleinman, L. Elperin et al. (1992). The effectiveness of cerebral imaging in the diagnosis of chronic headache: A reappraisal. *Arch. Intern. Med.* 152:2457–2462.

Weir, B. (1994). Headaches from aneurysms. *Cephalalgia* 14:79–87.

Wilterdink, J.L. (1994). Sentinel headaches and aneurysmal subarachnoid hemorrhage. In *Current Diagnosis in Neurology* (E. Feldmann, ed.), pp. 62–67. Mosby, St. Louis.

Wöber-Bingöl, C., C. Wöber, D. Prayer et al. (1996). Magnetic resonance imaging for recurrent headache in childhood and adolescence. *Headache 36*:83–90.

Wolpert, S.M. and L.R. Caplan. (1992). Current role of cerebral angiography in the diagnosis of cerebrovascular diseases. *AJR Am. J. Roentgenol. 159*:191–197.

Woolf, S.H. and D.B. Kamerow. (1990). Testing for uncommon conditions. The heroic search for positive test results. *Arch. Intern. Med. 15*: 2451–2458.

Yuichi, I., S. Shigeo, M. Takeshi et al. (1981). Postcontrast computed tomography in subarachnoid hemorrhage from ruptured aneurysms. *J. Comput. Assist. Tomogr. 5*:341–344.

Ziegler, D.K., S. Batnitzky, R. Barter et al. (1991). Magnetic resonance image abnormality in migraine with aura. *Cephalalgia 11*:147–150.

4

Pain-Sensitive Cranial Structures: Chemical Anatomy

F. MICHAEL CUTRER

The foundation of our current understanding of the anatomy of headache was laid over half a century ago by the work of Harold Wolff, Bronson Ray, and Wilder Penfield. They observed that mechanical stimulation of the brain parenchyma did not cause pain in awake patients who were undergoing craniotomies but that similar stimulation of the meninges and cerebral and meningeal blood vessels produced severe, penetrating, ipsilateral headache (Ray and Wolff, 1940; Penfield, 1935). They identified intracranial pain-sensitive components, including portions of the meninges, such as the basal dura and the venous sinuses and their tributaries; neural structures, such as the glossopharyngeal, vagus, and trigeminal cranial nerves as well as the upper cervical spinal nerves; and vascular structures, such as dural arteries, the carotid, vertebral and basilar arteries, the circle of Willis, and proximal portions of cerebral, vertebral, and basilar branches. The finding that intracranial vascular structures are pain-sensitive was consistent with centuries-old observations that extracranial vessels become sensitized and distended during headache attacks. These observations also formed one of the major underpinnings of the vasogenic theory of migraine: nociceptive axons have extensive branches, and one trigeminal ganglion cell may project to more than one large cerebral artery. In humans, the anatomy of the projections of trigeminal afferents to the dura mater has been well described (Moskowitz et al., 1987) but that to the major arteries of the circle of Willis has not. Anatomical dissection in primates suggests that trigeminal afferents from the first division join the carotid artery within its cavernous segment and subsequently project to the circle of Willis. Two neurophysiological studies (Bove and Moskowitz, 1997; Strassman et al., 1996) indicate that the primary afferent fibers that innervate the dura mater are activated by mechanical, thermal, and chemical stimulation. These high-threshold polymodal nociceptors may become sensitized by exposure to solutions of low pH and exhibit properties similar to those of the small, unmyelinated fibers that innervate other tissues.

TRIGEMINOVASCULAR SYSTEM: PRIMARY AFFERENT SENSORY NEURONS

The important role that vascular and meningeal structures play in headache initiation is related to their rich innervation by the primary afferent neurons that originate within the trigeminal ganglia (primarily the first division) (Mayberg et al., 1984) and dorsal root ganglia of the upper cervical spinal nerves (Arbab et al., 1986). Three types of nociceptive neurons that may be important in various types of head pain have been identified: small-caliber, unmyelinated, slow-conducting, pseudounipolar neurons called C fibers; small-diameter, lightly myelinated, more rapid-conducting fibers called A delta nociceptors; and a more recently discovered class of small-caliber fibers called "silent nociceptors" because they remain quiet during more normal nociceptive processes and fire only in response to high-intensity noxious stimulation (Handwerker et al., 1991; Schmidt et al., 1995). Stimulation of the small-caliber, unmyelinated C fibers results in the slow build-up of an aching, throbbing, or burning pain, while the faster-conducting A delta fibers probably transmit sharper initial pain sensations (Merrill, 2000). Upon activation, primary afferent neurons transmit nociceptive information from perivascular terminals through the trigeminal (Mayberg et al., 1984) and first and second spinal (Arbab et al., 1986) ganglia to enter the brain stem at the level of the pons. The nociceptive fibers then descend to project centrally across synapses on to second-order neurons within ventrolateral (Burstein et al., 1998) regions of the trigeminal nucleus caudalis (TNC) (Lisney, 1983) and the dorsal horn of the upper cervical spinal cord.

PAIN TRANSMISSION WITHIN THE CENTRAL NERVOUS SYSTEM

A large number of C-fiber afferent fibers contain substance P (Messlinger et al., 1993), calcitonin gene–related peptide (Nozaki et al., 1990), and neurokinin A, as well as other neurotransmitters and neuromodulators, in their central and peripheral (e.g., meningeal) axons. These neuropeptide-containing neurons express a tyrosine kinase receptor (Merrill, 2000). C fibers that do not contain neuropeptides express a surface lectin epitope that can be stained with IB4 (Bennett et al., 1996). Neuropeptide-containing trigeminovascular afferents terminate within the superficial lamina (I and II) of the TNC (Schaible et al., 1997), where many of them synapse on projection neurons to other brain stem sites or

the thalamus. C fibers that do not contain neuropeptides terminate within inner portions of lamina II and are thought to be heat nociceptors (Merrill, 2000).

Glutamate is the primary neurotransmitter in C fibers and is co-stored with substance P, neurokinin A, and calcitonin gene–related peptide. Activation of the peripheral nociceptor results in the generation of a depolarizing current that moves along the C fiber to cause the central release of glutamate and neuropeptides into the synaptic cleft. Glutamate in turn binds as an agonist to both prejunctional and postjunctional glutamate receptors (Basbaum, 1999). Glutamate receptors fall into two categories: ionotropic receptors, which are directly linked to calcium and sodium ion channels, and metabotropic receptors, which exert their effect via G-protein linkage to protein kinase second messengers. The ionotropic receptors include the N-methyl-D-aspartate (NMDA), kainate, and α-2-amino-3-[hydroxy-5-methylisoxazole-4yl] receptors and are associated with nociceptive transmission at fast excitatory synapses within the dorsal horn and the TNC. Postsynaptic excitation results from the influx of extracellular calcium ions after glutamate binding of the ionotropic receptors. Activation of certain metabotropic glutamate receptors (mGluR) by either glutamate or substance P results in the release of calcium from intracellular stores (Mayer and Miller 1990). The increase in intracellular calcium activates protein kinase C, which in turn, through NMDA receptor phosphorylation, causes displacement of the Mg^{2+} ion that normally blocks the NMDA receptor–linked ion channel. After displacement of the Mg^{2+} ion, the binding of glutamate to the NMDA receptor at resting membrane potentials results in inward Na^+ and Ca^{2+} currents and increased excitation of the postsynaptic neuron (Mayer et al., 1984). Although substance P also activates these metabotropic glutamate receptors, higher intensities of stimulation are needed to affect its release from prejunctional neurons (Bausbaum, 1999) than are required to cause prejunctional glutamate release. Although NMDA receptors have a fast excitatory response, NMDA receptor antagonists thus far have not been shown to reduce afferent excitation or to block acute nociception (Chaplan et al., 1997).

Second-order neurons within the TNC project and transmit nociceptive information to numerous subcortical sites, including the more rostral portions of the trigeminal complex (Stewart and King, 1963; Jacquin et al., 1990), the hypothalamus (Malick and Burstein, 1998), the nucleus of the solitary tract (Marfurt and Rajchert, 1991), the brain stem reticular formation (Renehan et al., 1986), the midbrain and pontine parabrachial nuclei (Bernard et al., 1989; Hayashi and Tabata, 1990), and the ipsilateral cerebellum (Huerta et al., 1983; Mantle St. John and Tracey, 1987). The TNC also sends projections to the ventrobasal thalamus (Huang, 1989; Jacquin et al., 1990; Kemplay and Webster, 1989; Mantle St. John and Tracey, 1987), the posterior thalamus (Peschanski et al., 1985; Shigenaga et al., 1983), and the medial thalamus (Craig and Burton, 1981). Nociceptive information is transmitted from the rostral brain stem to other areas of the brain (e.g., the limbic areas) that are thought to be involved in the emotional and vegetative responses to pain (Bernard et al., 1989).

Although it has been difficult to demonstrate areas of direct cortical activation after meningeal stimulation (Goadsby et al., 1991), there is increasing proof that trigemino-thalamo-cortical projections exist (Barnett et al., 1995). Most of the information relating to cerebral cortical activation in headache comes from functional blood-flow imaging studies performed in humans during unilateral headache attacks. In one study that employed positron emission tomography (PET), activation in the cingulate cortex and in the auditory and visual association areas was observed several hours into spontaneous unilateral attacks of migraine without aura (Weiller et al., 1995). These areas of increased cortical blood flow resolved after the headache was effectively treated with an abortive agent. Functional activation in the cingulate gyrus also occurs in other painful conditions and is related to the arousal, motor, and affective components of pain (Kwan et al., 2000). In another series of studies employing PET, areas of increased blood flow were seen in the

anterior cingulate and insular cortices after activation of V1 C fibers using a subcutaneous injection of capsaicin into the forehead (May et al., 1998). It has been hypothesized that two distinct populations of cortical neurons exist: one receives projections from the ventrobasal complex of the thalamus and subserves localization and discrimination of pain, and the other, which arises from the medial thalamus, is involved in the affective response to pain. The medial thalamus may participate in the transmission of both the discriminative and affective components of pain (Bushnell and Duncan, 1989), suggesting that these two pathways may not be distinct.

Information related to nociception can be modulated at sites extending from the TNC to the cortex. Modulation of the nociceptive signal, both sensitizing and suppressive, is likely to be very important in determining both the clinical features and the potential treatment of headache syndromes.

CENTRAL SENSITIZATION AND THE TRIGEMINAL SYSTEM

Activation of nociceptive primary afferent fibers increases the excitability of higher-order neurons within the TNC (Burstein et al., 1998). In nontrigeminal pain models, depolarization of C fibers with chemical and inflammatory stimuli has resulted in several state changes. These include expansion of receptive field size (Woolf and King, 1990), lowering of thresholds for second-order neuronal activation in the dorsal horn (Woolf, 1984), recruitment of inputs from normally non-nociceptive fibers (Woolf and King, 1990), and heightened response to suprathreshold stimuli. Collectively, these changes are referred to as "central sensitization" and are reflected clinically in the pain-associated phenomena of spread of cutaneous sensitivity to uninjured areas, *hyperalgesia* (lowered pain threshold), and *cutaneous allodynia* (generation of a painful response by normally innocuous stimuli).

Features of central sensitization are observed in headache syndromes and probably contribute to the intensification and prolongation of head pain. For example, migraine pain frequently expands, as the headache develops, to involve half or at times the whole head. In addition, small, usually innocuous head movements (e.g., coughing or straining) become painful during and in the hours after resolution of a migraine attack. Chemical stimulation of nociceptors within the meninges lowers the activation threshold of second-order neurons to low-intensity mechanical and thermal stimuli (Burstein et al., 1998). In addition, noxious chemical dural stimulation lowers the threshold for generation of cardiovascular responses (such as blood pressure elevation) by previously innocuous skin stimulation (Yamamura et al., 1999). Evidence of central sensitization may be seen in humans as well. In a recent study of 42 migraine patients, repeated measurements of mechanical and thermal pain thresholds were performed in periorbital and forearm skin during and between acute headache attacks; 79% of subjects exhibited cutaneous allodynia (Burstein et al., 2000).

CENTRAL INHIBITORY MODULATION OF TRIGEMINAL NOCICEPTION

Modulation within the central nervous system may be inhibitory as well. Defects of the intrinsic inhibitory system may also be important in the clinical evolution of chronic headache disorders. Within the TNC, the nociceptive signal can be modulated by inhibitory interneurons, within lamina II by projections from more rostral trigeminal nuclei (Kruger and Young, 1981) and the nucleus raphae magnus (Sessle et al., 1981), as well as by descending cortical inhibitory systems (Sessle et al., 1981; Wise and Jones, 1977). Inhibitory GABAergic and enkephalinergic interneurons are likely to act not only on projection neurons (Fields and Basbaum, 1994) but also on the glutamate-containing terminals of primary afferent neurons, where they affect presynaptic inhibition (Iliakis et al., 1996). The most powerful descending inhibitory system is likely to involve projections from insular cortical and hypothalamic areas

through the periaqueductal gray matter, and rostral ventral medial medulla to the superficial lamina of the TNC and the upper cervical dorsal horn (Messlinger and Burstein, 2000; Fields and Basbaum, 1994). Stimulation of the periaqueductal gray matter (Morgan et al., 1992), rostral ventral medial medulla (Lovick and Wolstencroft, 1979), areas of somatosensory cortex (Chiang et al., 1990), and hypothalamus (Rhodes and Liebeskind, 1978) suppresses nociceptive responses. The inhibitory interneurons within lamina II of the TNC receive input from descending excitatory serotonergic neurons from the periaqueductal gray matter and rostral ventral medial medulla (Fields and Basbaum, 1994). Morphine administration increases the release of serotonin in the superficial lamina of the TNC and decreases presynaptic release of substance P. This is consistent with the hypothesis that morphine may activate the 5-hydroxytryptamine–mediated inhibition of nociception in the TNC and dorsal horn (Yonehara et al., 1990). Parabrachial areas (ventrolateral nuclei) also have direct and bilateral projections to all the subnuclei of the trigeminal brain stem nuclear complex (Yoshida et al., 1997). Stimulation of the parabrachial area suppresses both spontaneous and evoked firing in TNC nociceptive neurons (Chiang et al., 1994).

CONCLUSIONS

The neuroanatomical substrates of head pain are quite complex and still incompletely characterized. Headaches appear to develop through a cascade of events that are modulated by both suppressive and sensitizing systems. Derangement in these modulatory systems may underlie the development of chronic headache syndromes. A greater understanding of the functional anatomy and physiology of head pain holds the key to more specific and effective treatments.

REFERENCES

Arbab, M.A.R., L. Wiklind, and N.A. Scendgaard. (1986). Origin and distribution of cerebral vascular innervation from superior cervical, trigeminal and spinal ganglia investigated with retrograde and anterograde WGA-HRP tracing in the rat. *Neuroscience 19*:695–708.

Barnett, E.M., G.D. Evans, N. Sun et al. (1995). Anterograde tracing of trigeminal afferent pathways from the murine tooth pulp to cortex using herpes simplex virus type 1. *J. Neurosci. 15*: 2972–2984.

Basbaum, A.I. (1999). Distinct neurochemical features of acute and persistent pain. *Proc. Natl. Acad. Sci. USA 96*:7739–7742.

Bennett, D., N. Dmietrieva, J.V. Priestley et al. (1996). trkA CGRP and IB4 expression in retrogradely labelled cutaneous and visceral primary sensory neurones in the rat. *Neurosci. Lett. 206*:33–36.

Bernard, J.F., M. Peschanski, and J.M. Besson. (1989). A possible spino-(trigemino)-ponto amygdaloid pathway for pain. *Neurosci. Lett. 100*:83–88.

Bove, G.M. and M.A. Moskowitz. (1997). Primary afferent neurons innervating guinea pig dura. *J. Neurophysiol. 77*:299–308.

Burstein, R., H. Yamamura, A. Malick et al. (1998). Chemical stimulation of the intracranial dura induces enhanced responses to facial stimulation in brain stem trigeminal neurons. *J. Neurophysiol. 79*:964–982.

Burstein, R., D. Yarnitsky, I. Goor-Aryeh et al. (2000). An association between migraine and cutaneous allodynia. *Ann. Neurol. 47*:614–624.

Bushnell, M.C. and G.H. Duncan. (1989). Sensory and affective aspects of pain perception: Is medial thalamus restricted to emotional issues? *Exp. Brain Res. 78*:415–418.

Chaplan, S.R., A.B. Malmberg, and T.L. Yaksh. (1997). Efficacy of spinal NMDA receptor antagonism in formalin hyperalgesia and nerve injury evoked allodynia in the rat. *J. Pharmacol. Exp. Ther. 280*:829–838.

Chiang, C.Y., J.O. Dostrovsky, and B.J. Sessle. (1990). Role of anterior pretectal nucleus in somatosensory cortical descending modulation of jaw-opening reflex in rat. *Brain Res. 515*:219–226.

Chiang, C.Y., J.W. Hu, and B.J. Sessle. (1994). Parabrachial area and nucleus raphe magnus–induced modulation of nociceptive and non-nociceptive trigeminal subnucleus caudalis neurons activated by cutaneous or deep inputs. *J. Neurophysiol. 71*:2430–2445.

Craig, A.D., Jr. and H. Burton. (1981). Spinal and medullary lamina I projection to nucleus submedius in medial thalamus: A possible pain center center. *J. Neurophysiol. 45*:443–466.

Fields, H.L. and A.I. Basbaum. (1994). Central nervous system mechanisms of pain modulation. In *Textbook of Pain* (P.D. Wall and R. Melzack,

eds.), pp. 243–257. Churchill Livingstone, Edinburgh.

Goadsby, P.J., A.S. Zagami, and G.A. Lambert. (1991). Neural processing of craniovascular pain: A synthesis of the central structures involved in migraine. *Headache 31*:365–371.

Handwerker, H.O., S. Kilo, and P.W. Reeh. (1991). Unresponsive afferent nerve of the rat. *J. Physiol. (Lond.) 435*:229–242.

Hayashi, H. and T. Tabata. (1990). Pulpal and cutaneous inputs to somatosensory neurons in the parabrachial area of the cat. *Brain Res. 511*: 177–179.

Huang, L.-Y.M. (1989). Origin of thalamically projecting somatosensory relay neurons in the immature rat. *Brain Res. 495*:108–114.

Huerta, M.F., A. Frankfurter, and J.K. Harting. (1983). Studies of the prinicipal sensory and spinal trigeminal nuclei of the rat: Projections to the superior colliculus, inferior olive, and cerebellum. *J. Comp. Neurol. 220*:147–167.

Iliakis. B., N.L. Anderson, P.S. Irish et al. (1996). Electron microscopy of immunoreactivity patterns for glutamate and gamma-aminobutyric acid in synaptic glomeruli of the feline spinal trigeminal nucleus (subnucleus caudalis). *J. Comp. Neurol. 366*:465–477.

Jacquin, M.F., N.L. Chiaia, J.H. Haring et al. (1990). Intersub-nuclear connections within the rat trigeminal brainstem complex. *Somatosen. Mot. Res. 7*:399–420.

Kemplay, S. and K.E. Webster. (1989). A quantitative study of the projections of the gracile, cuneate and trigeminal nuclei and of the medullary reticular formation to the thalamus in the rat. *Neuroscience 32*:153–167.

Kruger, L. and R.F. Young. (1981). Specialized features of the trigeminal nerve and its central connections. In *The Cranial Nerves* (M. Samii and P.J. Janetta, eds.), pp. 273–301. Springer-Verlag, Berlin.

Kwan, C.L., A.P. Crawley, D.J. Mikulis et al. (2000). An fMRI study of the anterior cingulate cortex and surrounding medial wall activations evoked by noxious cutaneous heat and cold stimuli. *Pain 85*:359–374.

Lisney, S.J.W. (1983). Some current topics of interest in the physiology of trigeminal pain: A review. *J. R. Soc. Med. 76*:292–296.

Lovick, T.A. and J.H. Wolstencroft. (1979). Inhibitory effects of nucleus raphe magnus on neuronal responses in the spinal trigeminal nucleus to nociceptive compared with non-nociceptive inputs. *Pain 7*:135–145.

Malick, A. and R. Burstein. (1998). Cells of origin of the trigeminohypothalamic tract in the rat. *J. Comp. Neurol. 400*:125–144.

Mantle St. John, L.A. and D.J. Tracey. (1987). Somatosensory nuclei in the brainstem of the rat:

Independent projections to the thalamus and cerebellum. *J. Comp. Neurol.* 255:259–271.

Marfurt, C.F. and D.M. Rajchert. (1991). Trigeminal primary afferent projections to "non-trigeminal" areas of the rat central nervous system. *J. Comp. Neurol.* 303:489–511.

May, A., H. Kaube, C. Buchel et al. (1998). Experimental cranial pain elicited by capsaicin: A PET study. *Pain* 74:61–66.

Mayberg, M.R., N.T. Zervas, and M.A. Moskowitz. (1984). Trigeminal projections to supratentorial pial and dural blood vessels in cats demonstrated by horseradish peroxidase histochemistry. *J. Comp. Neurol.* 223:46–56.

Mayer, M., G. Westbrook, and P.B. Guthrie. (1984). Voltage-dependent block by Mg^{2+} of NMDA responses in spinal cord neurones. *Nature* 309:261–263.

Mayer, M.L. and R.J. Miller. (1990). Excitatory amino acid receptors, second messengers and regulation of intracellular Ca^{2+} in mammalian neurons. *Trends Pharmacol. Sci.* 11:254–260.

Merrill, R.L. (2000). Neurophysiology of orofacial pain. *Oral Maxillofac. Surg. Clin. North Am.* 12:165–179.

Messlinger, K., and R. Burstein. (2000). Anatomy of central nervous system pathways related to head pain. In *The Headaches*, 2nd ed., (J. Olesen, P. Tfelt-Hansen, and K.M.A. Welch, eds.), pp. 77–86. Lippincott Williams & Wilkins, Philadelphia.

Messlinger, K., U. Hanesch, M. Baumgaetel et al. (1993). Innervation of the dura mater encephali of cat and rat: Ultrastructure and calcitonin gene–related peptide-like and substance P-like immunoreactivity. *Anat. Embryol.* 188:219–237.

Morgan, M.M., M.M. Heinricher, and L.H. Fields. (1992). Circuitry linking opioid-sensitive nociceptive modulatory system in periaqueductal grey and spinal cord with rostral ventromedial medulla. *Neuroscience* 47:863–871.

Moskowitz, M.A., K. Saito, L. Brezina et al. (1987). Nerve fibers surrounding intracranial and extracranial vessels from human and other species contain dynorphin-like immunoreactivity. *Neuroscience* 23:731–737.

Nozaki, K., Y. Uemura, S. Okamoto et al. (1990). Origins and distribution of cerebrovascular nerve fibers showing calcitonin gene–related peptide-like immunoreacitivy in the major cerebral artery of the dog. *J. Comp. Neurol.* 297:219–226.

Penfield, W. (1935). A contribution to the mechanism of intracranial pain. *Assoc. Res. Nerv. Ment. Dis.* 15:399–416.

Peschanski, M., F. Roudier, H.J. Ralston, III et al. (1985). Ultrastructural analysis of the terminals of various somatosensory pathways in the ventrobasal complex of the rat thalamus: An electron-microscopic study using wheatgerm agglutinin conjugated to horseradish peroxidase as an axonal tracer. *Somatosens. Res.* 3:75–87.

Ray, B.S. and H.G. Wolff. (1940). Experimental studies on headache. Pain-sensitive structures of the head and their significance in headache. *Arch. Surg.* 41:813–856.

Renehan, W.E., M.F. Jacquin, R.D. Mooney et al. (1986). Structure–function relationship in rat medullary and cervical dorsal horns. II. Medullary dorsal horn cells. *J. Neurophysiol.* 55:1187–1201.

Rhodes, D.L. and J.C. Liebeskind. (1978). Analgesia from rostral brainstem stimulation in the rat. *Brain Res.* 143:521–532.

Schaible, H.-G., A. Ebersberger, P. Peppel et al. (1997). Release of immunoreactive substance P in the trigeminal brain stem nuclear complex evoked by chemical stimulation of the nasal mucosa and the dura mater encephali—A study with antibody microphobes. *Neuroscience* 76:273–284.

Schmidt, R.F., M. Schmelz, C. Forester et al. (1995). Novel classes of responsive and unresponsive C nociceptors in human skin. *J. Neurosci.* 15:333–341.

Sessle, B.J., J.W. Hu, R. Dubner et al. (1981). Functional properties of neurons in trigeminal subnucleus caudalis of the cat. II. Modulation of responses to noxious and non-noxious stimulation by periaqueductal gray, nucleus raphe magnus, cerebral cortex and afferent influences, and effect of nalaxone. *J. Neurophysiol.* 45:193–207.

Shigenaga, A., Nakatani, T. Nishimori et al. (1983). The cells of origin of cat trigeminothalamic projections: Especially in the caudal medulla. *Brain Res.* 277:201–222.

Stewart, W.A. and R.B. King. (1963). Fiber projections from the nucleus caudalis of the spinal trigeminal nucleus. *J. Comp. Neurol.* 121:271–286.

Strassman, A.M., S.A. Raymond, and R. Burstein. (1996). Sensitization of meningeal sensory neurons and the origin of headaches. *Nature* 384:560–564.

Weiller, C., A. May, V. Limmroth et al. (1995). Brain stem activation in spontaneous human migraine attacks. *Nat. Med.* 1:658–660.

Wise, S.P. and E.G. Jones. (1977). Cells of origin and trigeminal distribution of descending projections of the rat somatic sensory cortex. *J. Comp. Neurol.* 175:129–158.

Woolf, C.J. (1984). Long term alterations in the excitability of the flexion reflex produced by peripheral tissue injury in the chronic decerebrate rat. *Pain* 18:325–343.

Woolf, C.J. and A.E. King. (1990). Dynamic alterations in the cutaneous mechanosensitive receptive fields of dorsal horn neurons in the rat spinal cord. *J. Neurosci.* 10:2717–2726.

Yamamura, H., A. Malick, N.L. Chamberlin et al. (1999). Cardiovascular and neuronal responses to head stimulation reflect central sensitization and cutaneous allodynia in a rat model of migraine. *J. Neurophysiol.* 81:479–493.

Yonehara, N., T. Shibutani, Y. Imai et al. (1990). Involvement of descending monoaminergic systems in the transmission of dental pain in the trigeminal nucleus caudalis of the rabbit. *Brain Res.* 508:234–240.

Yoshida, A., K. Chen, M. Moritani et al. (1997). Organization of the descending projections from the parabrachial nucleus to the trigeminal sensory nuclear complex and spinal dorsal horn in the rat. *J. Comp. Neurol.* 383:94–111.

5

Pathophysiology of Headache

PETER J. GOADSBY

Headache has come a long way during the seven editions of this book, in part because of the issues raised by its first author. Understanding headache is a challenging task given the large number of headache syndromes; the current International Headache Society (IHS) classification runs to 96 pages (Headache Classification Committee of the International Headache Society, 1988). However, understanding the mechanisms of headache is time well spent given the common nature of headache problems (Rasmussen, 1995; Stewart et al., 1992) and the expansion of treatments, particularly for migraine, that has taken place in the last few years (Goadsby and Silberstein, 1997). The emphasis in this chapter is on the primary headache syndromes, which are very common and, while not life-threatening, are lifestyle-disabling (see Chapter 7). After dealing specifically with migraine and cluster headache, the issues of the blood vessels, so close to Wolff's interests (Graham and Wolff, 1938, 1966; Ray and Wolff, 1940; Tunis and Wolff, 1953), and tension-type headache will be addressed.

GENERAL PRINCIPLES

Headache is an excellent example of a problem that spans the breadth of medicine. It can be at once a major symptom, such as in subarachnoid hemorrhage, and the most disabling aspect of a primary syndrome, such as in cluster headache. Headache may be divided into *primary headache*, in which the headache and any associated features are themselves the disease processes, and *secondary headaches*, in which the headache is a symptom of an underlying disorder. Much of the basic anatomy of all types of headache must be shared, since ultimately the trigeminal nucleus transduces nociceptive information from the head prior to its distribution within the brain. The best described anatomy and physiology have been developed in the investigation of migraine, but much of this substrate must be shared. Since secondary headache processes entrain very similar mechanisms for the expression of pain or even trigger primary headache mechanisms, it is not surprising that a secondary headache can mimic a primary headache phenotype and provide a very substantial diagnostic challenge, as described in Chapter 3.

MIGRAINE

Migraine is, in essence, an episodic headache that has certain associated features (Table 5–1), which give the clues to its pathophysiology (Table 5–2). In addition the term migraine is often used in two ways: first, to refer to the phenotype attacks, and secondly, to imply the underlining biotype of a headache disorder. It is interesting to compare the features of migraine and tension-type headache and to

Table 5–1 Simplified diagnostic criteria for migraine: comparison with tension-type headache (repeated attacks of headache lasting 4 to 72 hours or 30 minutes to 7 days for tension-type headache, which have these features)

Migraine	Tension-type headache
At least 2 of the following	
• Unilateral pain	• Bilateral pain
• Throbbing pain	• Nonthrobbing pain
• Aggravation by movement	• No effect of movement
• Moderate or severe intensity	• Mild or moderate intensity
At least 1 of the following	
• Nausea/vomiting	• No nausea/vomiting
• Photophobia and phonophobia	• Photophobia or phonophobia but not both

Adapted from the Headache Classification Committee of the International Headache Society (1988). Permission from Goadsby, P.J. and J. Olesen (1996). Diagnosis and Management of Migraine. *BMJ* 312:1279–1282.

ask "What is quintessentially migrainous?" How can we make the diagnosis based on understanding the elements that contribute to the dysfunction?

The essential aspects to be considered in understanding migraine are as follows:

• Anatomy of the large intracranial vessels and dura mater and their neural connections, which are known as the trigeminovascular system
• The physiology and pharmacology of activation of the peripheral branches of the ophthalmic branch of the trigeminal nerve as marked by plasma protein extravasation and neuropeptide release
• The physiology and pharmacology of the trigeminal nucleus, in particular its caudalmost part, the trigeminocervical complex
• The brain stem and diencephalic modula-

tory systems, which control trigeminal pain processing

Anatomy

Surrounding the large cerebral vessels, pial vessels, large venous sinuses, and dura mater is a plexus of largely unmyelinated fibers, which arise from the ophthalmic division of the trigeminal ganglion and, in the posterior fossa, from the upper cervical dorsal roots. The trigeminal fibers that innervate the cerebral vessels arise from neurons in the trigeminal ganglion which contain substance P (SP) and calcitonin gene–related peptide (CGRP) (Uddman et al., 1985), both of which can be released when the trigeminal ganglion is stimulated in either humans or cats (Goadsby et al., 1988). Stimulation of the cra-

Table 5–2 Possible substrates for the clinical features of migraine

Clinical feature	Possible pathophysiological substrate
Pain	Trigeminovascular system
Throbbing	pain-producing innervation of the large cranial vessels
Unilateral	trigeminal nerve/nucleus processing
Nausea	Trigeminal connections with caudal medial nucleus tractus solitarius
Sensory sensitivity	
Head movement	
Light	Abnormal brain stem modulation of sensory input, e.g., locus coeruleus
Sound	
Smells	
Episodic attacks	Channelopathic dysfunction in brain stem aminergic nociceptive control systems with trigeminovascular connections

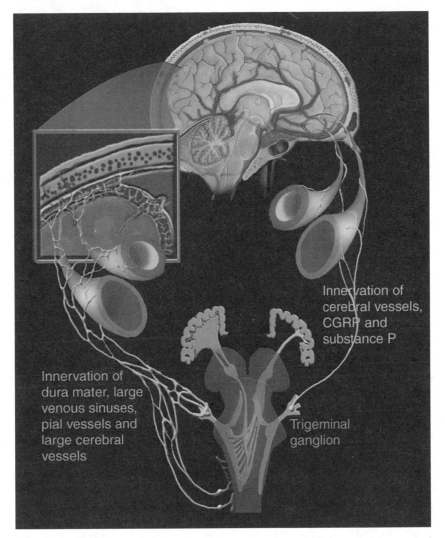

Figure 5–1 Craniovascular innervation by trigeminal, sympathetic, and cranial parasympathetic nerves. The large cerebral vessels, pial vessels, large venous sinuses, and dura mater are surrounded by a plexus of largely unmyelinated fibers that arise from the trigeminal ganglion and in the posterior fossa from the upper cervical dorsal roots. Fibers innervating cerebral vessels arise from within the trigeminal ganglion from neurons that contain substance P and calcitonin gene–related peptide (*CGRP*). (Reproduced with permission from Neurology Ambassador Programme, American Headache Society.)

nial vessels, such as the superior sagittal sinus, is certainly painful in humans (Feindel et al., 1960). In humans, the dural nerves that innervate the cranial vessels consist largely of small-diameter myelinated and unmyelinated fibers which almost certainly subserve a nociceptive function (Fig. 5–1).

What then is the source of pain in migraine? It must be borne in mind that the pain process is likely to be a combination of direct factors, i.e., activation of the nociceptors of pain-producing intracranial structures in concert with a reduction in the function of the endogenous pain-control pathways that normally gate that pain (Goadsby et al., 1991). If the carotid artery is occluded ipsilateral to the side of headache in migraineurs, two-thirds of them will experience relief, although this does not account for the other one-third (Drummond and Lance, 1983).

Moreover, distension of major cerebral vessels by balloon dilation leads to pain being referred to the ophthalmic division of the trigeminal nerve (Martins et al., 1993; Nichols et al., 1990, 1993).

Physiology of Peripheral Connections

Plasma Protein Extravasation

Moskowitz (1990) has provided an elegant series of experiments to suggest that the pain of migraine may be a form of sterile neurogenic inflammation. These are covered here briefly for continuity but are addressed in greater detail in Chapter 4. Neurogenic plasma extravasation can be seen during electrical stimulation of the trigeminal ganglion in the rat (Markowitz et al., 1987). Plasma extravasation can be blocked by ergot alkaloids, indomethacin, acetylsalicylic acid, and the serotonin [5-hydroxytryptamine (5HT)]-1-like agonist sumatriptan (Moskowitz and Cutrer, 1993). In addition, structural changes in the dura mater are seen with trigeminal ganglion stimulation; these include mast cell degranulation and changes in postcapillary venules, including platelet aggregation (Dimitriadou et al., 1991).

While it is generally accepted that such changes, particularly the initiation of a sterile inflammatory response, would cause pain (Burstein et al., 1998; Strassman et al., 1996), it is not clear whether this is sufficient or requires other stimulators or promoters, with some recent clinical data demanding that the role of plasma protein extravasation be reexamined. Moreover, although the plasma extravasation in the retina that is blocked by sumatriptan is seen after trigeminal ganglion stimulation in the rat, no changes are seen with retinal angiography during acute attacks of migraine or cluster headache (May et al., 1998c). Clearly, blockade of neurogenic plasma protein extravasation is not completely predictive of antimigraine efficacy in humans, as evidenced by the failure in clinical trials of SP, neurokinin-1 antagonists (Connor et al., 1998; Diener, 1996; Goldstein et al., 1997; Norman et al., 1998), specific plasma protein extravasation blockers, CP122,288

(Roon et al., 1997), 4991w93 (Earl et al., 1999), an endothelin antagonist (May et al., 1996), and a neurosteriod ganaxolone (Data et al., 1998).

Neuropeptide Studies

Electrical stimulation of the trigeminal ganglion in both humans and cats leads to increases in extracerebral blood flow and local release of both CGRP and SP (Goadsby et al., 1988). In the cat, trigeminal ganglion stimulation also increases cerebral blood flow by a pathway traversing the greater superficial petrosal branch of the facial nerve, again releasing a powerful vasodilator peptide, vasoactive intestinal polypeptide (Goadsby and Duckworth, 1987). Stimulation of the more specifically vascular pain-producing superior sagittal sinus increases cerebral blood flow (Lambert et al., 1988) and jugular vein CGRP levels (Zagami et al., 1990). Human evidence that CGRP is elevated in the headache phase of migraine (Gallai et al., 1995; Goadsby et al., 1990), cluster headache (Fanciullacci et al., 1995; Goadsby and Edvinsson, 1994), and chronic paroxysmal hemicrania (Goadsby and Edvinsson, 1996) supports the view that the trigeminovascular system may be activated in a protective role in these conditions. Furthermore, CGRP infusion will trigger headache, some clearly migrainous, in humans (Lassen et al., 1998). It is of interest in this regard that compounds that have not shown activity in human migraine, notably the conformationally restricted analogue of sumatriptan CP122,288 (Knight et al., 1999b) and the conformationally restricted analogue of zolmitriptan 4991w93 (Knight et al., 1999a), were ineffective inhibitors of CGRP release after superior sagittal sinus stimulation in the cat.

Physiology of Central Connections

The Trigeminocervical Complex

Using Fos immunohistochemistry, a method for detecting activated cells, Fos-like immunoreactivity is seen in the trigeminal nucleus caudalis and in the dorsal horn at the C_1 and C_2 levels, after stimulation of the superior sagittal sinus in the cat (Kaube et al., 1993c) and monkey (Goadsby and Hoskin, 1997). Using 2-deoxyglucose measurements after superior sagittal sinus stimulation, it has also been shown that neuronal activity is increased in the trigeminal nucleus caudalis and in the dorsal horn at the C_1 and C_2 levels (Goadsby and Zagami, 1991). It is likely that the trigeminal nucleus extends beyond the traditional nucleus caudalis to the dorsal horn of the high cervical region in a functional continuum that could be regarded as a *trigeminocervical complex*. This structure provides second-order neurons for the entire set of intracranial pain-producing structures (Fig. 5–2). This arrangement explains why patients with primary headache complain of pain in the head that does not respect the cutaneous distribution of either the trigeminal or cervical nerve pain all over the head. Moreover, stimulation of a lateralized structure, the middle meningeal artery, produces Fos expression bilaterally in both the cat and the monkey brain (Hoskin et al., 1999), a finding that is consistent with the observation that up to one-third of patients complain of bilateral pain. Experimental pharmacological evidence suggests that some abortive antimigraine drugs, such as ergots (Hoskin et al., 1996), acetylsalicylic acid (Kaube et al., 1993a), sumatriptan after blood–brain barrier disruption (Kaube et al., 1993b), eletriptan (Goadsby and Hoskin, 1999), naratriptan (Cumberbatch et al., 1998; Goadsby and Knight, 1997), rizatriptan (Cumberbatch et al., 1997), and zolmitriptan (Goadsby and Hoskin, 1996), can have actions at these second-order neurons that reduce cell activity

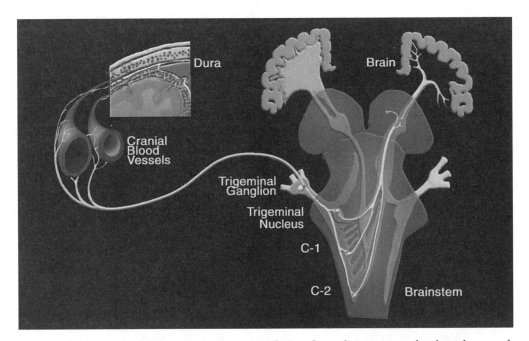

Figure 5–2 The central concepts in our current understanding of migraine pathophysiology are based on the anatomical and physiological relationships of the trigeminovascular system. The key aspects of the trigeminovascular system are (1) the pain-producing cranial vessels and dura mater, which refer pain mainly to the first (ophthalmic) division of the trigeminal nerve; (2) the peripheral branches of the trigeminal nerve, which are activated during migraine and have been modeled using studies of neurogenic plasma protein extravasation and neuropeptide release; (3) the central processing of pain signals in the trigeminocervical complex, in which second-order neurons receive input and project rostrally to transmit the pain signal within the central nervous system. These three aspects serve as the basis for understanding the pain and, thus, how acute anti-migraine drugs might act. (Reproduced with permission from Neurology Ambassador Programme, American Headache Society.)

and suggest a further possible site for therapeutic intervention in migraine. The pharmacology of these compounds (Goadsby, 1998) suggests that there is a $5HT_{1B/1D}$ inhibitory receptor within the trigeminal nucleus that may be a useful therapeutic target in migraine.

Higher-Order Processing

Following transmission in the caudal brain stem and high cervical spinal cord, information is relayed in a group of fibers (the quintothalamic tract) to the thalamus (Table 5–3). Vascular pain processing in the thalamus occurs in the ventroposteromedial thalamus, medial nucleus of the posterior complex and intralaminar thalamus in experimental animals (Zagami and Goadsby, 1991). Zagami and Lambert (1991), by application of capsaicin to the superior sagittal sinus, has shown that trigeminal projections with a high degree of nociceptive input are processed in neurons, particularly in the ventroposteromedial thalamus and its ventral periphery. Human imaging studies have confirmed activation of the thalamus contralateral to pain in acute cluster headache (May et al., 1998a) and in short-lasting unilateral neuralgiform headache with conjunctival injection and tearing (SUNCT) (May et al., 1999b). The properties and further higher-center connections of these neurons are the subject of ongoing studies that will allow us to build a more complete picture of the trigeminovascular pain pathways (Table 5–2).

Central Modulation Defining the Syndrome

In one of the most interesting studies done in recent years, activation of the rostral brain stem was seen using positron emission tomography (PET) during migraine without aura (Weiller et al., 1995). The brain stem areas were active immediately after successful treatment of the headache but were not active interictally, whereas the cingulate cortex and visual and auditory association cortex were active only during the headache and not after treatment. This differentiation suggests that the brain stem activation represented some fundamental part of the disorder and was not simply a response to pain. The activation corresponds with the brain region that Raskin et al. (1987) initially reported and Veloso et al. (1998) confirmed to cause migraine-like headache when stimulated in patients who had electrodes implanted for pain control.

Stimulation of a discrete nucleus in the brain stem that is included in the area activated on PET, the nucleus locus coeruleus (the main central noradrenergic nucleus), reduces cerebral blood flow in a frequency-dependent manner in experimental animals (Goadsby et al., 1982) through an α_2-adrenoceptor-linked mechanism (Goadsby et al., 1985). This reduction is maximal in the occipital cortex (Goadsby and Duckworth, 1989). While a 25% overall reduction in cerebral blood flow is seen, extracerebral vasodilation occurs in parallel (Goadsby et al., 1982). In addition, the main serotonin-

Table 5–3 Neuroanatomical processing of vascular head pain

Target innervation	Structure	Comments
Cranial vessels	Ophthalmic branch of trigeminal nerve	
Dura mater		
1st	Trigeminal ganglion	Middle cranial fossa
2nd	Trigeminal nucleus (quintothalamic tract)	Trigeminal nerve caudalis and C_1/C_2 dorsal horns
3rd	Thalamus	Ventrobasal complex, medial nerve of posterior group, intralaminar complex
Final	Cortex	Insulae, frontal cortex, anterior cingulate cortex, basal ganglia

containing nucleus in the brain stem, the midbrain dorsal raphe nucleus, can increase cerebral blood flow when activated (Goadsby et al., 1991). Stimulation of this ventrolateral periaqueductal gray region inhibits sagittal sinus-evoked trigeminal neuronal activity in the cat (Knight and Goadsby, 1999). Taken together, it seems entirely plausible to consider that rostral brain stem areas play a pivotal, if not defining, role in migraine (Fig. 5–3).

CLUSTER HEADACHE AND RELATED CONDITIONS

Cluster headache is a clinically well-defined disorder in which patients suffer extremely painful headaches with clock-like regularity one to three times or more a day for perhaps several months, usually followed by a period of remission (Headache Classification Committee of the International Headache Society, 1988). Cluster headache has been recognized for at least 250 years (Isler, 1993), yet until recently its mechanism has been poorly understood. Closely related conditions include paroxysmal hemicrania and the SUNCT syndrome, which also feature relatively short-lasting headaches with evidence of activation of the cranial parasympathetic outflow (Goadsby and Lipton, 1997).

The three major aspects of the pathophysiology of cluster headache are as follows: the trigeminal distribution of the pain, the autonomic features, and the episodic pattern of the attacks (which are in many ways the de-

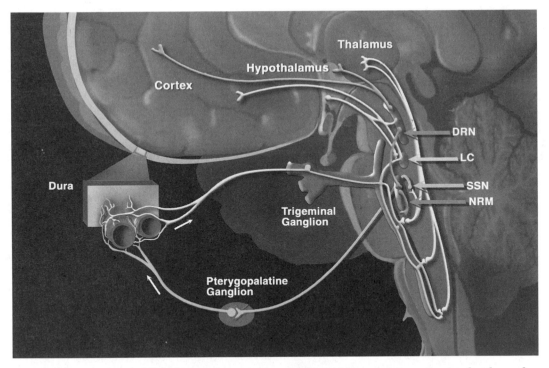

Figure 5–3 Activation of the rostral brain stem in patients with spontaneous migraine has been demonstrated using positron emission tomography. This region (*red area*) was active during the acute attack, and activation persisted after successful treatment but was not present between attacks (Weiller et al., 1995). These findings suggest that there are brain stem regions that play a pivotal role in either initiation or termination of the acute attack of migraine. Indeed, migraine may well be a defect of normal control mechanisms for suppressing input because similar regions in the experimental animal gate trigeminal nociceptive information (Knight and Goadsby, 1999). Key to abbreviations: *DRN*, dorsal raphe nucleus; *LC*, locus coeruleus; *NRM*, nucleus raphe magnus; *SSN*, superior salivatory nucleus. (Reproduced with permission from Neurology Ambassador Programme, American Headache Society.)

fining clinical signature of the disorder compared to migraine) (Lance and Goadsby, 1998). These features raise the classic issues of the location of the lesion and the generic terminology that should be applied to these and related headaches, such as migraine. The classic observation during angiography of a patient suffering an acute cluster headache demonstrating changes in the internal carotid artery (Ekbom and Greitz, 1970) suggested a pathological focus in the region of the cavernous sinus. The arguments for this locus for the disease have been set out elsewhere (Hardebo, 1994; Moskowitz, 1988). By outlining what is known about cluster headache, I will make an argument for it to be considered as a central nervous system disorder involving the posterior hypothalamic circadian cycling mechanisms.

Neuroendocrine Changes

Perhaps the key feature of cluster headache is the cycling of short-lasting attacks of pain or cycling between bouts of pain and periods of complete freedom from attacks. Kudrow (1976, 1977) was the first to point out that testosterone levels were altered in cluster headache patients during bouts; this implicated hypothalamic dysfunction. Nelson (1978) could not confirm this result. Leone and colleagues (1990) identified reduced responses to stimulation by thyrotropin-releasing releasing hormone, and there are interesting observations of disordered circadian rhythm for cortisol, growth hormone, lutenizing hormone, and prolactin (Chazot et al., 1984; Leone and Bussone, 1993; Leone et al., 1995). One area involved in human clock systems is the suprachiasmatic nucleus in the hypothalamic gray, which sits at the base of the third ventricle (Moore-Ede, 1983). Melatonin is produced by the pineal gland and has a strong circadian rhythm that is regulated by the suprachiasmatic nucleus (Moore, 1997). Connections between the retina and the hypothalamus are thought to provide light cues for the circadian rhythm (Hofman et al., 1996). The characteristic nocturnal peak of melatonin secretion is blunted during the active phase of cluster headache

(Waldenlind et al., 1987). Neuroendocrine changes in cluster headache have, therefore, implicated this region of the brain in the pathophysiology of the disorder.

Imaging Studies

Cluster headache attacks can be triggered with nitroglycerin spray (Ekbom, 1968), and recent PET scan studies in patients with cluster headache have taken advantage of this fact, although the pattern of activation in the brain is no different from that of spontaneous attacks (May et al., 2000). The areas that were observed to be activated fell into three categories: areas generally associated with pain, an area that seems specific to cluster headache, and vascular structures (May et al., 1998a).

Pain

The anterior cingulate was significantly activated during acute cluster headache, as would be expected since in most human PET studies with pain, activation of the anterior cingulate is observed, perhaps as a part of the affective response (Derbyshire et al., 1997). Activation was also observed in the frontal cortex and insulae and the thalamus contralateral to the side of the pain. In addition, there was activation in the ipsilateral basal ganglia. This is not the first observation of basal ganglia changes associated with pain (Chudler and Dong, 1995; Derbyshire et al., 1997), and it may simply relate to movement or the wish to move, which is common in cluster patients, or even some deliberate inhibition of movement.

Cluster Headache

The only activated area that is particular to cluster headache is the ipsilateral hypothalamic gray. This is in contrast to the results of Hsieh et al. (1996), who did PET scans on four cluster headache patients, two with right-sided and two with left-sided headaches. They observed cingulate cortex and frontal activation but not hypothalamic activation or thalamic activation. The data were not mirrored in that study. May and colleagues (1998a) observed ipsilateral activation at the base of the third ventricle in the hypothalamic gray. This area is of obvious interest because of its role in the control of the circadian rhythm of neurons, as outlined above. Moreover, voxel-based morphometry, a method of comparing sets of brains for subtle differences, demonstrated a small enlargement of the grey matter region of the posterior hypothalamus in patients with cluster headache (May et al., 1999a), which is totally consistent with the functional imaging data.

Vascular Change

In the PET study of acute cluster headache, pooling of tracer in the region of the cavernous sinus/internal carotid artery was noted. This suggests vasodilation and, in view of classical ideas concerning cluster headache pathophysiology, is dealt with below, specifically in the vascular section. Suffice to say that pooling is in no way specific to cluster headache and suggests that the disorder is neurovascular, not primarily vascular, in nature.

NEUROVASCULAR HEADACHE: WHAT HAPPENED TO THE BLOOD VESSELS?

In a study of experimental head pain in which capsaicin was injected into the forehead of volunteers without headache (May et al., 1998b), there was a bilateral activation pattern in midline structures over several planes, slightly lateralized to the left, anterior to the brain stem and posterior to the chiasmatic region. Superimposed on a magnetic resonance imaging template, the location of the activation covers intracranial arteries as well as the region of the cavernous sinus bilaterally but more marked on the ipsilateral side.

Similarly, strong activation was observed in the same region in the cluster headache study (the cavernous sinus) (May et al., 1998a). This change might be interpreted as increased venous inflow from the superior ophthalmic vein, which drains the ophthalmic artery (Waldenlind et al., 1993), or a longer transit time for the tracer in this region, which could be due to impeded venous drainage. Another, more exciting possibility is that the observed increase in activation is due to bilateral dilation of the internal carotid artery, since such a change would suggest vasodilation mediated by the ophthalmic division of the trigeminovascular system, a neurally driven vasodilation. It is difficult to assess the contribution of these two sources to the activity measured using PET.

To further address this question, magnetic resonance angiography was performed using the same design as the PET study (May et al., 1998a). Using an image calculation tool, the angiographies were subtracted from each other, leaving only structural changes between conditions. It was demonstrated that in the condition nitroglycerine (NTG) inhalation without headache there was dilation of the basilar artery and the internal carotid arteries bilaterally compared to the rest state (May et al., 1999c). These vessels stayed dilated during the third condition (cluster headache attack), some 20 to 30 minutes later. Given that we have observed vasodilation in large vessels in cluster headache and increased signal in the region of the cavernous sinus after capsaicin injection to the forehead in a PET study (May et al., 1998b), it seems clear that the vascular changes are an epiphenomenon of activation of the trigeminovascular system (Goadsby and Duckworth, 1987) and that cluster headache is not a disorder of the carotid vasculature or cavernous sinus. We have recently seen the very same change in this region in acute migraine studied with PET (Bahra et al., unpublished data). The data suggest that activation of the trigeminal system, as such, triggers the impeded arterial or venous drainage or increases flow in the region of these vessels. At the physiological level, the common link is the involvement of the ophthalmic division of the trigeminal nerve by a neurally driven dilation of the carotid vessels; on the basis of the data, these headaches should be regarded as neurovascular since vessel change occurs generically with first division of trigeminal pain.

TENSION-TYPE HEADACHE

While most people probably think that they understand tension-type headache (TTH), it seems to the author that this is one of the greatest obstacles to its study. One is generally less questioning about what is true than about what is not thought to be true; TTH implies a process underlying the syndrome, but is this accurate?

The Clinical Problem

Perhaps one of the main stumbling blocks to the study of TTH is the clinical definition. The definition is as much about what TTH is not as what it is. It should not be pulsating, should not be severe, should not be unilateral, should not be aggravated by physical activity, and should have no nausea. It may have photophobia or phonophobia, but not both. Yet are any of these so-called features distinguishing, when they may be seen in migraine. Moreover, chronic TTH offers the possibility of nausea or photophobia or phonophobia but is otherwise phenotypically the same. What is the rationale to allow nausea in chronic TTH but not episodic? What is the possible reason to allow either photophobia or phonophobia in TTH but not both? There are no answers, and there can be no answers until the study of TTH parcels out all of the features prospectively. The phenotype TTH can probably be produced by a number of biological changes. The fundamental clinical difference between TTH and migraine is that TTH lacks features of sensory sensitivity of any description, so absolutely no nausea and no sensitivity to light, sound, or movement should be permitted; also, it lacks the usual triggering associations of migraine, such as aggravation by menses, skipping meals, or changing sleep patterns. One must ask, how many patients who have contributed to the TTH literature have migrainous biology? This issue must be resolved if we are to understand TTH.

Mechanisms

Given our current knowledge of TTH, it is useful to talk about possible mechanisms rather than identifying one primary factor as causative. It is worth setting out what has been noted as a basis for thinking about the disorder. What follows uses the IHS system, and readers should evaluate the data in light of the clinical remarks above.

Epidemiology and Genetics

The 1-year prevalence of TTH is somewhere between 30% and 80%, most likely on the higher end. In a very thorough general population-based study in Denmark, Rasmussen and colleagues (1991) found a 1-year prevalence of TTH of 69% for men and 88% for women, giving a slight predominance in women. In a telephone-based population sample in the United States, TTH was less common, running at 38% of the population (Schwartz et al., 1998). Chronic TTH is seen in about 2% of the population (Castillo et al., 1999; Scher et al., 1998). In a general population, most patients with TTH do not consult their physicians (Rasmussen et al., 1992). One study suggests that there are some genetic factors at play in chronic TTH (Ostergaard et al., 1997). Stress is just as often identified as a trigger for migraine as TTH (Scharff et al., 1995) and as such has no diagnostic utility when patients report the symptom.

Muscle Mechanisms

The dull, bilateral, generalized nature of typical TTH provides the impetus to study peripheral sources for the pain. Indeed, TTH has been called "muscle contraction headache." Injection of saline into cranial muscles certainly induces pain (Kellgren, 1938), and this usually takes 10 to 15 seconds to build up (Jensen and Norup, 1992). Pain from muscle injection is not necessarily restricted to the muscle injected, so injections into the temporalis muscle can cause pain in neck muscles (Simmons et al., 1943). Alogenic substances, such as bradykinin and serotonin, have been injected into human cranial muscles, with minimal pain from the bradykinin and no pain from the serotonin, although together they are more painful than isotonic saline (Jensen et al., 1990). Direct electrical stimulation of muscle causes cramp-like local pain (Laursen et al., 1997), while a combination of chewing and temporal artery ischemia will produce a dull bifrontal headache (Gobel and Cordes, 1990).

Consistent with these observations, pericranial muscles in patients with TTH are more tender than in healthy controls when studied blinded, although this was found mainly for patients with frequent headache of greater than 25 days a month (Langemark and Olesen, 1987). Later studies have shown tenderness in both episodic and chronic TTH (Jensen et al., 1993, 1998). Pressure pain detection thresholds have been used to study whether this cranial pain is due to some local factor or associated with a more generalized disorder. Pressure pain detection thresholds are normal in episodic TTH (Jensen et al., 1993), whereas they are abnormal in chronic TTH (Bendtsen et al., 1996; Schoenen et al., 1991a). Moreover, patients with chronic TTH are more sensitive to other stimuli, such as thermal stimuli (Langemark et al., 1989). Muscle hardness, which has recently begun to be measured with an ingenious noninvasive technique (Sakai et al., 1995), requires further study. Whether changes represent local pathology or reflexly induced change needs consideration.

Given the very interesting role of nitric oxide generation in spinal cord nociception (Meller and Gebhart, 1993), the recent result of a double-blind study that showed reduction in pain intensity in chronic TTH when the nitric oxide synthase inhibitor L-N^G-methylarginine hydrochloride was given (Ashina et al., 1999) suggests a central mechanism for some part of this tenderness.

Neurophysiological Findings

Because muscle contraction has been thought to play a key role in TTH and is indeed enshrined in the current IHS classification, electromyography (EMG) has been of interest in the condition. A review of the data to the mid-1980s (Pikoff, 1984) concluded that in about half of the studies the muscles were normal and in the other half muscular activity was increased. In chronic TTH, EMG activity tends to be higher in patients than controls, but this is unrelated to headache severity or

pressure pain thresholds (Schoenen et al., 1991b). Similarly, there is no increase in EMG activity during a headache compared with EMG activity in the absence of a headache (Clark et al., 1995; Jensen, 1995).

Neurophysiological methods have allowed the study of brain stem pathways that have processing functions in headache. The most extensively studied reflex has been that involving exteroceptive suppression produced as a suppression of voluntary masseter and temporalis contraction with electrical stimulation of trigeminal nerve fibers. Exteroceptive suppression is divided into two periods, the early period ES_1, mediated by an oligosynaptic pathway, and the late period ES_2, mediated by a polysynaptic pathway (Desmedt and Godaux, 1976). The interneurons responsible for ES_2 are likely to be part of the bulbar reticular formation (Hopf, 1994) and receive modulatory projections from limbic structures and the periaqueductal gray matter (Schoenen, 1993b). The ES_2 duration is reduced in chronic TTH (Schoenen et al., 1987) but normal in episodic TTH and migraine (Schoenen, 1993a). The conventional blink reflex is normal in TTH (Sand and Zwart, 1994), although the modified nociceptive-specific reflex has not been studied (Kaube et al., 2000). Contingent negative variation, an event-related potential that is recorded over the frontal cortex, is normal in TTH (Schoenen and Timsit-Berthier, 1993).

Given the changes described and the biochemical changes that revolve around central opiate activity (Langemark et al., 1995), its seems that the bulk of the pathophysiological processes in TTH fall within the central nervous system. A vicious cycle of peripheral activation with sensitization and further peripheral activation may underlie some of the muscle observations. Until the clinical material is clarified more closely, our understanding of TTH will progress very slowly.

REFERENCES

Ashina, M., L.H. Lassen, L. Bendtsen et al. (1999). Effect of inhibition of nitric oxide synthase on chronic tension-type headache. *Lancet* 353:287–289.

Bendtsen, L., R. Jensen, and J. Olesen. (1996). Decreased pain detection and tolerance thresholds in chronic tension-type headache. *Arch. Neurol.* 53:373–376.

Burstein, R., H. Yamamura, A. Malick et al. (1998). Chemical stimulation of the intracranial dura induces enhanced responses to facial stimulation in brain stem trigeminal neurons. *J. Neurophysiol.* 79:964–982.

Castillo, J., P. Muqoz, V. Guitera et al. (1999). Epidemiology of chronic daily headache in the general population. *Headache* 39:190–196.

Chazot, G., B. Claustrat, J. Brun et al. (1984). A chronobiological study of melatonin, cortisol, growth hormone and prolactin secretion in cluster headache. *Cephalalgia* 4:213–220.

Chudler, E.H. and W.K. Dong. (1995). The role of the basal ganglia in nociception and pain. *Pain* 60:33–38.

Clark, G.T., S. Sakai, R. Merrill et al. (1995). Cross-correlation between stress, pain, physical activity, and temporalis muscle EMG in tension-type headache. *Cephalalgia* 15:511–518.

Connor, H.E., L. Bertin, S. Gillies et al. (1998). Clinical evaluation of a novel, potent, CNS penetrating NK_1 receptor antagonist in the acute treatment of migraine. *Cephalalgia* 18:392.

Cumberbatch, M.J., R.G. Hill, and R.J. Hargreaves. (1997). Rizatriptan has central antinociceptive effects against durally evoked responses. *Eur. J. Pharmacol.* 328:37–40.

Cumberbatch, M.J., R.G. Hill, and R.J. Hargreaves. (1998). Differential effects of the $5HT_{1B/1D}$ receptor agonist naratriptan on trigeminal versus spinal nociceptive responses. *Cephalalgia* 18:659–664.

Data, J., K. Britch, N. Westergaard et al. (1998). A double-blind study of ganaxolone in the acute treatment of migraine headaches with or without an aura in premenopausal females. *Headache* 38:380.

Derbyshire, S.W.G., A.K.P. Jones, F. Gyulai et al. (1997). Pain processing during three levels of noxious stimulation produces differential patterns of central activity. *Pain* 73:431–445.

Desmedt, J.E. and E. Godaux. (1976). Habituation of exteroceptive suppression and of exteroceptive reflexes in man as influenced by voluntary contraction. *Brain Res.* 106:21–29.

Diener, H.C. (1996). Substance-P antagonist RPR100893-201 is not effective in human migraine attacks. *Proceedings of the VIth International Headache Seminar* (J. Olesen and P. Tfelt-Hansen, eds.). Lippincott-Raven, New York.

Dimitriadou, V., M.G. Buzzi, M.A. Moskowitz et al. (1991). Trigeminal sensory fiber stimulation induces morphological changes reflecting secretion in rat dura mater mast cells. *Neuroscience* 44:97–112.

Drummond, P.D. and J.W. Lance. (1983). Extracranial vascular changes and the source of pain in migraine headache. *Ann. Neurol.* 13:32–37.

Earl, N.L., S.A. McDonald, M.T. Lowy, and the 4991W93 Investigator Group. (1999). Efficacy and tolerability of the neurogenic inflammation inhibitor, 4991W93, in the acute treatment of migraine. *Cephalalgia* 19:357.

Ekbom, K. (1968). Nitroglycerin as a provocative agent in cluster headache. *Arch. Neurol.* 19:487–493.

Ekbom, K. and T. Greitz. (1970). Carotid angiography in cluster headache. *Acta Radiol.* 10:177–186.

Fanciullacci, M., M. Alessandri, M. Figini et al. (1995). Increases in plasma calcitonin gene–related peptide from extracerebral circulation during nitroglycerin-induced cluster headache attack. *Pain* 60:119–123.

Feindel, W., W. Penfield, and F. McNaughton. (1960). The tentorial nerves and localisation of intracranial pain in man. *Neurology* 10:555–563.

Gallai, V., P. Sarchielli, A. Floridi et al. (1995). Vasoactive peptide levels in the plasma of young migraine patients with and without aura assessed both interictally and ictally. *Cephalalgia* 15:384–390.

Goadsby, P.J. (1998). 5-$HT_{1B/1D}$ agonists in migraine: Comparative pharmacology and its therapeutic implications. *CNS Drugs* 10:271–286.

Goadsby, P.J. and J.W. Duckworth. (1987). Effect of stimulation of trigeminal ganglion on regional cerebral blood flow in cats. *Am. J. Physiol.* 253:R270–R274.

Goadsby, P.J. and J.W. Duckworth. (1989). Low frequency stimulation of the locus coeruleus reduces regional cerebral blood flow in the spinalized cat. *Brain Res.* 476:71–77.

Goadsby, P.J. and L. Edvinsson. (1994). Human in vivo evidence for trigeminovascular activation in cluster headache. *Brain* 117:427–434.

Goadsby, P.J. and L. Edvinsson. (1996). Neuropeptide changes in a case of chronic paroxysmal hemicrania—Evidence for trigemino-parasympathetic activation. *Cephalalgia* 16:448–450.

Goadsby, P.J., L. Edvinsson, and R. Ekman. (1988). Release of vasoactive peptides in the extracerebral circulation of man and the cat during activation of the trigeminovascular system. *Ann. Neurol.* 23:193–196.

Goadsby, P.J., L. Edvinsson, and R. Ekman. (1990). Vasoactive peptide release in the extracerebral circulation of humans during migraine headache. *Ann. Neurol.* 28:183–187.

Goadsby, P.J. and K.L. Hoskin. (1996). Inhibition of trigeminal neurons by intravenous administration of the serotonin (5HT)-1-D receptor agonist zolmitriptan (311C90): Are brain stem sites a therapeutic target in migraine? *Pain* 67:355–359.

Goadsby, P.J. and K.L. Hoskin. (1997). The distribution of trigeminovascular afferents in the non-human primate brain *Macaca nemestrina*: A c-fos immunocytochemical study. *J. Anat. 190*:367–375.

Goadsby, P.J. and K.L. Hoskin. (1999). Differential effects of low dose CP122,288 and eletriptan on Fos expression due to stimulation of the superior sagittal sinus in the cat. *Pain 82*:15–22.

Goadsby, P.J. and Y.E. Knight. (1997). Naratriptan inhibits trigeminal neurons after intravenous administration through an action at the serotonin ($5HT_{1B/1D}$) receptors. *Br. J. Pharmacol. 122*: 918–922.

Goadsby, P.J., G.A. Lambert, and J.W. Lance. (1982). Differential effects on the internal and external carotid circulation of the monkey evoked by locus coeruleus stimulation. *Brain Res. 249*:247–254.

Goadsby, P.J., G.A. Lambert, and J.W. Lance. (1985). The mechanism of cerebrovascular vasoconstriction in response to locus coeruleus stimulation. *Brain Res. 326*:213–217.

Goadsby, P.J. and R.B. Lipton. (1997). A review of paroxysmal hemicranias, SUNCT syndrome and other short-lasting headaches with autonomic features, including new cases. *Brain 120*:193–209.

Goadsby, P.J. and J. Olesen. (1996). Diagnosis and management of migraine. *BMJ 312*:1279–1282.

Goadsby, P.J. and S.D. Silberstein, eds. (1997). *Headache*. Butterworth-Heinemann, New York.

Goadsby, P.J. and A.S. Zagami. (1991). Stimulation of the superior sagittal sinus increases metabolic activity and blood flow in certain regions of the brainstem and upper cervical spinal cord of the cat. *Brain 114*:1001–1011.

Goadsby, P.J., A.S. Zagami, and G.A. Lambert. (1991). Neural processing of craniovascular pain: A synthesis of the central structures involved in migraine. *Headache 31*:365–371.

Gobel, H. and P. Cordes. (1990). Circadian variation of pain sensitivity in pericranial musculature. *Headache 30*:418–422.

Goldstein, D.J., O. Wang, J.R. Saper et al. (1997). Ineffectiveness of neurokinin-1 antagonist in acute migraine: A crossover study. *Cephalalgia 17*:785–790.

Graham, J.R. and H.G. Wolff. (1938). Mechanism of migraine headache and action of ergotamine tartrate. *Arch. Neurol. Psychiatry 39*:737–763.

Graham, J.R. and H.G. Wolff. (1966). Mechanism of migraine headache and action of ergotamine tartrate. In *The Circulation of the Brain and Spinal Cord*, Vol. 18, pp. 638–669. Hafner, New York.

Hardebo, J.E. (1994). How cluster headache is explained as an intracavernous inflammatory process lesioning sympathetic fibres. *Headache 34*: 125–131.

Headache Classification Committee of the International Headache Society. (1988). Classification and diagnostic criteria for headache disorders, cranial neuralgias and facial pain. *Cephalalgia 8*(Suppl. 7):1–96.

Hofman, M.A., J.N. Zhou, and D.F. Swaab. (1996). Suprachiasmatic nucleus of the human brain: An immunocytochemical and morphometric analysis. *J. Comp. Neurol. 305*:552–556.

Hopf, H.C. (1994). Topodiagnostic value of brain stem reflexes. *Muscle Nerv. 17*:475–484.

Hoskin, K.L., H. Kaube, and P.J. Goadsby. (1996). Central activation of the trigeminovascular pathway in the cat is inhibited by dihydroergotamine: A c-*fos* and electrophysiology study. *Brain 119*:249–256.

Hoskin, K.L., A. Zagami, and P.J. Goadsby. (1999). Stimulation of the middle meningeal artery leads to bilateral Fos expression in the trigeminocervical nucleus: A comparative study of monkey and cat. *J. Anat. 194*:579–588.

Hsieh, J.C., J. Hannerz, and M. Ingvar. (1996). Right-lateralized central processing for pain of nitroglycerin-induced cluster headache. *Pain 67*:59–68.

Isler, H. (1993). Episodic cluster headache from a textbook of 1745: Van Swieten's classic description. *Cephalalgia 13*:172–174.

Jensen, K. and M. Norup. (1992). Experimental pain in human temporal muscle induced by hypertonic saline, potassium and acidity. *Cephalalgia 12*:101–106.

Jensen, K., U. Pedersen-Bjergaard, C. Tuxen et al. (1990). Pain and tenderness in human temporal muscle induced by bradykinin and 5-hydroxytryptamine. *Peptides 11*:1127–1132.

Jensen, R. (1995). Mechanisms of spontaneous tension-type headache: An analysis of tenderness, pain thresholds and EMG. *Pain 64*:251.

Jensen, R., L. Bendtsen, and J. Olesen. (1998). Muscular factors are of importance in tension-type headache. *Headache 38*:10–17.

Jensen, R., B.K. Rasmussen, B. Pedersen et al. (1993). Muscle tenderness and pressure pain thresholds in headache: A population study. *Pain 52*:193–199.

Kaube, H., K.L. Hoskin, and P.J. Goadsby. (1993a). Intravenous acetylsalicylic acid inhibits central trigeminal neurons in the dorsal horn of the upper cervical spinal cord in the cat. *Headache 33*:541–550.

Kaube, H., K.L. Hoskin, and P.J. Goadsby. (1993b). Sumatriptan inhibits central trigeminal neurons only after blood–brain barrier disruption. *Br. J. Pharmacol. 109*:788–792.

Kaube, H., Z. Katsarava, T. Kaufer et al. (2000). A new method to increase the nociception specificity of the human blink reflex. *Clin. Neurophysiol. 111*:413–416.

Kaube, H., K. Keay, K.L. Hoskin et al. (1993c). Expression of c-fos-like immunoreactivity in the trigeminal nucleus caudalis and high cervical cord following stimulation of the sagittal sinus in the cat. *Brain Res. 629*:95–102.

Kellgren, J.H. (1938). Observations on referred pain arising from muscle. *Clin. Sci. (Colch.) 3*: 175–190.

Knight, Y.E., H.E. Connor, L. Edvinsson et al. (1999a). Only 5HT$_{1B/1D}$ agonist doses of 4991W93 inhibit CGRP release in the cat. *Cephalalgia 19*:401.

Knight, Y.E., L. Edvinsson, and P.J. Goadsby. (1999b). Blockade of CGRP release after superior sagittal sinus stimulation in cat: A comparison of avitriptan and CP122,288. *Neuropeptides 33*:41–46.

Knight, Y.E. and P.J. Goadsby. (1999). Brainstem stimulation inhibits trigeminal neurons in the cat. *Cephalalgia 19*:315.

Kudrow, L. (1976). Plasma testosterone levels in cluster headache preliminary results. *Headache 16*:228–231.

Kudrow, L. (1977). Plasma testosterone and LH levels in cluster headache. *Headache 17*:91–92.

Lambert, G.A., P.J. Goadsby, A.S. Zagami et al. (1988). Comparative effects of stimulation of the trigeminal ganglion and the superior sagittal sinus on cerebral blood flow and evoked potentials in the cat. *Brain Res. 453*:143–149.

Lance, J.W. and P.J. Goadsby. (1998). *Mechanism and Management of Headache*, 6th ed. Butterworth-Heinemann, London.

Langemark, M., F.W. Bach, R. Ekman et al. (1995). Increased cerebrospinal fluid metenkephalin immunoreactivity in patients with chronic tension-type headache. *Pain 63*:103–107.

Langemark, M., K. Jensen, T.S. Jensen et al. (1989). Pressure pain thresholds and thermal nociceptive thresholds in chronic tension-type headache. *Pain 38*:203–210.

Langemark, M. and J. Olesen. (1987). Pericranial tenderness in tension headache. A blind, controlled study. *Cephalalgia 7*:249–255.

Lassen, L.H., V.B. Jacobsen, P. Petersen et al. (1998). Human calcitonin gene–related peptide (hCGRP)–induced headache in migraineurs. *Eur. J. Neurol. 5*(Suppl. 3):S63.

Laursen, R.J., T. Graven-Nielsen, T.S. Jensen et al. (1997). Quantification of local and referred pain in humans by intramuscular electrical stimulation. *Eur. J. Pain 1*:105–113.

Leone, M. and G. Bussone. (1993). A review of hormonal findings in cluster headache. Evidence for hypothalamic involvement. *Cephalalgia 13*:309–317.

Leone, M., V. Lucini, D. D'Amico et al. (1995). Twenty-four-hour melatonin and cortisol plasma levels in relation to timing of cluster headache. *Cephalalgia 15*:224–229.

Leone, M., G. Partuno, A. Vescovi et al. (1990).

Neuroendocrine dysfunction in cluster headache. *Cephalalgia 10*:235–239.

Markowitz, S., K. Saito, and M.A. Moskowitz. (1987). Neurogenically mediated leakage of plasma proteins occurs from blood vessels in dura mater but not brain. *J. Neurosci. 7*:4129–4136.

Martins, I.P., E. Baeta, T. Paiva et al. (1993). Headaches during intracranial endovascular procedures: A possible model of vascular headache. *Headache 33*:227–233.

May, A., J. Ashburner, C. Buchel et al. (1999a). Correlation between structural and functional changes in brain in an idiopathic headache syndrome. *Nat. Med. 5*:836–838.

May, A., A. Bahra, C. Buchel et al. (1998a). Hypothalamic activation in cluster headache attacks. *Lancet 351*:275–278.

May, A., A. Bahra, C. Buchel et al. (1999b). Functional MRI in spontaneous attacks of SUNCT: Short-lasting neuralgiform headache with conjunctival injection and tearing. *Ann. Neurol. 46*: 791–793.

May, A., C. Buchel, A. Bahra et al. (1999c). Intracranial vessels in trigeminal transmitted pain: A PET study. *Neuroimage 9*:453–460.

May, A., A. Bahra, C. Buchel et al. (2000). PET and MRA findings in cluster headache and MRA in experimental pain. *Neurology 55*:1328–1335.

May, A., H.J. Gijsman, A. Wallnoefer et al. (1996). Endothelin antagonist bosentan blocks neurogenic inflammation, but is not effective in aborting migraine attacks. *Pain 67*:375–378.

May, A., H. Kaube, C. Buechel et al. (1998b). Experimental cranial pain elicited by capsaicin: A PET-study. *Pain 74*:61–66.

May, A., S. Shepheard, A. Wessing et al. (1998c). Retinal plasma extravasation can be evoked by trigeminal stimulation in rat but does not occur during migraine attacks. *Brain 121*:1231–1237.

Meller, S.T. and G.F. Gebhart. (1993). Nitric oxide (NO) and nociceptive processing in the spinal cord. *Pain 52*:127–136.

Moore, R.Y. (1997). Circadian rhythms: Basic neurobiology and clinical applications. *Annu. Rev. Med. 48*:253–266.

Moore-Ede, M.C. (1983). The circadian timing system in mammals: Two pacemakers preside over many secondary oscillators. *Fed. Proc. 42*: 2802–2808.

Moskowitz, M.A. (1988). Cluster headache—Evidence for a pathophysiologic focus in the superior pericarotid cavernous sinus plexus. *Headache 28*:584–586.

Moskowitz, M.A. (1990). Basic mechanisms in vascular headache. *Neurol. Clin. 8*:801–815.

Moskowitz, M.A. and F.M. Cutrer. (1993). Sumatriptan: A receptor-targeted treatment for migraine. *Annu. Rev. Med. 44*:145–154.

Nelson, R.F. (1978). Testosterone levels in cluster and non-cluster migrainous patients. *Headache* 18:265–267.

Nichols, F.T., M. Mawad, J.P. Mohr et al. (1993). Focal headache during balloon inflation in the vertebral and basilar arteries. *Headache* 33: 87–89.

Nichols, F.T., M. Mawad, J.P. Mohr et al. (1990). Focal headache during balloon inflation in the internal carotid and middle cerebral arteries. *Stroke* 21:555–559.

Norman, B., D. Panebianco, and G.A. Block. (1998). A placebo-controlled, in-clinic study to explore the preliminary safety and efficacy of intravenous L-758,298 (a prodrug of the NK_1 receptor antagonist L-754,030) in the acute treatment of migraine. *Cephalalgia* 18:407.

Ostergaard, S., M.B. Russell, L. Bendtsen et al. (1997). Comparison of first degree relatives and spouses of people with chronic tension-type headache. *BMJ* 314:1092–1093.

Pikoff, H. (1984). Is the muscular model of headache still viable? A review of conflicting data. *Headache* 24:186–198.

Raskin, N.H., Y. Hosobuchi, and S. Lamb. (1987). Headache may arise from perturbation of brain. *Headache* 27:416–420.

Rasmussen, B.K. (1995). Epidemiology of headache. *Cephalalgia* 15:45–68.

Rasmussen, B.K., R. Jensen, and J. Olesen. (1992). Impact of headache on sickness absence and utilisation of medical services: A Danish population study. *J. Epidemiol. Community Health* 46:443–446.

Rasmussen, B.K., R. Jensen, and M. Schroll. (1991). Epidemiology of headache in the general population: A prevalence study. *J. Clin. Epidemiol.* 44:1147–1157.

Ray, B.S. and H.G. Wolff. (1940). Experimental studies on headache. Pain sensitive structures of the head and their significance in headache. *Arch. Surg.* 41:813–856.

Roon, K., H.C. Diener, P. Ellis et al. (1997). CP-122,288 blocks neurogenic inflammation, but is not effective in aborting migraine attacks: Results of two controlled clinical studies. *Cephalalgia* 17:245.

Sakai, F., S. Ebihara, M. Akiyama et al. (1995). Pericranial muscle hardness in tension-type headache: A non-invasive measurement method and its clinical application. *Brain* 2:523–531.

Sand, T. and J.A. Zwart. (1994). The blink reflex in chronic tension-type headache, migraine and cervicogenic headache. *Cephalalgia* 14:447–450.

Scharff, L., D.C. Turk, and D.A. Marcus. (1995). Triggers of headache episodes and coping responses of headache diagnostic groups. *Headache* 35:397–403.

Scher, A., W.F. Stewart, J. Liberman et al. (1998).

Prevalence of frequent headache in a population sample. *Headache* 38:497–506.

Schoenen, J. (1993a). Exteroceptive suppression of temporalis muscle activity in patients with chronic headache and in normal volunteers: Methodology, clinical and pathophysiological relevance. *Headache* 33:3–17.

Schoenen, J. (1993b). Exteroceptive suppression of temporalis muscle activity: Methodological and physiological aspects. *Cephalalgia* 13:3–10.

Schoenen, J., D. Bottin, F. Hardy et al. (1991a). Cephalic and extra-cephalic pressure pain thresholds in chronic tension-type headache. *Pain* 47:145–149.

Schoenen, J., P. Gerard, V. De Pasqua et al. (1991b). Multiple clinical and paraclinical analyses of chronic tension-type headache associated or unassociated with disorder of pericranial muscles. *Cephalalgia* 11:135–139.

Schoenen, J., B. Jamart, P. Gerard et al. (1987). Exteroceptive suppression of temporalis muscle activity in chronic headache. *Neurology* 37: 1834–1836.

Schoenen, J. and M. Timsit-Berthier. (1993). Contingent negative variation: Methods and potential interest in headache. *Cephalalgia* 13:28–32.

Schwartz, B.S., W.F. Stewart, D. Simon et al. (1998). Epidemiology of tension-type headache. *JAMA* 279:381–383.

Simmons, D.J., E. Day, H. Goodell et al. (1943). Experimental studies on headache: Muscles of the scalp and neck as sources of pain. *Assoc. Res. Nerv. Ment. Dis.* 23:228–244.

Stewart, W.F., R.B. Lipton, D.D. Celentano et al. (1992). Prevalence of migraine headache in the United States: Relation to age, income, race and other sociodemographic factors. *JAMA* 267: 64–69.

Strassman, A.M., S.A. Raymond, and R. Burstein. (1996). Sensitization of meningeal sensory neurons and the origin of headaches. *Nature* 384: 560–563.

Tunis, M.M. and H.G. Wolff. (1953). Long term observations of the reactivity of the cranial arteries in subjects with vascular headache of the migraine type. *Arch. Neurol. Psychiatry* 70: 551–557.

Uddman, R., L. Edvinsson, R. Ekman et al. (1985). Innervation of the feline cerebral vasculature by nerve fibers containing calcitonin gene–related peptide: Trigeminal origin and coexistence with substance P. *Neurosci. Lett.* 62: 131–136.

Veloso, F., K. Kumar, and C. Toth. (1998). Headache secondary to deep brain implantation. *Headache* 38:507–515.

Waldenlind, E., K. Ekbom, and J. Torhall. (1993). MR-angiography during spontaneous attacks of cluster headache: A case report. *Headache* 33: 291–295.

Waldenlind, E., S.A. Gustafsson, K. Ekbom et al. (1987). Circadian secretion of cortisol and melatonin in cluster headache during active cluster periods and remission. *J. Neurol. Neurosurg. Psychiatry* 50:207–213.

Weiller, C., A. May, V. Limmroth et al. (1995). Brain stem activation in spontaneous human migraine attacks. *Nat. Med.* 1:658–660.

Zagami, A.S. and P.J. Goadsby. (1991). Stimulation of the superior sagittal sinus increases metabolic activity in cat thalamus. In *New Advances in Headache Research*, Vol. 2 (F.C. Rose, ed.), pp. 169–171. Smith-Gordon, London.

Zagami, A.S., P.J. Goadsby, and L. Edvinsson. (1990). Stimulation of the superior sagittal sinus in the cat causes release of vasoactive peptides. *Neuropeptides* 16:69–75.

Zagami, A.S. and G.A. Lambert. (1991). Craniovascular application of capsaicin activates nociceptive thalamic neurons in the cat. *Neurosci. Lett.* 121:187–190.

6

Genetics of Headache

MICHEL D. FERRARI
JOOST HAAN

Recent investigations have shown that genetic factors play an important role in the three most prevalent primary headache syndromes: migraine, cluster headache, and tension-type headache. In other, less frequent primary headache syndromes, such as chronic paroxysmal hemicrania, hemicrania continua, and short-lasting unilateral neuralgiform headache with conjunctival injection and tearing (SUNCT), a genetic cause is not evident.

In the past, genetic investigations have focused mainly on migraine, and only lately have they turned to cluster headache and tension-type headache. Thus, much is already known about the genetics of migraine, little about the genetics of cluster headache, and virtually nothing about the genetics of tension-type headache. Nevertheless, it is likely that the two latter syndromes will benefit from the knowledge gathered during the study of migraine genetics.

In this chapter, migraine, cluster headache, and tension-type headache will be described separately.

GENETICS OF MIGRAINE

Migraine is a chronic, paroxysmal, neurologic disorder with widely varying symptoms, affecting up to 16% of the general population. Women are affected more often than men. The disease can start at any age. The two major forms of migraine are migraine with aura (MA) and migraine without aura (MO) (Classification Committee of the International Headache Society, 1988).

The pathophysiology of parts of the migraine attack, notably the aura and headache phases, are at least partly understood (Ferrari, 1998). The true cause of migraine, i.e., why and how a migraine attack begins, is not known. Everyone may suffer from one or two migraine attacks in life, indicating that the migraine attack itself is not abnormal but that the tendency toward recurrent attacks is. It is commonly believed that there is an individual "threshold" to get migraine attacks. This threshold may be high so that migraine attacks occur seldom, e.g., only under unfavorable external conditions, or it may be low so that attacks occur frequently after common triggers or apparently spontaneously. There are many arguments in favor of the theory that the migraine threshold is determined by genetic factors (Table 6–1).

Genetic Investigations of Migraine

Genetic investigations of migraine have followed several lines: twin studies, family studies, study of rare genetic migraine variants, and association studies (reviewed in Haan et

Table 6–1 Arguments for the theory that migraine is hereditary

- Increased risk of migraine in first-degree relatives of migraine probands
- Higher concordance rate of migraine in monozygotic twins
- Rare, clearly autosomal dominant forms of migraine (e.g., FHM)
- Migraine is a prominent symptom of several hereditary disorders (CADASIL, MELAS, essential tremor, etc.)
- Sib-pair analyses show involvement of FHM p19 locus
- Association studies show possible involvement of several loci in MO and MA (see Table 6–2)
- Linkage of typical migraine families to FHM p19 locus and X chromosome

Key to abbreviations: FHM, familial hemiplegic migraine; CADASIL, cerebral autosomal dominant arteriopathy with subcortical infarcts and leukoencephalopathy; MELAS, mitochondrial encephalopathy with lactic acidosis and stroke-like episodes; MO, migraine without aura; MA, migraine with aura.

al., 1997; Russell, 1997; Ferrari and Russell, 1999).

Twin and family studies have been extensively reviewed elsewhere (Haan et al., 1997; Russell, 1997; Ferrari and Russell, 1999) and will not be discussed here in detail. Virtually all earlier twin and family studies had methodological flaws, but more recent ones have given sufficient evidence for a genetic etiology of migraine (Ferrari and Russell, 1999). For example, recent twin studies have proven a higher concordance rate for monozygotic twins compared to dizygotic twins, for twins reared both together and apart (Ziegler et al., 1998; Ulrich et al., 1999). From these studies it was calculated that approximately 50% of the variance in liability to MO and MA is attributable to genetic factors, with nonshared environmental factors. A recent family study found a relative risk of first-degree family members of patients with MO of 1.9 and of those with MA of 3.8 compared with the general population (Russell and Olesen, 1995). In another study, it was calculated that familial factors account for less than one-half of migraine cases in the population but the genetic risk increases with the degree of migraine disability (Stewart et al., 1997).

In studies of the mode of inheritance in migraine, maternal and X-linked transmission were excluded in the majority of pedigrees.

Most studies found evidence for multifactorial inheritance, which is a combination of environmental and (poly-)genetic factors (Russell and Olesen, 1993; Ferrari and Russell, 1999).

Familial Hemiplegic Migraine

The most fruitful line of genetic research on migraine is the investigation of families with familial hemiplegic migraine (FHM), a rare autosomal-dominant form of MA (Classification Committee of the International Headache Society, 1988). Attacks are characterized by migrainous headache with photophobia, phonophobia, and nausea and vomiting. They are preceded or accompanied by hemiparesis. The attack onset is usually in childhood, virtually always before 30 years of age. The hemiparesis may last from minutes to weeks and always resolves without sequellae. Patients with coma during the attacks have been described. In approximately 20% of FHM families, progressive cerebellar ataxia occurs next to the migraine and cerebellar atrophy on magnetic resonance imaging is evident. Patients may also have attacks of "nonhemiplegic" typical MO or MA. Individuals with FHM and with nonhemiplegic typical migraine can be found in FHM families. These observations strongly suggest that FHM is part of the migraine spectrum and that genes involved in FHM are candidates for nonhemiplegic typical MO and MA (Haan et al., 1997).

Linkage studies have shown that approximately 50% of the reported FHM families are linked to chromosome 19p13 markers (Joutel et al., 1993, 1994; Ophoff et al., 1994). All FHM families with associated ataxia are linked to chromosome 19p13. Recently, two groups found linkage in three FHM families without ataxia to chromosome 1 markers (Ducros et al., 1997; Gardner et al., 1997). There remain FHM families that could not be linked to either chromosome 19 or chromosome 1, indicating that at least a third gene must be involved in FHM (Ducros et al., 1997). Except for progressive ataxia, no clinical differences are apparent between chromosome 19–linked, chromosome 1–

linked, and nonlinked FHM patients (Terwindt et al., 1996).

Familial Hemiplegic Migraine and the P/Q-Type Ca²⁺ Channel

In 1996, a voltage-gated P/Q-type calcium channel α_{1A}-subunit gene (*CACNA1A*) was identified in the FHM candidate region on chromosome 19 (Ophoff et al., 1996). The gene is transcribed specifically in the cerebellum, the cerebral cortex, the thalamus, and the hypothalamus. Four different missense mutations were identified in five unrelated FHM families (Ophoff et al., 1996). Mutations in the same gene were subsequently found in several other FHM families from different countries (Fig. 6–1). Now, several different missense mutations in *CACNA1A* have been associated with FHM (Ophoff et al., 1996; Ducros et al., 1999; Gardner et al., 1999; Carrera et al., 1999; Battistini et al., 1999; Vahedi et al., 1999). The T666M mutation seems to be the most prevalent, being detected so far in ten FHM families and one sporadic FHM patient (Ophoff et al., 1996; Ducros et al., 1999).

Interestingly, the second FHM locus on chromosome 1q is near a brain-specific R/T calcium channel α_{1E}-subunit gene (*CACNA1E*) (Ducros et al., 1997; Gardner et al., 1997). Mutation analysis should disclose whether this gene is involved in chromosome 1–linked FHM families.

Calcium Channel Genes

Calcium is an essential signaling molecule in many biological systems, the intracellular level being 20,000-fold lower than the extracellular concentration. Sustained rises in intracellular calcium result in cell death. Therefore, homeostatic mechanisms to control calcium inflow and outflow are very important. Voltage-gated calcium channels are key regulators of intracellular calcium concentration (reviewed in Cooper and Jan, 1999). They consist of several subunits, of which the α_1 subunit is the most important for migraine. Six genes (A, B, C, D, E, and S) that encode

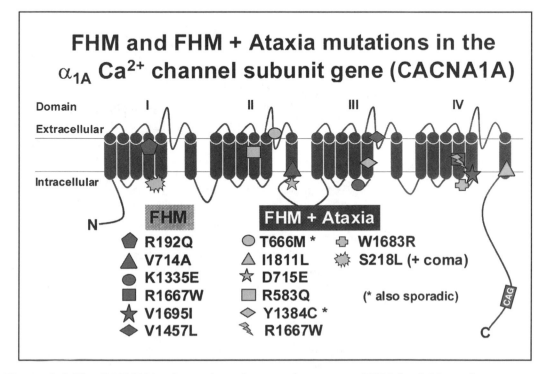

Figure 6–1 The *CACNA1A* calcium channel gene with mutations. *FHM*, familial hemiplegic migraine.

α_1 subunits have been identified. The α_1 subunit consists of four internal homologous repeats (I–IV), each containing six putative α-helical membrane-spanning segments (S1–S6) and one pore-forming (P) segment between S5 and S6 that spans only the outer part of the transmembrane region. The S4 segment contains a positively charged amino acid in every third or fourth position and is the voltage sensor for the voltage-gated ion channels. The β subunits are cytoplasmic proteins capable of modulating current amplitude, activation and inactivation kinetics, and voltage dependence when coexpressed with α_1 subunits. The β subunits are encoded by four different genes, all expressed in the brain. The $\alpha_2\delta$ subunit is encoded by a single gene and consists of glycosylated α_2 and δ proteins linked together by disulfide bonds, with δ as the transmembrane protein anchor and α_2 extracellular.

Additional molecular diversity arises from alternative splicing of the α, β, and $\alpha_2\delta$ transcripts. The characteristics of the different calcium channel types are primarily correlated with the different α_1 isoforms. The α_{1A} subunit encodes P- and Q-type calcium channels, which were originally identified in cerebellar Purkinje cells and granule cells. P- and Q-type calcium channels differ in inactivation kinetics, possibly due to α_{1A}-subunit splice variants, post-translational modification, or the influence of an auxiliary subunit.

Functional Studies of Mutated P/Q-Type Ca²⁺ Channels

In one study, FHM mutations were introduced into rabbit α_1 subunits, which show 94% sequence identity with the human gene (Kraus et al., 1998). The mutant subunits were functionally expressed in *Xenopus laevis* oocytes, and three of the four FHM mutations studied (T666M, V714A, I1819L) altered the inactivation gating of the calcium channels, increasing or decreasing their functional availability. When studied in human embryonic kidney 293 cells containing human α_{1A} and other regulatory subunits, FHM mutations affected the biophysical properties

and density of functional calcium channels (Pietrobon et al., 1998; Hans et al., 1999). These mutations were shown to lead to both gain and loss of function of human P/Q-type calcium channels (Hans et al., 1999).

The Chromosome 19 Familial Hemiplegic Migraine Locus and "Normal" Migraine

Several studies have demonstrated the involvement of the *CACNA1A* gene in typical MO and MA. First, an affected sib-pair analysis showed that the *CACNA1A* gene is likely involved in the common types of migraine, with a stronger effect in MA (May et al., 1995). Second, a classical linkage study in one large family including 17 available affected members with typical migraine demonstrated linkage to the chromosome 19 locus (Nyholt et al., 1998b). Third, in a study of FHM families, two family members with typical (nonhemiplegic) migraine had the I1811L mutation in the *CACNA1A* gene (Terwindt et al., 1998). Thus, the chromosome 19p FHM locus appears to be involved in normal, nonhemiplegic MO and MA. Direct mutation analysis in migraine patients, however, will be required to fully establish the specific role of the calcium channel gene.

Episodic Ataxia

Episodic ataxia (EA) is characterized by recurrent attacks of generalized ataxia and other signs of cerebellar dysfunction. The disease is heterogeneous, and at least two autosomal-dominantly inherited types have been distinguished. Episodic ataxia type 1 (EA-1) is characterized by brief episodes of ataxia and dysarthria lasting seconds to minutes and is associated with interictal myokymia. It is caused by missense mutations in a potassium channel gene (*KCNA1*) on chromosome 12p14 (Browne et al., 1994). Episodic ataxia type 2 (EA-2) is also referred to as acetazolamide-responsive paroxysmal cerebellar ataxia, paroxysmal vestibulocerebellar ataxia, or hereditary paroxysmal cerebellar ataxia. It is characterized by attacks of generalized ataxia, usually associated with an interictal nystagmus. Treatment with acetazolamide is often effective at preventing attacks. Attacks typically last a few hours and can be precipitated by emotional stress, exercise, or alcohol. Patients may have migraine-like symptoms both in between and during the attacks of ataxia. Magnetic resonance imaging may show cerebellar atrophy. The clinical onset of EA-2 generally occurs in childhood or early adulthood.

Studies have linked EA-2 to the same interval on chromosome 19p as FHM (Kramer et al., 1995; Vahedi et al., 1995; Von Brederlow et al., 1995; Teh et al., 1995). Subsequent mutation analysis has revealed several different truncating mutations in the CACNA1A calcium channel gene in unrelated EA-2 families from different countries (Ophoff et al., 1996; Yue et al., 1998; Denier et al., 1999) (Fig. 6–1). All EA2 mutations result in truncated α_{1A} subunits that are unlikely to form functional calcium channels and may either degrade, resulting in haploinsufficiency, or negatively influence channel assembly in the membrane.

Chronic Ataxia

The autosomal-dominant spinocerebellar ataxias (SCAs) are a clinically and genetically heterogeneous group of disorders with many possible accompanying features in addition to the ataxia, such as ophthalmoplegia, pyramidal and extrapyramidal signs, neuropathy, dysarthria, amyotrophy, and pigmentary retinopathy (Klockgether and Evert, 1998). Genes are located on chromosomes 6p22-p23 (SCA1), 12q23-24.1 (SCA2), 14q32.1 (SCA3, also Machado-Joseph disease), 16q24-ter (SCA4), 11 (SCA5), and 3p12-p21.1 (SCA7). For several SCAs, the disease-causing mutations have been identified as expanded and unstable CAG trinucleotide repeats.

Six different cDNA isoforms of the CACN1A1 gene have been reported, of which three contained a five-nucleotide insertion prior to the previously described stop codon, resulting in a shift of the open reading frame in which the CAG repeat is predicted to encode a polyglutamine stretch. Small triplet expansions of the intragenic CAG repeat

ranging from 21 to 30 repeat units were observed in patients with SCA6, whereas normal chromosomes displayed 4 to 20 repeats (Zhuchenko et al., 1997). The CAG repeat length is inversely correlated with age at onset of ataxia. Anticipation of the disease was observed clinically, but no detectable intergenerational allele size change was seen, in contrast to other SCAs. The proportion of SCA6 in the total group of SCA patients differs between populations: 0% in Portugal, 13% in Germany, and 30% in Japan. Homozygous cases have been described, however, with the same severity of ataxia as heterozygous patients.

As both chromosome 19–linked FHM and EA-2 may be accompanied by progressive cerebellar ataxia and atrophy, screening for CAG repeat expansion in FHM and EA-2 families with chronic cerebellar ataxia is important. So far, however, these studies have shown no evidence for CAG repeat expansions (Terwindt et al., 1998a; Denier et al., 1999), suggesting that FHM missense mutations and EA-2 truncating mutations suffice to cause cerebellar atrophy and ataxia.

CACNA1A Mutation: Missense, Truncating, or CAG Expansion

There seems to be a strong genotype–phenotype correlation of the mutations in the CACNA1A gene. It can be generally said that FHM is caused by missense mutations, EA-2 by more severe truncating mutations, and SCA6 by CAG repeat expansions (Tournier-Lasserve, 1999). The functional consequences of the different types of mutation are very important for our knowledge of how abnormalities in the CACNA1A gene cause certain symptoms. There are, however, several exceptions to the above-mentioned genotype–phenotype correlation. Several families with small SCA6 CAG expansions have been described, with a clinical course characterized by episodic, and not chronic, ataxia (Jodice et al., 1997; Jen et al., 1998). In one of these families, an intergenerational allele size change showed that a CAG_{20} allele was associated with an EA-2 phenotype and a CAG$_{25}$ allele with progressive cerebellar ataxia (Jodice et al., 1997).

A family with progressive ataxia (resembling SCA6) was described with a missense mutation instead of a CAG repeat expansion (Yue et al., 1997). Recently, an EA-2 family with a truncating mutation was described in which two members suffered from episodes of hemiplegia (resembling FHM) next to episodic ataxia (Jen et al., 1999).

These observations suggest that FHM, EA-2, and SCA6 are part of a spectrum of *CACNA1A* diseases, in which a certain type of mutation can lead to a number of possible symptoms.

CACNA1A and Other Calcium Channel Subunit Mutations in Mice

Simultaneously with the identification of *CACNA1A* mutations in FHM and EA-2, mutations in the *CACNA1A* gene were found in the tottering (*tg*) and leaner (*tg^{la}*) mouse phenotypes (Fig. 6–1) (Fletcher et al., 1996; Doyle et al., 1997). These recessive tottering mice have been studied extensively as models for human epilepsy. The mutation in the tottering mouse is a missense mutation close to the pore-forming P loop of the second transmembrane domain, very similar to one of the FHM missense mutations, and most likely affects the pore function of the P/Q-type calcium channel. The more severe leaner mouse is associated with a splice site mutation, producing an aberrant intracellular terminus, and resembles the mutations found in two EA-2 families. Mutations at the mouse tottering locus result in intermittent convulsions similar to human absence epilepsy, motor seizures, and mild ataxia. The leaner (*tg^{la}*) mouse suffers from absence seizures but no motor seizures. The *tg^{la}* mutants are more ataxic and often do not survive past weaning. The profound chronic ataxia is associated with pervasive Purkinje and granule cell loss throughout the anterior cerebellum and reduced cerebellar size. Recent whole-cell and single-channel patch-clamp recordings have shown that leaner mutant mice have significantly altered P-type calcium channel currents (Dove et al., 1998; Lorenzon et al., 1998).

The lethargic mouse (*lh*) is another naturally occurring mutant associated with ataxia and seizures. Homozygotes of the *lh* mouse are characterized by ataxia, lethargic behavior, motor seizures, and seizures resembling the absence seizures of human petit mal epilepsy. It has been shown to be due to a mutation in the calcium channel β_4-subunit gene (Burgess et al., 1997). Stargazer mice have spike-wave seizures characteristic of absence epilepsy. Recently, mutations have been found in a neuronal Ca^{2+}-channel γ-subunit gene as a cause of the phenotype in these spontaneously occurring mouse mutants (Letts et al., 1998).

Other Hereditary Diseases Associated with Migraine

There are several hereditary diseases in which migraine is a prominent symptom: epilepsy, cluster headache (see below), a new syndrome characterized by autosomal-dominant vascular retinopathy and Raynaud's phenomenon (Terwindt et al., 1998b), familial migraine with vertigo and essential tremor (Baloh et al., 1996), dyslipoproteinemias, hereditary hemorrhagic telangiectasia, Tourette's syndrome, alternating hemiplegia of childhood, several psychiatric disorders, Stormorken syndrome, hereditary essential tremor, cerebral cavernous malformations, hereditary cerebral amyloid angiopathy, cerebral autosomal-dominant arteriopathy with subcortical infarcts and leukoencephalopathy (CADASIL), and several movement disorders. Most of these diseases and their relationship to migraine are reviewed elsewhere (Haan et al., 1997). Further study of these diseases might give new clues to the genetic cause of migraine, but there is no evidence of a contribution to MO or MA of the genes involved in these disorders at present.

Other Genes Associated with Migraine

The results of association studies are difficult to interpret. Every positive association between locus markers and a disease must be confirmed in large independent samples,

Many association studies have been performed in migraine (Table 6–2). Definitive positive or negative conclusions, however, cannot be drawn from them.

Several arguments suggest that dopamine plays a role in migraine pathophysiology (Peroutka et al., 1997). In a case-control study, a significantly increased frequency of the dopamine D2 receptor NCI C allele of the polymorphism in exon 6 was observed among MA patients but not in those with MO (Peroutka et al., 1997, 1998). This finding could not be reproduced in a small uncontrolled association study of 47 MA and 55 MO patients in Germany (Dichgans et al., 1998). In an association study in the isolated population of Sardinia, the DRD2 allele showed an increase in a subgroup of dopaminergic migraineurs, who were selected because of the presence of both nausea and yawning immediately before or during the pain phase of migraine (Del Zompo et al., 1998). In another study, preliminary evidence of serotonin transporter gene involvement in migraine patients was found (Ogilvie et al., 1998).

X-linked Inheritance

There is a strong female preponderance among migraineurs. Evidence of significant excess allele sharing to chromosome Xq markers was found in two families with typical migraine (Nyholt et al., 1998a), suggesting that X-linked genetic factors may be associated with an increased risk of migraine with and without aura in some families.

Mitochondrial Involvement

Mitochondrial DNA (mtDNA) is exclusively maternally transmitted. As many migraine families show a predominantly maternal inheritance pattern, it has been postulated that migraine is caused by mitochondrial dysfunction.

There are several indications that mitochondrial dysfunction plays a role in migraine pathophysiology: abnormal brain energy metabolism was evidenced in migraineurs by ^{31}P- and ^{1}H-magnetic resonance spectroscopy; elevated blood lactate was found during effort in patients with migrainous stroke, migraine with aura, and FHM; ragged red fibers were found in muscle biopsies of patients with migrainous stroke and FHM; and decreased mitochondrial enzyme activity was found in platelets of MA and MO patients (Welch and Ramadan, 1995).

It is not known whether the mitochondrion (encoded by the nuclear and mitochondrial

Table 6–2 Genetic studies of migraine

Author	Gene or locus investigated	Results
Hovatta et al., 1994	FHM 19p locus	No involvement in 4 migraine families
Pardo et al., 1995	Various markers	Association of Group Component locus, association of Esterase D locus, no association with various other markers
Buchwalder et al., 1996	5-HT$_{2a}$ and 5-HT$_{2c}$ receptor genes	No association with MO and MA
Nyholt et al., 1996	5-HT$_{2a}$ receptor gene	No association with MO and MA
Burnett et al., 1997	5-HT$_{2c}$ receptor gene	No association with MO and MA
Griffiths et al., 1997	Endothelial NO synthetase gene	No association with migraine
Paterna et al., 1997	ACE gene deletion	Possible association with MO
Monari et al., 1997	5-HT$_{1d}$, 5-HT$_{1b}$, 5-HT$_{2a}$, 5-HT transporter, CACNLB1, FHM 19p locus	No association or linkage in 14 migraine families
Peroutka et al., 1997	Dopamine D2 receptor gene	Involvement of DRD2 in MA
Dichgans et al., 1998	Dopamine D2 receptor gene	No involvement
Peroutka et al., 1998	Dopamine D2 receptor gene	Association with MA, anxiety, depression
Ogilvie et al., 1998	Serotonin transporter gene	Involvement in MO and MA
Del Zompo et al., 1998	Dopamine receptor genes	Involvement of DRD2 locus in MO
Nyholt et al., 1998a	Xq markers	Excess allele sharing in 2 migraine families
Nyholt et al., 1998b	FHM 19p13 locus	Linkage in 1 large typical migraine family

Key to abbreviations: FHM, familial hemiplegic migraine; 5-HT, 5-hydroxytryptamine; NO, nitric oxide; MO, migraine without aura; MA, migraine with aura.

genomes) is the primary site of the dysfunction or whether the mitochondrial disturbance occurs secondary to another cause. There are some indications that mtDNA mutations are related to migraine: one patient suffered from recurrent migrainous strokes and had a muscle mtDNA deletion (Bresolin et al., 1991). Furthermore, virtually all patients with mitochondrial encephalomyopathy with lactic acidosis and stroke-like episodes (MELAS) suffer from migraine, as do many of their family members. Migraine also occurs frequently in patients with Leber's hereditary optic neuropathy (LHON); in patients with neuropathy, ataxia, and retinitis pigmentosa (NARP); and in patients with myoclonic epilepsy with ragged red fibers (MERFF).

There have been only a few studies of mtDNA mutations in migraine patients. In five related FHM patients ^{31}P-magnetic resonance spectroscopy showed abnormalities, ragged red fibers, and elevated serum lactate but the MELAS 3243 and 3271 mutations were not present in muscle DNA (Uncini et al., 1995). In a study of 53 Japanese patients with migraine, 13 harbored a 11084 mutation (Shimomura et al., 1995). This finding could not, however, be confirmed in Danish patients with migraine (Russell et al., 1997). Since the mutation was absent in Danish controls, it can be concluded that this mutation is rare in non-Japanese populations and does not play a significant role in the Danish migraineurs. It is likely that this mutation is a polymorphism that occurs in the Japanese population (Sakuta et al., 1993).

In a German study, no large-scale deletions or MELAS 3243 or MERFF 8344 mutations were found in 23 MA patients (Klopstock et al., 1996). The results of a Finnish study suggest that occipital stroke in migraine is associated with mtDNA haplogroup U (Majamaa et al., 1998). These results remain to be confirmed. In the same study, mtDNA 8344, 8993, and 11778 mutations and the common 4977 bp deletion were absent. Another study found no mtDNA 3243, 4136, 5244, 5460, 7444, 15257, 15612, 8344, 3460, 4160, or 11778 mutations in patients with MA (Ojaimi et al., 1998). Some patients with MA carried a "secondary Leber hereditary opticus neu-

ropathy" mutation (mtDNA 4216 or 13708), but this was not statistically significantly different from controls. We found no mtDNA mutations in a series of patients with migrainous stroke (Haan et al., 1999).

GENETICS OF CLUSTER HEADACHE

The pathogenesis of cluster headache (CH) is unknown. It was long thought that the most likely cause of CH attacks was abnormal vasodilation of the internal carotid artery in the region of the cavernous sinus, but recent investigations have shown that central structures are also involved (May et al., 1998; Goadsby et al., 1999). A genetic predisposition underlying the vascular and/or central disturbances of CH attacks is likely: CH has been described in several monozygotic twin pairs and multiple members of some families (reviewed in Haan et al., 1997; Montagna et al., 1998). Besides, family studies have shown an increased risk for CH in first- and second-degree family members of probands with CH (Russell et al., 1995a,b).

Investigation of the genetic cause of CH is difficult for several reasons. First, virtually all CH pedigrees are too small for linkage studies. Second, for allele-sharing studies such as sib-pair analysis, a great number of families with multiple affected sibs is needed, which will be difficult to find in CH. Furthermore, it is difficult to propose candidate genes in CH as this headache syndrome is seldom described in association with other (hereditary) disorders and virtually no clues to an underlying metabolic disturbance exist.

The only disease described to be in familial association with CH is migraine (Kudrow and Kudrow, 1994; D'Amico et al., 1997; Colantoni et al., 1999). The two genetic sites involved in FHM (*CACNA1A* and the chromosome 1 locus) have not been studied in cluster headache so far.

In the only previous molecular analysis of CH, a point mutation was found in platelet mitochondrial tRNA$^{\text{Leu(UUR)}}$ in one CH patient (Shimomura et al., 1994). Subsequent studies could not confirm this finding (Cortelli et al., 1995; Seibel et al., 1996).

When looking at the reported pedigrees with multiple CH patients, it is clear that an autosomal-dominant mode of inheritance (probably with incomplete penetrance) is more likely than mitochondrial inheritance since transmission from father to offspring is seen in several families. This was confirmed in a complex segregation analysis, which shows that CH is an autosomal-dominant inherited disorder (Russell et al., 1995a,b).

GENETICS OF TENSION-TYPE HEADACHE

Chronic tension-type headache (TTH) is a common chronic disorder that affects up to 3% of the population. Although TTH is often regarded as being caused predominantly by external factors, such as stress and abnormal posture, many patients report complaints of TTH in their family members. In a family study of probands with chronic TTH, the population relative risk of first-degree family members in a 1-year period was estimated to be 3.18 and in spouses, 1.23. The lifetime risk was 3.14 for first-degree relatives and 0.82 for spouses (Russell et al., 1998; Ostergaard et al., 1998). As probands and spouses share a part of their environment but differ in genetic constitution, the higher risk of chronic TTH in first-degree family members was attributed to genetic factors. The mode of inheritance, assessed by complex segregation analysis, was found to be multifactorial (Russell et al., 1998). Whether this phenomenon is due to genetic heterogeneity or a combination of genetic and environmental factors remains to be determined.

REFERENCES

Baloh, R.W., C.A. Foster, M.D. Qing Yue et al. (1996). Familial migraine with vertigo and essential tremor. *Neurology* 46:458–460.

Battistini, S., S. Stenirri, M. Piatti et al. (1999). A new CACNA1A gene mutation in acetazolamide-responsive familial hemiplegic migraine and ataxia. *Neurology* 53:38–43.

Bresolin, N., P. Martinelli, B. Barbirolli et al. (1991). Muscle mitochondrial DNA deletion and ³¹P-NMR spectroscopy alterations in a migraine patient. *J. Neurol. Sci.* 104:182–189.

Browne, D.L., S.T. Gancher, J.G. Nutt et al. (1994). Episodic ataxia/myokymia syndrome is associated with point mutations in the human potassium channel gene, *KCNA1*. *Nat. Genet.* 8:136–140.

Buchwalder, A., S.K. Welch, and S.J. Peroutka (1996). Exclusion of 5-HT2a and 5-HT2c receptor genes as candidate genes for migraine. *Headache* 36:254–258.

Burgess, D.L., J.M. Jones, M.H. Meister et al. (1997). Mutation of the Ca^{2+} channel β subunit gene *Cchb4* is associated with ataxia and seizures in the lethargic (lh) mouse. *Cell* 88:385–392.

Burnett, P.W.J., P.J. Harrison, G.M. Goodwin et al. (1997). Allelic variation in the serotonin 5-HT2c receptor and migraine. *Neuroreport* 8:2651–2653.

Carrera, P., M. Piatti, S. Stenirri et al. (1999). Genetic heterogeneity in Italian families with familial hemiplegic migraine. *Neurology* 53:26–32.

Classification Committee of the International Headache Society. (1988). Classification and diagnostic criteria for headache disorders, cranial neuralgias and facial pain. *Cephalagia* 8(Suppl. 7):1–96.

Colantoni O., P. Geppetti, and A. Bianchi (1999). Re-occurrence of cluster headache in two families with significant migraine frequency. *Cephalagia* 19:423–424.

Cooper, E.C. and L.Y. Jan (1999). Ion channel genes and human neurological disease: Recent progress, prospects, and challenges. *Proc. Natl. Acad. Sci. USA* 96:4759–4766.

Cortelli P., A. Zacchini, P. Barboni et al. (1995). Lack of association between mitochondrial tRNA^Leu(UUR) point mutation and cluster headache. *Lancet* 345:1120–1121.

D'Amico, D., V. Centonze, L. Grazzi et al. (1997). Coexistence of migraine and cluster headache: Report of 10 cases and possible pathogenetic implications. *Headache* 37:21–25.

Del Zompo, M., A. Cherchi, M.A. Palmas et al. (1998). Association between dopamine receptor genes and migraine without aura in a Sardinian sample. *Neurology* 51:781–786.

Denier, C., A. Ducros, K. Vahedi et al. (1999). High prevalence of CACNA1A truncations and broader clinical spectrum in episodic ataxia type 2. *Neurology* 52:1816–1821.

Dichgans, M., S. Förderreuther, M. Deiterich et al. (1998). The D2 receptor NciI allele: Absence of allelic association with migraine with aura. *Neurology* 51:928.

Dove, L.S., L.C. Abbott, and W.H. Griffith (1998). Whole-cell and single-channel analysis of P-type calcium currents in cerebellar Purkinje cells of leaner mutant mice. *J. Neurosci.* 18:7687–7699.

Doyle, J., X.J. Ren, G. Lennon et al. (1997). Mutations in the *CACNL1A4* calcium channel gene are associated with seizures, cerebellar degeneration, and ataxia in tottering and leaner mutant mice. *Mamm Genome* 8:113–120.

Ducros, A., C. Denier, A. Joutel et al. (1999). Recurrence of the T666M calcium channel *CACNA1A* gene mutation in familial hemiplegic migraine with progressive cerebellar ataxia. *Am. J. Hum. Genet.* 64:89–98.

Ducros, A., A. Joutel, K. Vahedi et al. (1997). Mapping of a second locus for familial hemiplegic migraine to 1q21-q23 and evidence of further heterogeneity. *Ann. Neurol.* 42:885–890.

Ferrari, M.D. (1998). Migraine. *Lancet* 351:1043–1051.

Ferrari, M.D. and M.B. Russell (1999). Genetics of migraine. Is migraine a genetically determined channelopathy? In *The Headaches*, 2nd ed. (J. Olesen, P. Tfelt-Hansen, and K.M.A. Welch, eds.). Raven Press, New York. Chapter 30, 241–254.

Fletcher, C.F., C.M. Lutz, T.N. O'Sullivan et al. (1996). Absence epilepsy in tottering mutant mice is associated with calcium channel defects. *Cell* 87:607–617.

Gardner, K., M. Barmada, L.J. Ptacek et al. (1997). A new locus for hemiplegic migraine maps to chromosome 1q31. *Neurology* 49:1231–1238.

Gardner, K., O. Bernal, M. Keegan et al. (1999). A new mutation in the Chr19p calcium channel gene *CACNL1A4* causing hemiplegic migraine with ataxia. *Neurology* 52(Suppl. 2):A115–A116.

Goadsby, P.J., A. Bahra, and A. May (1999). Mechanisms of cluster headache. *Cephalalgia* 19(Suppl. 23):19–23.

Griffiths, L.R., D.R. Nyholt, R.P. Curtain et al. (1997). Migraine association and linkage studies of an endothelial nitric oxide synthase (*NOS3*) gene polymorphism. *Neurology* 49:614–617.

Haan, J., G.W. Terwindt, and M.D. Ferrari (1997). Genetics of migraine. *Neurol. Clin.* 15:43–60.

Haan, J., G.M. Terwindt, J.A. Maassen et al. (1999). Search for mitochondrial DNA mutations in migraine subgroups. *Cephalalgia* 19:20–22.

Hans, M., S. Luvisetto, M.E. Williams et al. (1999). Functional consequences of mutations in the human alpha1a calcium channel subunit linked to familial hemiplegic migraine. *J. Neurosci.* 19:1610–1619.

Hovatta, I., M. Kallela, M. Farkkila et al. (1994). Familial migraine: Exclusion of the susceptibility gene from the reported locus of familial hemiplegic migraine on 19p. *Genomics* 23:707–709.

Jen, J., Q. Yue, S.F. Nelson et al. (1999). A novel nonsense mutation in CACNA1A causes episodic ataxia and hemiplegia. *Neurology* 53:34–37.

Jen, J.C., Q. Yue, J. Karrim et al. (1998). Spinocerebellar ataxia type 6 with positional vertigo and acetazolamide responsive episodic ataxia. *J. Neurol. Neurosurg. Psychiatry* 65:565–568.

Jodice, C., E. Mantuano, L. Veneziano et al. (1997). Episodic ataxia type 2 (EA2) and spinocerebellar taxia type 6 (SCA6) due to CAG repeat expansion in the *CACNA1A* gene on chromosome 19p. *Hum. Mol. Genet.* 11:1973–1978.

Joutel, A., M.G. Bousser, V. Biousse et al. (1993). A gene for familial hemiplegic migraine maps to chromosome 19. *Nat. Genet.* 5:40–45.

Joutel, A., A. Ducros, K. Vahedi et al. (1994). Genetic heterogeneity of familial hemiplegic migraine. *Am. J. Hum. Genet.* 55:1166–1172.

Klockgether, T. and B. Evert (1998). Genes involved in hereditary ataxias. *Trends Neurosci.* 21:412–418.

Klopstock, T., A. May, P. Seibel et al. (1996). Mitochondrial DNA in migraine with aura. *Neurology* 46:1735–1738.

Kramer, P.L., Q. Yue, S.T. Gancher et al. (1995). A locus for the nystagmus-associated form of episodic ataxia maps to an 11-cM region on chromosome 19p. *Am. J. Hum. Genet.* 57:182–185.

Kraus, R.L., M.J. Sinegger, H. Glossmann et al. (1998). Familial hemiplegic migraine mutations change α_{1A} Ca^{2+} channel kinetics. *J. Biol. Chem.* 273:5586–5590.

Kudrow, L. and D.B. Kudrow (1994). Inheritance of cluster headache and its possible link to migraine. *Headache* 34:400–407.

Letts, V.A., R. Felix, G.H. Biddlecome et al. (1998). The mouse stargazer gene encodes a neuronal Ca^{2+}-channel gamma subunit. *Nat. Genet.* 19:340–347.

Lorenzon, N.M., C.M. Lutz, W.N. Frankel et al. (1998). Altered calcium channel currents in Purkinje cells of neurological mutant mouse *leaner*. *J. Neurosci.* 18:4482–4489.

Majamaa, K., S. Finnila, J. Turkka et al. (1998). Mitochondrial DNA haplogroup U as a risk factor for occipital stroke in migraine. *Lancet* 352:455–456.

May, A., A. Bahra, C. Büchel et al. (1998). Hypothalamic activation in cluster headache attacks. *Lancet* 352:275–278.

May, A., R.A. Ophoff, G.M. Terwindt et al. (1995). Familial hemiplegic migraine locus on 19p13 is involved in the common forms of migraine with and without aura. *Hum. Genet.* 96:604–608.

Monari, L., M. Mochi, M.L. Valentino et al. (1997). Searching for migraine genes: Exclusion of 290 cM out of the whole human genome. *Ital. J. Neurosci.* 18:277–282.

Montagna, P., M. Mochi, G. Prologo et al. (1998). Heritability of cluster headache. *Eur. J. Neurol.* 5:343–345.

Nyholt, D.R., R.P. Curtain, P.T. Gaffney et al.

(1996). Migraine association and linkage analyses of the human 5-hydroxytryptamine ($5HT_{2A}$) receptor gene. *Cephalalgia* 16:463–467.

Nyholt, D.R., J.L. Dawkins, P.J. Brimage et al. (1998a). Evidence for an X-linked genetic component in familial typical migraine. *Hum. Mol. Genet.* 7:459–463.

Nyholt, D.R., R.A. Lea, P.J. Goadsby et al. (1998b). Familial typical migraine. Linkage to chromosome 19p13 and evidence for genetic heterogeneity. *Neurology* 50:1428–1432.

Ogilvie, A.D., M.B. Russell, P. Dhall et al. (1998). Altered allelic distributions of the serotonin transporter gene in migraine with and without aura. *Cephalalgia* 18:23–26.

Ojaimi, J., S. Katsbanis, S. Bower et al. (1998). Mitochondrial DNA in stroke and migraine with aura. *Cerebrovasc. Dis.* 8:102–106.

Ophoff, R.A., G.M. Terwindt, M.N. Vergouwe et al. (1996). Familial hemiplegic migraine and episodic ataxia type-2 are caused by mutations in the Ca^{2+} channel gene *CACNL1A4*. *Cell* 87:543–552.

Ophoff, R.A., R. Van Eijk, L.A. Sandkuijl et al. (1994). Genetic heterogeneity of familial hemiplegic migraine. *Genomics* 22:21–26.

Østergaard, S., M.B. Russell, L. Berndtsen et al. (1998). Comparison of first degree relatives and spouses of people with chronic tension headache. *BMJ* 314:1092–1093.

Pardo, J., A. Carracedo, I. Munoz et al. (1995). Genetic markers: Association study in migraine. *Cephalalgia* 15:200–204.

Paterna, S., P. Di Pasquale, C. Cottone et al. (1997). Migraine without aura and ACE-gene deletion polymorphism: Is there a correlation? Preliminary findings. *Cardiovasc. Drugs Ther.* 11:603–604.

Peroutka, S.J. (1997). Dopamine and migraine. *Neurology* 49:650–656.

Peroutka, S.J., S.C. Price, T.L. Wilhoit et al. (1998). Comorbid migraine with aura, anxiety, and depression is associated with dopamine D2 receptor (DRD2) NcoI alleles. *Mol. Med.* 4:14–21.

Peroutka, S.J., T. Wilhoit, and K. Jones (1997). Clinical susceptibility to migraine with aura is modified by dopamine D2 receptor (DRD2) NcoI alleles. *Neurology* 49:201–206.

Pietrobon, S., S. Luvisetto, M. Spagnolo et al. (1998). Effect of mutations linked to familial hemiplegic migraine on the biophysical properties of human α_{1A}-containing calcium channels. *Soc. Neurosci.* 24:21.

Russell, M.B. (1997). Genetic epidemiology of migraine and cluster headache. *Cephalalgia* 17:683–701.

Russell, M.B., P.G. Andersson, and L.L. Thomsen (1995a). Familial occurrence of cluster headache. *J. Neurol. Neurosurg. Psychiatry* 58:341–343.

Russell, M.B., P.G. Andersson, L.L. Thomsen et al. (1995b). Cluster headache is an autosomal dominantly inherited disorder in some families: A complex segregation analysis. *J. Med. Genet.* 32:954–956.

Russell, M.B., M. Diamant, and S. Norby (1997). Genetic heterogeneity of migraine with and without aura in Danes cannot be explained by mutation in mtDNA nucleotide pair 11084. *Acta. Neurol. Scand.* 96:171–173.

Russell, M.B., L. Iselius, S. Østergaard et al. (1998). Inheritance of chronic tension-type headache investigated by complex segregation analysis. *Hum. Genet.* 102:138–140.

Russell, M.B. and J. Olesen (1993). The genetics of migraine without and migraine with aura. *Cephalalgia* 13:245–248.

Russell, M.B. and J. Olesen (1995). Increased familial risk and evidence of genetic factor in migraine. *BMJ* 311:541–544.

Sakuta, R., Y. Goto, I. Nonaka et al. (1993). An A-to-G transition at nucleotide pair 11084 in the *ND4* gene may be an mtDNA polymorphism. *Am. J. Hum. Genet.* 57:964–965.

Seibel, P., T. Grunewald, A. Gundolla et al. (1996). Investigation on the mitochondrial transfer $RNA^{Leu(UUR)}$ in blood cells from patients with cluster headache. *J. Neurol.* 243:305–307.

Shimomura, T., A. Kitano, H. Marukawa et al. (1994). Point mutation in platelet mitochondrial $tRNA^{Leu(UUR)}$ in patient with cluster headache. *Lancet* 344:625.

Shimomura, T., A. Kitano, H. Marukawa et al. (1995). Mutation in platelet mitochondrial gene in patients with migraine. *Cephalalgia* 15(Suppl. 14):10.

Stewart, W.F., J. Staffa, R.B. Lipton et al. (1997). Familial risk of migraine: A population-based study. *Ann. Neurol.* 41:166–172.

Teh, B.T., P. Silburn, K. Lindblad et al. (1995). Familial periodic cerebellar ataxia without myokymia maps to a 19-cM region on 19p13. *Am. J. Hum. Genet.* 56:1443–1449.

Terwindt, G.M., R.A. Ophoff, J. Haan et al. (1996). Familial hemiplegic migraine: A clinical comparison of families linked and unlinked to chromosome 19. *Cephalalgia* 16:153–155.

Terwindt, G.M., R.A. Ophoff, J. Haan et al. (1998a). Variable clinical expression of mutations in the P/Q type calcium channel gene in familial hemiplegic migraine. *Neurology* 50:1105–1110.

Terwindt, G.M., J. Haan, R.A. Ophoff et al. (1998b). Clinical and genetic analysis of a large Dutch family with autosomal dominant vascular retinopathy, migraine and Raynaud's phenomenon. *Brain* 121:303–316.

Tournier-Lasserve, E. (1999). *CACNA1A* mutations. Hemiplegic migraine, episodic ataxia type 2, and the others. *Neurology* 53:3–4.

Ulrich, V., M. Gervil, K.O. Kyvik et al. (1999). Evidence of a genetic factor in migraine with aura:

A population based Danish twin study. *Ann. Neurol. 45*:241–246.

Uncini, A., R. Lodi, A. Di Muzio et al. (1995). Abnormal brain and muscle energy metabolism shown by ^{31}P-MRS in familial hemiplegic migraine. *J. Neurol. Sci. 129*:214–222.

Vahedi, K., C. Denier, A. Ducros et al. (1999). Sporadic hemiplegic migraine with de novo CACNA1A missense mutation. *Neurology 52*(Suppl. 2):A274.

Vahedi, K., A. Joutel, P. van Bogaert et al. (1995). A gene for hereditary paroxysmal cerebellar ataxia maps to chromosome 19p. *Ann. Neurol. 37*:289–293.

Von Brederlow, B., A.F. Hahn, W.J. Koopman et al. (1995). Mapping the gene for acetazolamide responsive hereditary paroxysmal cerebellar ataxia to chromosome 19p. *Hum. Mol. Genet. 4*: 279–284.

Welch, K.M.A. and N.M. Ramadan (1995). Mitochondria, magnesium and migraine. *J. Neurol. Sci. 134*:9–14.

Yue, Q., J.C. Jen, S.F. Nelson et al. (1997). Progressive ataxia due to a missense mutation in a calcium-channel gene. *Am. J. Hum. Genet. 61*: 1078–1087.

Yue, Q., J.C. Jen, M.W. Thwe et al. (1998). De novo mutation in CACNA1A caused acetazolamide-responsive episodic ataxia. *Am. J. Med. Genet. 77*:298–301.

Zhuchenko, O., J. Baily, P. Bonnen et al. (1997). Autosomal dominant cerebellar ataxia (SCA6) associated with small polyglutamine expansions in the alpha 1A-voltage-dependent calcium channel. *Nat. Genet. 15*:62–69.

Ziegler, D.W., Y.M. Hur, T.J. Bouchard et al. (1998). Migraine in twins raised together and apart. *Headache 38*:417–422.

7

Epidemiology and Impact of Headache

RICHARD B. LIPTON
SANDRA W. HAMELSKY
WALTER F. STEWART

Headache is a symptom that has many causes (Classification Committee of the International Headache Society, 1988). In epidemiologic studies, one must define the disorder of interest (i.e., migraine, brain-tumor headache) before one can study its distribution in the general population. Recent epidemiologic studies have clarified our understanding of the scope and distribution of the public health problem imposed by various headache disorders (Rasmussen et al., 1991a,b; Wong et al., 1995; Barea et al., 1996; Lavados and Tenhamm, 1998; Pryse-Phillips et al., 1992; Wang et al., 1997; Schwartz et al., 1998; Stewart et al., 1992; Lipton and Stewart, 1993; Silberstein et al., 1998; Rasmussen, 1995; Scher et al., 1999). These findings have implications for both clinical practice and public health policy (Lipton et al., 1994).

Epidemiologic studies can add to our understanding of headache disorders from a number of perspectives. They can be used to assess the reliability, validity, and generalizability of various case definitions for headache disorders within and outside of the classification system of the International Headache Society (IHS) (Lipton et al., 1993; Merikangas et al., 1993; Merikangas and Frances, 1993; Mortimer et al., 1992; Metsahonkala

and Sillanpaa, 1994). They can help clarify the demarcation between migraine and other primary headache disorders (Rasmussen, 1995; Schwartz et al., 1997). Prevalence studies provide one measure of the scope of the public health problem for a particular headache disorder. The impact of illness on individuals and on society can be addressed by measuring health-related quality of life, work loss, and health care use in population-based samples (Lipton et al., 2000b; Stewart et al. 1996b). Examining sociodemographic, familial, and environmental risk factors helps to identify groups at highest risk for various headache disorders and may ultimately provide clues to disease mechanisms or preventive strategies. Epidemiologic studies are also necessary to study comorbidity (Lipton and Silberstein, 1994). Finally, epidemiologic studies are a prelude to public health interventions designed to improve the diagnosis and treatment of particular headache disorders (Stewart et al., 1992; Lipton et al., 1994).

Population-based studies identify people with various headache disorders whether or not they are currently seeking medical care for their headaches. In epidemiologic studies, the population is actively assessed to identify individuals with headache and to determine the types and whether or not headache treatment has been sought (Lipton et al., 1998). For example, only half of active migraine sufferers see a doctor specifically for headache each year (Lipton and Stewart, 1993). Many migraine studies are conducted in subspecialty practices, yet fewer than 15% of migraine sufferers ever consult neurologists and fewer than 2% consult headache specialists (Stewart et al., 1992; Lipton et al., 1998). As a consequence, clinic-based studies may suffer from substantial selection bias (Rasmussen, 1995; Linet and Stewart, 1984). Factors that predispose individuals to consult specialists may be mistaken for attributes of the disease.

Recent epidemiologic studies of the primary headache disorders have employed the criteria of the IHS (Classification Committee of the International Headache Society, 1988; Rasmussen, 1995; Scher et al., 1999). These criteria are more complete, explicit, and rigorous than those used in past studies (Classification Committee of the International Headache Society, 1988; Silberstein et al., 1998; Scher et al., 1999). This chapter reviews the epidemiology of migraine and tension-type headache, emphasizing the population-based studies that use the criteria proposed by the IHS. The epidemiology of very frequent and chronic daily headache disorders is included in Chapter 11.

METHODOLOGIC ISSUES

Case Definitions

For clinical practice and epidemiologic research, it is important to have a reliable and valid case definition of primary headache disorders (Lipton et al., 1993; Merikangas et al., 1993; Merikangas and Frances, 1993). *Reliability* implies that independent diagnostic evaluations yield consistent diagnostic results (Lipton et al., 1993). *Validity* refers to the relationship between the assigned diagnosis and the underlying biology of the disorder. In the absence of a true diagnostic gold standard, validity is supported if diagnostic groups

include members with common risk factors, natural histories, treatment response profiles, and biological markers (Merikangas et al., 1993; Merikangas and Frances, 1993).

Many case definitions for migraine and tension-type headache have been proposed. Different definitions have emphasized different features, and some criteria have been poorly specified. Rather than specifying the features or combinations of features required to establish or exclude a diagnosis, prior criteria listed the features that are usually present (Friedman et al., 1962). Lack of clarity in case definition inevitably leads to unreliability in diagnosis (Lipton et al., 1993).

Efforts to define migraine empirically have attempted to distinguish it from tension-type headache based on specific symptom constellations. Such work is often intended to test the "spectrum" or "continuum" concept, the idea that migraine and tension-type headache exist as polar ends on a continuum of severity, varying more in degree than in kind (Featherstone, 1985; Raskin, 1988; Waters, 1986). The alternative model views migraine and tension-type headache as nosologically distinct entities that differ in severity.

Waters (1972, 1986) examined the associations between three "key features" of migraine (warning, unilateral pain, and nausea or vomiting) in a sample of women between the ages of 20 and 64 and found that as headache intensity increased, migrainous symptoms occurred together more frequently. He concluded: "The distribution of headache severity extends as a continuous spectrum from mild attacks, which usually have neither unilateral distribution nor warning nor nausea, to severe headaches which are frequently accompanied by the three migraine features." Other authors have offered some empirical support for the continuum concept (Featherstone, 1985; Celentano et al., 1990).

The debate regarding the relationship between migraine and tension-type headache is ongoing. Progress requires the development of testable predictions that are compatible with only one model. Recent evidence based on treatment response to sumatriptan suggests that migraine and tension-type headaches are distinct, as migraine responds to sumatriptan while tension-type headaches respond at placebo rates (Lipton et al., 2000d). However, among individuals with IHS migraine, attacks of episodic tension-type headache respond to sumatriptan (Lipton et al., 2000d). Thus, in individuals with migraine, phenotypic episodic tension-type headache appears to have a triptan-responsive mechanism. We suggest that migraine and episodic tension-type headache are nosologically distinct but that, among migraine sufferers, individual attacks of migraine and tension-type headache may be part of a spectrum of severity.

To improve the classification, the IHS published criteria for a broad range of headache disorders (Classification Committee of the International Headache Society, 1988). The criteria, based on international expert consensus, are more explicit and better operationalized than the prior consensus criteria. They clearly indicate the features required to confirm or exclude particular headache diagnoses. Empirical assessment of the criteria is an area of active research. In one study, four clinicians reviewed videotapes of structured patient interviews and then assigned diagnoses based on IHS criteria. The good overall level of agreement is reflected by the kappa statistic of 0.74 (Granella et al., 1994).

Other studies have also examined the performance of the IHS criteria (Rasmussen, 1995; Mortimer et al., 1992; Metsahonkala and Sillanpaa, 1994). Conflicting results have been obtained with respect to the comprehensiveness of the criteria. Analysis of a population-based study revealed the criteria to be comprehensive in that virtually all headache types could be classified (Rasmussen et al., 1992). In contrast, in clinic-based studies, substantial numbers of patients could not be classified. Particularly problematic for the IHS criteria is the classification of chronic daily headaches (Solomon et al., 1992; Sandrini et al., 1993; Mathew, 1993; Silberstein et al., 1994). Based on emerging data, the IHS criteria are currently being revised. The IHS criteria represent an enormous advance in headache classification and have provided a firm diagnostic foundation for epidemiologic research. Diagnostic criteria for the various headache disorders are discussed in the respective chapters.

Some Epidemiologic Terms

Many epidemiologic studies have examined migraine prevalence. *Prevalence* refers to the proportion of a given population that has a disease over a defined period of time. For example, *lifetime prevalence* refers to the proportion of individuals who have ever had a condition. *Period prevalence* refers to the proportion of individuals who have had the condition over some defined interval. The most common period selected for study is 1 year. As the period selected for study increases, prevalence increases. Prevalence is an important measure of the burden of disease.

Incidence refers to the rate of onset of new cases of a disease in a defined population over a given period of time. To conduct a migraine incidence study, one must first eliminate anyone in the population who currently has a diagnosis of migraine. Migraine-free individuals are then followed to determine the rate of development of new cases. Incidence is usually expressed as the number of new cases per 1,000 person-years of follow-up. An incidence of 15 per 1,000 person-years of follow-up means that if 1,000 migraine-free individuals are followed for 1 year, 15 will develop new-onset migraine.

There is a mathematical relationship between incidence and prevalence. Prevalence is determined by the product of average incidence and average duration of disease. In a given population, the prevalence of migraine may increase because either incidence or duration of disease increases.

MIGRAINE

Incidence

Few studies of migraine incidence have been performed, and none has systematically followed a large sample of migraine-free individuals across a broad range of ages to ascertain new cases of IHS migraine. Estimating the incidence of a chronic disorder with episodic manifestations, such as migraine, is challenging (Cummings et al., 1990). Since diagnostic criteria for migraine without aura require at least five lifetime attacks, should incidence be estimated using the time of the first or the fifth attack? Further, the disease affects individuals of all ages and the incidence rate varies substantially by age. To accurately describe incidence, there must be a large cohort study of initially migraine-free individuals across the lifespan.

Breslau et al. (1996) conducted a prospective study in a large health maintenance organization. The inception cohort of 1,007 individuals ranged in age from 21 to 30 years. Most of the sample (972/1,007) completed follow-up interviews 3.5 and 5.5 years after enrollment. The at-risk population comprised the 848 participants who did not meet the criteria for migraine at baseline. Over 5.5 years of follow-up, the cumulative incidence of migraine was 8.4% (71/848, 60 women and 11 men), for a rate of 17.0 per 1,000 person-years (24.0 women, 6.0 men). This excellent study is limited by the relatively narrow age range of the inception cohort.

In addition to this longitudinal study, two population-based studies estimated the incidence of migraine using the participants' recall of age at migraine onset. In Washington County, Maryland, telephone interviews conducted with 10,169 residents between the ages of 12 and 29 identified 392 men and 1,018 women with migraine (Stewart et al., 1991). This study used a case definition that differed slightly from the IHS definition. In both men and women, the incidence rate of migraine with aura peaks 3 to 5 years earlier than migraine without aura (Fig. 7–1). In addition, the incidence of migraine in women peaked at a later age than in men. *Telescoping*, which is the tendency to report events that occurred in the past as having occurred closer to the present (Brown et al., 1985), complicates incidence estimates based on retrospectively reported age at onset. Studies that estimate the age-specific incidence of migraine based on recall would probably be biased toward older ages at headache onset as current migraine sufferers report the age at onset to be closer to the present than it actually was (Cummings et al., 1990; Brown et al., 1985). To adjust for telescoping, the Washington County study adjusted the age-specific incidence rates for the time interval between the reported age at onset and the age at interview (Stewart et al., 1991). This study was limited by the age range of participants as individuals over 30 years of age were not enrolled. Peak incidence rates for migraine with aura were 6.6/1,000 person-years for men and 14.1/1,000 person-years for women. The peak incidence of migraine without aura was 10.1/1,000 person-years in men and 18.9/1,000 person-years in women. These incidence estimates are somewhat higher than those reported by Breslau et al. (1996), perhaps because of the younger age distribution of the Washington County sample.

A population-based study conducted by Rasmussen (1995) showed the age-adjusted annual incidence of migraine to be 3.7 per 1,000 person-years (women 5.8, men 1.6).

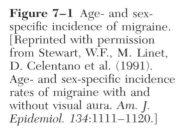

Figure 7–1 Age- and sex-specific incidence of migraine. [Reprinted with permission from Stewart, W.F., M. Linet, D. Celentano et al. (1991). Age- and sex-specific incidence rates of migraine with and without visual aura. *Am. J. Epidemiol. 134*:1111–1120.]

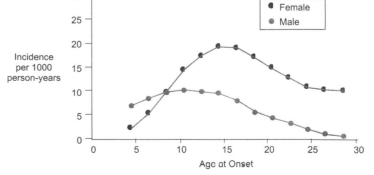

Neither age-specific incidence nor incidence by migraine subtypes was reported. This sample had a much older age distribution, perhaps accounting for the lower rates.

As an alternative approach to estimating migraine incidence, the linked medical records system in Olmstead County, Minnesota, was used. A review of 6,400 patient records yielded 629 individuals who fulfilled criteria for migraine (Stang et al., 1992). Age-adjusted incidence rates were 1.37 per 1,000 person-years for men and 2.94 per 1,000 person-years for women. In this study, the incidence rates were lower than in the aforementioned studies, perhaps because only individuals who consulted a health care provider for headache and provided a detailed medical history that was recorded in the medical record were eligible for inclusion in the numerator of the incidence estimate.

Prevalence

Prevalence estimates for migraine have varied widely, largely because of differences in case definitions and demographic features of study populations. Since migraine prevalence varies by age, gender, race, geography, and socioeconomic status, prevalence differences among studies may be influenced by these factors (Scher et al., 1999; Stewart et al., 1995). We conducted meta-analyses of published population-based studies in 1995 and 1998; in each case, our purpose was to explain the variation in migraine prevalence estimates among studies and to develop summary measures of prevalence.

In 1995, the meta-analysis included 24 studies published prior to 1994, only five of which used the IHS diagnostic criteria (Stewart et al., 1995). Over 65% of the variation in prevalence estimates among studies was explained by only a few factors. The single most important factor, case definition, accounted for the largest portion of variation in prevalence (36.1%) among studies. Another important factor was the gender distribution of the study sample, which accounted for 14.5% of the variation among studies; migraine was more prevalent among women than men. Linear and quadratic terms for age accounted

for 16.4% of variance. Methodologic factors, such as the source of the population, the response rate, and whether diagnoses were confirmed by a clinical examination, did not have substantial incremental explanatory power. This model left about one-third of the variance among studies unexplained.

We reasoned that if case definition was held constant, we might identify other important factors that explain variation among studies. In 1998, we conducted a second meta-analysis that included 18 population-based studies based on the IHS criteria (Scher et al., 1999). In this meta-analysis, case definition was held relatively constant. In addition, we conducted separate meta-analyses for men and women. Therefore, two of the most important explanatory factors in the first meta-analysis (case definition and gender) were eliminated. In this second meta-analysis, prevalence peaked during the third and fourth decades of life among men and women (Figure 7–2). Age (age and age squared) and geographic location of the study population accounted for 74% of the variation in migraine prevalence in women and 58% in men. Prevalence was highest in North America, South America, and Western Europe; intermediate in Africa; and lowest in Asia. Once again, methodologic factors such as sampling method, response method, response rate, and recall period had modest explanatory power.

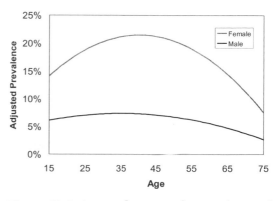

Figure 7–2 Age- and sex-specific prevalence of migraine based on a meta-analytic summary of 18 population-based studies. [Reprinted with permission from Scher, A.I., W.F. Stewart, and R.B. Lipton (1999). Migraine and headache: A meta-analytic approach. In *Epidemiology of Pain* (I. Crombie, ed.), pp. 159–170. IASP Press, Seattle.]

Using the IHS case definition, a substantial proportion of the variation in migraine prevalence can be explained by remarkably few factors. However, some of the variation remains unexplained. Socioeconomic status, cultural differences in symptom reporting, or other unmeasured factors may account for part of the residual variation in migraine prevalence (Scher et al., 1999; Stewart et al., 1995).

Prevalence by Age and Gender

As noted in the meta-analyses, migraine prevalence varies by age and gender. At postpubertal ages, migraine prevalence is consistently higher in women than men (Scher et al., 1999). The prevalence of migraine varies with age, peaking between the ages of 35 to 45 years (Fig. 7–2). Overall, prevalence is highest from ages 25 to 55, the years of peak productivity. This age distribution helps to explain the enormous economic impact of migraine; as discussed below, migraine is an important cause of absenteeism and reduced productivity at work.

Prevalence by Race and Geographic Region

Race and geographic region contribute to variation in migraine prevalence. A population-based study in the United States compared the prevalence of migraine among Caucasians, African-Americans, and Asian-Americans living in Baltimore County, Maryland (Stewart et al., 1996a). After adjusting for sociodemographic covariates, prevalence of migraine was lowest in Asian-Americans (women 9.2%, men 4.8%), intermediate in African-Americans (women 16.2%, men 7.2%), and highest in Caucasians (women 20.4%, men 8.6%). These results mirror the meta-analytic finding that prevalence is lowest in Asia and Africa, with considerably higher prevalence in Europe, Central and South America, and North America (Scher et al., 1999).

What accounts for the variation in migraine prevalence by race and geographic region? Sociocultural factors such as diet, stress, and the environment contribute and differences in genetic susceptibility may play a role. The relative contribution of genetic and environmental risk factors or their interaction remains to be determined.

Prevalence by Education and Income

Population-based studies conducted in North America indicate that migraine prevalence is inversely related to socioeconomic status (SES), as measured by household income or education (Stewart et al., 1992; Lipton and Stewart, 1993; Stewart et al., 1996a; Kryst and Scherl, 1994); i.e., as income or education increases, migraine prevalence declines. This population finding contradicts prior beliefs regarding a direct relationship between migraine prevalence and income. This discrepancy may be explained by perceptions about migraine that arise in those who seek medical care. In the doctor's office, migraine may appear to be a disease of high-income individuals because medical diagnosis of migraine is more common among high-income groups (Lipton et al., 1992; Stang and Osterhaus, 1993). Studies outside the United States have not reported the inverse relationship between migraine prevalence and SES (Abu-Arefeh and Russell, 1994; Gobel et al., 1994; O'Brien et al., 1994; Rasmussen, 1992). Reasons for these discrepant results remain unclear.

INDIVIDUAL IMPACT: FREQUENCY AND SEVERITY OF ATTACKS

The individual impact of migraine is measured by assessing the pattern of symptoms as well as the frequency and severity of attacks. Factors such as the level of pain intensity, the presence and severity of associated symptoms (nausea, vomiting, photophobia, phonophobia), and the attack duration are important determinants of the severity of an individual attack; but migraine also has a cumulative impact over time. The aggregate impact of the illness is determined not just by attack characteristics, but also by attack frequency, comorbid illnesses, psychological factors, and coping strategies, including pharmacotherapy (Stewart et al., 1994).

A recent population-based telephone interview survey involving 1,748 migraine sufferers reported the prevalence of specific migraine characteristics (Stewart et al. 1996b). Approximately 80% of subjects reported pain that was severe (women 38.9%, men 46.0%) or very severe (women 43.3%, men 31.8%). The remainder of the subjects reported mild to moderate pain. Approximately 82% of migraine sufferers reported photophobia (overall 81.9%, women 83.5%, men 76.5%), while about 78% reported phonophobia (overall 77.9%, women 79.3%, men 72.9%). More than half (58.8%) of migraine participants reported that nausea accompanies their migraine headache half of the time or more (women 62.1%, men 47.3%), while only a small proportion reported vomiting. The median attack frequency for migraine sufferers was one to two migraine attacks per month. Duration of untreated attacks varies onsiderably by gender. Among women, approximately 71% of attacks last longer than 24 hours. In contrast, 48% of men reported attacks that last longer than 24 hours. These findings are similar to those reported in earlier studies (Rasmussen et al, 1991; Rasmussen, 1995; Gobel et al., 1994).

HEALTH-RELATED QUALITY-OF-LIFE STUDIES

Quality of life refers to individuals' perceptions of their general well-being and life position in the context of their culture and value systems and in relation to their goals, standards, and concerns. Quality of life is influenced by a range of variables, including environmental, economic, social, health-related, spiritual, and political factors. Health-related quality of life (HRQoL) is one component of overall quality of life and encompasses individuals' health states, functional status, and well-being (Tarlov et al., 1989). The fundamental domains of HRQoL include physical, psychological, and social areas; role-functioning; and general well-being. Measures of HRQoL can provide a more global

and qualitative assessment of an individual's status and of the aggregate burden imposed by migraine and other health conditions.

Both generic and disease-specific measures have been used to measure HRQoL among migraine sufferers. Generic HRQoL instruments are designed to measure the impact of a range of illnesses using a common scale; this facilitates comparisons of the HRQoL impact across various medical conditions. The most commonly used generic measures of HRQoL in migraine are the Medical Outcomes Study (MOS) instruments developed by the Rand Corporation. The MOS instruments include the Short Form 20 (SF-20) (Stewart et al., 1988), the Short Form 36 (SF-36) (McHorney et al., 1993), and the Short Form 12 (SF-12) (Ware et al., 1996), all of which have been used in migraine studies. Other generic HRQoL scales used in migraine studies include the Sickness Impact Profile (SIP) (Damiano, 1996), the Nottingham Health Profile (NHP) (McEwen and McKenna, 1996), and the Psychological General Well-Being (PGWB) index (Dahlof and Dimenas, 1995). In contrast to generic HRQoL measures, disease-specific instruments contain questions that address the impact of a specific illness. By focusing on the impact of particular illnesses, disease-specific HRQoL measures may provide more precise measurement and greater sensitivity to change over time than generic measures (Hurst et al., 1998). However, disease-specific HRQoL measures cannot be used to compare HRQoL across disease categories.

Disease-specific HRQoL measures for migraine fall into two broadly defined categories: those that measure HRQoL for a single migraine attack (Hartmaier et al., 1995; Santanello et al., 1995) and those that measure HRQoL over a period of weeks or months (Adelman et al., 1996; Wagner et al., 1996). The single attack measures summarize the impact of a single migraine attack (with or without therapy) over 24 hours. This measure can be used in randomized, placebo-controlled trials and is highly sensitive to treatment effects (Santanello et al., 1997). The idea that HRQoL can be measured over a 24-hour period has been challenged (Steiner, 1998).

Disease-specific measures that evaluate HRQoL over weeks or months have been applied to studies that compare HRQoL before and after treatment (Adelman et al., 1996; Gross et al., 1996; Mushet et al., 1996) and in randomized trials comparing a novel therapy with usual care (Block et al., 1998).

Clinic-based Studies

Most studies of HRQoL in migraine have been conducted in clinic-based samples or in the context of clinical trials. On average, migraine sufferers visiting a clinic or participating in a clinical trial have more severe disease than the general population (Lipton et al., 1998). Factors that lead to seeking care, including severity of illness and comorbid conditions, may influence HRQoL measurement, limiting the generalizability of results to broader populations. In addition, in clinic-based studies of HRQoL, it is difficult to define appropriate nonmigraine controls. In studies that assess response to treatment, the lack of a control group may overestimate the benefits of treatment because of regression toward the mean. Trials that include a usual-care arm or placebo group address this issue (Adelman et al., 1996; Gross et al., 1996; Mushet et al., 1996; Santanello et al., 1997; Block et al., 1998).

In clinic-based samples, migraine sufferers have lower HRQoL than reference samples from the US population (Solomon et al., 1993; Osterhaus et al., 1994). For example, Solomon et al. (1993) administered the SF-20 to 208 patients attending a headache clinic to measure the HRQoL of chronic headache patients. In this clinic-based sample, HRQoL was significantly reduced relative to published population norms and relative to patients with other chronic conditions, such as arthritis, diabetes, and back problems. Osterhaus et al. (1994) reported similar results in a sample of migraine clinical trial participants using the SF-36; the HRQoL domains that were most affected included bodily pain and role disability due to physical health.

Dahlof and Dimenas (1995) compared the well-being of migraine sufferers with an age- and sex-matched control group using three measures: Minor Symptoms Evaluation Profile (MSEP), Subjective Symptoms Assessment Profile (SSAP), and the PGWB Index. To assess HRQoL between attacks, migraine sufferers were asked to complete the questionnaire at least 1 week following their last migraine attack. The investigators found that, even between attacks, migraine sufferers reported more symptoms and greater emotional distress as well as disturbed contentment, vitality, and sleep relative to the control population.

Population-based Studies

At least three studies have assessed HRQoL in a population-based sample of migraine sufferers and a contemporaneous control population (Lipton et al., 1999, 2000b; Terwindt et al., 2000c). Each of these studies used a variation of the MOS instrument, including the SF-36 (Terwindt et al., 2000; Lipton et al., 1999) and the SF-12 (Lipton et al., 2000b). All of these studies screened the general population to identify migraine cases and nonmigraine control subjects. The HRQoL scores in the migraine population were significantly lower than those in the control population in all three studies. These studies also described the relationships between HRQoL and migraine frequency, disability, and depression. As migraine frequency and disability increased, HRQoL decreased (Lipton et al., 2000b; Terwindt et al., 2000). One study found that migraine and depression are comorbid but that each disorder has an independent influence on HRQoL (Lipton et al., 2000b).

Effect of Headache Therapy on Health-related Quality of Life

A growing number of studies have assessed the effects of headache therapy on generic and disease-specific HRQoL measures. Most of the migraine-specific instruments were designed and validated by pharmaceutical companies. Therefore, the choice of a migraine-specific instrument is often determined by the study sponsor. As a result, it is difficult to compare the effects of different drugs on migraine-specific quality of life.

The effect of sumatriptan on HRQoL has been studied extensively, using both a generic HRQoL measure (i.e., SF-36) and the Migraine-Specific Quality of Life Questionnaire (MSQoL). Treatment with sumatriptan consistently improved HRQoL scores (Adelman et al., 1996; Gross et al., 1996; Mushet et al., 1996; Solomon et al., 1993; Jhingran et al., 1996; Lofland et al., 1998, 1999). These studies often compared HRQoL after treatment with the pretreatment baseline, a design that does not support rigorous inferences. A stronger design uses random allocation of patients to treatment groups.

As early as 3 months after beginning therapy, significant improvements in HRQoL were observed in physical role functioning, bodily pain, general health perception, vitality, emotional role functioning, and mental health domains (Adelman et al., 1996; Gross et al., 1996; Cohen et al., 1996; Jhingran et al., 1996). Patients treated with sumatriptan also had improvement in HRQoL as measured by the MSQoL. Across studies, patients consistently reported significant improvements on all three scales of the MSQoL: role-restrictive, role-preventive, and emotional. Improvements in HRQoL often accrue over 6 months of treatment, while the benefits for individually treated attacks are immediate. Since HRQoL captures the burden of disease both during and between attacks, we suggest that HRQoL improves over multiple attacks as patients learn that they have a reliable treatment.

HRQol scores showed improvement after treatment with more recently developed 5-hydroxytryptamine type 1 (5-HT$_1$) agonists (rizatriptan and zolmitriptan) (Santanello et al., 1997; Schoenen and Sawyer, 1997). Using the 24-hour Migraine Quality of Life Questionnaire (MQoLQ), Santanello et al. (1997) assessed the impact of migraine and migraine therapy (rizatriptan) on HRQoL during an acute migraine attack. The rizatriptan-treated group showed significant improvements in quality of life compared with the placebo-treated group in three of the five measured domains: social functioning, migraine symptoms, and feelings/concerns. Significant improvement was not observed in energy/vitality or work functioning.

Health-related Quality of Life and Disability

In headache research, disability scales and HRQoL instruments are used to measure various aspects of the burden of disease. These two types of instruments measure impact differently and have different interpretations. Generally, HRQoL is scaled in a positive direction, with higher scores reflecting better HRQoL (i.e., better outcome). For disability measures, higher scores reflect greater levels of activity limitations (i.e., worse outcome). Disability measures assess impairment in role functioning, i.e., reduced ability to function in defined roles, such as paid work. Disability measures are often scored in intuitively meaningful units (i.e., lost hours or lost days due to illness). However, HRQoL reflects an individual's qualitative assessment of role functioning as well as his or her perceptions about bodily pain, general health, vitality, and other issues. Often, HRQoL is measured in arbitrary, constructed units; scales often have a mean score of 50 and standard deviation of 10.

The Henry Ford Hospital Disability Inventory (HDI) is a valid and reliable tool that was designed to evaluate self-perceived disabling effects of headache (Jacobson et al., 1994). The instrument contains 25 questions subgrouped into emotional and functional domains and has much in common with disease-specific HRQoL instruments.

Another disability instrument, the Migraine Disability Assessment Scale (MIDAS), consists of five questions that focus on lost time in three domains: school work or work for pay; household work or chores; and family, social, and leisure activities. Respondents report the number of lost workdays and number of days with significant limitations in activity ($\geq 50\%$ reduced productivity) due to headache that occurred over the previous 3 months. The MIDAS questionnaire has demonstrated reliability (Stewart et al., 1999), as reported in two separate population-based studies in the United States and United Kingdom, and validity, using a 3-month daily diary study as the gold standard (Stewart et al., 2000). Scores on the MIDAS are highly correlated with physician judgments about the severity of illness and need for treatment (Lipton et al., 2000a). The MIDAS score can be used to classify migraine sufferers into four disability grades that predict treatment needs. A recent randomized, placebo-controlled trial showed that MIDAS grade provides a basis for selecting initial treatment in stratified care (Lipton et al., 2000e).

SOCIETAL IMPACT

Direct Costs

Direct costs include all of the costs of diagnosing and treating a particular disorder. Drivers of the cost of treatment vary from condition to condition and may include outpatient visits, diagnostic and laboratory procedures, the use of emergency department services, hospitalization, and the cost of treatment, including prescriptions. Most of migraine's direct costs result from outpatient visits and prescription medications.

A recent study of the epidemiology and patterns of health care use for migraine in the United States found that the patterns of health-care utilization are changing (Lipton et al., 2000c). Thirty-four percent of migraine sufferers had never consulted a doctor for headache, 19% had not consulted a doctor for at least 1 year (lapsed consulters), and 47% had seen a doctor for headache within the last year (current consulters). In comparison with the American Migraine Study conducted in 1989 (Stewart et al., 1992), the self-reported rates of current consultation have tripled.

Several studies have reported that certain demographic features and headache characteristics are associated with physician consultation. For example, consultation is more common among women than men and increases with increasing age (Lipton et al., 1998, 2000c). In addition, individuals with higher pain intensity, longer attacks, greater disability, and more associated symptoms are more likely to consult a doctor about their migraine (Lipton et al., 1998, 2000c).

Patients with migraine have higher overall medical consultation rates than people without migraine (Clouse and Osterhaus, 1994). To assess health-care resource use, migraine sufferers enrolled in a United Healthcare affiliated plan were reviewed. Eligible subjects were enrolled in the health plan for at least 1 year, had a medical claim for migraine, and had a pharmacy claim for a medication potentially used for migraine treatment. During an 18-month follow-up period, the consultation rates of migraine sufferers (n = 1,336) were compared with nonmigraine sufferers (n = 1,336) matched on the basis of age, sex, duration of enrollment, and subscriber or dependent status. Migraine sufferers made 2,616 visits for migraine and 19,971 visits for reasons other than migraine. In contrast, nonmigraine sufferers made a total of 13,072 visits during the same period. Interestingly, a small proportion of migraine sufferers account for the majority of physician visits. While most migraine sufferers report one to four physician visits a year, only a small proportion (7.6%) report more than 12 visits (Osterhaus et al., 1992). An important limitation of this study is the selected study population: only migraine sufferers who sought treatment and received a migraine diagnosis were included.

Emergency department (ED) use is not common among migraine sufferers. Population-based 1-year estimates of ED use were approximately 5% in men and 3% in women in a US study (Linet et al., 1989). Michel et al. (1996) reported similar 6-month ED rates among a population-based group of migraine sufferers in France. Lifetime hospitalization rates of population-based samples range from 13% to 20% (Celentano et al., 1992; Edmeads et al., 1993). Use of the ED is more common among users of prescription medication (Celentano et al., 1992). In this study, the highest rates were reported among migraine sufferers using prescription medication (women 33%, men 27%); these rates were three times higher than those of nonprescription medication users.

Hospitalization rates among headache sufferers specifically for headache are low (Stang and Osterhaus, 1993; Clouse and Osterhaus, 1994; Osterhaus et al., 1992; Michel et al., 1996). However, overall hospitalization rates among migraine sufferers are reported to be twice as high as those in a healthy population (Clouse and Osterhaus, 1994).

Lofland et al. (1998, 1999) conducted a study among migraine sufferers enrolled in a mixed-model independent practice association/managed care organization to assess changes in health-care utilization before and after treatment with sumatriptan. Subjects were identified when they filled a new prescription for sumatriptan. The study showed that treatment with sumatriptan decreases health-care utilization rates. In the 6 months before treatment with sumatriptan, 178 patients had a total of 260 migraine-related medical claims (physician office visits, ED visits, and medical procedures). However, after 6 months of sumatriptan use, migraine-related medical claims decreased by 34%, to only 172. The number of migraine claims reported in this study is probably overestimated relative to migraine sufferers in the general community since study subjects were selected based on their utilization of the health-care system.

Three studies have translated health care use into direct costs (Clouse and Osterhaus, 1994; Osterhaus et al., 1992; Hu et al., 1999). Clouse and Osterhaus (1994) estimated that the average claim per member per month was $145; however, this figure includes migraine as well as nonmigraine costs. Osterhaus et al. (1992) reported that yearly direct medical costs were $817 per migraine sufferer. This figure is probably higher than what would be found in a population-based sample of migraine sufferers; the investigators studied a sample of clinical trial participants.

In contrast to these reports, Hu et al. (1999) reported the direct costs of migraine based on a US population-based sample. In this study, the annual treatment costs of migraine were estimated to be over $1 billion, about $100 per migraine sufferer per year. Physician visits (60%) and prescription drugs (30%) accounted for the majority of treatment-related costs. Visits to the ED accounted for a small proportion of total costs (1%). Because this study was based on 1994 data, before triptan use became widespread, the results undoubtedly substantially underestimate the current direct costs.

Headache severity is directly related to direct costs (Lipton et al., 1997; Von Korff et al., 1994). Von Korff et al. (1994) assigned headache sufferers to one of four severity grades based on a composite of pain and disability (activity limitations). Grade 1 patients were defined by relatively low or moderate pain intensity without activity limitations. Grade 2 patients were defined by high pain intensity without activity limitations. Grade 3 patients were defined by moderate activity limitations. Grade 4 patients were defined by severe activity limitations. Members of a managed care organization, Group Health of Puget Sound, were classified into the four grades based on a self-administered questionnaire and then followed for 2 years. Claims data for these patients indicated that as headache severity grade increased, so did headache treatment costs (Lipton et al., 1997). Among grade 1 patients, treatment costs were $200 per patient per year. In contrast, the headache treatment costs of grade 4 patients were $800 per patient per year. The estimate for grade 4 patients approximates estimates provided by Osterhaus et al. (1992) for clinical trial participants.

Indirect Costs

While the direct costs of migraine are substantial, the indirect costs are even greater. Indirect costs include the aggregate economic effects of migraine on productivity at work, at home, and in other roles. We emphasize the substantial burden of migraine at work. Migraine sufferers may miss work because of their headaches or be less productive while at work with a headache. Studies of direct costs must measure reduced productivity as well as absenteeism. Many studies examine actual days of missed work, time at work with headache, and percent effectiveness while at work with a headache. The components are sometimes combined in an index termed lost workday equivalents (LWDEs), which equals actual days of missed work plus days at work with headache times 1 minus percent effectiveness while at work with headache (Osterhaus et al., 1992).

Productivity losses due to migraine are difficult to measure. The ideal study would include representative samples of migraine sufferers, complete case ascertainment, and objective daily measurements of productivity. Some investigations have included biased populations (Stang and Osterhaus, 1993; Osterhaus et al., 1992), which limits generalizability. Other studies in population-based samples used relatively long recall intervals (Rasmussen et al., 1992; Stewart et al., 1996b; Schwartz et al., 1997), generating reports of uncertain validity. At least two studies have been conducted in population-based samples of migraine sufferers (to maximize generalizability) using daily disability diaries to minimize recall bias (Von Korff et al., 1998; Michel et al., 1999).

Von Korff et al. (1998) estimated the number of LWDEs in a population-based sample of employed migraine sufferers who completed a daily diary for 3 months. (The daily diary was used to improve the accuracy of the work-loss data.) During the 3-month period, migraine sufferers missed an average of 1.1 days due to headache. Subjects who continued to work during a headache attack reported work effectiveness that was reduced by 41%. Migraine sufferers reported an average of three LWDEs.

In this study, the most severely affected migraine sufferers accounted for most of the work loss and reduced work performance. The most disabled 20% of the participants accounted for 77% of work-loss; 40% of subjects accounted for 75% of the LWDEs.

The lost workday and LWDE figures reported by Von Korff et al. (1998) are higher than those reported in most other population-based studies (Stang and Osterhaus, 1993; Osterhaus et al., 1992; Stewart et al., 1996b; van Roijen et al., 1995). The use of a daily diary probably improved recall and, thus, the accuracy of data collection.

Michel et al. (1999) conducted a 3-month prospective daily diary study examining work-loss data among 231 migraine sufferers and 188 nonheadache-prone control subjects. Over a 3-month period, participants used a daily diary to record the presence or absence of headache and the work situation that day (unemployment, holiday, weekend, medical reason, nonmedical reason). Absenteeism was classified into two groups: sickness-related absenteeism (i.e., number of workdays missed or interrupted for medical reasons) and headache-related absenteeism (i.e., number of workdays missed or interrupted on days with headache). In this study, migraine sufferers reported an average of 1.45 missed days due to medical reasons, 0.25 of which were due to headache. Sickness-related absenteeism was statistically higher in migraine sufferers than in control subjects. The control population, however, reported 0.96 sickness-related days, 0.07 of which were due to headache. Interestingly, in this study, the higher absenteeism was related to comorbid medical conditions, not headaches.

Since migraine sufferers avoid sick leave for headache, it is important to measure time lost due to reduced productivity while working with a headache; however, Michel et al. (1999) did not report LWDE data. The amount of lost work time due to LWDEs is significant. For example, as Von Korff et al. (1998) reported, over a 3-month period, migraine sufferers lost only 1.1 days due to headache but 3 days due to headache-related reduced productivity. Not including reduced productivity time is one weakness of the Michel et al. (1999) study and may help to explain the low missed work-time rates reported therein. Additionally, some of the variation in work-loss data may be due to cultural differences in the acceptability of medically related absences.

Both Michel et al. (1999) and Von Korff et al. (1998) studied work loss in an employed population. However, frequent headache can result in reduced labor force participation (Stang et al., 1998). Therefore, to understand migraine's impact on productivity, further research is needed on the effects of headache on labor force participation as well as reduced productivity among those in the labor force.

While several studies have estimated lost workdays and reduced effectiveness at work, only a few studies have estimated the costs associated with lost productivity. Some of these studies evaluate self-identified migraine sufferers (Stang and Osterhaus, 1993). Since disease awareness is greatest among severe sufferers, they most likely overestimated disability at the individual level. Because they excluded sufferers who did not know they had migraine, they dramatically underestimated prevalence. Osterhaus et al. (1992), derived estimates of disability from clinical-trial participants, a sample that most likely overestimates the severity of disease in the general population. Studies of more representative populations are discussed below.

Hu et al. (1999) estimated the indirect costs of migraine in a population-based sample of migraine sufferers. In this study, prevalence estimates were derived from two existing population-based databases: the American Migraine Study and the Baltimore County survey (Stewart et al., 1992, 1996a). The American Migraine Study was a national probability sample of over 20,000 individuals, while the Baltimore County survey was comprised of over 13,000 participants. The authors estimate that migraine costs American employers over $13 billion per year due to absenteeism and reduced effectiveness at work (Hu et al., 1999). Assuming that the percentage of people working for pay among migraine sufferers is the same as in the general population (i.e., 73% of men and 57% of women), lost productivity costs in this study were $690 for men and $1,127 for women.

Michel et al. (1999) reported the indirect costs of migraine in a population-based sample, but they reported much lower cost estimates. The total indirect costs reported in this study were $240 per migraine sufferer per year. This estimate is lower because the number of lost workdays reported by this population was relatively low and the investigators did not account for reduced productivity while at work. Furthermore, the scale on which the wages were calculated was not specified. However, since this was a French study, the wages may be different from those in the US studies.

Human capital studies assume that the economic value of a missed hour of work is equivalent to the wages for that hour. This methodology has several potential pitfalls. Human capital methodology overestimates the monetary impact of reduced effectiveness or absenteeism if coworkers or employees with migraine compensate for the time loss. In contrast, if costly errors are made during an attack, the wages for that time may underestimate the cost of that error. Although human capital studies account for the value of time lost by the working population, they do not assess the value of time lost by caregivers or homemakers. Since migraine prevalence peaks during the childbearing and family-caregiving years, it can have a substantial impact in family functioning when a caregiver's role is repeatedly disrupted.

TENSION-TYPE HEADACHE

Prevalence

Published estimates for the 1-year period prevalence for episodic and chronic tension-type headache (CTTH) vary widely (Table 7–1). Lifetime prevalences are higher than 1-year period prevalences. Variation in prevalence estimates may be due to differences in study methodology, including case definition as well as demographic factors, such as age of the population. Studies differ in level of diagnostic specificity; some studies group all TTH (IHS 2.0) subjects together, while others distinguish ETTH (IHS 2.1), CTTH (IHS 2.2), and headaches of the tension type that fulfill all criteria except one (IHS 2.3). These criteria are discussed in Chapter 2.

Data collection methods may also influence prevalence estimates. Methods of data collection (e.g., self-administered questionnaires, telephone interviews, and clinical examinations) as well as the quality of data collection contribute to variations in diagnostic accuracy. The source of the study population may contribute to variation in prevalence estimates. A meta-analysis might help to explain how much each of these factors contributes to the variation in prevalence among studies.

Table 7–1 Prevalence of episodic tension-type headache (ETTH) and chronic tension-type headache (CTTH) as reported in studies from well-defined populations

Author, country	Population type	Response method	Sample size	Headache type	Prevalence period	Age range (years)	Women	Men	Overall
Abu-Arefeh (UK)	Community	Mail SAQ, clinical exam	2,165	Unspecified	1 year	5 to 15			0.9
Barea (Brazil)	School survey	In-person interview, clinical exam	538	ETTH + CTTH + other TTH (2.3)	1 year	5th to 8th grade	76.7	68.3	72.3
					1 week	5th to 8th grade	35.3	16.1	25.6
					24 hours	5th to 8th grade	10.1	5.1	7.6
Castillo (Spain)	Community	SAQ, clinical exam	1,883	CTTH	1 month	18 to 89	2.0	0.2	2.2
Franceschi (Italy)	Community	In-person interview, clinical exam	312	Unspecified	Lifetime	"Elderly"	4.0	4.3	4.1
					1 year	"Eldely"	4.0	1.2	2.6
Gobel (Germany)	Community	Mail SAQ	4,061	ETTH	Lifetime	18 to 35			12.0
						36 to 55			14.0
						56			12.0
						All ages (18)	13.0	13.0	13.0
				CTTH	Lifetime	18 to 35			0.0
						36 to 55			1.0
						56			1.0
						All ages (18)			1.0
Tekle Haimanot (Ethiopia)	Community	In-person interview	15,000	CTTH	1 year	20 to 29	1.0	0.0	
						30 to 39	0.0	0.4	
						40 to 49	0.7	0.4	
						50 to 59	4.3	0.9	
						60 to 69	8.1	2.0	
						70 to 79	3.9	2.8	
						80 to 89	0.0	1.9	
						All ages (20 to 89)	1.7	0.0	
Jabbar (Saudi Arabia)	Community	In-person interview	5,891	Unspecified	Lifetime	16 to 19	2.3	0.1	1.7
						20 to 29			2.1
						30 to 39			1.8
						40 to 49			2.9
						50 to 59			3.9
						60			6.0
									6.3
						All ages (16)			3.1

Author (country)	Sample	Method	No.	Headache type	Duration	Age (years)			
Lavados (Chile)	Community	In-person interview	1,385	ETTH	1 year	15 to 29	30.5	16.5	23.7
						30 to 39	34.8	17.4	26.4
						40 to 49	33.0	21.0	27.5
						50 to 59	32.1	16.1	25.9
						60	23.2	14.3	19.6
						All ages (15)			24.3
				CTTH	1 year	15 to 29	1.6	0.8	1.2
						30 to 39	2.6	1.4	2.0
						40 to 49	7.3	0.0	3.9
						50 to 59	5.9	1.1	3.7
						60	6.2	2.6	4.8
						All ages (15)			2.6
Merikangas (Switzerland)	Community	In-person interview	379	ETTH + CTTH	1 year	28 to 29	18.0	13.5	15.8
				ETTH	1 year	28 to 29			15.3
				CTTH	1 year	28 to 29			0.5
Mitsikostas (Greece)	Monks	SAQ, clinical exam	449	ETTH	Lifetime	>50		2.0	
				CTTH	Lifetime	>50		1.3	
Pereira Monteiro (Portugal)	Medical school students	In-person SAQ	491	ETTH + CTTH	Unknown	18 to 32			16.0
				ETTH					15.5
				CTTH					0.4
Pryse-Phillips (Canada)	Community	Telephone interview	1,573	ETTH + CTTH	Unspecified	15 to 24			20.0
						25 to 34			33.0
						25 to 44			23.0
						45 to 54			12.0
						55 to 65			7.0
						>65			5.0
Rasmussen (Denmark)	Community	Clinical exam	740	ETTH	1 year	All ages (15)	64.0	36.0	
						25 to 34	93.0	68.0	81.0
						35 to 44	92.0	63.0	77.0
						45 to 54	82.0	70.0	75.0
						55 to 64	74.0	49.0	61.0
						All ages (25 to 64)	86.0	63.0	74.0
				CTTH	Lifetime	All ages (25 to 64)	88.0	69.0	78.0
					1 year	All ages (25 to 64)			3.0

Table continues on following page

Table 7–1 *Continued*

Author, country	Population type	Response method	Sample size	Headache type	Prevalence period	Age range (years)	Women	Men	Overall
Roh (South Korea)	Community	Telephone interview, mail SAQ	2,500	ETTH + CTTH + other TTH (2.3)	1 year	0 to 9			3.8
						10 to 19			29.8
						20 to 29			27.2
						30 to 39			22.2
						40 to 49			10.1
						50 to 59			4.4
						60			2.5
Schwartz (USA)	Community	Telephone interview	13,345	ETTH	1 year	All ages	14.7	17.8	16.2
						18 to 29	40.8	34.5	
						30 to 39	46.9	42.3	
						40 to 49	46.5	39.4	
						50 to 59	40.6	31.5	
						60 to 65	27.1	25.6	
						All ages (18 to 65)			38.3
				CTTH	1 year	18 to 29	2.6	1.7	
						30 to 39	2.5	1.0	
						40 to 49	2.9	1.9	
						50 to 59	4.2	1.1	
						60 to 65	2.7	1.5	
						All ages (18 to 65)			2.2
S-ikiatkhachorn (Thailand)	Old-age home	In-person interview	241	ETTH	1 year	61 to 98			16.2
				CTTH	1 year	61 to 98			2.1
Wang (China)	Community	In-person interview, clinical exam	1,533	2.1, 2.2, 2.3	1 year	65 to 69	45.0	17.0	32.0
						70 to 74	44.0	22.0	33.0
						75 to 79	47.0	20.0	37.0
						80	48.0	22.0	39.0
				ETTH	1 year	All ages (65)	46.0	20.0	35.0
				CTTH	1 year	All ages (65)			23.0
				2.3	1 year	All ages (65)			2.4
						All ages (65)			8.8
Wong (Hong Kong)	Community	Telephone interview	7,356	ETTH + CTTH + other TTH (2.3)	1 year	15 to 24	1.82	1.30	1.55
						25 to 34	2.96	1.41	2.13
						35 to 44	5.78	2.09	3.87
						45 to 54	2.33	1.24	1.75
						55 to 64	2.11	1.07	1.59
						>65	0.73	—	0.40
						All ages (15)	2.68	1.27	1.96

Key to abbreviations: SAQ, self-administered questionnaire; ETTH, episodic tension type headache; CTTH, chronic tension type headache; other TTH, TTH missing a scizlo diagnostic feature; TTH (2.3), IHS defered TTH (2.3).

Following is a summary of several major TTH studies that were conducted in representative samples and used the IHS criteria.

The first population study that examined ETTH prevalence using the IHS criteria was conducted in Denmark (Rasmussen et al., 1991a). Potential participants were identified from the Danish National Central Person Registry and invited to a general health examination, with an emphasis on headache. In this study of 740 subjects, the 1-year period prevalence of ETTH was 74.0%. Since potential subjects were invited to a health exam with an emphasis on headache, individuals who had headaches may have been more likely to participate.

There has been one large-scale population survey in the United States describing the epidemiology of IHS-defined ETTH and CTTH (Schwartz et al., 1998). Data from a telephone interview survey of 13,345 residents of Baltimore County, Maryland, were used to estimate the 1-year period prevalence of ETTH and CTTH by sex, age, education, and race. The 1-year period prevalence of ETTH was 38.3%, substantially lower than in the Danish study (Rasmussen et al., 1991b; Rasmussen, 1992).

In Santiago, Chile, Lavados and Tenhamm (1998) conducted in-person interviews in a representative sample of 1,385 adults. Subjects reported details about the type of headache that they suffered most often. The 1-year prevalence of ETTH was 24.3%. The lower prevalence in this study compared with the US study (Schwartz et al., 1998) may be explained by differences in case definition. In Santiago, only the most common type of headache was eligible for classification. In the US study, classification based on a single headache type yielded lower prevalence estimates than classification regarding all headache types.

The prevalence of CTTH is markedly lower than that of ETTH. Across studies, 1-year period prevalence estimates range from 1.7% to 2.2% (Rasmussen et al., 1991b; Lavados and Tenhamm, 1998; Schwartz et al., 1998; Tekle Haimanot et al., 1995; Castillo et al., 1999). Overall, 4% to 5% of the population report headaches 15 or more days per month (Rasmussen et al., 1991b; Lavados and Tenhamm, 1998; Schwartz et al., 1998; Tekle Haimanot et al., 1995; Castillo et al., 1999).

Prevalence by Gender and Age

The prevalence of ETTH and CTTH varies with gender and age. Tension-type headache is slightly more common among women than men. For example, in the United States, 42% of women and 36% of men have ETTH, yielding an overall gender prevalence ratio of 1.16 (Schwartz et al., 1998). The female preponderance occurs at all age, race, and educational levels. Most studies report a higher prevalence of TTH among women (Rasmussen et al., 1991b; Wong et al., 1995; Barea et al., 1996; Lavados and Tenhamm, 1998; Pryse-Phillips et al., 1992; Wang et al., 1997), with female to male gender ratios ranging from 1.16 (Schwartz et al., 1998) to 1.9 (Lavados and Tenhamm, 1998).

The female preponderance for CTTH is substantially greater than that of ETTH. For example, in the United States, the prevalence of CTTH was reported to be 2.8 in women and 1.4 in men, with an overall gender prevalence ratio of 2.0 (Schwartz et al., 1998). Other studies have also reported a female preponderance in CTTH (Lavados and Tenhamm, 1998; Tekle Haimonot et al., 1995; Castillo et al., 1999). Schwartz et al. (1998) noted that the female preponderance in CTTH falls between that of ETTH and migraine and suggested that the gender ratio may imply a biological link to migraine.

The prevalence of TTH may vary by age, although results are inconsistent across studies. Several studies show that prevalence peaks in the 30s and 40s, with a decline thereafter (Wong et al., 1995; Lavados and Tenhamm, 1998; Pryse-Phillips et al., 1992, Schwartz et al., 1998). One study suggested that prevalence decreases with age (Rasmussen et al., 1991b). Gobel et al. (1994) found no difference in prevalence by age. Their lack of association with age may be attributed to the use of very wide age intervals; in most studies, age is categorized into 10-year intervals (Rasmussen et al., 1991b; Wong et al., 1995; Lavados and Tenhamm, 1998; Pryse-

Phillips et al., 1992, Schwartz et al., 1998); the 20-year age groupings in this study may have attenuated the relationship to age.

Several authors report that the prevalence of CTTH increases with age (Lavados and Tenhamm, 1998; Schwartz et al., 1998; Tekle Haimanot et al., 1995). Some individuals may begin with ETTH; headaches may gradually increase over time until criteria for CTTH are met (Merikangas and Frances, 1993; Lange-mark et al., 1988).

Prevalence by Race and Geographic Region

Geographic and racial differences may account for part of the variation in the prevalence of TTH among studies. Studies have shown prevalence to be highest in the Western Hemisphere (Rasmussen et al., 1991b; Lavados and Tenhamm, 1998; Pryse-Phillips et al., 1992; Schwartz et al., 1998) and lowest in Asian countries (Wong et al., 1995).

A US study examined TTH prevalence by race (Schwartz et al., 1998). The prevalence of ETTH was significantly higher in Caucasians than in African-Americans in both men (40.1% vs. 22.8%) and women (46.8% vs. 30.9%). The prevalence of CTTH by race paralleled the observations for ETTH: prevalence was higher in Caucasians than in African-Americans in both men (1.6% vs. 1.0%) and women (3.0% vs. 2.2%). The explanation for these racial patterns remains undetermined.

Prevalence by Socioeconomic Status

The relationship between SES and TTH prevalence varies among studies. Schwartz et al. (1998) used educational level as a measure of SES. The prevalence of ETTH was directly related to education, peaking in individuals who had a graduate-level education (men 48.5%, women 48.9%). Similarly, Lavados and Tenhamm (1998) found a direct relation between ETTH prevalence and SES. Other studies, including a German study that used only two educational categories (i.e., basic and secondary) (Gobel et al., 1994), have not found this direct association (Pryse-Phillips et

al., 1992; Gobel et al., 1994). Perhaps their analysis lacked sensitivity because they used only two categories. The influence of SES may also vary by country. While migraine prevalence declines with SES, the prevalence of ETTH increases, at least in the United States. These discrepant epidemiologic patterns support the view that migraine and ETTH are nosologically distinct.

The relationship of SES to CTTH is different from that of SES to ETTH. Two studies reported that the prevalence of CTTH declines with increasing educational level, especially among women (Lavados and Tenhamm, 1998; Schwartz et al., 1998). Though one study found no association (Gobel et al., 1994), this pattern of an inverse relationship is similar to findings in migraine, not ETTH. Schwartz et al. (1998) point out that CTTH, with its higher risk in women and strong relationship to SES, has an epidemiologic profile intermediate between that of ETTH and migraine.

Headache Characteristics

Most subjects with ETTH (90%) report mild to moderate headache pain and attacks that typically occur three times a month (Rasmussen et al., 1991b; Lavados and Tenhamm, 1998; Schwartz et al., 1998; Gobel et al., 1994). However, CTTH is associated with higher pain intensity and more frequent attacks (Schwartz et al., 1998). In one study, 86% of subjects reported moderate or severe pain (moderate 44%, severe 42%) (Gobel et al., 1994). Using a ten-point pain scale, Schwartz et al. (1998) found that pain intensity ratings were significantly higher in subjects with CTTH than in those with ETTH (CTTH 5.55, ETTH 4.98; $p < 0.001$). By definition, CTTHs occur 15 or more days per month (Classification Committee of the International Headache Society, 1988; Schwartz et al., 1998; Gobel et al., 1994).

The clinical profile of TTH varies by gender. Bilateral pain occurs in the majority of TTH sufferers, but it occurs with greater frequency in women than men (Lavados and Tenhamm, 1998). Throbbing pain is common in men (66.4%) and women (56.8%) with

ETTH; this feature, often viewed as a hallmark of migraine, poorly discriminates the two disorders. Pressing pain is also frequently reported. Many subjects with TTH report that pain is exacerbated with movement (men 69.8%, women, 75.5%; p = 0.4), which is surprising since pain that is exacerbated by movement is normally associated with migraine rather than TTH. Photophobia or phonophobia was common, especially in women. If both features were present, a diagnosis was not possible; but each feature occurred in isolation with surprising frequency.

The proportions of subjects with CTTH and ETTH who reported lost and reduced-effectiveness days were similar: 11.8% of CTTH sufferers reported lost workdays and 46.5% reported reduced-effectiveness days (Schwartz et al., 1997). Sufferers of CTTH reported more frequent lost workdays and reduced-effectiveness days than ETTH sufferers. Subjects with lost workdays reported an average of 27.4 lost workdays per person; subjects with reduced-effectiveness days reported approximately 20.4 reduced-effectiveness days per person.

Economic Impact

The first population-based study to examine work-loss data in ETTH was reported by Rasmussen et al. (1992) in Denmark. Twelve percent of employed participants were absent from work at least once during the previous year because of ETTH. The majority of those who missed work (68%) were absent for 1 to 7 days during the previous year. Twenty-five percent were absent between 8 and 14 days during the year, and only 16% were absent more than 14 days during the previous year.

Schwartz et al. (1997, 1998) also measured the impact of headache in the workplace in a study conducted in Baltimore County, Maryland. Inability to function (actual missed work) and reduced ability to function were measured separately. Of the lost work time associated with headache, 19% of the missed workdays and 22% of the reduced-effectiveness days were specifically due to ETTH (Schwartz et al., 1997). Among subjects with ETTH, 8.3% reported missed workdays (absenteeism), while 43.6% reported reduced-effectiveness days at work due to headache. Among those with missed workdays, an average of 8.9 missed workdays were reported, while subjects with reduced-effectiveness days reported approximately 5.0 reduced-effectiveness days per person. Lavados and Tenhamam (1998) found higher levels of missed work among their sample of TTH sufferers: 25% of men and 38.9% of women reported missed work due to headaches.

CONCLUSION

Headache is a very common symptom with a broad range of causes. The 1-year period prevalence of ETTH is approximately 36% for men and 42% for women (Schwartz et al., 1998). The 1-year period prevalence of migraine is 15% to 19% in women and 6% in men (Stewart et al., 1992; Lipton and Stewart, 1993). These disorders impose a substantial burden on the individual headache sufferers, their families, and society.

Migraine sufferers report frequent, painful, and temporarily disabling attacks. Migraine sufferers experience notable decrements in HRQoL that are not accounted for by comorbid depression and are equivalent to those of asthma. In addition, Hu et al. (1999) conservatively estimated that the annual direct costs for migraine were over $1 billion per year in the United States and that migraine costs American employers $13 billion per year due to absenteeism and reduced effectiveness at work.

In comparison with migraine, ETTH has a modest impact on the individual sufferer. It is generally less painful than migraine and less likely to impose activity limitations (Schwartz et al., 1997, 1998). However, the aggregate societal impact is large because the disorder is highly prevalent. The individual impact of CTTH is greater than that of ETTH, but the disorder is less common. Frequent primary headaches impose an enormous burden.

Measuring the burden of migraine and TTH helps to define the opportunity provided by effective treatment. Barriers to care occur at the levels of consultation, initial diagnosis, treatment, and follow-up.

REFERENCES

Abu-Arefeh, I. and G. Russell (1994). Prevalence of headache and migraine in schoolchildren. *BMJ* 309:765–769.

Adelman, J., M. Sharfman, R. Johnson et al. (1996). Impact of oral sumatriptan on workplace productivity, health-related quality of life, healthcare use, and patient satisfaction with medication in nurses with migraine. *Am. J. Managed Care* 2:1407–1416.

Barea, L., M. Tannhauser, and N. Rotta (1996). An epidemiologic study of headache among children and adolescents of southern Brazil. *Cephalalgia* 16:545–549.

Block, G., J. Goldstein, A. Polis et al. (1998). Efficacy and safety of rizatriptan versus standard care during long-term treatment for migraine. *Headache* 38:764–771.

Breslau, N., H. Chilcoat, and P. Andreski (1996). Further evidence on the link between migraine and neuroticism. *Neurology* 47:663–667.

Brown, N., L. Rips, and S. Shevell (1985). The subjective dates of natural events in very long-term memory. *Cognit. Psychol.* 17:139–177.

Castillo, J., P. Munoz, V. Guitera et al. (1999). Epidemiology of chronic daily headache in the general population. *Headache* 39:190–196.

Celentano, D., W. Stewart, R. Lipton et al. (1992). Medication use and disability among migraineurs: A national probability sample survey. *Headache* 32:223–228.

Celentano, D.D., W.F. Stewart, and M.S. Linet (1990). The relationship of headache symptoms with severity and duration of attacks. *J. Clin. Epidemiol.* 43:983.

Classification Committee of the International Headache Society. (1988). Classification and diagnostic criteria for headache disorders, cranial neuralgias and facial pain. *Cephalalgia* 8(Suppl. 7):1–96.

Clouse, J. and J. Osterhaus (1994). Healthcare resource use and costs associated with migraine in a managed healthcare setting. *Ann. Pharmacother.* 28:659–664.

Cohen, J., D. Beall, D. W. Miller et al. (1996). Subcutaneous sumatriptan for the treatment of migraine: humanistic, economic, and clinical consequences. *Fam. Med.* 28:171–177.

Cummings, R., J. Kelsey, and M. Nevitt (1990). Methodologic issues in the study of frequent and recurrent health problems. *Ann. Epidemiol.* 1:49–56.

Dahlof, C. and E. Dimenas (1995). Migraine patients experience poorer subjective well-being/quality of life even between attacks. *Cephalalgia* 15:31–36.

Damiano, A. (1996). The sickness impact profile. In *Quality of Life and Pharmacoeconomics in Clinical Research* (B. Spilker, ed.), pp. 347–354. Lippincott-Raven, Philadelphia.

Edmeads, J., H. Findlay, P. Tugwell et al. (1993). Impact of migraine and tension-type headache on life-style, consulting behavior, and medication use: A Canadian population survey. *Can. J. Neurol. Sci.* 20:131–137.

Featherstone, H.J. (1985). Migraine and muscle contraction headaches: A continuum. *Headache* 24:194.

Friedman, A.P., K.H. Finley, and J.R. Graham (1962). Classification of headache. *Arch. Neurol.* 6:173.

Gobel, H., M. Petersen-Braun, and D. Soyka (1994). The epidemiology of headache in Germany: A nationwide survey of a representative sample on the basis of the headache classification of the International Headache Society. *Cephalalgia* 14:97–106.

Granella, E., R. D'Alessandro, and G.C. Manzoni et al. (1994). International Headache Society classification: Interobserver reliability in the diagnosis of primary headaches. *Cephalalgia* 14:16.

Gross, M., A. Dowson, L. Deavy et al. (1996). Impact of oral sumatriptan 50 mg in work productivity and quality of life in migraineurs. *Br. J. Med. Econ.* 19:231–246.

Hartmaier, S., N. Santanello, R.S. Epstein et al. (1995). Development of a brief 24-hour migraine specific quality of life questionnaire. *Headache* 35:320–329.

Hu, X., L. Markson, R.B. Lipton et al. (1999). Disability and economic costs of migraine in the United States: A population-based approach. *Arch. Intern. Med.* 159:813–818.

Hurst, B., U. Macclesfield et al. (1998). Assessing outcomes of treatment for migraine headache using generic and specific measures. *Neurology* 50(Suppl. 4):A180–A181.

Jacobson, G., N. Ramadan, S.K. Aggarwal et al. (1994). The Henry Ford Hospital Headache Disability Inventory (HDI). *Neurology* 44:837–842.

Jhingran, P., R. Cady, J. Rubino et al. (1996). Improvements in health-related quality of life with sumatriptan treatment for migraine. *J. Fam. Pract.* 42:36–42.

Kryst, S. and E. Scherl (1994). A population-based survey of the social and personal impact of migraine. *Headache* 34:344–350.

Langemark, M., J. Olesen, D. Poulsen et al. (1988). Clinical characterization of patients with chronic tension headache. *Headache* 28:590–596.

Lavados, P. and E. Tenhamm (1998). Epidemiology of tension-type headache in Santiago, Chile: A prevalence study. *Cephalalgia* 18:552–558.

Linet, M.S. and W.F. Stewart (1984). Migraine headache: Epidemiologic perspectives. *Epidemiol. Rev.* 6:107.

Linet, M.S., W.F. Stewart, D.D. Celentano et al. (1989). An epidemiologic study of headache among adolescents and young adults. *JAMA* 261:2211.

Lipton, R.B., J.C. Amatniek, M.D. Ferrari et al. (1994). Migraine: identifying and removing barriers to care. *Neurology* 44(Suppl. 6):56.

Lipton, R.B., P.J. Goadsby, J.P.C. Sawyer et al. (2000a). Migraine: Diagnosis and assessment of disability. *Rev. Contemp. Pharmacother.* 11:63–73.

Lipton, R.B., S. Hamelsky, K.B. Kolodner et al. (2000b). Migraine, quality of life, and depression: A population-based case-control study. *Neurology* 55:629–635.

Lipton, R.B., J. Liberman, K. Kolodner et al. (1999). Migraine headache disability and quality-of-life: A population-based case-control study. *Headache* 39:365.

Lipton, R.B., A.I. Scher, W.F. Stewart et al. (2000c). Patterns of healthcare utilization for migraine: A comparative study in the United States and United Kingdom.

Lipton, R.B. and S.D. Silberstein (1994). Why study the comorbidity of migraine? *Neurology* 44(Suppl. 7):4–5.

Lipton, R.B. and W.F. Stewart (1993). Migraine in the United States: A review of epidemiology and health care use. *Neurology* 43(Suppl. 3): S6–S10.

Lipton, R.B., W.F. Stewart, R.K. Cady et al. (2000d). Sumatriptan effectively treats the full spectrum of headaches in migraineurs: Results from the Spectrum Study. *Headache* 40:783–791.

Lipton, R., W. Stewart, D. Celentano et al. (1992). Undiagnosed migraine headaches: A comparison of symptom-based and reported physician diagnosis. *Arch. Intern. Med.* 152:1273–1278.

Lipton, R.B., W.F. Stewart, and K. Merikangas (1993). Reliability in headache diagnosis. *Cephalalgia* 13(Suppl. 12):29.

Lipton, R., W. Stewart, and D. Simon (1998). Medical consultation for migraine: Results of the American Migraine Study. *Headache* 38:87–90.

Lipton, R.B., W.F. Stewart, A.M. Stone et al. (2000e). Stratified care is more effective than step care strategies for migraine: Results of the Disability in Strategies of Care (DISC) study. *JAMA* 284:2599–2605.

Lipton, R.B., W.F. Stewart, and M. Von Korff (1997). Burden of migraine: Societal costs and therapeutic opportunities. *Neurology* 48(Suppl. 3):S4–S9.

Lofland, J., N. Johnson, D. Nash et al. (1998). Improvements in managed care patients' health-related quality of life after sumatriptan (Imitrex). *Headache* 38:391.

Lofland, J.H., N.E. Johnson, A.S. Batenhorst et al. (1999). Changes in resource use and outcomes for patients with migraine treated with sumatriptan. *Arch. Intern. Med.* 159:857–863.

Mathew, N.T. (1993). Transformed migraine. *Cephalalgia* 13(Suppl. 2):78.

McEwen, J. and S. McKenna (1996). Nottingham Health Profile. In *Quality of Life and Pharmacoeconomics in Clinical Research* (B. Spilker, ed.), pp. 281–286. Lippincott-Raven, Philadelphia.

McHorney, C., J. Ware, and A.E. Raczek (1993). The MOS 36-item short form health survey (SF-36): II. Psychometric and clinical tests of validity in measuring physical and mental health constructs. *Med. Care* 31:247–263.

Merikangas, K.R. and A. Frances (1993). Development of diagnostic criteria for headache syndromes: Lessons from psychiatry. *Cephalalgia* 13(Suppl. 12):34.

Merikangas, K.R., A.E. Whitaker, and J. Angst (1993). Validation of diagnostic criteria for migraine in the Zurich Longitudinal Cohort Study. *Cephalalgia* 13(Suppl. 12):47.

Metsahonkala, L. and M. Sillanpaa (1994). Migraine in children: An evaluation of the IHS criteria. *Cephalalgia* 14:285.

Michel, P., J. Dartigues, G. Duru et al. (1999). Incremental absenteeism due to headache in migraine: Results from the Mig-Access French National Cohort. *Cephalalgia* 19:503–510.

Michel, P., P. Pariente, G. Duru et al. (1996). MIG ACCESS: A population-based, nationwide, comparative survey of access to care in migraine in France. *Cephalalgia* 16:50–55.

Mortimer, J., J. Kay, and A. Jaron (1992). Epidemiology of headache and childhood migraine in an urban general practice using ad hoc, Vahlquist, and IHS criteria. *Dev. Med. Child. Neurol.* 34:1095.

Mushet, G., D. Miller, B. Clements et al. (1996). Impact of sumatriptan on workplace productivity, nonwork activities, and health-related quality of life among hospital employees with migraine. *Headache* 36:137–143.

O'Brien, B., R. Goeree, and D. Steiner (1994). Prevalence of migraine headache in Canada: A population-based survey. *Int. J. Epidemiol.* 23:1020–1026.

Osterhaus, J.T., D.L. Gutterman, and J.R. Plachetka (1992). Healthcare resource and lost labour costs of migraine headache in the US. *Pharmacoeconomics* 1:67–76.

Osterhaus, J., R. Townsend, B. Gandek et al. (1994). Measuring functional status and well-being of patients with migraine headache. *Headache* 34:337–343.

Pryse-Phillips, W., H. Findlay, P. Tugwell et al. (1992). A Canadian population survey on the clinical, epidemiologic and societal impact of migraine and tension-type headache. *Can. J. Neurol. Sci. 19*:333–339.

Raskin, N.H. (1988). *Headache*, 2nd ed. Churchill Livingstone, New York.

Rasmussen, B. (1992). Migraine and tension-type headache in a general population: Psychosocial factors. *Int. J. Epidemiol. 21*:1138–1143.

Rasmussen, B. (1995). Epidemiology of headache. *Cephalalgia 15*:45–68.

Rasmussen, B., R. Jensen, and J. Olesen (1991a). A population-based analysis of the diagnostic criteria of the International Headache Society. *Cephalalgia 11*:129.

Rasmussen, B., R. Jensen, and J. Olesen (1992). Impact of headache on sickness absence and utilisation of medical services: A Danish population study. *J. Epidemiol. Community Health 46*:443–446.

Rasmussen, B., R. Jensen, M. Schroll et al. (1991b). Epidemiology of headache in a general population: A prevalence study. *J. Clin. Epidemiol. 44*:1147–1157.

Sandrini, G., G.C. Manzoni, C. Zanferrari et al. (1993). An epidemiologic approach to nosography of chronic daily headache. *Cephalalgia 13*(Suppl. 12):72.

Santanello, N., S. Hartmaier et al. (1995). Validation of a new quality of life questionnaire for acute migraine headache. *Headache 35*:330–337.

Santanello, N., A. Polis et al. (1997). Improvement in migraine-specific quality of life in a clinical trial of rizatriptan. *Cephalalgia 17*:867–872.

Scher, A.I., W.F. Stewart, and R.B. Lipton (1999). Migraine and headache: A meta-analytic approach. In *Epidemiology of Pain* (I. Crombie, ed.), pp. 159–170. IASP Press, Seattle.

Schoenen, J. and J. Sawyer (1997). Zolmitriptan (Zomig, 311C90), a novel dual central and peripheral 5HT1B/1D agonist: An overview of efficacy. *Cephalalgia 17*(Suppl. 18):28–40.

Schwartz, B.S., W.F. Stewart, and R.B. Lipton (1997). Lost workdays and decreased work effectiveness associated with headache in the workplace. *J. Occup. Environ. Med. 39*:320–327.

Schwartz, B.S., W.F. Stewart, D. Simon et al. (1998). Epidemiology of tension-type headache. *JAMA 279*:381–383.

Silberstein, S., R. Lipton, and P. Goadsby (1998). *Headache in Clinical Practice*. Isis Medical Media, Oxford.

Silberstein, S.D., R.B. Lipton, S. Solomon et al. (1994). Transformed migraine: Proposed criteria. *Headache 34*:1.

Solomon, G., F. Skobieranda, and L. Gragg (1993). Quality of life and well-being of headache patients: Measurement by the Medical

Outcomes Study instrument. *Headache 33*:351–358.

Solomon, S., R.B. Lipton, and L.C. Newman (1992). Evaluation of chronic daily headache: Comparison to criteria for chronic tension-type headache. *Cephalalgia 12*:365.

Stang, P. and J. Osterhaus (1993). Impact of migraine in the United States: Data from the National Health Interview Survey. *Headache 33*: 29–35.

Stang, P., M. Von Korff, and B.S. Galer (1998). Reduced labor force participation among primary care patients with headache. *J. Gen. Intern. Med. 13*:296–302.

Stang P., T. Yanagihara, J. Swanson et al. (1992). Incidence of migraine headache: A population-based study in Olmstead County, Minnesota. *Neurology 42*:1657–1662.

Steiner, T. (1998). Please don't hijack "quality of life". *Cephalalgia 18*:227–228.

Stewart, A., R. Hays et al. (1988). The MOS Short Form General Health Survey: Reliability and validity in a patient population. *Med. Care 26*: 724–735.

Stewart, W.F., M. Linet, D. Celentano et al. (1991). Age- and sex-specific incidence rates of migraine with and without visual aura. *Am. J. Epidemiol. 134*:1111–1120.

Stewart, W.F., R.B. Lipton, D.D. Celentano et al. (1992). Prevalence of migraine headache in the United States: Relation to age, income, race, and other sociodemographic factors. *JAMA 267*: 64–69.

Stewart, W.F., R.B. Lipton, K. Kolodner et al. (1999). Reliability of the Migraine Disability Assessment (MIDAS) score in a population based sample of headache sufferers. *Cephalalgia 19*: 107–114.

Stewart, W.F., R.B. Lipton, K.B. Kolodner et al. (2000). Validity of the Migraine Disability Assessment (MIDAS) score in comparison to a diary-based measure in a population sample of migraine sufferers. *Pain 88*(1):41–52.

Stewart, W.F., R.B. Lipton, and J. Liberman (1996a). Variation in migraine prevalence by race. *Neurology 16*:231–238.

Stewart, W.F., R.B. Lipton, and D. Simon (1996b). Work-related disability: Results from the American Migraine Study. *Cephalalgia 16*:231–238.

Stewart, W.F., A. Schechter, and R.B. Lipton (1994). Migraine heterogeneity: Disability, pain intensity, and attack frequency and duration. *Neurology 44*(Suppl. 4):S24–S39.

Stewart, W.F., D. Simon, A. Schechter et al. (1995). Population variation in migraine prevalence: A meta-analysis. *J. Clin. Epidemiol. 48*: 269–280.

Tarlov, A., J. Ware, S. Greenfield et al. (1989). The Medical Outcomes Study: An application of methods for monitoring the results of medical care. *JAMA 262*:925–930.

Tekle Haimanot, R., B. Seraw, L. Forsgren et al. (1995). Migraine, chronic tension-type headache, and cluster headache in an Ethiopian rural community. *Cephalalgia* 15:482–488.

Terwindt, G., L. Launer, and M. Ferrari (2000). The impact of migraine on quality of life in the general population: The GEM study. *Neurology* 55:624–629.

Van Roijen, L., M. Essink-Bot, M. Koopmanschap et al. (1995). Societal perspective on the burden of migraine in the Netherlands. *Pharmacoeconomics* 7:170–179.

Von Korff, M., W.F. Stewart et al. (1994). Assessing headache severity: New directions. *Neurology* 44(Suppl. 4):40–46.

Von Korff, M., W.F. Stewart, D.S. Simon et al. (1998). Migraine and reduced work performance: A population-based diary study. *Neurology* 50:1741–1745.

Wagner, T., D. Patrick et al. (1996). A new instrument to assess the long-term quality of life effects from migraine: Development and psychometric testing of the MSQOL. *Headache* 36:484–492.

Wang, S., H. Liu, J. Fuh et al. (1997). Prevalence of headaches in a Chinese elderly population in Kinmen: Age and gender effect and cross-cultural comparisons. *Neurology* 49:195–200.

Ware, J., M. Kosinski et al. (1996). A 12-item short form health survey: construction of scales and preliminary tests of reliability and validity. *Med. Care* 34:220–233.

Waters, W.E. (1986). *Headache*. (Series in Clinical Epidemiology). PSG Publishing Company, Littleton, Massachusetts.

Wong, T., K. Wong, T. Yu et al. (1995). Prevalence of migraine and other headaches in Hong Kong. *Neuroepidemiology* 14:82–91.

8

Migraine Comorbidity

AARON L. SHECHTER
RICHARD B. LIPTON
STEPHEN D. SILBERSTEIN

Migraine is associated with a number of neurologic and psychiatric disorders, including stroke, epilepsy, depression, and anxiety disorders. Feinstein (1970) coined the term "comorbidity," which now refers to a greater than coincidental association of two conditions in the same individual (Lipton and Silberstein, 1994). Possible explanations for comorbidity include the following: (1) shared environmental or genetic risk factors; (2) one condition causing the other; and (3) the random co-occurrence of the two disorders. The nonrandom co-occurrence of two conditions may be attributable to methodologic artifacts, including *sampling bias*, in which samples are from clinical populations that are not representative of disease in the general population, and *assessment bias*, in which the co-occurrence of the two conditions is an artifact of overlapping diagnostic criteria and lack of an appropriate comparison group to control for factors that may confound the association.

Understanding the comorbidity of migraine is important from both clinical and research perspectives (Lipton and Silberstein, 1994). Comorbidity has implications for headache diagnosis. Migraine has substantial symptomatic overlap with several of the conditions comorbid with it. For example, both migraine and epilepsy can cause transient alterations of consciousness as well as headache. This problem of differential diagnosis is well recognized. Less well recognized is the problem of concomitant diagnosis. For conditions that are comorbid with migraine, the presence of migraine should increase, not reduce, the index of diagnostic suspicion. Comorbidity also has important implications for treatment. Comorbid conditions may impose therapeutic limitations but may also create therapeutic opportunities. For example, when migraine and depression occur together, an antidepressant may successfully treat both. Antiepileptic agents, such as divalproex sodium, gabapentin, and topiramate, may prevent attacks of both migraine and epilepsy. Additionally, the study of comorbidity may provide epidemiologic clues to the fundamental mechanisms of migraine.

Many studies of comorbidity have methodologic limitations. Studies of comorbidity require reliable and valid definitions and systematic ascertainment of the conditions being studied. Some studies conducted prior to the introduction of the International Headache Society (IHS) diagnostic criteria for migraine (Headache Classification Committee of the International Headache Society, 1988) used idiosyncratic definitions of migraine (i.e., frequent headache, classical migraine with neurologic prodromes). Clinic-based studies often used thorough clinical evaluations, but selection or ascertainment bias may have influenced measures of comorbidity. Epidemiologic studies often rely on systematic screening of large populations. These studies generally use validated methods to ascertain case status, which are less labor-intensive than clinic-based evaluations. We believe that definitive comorbidity studies must be conducted in population samples to avoid the influence of selection or ascertainment bias. In this chapter, we consider the conditions whose comorbidity with migraine is supported by population studies: stroke, epilepsy, psychiatric disease, and Raynaud's syndrome. We also briefly review the evidence linking migraine and essential tremor.

MIGRAINE AND STROKE

Both migraine and stroke are chronic neurologic disorders associated with focal neurologic deficits, alterations in cerebral blood flow, and headache. The relationships between migraine and stroke are complex. Headaches have been associated with stroke as ictal, preictal, or postictal phenomena (Welch, 1994). The association between migraine and stroke is strongest for migraine with aura and for stroke within the posterior circulation (Tatemichi and Mohr, 1986; Bougousslavsky and Reglli, 1987; Rothrock et al., 1993). Migraine aura, if sufficiently prolonged, may give rise to stroke, a condition that is termed "true migrainous infarction" (Headache Classification Committee of the International Headache Society, 1988; Welch, 1994).

A number of hospital case series have estimated the proportion of strokes attributable to migraine using case-by-case clinical review. In adult patients under 50 years of age, 1% to 17% of strokes have been attributed to migraine (Welch, 1994; Alvarez et al., 1989; Tatemichi and Mohr, 1986). Bougousslavsky et al. (1987) reported that if stroke occurred during a migraine attack, only 9% of patients had an arterial lesion; if the stroke was remote from the migraine attack, 91% had an arterial lesion. Mechanisms other than tradi-

tional arterial disease may underlie migrainous infarction.

A number of case-control studies have examined migraine as a risk factor for stroke. The Collaborative Group for the Study of Stroke in Young Women (1975) compared hospitalized stroke patients with both hospital-based and community controls. There was a twofold increase in the risk of stroke for women with migraine when compared with community controls but not hospital controls (Collaborative Group for the Study of Stroke in Young Women, 1975). Henrich and Horowitz (1989) found an association between migraine and stroke in a hospital-based case-control study, but differences disappeared after adjusting for stroke risk factors.

In case-control studies of young women, patients with stroke were compared to patients without stroke. Four of these studies were hospital-based, with the number of cases varying from 20 to 146 (Batista et al., 1989; Brody and Kadowitz, 1974; Ettinger et al., 1996; Welch et al., 1976). All of the studies showed increased risk of ischemic stroke in migraine patients, with odds ratios (ORs) ranging from 1.9 to 4.3. Tzourio et al. (1993, 1995) reported that migraine was associated with a fourfold increased risk of stroke in women under 45 years of age, with an even greater risk in women who smoked. There was a greater risk among women under 45 years of age who reported a history of migraine with aura. In none of these epidemiologic studies, however, were details available regarding attack, the cause of stroke, or whether the stroke was induced by the migraine attack characteristics. In the largest study, 497 cases were recruited from Danish population-based registries in which all hospitalized cases are registered. Controls were also selected through a national register, and the participation rate was high for both cases and controls (85% and 88%, respectively) (Lindegaard, 1995).

In a longitudinal study, Henrich et al. (1986) estimated that the incidence of cerebral "migrainous infarction" was 3.36/100,000; when subjects with other stroke risk factors were excluded, the estimate decreased to 1.44/100,000. To place this in context, the overall rates of ischemic stroke in the general population under 50 years of age range from 6.5/100,000 to 22.8/100,000 (Kittner et al., 1993). To interpret these data, one must estimate the relative risk (RR) in migraine populations, with and without aura, stratified by migraine type (with and without aura) and adjust for potential confounders.

The association between migraine and hemorrhagic stroke has not been extensively studied. Whereas the Collaborative Group for the Study of Stroke in Young Women (1975) found that migraine was similarly associated with both ischemic and hemorrhagic stroke in the recent European World Health Organization, no association [OR, 1.10, 95% confidence interval (CI) 0.63–1.94] with migraine was found (Chang et al., 1999). In the pooled analysis of data from two recent US population-based case-control studies conducted by Kaiser Permanente and the University of Washington, the crude OR was 1.45 (95% CI 1.01–2.08). In all three reports, most hemorrhagic stroke cases were subarachnoid hemorrhage (Tzourio et al., 2000).

To better understand the relationship between migraine and stroke, Welch (1994) proposed a classification system that recognizes four types of relationship between migraine and stroke: coexistent stroke and migraine, stroke with clinical features of migraine, migraine-induced stroke, and uncertain classification.

For stroke and migraine to be coexistent, "a clearly defined stroke syndrome must occur remotely in time from a typical migraine attack" (Welch, 1994). It may not be possible to establish the presence or absence of a causal relationship in an individual case. At least some cases may be coincidentally related. Some cases may be linked by underlying risk factors, such as mitral valve prolapse (Gamberini et al., 1984).

In stroke with clinical features of migraine, Welch (1994) indicates that "a structural lesion that is unrelated to migraine pathogenesis presents with clinical features of a migraine attack." He identifies two subtypes: symptomatic and migraine mimics. In the symptomatic group, an established structural disease causes episodes typical of migraine with aura, an example of which is an arteriovenous malformation that masquerades as migraine. For migraine mimic, stroke is accompanied by headache and other neurologic symptoms and signs that resemble migraine.

In migraine-induced stroke, the neurologic deficit of the stroke must be identical to the neurologic symptoms of prior migraine attacks. In addition, the stroke must occur in the course of a typical migraine attack, and other causes of stroke must be excluded.

When classification is uncertain, migraine and stroke appear to be related, but causal attribution is difficult. For example, a patient may have a typical migraine with aura, take a vasoactive drug such as ergotamine, and then have a cerebral infarction. When this rare sequence occurs, it is not clear if the stroke is a consequence of the migraine itself, of the treatment, or of an interaction between the two factors. To clarify the causal mechanisms, one would need to compare the rates of stroke that occur in close proximity to migraine with aura with and without vasoactive treatment. Migraine-like headaches and stroke may be associated with systemic vasculitis, antiphospholipid antibody syndrome, mitochondrial encepholopathies, and oral contraceptive use. Classifying stroke and migraine in these settings is difficult.

The overall pattern of results is consistent as all studies found an association between migraine and ischemic stroke in women under 45 years of age. However, all of the studies are observational; therefore, the association could be an artifact of some potential bias related to study design. These biases may include patient selection, diagnosis of stroke or migraine, recall bias, or other confounding variables, such as smoking or oral contraceptive use.

MIGRAINE AND EPILEPSY

Migraine and epilepsy are comorbid. Andermann and Andermann (1987) reported a median epilepsy prevalence of 5.9% (range 1% to 17%) in migraineurs, which greatly exceeds the population prevalence of 0.5% (Hauser et al., 1991). The reported migraine prevalence in epileptics ranges from 8% to 23% (Olesen, 1993). Methodologic problems make these studies difficult to interpret (Olesen, 1993).

The comorbidity of migraine and epilepsy was studied using Columbia University's Epilepsy Family Study (Ottman and Lipton, 1994, 1996; Lipton et al., 1994). Among subjects with epilepsy (probands), the prevalence of a migraine history was 24%. Among relatives with epilepsy, 26% had a history of migraine. In control relatives without epilepsy, the prevalence of a migraine history was 15%. The relative risk of migraine in persons with epilepsy was 2.4, for both probands and their epileptic relatives. Migraine risk was not related to age at epilepsy onset (partial vs. generalized) but was highest in post-traumatic epileptics (RR = 4.1).

Using reconstructed cohort methods, migraine risk is elevated both before and after seizure onset; therefore, it cannot be accounted for solely as a cause or solely as a consequence of epilepsy (Ottman and Lipton, 1994, 1996; Lipton et al., 1994). Because migraine risk is particularly elevated in post-traumatic epileptics and head injury is also a risk factor for both disorders, shared environmental risk factors may contribute to their comorbidity (Shechter et al., 1990; Annergers et al., 1980). However, known environmental risk factors cannot fully account for this comorbidity because migraine risk is also elevated in individuals with idiopathic epilepsy. Shared genetic risk factors cannot completely account for comorbidity as migraine risk is elevated in probands with and without a positive family history of epilepsy.

Perhaps an altered brain state increases the risk of both migraine and epilepsy and, thus, accounts for the comorbidity of these disorders (Welch, 1994; Hauser et al., 1991). Genetic or environmental risk factors may increase neuronal excitability or decrease the threshold to both types of attack. A reduction in brain magnesium (Welch et al., 1991) or alterations in neurotransmitters provide plausible potential substrates for this alteration in neuronal excitability (Welch, 1987; Welch et al., 1991; Olesen, 1993).

The association between migraine and epilepsy has implications for clinical practice.

When treating patients for one disorder, it is important to maintain a heightened index of suspicion for the other disorder. Differentiating migraine and epilepsy can be difficult (Andermann and Andermann, 1987; Marks and Ehrenberg, 1993) as both conditions are characterized by episodes of neurologic dysfunction. Headache without other neurologic features is rare as a manifestation of epilepsy. The most difficult diagnostic issue is differentiating migraine with aura from partial complex seizure. If the aura is brief (less than 5 minutes) and associated with alteration of consciousness, automatisms, and other positive motor features (tonic–clonic movements), epilepsy is more likely. If the aura is of long duration (more than 5 minutes) and has a mix of positive (scintillations, tingling) and negative (visual loss, numbness) features, migraine is more likely.

Treatment strategies for patients with comorbid migraine and epilepsy should be governed by the presence of comorbid disease. For example, drugs that lower seizure threshold should be used cautiously. Examples of such drugs include tricyclic antidepressants, selective serotonin reuptake inhibitors, and neuroleptics. However, it is sometimes advantageous to treat both migraine and epilepsy with a single drug, such as divalproex sodium (Jensen et al., 1994), gabapentin, or topiramate.

MIGRAINE AND PSYCHIATRIC DISEASE

Headache and psychiatric disorders have many links and parallels in their classification, diagnosis, comorbidity, mechanisms, and treatment. Silberstein et al. (1995) reviewed a number of studies that examined the relationship of migraine to specific psychiatric disorders. Several clinic-based studies have reported an increased prevalence of migraine in patients with major depression and an increased prevalence of major depression in patients with migraine (Marchesi et al., 1989; Merikangas et al., 1988; Morrison and Price, 1989). Three population-based studies have examined a wide range of psychiatric disorders in addition to major depression (Breslau et al., 1991; Merikangas, 1990, 1993; Stewart et al., 1989, 1992).

Merikangas et al. (1990) reported on the association of migraine with specific psychiatric disorders in a random sample of 457 adults between 27 and 28 years of age in Zurich, Switzerland. Persons with migraine (n = 61) were found to have increased 1-year rates of affective and anxiety disorders. Specifically, the OR for major depression (OR = 2.2, 95% CI 1.1–4.8), bipolar spectrum disorders (OR = 2.9, 95% CI 1.1–8.6), generalized anxiety disorder (OR = 2.7, 95% CI 1.5–5.1), panic disorder (OR = 3.3, 95% CI 0.8–13.8), simple phobia (OR = 2.4, 95% CI 1.1–5.1), and social phobia (OR = 3.4, 95% CI 1.1–10.9) were significantly higher in persons with migraine than in persons without migraine.

Migraine with major depression is frequently complicated by an anxiety disorder. In persons with all three disorders, Merikangas et al. (1990) suggest that the onset of anxiety generally precedes the onset of migraine, whereas the onset of major depression usually follows the onset of migraine (Silberstein et al., 1995).

Stewart et al. (1989) studied the relationship of migraine to panic disorder and panic attacks in a population-based telephone interview survey of 10,000 residents of Washington County, Maryland, who were between the ages of 12 and 29. The highest rates of migraine headaches occurring in the preceding week were reported by men and women with a history of panic disorder. The RR of migraine headache occurring during the previous week and associated with a history of panic disorder was 6.96 in men and 3.70 in women.

In a follow-up analysis of the same sample, Stewart et al. (1992) found that 14.2% of women and 5.8% of men who had experienced headache in the previous 12 months had consulted a physician for the problem. An unexpectedly high proportion of those who had consulted a physician for headache had a history of panic disorder. Of those who had recently seen a physician, 15% of women and 12.8% of men between 24 and 29 years of age had a panic disorder. This suggests that

comorbid psychiatric disease is associated with seeking care for headache disorders.

Breslau et al. (1991) studied the association of IHS-defined migraine with specific psychiatric disorders in a sample of 1,007 young adults between 21 and 30 years of age in southeast Michigan. Persons with a history of migraine (n = 128) had significantly higher lifetime rates of affective disorder, anxiety disorder, illicit drug disorder, and nicotine dependence. Sex-adjusted ORs were 4.5 (95% CI 3.0–6.9) for major depression, 6.0 (95% CI 2.0–18.0) for manic episode, 3.2 (95% CI 2.2–4.6) for any anxiety disorder, and 6.6 (95% CI 3.2–13.9) for panic disorder (Breslau and Davis, 1993). The psychiatric comorbidity odds associated with migraine with aura were generally higher than those associated with migraine without aura (Breslau et al., 1991). Migraine with aura was associated with an increased lifetime prevalence of both suicidal ideation and suicide attempts, after controlling for the factors of sex, major depression, and other concurring psychiatric disorders (Breslau, 1992).

Using follow-up data gathered 3.5 years after baseline, Breslau et al. (1994a) reported on the prospective relationship between migraine and major depression in a cohort of young adults. The RR for the first onset of major depression during the follow-up period in persons with prior migraine vs. those with no prior migraine was 4.1 (95% CI 2.2–7.4). The RR for the first onset of migraine during the follow-up period in persons with prior major depression vs. those with no history of major depression was 3.3 (95% CI 1.6–6.6).

In summary, recent epidemiologic studies support the association between migraine and major depression previously reported in clinic-based studies. The prospective data indicate that the observed cross-sectional or lifetime association between migraine and major depression could result from a bidirectional influence, from migraine to subsequent onset of major depression and from major depression to first migraine attack. Furthermore, these epidemiologic studies indicate that persons with migraine have increased prevalence of bipolar disorder, panic disorder, and one or more anxiety disorders (Silberstein et al., 1995; Breslau and Davis, 1992; Breslau et al., 1994a,b).

Major depression in persons with migraine might represent a psychologic reaction to repeated, disabling migraine attacks. Migraine has an earlier mean age at onset than major depression, both in the general population and in persons with comorbid disease. Nonetheless, the bidirectional influence of each condition on the risk for the onset of the other is incompatible with the simple causal model (Breslau et al., 1994a,b, 2000). Furthermore, Breslau and Davis (1992) reported that the increased risk for a first episode of major depression (and/or panic disorder) did not vary by the proximity of migraine attacks. These findings lessen the plausibility that the migraine–depression association results from the demoralizing experience of recurrent and disabling headaches, suggesting instead that their association might reflect shared etiologies.

Breslau et al. (2000) examined the migraine–depression comorbidity in a large-scale epidemiologic study, the Detroit Area Study of Headache. The study comprised three groups: persons with migraine (n = 536), persons with other severe headaches of comparable pain severity and disability (n = 162), and matched controls with no history of severe headache (n = 586). These three representative samples of the population were identified by a random-digit dialing telephone survey of 4,765 persons 25 to 55 years of age. The lifetime prevalence of major depression was 40.7% in persons with migraine, 35.8% in those with other severe headaches, and 16.0% in controls. Sex-adjusted ORs in the two headache groups, relative to controls, were approximately of the same magnitude, 3.5 and 3.2. However, examination of the bidirectional relationship between major depression and each headache type yielded different results. A bidirectional relationship was observed with respect to migraine: migraine signaled an increased risk for the first onset of major depression and major depression signaled an increased risk for the first occurrence of migraine. Sex-adjusted hazard ratios were 2.4 and 2.8, respectively (both statistically significant). In contrast, severe nonmi-

graine headache signaled an increased risk for major depression, but there was no evidence of a significant influence in the reverse direction, i.e., from major depression to severe headache. Sex-adjusted hazard ratios were 3.6 and 1.6, respectively (only the first statistically significant).

The pattern of the results suggests that different causal pathways might account for the comorbidity of major depression in these two headache categories. The results for migraine suggest shared causes, whereas those for other headache of comparable severity suggest a causal effect of headache on depression.

Another line of evidence comes from a study of a biologic marker of depression in migraineurs. Jarman et al. (1990) administered the tyramine test to 40 migraine patients, 16 of whom had a lifetime history of major depression. Low tyramine conjugation, a trait marker for endogenous depression, was strongly associated with a lifetime history of major depression in subjects with comorbid disease, regardless of their current psychiatric status. The authors argued that the association of the trait marker with major depression in migraineurs ruled out the possibility that the depression was a psychologic reaction to migraine attacks (Silberstein et al., 1995).

PSYCHOPATHOLOGY OF MIGRAINE AND PERSONALITY CHARACTERISTICS

The relationship between migraine and psychopathology has been discussed far more often than it has been systematically studied (Silberstein et al., 1995). Over the years, many studies have focused on particular personality traits of migraineurs. The basic assumptions are that (1) migraineurs share personality traits, (2) these traits are enduring and measurable, and (3) these traits differentiate migraineurs from control subjects (Schmidt et al., 1986). The notion of a "migraine personality" first grew out of clinical observations of highly selected patients seen in subspecialty clinics (Silberstein et al., 1995).

Touraine and Draper (1934) reported that migraineurs were deliberate, hesitant, insecure, detailed, perfectionistic, sensitive to criticism, and deeply frustrated emotionally. They were said to lack warmth and to have difficulty making social contacts. Wolff (1937) found migraineurs to be rigid, compulsive, perfectionistic, ambitious, competitive, chronically resentful, and unable to delegate responsibility.

Most investigations have used psychometric instruments such as the Minnesota Multiphasic Personality Inventory (MMPI) (Hathaway and McKinley, 1943) or the Eysenck Personality Questionnaire (EPQ) (Eysenck and Eysenck, 1975). The EPQ is a well-standardized measure that includes four scales: (1) psychoticism (P), (2) extroversion (E), (3) neuroticism (N), and (4) lie (L).

Brandt et al. (1990) used the Washington County Migraine Prevalence Study to conduct the first population-based case-control study of personality in patients with migraine. More than 10,000 12- to 29-year-olds who were selected through random-digit dialing received a diagnostic telephone interview. Subjects who met the criteria for migraine with or without aura (n = 162) were compared with subjects without migraine. Each subject received the EPQ, the 28-item version of the General Health Questionnaire (Goldberg, 1975), and a question about headache laterality.

Subjects with migraine scored significantly higher than control subjects on the neuroticism scale of the EPQ, indicating that they were more tense, anxious, and depressed than the control group. In addition, women with migraine scored significantly higher than control subjects on the psychoticism scale of the EPQ, indicating that they were more hostile, less interpersonally sensitive, and out of step with their peers. Rasmussen (1992) screened a population-based sample to identify patients with migraine and those with tension-type headache (TTH). Tension-type headache occurring alone was associated with high neuroticism scores on the EPQ. Persons with pure migraine (i.e., without TTH) did not score above the norms on the neuroticism scale, although persons with migraine, with and without TTH, tended to score above the norms on the neuroticism scale.

Merikangas et al. (1993) investigated the cross-sectional association between personality, symptoms, and headache subtypes as part of a prospective longitudinal study of 19- and 20-year-olds in Zurich, Switzerland. Subjects with migraine scored higher on indicators of neuroticism than subjects without migraine.

In summary, studies that used the EPQ or similar personality measures and compared persons with migraine to control subjects without migraine have generally reported an association between migraine and neuroticism (Passchier et al., 1984; Passchier and Orlebeke, 1985; Phillips, 1976; Rasmussen, 1992; Silberstein et al., 1995).

Many investigators (Invernizzi et al., 1989; Kudrow and Sutkus, 1979; Sternbach, 1980; Weeks et al., 1983) have used the MMPI to investigate the personalities of migraineurs. These studies have been limited by several factors (Stewart et al., 1991). The MMPI studies have usually been clinic-based, limiting their generalizability and creating opportunities for selection bias. Most have not used control groups, relying instead on historical norms. Many have not used explicit diagnostic criteria for migraine. Despite these limitations, most studies have shown elevation of the neurotic triad, although this is not statistically significant (Silberstein et al., 1995).

Studies of migraine and personality have generally not controlled for drug use, headache frequency, and headache-related disability. Furthermore, they have not controlled for major psychiatric disorders (such as major depression or panic disorder), which occur more commonly in migraineurs. The association between major psychiatric disorders and personality disorders may confound the assessment of the relationships between these disorders and migraine. Neuroticism, in particular, is associated with depression and anxiety, which occur with increased prevalence in migraineurs. Differences in neuroticism across studies might reflect variations in the role of comorbid psychiatric disease. The available data suggest that subjects with migraine may be more neurotic than those without migraine. The stereotypical rigid, obsessional migraine personality might reflect the selection bias of a distinct subtype of migraine that is more likely to be seen in the clinic.

Breslau and Andreski (1995) examined the association between migraine and personality, taking into account a history of concurring psychiatric disorders. Data came from their epidemiologic study of young adults in Detroit, Michigan. Migraine was associated with neuroticism but not with extroversion or psychoticism, as measured by the EPQ. The association remained significant when the authors controlled for sex and history of major depression and anxiety disorders. More than 25% of persons with migraine alone, uncomplicated by psychiatric comorbidity, scored in the highest quartile of neuroticism. The results suggest that subjects with migraine are more likely to have psychopathology and to adjust poorly to their medical condition. The findings also suggest that the association between migraine and neuroticism is not attributable to comorbid depression or anxiety disorders.

Breslau et al. (1996) presented findings from prospective data on the migraine–neuroticism association from their epidemiologic study of young adults. In women, neuroticism measured at baseline predicted the first incidence of migraine during the 5-year follow-up. Specifically, controlling for major depression and anxiety disorders at baseline, women scoring in the highest quartile of the neuroticism scale were nearly three times more likely to develop migraine than those scoring in the lowest quartile. In men, neuroticism did not predict migraine, although the small number of cases in men precluded reliable estimates of the risk for migraine associated with neuroticism.

MIGRAINE AND RAYNAUD'S SYNDROME

There is increased prevalence of migraine in individuals who have rheumatologic disorders, including Sjögren's syndrome (Pal et al., 1989) and systemic lupus erythematosus (Isenberg et al., 1982). Several case series (Mil-

ler et al., 1981; Atkinson and Appenzeller, 1976; O'Keeffe et al., 1992, 1993; Pal et al., 1989; Isenberg et al., 1982; Leppert et al., 1987; Zahavi et al., 1984) have suggested that migraine is comorbid with Raynaud's phenomenon (RP). Zahavi et al. (1984) found an increased prevalence of RP in migraineurs. O'Keeffe et al. (1992) found an increased prevalence of migraine and chest pain in a sample of patients with primary RP. In a follow-up study, O'Keeffe et al. (1993) found an increased prevalence of migraine in a group of patients with RP compared with controls. Miller et al. (1981) found an increased prevalence of both migraine and RP in patients with variant angina. Leppert et al. (1987) found a high prevalence of recurrent headaches in a population of women with RP. Terwindt et al. (2000) found a genetic link between migraine, RP, and vascular retinopathy in one extended Dutch family. Finding a gene for this family may help to elucidate the genetic background of migraine and other vascular disorders indicating RP.

MIGRAINE AND ESSENTIAL TREMOR

A cross-sectional study conducted by Biary et al. (1990) found a relationship between essential tremor and migraine. Patients were identified from either a movement disorder clinic or a headache clinic. Controls were selected from students, hospital staff, and visitors. The prevalence of migraine among patients with essential tremor was 36% compared with 23% in the control group. The prevalence of essential tremor was 17% among patients with migraine compared with 6% in the control group. In a regression analysis controlling for age and gender, the odds of migraine were 12.1 times higher in essential tremor patients compared with controls. A similar regression analysis found the odds of essential tremor to be 16.2 times greater among migraine patients compared with controls. This one small study, while limited, suggests that two common neurologic disorders, migraine and essential tremor, may be associated. Beta blockers have been effective at treating both conditions (Winkler and Young, 1974; Weber and Reinmuth, 1972).

CONCLUSIONS

Several disorders are strongly associated with migraine headache in both clinical samples and the general population. The strongest associations have been observed between migraine and stroke, migraine and epilepsy, and migraine and psychiatric disease. Studies of comorbidity are important in clinical practice because they enforce the need for heightened diagnostic suspicion. In addition, comorbidity influences choice of therapy, imposing limitations due to contraindications and opportunities to treat two conditions with a single agent. Future studies need to be designed to specifically investigate patterns and causes of comorbidity in migraine and other diseases using standardized diagnostic definitions and reliable methods of ascertainment of both migraine and the comorbid condition. Ultimately, identification of comorbidities should yield insights into the pathophysiology of migraine.

REFERENCES

Alvarez, J., J. Matias-Guiu, and J. Sumalla (1989). Ischemic stroke in young adults: Analysis of etiological subgroups. *Acta. Neurol. Scand.* 80:29–34.

Andermann, E. and F.A. Andermann (1987). Migraine–epilepsy relationships: Epidemiological and genetic aspects. In *Migraine and Epilepsy* (F.A. Andermann and E. Lugaresi, eds.), pp. 281–291. Butterworths, Boston.

Annergers, J.F., J.D. Grabow, and R.V. Groover (1980). Seizures after head trauma: A population study. *Neurology* 30:683–689.

Atkinson, R.A. and O. Appenzeller (1976). Hemicrania and Raynaud's phenomenon; manifestations of the same disease? *Headache* 16:1–3.

Batista, M.D., T.P. Cartledge, A. Zellmer et al. (1989). The antiprogesterone RU 486 delays ovulation in spontaneous and GnRH induced menstrual cycles [Abstract]. In *Endocrine Society 71st Annual Meeting*, p. 431. Endocrine Society, Bethesda, MD.

Biary, N., W. Koller, and P. Langenberg (1990). Correlation between essential tremor and migraine headache. *J. Neurol. Neurosurg. Psychiatry* 53:1060–1062.

Bogousslavsky, J., P.A. Despland, and F. Regli (1987). Spontaneous dissection with acute stroke. *Arch. Neurol.* 44:137–140.

Bougousslavsky, J. and F. Reglli (1987). Ischemic stroke in adults younger than 30 years of age: Cause and prognosis. *Arch. Neurol.* 44:479–482.

Brandt, J., D. Celentano, and W.F. Stewart (1990). Personality and emotional disorder in a community sample of migraine headache sufferers. *Am. J. Psychiatry* 147:303–308.

Breslau, N. (1992). Migraine, suicidal ideation, and suicide attempts. *Neurology* 42:392–395.

Breslau, N. and P. Andreski (1995). Migraine, personality, and psychiatric comorbidity. *Headache* 35:382–386.

Breslau, N., H.D. Chilcoat, and P. Andreski (1996). Further evidence on the link between migraine and neuroticism. *Neurology* 47:663–667.

Breslau, N. and G.C. Davis (1992). Migraine, major depression and panic disorder: A prospective epidemiologic study of young adults. *Cephalalgia* 12:85–89.

Breslau, N. and G.C. Davis (1993). Migraine, physical health and psychiatric disorders: A prospective epidemiologic study of young adults. *J. Psychiatr. Res.* 27:211–221.

Breslau, N., G.C. Davis, and P. Andreski (1991). Migraine, psychiatric disorders and suicide attempts: An epidemiological study of young adults. *Psychiatry Res.* 37:11–23.

Breslau, N., G.C. Davis, L.R. Schultz, and E.L. Peterson (1994a). Migraine and major depression: A longitudinal study. *Headache* 34: 387–393.

Breslau, N., K. Merikangas, and C.L. Bowden (1994b). Comorbidity of migraine and major affective disorders. *Neurology* 44:17–22.

Breslau, N., L.R. Schultz, W.F. Stewart et al. (2000). Headache and major depression: Is the association specific to migraine? *Neurology* 54: 308–313.

Brody, M.J. and P.J. Kadowitz (1974). Prostaglandins as modulators of the autonomic nervous system. *Fed. Proc.* 33:48–60.

Chang, C.L., M. Donaghy, and N. Poulter (1999). Migraine and stroke in young women: Case-control study. The World Health Organization Collaborative Study of Cardiovascular Disease and Steroid Hormone Contraception. *BMJ 318:* 13–18.

Collaborative Group for the Study of Stroke in Young Women. (1975). Oral contraceptives and stroke in young women. *JAMA 231:*718–722.

Ettinger, B., G.D. Friedman, T. Bush, and C.P. Quesenberry (1996). Reduced mortality associated with long-term postmenopausal estrogen therapy. *Obstet. Gynecol.* 87:6–12.

Eysenck, H.J. and S.B. Eysenck (1975). *Manual of the Eysenck Personality Questionnaire*. Educational and Industrial Testing Service, San Diego.

Feinstein, A.R. (1970). The pretherapeutic classification of comorbidity in chronic disease. *J. Chronic Dis.* 23:455–468.

Gamberini, G., R. D'lessandro, E. Labriola et al. (1984). Further evidence on the association of mitral valve prolapse and migraine. *Headache* 24:39–40.

Goldberg, D. (1975). *Manual of the General Health Questionnaire*. Educational and Industrial Testing Service, San Diego.

Hathaway, S.R. and J.C. McKinley (1943). *Minnesota Multiphasic Personality Inventory*. University of Minnesota, Minneapolis.

Hauser, W.A., J.F. Annergers, and L.T. Kurland (1991). Prevalence of epilepsy in Rochester, Minnesota. *Epilepsia* 32:429–445.

Headache Classification Committee of the International Headache Society. (1988). Classification and diagnostic criteria for headache disorders, cranial neuralgia, and facial pain. *Cephalalgia* 8:1–96.

Henrich, J.B. and R.I. Horowitz (1989). A controlled study of ischemic stroke risk in migraine patients. *J. Clin. Epidemiol.* 42:773–780.

Henrich, J.B., P.A.G. Sandercock, C.P. Warlow et al. (1986). Stroke and migraine in the Oxfordshire Community Stroke Project. *J. Neurol.* 233:257–262.

Invernizzi, G., C. Gala, and M. Buono (1989). Neurotic traits and disease duration in headache patients. *Cephalalgia* 9:173–178.

Isenberg, D.A., D.M. Thomas, M.L. Snaith et al. (1982). A study of migraine in systematic lupus erythematosis. *Ann. Rheum. Dis.* 41:30–32.

Jarman, J., M. Fernandez, P.T. Davies et al. (1990). High incidence of endogenous depression in migraine: Confirmation of tyramine test. *J. Neurol. Neurosurg. Psychiatry* 53:573–575.

Jensen, R., T. Brinck, and J. Olesen (1994). Sodium valproate has a prophylactic effect in migraine without aura. *Neurology* 44:647–651.

Kittner, S.J., R.J. McCarer, and R.W. Sherwin (1993). Black–white differences in stroke among young adults. *Stroke* 24:113–115.

Kudrow, L. and G.J. Sutkus (1979). MMPI pattern specificity in primary headache disorders. *Headache* 19:18–24.

Leppert, J., H. Aberg, I. Ringqvist et al. (1987). Raynaud's phenomenon in a female population: Prevalence and association with other conditions. *J. Vasc. Dis.* 38:871–877.

Lindegaard, O. (1995). Oral contraceptives, pregnancy and the risk of cerebral thromboembolism: The influences of diabetes, hypertension, migraine, and previous thrombotic disease. *Br. J. Obstet. Gynaecol.* 102:1–3.

Lipton, R.B., R. Ottman, B.L. Ehrenberg et al. (1994). Comorbidity of migraine: The connection between migraine and epilepsy. *Neurology* 44:28–32.

Lipton, R.B. and S.D. Silberstein (1994). Why study the comorbidity of migraine? *Neurology* 44:4–5.

Marchesi, C., A. De Ferri, and N. Petrolini (1989). Prevalence of migraine and muscle tension headache in depressive disorders. *J. Affect. Disord.* 16:33–36.

Marks, D.A. and B.L. Ehrenberg (1993). Migraine related seizures in adults with epilepsy, with EEG correlation. *Neurology* 43:2476–2483.

Merikangas, K.R. (1990). Genetic epidemiology of migraine. In *Migraine: A Spectrum of Ideas* (M. Sandler and G.M. Collins, eds.), pp. 40–47. Oxford University Press, Oxford.

Merikangas, K.R., J. Angst, and H. Isler (1990). Migraine and psychopathology: Results of the Zurich cohort study of young adults. *Arch. Gen. Psychiatry* 47:849–853.

Merikangas, K.R., J.R. Merikangas, and J. Angst (1993). Headache syndromes and psychiatric disorders: Associations and familial transmission. *J. Psychiatr. Res.* 27:197–210.

Merikangas, K.R., N.J. Risch, J.R. Merikangas et al. (1988). Migraine and depression: Association and familial transmission. *J. Psychiatr. Res.* 22:119–129.

Merikangas, K.R., D.E. Stevens, and J. Angst (1993). Headache and personality: Results of a community sample of young adults. *J. Psychiatr. Res.* 27:187–196.

Miller, D., D.D. Waters, W. Warnica et al. (1981). Is variant angina the coronary manifestation of a generalized vasospastic disorder? *N. Engl. J. Med.* 304:763–766.

Morrison, D.P. and W.H. Price (1989). The prevalence of psychiatric disorder among female new referrals to a migraine clinic. *Psychol. Med.* 19:919–925.

O'Keeffe, S.T., N.P. Tsapatsaris, and W.P. Beetham (1992). Increased prevalence of migraine and chest pain in patients with primary Raynaud disease. *Ann. Intern. Med.* 116:985–989.

O'Keeffe, S.T., N.P. Tspatsaris, and W.P. Beetham (1993). Association between Raynaud's phenomenon and migraine in a random population of hospital employees. *J. Rheumatol.* 20:1187–1188.

Olesen, J. (1993). Synthesis of migraine mechanisms. In *The Headaches* (J. Olesen, P. Tfelt-Hansen, and K.M.A. Welch, eds.), pp. 247–253. Raven Press, New York.

Ottman, R. and R.B. Lipton (1994). Comorbidity of migraine and epilepsy. *Neurology* 44:2105–2110.

Ottman, R. and R.B. Lipton (1996). Is the comorbidity of epilepsy and migraine due to a shared genetic susceptibility? *Neurology 47*: 918–924.

Pal, B., C. Gibson, J. Passmore et al. (1989). A study of headaches and migraine in Sjogren's syndrome and other rheumatic disorders. *Ann. Rheum. Dis. 48*:312–316.

Passchier, J., H. Hylkema, and J.F. Orlebeke (1984). Personality and headache type: A controlled study. *Headache 24*:140–146.

Passchier, J. and J.F. Orlebeke (1985). Headaches and stress in school children: An epidemiological study. *Cephalalgia 5*:167–176.

Phillips, C. (1976). Headache and personality. *J. Psychosom. Res. 20*:535–542.

Rasmussen, B.K. (1992). Migraine and tension-type headache in a general population: Psychosocial factors. *Int. J. Epidemiol. 21*:1138–1143.

Rothrock, J., J. North, K. Madden et al. (1993). Migraine and migrainous stroke: Risk factors and prognosis. *Neurology 43*:2473–2476.

Schmidt, F.N., P. Carney, and G. Fitzsimmons (1986). An empirical assessment of the migraine personality type. *J. Psychosom. Res. 30*:189–197.

Shechter, A., W.F. Stewart, and D.D. Celentano (1990). An epidemiologic study of migraine and head injury [Abstract]. *Neurology 40*:245.

Silberstein, S.D., R.B. Lipton, and N. Breslau (1995). Migraine: Association with personality characteristics and psychopathology. *Cephalalgia 15*:337–369.

Sternbach, R.A. (1980). MMPI pattern in common headache disorders. *Headache 20*:311–315.

Stewart, W.F., M.S. Linet, and D.D. Celentano (1989). Migraine headaches and panic attacks. *Psychosom. Med. 51*:559–569.

Stewart, W.F., M.S. Linet, D.D. Celentano et al. (1991). Age and sex-specific incidence rates of migraine with and without visual aura. *Am. J. Epidemiol. 34*:1111–1120.

Stewart, W.F., A. Shechter, and J. Liberman. (1992). Physician consultation for headache pain and history of panic: Results from a population-based study. *Am. J. Med. 92*:35S–40S.

Tatemichi, T.K. and J.P. Mohr (1986). Migraine and stroke. In *Stroke: Pathophysiology, Diagnosis and Management* (H.J.M. Barnett, B.M. Stein, J.P. Mohr et al., eds.), pp. 845–863. Churchill Livingstone, New York.

Terwindt, G.M., J. Haan, R.A. Ophoff et al. (2000). Clinical and genetic analysis of a large Dutch family with autosomal dominant vascular retinopathy, migraine, and Raynaud's phenomenon. *Brain 121*:303–316.

Touraine, G.A. and G. Draper (1934). The migrainous patient: A constitutional study. *J. Nerv. Ment. Dis. 80*:183–204.

Tzourio, C., S.J. Kittner, M.G. Bousser et al. (2000). Migraine and stroke in young women. *Cephalalgia 20*:190–199.

Tzourio, C. and A. Tehindrazanarivelo (1993). Case-control study of migraine and risk of ischemic stroke. *BMJ 307*:289–292.

Tzourio, C., A. Tehindrazanarivelo, S. Iglesias et al. (1995). Case-control study of migraine and risk of ischemic stroke in young women. *BMJ 310*:830–833.

Weber, R.B. and O.M. Reinmuth (1972). The treatment of migraine with propranolol. *Neurology 22*:366–369.

Weeks, R., S. Baskin, and F. Sheftell (1983). A comparison of MMPI personality data and frontalis electromyographic readings in migraine and combination headache patients. *Headache 23*:75–82.

Welch, K.M.A. (1987). Migraine: A behavioral disorder. *Arch. Neurol. 44*:323–327.

Welch, K.M.A. (1994). Relationships of stroke and migraine. *Neurology 44*:33–36.

Welch, K.M.A., G.L. Barkley, N. Tepley et al. (1991). Magnetoencephalographic studies of migraine: Evidence for central neuronal hyperexcitability. In *New Advances in Headache Research* (F.C. Rose, ed.), pp. 127–130. Smith Gordon, London.

Welch, K.M.A., E. Chabi, J.H. Nell et al. (1976). Biochemical comparison of migraine and stroke. *Headache 6*:160.

Winkler, G.J. and R.R. Young (1974). Efficacy of chronic propranolol therapy in action tremors of the familial, senile, or essential varieties. *N. Engl. J. Med. 290*:984–988.

Wolff, H.G. (1937). Personality features and reactions of subjects with migraine. *Arch. Neurol. Psychiatry 37*:895–921.

Zahavi, I., A. Chagnac, R. Hering et al. (1984). Prevalence of Raynaud's phenomenon in patients with migraine. *Arch. Intern. Med. 144*: 742–744.

Diagnosis and Treatment of Primary Headache Disorders

Migraine: Diagnosis and Treatment

STEPHEN D. SILBERSTEIN
JOEL R. SAPER
FREDERICK G. FREITAG

Migraine is a common episodic headache disorder with a 1-year prevalence of approximately 18% in women, 6% in men, and 4% in children. It is characterized by attacks consisting of various combinations of headache and neurologic, gastrointestinal, and autonomic symptoms. Most patients develop migraine in the first three decades of life, but in some it develops in the fourth or even the fifth decade (see Chapter 7). The term "migraine" is derived from the Greek word *hemicrania*, introduced by Galen in approximately 200 A.D. (Critchley, 1967).

CLASSIFICATION

Most migraine descriptions stress three features: the unilateral distribution of the headache; the presence of a warning (often visual); and nausea or vomiting (Waters, 1986). The Ad Hoc Committee on Classification of Headache (Friedman et al., 1962) described vascular headache of migraine type as follows:

Recurrent attacks of headache, widely varied in intensity, frequency, and duration. The attacks are commonly unilateral in onset; are usually associated with anorexia and sometimes with nausea and vomiting; in some are preceded by, or associated with, conspicuous sensory, motor, and mood disturbances; and are often familial. (p. 14)

In an attempt to increase precision, the International Headache Society (IHS) proposed and published its classification of headache disorders (Headache Classification Committee of the International Headache Society, 1988) (see Chapter 2). While the old ad hoc criteria were not sufficiently specific, the new IHS classification system has raised many areas of dispute. Some believe it to be too complex and arbitrary. Others believe that it is not useful in primary-care settings and fails to adequately address chronic daily headache. Nonetheless, it has served to provide a highly uniform tool for conducting clinical trials (Solomon and Lipton, 1991; Rapoport, 1992). The IHS criteria attempt to diagnose headache types rather than headache syndromes yet require a number of attacks over a period of time before a diagnosis can be made. They are currently undergoing revision.

Migraine headaches were formerly divided into two varieties: classic and common (Silberstein, 1984). The IHS calls the common type "migraine without aura" (1.1) and the classic type "migraine with aura" (1.2), the aura being the complex of focal neurologic symptoms that precedes or accompanies an attack (Headache Classification Committee of the International Headache Society, 1988). At most, only 30% of migraine headaches are "classic" (Ziegler and Hassanein, 1990). The same patient may have migraine headache without aura, migraine headache with aura, and migraine aura without headache.

To establish a diagnosis of migraine under the IHS classification, certain clinical features must be present and organic disease must be excluded (Table 9–1). To diagnosis migraine without aura (1.1), five attacks are needed, each lasting 4 to 72 hours and having two of the following four characteristics: unilateral location, pulsating quality, moderate to severe intensity, and aggravation by routine physical activity. In addition, the attacks must have at least one of the following: nausea and/or vomiting and/or photophobia and phonophobia (Table 9–2). Using these criteria, no single associated feature is mandatory for diagnosing migraine, although recurrent episodic attacks must be documented. A patient who has pulsatile pain aggravated by routine activity, photophobia, and phonophobia meets the criteria, as does the more typical patient with unilateral throbbing pain and nausea (Headache Classification Committee of the International Headache Society, 1988). If one of the criteria is missing, the headache is called *migrainous* (1.7).

A migraine attack usually lasts less than a day; when it persists for more than 3 days, the term "status migrainosus" is applied. Although migraine often begins in the morning, sometimes awakening the patient from sleep at dawn, it can begin at any time of the day or night. The frequency of attacks is extremely variable, from a few in a lifetime to several a week. The median frequency is 1.5 attacks per month; 10% of migraineurs have one attack per week (Stewart et al., 1994b).

To diagnose IHS migraine with aura (1.2) (Table 9–3), at least two attacks with three of the following four features are required: one or more fully reversible aura symptoms, aura developing over more than 4 minutes, aura lasting less than 60 minutes, and headache following the aura with a free interval of less than 60 minutes. Migraine with aura is subdivided into migraine with typical aura (1.2.1)

Table 9–1 International Headache Society migraine classification

1	Migraine
	1.1 Migraine without aura
	1.2 Migraine with aura
	1.2.1 Migraine with typical aura
	1.2.2 Migraine with prolonged aura
	1.2.3 Familial hemiplegic migraine
	1.2.4 Basilar migraine
	1.2.5 Migraine aura without headache
	1.2.6 Migraine with acute onset aura
	1.3 Ophthalmoplegic migraine
	1.4 Retinal migraine
	1.5 Childhood periodic syndromes that may be precursors to or associated with migraine
	1.5.1 Benign paroxysmal vertigo of childhood
	1.5.2 Alternating hemiplegia of childhood
	1.6 Complications of migraine
	1.6.1 Status migrainosus
	1.6.2 Migrainous infarction
	1.7 Migrainous disorder not fulfilling above criteria

Table 9–2 Migraine without aura

Diagnostic criteria

A. At least 5 attacks fulfilling B–D
B. Headache lasting 4 to 72 hours (untreated or unsuccessfully treated)
C. Headache has at least 2 of the following characteristics:
   1. Unilateral location
   2. Pulsating quality
   3. Moderate or severe intensity (inhibits or prohibits daily activities)
   4. Aggravation by walking stairs or similar routine physical activity
D. During headache at least 1 of the following:
   1. Nausea and/or vomiting
   2. Photophobia and phonophobia
E. No evidence of organic disease

*Previously used terms: common migraine, hemicrania simplex.

Table 9–3 Migraine with aura (classic migraine)

Diagnostic criteria

A. At least 2 attacks fulfilling B
B. At least 3 of the following characteristics:
   1. One or more fully reversible aura symptoms indicating brain dysfunction
   2. At least 1 aura symptom develops gradually over more than 4 minutes or 2 or more symptoms occur in succession
   3. No single aura symptom lasts more than 60 minutes
   4. Headache follows aura with a free interval of less than 60 minutes (it may also begin before or simultaneously with the aura)
C. History, physical examination, and, where appropriate, diagnostic tests exclude a secondary cause

(homonymous visual disturbance, unilateral numbness or weakness, or aphasia), migraine with prolonged aura (1.2.2) (aura lasting more than 60 minutes), familial hemiplegic migraine (1.2.3), basilar migraine (1.2.4), migraine aura without headache (1.2.5), and migraine with acute-onset aura (1.2.6). Other varieties of migraine include ophthalmoplegic migraine (1.3), retinal migraine (1.4), and childhood periodic syndromes (1.5). The IHS classification system does not have specific criteria for the headache of migraine with aura, but it is reasonable to expect that it would be similar to that of migraine without aura. Most migraine-with-aura sufferers also have attacks without aura. The aura usually lasts 20 to 30 minutes and typically precedes the headache, but occasionally it occurs with the headache or only during the headache. In contrast to a transient ischemic attack (TIA), the aura of migraine evolves gradually and consists of both positive (e.g., scintillations, tingling) and negative (e.g., scotoma, numbness) features. If the aura is stereotypical, the diagnosis of migraine with aura is warranted, even if the subsequent headache does not have typical migrainous features. Almost any symptom or sign of brain dysfunction may be a feature of the aura, but the most common aura is a visual phenomenon.

Focal symptoms and signs of the aura may persist beyond the headache phase. Formerly termed "complicated migraine," the IHS classification has introduced two more specific labels. If the aura lasts for more than 1 hour but less than 1 week, the term "migraine with prolonged aura" is applied. If the signs persist for more than 1 week or a neuroimaging procedure demonstrates a stroke, a *migrainous infarction* (IHS 1.6.2) has occurred. Particularly in mid- or late life, the aura may not be followed by the headache (migraine equivalent or late-life migraine accompaniment).

CLINICAL FEATURES OF MIGRAINE

The migraine attack can be divided into four phases: premonitory (prodrome), which occurs hours or days before the headache; the aura, which immediately precedes the head-

Table 9–4 Migraine attack

I.	Premonitory phase
II.	Aura
III	Headache
IV.	Postdrome

ache; the headache itself; and the postdrome (Table 9–4). Migraine without aura consists of at least the headache and possibly the postdrome. Migraine with aura consists of at least the aura and the headache. If the headache is absent, it is migraine aura without headache. Both may be associated with premonitory symptoms.

Premonitory Phase (Prodrome)

Premonitory phenomena occur hours to days before headache onset in about 60% of migraineurs and can consist of psychologic, neurologic, or general (constitutional, autonomic) symptoms (Table 9–5). Psychologic symptoms include depression, euphoria, irritability, restlessness, mental slowness, hyperactivity, fatigue, and drowsiness. Neurologic phenomena include photophobia, phonophobia, and hyperosmia, among others. General symptoms include a stiff neck, a cold feeling, sluggishness, increased thirst, increased urination, anorexia, diarrhea, constipation, fluid retention, and food cravings.

Two types of migraine prodromes are described: *nonevolutive*, which precedes the attack by up to 48 hours, and *evolutive*, which starts approximately 6 hours before the attack, gradually increasing in intensity and culminating in the attack. A dopaminergic mechanism has been suggested (Amery et al., 1986a,b). Premonitory symptoms are common: Blau (1980) found them in 28/50 migraineurs, while Isler (1986) found them in 65/100 migraineurs, with equal frequency in migraine with or without aura.

Aura

The migraine aura is comprised of focal neurologic phenomena that precede or accompany an attack. Most aura symptoms develop over 5 to 20 minutes and usually last less than

Table 9–5 Premonitory phenomena (prodrome)

Psychologic	Neurologic	General
Depression	Photophobia	Stiff neck
Hyperactivity	Difficulty concentrating	Food cravings
Euphoria	Phonophobia	Cold feeling
Talkativeness	Dysphasia	Anorexia
Irritability	Hyperosmia	Sluggishness
Drowsiness	Yawning	Diarrhea or constipation
Restlessness		Thirst
		Urination
		Fluid retention

60 minutes (Headache Classification Committee of the International Headache Society, 1988). The aura can be characterized by visual, sensory, or motor phenomena and may involve language or brain stem disturbances (Table 9–6). If it occurs, the headache usually begins within 60 minutes of the end of the aura. In one prospective study, headache followed the aura only 80% of the time (Jensen et al., 1986). If the headache is delayed, most patients do not return to a normal sense between the end of the aura and the onset of the headache. Fears, somatic complaints, alterations in mood, disturbances of speech or thought, or detachment from the environment or from other people may occur. The headache may begin before or simultaneously with the aura, or the aura may occur in isolation. Rarely, auras may occur repeatedly. This may be many times an hour for as long as several months. These have been termed "migraine aura status," but other organic causes must be considered (Silberstein and Young, 1995a). Sacks (1985) described two variations: scotomata occurring repeatedly, even alternating sides, and closely repeating cycles of migrating sensory auras occurring for hours on end. Patients may experience more than one type of aura, with a progression from one symptom to another. Most patients with a sensory aura also have a visual aura (Ziegler and Hassanein, 1990) (Fig. 9–1).

Visual aura is the most common of the neurologic events; it occurs in 99% of patients who have an aura and often has a hemianoptic distribution (Russell and Olesen, 1996). The aura may consist of *photopsia* (the sensation of unformed flashes of light before the eyes), *scotoma* (partial loss of sight) (Lance and Anthony, 1966; Wilkinson, 1986; Hupp et al., 1989; Hachinski et al., 1973), or the almost diagnostic aura of migraine, the fortification spectrum (Wilkinson, 1986; Hachinski et al., 1973).

Auras vary in complexity. Elementary visual disturbances include scotomata, simple flashes (phosphenes), specks, or geometric forms. They may move across the visual field, sometimes crossing the midline. Shimmering or undulations in the visual field may also occur and may be described by patients as "heat waves." These "minor visual disorders" are more likely to occur during than before the headache (Selby and Lance, 1960). Because they are bilateral, they are believed to arise from the occipital cortex. More complicated auras include *teichopsia* (Greek: "town wall" and "vision") or fortification spectrum, the most characteristic visual aura of migraine. An arc of scintillating lights, usually but not always beginning near the point of fixation, may form into a herringbone-like pattern that expands to encompass an increasing portion

Table 9–6 Aura

Visual: scotoma; photopsia or phosphenes; geometric forms; fortification spectra; objects may rotate, oscillate, or shimmer; brightness appears often very bright

Visual hallucinations or distortions: metamorphopsia; macropsia; zoom or mosaic vision

Sensory: paresthesias, often migrating, often lasting for minutes (cheiro-oral), and can become bilateral olfactory hallucinations

Motor: weakness or ataxia

Language: dysarthria or aphasia

Delusions and disturbed consciousness: déjà vu, multiple conscious trance-like states

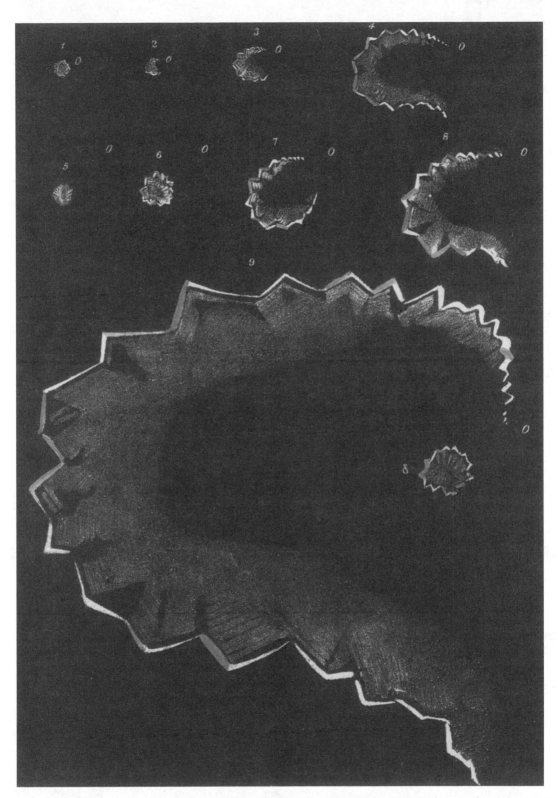

Figure 9–1 Migraine aura. 1–4. Early stages of sinistral Teichopsia beginning close to the sight-point, as seen in the dark. The letter O marks the sight-point in every figure. 5–8. A similar series of the early stages of sinistral Teichopsia beginning a few degrees below and to the left of the sight-point. 9. Sinistral Teichopsia fully developed. § Beginning of a secondary attack, which never attains full development, unless it arises on the opposite side. [From Airy H (1871) *On a Distinct Form of Transient Hemiopsia. Phil. Transact. for 1870*, p. 247.]

of a visual hemifield. It migrates across the visual field with a scintillating edge of often zigzag, flashing, or occasionally colored phenomena. The visions of Hildegard of Bingen, a 12th century abbess, have been attributed in part to her migrainous auras. Characteristic of the visions that she and other visionary prophets, including Ezekiel, experienced were working, boiling, or fermenting lights.

Visual distortions and hallucinations, speculated to represent Lewis Carroll's descriptions in *Alice in Wonderland*, can occur. These phenomena are more common in children, usually followed by a headache, and characterized by a complex disorder of visual perception that may include metamorphopsia, micropsia, macropsia, and zoom or mosaic vision (Hosking, 1988; Sacks, 1985). Nonvisual symptoms can occur and include complex difficulties in the perception and use of the body (*apraxia* and *agnosia*); speech and language disturbances; states of double or multiple consciousness associated with *déjà vu* or *jamais vu*; and elaborate dreamy, nightmarish, trance-like, or delirious states. Olfactory hallucinations may also occur (Diamond et al., 1985).

Paresthesias characterize the second most common aura and occur in about one-third of migraineurs with aura. They are typically cheiro-oral, with numbness starting in the hand, migrating up the arm, and then jumping to involve the face, lips, and tongue (Russell and Olesen, 1996). The leg is occasionally involved (Manzoni et al., 1985). As with visual auras (with positive, followed by negative, symptoms), paresthesias may be followed by numbness and, in a few cases, loss of position sense. Paresthesias begin bilaterally or become bilateral in half of patients. Sensory auras rarely occur in isolation and usually follow a visual aura (Silberstein and Lipton, 1994; Silberstein and Young, 1995a).

Motor symptoms may occur in up to 18% of patients, often in association with sensory symptoms (Jensen et al., 1986); however, true weakness is rare and always unilateral (Manzoni et al., 1985). Sensory ataxia is often reported as weakness (Manzoni et al., 1985); hyperkinetic movement disorders, including chorea, have been reported (Silberstein and

Young, 1995a). Aphasic auras have been reported in 17% to 20% of patients (Jensen et al., 1986; Manzoni et al., 1985). However, since patients are rarely examined during an aura, many of the reported cases may be dysarthria and not aphasia (Manzoni et al., 1985).

Migraine Aura without Headache

Periodic neurologic phenomena, which may be the aura of migraine, can occur in isolation without the headache (Whitty, 1967). These phenomena (scintillating scotoma, recurrent sensory, motor, and mental phenomena) must be differentiated from TIAs and focal seizures and are diagnosed as migraine only after full investigation and reasonable follow-up. Transient visual disturbances (TVDs), with flickering or scintillating phenomena, also occur with numerous other conditions, including blood cell diseases, retinal detachment, cluster headaches, trauma, and syncope, but are not generally associated with cerebrovascular embolic or thrombotic disease (Mattsson and Lundberg, 1999). Headache occurring in association with the symptoms of aura will help to confirm the diagnosis but does not exclude TIA. Ziegler and Hassanein (1990) reported that 44% of their patients who had headache with aura had aura without headache at some time.

Levy (1988) found that 32% of Cornell neurologists had a history of transient neurologic loss, most commonly visual (field cuts, obscurations, scotomata) and less commonly nonvisual (hemiparesis, clumsiness, paresthesias, dysarthria) symptoms. Migraine was reported in 29%, occurring in 44% of those reporting and 22% of those not reporting transient central nervous system (CNS) dysfunction. None developed any residual deficit or chronic neurologic disorder at 5-year follow-up, suggesting that these are benign migrainous accompaniments.

Fisher (1980) described transient neurologic phenomena characteristically not associated with headache (late-life migrainous accompaniments or transient migrainous accompaniments) in 188 patients over the age of 40; 60% were men and 57% had a history of recurrent headache. Attacks of episodic neurologic dysfunction lasted from 1 minute to 72 hours and had variable recurrence rates (one attack 27%, two to ten attacks 45%, more than ten attacks 28%). Scintillating scotoma was considered to be diagnostic of migraine even when it occurred in isolation, whereas other episodic neurologic symptoms (paresthesias, aphasia, and sensory and motor symptoms) needed more careful evaluation.

Wijman et al. (1998) determined the frequency, characteristics, and stroke outcome of subjects with migrainous visual symptoms in the Framingham study. Visual symptoms occurred in 186 subjects. Visual symptoms that corresponded to the visual aura of migraine were reported by 26/186 subjects (14%), with a prevalence of 1.23% overall (1.33% in women and 1.08% in men). Numbers ranged from 1 to 500 (ten or more in 69% of subjects) and lasted 15 to 60 minutes in 50% of subjects. In 65% of subjects, the episodes were stereotypical. They began after age 50 in 77%. The pattern of visual manifestations varied widely among subjects. Episodes were never accompanied by headaches in 58%, and 42% had no headache history. Only in 19% of subjects did the migrainous visual episodes meet the IHS criteria for migraine aura, usually because one of the criteria ("at least one aura symptom develops gradually over more than four minutes") could not be reliably ascertained.

Three of 26 subjects (11.5%) had a stroke 1 or more years later; one had a subarachnoid hemorrhage 1 year later; one had a brainstem infarct 3 years later; and one had a cardioembolic stroke secondary to atrial fibrillation 27 years later. This stroke incidence rate of 11.5% was significantly lower than that of 33.3% of subjects with TIAs in the same cohort (p = 0.030) (these usually occurred within 6 months) and did not differ from that of 13.6% of those without migrainous phenomena or TIAs.

O'Connor and Tredici (1981) described 61 cases of transient neurologic dysfunction in men seen during a 15-year period at the United States Air Force School of Aerospace Medicine. These cases were derived from a selected group of highly trained young men whose profession required outstanding visual abilities. Age at onset was 12 to 44 years. Family history was present in 15 (24.6%), and a personal history of migraine was present in only two (3.3%). Eighteen subjects (29.5%) had nonvisual neurologic deficits during the episodes. Permanent neurologic deficiency occurred in one patient.

Cohen et al. (1984) reported 31 cases of TVD attributed to migraine. Headache was present in 20 patients (64.5%). A family history of migraine was found in 61%; and 57% had a personal history of migraine. After approximately 2 years, one patient died of cardiac disease, none had a stroke, one developed amaurosis fugax, and one developed transient global amnesia.

Mattsson and Lundberg (1999) estimated the prevalence and characteristics of TVD of possible migraine origin in both a clinical and a general population. One hundred consecutive female migraine patients (17 to 69 years) and 245 women from the general population (40 to 75 years) were interviewed. Lifetime prevalence was 37% in migraine patients and 13% in the general population. There were no differences in the TVD characteristics between the groups. Slightly less than half of each group had a gradual onset of 5 or more minutes (45% and 46% of the groups, respectively). Headache following TVDs had more migrainous features in patients than in controls. The TVDs that did not fulfill the IHS criteria for migraine with aura probably represented abortive migraine phenomena.

Visual migrainous phenomena are not rare since they occur in 1.33% of women and in 1.08% of men in a general population sample and are usually benign. Transient migrainous accompaniments (scintillating scotomata, numbness, aphasia, dysarthria, and motor weakness) may occur for the first time after the age of 45 and may be easily confused with TIAs of cerebrovascular origin. Diagnosis in all but the most classical cases is still by exclusion (Table 9–7).

Headache

A migraine headache is typically unilateral, throbbing, moderate to marked in severity, and aggravated by routine physical activity.

Table 9–7 Migraine equivalents

Scintillating scotoma
Paresthesias
Aphasia
Dysarthria
Hemiplegia
Blindness
Blurring of vision
Hemianopia
Transient monocular blindness
Ophthalmoplegia
Oculosympathetic palsy
Mydriasis
Confusion-stupor
Cyclical vomiting
Seizures
Diplopia
Deafness
Recurrence stroke deficit
Chorea

Not all of these features are required by the IHS: pain may be bilateral and throbbing or unilateral and achy. The headache of migraine can occur at any time of day or night but occurs most frequently on arising in the morning (Selby and Lance, 1960). Onset is usually gradual; the pain peaks, then subsides, and usually lasts less than 24 hours, with a range of 4 to 72 hours in adults and 2 to 48 hours in children (Headache Classification Committee of the International Headache Society, 1988). The headache is bilateral in 40% and unilateral in 60% of cases; it consistently occurs on the same side in 20% of patients (Selby and Lance, 1960). Migraineurs whose headaches alternate sides do not develop more consistently lateralized headache with the passage of time.

The pain varies greatly in intensity, ranging from annoying to incapacitating, although most migraineurs report at least moderate pain (Stewart et al., 1994a,b). The pain has a throbbing quality, particularly when severe, but can be tight or bandlike (Selby and Lance, 1960). During an attack, pain may move from one part of the head to another and may radiate down the neck into the shoulder. The pain is commonly aggravated by physical activity or simple head movement. Patients prefer to lie down in a dark, quiet room. Scalp tenderness occurs in many patients during or after the headache. This ten-

derness may involve the head and neck and prevent the patient from lying on the affected side (Drummond, 1987).

Many migraineurs have headache profiles that do not meet the IHS criteria for migraine (Olesen, 1978). Some are migrainous (1.7), missing one criterion; others are shorter and less severe and often meet the IHS criteria for episodic tension-type headache (TTH). Some patients note that their headache begins as a TTH and builds into a migraine (Olesen, 1978; Drummond and Lance, 1984). We believe these phenomenologic TTHs are migrainous in nature, have more migraine features than TTH features, and, unlike typical TTH occurring in nonmigraineurs, respond to specific migraine drugs (Silberstein, 1993a; Cady et al., 1997; Lipton et al., 1999).

Migraineurs may also experience short-lived jabs of pain, which last for seconds and occur between more characteristic migraine attacks (so-called idiopathic stabbing headache). The pain is described as an "icepick," "needle," "nail," "jabs and jolts," or "pinprick" headache and occurs in about 40% of migraineurs (Raskin and Schwartz, 1980).

Associated Phenomena

Migraine attacks are characteristically accompanied by other associated symptoms that often contribute to migraine-related disability. Their type and prevalence are detailed in Table 9–8. Gastrointestinal disturbances are often the most distressing symptoms. Anorexia is common, but food cravings can occur; nausea occurs in 90% of patients and vomiting in about one-third (Selby and Lance, 1960; Olesen, 1978; Silberstein, 1995). Gastroparesis contributes to gastrointestinal distress and poor absorption of oral medication (Volans, 1978; Saper, 1983; Boyle et al., 1990). Diarrhea occurs in about 16% of patients (Selby and Lance, 1960; Russell et al., 1992; Olesen, 1978; Anthony and Rasmussen, 1993; Rasmussen et al., 1991a). Many migraineurs have enhanced sensory perception or sensitivity manifested by photophobia, phonophobia, and osmophobia and seek a dark, quiet room (Selby and Lance, 1960; Drummond, 1986).

Table 9–8 Associated phenomena

Reference	Study type	No. of patients	Nausea	Vomiting	Photophobia	Phonophobia	Visual disturbances	Dizziness
Selby and Lance, 1960	C	500	87	55	82	NR[a]	41	72
Lance and Anthony, 1966	C	500	93	55	49	NR	33	NR
Olesen, 1978	C	750	86	47	NR	NR	20	NR
Iversen et al., 1990	C	30	90	NR	95	97	NR	NR
Davies et al., 1991	C	354						
w/o aura			89	60	NR	NR	NR	NR
w/aura			85	60	NR	NR	NR	NR
Rasmussen et al., 19917	P	740	82	50	83	86	NR	NR
Lipton et al., 1992	P	2,479						
physician-diagnosed			74(F) 66(M)	39(F) 63(M)	72(F) 63(M)	68(F) 61(M)	56(F) 45(M)	NR
nonphysician-diagnosed			60(F) 49(M)	18(F) 18(M)	63(F) 61(M)	65(F) 63(M)	30(F) 29(M)	NR
Rasmussen and Olesen, 1992	P	58	95	62	95	98	NR	NR
Russell et al., 1992	C	61, clinical interview						
w/o aura			85	NR	98	82	NR	NR
w/aura			100	NR	100	100	NR	NR
		61, headache diary						
w/o aura			80	NR	82	75	NR	NR
w/aura			53	NR	68	60	NR	NR

[a]NR, not reported.

Others have lightheadedness and vertigo (Kuritzky et al., 1981). Premonitory symptoms, such as exhilaration, agitation, fatigue, lethargy, disorientation, hypomania, anger, rage, or depression, can continue into the headache. Constitutional, mood, and mental changes are almost universal. Blurry vision, nasal stuffiness, pallor or redness, and sensations of heat, cold, or sweating may occur. Fluid retention can develop hours to days before the headache. Frank edema may precede, accompany, or follow the headache, with resolution of the fluid retention after the headache resolves (Dalessio, 1980).

The prevalence of associated symptoms is higher in clinic-based than population-based studies, probably because more effective interviewing techniques and more definitive criteria are used in the clinic. In addition, a selection bias toward patients with more severe headache may result in more symptoms being reported (Silberstein, 1995). Studies that graded the severity of nausea, photophobia, and phonophobia have improved the dif-

ferentiation of migraine from TTH; by definition, these symptoms were more prevalent and more severe in migraineurs (Silberstein, 1995).

Celentano et al. (1990), using a population-based telephone interview, estimated the prevalence of severe headaches in adolescents and young adults. Symptoms usually considered diagnostic of migraine (nausea and/or vomiting, visual disturbances, and photophobia) were significantly associated with prolonged duration and more severe pain; although these symptoms were reported relatively infrequently in the study population, they were associated with headaches that caused the greatest impairment (Silberstein, 1995).

The prevalence of migraine-associated symptoms, particularly nausea and vomiting, has also been estimated by placebo-controlled drug studies (Cady et al., 1991; Friedman et al., 1989; Cerenex Pharmaceuticals, 1993; Chabriat et al., 1994; Tfelt-Hansen, 1993; Tfelt-Hansen and Olesen,

1984; Ziegler et al., 1994). Forty-five percent to 100% of patients had nausea prior to treatment, which was similar to prevalence rates observed in other studies of adult migraineurs. The prevalence of vomiting was much lower but varied dramatically from study to study, as might be anticipated as a result of treatment of the acute migraine attack. Photophobia, when analyzed, occurred in 86% to 97% of patients, while phonophobia was rarely analyzed (Silberstein, 1995).

Silberstein (1995) performed a telephone interview survey of 500 self-reported migraine sufferers. The most commonly reported symptoms associated with migraine, in addition to pain, were nausea, visual problems, and vomiting. Nausea occurred in more than 90% of all migraineurs; nearly one-third of these experienced nausea during every attack. Vomiting occurred in almost 70% of all migraineurs; nearly one-third of these vomited in the majority of attacks. Thirty percent of those who experienced nausea and 42% of those with vomiting indicated that the symptom interfered with their ability to take oral migraine medication. Visual problems and vomiting were also reported to occur in most attacks by 70% and 32% of respondents, respectively. The only other symptom that occurred in more than 20% of respondents in a majority of attacks was sound sensitivity or auditory problems. Some symptoms reported by 10% or less of respondents (light sensitivity, dizziness, neck pain) occurred in a high percentage of their attacks, suggesting that these symptoms may be specific but not sensitive indicators of migraine. Most of the commonly associated symptoms were most often rated as moderate to severe, consistent with the increased severity that would be expected with the more severe headaches in this study (as a result of selection criteria) (Silberstein, 1995).

Nausea and/or vomiting, photophobia, and phonophobia are important criteria for migraine diagnosis, particularly if the headache is not accompanied by aura. Nausea and vomiting also interfere with medication ingestion and were among the principal reasons for a patient discontinuing a specific migraine medication. Gastric emptying can be delayed and oral drug absorption impaired during an attack of migraine (Boyle et al., 1990; Volans, 1978), and vomiting may result in drug loss, thereby compromising the therapeutic effectiveness of orally administered drugs (Silberstein, 1995).

Postdrome

Following the headache, the patient may have impaired concentration or feel tired, washed out, irritable, and listless. Some people feel unusually refreshed or euphoric after an attack. Muscle weakness, aching, and anorexia or food cravings can occur (Blau, 1982).

MIGRAINE VARIANTS

Basilar Migraine

Basilar migraine (1.2.4) was originally called "basilar artery migraine" (Headache Classification Committee of the International Headache Society, 1988) or "Bickerstaff's syndrome" (Bickerstaff, 1987). Although originally believed to be mainly a disorder of adolescent girls, it affects all age groups and both sexes, with the usual female predominance. The aura generally lasts less than 1 hour and is usually followed by a headache that may be occipital. The headache can be associated with nausea and even projectile vomiting. A typical hemianoptic field disturbance can rapidly expand to involve all visual fields, leading at times to temporary blindness. A distinguishing characteristic of basilar migraine is the bilateral nature of many of the associated neurologic events, which helps to differentiate it from more typical migraine. The visual aura is usually followed by one or more of the following symptoms: dysarthria, vertigo, tinnitus, decreased hearing, diplopia, ataxia, bilateral paresthesia, bilateral paresis, and impaired cognition, which, when marked, define confusional migraine. The IHS criteria for basilar migraine require the presence of one or more of the preceding aura symptoms.

Confusional migraine (Hosking, 1988) occurs more commonly in boys than girls, with an incidence of about 5%. It is characterized by a typical aura; a headache, which may be insignificant; and confusion, which may precede, occur with, or follow the headache. The confusion is characterized by inattention, distractibility, and difficulty maintaining speech and other motor activities. Agitation, memory disturbances, obscene utterances, violent behavior, and sedation or a drugged feeling can occur. The electroencephalogram (EEG) may be abnormal during the attack. Single attacks are most common, multiple attacks are rare, and attacks can be triggered by mild head trauma. If the level of consciousness is more profoundly disturbed, migraine stupor lasting 2 to 5 days can occur (Saper and Lossing, 1974). The differential diagnosis includes drug ingestion, metabolic encephalopathies (Reye's syndrome, hypoglycemia), viral encephalitis, the postictal state, and acute psychosis. Confusional migraine is part of the syndrome of migraine, with white matter abnormality linked to chromosome 19 (Chabriat et al., 1995a).

Ophthalmoplegic migraine (1.3) is characterized by at least two attacks associated with ocular cranial nerve palsy (usually the third cranial nerve with a dilated pupil) and unilateral migrainous eye pain. Rarely, the fourth and sixth cranial nerves are involved. The duration of ophthalmoplegia is variable, from hours to months. By definition, a parasellar, retro-orbital cavernous sinus or midcranial fossa lesion must be ruled out. The differential diagnosis includes berry aneurysm, acute sphenoid sinusitis, or sphenoid mucocele. Some cases of ophthalmoplegic migraine fit the criteria for Tolosa-Hunt syndrome of painful ophthalmoplegia (Hansen et al., 1990): steady, gnawing, boring eye pain; involvement of nerves of the cavernous sinus; symptoms lasting days or weeks; spontaneous remission, with recurrent attacks occurring after months or years; computed tomography (CT) or magnetic resonance imaging (MRI) demonstrating confinement to the cavernous sinus; and steroid responsiveness. Mark et al. (1998) reported six patients with typical clinical features of ophthalmoplegic migraine who had enhancement of the cisternal segment of the oculomotor nerve during the acute phase. This was followed by resolution of the enhancement over several weeks as the symptoms resolved. Enhancement can occur in a variety of infectious (Nelson et al., 1992; Pachner et al., 1989; Blake et al., 1995; Schmitt et al., 1993) (Lyme disease, syphilis, coccidioidomycosis, human immunodeficiency virus) and noninfectious (lymphoma, leukemia, sarcoid, Tolosa-Hunt syndrome, Fisher syndrome) inflammatory conditions. A lumber puncture is needed to rule out infections and neoplastic causes. This disorder may be due to a viral infection of the oculomotor nerve similar to Bell's palsy (a viral neuritis with nerve enhancement) (May, 1986). Contrast-enhanced MRI and magnetic resonance angiography (MRA) are the procedures of choice in evaluating patients with oculomotor palsy. If magnetic resonance shows enhancement of the cisternal portion of the oculomotor nerve and lumbar puncture is negative, a presumptuous diagnosis of ophthalmoplegic migraine can be made; but follow-up is necessary to be sure the symptoms resolve. If the magnetic resonance and lumbar puncture are negative, a conventional angiogram may still be necessary to rule out an aneurysm (Mark et al., 1998).

Tolosa-Hunt syndrome (12.1.5) (Headache Classification Committee of the International Headache Society, 1988) is a rare, painful ophthalmoplegia due to a granulomatous inflammation of the cavernous sinus. Diagnosis is based on the combination of one or more episodes of painful ophthalmoplegia with paralysis of the third, fourth, and/or sixth cranial nerves and exclusion of other causes, including aneurysm, diabetes mellitus, paranasal mucocele, parasellar neoplasm, carotid cavernous fistula, sphenoid sinusitus, and other disorders of the cavernous sinus. It lasts an average of 8 weeks untreated, and pain is relieved by corticosteroids within 72 hours. de Arcaya et al. (1999) analyzed CTs and MRIs, with and without contrast enhancement, of the cranium and orbits of patients fulfilling IHS criteria for Tolosa-Hunt syndrome. Computed tomographic scan, with and without contrast enhancement, showed an enlarged cavernous sinus in only one of five patients. In all four patients, MRI was abnormal, showing a convex enlargement of the symptomatic cavernous sinus by an abnormal tissue isointense with gray matter on short TR/TE images and isohypointense on long TR/TE scans. It markedly enhanced after contrast injection and, in two patients, extended into the orbital apex and subtemporal fossa ipsilaterally. Three months after successful treatment with corticosteroids, the abnormal tissue, although diminished in size, was still visible on MRI. It disappeared only after 6 months of treatment. Painful ophthalmoplegia, cavernous sinus enlargement on MRI, and slow resolution with corticosteroid treatment are highly suggestive of Tolosa-Hunt syndrome (de Arcaya et al., 1999).

Hemiplegic Migraine

The IHS (Headache Classification Committee of the International Headache Society, 1988) has subdivided hemiplegic migraine into sporadic and familial forms (1.2.3.), both of which typically begin in childhood and cease with adulthood. This separation may not be justified (Whitty, 1986; Bradshaw and Parsons, 1965). Forty-seven percent of Bradshaw and Parsons' (1965) patients had a family history of migraine; 18% had a family history of hemiplegic migraine. Average age at onset of hemiplegic migraine may be earlier than that of migraine without aura, while the attacks themselves are frequently precipitated by minor head injury. Changes in consciousness ranging from confusion to coma are a feature, especially in childhood, and occurred in 23% of Bradshaw and Parsons' series (1965). The prevalence of hemiplegic migraine is uncertain, varying from 4% to 30% (Whitty, 1986; Selby and Lance, 1960). The differential diagnosis of hemiplegic migraine includes focal seizures, stroke, homocystinuria, and MELAS (mitochondrial encephalopathy, lactic acidosis, and stroke-like episodes) syndrome (Hosking, 1988).

Familial hemiplegic migraine (FHM) is an autosomal dominant, genetically heterogenous form of migraine with aura, with variable penetration (Table 9–9). The aura is characterized by motor weakness of variable intensity. The syndrome includes attacks of

Table 9–9 Familial hemiplegic migraine[a]

Diagnostic criteria
A. Fulfills criteria for 1.2
B. Aura includes some degree of hemiparesis and may be prolonged
C. At least one first-degree relative has identical attacks

[a]Migraine with aura including hemiparesis and where at least one first-degree relative has identical attacks.

migraine without aura, migraine with typical aura, severe episodes with prolonged aura (up to several days or weeks), fever, meningismus, and impaired consciousness ranging from confusion to profound coma. Headache may precede the hemiparesis or be absent. The onset of the hemiparesis may be abrupt and may simulate a stroke (Whitty, 1986). All of Bradshaw and Parsons' (1965) patients had associated paresthesias; 88% had visual auras, and 44% had speech disturbances. Weakness lasted less than 1 hour in 58% of patients; however, it lasted 1 to 3 hours in 14%, 3 to 24 hours in 12%, and between 1 day and 1 week in 16% of patients. The syndrome can change in an affected individual over his or her lifetime. A person who has FHM in adolescence may develop migraine with aura as an adult and migraine without aura later in life (Stewart et al., 1994b).

The headache can be generalized (29%), contralateral (47%), or ipsilateral (22%) to the hemiparesis. Before assessment, 17% of Bradshaw and Parsons' (1965) patients had a single neurologic episode, 37% had between two and six episodes, and the remainder had more than seven attacks. The longer-lasting episodes were associated with more profound weakness and tended to recur less frequently.

In 20% of unselected FHM families, patients can have fixed cerebellar symptoms and signs such as nystagmus and progressive ataxia. Cerebellar ataxia may occur before the first hemiplegic migraine attack and progress independently of the frequency or severity of hemiplegic migraine attacks. All of these families have been linked to chromosome 19 (Tournier-Lasserve, 1999).

Episodic ataxia type 2 (EA2) is also an autosomal dominant disorder, characterized by paroxysmal attacks of ataxia that last 15 minutes to hours or days; provoked by emotional or physical stress, alcohol, or coffee but not by startle; and associated with interictal nystagmus and acetazolamide responsiveness. The gene for 60% of affected families has been localized to the short arm of chromosome 19p13 and cloned (Ophoff et al., 1996). Mutations within CACNA1A, a gene encoding for the α_{1A} subunit of a neuronal P/Q-type calcium channel, cause both FHM and EA2. Another gene for FHM has been mapped to chromosome 1 (Gardner et al., 1997). All EA2 families have been linked to chromosome 19 (Ducros et al., 1997).

Two distinct types of CACNA1A mutation were identified in hemiplegic migraine (missense) and EA2 (truncating). However, Jen et al. (1999) suggest that truncating mutations within CACNA1A may, in some EA2 patients, cause paroxysmal episodes combining ataxia and hemiplegia. Indeed, two of the 13 patients in the pedigree experienced hemiparesis during their ataxic spells. One of these patients had complained since infancy of paroxysmal attacks of vertigo and ataxia accompanied by headaches with nausea and photophobia (Tournier-Lasserve, 1999).

Cerebral Autosomal Dominant Arteriopathy with Subcortical Infarcts and Leukoencephalopathy

Cerebral autosomal dominant arteriopathy with subcortical infarcts and leukoencephalopathy (CADASIL) is an inherited arterial disease of the brain that was originally mapped to chromosome 19 in two unrelated French families (Tournier-Lasserve et al., 1993) and has since been reported in more than 200 families worldwide (Joutel et al., 1996). The complete CADASIL phenotype consists of more than just recurrent episodes of focal brain deficits (recurrent strokes) starting in midadult life, often leading to dementia, residual motor disability, and pseudobulbar palsy. Attacks of migraine with aura occur in 30% and mood disorders in 20% of patients (Ducros et al., 1995; Chabriat et al., 1995a). Most of the strokes are classic lacunar infarcts. All individuals with symptoms have abnormal MRIs with extensive symmetrical areas of increased T2 signals in the white matter and well-delineated hypointense lesions on T1-weighted images suggestive of small infarcts in the deep white matter and basal ganglia (Joutel et al., 1996). Earlier onset, benign prognosis, and normal MRI findings distinguish FHM from CADASIL.

The main clinical feature of CADASIL is recurrent subcortical events, either transient or (more often) permanent, that occur at a mean age of 45 years. However, the vascular presentation is not constant, and other symptoms, such as dementia or migraine with aura and depression, can occur. Although these symptoms are usually associated with a history of recurrent strokes, they may be prominent or only a manifestation of the disease. Subcortical dementia associated with pseudobulbar palsy is the second most common manifestation of CADASIL, occurring in one-third of affected family members and in 90% of subjects before death. It is characterized by frontal-like symptoms, memory impairment, gait disturbances, pyramidal signs, pseudobulbar palsy, and sphincter incontinence. Attacks of migraine with aura were observed in 22% of cases. Its prevalence in the general population is about 6%.

Characteristic MRI abnormalities can be detected before the appearance of symptoms and used to diagnose CADASIL in genetically at-risk family members who have a pattern of autosomal dominant inheritance (Hutchinson et al., 1995).

Chabriat et al. (1995b) used MRI and genetic linkage analysis to study 148 subjects belonging to seven families with CADASIL. Forty-five family members (23 men and 22 women) were clinically affected. The most frequent symptoms included recurrent subcortical ischemic events (84%), progressive or stepwise subcortical dementia with pseudobulbar palsy (31%), migraine with aura (22%), and mood disorders with severe depressive episodes (20%). All symptomatic subjects had prominent signal abnormalities on MRI, with hyperintense lesions on T2-weighted images in the subcortical white matter and basal ganglia (which were also present in 19 asymptomatic subjects). Mean age at onset of symptoms ± standard deviation (SD) was 45 ± 10.6 years, with attacks of migraine with aura occurring earlier in life (38.1 ± 8.03 years) than ischemic events (49.3 ± 10.7 years). Mean age at death was 64.5 ± 10.6 years. On the basis of MRI data, the penetrance of the disease appears to be complete between 30 and 40 years of age.

The arteriopathy underlying the disorder is neither atherosclerotic nor amyloid and involves the media of small cerebral arteries. However, lesions may be observed to a lesser extent in extracerebral arteries, including skin arterioles. Ultrastructural examination reveals abnormal patches of agranular osmiophilic material within the basal membranes of vascular smooth-muscle cells (Joutel et al., 1997). Skin biopsy can be diagnostic.

Joutel et al. (1997) identified *Notch3* as the defective gene in CADASIL. Members of the *Notch* gene family encode evolutionarily conserved transmembrane receptors and are involved in cell fate specification during embryonic development. The *Notch3* gene includes 33 exons encoding a protein of 2,321 amino acids. Its extracellular domain contains 34 epidermal growth factor-like repeats. From data on *Drosophila*, this extracellular domain seems to be involved in ligand binding, whereas the intracellular domain carries the intrinsic signal-transducing activity. Identification of the CADASIL gene provided the basic information needed to set up a direct genotypic diagnostic test (Joutel et al., 1997).

Fifty unrelated patients with CADASIL and 100 healthy controls were screened for mutations along the entire *Notch3* sequence by means of single-strand conformation polymorphism, heteroduplex, and sequence analyses. Strongly stereotyped missense mutations, located within the epidermal growth factor-like repeats in the extracellular domain of *Notch3*, were detected in 45 patients. Clustering of mutations within the two exons encoding the first five epidermal growth factor-like repeats was observed in 32 patients. All of these mutations led to loss or gain of a cysteine residue and, therefore, to an unpaired number of cysteine residues within a given epidermal growth factor-like domain.

None of these mutations was found in the 100 controls (Joutel et al., 1996).

Chabriat et al. (1995a) described one family without evidence of migrainous infarct or prolonged aura in which eight of the 12 examined members of the pedigree had throbbing headache. The disorder is characterized by recurrent headache attacks with many features of migraine. Attacks usually lasted 2 to 48 hours (patients were asymptomatic between attacks) and were preceded by focal neurologic symptoms that developed gradually over 5 to 15 minutes and usually resolved in less than 60 minutes. Paresthesias and unilateral or bilateral blurring of vision were the most frequent of these symptoms. Six patients satisfied the IHS diagnostic criteria for migraine with typical aura, one for a migrainous disorder with aura and one for migraine without aura. Some subjects had unusual and severe attacks on occasion. One had hyperthermia and stupor that resolved in less than 24 hours and was suggestive of basilar migraine. Another had headache, coma, fever, and aseptic meningitis that resolved within 15 days. Most, but not all, of the subjects had striking MRI abnormalities. Numerous areas of decreased signal intensity on T1-weighted images and of increased signal intensity were found in the basal ganglia and the subcortical white matter.

White matter abnormalities (WMAs) have been reported in migraine, particularly migraine with aura. Some believe this results from repeated ischemic insults that could occur during the migrainous auras. However, WMAs were also found in the family described by Chabriat et al. (1995a). Another explanation is that migraine with aura and WMA could be consequences of the same underlying vascular disorder that is present in mitochondrial diseases or antiphospholipid antibody syndrome. A mutation near the CADASIL locus could thus be a new cause of migraine associated with WMA on MRI.

Alternating Hemiplegia of Childhood

Alternating hemiplegia (AH) is a rare disease that begins in infancy (before 18 months of age). The disorder is characterized by sudden, repeated attacks of hemiplegia involving each side alternately, lasting hours to days and associated with dystonic features. During an attack, the child is acutely uncomfortable and has signs of autonomic disturbance. Other paroxysmal phenomena, such as tonic spells, dystonic posturing, choreoathetosis, and nystagmus, can occur with the hemiplegia or independently. This is a progressive disorder that produces a fixed motor deficit, retardation, and dyskinesias. Fifty percent of patients with AH have a family history of migraine. In contrast to AH, hemiplegic migraine is not a progressive disorder and is not associated with dystonia or retardation. Flunarizine was shown to be effective in AH in a double-blind controlled study (Casaer, 1989).

Migraine in Children

Children frequently have migraine or TTH. Bille (1962) studied the occurrence of headache in 8,993 school children in Uppsala, Sweden, and found that headache prevalence increased from 39% at age 6 to over 70% by age 15. Migraine prevalence (probably underestimated by overstrict criteria), equal in boys and girls, was 3.9%. Goldstein and Chen (1982) reviewed a number of reports of migraine prevalence in children and adults. Migraine prevalence was equal in boys and girls prior to puberty. After puberty, the expected female predominance was observed. This will be covered in Chapter 25.

TREATMENT OF MIGRAINE

Principles of Care and General Approach

Effective migraine treatment begins with making an accurate diagnosis, ruling out alternate causes, ordering appropriate studies, and addressing the headache's impact. An accurate diagnosis should be established prior to instituting treatment because a medication specific for migraine may be without value or even harmful if used to treat a condition that looks like, but is not, migraine. For example, a patient with an acute symptomatic head-ache due to a stroke or SAH may respond to a triptan but the neurologic deficit may be adversely influenced.

Once a diagnosis has been made, patients benefit from a full explanation. Patients with recurrent headache often believe that their complaints have not been taken seriously. They are often worried that they have a life-threatening condition, such as a brain tumor or an aneurysm. Just as they want headache relief, patients want to know what is wrong with them (Packard, 1979) and to be assured that the physician is committed to relieving their distress. Patients are relieved to find out that their headache is neither secondary to an organic disorder nor psychogenic.

Migraine varies widely in its frequency, severity, and impact on the patient's quality of life. A treatment plan should consider not only the patient's diagnosis, symptoms, and any coexistent or comorbid conditions, but also the patient's expectations, needs, and goals. Deal with the patient's most disturbing symptoms in the most appropriate way (Lipton and Silberstein, 1994). Patients have the expectation and the right to participate in their treatment. Patient commitment improves compliance and fosters the patient–physician relationship. Patients need to be informed of the goals of treatment, the purpose of the various components of their treatment plan, the need for follow-up care, and the adverse effects of the medication. Meeting treatment needs and patient preferences may not always be possible. It is often not possible to fulfill the goals of both complete relief and maintenance of normal function. Patients may prefer one to the other depending on the situation; i.e., they might accept sedation from a rescue medication but not from a first-line therapy.

Comorbidity is the presence of two or more disorders, the association of which is more likely than chance. Conditions that occur in migraineurs with a higher prevalence than coincidence include stroke, epilepsy, mitral valve prolapse, Raynaud's syndrome, and certain psychologic disorders, including depression, mania, anxiety, and panic (Table 9–10). Co-occurring (any other disorder present) and comorbid disease and the presence

Table 9–10 Migraine comorbid disease

Cardiovascular
   Hyper- or hypotension
   Raynaud's disease
   Mitral valve prolapse
   Angina/myocardial infarction
   Stroke
Psychiatric
   Depression
   Mania
   Panic disorder
   Anxiety disorder
Neurologic
   Epilepsy
   Positional vertigo
Gastrointestinal
   Functional bowel disorders
Other
   Asthma
   Allergies

of nonheadache symptoms present both therapeutic opportunities and limitations. For example, if nausea and vomiting (both migraine-associated symptoms) are prominent, a non-oral route of drug administration is needed.

Migraineurs should be educated about their condition and its treatment and encouraged to participate in their own management. Patients are given a headache calendar to accurately establish the frequency, intensity, and duration of headache and the presence of associated symptoms such as aura or nausea and vomiting. Provoking factors, such as menses, missed meals, or too little sleep, can be identified. Once a treatment program has been prescribed, the calendar can be used to show the effectiveness of both acute and preventive treatments (Dalessio, 1987).

A comprehensive headache treatment plan includes the following: (1) education and reassurance; (2) prevention of attacks by avoidance of triggers; (3) use of nonpharmacologic treatments such as relaxation, biofeedback, and lifestyle regulation (maintaining a regular schedule, getting adequate sleep and exercise, and stopping smoking); (4) treatment of the acute attack to relieve pain and impairment and stop progression; (5) long-term preventive therapy to reduce attack frequency, severity, and duration; (6) use of physical and alternative medicine when appropriate; and (7) periodic reassessment and reconsideration of the treatment plan.

Avoidance of Provoking/Activating Factors (Triggers)

Migraineurs are physiologically and perhaps psychologically hyperresponsive to a variety of internal and external stimuli, including hormonal changes, dietary factors, environmental changes, sensory stimuli, and stress (Saper, 1983; Silberstein and Silberstein, 1990b) (Table 9–11). Too much or too little sleep, missed or delayed meals, menstruation, alcohol, food and food additives, chemical and drug ingestion and withdrawal, light glare, and odors have been reported to provoke or activate migraine in susceptible individuals. Their association is based on anecdotal data and reports of adverse drug reactions. The fact that these stimuli are associated with headache does not prove causality or eliminate the need to consider other etiologies. Premonitory symptoms of migraine (chocolate craving, anxiety, exhilaration, or depression) can be mistaken for migraine triggers. Putative migraine triggers may not consistently incite a migraine attack because the migraine threshold may vary with time, depending on intrinsic or extrinsic factors not yet fully understood. This variability may make a migraineur more sensitive to trig-

Table 9–11 Migraine triggers

Diet
   Hunger
   Alcohol
   Additives
   Certain foods
Chronobiologic
   Sleep (Too much or too little)
   Schedule change
Hormonal changes
   Menstruation
Environmental factors
   Light glare
   Odors
   Altitude
   Weather change
Head or neck pain
   Of another cause
Physical exertion
   Exercise
   Sex
Stress and anxiety
   Letdown
Head trauma

ger factors at certain times than at others. Several trigger factors occurring within close proximity may be more likely to elicit a migraine than a single trigger factor.

Van den Bergh et al. (1987) collected information on provoking factors in 217 migraineurs. Most patients (85%) were aware of the presence of one or more factors. The most prevalent activating factors were specific foods (44.7%), menstruation (49%), alcoholic beverages (51.0%), and stress (48.8%). Because common events happen frequently, the association between a headache and an exposure to a substance may be mere coincidence.

Coincidental Headache

Coincidental headaches occur on the basis of chance. In a population-based study, 1-day point prevalence for any headache was 11% in men and 22% in women (Rasmussen et al., 1991b). Headache can be a symptom of a systemic disease, and drugs given to treat the condition will be associated with headache. For example, drugs used to treat the common cold may have headache identified incorrectly as an adverse drug reaction since headache can be a symptom of a cold. In acute migraine drug trials, headache as well as other associated symptoms are listed as adverse drug reactions despite the fact that they are symptoms of the disorder and not the result of treatment (Silberstein, 1998a).

Reverse Causality

Premonitory symptoms of migraine (chocolate craving, anxiety, exhilaration, or depression) can mistakenly be believed to be migraine triggers. Thus, the desire for and the consumption of the food may be part of the migraine complex and not a migraine trigger (Silberstein, 1998a; Saper, 1983).

Interaction Headache

Some disorders might predispose to drug-, food-, or chemical-related headache or other adverse drug reaction. Alone, neither the drug nor the condition would produce head-

ache. A nonsteroidal anti-inflammatory drug (NSAID) may produce headache by inducing aseptic meningitis in susceptible individuals; a lactose-intolerant individual might develop a headache after drinking milk (Silberstein, 1998a).

Causal

Acute or chronic drug, food, or chemical exposure may be causally related to the headache (Silberstein, 1998a).

Diet

The role that food allergy plays in migraine is undetermined. The most common cause of what patients commonly call "food allergy" is food *aversion*, a psychologic response to the food itself (Bix et al., 1984). Most food reactions are chemically mediated, e.g., lactose intolerance (Bayless et al., 1975); nitrites ("hot dog headache") (Raskin, 1981); monosodium glutamate, which is believed to be responsible for Chinese restaurant syndrome (Schaumberg et al., 1969); red wine (Littlewood et al., 1988); other alcohol (Raskin, 1981); and perhaps aspartame (Koehler and Glaros, 1988; Schiffman et al., 1987). Chocolate is probably not a migraine-provoking factor (Moffett et al., 1974) and in a recent double-blind study was not found to be more likely to provoke a migraine headache than carob (Marcus et al., 1997).

Ethanol, alone or in combination with congeners (as in wine or liquor), can induce headache in susceptible individuals, often within hours of ingestion (Olesen, 1984). In the United Kingdom, red wine is more likely to trigger migraine than white, while in France and Italy white wine is more likely to produce headache than red. Headaches are more likely to develop in response to white wine if red coloring matter has been added (Masyczek and Pugh, 1983). Migraineurs who believed that red wine (but not plain alcohol) provoked their headaches were challenged either with red wine or a vodka mixture of equivalent alcoholic content. Red wine provoked migraine in 9/11 subjects, vodka in 0/11. Neither provoked headache in other migraine subjects or controls (Littlewood et al., 1988). It is not known which component of red wine triggers headache. Some have suggested that the specific phenolic flavonoids may be the trigger (Littlewood et al., 1987). Headache related to red wine may be blocked by prostaglandin synthesis inhibitors (Kaufman and Starr, 1991).

The use of elimination diets and clinical ecology is controversial (Egger et al., 1983; MacDonald et al., 1989; Ferguson, 1990; Jewett et al., 1990). Most diet-restriction studies have lacked adequate control groups. Rather than having a "placebo" diet to control for expectation, they have used the patient's usual diet as a baseline control (Salfield et al., 1987). These studies frequently show that headaches are decreased on the restrictive diet compared to baseline (Scharff and Marcus, 1999; Applebaum, 1984; Bentley et al., 1984; Podell, 1984). Protein-, tryptophan-, and carbohydrate-rich diets have been recommended (Hasselmark et al., 1987; Carter et al., 1985).

Medina and Diamond (1978) compared an ad libitum diet to a diet high in vasoactive amines and to a diet low in vasoactive amines in 41 migraineurs. They found no differences in headache indices between these diets or between a free diet, a tyramine-free diet, and a tyramine-containing diet (24 migraineurs) (Medina and Diamond, 1977).

Dietary manipulation can result in headache improvement, regardless of the type of diet used. Controlled draconian studies have identified differences between restricted and control diets. Ninety-five migraineurs from a neurology clinic were placed on a strict elimination diet (McQueen et al., 1989). Thirty-six (37.9%) dropped out and 37 became headache-free for at least 2 weeks. Nineteen of these 37 individuals then participated in double-blind challenges and went on to the test diet. Response rates to the dietary challenges varied from 21% to 58%. The response to the two placebos was 20% (sucrose) and 32% (starch), respectively. An appropriate diet based on the challenge was then administered to the 19 subjects, this time with a control diet consisting of trigger foods to which the individuals had responded during

the challenges. Subjects were randomly assigned to either the approved diet or the trigger diet and crossed over to the other diet after 4 weeks. A 50% reduction in headache occurred in nine subjects in the trigger-elimination diet and in three subjects in the trigger-inclusion diet. Thus, only a small subset of migraineurs could benefit from a strict diet.

Egger et al. (1983) studied 99 children with severe, frequent migraine who had been referred to a tertiary-care center. Eighty-eight were able to complete an oligoantigenic diet; of these, 48 were atopic, 41 were hyperactive, and 14 had seizures. Only 40/74 completed a double-blind trial. Twenty-six of 40 responded to a previously identified food. However, the challenges were not carried out under medical supervision and not all of the 40 subjects developed headaches.

MacDonald et al. (1989) used an elimination diet in 60 children with migraine. At most, 15% of the children were found to be food-intolerant. Twenty-three percent showed no benefit from the diet, 28% were noncompliant, 13% had a spontaneous remission as soon as they were given details of the diet, and 17% had a remission while on the diet but did not respond to food challenges. MacDonald et al. (1989) felt that the diet was expensive, difficult to administer, nutritionally inadequate, and not of major benefit in treating migraine.

Practitioners have diagnosed food intolerance by unusual techniques of laboratory and clinical investigation, such as hair analysis, cytotoxic blood tests, iridology, and sublingual and injection provocation tests. Jewett et al. (1990), in a double-blind manner, attempted to reproduce allergic symptoms, including headache, by intradermally injecting extracts of suspected allergens. They found that the diagnostic and neutralization procedures, which had been assumed to be fully effective in unblinded use, were due to the placebo response.

It had been believed that vasoactive amines, such as tyramine and phenylethylamines, were responsible for triggering migraine in certain patients. It was suggested that a tyramine metabolism–conjugating defect was present in some migraine patients (Glover et al., 1983; Youdim et al., 1971). A clinical trial was devised to determine if dietary triggers in migraine and other headaches could be related to patient suggestibility or allergic mechanisms. While a subset of migraine-with-aura patients did have headaches related to specific foods, this did not correlate with apparent allergy mediation (Nattero et al., 1991).

Previous studies had suggested a correlation between foods that reportedly triggered attacks in migraineurs and the levels of the vasoactive amines present. However, recent work utilizing current technology suggests that there is no link between foods that trigger migraine and their vasoactive amine content. Any effect seen by foods as a trigger is probably coincidental or purely idiosyncratic (Mosniam et al., 1996; Shulman and Walker, 1999).

Thus, based upon current data, most migraineurs do not require severely restricted diets but they should avoid foods or additives that they feel might provoke their headaches. Migraineurs should consume alcohol, particularly red wine, with caution. They should avoid large amounts of monosodium glutamate, aspartamine, and perhaps cured meats (nitrites). They should not skip meals. The value of avoiding strong cheeses, pickled herring, chicken liver, and chocolate is unproven; these should be restricted only when patients demonstrate a reliable pattern of migraine in conjunction with eating these foods. Patients with a lactase deficiency should use supplemental lactase (Lactaid). Elimination diets are rarely necessary.

Sleep

Alterations in chronobiology, such as too much or too little sleep, can provoke migraine, as can shift work or jet lag. Patients with migraine need to maintain proper sleep practices; i.e., keep a regular bedtime and avoid sleeping in on weekends. It has been theorized that migraineurs have a defect in chronobiologic synchronizing systems (Saper et al., 1993).

Hormonal Factors and Migraine

MENSTRUAL MIGRAINE

Menstrual migraine is defined as an attack occurring 1 day before and up to 4 days after the onset of menses. Premenstrual migraine occurs 7 days to 1 day before the onset of menses. Migraine attacks occur around the menses in 60% of women and exclusively during this period (true menstrual migraine) in 14% (Epstein et al., 1975). Premenstrually, it may be accompanied by other features of premenstrual dysphoric disorder (PMDD), including mood changes, backache, nausea, and breast tenderness and swelling (American Psychiatric Association, 1994). During menstruation, migraine is often associated with dysmenorrhea. Menstrual migraine is most likely due to estrogen withdrawal, which may trigger migraine attacks in susceptible women (Silberstein and Merriam, 1997; Somerville, 1971).

MIGRAINE AND PREGNANCY

Migraine may worsen in the first trimester of pregnancy but significantly improve during later pregnancy. Twenty-five percent of women have no change. Women with a history of menstrual migraine typically have an improvement of all of their migraine types with pregnancy, perhaps due to sustained high estrogen levels (Lance and Anthony, 1966; Somerville, 1972; Bousser et al., 1990; Ratinahirana et al., 1990; Silberstein and Lipton, 1996).

MIGRAINE AND MENOPAUSE

Migraine prevalence decreases with advancing age (Goldstein and Chen, 1982). Menopause may bring regression, worsening, or no change in migraine. Estrogen replacement therapy can exacerbate migraine or prevent natural improvement (Silberstein and Merriam, 1997). Women with natural menopause often show improvement in their migraines, while women with surgical menopause often worsen (Neri et al., 1993).

MIGRAINE AND HORMONAL CONTRACEPTION

The oral contraceptives (OCs) that are most commonly used in the United States contain combinations of estrogen and progestin and are taken 21 days each month. The older high-estrogen OCs had an increased risk of stroke, but this risk has been significantly reduced with the new low-estrogen formulations. Progestin-only OCs are also available, as are implantable and injectable progestins (Silberstein and Merriam, 1997).

Combination OCs can induce, change, or alleviate headache. A first migraine attack can be provoked by OCs, most often in women with a family history of migraine. Existing migraine may be exacerbated, and headaches may predictably occur on days off the OC. Headaches may become more severe and/or frequent and may be associated with neurologic symptoms. They may become refractory to standard treatment. Generally, data from neurologic or migraine clinics show increased incidence, severity, and refractoriness of migraine in OC users; however, results from contraceptive clinics and general practitioners are more favorable (Silberstein and Merriam, 1997).

Women with cardiovascular or cerebrovascular risk factors or moderate to severe neurologic events in migraine, especially those who smoke, should avoid OCs. Progestin-only hormonal contraception may be safer but probably aggravates headache (Silberstein and Merriam, 1997).

Other Provoking Phenomena

Environmental factors, including weather or temperature change, light glare, pungent odors, and high altitude are cited as provoking migraine headaches in susceptible individuals (Van den Bergh et al., 1987). Head and neck pain of another cause may also provoke migraine. Physical exertion from exercise or sexual activity can incite headaches (Blau, 1987). Stress and anxiety, particularly the poststress letdown phase, can precipitate a migraine headache, as can head trauma (Saper, 1983; Diamond, 1964; Raskin, 1988; Blau, 1987; Van den Bergh et al., 1987; Speed, 1989; Lance, 1982). Some headache experts believe that most migraine attacks oc-

cur from intrinsic provocation or timing not related to external events.

Nonpharmacologic Treatment

Behavioral interventions that we believe are of benefit for migraineurs include regular exercise, good health practices, regular mealtimes, adequate sleep, and maintaining accustomed patterns of activity (Saper, 1983). Chronobiologic phenomena may play an important role in provoking migraine. Migraineurs are less capable of adjusting to changes in expected external stimuli, such as mealtimes, stress, or awakening and retiring times. Attempt to regulate the patient's daily activities of living. Meals should be at approximately the same time every day, as should retiring and awakening times. Weekends should approximate the rest of the week, including breakfast time and the amount of food taken early in the morning.

Nonpharmacologic techniques of relaxation training, biofeedback, and formal psychotherapy are useful in selected patients. Biofeedback and relaxation therapy also serve to engage patients in cognitive behavioral therapy. These techniques are especially useful in children, pregnant women, and individuals in whom stress is a trigger. With an acute attack, the patient should avoid uncomfortable sensory stimuli and, if possible, retire to a dark, quiet room. Ice packs or heat may be useful adjuncts.

Biofeedback using electromyography (EMG) and thermal and hand-warming techniques may be helpful for some migraineurs. Patients who are not depressed, do not have chronic daily headache or medication-overuse headache, and are well motivated can use these techniques with trained technicians and will probably benefit from them (Diamond et al., 1979; Duke University and Center for Clinical Health Policy Research, 1999; Diamond and Montrose, 1984).

Since migraine is a recurrent episodic disorder, periodic follow-up medical management is required. At each visit, the benefits and detrimental effects of treatments should be reviewed and the headache calendar examined. Routine blood work, blood levels of medication, and drug screens can be obtained if necessary (Dalessio, 1987).

Pharmacotherapy

General Considerations

The pharmacologic treatment of migraine may be acute (abortive) or preventive (prophylactic), and patients with frequent severe headaches often require both approaches. Acute treatment attempts to relieve or stop the progression of an attack or the pain and impairment once an attack has begun. Preventive therapy is given, even in the absence of a headache, in an attempt to reduce the frequency and severity of anticipated attacks. Acute treatment is appropriate for most attacks and should be used a maximum of 2 to 3 days a week. Preventive therapy is used more selectively. Before starting a fertile woman on any medication, it is important to discuss pregnancy and the need for effective means of birth control.

Neuropharmacology of Migraine Treatment

SEROTONIN

Serotonin, or 5-hydroxytryptamine (5-HT), is widely distributed throughout the body, with major concentrations in the gastrointestinal tract (90%), the platelets (8%), and the brain. At least three distinct types of molecular structure are "recognized" by 5-HT: seven guanine nucleotide–binding G protein–coupled receptors, one ligand-gated ion channel, and one transporter (Table 9–12) (Silberstein, 1994; Mamounas et al., 1992; Hoyer et al., 1994; Miguel and Hamon, 1992; Weinshank et al., 1992; Waeber and Palacios, 1991; Palacios et al., 1991).

The 5-HT$_1$ family of inhibitory G protein–linked receptors has five heterogeneous subtypes: A, B, D, E, and F. The 5-HT$_2$ G protein–linked receptors stimulate phosphoinositol hydrolysis. Other G protein–coupled receptors are 5-HT$_4$, 5-HT$_5$, 5-HT$_6$, and

Table 9–12 Serotonin (5-HT) Receptors

G protein–coupled receptors
  5-HT$_1$
  5-HT$_2$
  5-HT$_3$
  5-HT$_4$
  5-ht$_5$
  5-ht$_6$
  5-ht$_7$
Ligand-gated ion channels
  5-HT$_3$
Transporters
  5-HT uptake site

5-HT$_7$. The 5-HT$_3$ receptor is coupled to an ion channel (Silberstein, 1994; Branchek et al., 1991; Hoyer et al., 1994; Humphrey et al., 1993; Monsma et al., 1992; Ruat et al., 1993).

The 5-HT$_1$ family subtypes can be grouped together based on the absence of introns in the cloned genes, common G-protein transduction systems [including inhibition of adenylate cyclase, with a reduction in cyclic adenosine monophosphate (cAMP) production], elevation of intracellular calcium concentrations, and stimulation of phospholipase C in transfected cells.

The 5-HT$_{1A}$ receptor has a high selective affinity for 8-Hydroxy-2-2(di-n-propylamino) tetralin (8-OH-DPAT). Activated human 5-HT$_{1A}$ receptors expressed in HeLa cells inhibit forskolin-stimulated adenylate cyclase activity. Drugs such as buspirone act as agonists in cell lines with a large number of receptors and as antagonists in cell lines with few receptors, suggesting that this property of a ligand is dependent on receptor density (Humphrey et al., 1993; Peroutka, 1993).

The 5-HT$_{1D}$ receptor subfamily is comprised of two closely related subtypes, 5-HT$_{1D}$ and 5-HT$_{1B}$. Both human and rodent B and D receptors have been cloned. The rodent 5-HT$_{1B}$ receptor is 97% homologous to the 5-HT$_{1B}$ human receptor, which had been called the 5-HT$_{1D\beta}$ receptor, with the original 5-HT$_{1D}$ receptor being called 5-HT$_{1D\alpha}$.

Both 5-HT$_{1D}$ and 5-HT$_{1B}$ mRNA are expressed in human trigeminal ganglia. However, immunoreactivity to 5-HT$_{1D}$ receptors is present on trigeminal nerve endings, while

5-HT$_{1B}$ immunoreactivity is present on cranial blood vessels (Beer et al., 1993; Longmore et al., 1997). Triptans and ergot alkaloids have high affinity for both the human 5-HT$_{1B}$ and 5-HT$_{1D}$ receptors (Waeber and Palacios, 1991; Russell and Olesen, 1995).

The cloned human 5-HT$_{1E}$ receptor has low affinity for 5-carboxamidotriptamine (5-CT) and sumatriptan, unlike other 5-HT$_1$ receptors (McAllister et al., 1992; Zgombick et al., 1992). The cloned human 5-HT$_{1F}$ receptor, like its closest genetic relative the 5-HT$_{1E}$ receptor, has low affinity for 5-CT but differs in its high affinity for sumatriptan (Adham et al., 1993). The 5-HT$_{1F}$ receptor does not mediate vasoconstriction. The 5-HT$_{1F}$ receptor has been localized using autoradiography to areas of the human brain associated with pain transmission (trigeminal nucleus caudalis, substantia gelatinosa of the spinal cord). The density of 5-HT$_{1F}$ receptors in these areas is greater than that of 5-HT$_{1D}$ receptors (Connor and Beattie, 1999).

A selective 5-HT$_{1F}$ receptor agonist, LY334370, which shows about 100-fold selectivity for 5-HT$_{1F}$ over other 5-HT$_{1B}$ and 5-HT$_{1D}$ receptors, has been identified (Johnson et al., 1997). This compound inhibits dural plasma protein extravasation in guinea pigs at very low doses.

Alniditan has high affinity for 5-HT$_{1B}$ and 5-HT$_{1D}$ receptors but, in contrast to sumatriptan, relatively low 5-HT$_{1F}$ receptor affinity. Alniditan is more potent than sumatriptan at blocking neurogenic plasma protein extravasation in the dura of anesthetized rats (Limmroth et al., 1997). Thus, 5-HT$_{1F}$ receptor activity is not necessary but could be sufficient for antimigraine activity (Connor and Beattie, 1999).

The 5-HT$_2$ receptors (5-HT$_{2A}$, 5-HT$_{2B}$, 5-HT$_{2C}$) (Table 9–12) have close sequence homology, similar intron and exon gene products, the same G protein–linked transduction system (stimulation of phospholipase C), and similar operational profiles. The classic 5-HT$_2$ receptor is now called 5-HT$_{2A}$. The 5-HT$_{2B}$ receptor is the new name for the 5-HT$_{2F}$ fundus receptor. The 5-HT$_{1C}$ receptor, originally named a "1" receptor based on its high affinity for serotonin, has been renamed the 5-HT$_{2C}$ receptor because of its second-messenger and operational properties. The human 5-HT$_{2A}$, 5-HT$_{2B}$, and 5-HT$_{2C}$ receptors are found in the CNS.

The 5-HT$_3$ receptors are distinct as they belong to the ligand-gated ion channel receptor superfamily. Selective 5-HT$_3$ receptor antagonists are antiemetics and may be useful for irritable bowel syndrome (Humphrey et al., 1993; Peroutka, 1993; Fozard, 1992).

The 5-HT$_4$ receptors are G protein–coupled receptors positively linked to adenylate cyclase (Silberstein, 1994) and were first characterized in the CNS. Activation of 5-HT$_4$ receptors may have a role in learning and memory, anxiolysis, and analgesia, with proconceptive as well as antinociceptive effects. It has yet to be determined whether there is any role for 5-HT$_4$ receptors in migraine pathogenesis or for selective ligands in migraine treatment (Connor and Beattie, 1999).

The 5-HT$_5$ receptor is subdivided into 5-ht$_{5A}$ and 5-ht$_{5B}$ subtypes. Their signal-transduction pathway(s) and physiologic roles are unclear. The cloned 5-ht$_6$ receptor is positively coupled to adenylate cyclase and expressed within the CNS (Hoyer et al., 1994; Hoyer and Martin, 1997). It is abundant in extrapyramidal and limbic areas, consistent with a role in the serotonergic control of motor function and mood, respectively. The antipsychotic activity of some neuroleptic agents (e.g., clozapine) may be due to an interaction with 5-ht$_6$ receptors (Roth et al., 1994).

The 5-HT$_7$ receptor has now been cloned and sequenced and its functional properties characterized. It is positively coupled to adenylate cyclase in both neuronal and nonneuronal tissue. The 5-HT$_7$ receptor is the previously described "5-HT$_1$-like" receptor, mediating smooth-muscle relaxation. Activation of the 5-HT$_7$ may be involved in cranial vasodilation and nociceptive processing (Connor and Beattie, 1999; Watson and Girdlestone, 1996; Eglen et al., 1997).

SEROTONIN AND MIGRAINE

The evidence linking 5-HT to migraine is circumstantial. During a migraine attack, platelet 5-HT decreases, urinary 5-HT increases in some patients, and 5-hydroxyindole acetic acid (5-HIAA, a major metabolite of 5-HT) may increase (Ferrari et al., 1989). These changes in 5-HT are most likely epiphenomena since changes in plasma 5-HT levels are probably not of clinical significance in regulating cerebral arterial tone. Other supporting evidence is the observation that headache can be precipitated by reserpine, a 5-HT releaser; relieved by 5-HT or 5-HT$_1$ agonists; and blocked by pretreatment with methysergide, a 5-HT$_2$ antagonist (Silberstein, 1994; Anthony et al., 1967; Ferrari et al., 1989; Ferrari and Saxena, 1993b; Fozard, 1982; Kimball et al., 1960; Lance, 1992; Somerville, 1976).

Headaches similar to migraine can be triggered by 5-HT-releasing agents such as fenfluramine or reserpine and exacerbated by selective inhibition of 5-HT reuptake (Fozard, 1982). Metachlorophenylpiperazine (mCPP), a metabolite of trazodone, can trigger migraine, conceivably by activating the 5-HT$_{2B}$ or 5-HT$_{2C}$ receptors (Fozard and Gray, 1989). Infusion of 5-HT has been said to abort a migraine attack, but this could not be replicated by Somerville (1976). Agonists of 5-HT$_{1D}$ such as ergotamine, dihydroergotamine (DHE), and the triptans can abort an acute migraine attack. This is not evidence for 5-HT deficiency as their effectiveness is due in part to (1) agonism of 5-HT$_1$ inhibitory heteroreceptors on the trigeminal nerve blocking neurogenic inflammation and pain transmission (Moskowitz, 1990) and (2) their direct inhibitory effects on pain transmission in the trigeminal nucleus caudalis (Goadsby and Hoskin, 1996; Cumberbatch et al., 1997). The centrally penetrant triptans and DHE have been shown to bind to and inhibit the activity of the nucleus caudalis of the trigeminal complex in the brain stem (Goadsby and Gundlach, 1991). The drugs also are vasoconstrictors and close arteriovenous anastomoses (AVAs). The relevance of this to their mechanism of action is unclear.

Ergotamine, DHE, and the triptans have affinity for the 5-HT$_{1B}$ and 5-HT$_{1D}$ receptors. They have variable affinity for the 5-HT$_{1E}$ and 5-H$_{1F}$ receptors. Ergotamine and DHE also bind to the 5-HT$_2$, α_1- and α_2-noradrenergic, and dopamine receptors. The acute antimigraine action of both classes of drugs is probably related to their high affinity and agonism for the 5-HT$_1$ receptor. Some believe that a selective 1D neuronal mechanism is all that is needed, and others suggest that 1B agonism is required.

PNU 142633 is a highly selective 5HT$_{1D}$ agonist that has the expected pharmacologic effects on biochemical processes. However, the drug was comparable to placebo in a placebo-controlled double-blind trial (McCall, 1999). The 5-HT$_{1F}$ receptor agonists, which are devoid of vasoconstrictive activity, have antimigraine activity (Johnson et al., 1997).

Stimulation of trigeminal neurons results in the release of substance P, calcitonin gene–related peptide (CGRP), and neurokinin A and in neurogenically induced inflammation in the rat dura mater. Specific migraine drugs (ergotamine, DHE, and the triptans) that are agonists at presynaptic 5-HT$_{1D}$ and/or 5-HT$_{1F}$ receptors inhibit the release of these neuropeptides, blocking neurogenic inflammation (Saito et al., 1988a; Connor and Beattie, 1999). Methysergide works in this model only after chronic administration; this is consistent with its clinical usefulness as a prophylactic antimigraine drug (Moskowitz, 1990). The NSAIDs block neurogenic inflammation by a direct effect on dural blood vessels (see Chapter 5).

Dihydroergotamine (Goadsby and Gundlach, 1991) and the brain-penetrant triptans pass through the blood–brain barrier and label nuclei in the brain stem and spinal cord that are intimately involved in pain transmission and modulation. The trigeminal caudalis nucleus, the major relay nucleus for head and face pain, is activated by stimulation of the sagittal sinus; this activity is transmitted to the thalamus. Both ergots and the brain-penetrant triptans (and sumatriptan after disruption of the blood–brain barrier), in clinically relevant doses, suppress this activation. These data strongly suggest that the specific migraine drugs exert their antimigraine effect in part by a receptor-mediated neural pathway in the CNS with inhibition of pain transmission (Lance, 1986). (Sumatriptan may access the CNS through a more porous blood–

brain barrier during a migraine attack, see Chapter 5.)

Migraine-specific drugs constrict meningeal, dural, cerebral, and pial vessels by stimulating vascular 5-HT$_{1B}$ receptors (Ferrari and Saxena, 1993a; Longmore et al., 1997; Humphrey and Feniuk, 1991). They do not have an effect on cerebral hemispheric blood flow (Hachinski et al., 1978; Andersen et al., 1987), which suggests that their effect in migraine is independent of any cerebrovascular vasoconstrictive properties in the arterioles. The ergots and triptans close cerebral AVAs in cats and dogs. It has been proposed that migraine is due to the opening of these shunts in humans, but there are no strong supporting data for this theory (Spierings, 1984). The efficacy of the selective 5HT$_{1F}$ receptor agonists suggests that vasoconstriction is not necessary for migraine efficacy.

Before the characterization of 5-HT$_2$ subtypes, it was believed that 5-HT$_2$ (now 5-HT$_{2A}$) receptor antagonism was required for preventive drugs to be effective. The efficacy of the classic serotonin antagonist prophylactic drugs pizotifen, cyproheptadine, and methysergide had been ascribed to their 5-HT$_2$ receptor antagonism. However, there is no correlation between their 5-HT$_{2A}$ receptor affinity and clinical effectiveness. This suggests that 5-HT$_{2A}$ receptor binding is not relevant. Supporting evidence comes from the observation that some 5-HT$_{2A}$ receptor antagonists, such as mianserin, sergolexole, ketanserin, and ICI 169,369, are not effective migraine preventives (Silberstein, 1994; Fozard, 1982, 1990).

The antiserotonin migraine-preventive drugs are potent 5-HT$_{2B}$ and 5-HT$_{2C}$ receptor antagonists, while mCPP, a 5-HT$_{2B}$ and 5-HT$_{2C}$ receptor agonist, induces migraine in susceptible individuals (Brewerton et al., 1988; Gordon et al., 1993; Silberstein et al., 1992; Baxter et al., 1995). Methysergide, cyproheptadine, and pizotifen, effective migraine prophylactic drugs, are 5-HT$_{2B}$ and 5-HT$_{2C}$ receptor antagonists, while ketanserin, a selective 5-HT$_{2A}$ and a poor 5-HT$_{2B}$ and 5-HT$_{2C}$ receptor antagonist, is not (Fozard and Kalkman, 1994; Kalkman, 1999; Fozard, 1995). Methysergide, pizotifen, cy-

proheptadine, amitriptyline, propranolol, ketanserin, ritanserin, and mianserin do not discriminate between 5-HT$_{2B}$ and 5-HT$_{2C}$ sites (Kalkman, 1999). The average daily prophylactic human doses of the drugs correlate with their affinity for both 5-HT$_{2B}$ and 5-HT$_{2C}$ receptors (Fozard and Kalkman, 1994; Kalkman, 1999). Ketanserin (Winther, 1995), which lacks affinity for both the 5-HT$_{2B}$ and the 5-HT$_{2C}$ receptors, is not an effective preventive drug.

Brewerton et al. (1988) studied subjects with a prior personal or family history of migraine and found that mCPP, a major metabolite of the antidepressants trazodone and nefazodone, induces migraine hours after the immediate pharmacologic response to the drug (monitored by elevation of plasma cortisol and prolactin) is over. Gordon et al. (1993) used a lower dose of oral mCPP than Brewerton et al. (1988) and found a similar delay in headache onset. Gordon et al. (1993) found that mCPP induced headache in both migraineurs (five of eight) and nonmigraine controls (four of ten). No significant differences were found between the migraineurs and normal subjects in terms of their neuroendocrine or headache responses to mCPP, but there were highly significant associations between the cortisol responses and headache severity and duration. The increases in cortisol and body temperature induced by mCPP in humans can be abolished by 5-HT$_{2B/2C}$ receptor antagonists such as ritanserin (Seibyl et al., 1991), metergoline (Mueller et al., 1986; Kahn et al., 1990; Pigott et al., 1991), and methysergide (Kahn et al., 1990).

Pizotifen and methylergometrine are potent rabbit jugular vein endothelial cell 5-HT$_2$ receptor antagonists. The RNA for 5-HT$_{2B}$ receptors is expressed in the endothelial cells of human cerebral vessels (Bouchelet et al., 1996). Fozard (1990, 1995) has speculated that 5-HT$_{2B}$ or 5-HT$_{2C}$ receptor activation by mCPP or endogenously released 5-HT could dilate cerebral vessels. Vasodilation, however, is neither necessary nor sufficient to cause headache (Moskowitz, 1992a,b), but endothelium-derived nitric oxide (NO) can activate sensory trigeminovascular fibers resulting in CGRP release, which mediates pial artery vasodilation (Wei et al., 1992) and neurogenic inflammation (Fozard, 1990, 1995; Moskowitz, 1992b). In the dural membrane, mCPP itself can produce extravasation, which can be blocked by selective 5-HT$_{2B}$ antagonists (Nelson, 1996).

Fozard's (1995) speculations cannot explain the delay of head pain in humans following mCPP ingestion. Subjects experience the premonitory symptoms of migraine during the delay time: feelings of exhilaration, exhaustion, anxiety, depression, or cognitive difficulties. Rather than the headache, mCPP may induce the prodrome of migraine, which may be of hypothalamic origin.

Methysergide is also a 5-HT$_1$ receptor agonist, which contracts canine, bovine, and human cerebral arteries [the latter is a model for the human 5-HT$_{1B}$ receptor (Muller, 1986, 1992)]. Methysergide has lower affinity for the 5-HT$_1$ than for the 5-HT$_2$ binding site (Peroutka and Snyder, 1979). Methysergide-induced contraction of isolated dog saphenous vein is also mediated by 5-HT$_{1B}$ receptors (Saxena and DeVlaam, 1974). Mianserin, cyproheptadine, and to a large extent methysergide do not antagonize the serotonin-induced vasoconstriction in the canine carotid vascular bed (Saxena et al., 1971, 1986; Saxena, 1972; Saxena and DeVlaam, 1974). Methysergide selectively decreases carotid blood flow (Humphrey et al., 1990; Saxena et al., 1971; Saxena, 1974) by closing AVAs via 5-HT$_{1D/B}$ receptors (Saxena and Verdouw, 1984). This effect, in part due to its metabolite methylergometrine, is less marked than that of sumatriptan or ergotamine (Bom et al., 1989; DenBoer et al., 1991a,b; MacLennan and Martin, 1990).

Chronic, but not acute, treatment with methysergide attenuates dural plasma extravasation following electric stimulation of the rat trigeminal ganglion in the Moskowitz model (Saito et al., 1988b). The difference between acute and chronic drug administration could be due to accumulation of the active metabolite, methylergometrine. Moskowitz (1992b) has postulated that methysergide (or methylergometrine) presynaptically inhibits the release of CGRP from perivascular sensory nerves. However, functional antago-

nism (via vasoconstriction) of the vasodilator effects of CGRP also occurs (Krootila et al., 1992). In addition, there is an interaction with neuropeptide Y (NPY).

Saxena (1974) believes that methysergide's efficacy is due to its vasoconstrictor action within the carotid vascular bed, closing AVAs (Saxena and Verdouw, 1984). However, its carotid vasoconstrictor effect is less than that of ergotamine (Saxena, 1972; Bom et al., 1989; DenBoer et al., 1991a,b) or sumatriptan (DenBoer et al., 1991b), while its therapeutic effect may be due to its more potent vasoconstricting metabolite, methylergometrine (Muller, 1992; MacLennan and Martin, 1990).

The 36–amino acid peptide NPY is colocalized with norepinephrine in some sympathetic nerves. Both act as vasoconstrictors. In addition, it is one of the most abundant brain peptides, found in high concentration in the hypothalamus. It is involved in the control of body weight. It is a potent appetite stimulant, which also reduces energy expenditure by inhibiting the sympathetic nerves that stimulate brown adipose tissue. When acting via 5-HT$_{2B/2C}$ receptors, 5-HT is an anorectic agent; when stimulated, these receptors inhibit the production and release of NPY. Acting through the 5-HT$_{2B/2C}$ receptor, mCPP induces anorexia and reduces NPY levels in the paraventricular nucleus (Dryden et al., 1994). Methysergide blocks 5-HT$_{2B/2C}$ receptors, acutely increases NPY secretion, and chronically increases NPY mRNA levels. This may account in part for the weight gain seen with 5-HT$_2$ antagonists. Also, NPY blocks neurogenic inflammation. Could an increase in NPY, in the vicinity of trigeminal nerve endings, account in part for the preventive effect of 5-HT$_2$ antagonists (Dryden et al., 1995)?

OPIOID RECEPTORS

There are four distinct opioid receptor types: μ, δ, κ, and the "opioid-like orphan receptor" (Piros et al., 1996; Bovill, 1997; Darland et al., 1998) (Table 9–13). The μ receptor, important in sensory processing, including the modulation of nociceptive stimuli, extrapyramidal functioning, and limbic and neuroendocrine regulation, has three subtypes: the

Table 9–13 Opioids

Receptor	Endogenous ligand	Agonist	Antagonist
Mu (μ_1, μ_2, μ_3)	β-Endorphin	Morphine	Naloxone
Delta (δ_1, δ_2)	Enkephalin		Naloxone
Kappa (κ_1, κ_2, κ_3)	Dynorphin	Butorphanol	Naloxone
Orphan	OFQ/N		

high-affinity μ_1, the low-affinity μ_2, and the newly described μ_3 (Bovill, 1997). Morphine and other morphine-like opioid agonists produce analgesia primarily through μ-receptor activation, which also produces respiratory depression, miosis, reduced gastrointestinal motility, and feelings of well-being (euphoria) (Pasternak, 1993). The supraspinal mechanisms of analgesia produced by μ-opioid agonist drugs are thought to involve the μ_1 receptor, whereas spinal analgesia, respiratory depression, and the effects of opioids on gastrointestinal function are associated with the μ_2 receptor (Reisine and Pasternak, 1996). The μ_3 receptor binds opioid alkaloids, such as morphine, but has exceedingly low or no affinity for the naturally occurring endogenous opioid peptides. The μ_3 receptor occurs in macrophages, astrocytes, and endothelial cells and may be involved in immune processes. The endogenous ligand for this receptor may be morphine or codeine (Bovill, 1997).

There are three κ-receptor subtypes (Table 9–13). Dynorphin A is the natural ligand for the κ_1 receptor, which elicits spinal analgesia. The role of the κ_2 receptor is unknown. The κ_3 receptor is the dominant brain opioid receptor. Selective κ-receptor agonists continue to produce analgesia in animals that have been made tolerant to μ agonists. Agonists of κ_1 receptors act primarily in the spinal cord and cause less intense miosis and respiratory depression than do μ agonists. Analgesia of κ_3 receptors is mediated supraspinally. Instead of euphoria, κ agonists produce dysphoric, psychotomimetic effects (disoriented and/or depersonalized feelings) (Pfeiffer et al., 1986; Reisine and Pasternak, 1996).

Two subtypes of the δ receptor, whose natural ligand is the enkephalins, have been identified (Bovill, 1997). The novel opioid-like orphan receptor is coded by a gene (*LC132, ORL1, XOR, ROR-6, or KOR3*) that was originally identified because of its extensive nucleotide sequence homology with the δ receptor (Darland et al., 1998). The natural ligand for this receptor, an endogenous peptide (orphanin FQ/nociceptin, ORQ/N) has been identified as a part of a larger protein (preoORQ/N), whose gene maps to human chromosome 8p21 (Darland et al., 1998).

The opioids have been divided into three groups: morphine and related opioid agonists; opioids with mixed actions, such as nalorphine, butorphanol, and pentazocine, which are agonists at some receptors and antagonists or very weak partial agonists at others; and opioid antagonists, such as naloxone. Mixed agonist/antagonists, such as pentazocine and nalorphine, can produce disturbing psychotomimetic effects that are not effectively blocked by naloxone (Reisine and Pasternak, 1996; Pasternak, 1993).

Although there are many compounds that have pharmacologic properties similar to morphine, none is clinically superior at relieving pain. Morphine-like drugs produce analgesia without loss of consciousness and often without drowsiness, changes in mood, or mental clouding. Mixed agonist/antagonists and partial agonists differ from morphine in that they are not full agonists at all opioid-receptor subtypes. Nalorphine, cyclazocine, and nalbuphine are competitive μ antagonists but κ-receptor agonists. Pentazocine and butorphanol are weaker μ antagonists or partial μ- and κ-receptor agonists. The combination of μ antagonism and κ agonism is responsible for the designation of these drugs as mixed agonist/antagonist agents (Reisine and Pasternak, 1996).

SECOND MESSENGERS

The receptor is located on and in the plasma membrane. In order to transfer information, it is coupled to effectors located in the plasma membrane that include ion channels and multiple G proteins. The G proteins that function in transmembrane signaling are heteromers consisting of α, β, and γ subunits in increasing order of molecular weight (Gilman, 1989; Krebs, 1989; Berridge, 1989; Mikoshiba, 1993; Simon et al., 1991; Nishizuka, 1989). G proteins can be either stimulatory or inhibitory.

After an agonist binds to a G protein–coupled receptor, a complex rearrangement occurs. In the resting state, guanosine diphosphate (GDP) is bound to the α subunit. When an agonist binds to the receptor, signaling begins by activating the G protein. This results in the exchange of GDP for guanosine triphosphate (GTP) on the α subunit of the G protein and the dissociation of the α-GTP subunit from the β-γ dimer. A single receptor can activate multiple G-protein molecules. The α-GTP and β-γ subunits may then interact with ion channels or enzymes to generate or prevent generation of regulatory molecules or second messengers. The β-γ dimer functions as an anchor for the α subunit to the plasma membrane (Gilman, 1989; Simon et al., 1991).

Termination of the signal occurs when the GTP that is bound to the α subunit is hydrolyzed to GDP. The α subunit then reassociates with the β-γ dimer. Multiple distinct G proteins have been identified. Pertussis toxin uncouples the receptor from some G proteins by interacting with the α subunit, which blocks signal transduction. Some α subunits are activated by cholera toxin. Intestinal epithelial G-α is the natural target for the toxin: activation results in enhanced fluid secretion into the gut. Inhibitory α subunits (part of inhibitory G proteins) also exist, which when activated result in the inhibition of second-messenger production (Gilman, 1989; Simon et al., 1991).

The cell membrane is like a switchboard, with multiple receptors and different effectors. Ligands can both activate and inhibit receptors that are linked to excitatory and inhibitory G proteins. The G-protein α subunit cycles between an inactive, GDP-bound state to an active, GTP-bound state. The G-protein subunits modulate the activity of membrane and cytoplasmic enzymes. A single α subunit can interact with more than one effector. (1) G proteins can stimulate adenylate cyclase (AC) activity, leading to cAMP formation and enhanced activity of protein kinase A (PKA). (2) Other pertussis toxin–sensitive G-proteins inhibit AC activity. (3) Some G proteins can activate the enzyme phosphoinositidase, which hydrolyzes phosphatidylinositol 4,5-biphosphate (PIP_2) into two active messengers, diacylglycerol (DAG) and inositol 1,4,5-triphosphate (IP_3), which is water-soluble, diffuses into the cytosol, and results in the release of calcium. The membrane-bound DAG activates protein kinase C (PKC). (4) Some G proteins are directly linked to ion channels, including calcium channels (Gilman, 1989; Nishizuka, 1989).

Protein kinases are a large family of proteins with important roles in the regulation of cell function. Some are receptors for tumor promoters. One, PKA, is the effector for cAMP. Another, PKC, is a calcium- (Ca^{2+}) and phospholipid- (DAG) dependent serine/threonine protein kinase. Activation of PKC through signal transduction is mediated by DAG. Protein kinase C plays an important role in many physiological functions, including adhesion, secretion, exocytosis, modulation of ion conduction, downregulation of receptors, and gene expression. It activates the Ca^{2+} transport ATPase and Na^+/Ca^{2+} exchange protein, both of which remove Ca^{2+} from the cytosol. It is also involved in gene expression and C-fos activation, which may be responsible for its role in learning and long-term potentiation (Mikoshiba, 1993; Simon et al., 1991; Nishizuka, 1989).

Another second messenger, IP_3, releases calcium stores and results in intracellular calcium oscillations. Produced by the G-protein activation of phosphoinositidase, IP_3 is one part of a bifurcating signaling system, the other limb of which is controlled by DAG. Both are produced by the hydrolysis of PIP_2. Inositol triphosphate diffuses into the cytoplasm to release calcium. Its action is terminated by hydrolysis. Ultimately, free inositol, the precursor of PIP_2, is formed. Lithium lowers brain inositol levels by blocking the hydrolysis of inositol monophosphate, resulting in depletion of the PIP_2 precursor and producing receptor desensitization. Through one of at least two different high-affinity receptors linked to calcium channels, IP_3 releases calcium from an IP_3-sensitive, localized, nonmitochondrial pool (Mikoshiba, 1993). The IP_3 calcium signal often initiates within a discrete region of the cell and is followed at times by a wave of increased cellular calcium. In some tissues, the Ca^{2+} oscillation frequency is dependent on the external 5-HT concentration. The Ca^{2+} channel activity of the IP_3 receptor is modulated by PKA and PKC. The frequency, as opposed to the amplitude, of intracellular calcium oscillations, induced by pulse secretions of IP_3, may be the intracellular signal (Mikoshiba, 1993; Simon et al., 1991; Nishizuka, 1989).

Nitric oxide (NO) is a highly diffusible free radical gas, initially identified in macrophages and endothelial cells, where it is the vascular relaxing factor released in response to acetylcholine. It is synthesized from the guanidonitrogen of L-arginine by the enzyme NO synthetase (NOS). It activates soluble guanyl cyclase, resulting in increased intracellular cyclic guanosine monophosphate (cGMP). In the CNS, NOS is localized in neurons scattered throughout the brain and spinal cord. Following activation of the N-methyl-D-aspartate (NMDA) receptor, NO is formed in the postsynaptic neuron. Once formed, it can diffuse into the presynaptic neuron, acting as an intercellular messenger. It may induce changes in the synaptic contact between the pre- and postsynaptic neurons, creating synaptic memory. It may also be involved in the genesis of the headache caused by nitroglycerine. Nitroglycerine is metabolized to NO, which releases CGRP from certain neurons,

potentially producing vasodilation and headache. It may also be the link between neural activity and cerebral blood flow (Ferrari et al., 1989; Dawson et al., 1992; Ladecola, 1993).

Treatment of the Prodrome

Premonitory symptoms, such as elation, hunger, thirst, and drowsiness, that precede the headache by as much as 24 hours suggest a hypothalamic disturbance, perhaps mediated by dopamine and serotonin. The periodicity of migraine and the flow of symptoms from prodrome to aura to headache may be regulated by the hypothalamic arcuate nucleus (see Chapter 5).

Two studies examined the effect of administering domperidone (an antidopaminergic drug that is not known to pass the blood–brain barrier) during the migraine prodrome. No adverse events were reported when domperidone was administered during the prodrome. One study conducted among patients with migraine with aura found that domperidone, taken at the onset of premonitory symptoms, was significantly more effective than placebo at preventing the headache phase (Amery and Waelkens, 1983). A subsequent study found evidence of a dose-response relationship, with a 40 mg dose being significantly more effective than a 20 mg dose (Waelkens, 1984).

Domperidone, 30 mg taken at the earliest appearance of the premonitory symptoms, prevented 66% of headache attacks. For maximal efficacy, the drug must be taken at the first appearance of the nonevolutive premonitory symptoms (those that do not merge into the headache and that occur at least 6 hours before the attack). Taking the medication for evolutive prodromal symptoms (occurring within 6 hours of the attack) was not as effective. Spierings (1989) suggested that metoclopramide may be as effective as domperidone.

A single trial of DHE nasal spray (NS) during the migraine prodrome demonstrated statistically significant superiority over placebo at preventing the anticipated migraine attack (Massiou, 1987).

In an open trial, naratriptan given during the migraine prodrome prevented the subsequent headache (Luciani et al., 2000).

Treatment of the Aura

In migraine with aura, a wave of oligemia spreads forward from the occipital area, precedes the aura, and persists into the headache phase (Olesen and Edvinsson, 1988). The rate of progression of oligemia is the same as the rate of the spreading electrical depression measured by Leao (1944), who electrically stimulated exposed rabbit cortices and monitored the induced changes in electrical activity, which spread over the cortex at a rate of 2 to 3 mm/min.

Decreased cerebral blood flow (CBF) during acute migraine has been found using positron emission tomography (PET). Woods et al. (1994) reported a single case in which a volunteer control subject experienced the onset of a migraine attack while undergoing a series of blood-flow measurements using PET and oxygen-15-labeled water.

Subjects who had a spontaneous migraine visual aura have been studied with functional MRI (Cutrer et al., 1998). Interictally, using perfusion-weighted imaging, CBF, cerebral blood volume, and mean transit time were normal and symmetrical. During visual auras, CBF decreased 15% to 53%, cerebral blood volume decreased 6% to 33%, and mean transit time increased 10% to 54% in the occipital cortex gray matter contralateral to the affected visual hemifield. When multiple perfusion images were obtained during the same aura, the margin of the perfusion defect moved anteriorly. The absence of diffusion abnormalities in these patients suggests that ischemia does not occur during the migraine aura (Cutrer and O'Donnell, 1999).

Cao et al. (1997) visually triggered headache in six migraineurs (five with aura and one without). A wave of activated and then suppressed activity as measured by the blood oxygen level dependent (bold) technique propagated into the contiguous occipital cortex at a rate of 3 to 6 mm/min.

These recent PET and functional MRI studies and older magnetoencephalogram studies support the existence of the spreading phenomena in humans with migraine (Simkins et al., 1989), suggesting that spreading depression may be the mechanism that produces spreading oligemia and the aura (see Chapter 5) (Blau, 1984; Pearce, 1984; Raskin, 1990a; Welch et al., 1990).

Wolff found that inhalation of 10% CO_2 in air for 5 minutes was temporarily effective at decreasing the visual aura of migraine (Dalessio, 1980). Inhalation of 10% CO_2 with 90% O_2 was always effective at abolishing the aura of migraine and preventing the development of the expected headache. When headache was present, the effect of 10% CO_2 with 90% O_2 was unpredictable. Alvarez (1934) found that inhalation of 100% O_2 for 15 to 120 minutes produced relief in 42% of patients. The earlier the treatment, the better the result. Alvarez's patients had a more unpredictable result compared to Wolff's and required longer treatment.

Wolff concluded that the migraine aura was caused by a primary vasoconstriction that could be overridden by administration of the potent vasodilator arterial carbon dioxide (Dalessio, 1980). However, experimental studies on cortical spreading depression (CSD) offer another explanation. Hypercapnic hyperoxia inhibits the propagation of CSD. Thus, the effects of hypercapnia on the migraine aura may be mediated by CSD inhibition (Lauritzen, 1986).

Wolff found that inhalation of small amounts of amyl nitrite could temporarily reverse the preheadache scotoma in some subjects (Dalessio, 1980). Inhalation of larger amounts of amyl nitrite produced generalized vasodilation, hypotension, and enlargement of the scotoma.

Kupersmith et al. (1987) found that inhaling isoproterenol at the onset of the aura could abort the neurologic or visual deficit of migraine with aura and basilar migraine. In some cases, the resulting headache was unaffected; in others, it became more severe with the use of isoproterenol. Kunkel (1982) demonstrated the utility of vasodilators in a small number of patients who had migraine with aura. Administering nitroglycerin or amyl nitrate early in the aura phase of the attacks resulted in resolution of the neurologic symptoms in about half the cases. There was minimal impact on the headache phase or severity (Kunkel, 1982).

Sublingual nifedipine 10 mg was effective at reversing the focal neurologic symptoms of migraine with prolonged aura (including aphasia and a mild right hemianopia) (Goldner and Levitt, 1987; Miller and Santoro, 1985). The actual value of treatment for the aura is uncertain, as is the mechanism that causes the aura. Hoffer et al. (1992) found that nifedipine was not effective at treating the headache when given during the aura of migraine. Subcutaneous (SC) sumatriptan is not effective at treating the headache of migraine when given during the aura (Ensink, 1991).

We have anecdotally found that corticosteroids, neuroleptics, intravenous (IV) magnesium, and IV furosemide (Lasix) (Rozen, 1999) were effective at treating prolonged or continuous auras with the addition of concomitant preventive medication. Calcium channel antagonists (verapamil and flunarizine) and anticonvulsants (divalproex, lamotrigine, and gabapentin) may prevent the occurrence of the aura even in the absence of a headache (Lampl et al., 1999).

Treatment of Acute Migraine Headache

The type, severity, and frequency of a migraine determine its treatment. Acute medication is indicated even if patients are using preventive medication. It is important to treat the headache as early as possible, both to prevent its escalation and to increase the drug's effectiveness. Often, migraine begins with pain of mild to moderate severity and is described as similar to a tension-type headache. As the headache increases in severity, it takes on more migraine-like features. Mild and severe migraine forms respond, in migraineurs, to triptans (Lipton et al., 1999; Silberstein, 1984).

Medication for an acute attack can be specific or nonspecific. Nonspecific medications are used to control the pain and associated symptoms of migraine as well as other pain disorders, while specific medications control the migraine attack but are not useful for nonheadache pain disorders. Nonspecific acute headache medications include analgesics (NSAIDs and combination analgesics), antiemetics, opioids, corticosteroids, and dopamine antagonists. Specific acute headache medications include ergotamine, DHE, and the selective 5-HT$_1$ agonists (triptans). It is advisable to develop a treatment strategy for headaches of different severity, utilizing one or more of these drug classes (Silberstein, 1991), that includes initial treatment, a backup treatment, and a rescue treatment, taking into consideration the patient's age and any coexistent illnesses, the migraine type, and the severity, frequency, disability, and associated features (including nausea and vomiting) of the attack.

Several treatment tips are recommended. Treatment should be tailored to the attack and to the individual. Determine the response, if any, to previous treatment and the potential for drug overuse. Be aware of all of the drugs that the patient is using, both prescription and over-the-counter. Acute headache medication overuse often causes treatment failure. Headaches should be stratified primarily by severity and disability and treated with the medications most likely to be effective for that attack, taking into account the drug's efficacy, safety, and side effects. Maximize the chance that treatment will be effective by using the correct dose and appropriate formulation and treating the attack early.

The formulation and route of administration are based on the attack severity, how rapidly it escalates, the patient's preference, the presence or absence of severe nausea or vomiting, and the need for rapid relief. Use a nonoral route and consider an antiemetic when there is significant early nausea or vomiting. Do not restrict antiemetics to patients who are vomiting or likely to vomit. Nausea itself is one of the most disabling symptoms of migraine and should be treated appropriately (Silberstein, 1997b). Antiemetics, in combination with analgesics, are commonly used in European centers (Wilkinson, 1988a; Olesen et al., 1979). In general, for the same chemical entity, injections are faster and more effective than suppositories and nasal spray, which in turn are generally faster-acting and more effective than tablets.

Individualize treatment. Patients with mild to moderate attacks can use NSAIDs or combinations such as aspirin plus acetaminophen plus caffeine or acetaminophen plus isometheptene plus dichloralphenazone for initial therapy. Patients with more severe migraine and those whose headaches are known to respond poorly to simple NSAIDs and combination analgesics should be treated with specific agents (triptans, DHE, ergotamine). It is important to get the treatment "right" as soon as possible, to reduce pain, disability, and dropouts. Patients who had moderate or nonsevere headache and were stratified to a triptan based on a migraine disability assessment scale (MIDAS) score that showed moderate or severe disability did better than patients who were given aspirin and metoclopramide. There was less escalation of medication and higher efficacy (Lipton et al., 2000). Failure to use a more effective treatment early may increase the pain, impairment, and impact of the headache. A backup medication is needed in case initial treatment fails. Triptans or DHE can be used if analgesics fail; neuroleptics, parenteral ketorolac, or combination analgesics (with opioids or butalbital) can be used if triptans or ergots fail.

For severe migraine, a self-administered rescue medication is needed when other treatments fail. Rescue medications may not completely eliminate pain and return patients to normal activities, but they provide relief without the discomfort and expense of a visit to the physician's office or emergency department. Rescue medications include potent opioids, neuroleptics, and corticosteroids.

Acute headache medication is the best approach when attacks are infrequent or compliance is a problem. It is not advisable to give a preventive medication for infrequent headaches that are generally well controlled by acute headache treatment. It is most appropriate to treat at least two different attacks before deciding that a drug is ineffective. If there is no benefit from the drug, be sure the dose is adequate and that no other factors in-

terfere with its effect. It may be necessary to change formulation or route of administration or add an adjuvant. Consider changing the drug when the response is incomplete or too slow, the headache recurs, the results are inconsistent after an adequate trial at an adequate dose, or the side effects are bothersome. Guard against medication-overuse headache. In general, limit acute headache treatment to 2 to 3 days/week. Medication-overuse headache results from the too frequent use of acute headache medications, often resulting in more frequent headache refractory to treatment.

Overuse of Headache Medications

Patients with frequent disabling headaches often overuse analgesics, opioids, ergotamine, and triptans. Some believe that more than 2 to 3 treatment days/week constitutes overuse for any drug. Others differentiate between drug classes and believe that excessive use can be characterized by as little as three doses of simple analgesics or NSAIDs more than 5 days/week, combination analgesics containing barbiturates or sedatives more than 3 days/week, triptans more than 3 days/week, ergotamine tartrate more than 2 days/week, or opioids more than 2 times/week (Diamond and Dalessio, 1982; Wilkinson, 1988b; Mathew, 1990; Andersson, 1988; Silberstein and Lipton, 1997; Saper, 1983, 1987, 1989, 1990; Saper and Jones, 1986; Silberstein et al., 1996).

Medication overuse by headache-prone patients can incite chronic daily headache, with growing dependence and habituation to symptomatic medication (Saper, 1983, 1986) (see Chapter 11). Following discontinuation of acute medication, withdrawal symptoms (including increased headache) and refractoriness to preventive medications are characteristic (Saper, 1983, 1986; Mathew, 1990; Kudrow, 1982). In most patients, stopping the acute medication will result in headache improvement after a period of increased headache (analgesic washout period) (Saper, 1986; Rapoport and Weeks, 1988; Baumgartner et al., 1989; Silberstein et al., 1996). In addition to the induction of chronic refractory headache, each class of medication has unique side effects: ergotism, analgesic nephropathy, gastrointestinal problems (including dyspepsia and ulcers), and anemia.

Nonpharmacologic treatment can be helpful. At the first sign of the attack, patients should remove themselves from situations of sensory overstimulation; if possible, they should rest in a dark, quiet room, apply an ice pack, and use acute medication. Pressure over the superficial temporal artery on the affected side is often temporarily effective.

Dose limits for acute medications should be set below the dose that might incite "rebound." The actual limit and duration of symptomatic drug use beyond which rebound occurs are unknown. For practical purposes, we have provided general and arbitrary guidelines. To maintain a drug-free interval between the days of drug use, it is important to limit the number of treatment days/week the drug is used (events) as well as the maximum amount of drug used per month. Another empiric strategy to limit overuse is to use alternate classes of medications. For example, alternate an NSAID with a triptan or DHE with a neuroleptic. However, no evidence exists to prove that this strategy works.

Evidence Base

In this chapter, we have utilized, in part, the technical report created by Duke University and the American Academy of Neurology under contract to the Agency for Healthcare Policy and Research (AHCPR), in which evidence from controlled trials on the efficacy and tolerability of drug treatments for acute and preventive migraine headache was identified and summarized. Trials were sought with a strategy that combined the MESH term "headache" (exploded) and a previously published strategy for identifying randomized controlled trials on the January 1966 to December 1996 MEDLINE database. Other computerized bibliographic databases, textbooks, and experts were also utilized. Selection criteria included all English-language controlled trials involving patients with acute migraine headache in which at least one

treatment offered was a drug treatment (Gray et al., 1999a,c).

Data collection and analysis were based on the number of patients who obtained headache relief according to an a priori definition of at least a 50% reduction in pain severity. Results were recorded and used to calculate odds ratios for headache relief. Measures of pain severity reported as group means (and standard deviations) were used to calculate standardized mean differences (or effect sizes). Where similar trials provided data, meta-analysis of efficacy measures was performed. The identity and rates of adverse events were recorded and statistically compared (Gray et al., 1999a).

Analysis of preventive migraine therapies poses methodological issues (P. McCroy et al., 1999). Many early studies, done prior to the IHS headache classification (Headache Classification Committee of the International Headache Society, 1988) used loose criteria to define migraine. Long-term studies often have high dropout rates independent of treatment. Studies completed before 1991 used a "headache index" (derived from mathematical formulae that included headache frequency and some combination of intensity and/or duration). The AHCPR technical report relied on a headache index for effect-size analysis, despite the fact that this is confounded by acute and rescue therapies (Gray et al., 1999a). Other end points measured included headache frequency and headache intensity. Clinical trials completed after 1991 often used a reduction in the total number of headache attacks in a 28-day period or the proportion of patients with a reduction of greater than 50% in headache frequency as end points. When they were used, effect-size analysis was based on these end points. Most comparative trials of two or more active treatments did not include a placebo arm. Improvement over baseline could be a reflection of the natural history of the illness during treatment (Massiou et al., 1997; Spierings, 1996; Steiner, 1997).

Many preventive studies were poorly performed, did not provide adequate details of statistical methods, or were reported only as abstracts, making proper analysis of the evidence difficult (but the studies were included nonetheless).

Analgesics, Including Nonsteroidal Anti-inflammatory Drugs

Acute treatment of mild to moderate headache often begins with the use of analgesics. Most people obtain headache relief with a simple analgesic, such as aspirin (Murray, 1964) or acetaminophen, either alone or in combination with caffeine or other adjuvants. Combination analgesics have some advantages: (1) combining two analgesics with different mechanisms of action can enhance analgesia (Beaver, 1984; McQuay et al., 1999), (2) caffeine not only enhances the analgesia of aspirin and acetaminophen (140%) (Beaver, 1984) as well as ibuprofen (Forbes et al., 1991) but is itself analgesic (Ward et al., 1991), (3) lower doses of different drugs reduce side effects, (4) analgesic combination drugs also offer product convenience (Beaver, 1984). The use of barbiturates or benzodiazepam is controversial. Any value of the barbiturate may be via a central effect: sedation or pain modulation (Saper, 1990). Some physicians believe that these combinations are more likely to lead to overuse and dependence and may not offer enough additional pain control to justify their use.

At least five different chemical classes of NSAIDs (Pradalier et al., 1988) have been used for headache treatment (Table 9–14): salicylates, arylpropionic acids, aryl- and heterocyclic acids, fenamic acids, and enolic acids. The major mechanism of action of NSAIDs is the differential inhibition of one of the two subtypes of the enzyme cyclo-oxygenase (COX1 and COX2), preventing prostaglandin synthesis (Campbell, 1990). Now, NSAIDs can be distinguished on the basis of their relative inhibitory activity on COX1 and COX2. In addition, some NSAIDs (ketoprofen, indomethacin, diclofenac) decrease the synthesis of leukotrienes by inhibiting 5-lipo-oxygenase (Campbell, 1990; Brooks and Day, 1991). One NSAID (meclofenamate) may be a direct prostaglandin receptor antagonist. In addition, NSAIDs interfere with a variety of membrane-associated

Table 9–14 Nonsteroidal anti-inflammatory drugs: chemical classification

Salicylic acids
  Aspirin
  Choline magnesium salicylate
  Salsalate
  Sodium salicylate
Arylpropionic acids
  Ibuprofen
  Naproxen
  Fenoprofen
  Ketoprofen
  Flurbiprofen
  Oxaprozin
Indole/heteroaryl acetic acids
  Tolectin
  Indomethacin
  Diclofenac
  Sulindac
  Ketorolac
Fenamic acids
  Mefenamic acid
  Meclofenamate
Enolic acids
  Phenylbutazone
  Piroxicam

processes, including the activity of NADPH oxidase in neutrophils and phospholipase C in macrophages (Brooks and Day, 1991). Also, NSAIDs may interfere with cell-adhesion molecules and have direct antinociceptive effects on neurons (McCormack, 1994).

Von Euler (1937) coined the term "prostaglandin" to describe the semen extract that contracts uterine smooth muscle. The 20-carbon polyunsaturated essential fatty acid arachidonic acid is the major source of prostaglandins in mammalian tissues (Cashman and McAnulty, 1995).

Prostaglandin synthesis requires the release of arachidonic acid from cell membrane phospholipids by phospholipase. Arachidonic acid is the substrate for the COX enzymes, which are membrane-bound glycoproteins (Hemler et al., 1976). Cyclo-oxygenase catalyzes the oxidation of arachidonic acid to a cyclic (doperoxide, PGG_2) and in a peroxidase step reduces the C15 hydroperoxide to a hydroxy (PGH_2) (Frölich, 1997). Most prostanoids do not directly activate nociceptors but, rather, sensitize them. Prostaglandins of the E series are involved in the hyperalgesia seen in acute inflammation. The predominant eicosanoid in such inflammatory conditions is

PGE$_2$, which acts synergistically with other mediators to produce inflammatory pain. It sensitizes receptors on afferent nerve endings to bradykinin and histamine.

There are two different COX enzymes encoded by two genes: COX1, the constitutive, and COX2, the induced form. The first is produced in normal, quiescent conditions and is important when prostaglandins have a protective function, such as gastric mucus production and renal blood flow maintenance (Cashman and McAnulty, 1995). It is found in platelets, where it is essential for thromboxane A$_2$ synthesis. Inhibition of thromboxane synthesis leads to loss of normal platelet aggregation. Activation of COX1 leads to prostacyclin production, which is antithrombogenic in the endothelium and cytoprotective in the stomach. In the kidney, prostaglandins are synthesized in the renal medulla, the ascending loop of Henle, and the cortex (Frölich, 1997).

The COX2 isoenzyme is found in endothelial cells, macrophages, and synovial fibroblasts (Frölich, 1997). It is found in small amounts in normal human lung, rat kidney, and fetal membranes; but most is the result of induction. It can be induced by interleukin-1 (IL-1) and endotoxin, and its expression is unregulated at sites of inflammation, increasing more than 20-fold during inflammation (Frölich, 1997).

Among the most commonly prescribed drugs in the world are the NSAIDs; but their use as anti-inflammatory, antipyretic, antithrombotic, and analgesic is limited by their gastric toxicity secondary to the suppression of prostaglandin synthesis (mainly through inhibition of COX1 activity), although several NSAIDs also have topical irritant properties (Wallace and Cirino, 1994). The ratio of inhibition of COX1 to COX2 by NSAIDs determines the likelihood of adverse effects. High-ratio NSAIDs such as aspirin and indomethacin have more adverse effects than ibuprofen, which has a low ratio. Dexamethasone, at anti-inflammatory concentrations, inhibits COX2 (Wallace and Cirino, 1994).

Aspirin at very low doses is a selective COX1 platelet inhibitor. At moderate doses, the COX1 inhibition is generalized; and the active metabolite of aspirin, salicylate, adds to its overall anti-inflammatory effect. Salicylate is a fairly selective COX2 inhibitor. It does not block platelet aggregation in humans at anti-inflammatory concentrations, and it does not produce gastrointestinal blood loss (Wallace and Cirino, 1994).

Nonselective COX inhibitors inhibit both COX1 and COX2 and include aspirin, indomethacin, piroxicam, diclofenac, and ibuprofen. Selective COX2 inhibitors include meloxicam (a newly developed drug recently introduced in several European countries), salicylate, and nimesulide (Wallace and Cirino, 1994). Salicylates (sodium salicylate, salicylamide, and magnesium trisalicylate) can be used safely in patients with aspirin-induced asthma (Wallace and Cirino, 1994).

Highly selective COX2 inhibitors show COX2:COX1 ratios of <0.001 in intact cells and include celecoxib, rofecoxib, CGP28238, DuP697, and NS398 (Frölich, 1997).

If COX2 is primarily responsible for the production of prostanoids that mediate inflammation, pain, and fever, it is unlikely that highly selective COX2 inhibitors will be more therapeutically effective than existing NSAIDs, since many of the existing NSAIDs are very effective COX2 inhibitors and it is possible that prostanoids produced via COX1 contribute to the inflammation, pain, and fever (Wallace and Cirino, 1994).

Some of the adverse effects of NSAIDs may be related to their ability to suppress COX2 activity. It is possible that COX2 is constitutively expressed in some tissues and that the prostanoids produced via this enzyme are physiologically important (Wallace and Cirino, 1994). Unlike the damage NSAIDs produce in the stomach, NSAID-induced small intestinal injury may not be related to suppression of prostaglandin synthesis. Thus, the sparing of intestinal prostaglandin synthesis by a selective COX2 inhibitor would not necessarily result in reduced intestinal toxicity (Wallace and Cirino, 1994).

Gastrointestinal toxicity can be reduced by linking the NSAID to an NO-releasing moiety. Nitric oxide maintains gastric mucosal blood flow, prevents leukocyte adherence within the gastric microcirculation, and counteracts the detrimental effects of COX suppression. It produces markedly less gastric injury than the native NSAIDs after both acute and chronic administration and does not cause detectable small intestinal injury (Wallace and Cirino, 1994).

The AHCPR analyzed 33 controlled trials of NSAIDs and other nonopiate analgesics and found them to be consistently effective for acute migraine headache pain relief compared to placebo. Aspirin (Hakkarainen et al., 1979; Boureau et al., 1994; Tfelt-Hansen and Olesen, 1984), ibuprofen (doses >400 mg) (Havanka-Kanniainen, 1989; Kloster et al., 1992), tolfenamic acid (Hakkarainen et al., 1979; Tokola et al., 1984), and naproxen sodium (Sargent et al., 1988; Johnson et al., 1985b) were superior to placebo. Individual positive placebo-controlled studies of diclofenac-K (Dahlof and Bjorkman, 1993), flurbiprofen (Awidi, 1982), naproxen (Andersson et al., 1989), piroxicam SL (Nappi et al., 1993), pirprofen (Kinnunen et al., 1988), and proquazone (Diserio et al., 1989) exist. Intramuscular (IM) diclofenac sodium was superior to placebo (Delbene et al., 1987) and low doses of acetaminophen IM (Karachalios et al., 1992). Oral acetaminophen was not significantly more effective than placebo (Diamond, 1976). In comparative trials, tolfenamic acid was superior to acetaminophen (Larsen et al., 1990) but no different from aspirin (Hakkarainen et al., 1979) or ibuprofen (Pearce et al., 1983). In some trials, adding an antiemetic or caffeine had no additional effect (Tfelt-Hansen and Olesen, 1984; Tokola et al., 1984; Hakkarainen et al., 1982). Three trials that were not included in the AHCPR technical report showed that the combination of acetaminophen, aspirin, and caffeine (Excedrin) was significantly more effective for headache relief than placebo in migraineurs (Lipton et al., 1998). Approximately 66% of treated patients had migraine headache of moderate intensity.

Comparative trials showed that opiate-containing aspirin compounds were more efficacious than aspirin alone (Hakkarainen et al., 1978, 1980). Ergotamine was superior to aspirin in two trials (Hakkarainen et al., 1978, 1980). No significant differences were observed between ergotamine ($\pm$ caffeine) and ketoprofen PR (Kangasniemi and Kaaja, 1992), naproxen sodium (Sargent et al., 1988; Treves et al., 1992; Pradalier et al., 1985) or tolfenamic acid (Hakkarainen et al., 1979). Oral sumatriptan was not significantly different from either aspirin plus metoclopramide (Oral Sumatriptan and Aspirin-plus-Metoclopramide Comparative Study Group, 1992) or lysine acetylsalicylate plus metoclopramide (Tfelt-Hansen et al., 1995). The clinical efficacy of ketorolac IM in comparative trials was inconclusive (Shrestha et al., 1996; Duarte et al., 1992; Davis et al., 1995; Larkin and Prescott, 1992).

Side effects with all of the NSAIDs include gastrointestinal upset, peptic ulcers and bleeding, abdominal pain, constipation, diarrhea, nausea, occasional paradoxical headache, lightheadedness, dizziness, somnolence, tinnitus, and fluid retention. In the short-term trials reviewed in the AHCPR technical report (Gray et al., 1999d), aspirin was generally well tolerated. Other NSAIDs were associated with higher rates of gastric irritation/discomfort, nausea, and vomiting. The NSAIDs were consistently associated with lower overall adverse event rates when compared with ergotamine; in particular, lower rates of nausea and vomiting were noted. Antiemetics did not reduce the adverse gastrointestinal events typically associated with NSAIDs (Gray et al., 1999c,d). The more lipid-soluble NSAIDs penetrate the CNS more effectively and may have greater central effects (Brooks and Day, 1991). All NSAIDs, which are both COX1 and COX2 inhibitors, are associated with an increased risk of peptic ulcer disease, the risk increasing with the dosage (Griffin et al., 1991), and aggravation of existing gastrointestinal inflammatory disease. Selective COX2 inhibitors may not have this risk. Contraindications to NSAIDs include active ulcer disease, gastritis, kidney disease, and bleeding disorders.

The NSAIDs can be used symptomatically or preventively and should be considered a first-line choice for the treatment of chronic paroxysmal hemicrania, menstrual migraine, exertional migraine, benign orgasmic cephalgia, hemicrania continua, and ice-pick headache. In order to be effective, NSAIDs must be given in adequate doses. If one NSAID is ineffective, another should be tried.

The efficacy of acetaminophen has just been established in acute migraine treatment (Lipton et al., 2000a). The danger of Reye's syndrome makes acetaminophen preferable to aspirin in children younger than 15 years with nonspecific headache (Silberstein, 1990). Acetaminophen is an option to aspirin or the other NSAIDs in patients with gastritis or bleeding disorder.

The most consistent evidence for efficacy exists for aspirin, ibuprofen, naproxen sodium, tolfenamic acid, and the combination agent acetaminophen plus aspirin plus caffeine. Their low cost and favorable tolerability make them a first-line treatment choice for mild-to-moderate migraine attacks or severe attacks that have been responsive in the past to similar NSAIDs or nonopiate analgesics. The NSAIDs most commonly used for headache relief are listed in Table 9–14. The dose should not exceed the maximum for each drug. In some cases, it can be repeated in 1 to 2 hours (naproxen, ibuprofen) as long as the maximal dose is not exceeded (Silberstein, 2000b).

Indomethacin (Indocin) is available as a 50 mg rectal suppository, which is useful in patients with severe nausea and vomiting.

Ketorolac (Toradol) can be given by injection (available as 15, 30, and 60 mg Cartrix for IM injection). No placebo-controlled trials testing the efficacy of ketorolac IM for treatment of acute migraine attack have been performed. Small comparative trials suggest equivalence to some agents, and a single comparison trial with meperidine demonstrated inferiority. Ketorolac IM is an option that may be used in a physician-supervised setting, although conclusions regarding clinical efficacy cannot be made at this time.

Injectable lysine acetylsalicylate (iLAS) has been used in the acute treatment of migraine. In a double-blind, multicenter trial that included 278 patients, iLAS was compared to SC sumatriptan and placebo. Both drugs were superior to placebo. Two hours following the administration of sumatriptan, iLAS, and placebo, 76.3%, 43.7%, and 14.3% of the patients, respectively, were pain-free. Thus, iLAS was significantly better tolerated than sumatriptan: adverse events with iLAS occurred in 7.6% and with sumatriptan in 37.8% of patients (Diener, 1999).

While there is no scientific evidence regarding the efficacy of the selective COX2 inhibitors in migraine and other headache, they have been shown to be analgesic in dental pain models (Morrison et al., 1999).

Celecoxib is a 1,5-diaryl pyrazole-based compound that inhibits recombinant COX2 with a median inhibitory concentration (IC_{50}) of 4×10^{-8} mol/l compared with 1.5×10^{-5} mol/l for COX1. Single doses of celecoxib, 100 or 400 mg, were superior to placebo and as effective as aspirin for pain relief following dental extraction. Phase II studies have established dose ranges of 100 to 400 mg/day for osteoarthritis and 200 to 800 mg/day for rheumatoid arthritis. An acute endoscopic study showed that levels of gastric mucosal injury with celecoxib 100 or 200 mg twice daily for 7 days were similar to those with placebo and reduced compared with naproxen 500 mg twice a day.

A selectivity ratio of <800 has been observed in cell lines expressing human COX1 and COX2. Rofecoxib selectively inhibited recombinant COX2 with an IC_{50} of 1.8×10^{-5} mol/l for COX1. Rofecoxib 50 mg was superior to placebo and at least as good as ibuprofen 400 mg or naproxen 550 mg for relief of pain following dental extraction; it is also antipyretic in humans. Phase II efficacy studies established a dose range of 12.5 to 25 mg daily, which was more effective than 5 mg. The rate of gastric or duodenal ulcers was similar to that observed with placebo and significantly lower when compared with ibuprofen (2,400 mg/day).

Patients using NSAIDs other than acetaminophen and selective COX2 inhibitors should be monitored for gastrointestinal blood loss, renal dysfunction, worsening of hypertension, and aggravation of colitis. Peripmenstrual use should be limited to 1 week at a time or three times a week when used regularly. It is not known if NSAIDs can produce rebound headache, but some have implicated these drugs (Henry et al., 1985).

Barbiturate Hypnotics

The AHCPR technical report (McCrory et al., 1998) identified ten separate controlled trials of butalbital-containing agents for headache treatment. Only one was conducted among migraineurs, and it did not include a placebo arm. This trial compared butalbital plus aspirin plus caffeine plus codeine (Fiorinal with codeine) with butorphanol NS (Stadol NS) (Goldstein et al., 1988). Butorphanol was superior in efficacy to the butalbital combination with codeine at 2 hours, but differences between the two treatments were not significant at 4 hours. Butalbital combined with codeine (Fiorinal with codeine) was associated with significantly fewer adverse events than butorphanol NS (McCrory et al., 1998; Goldstein et al., 1988).

No randomized, placebo-controlled studies have established the efficacy of butalbital-containing agents in the treatment of acute migraine headaches. Because of concerns about overuse, medication-overuse headache, and withdrawal, the use of butalbital-containing analgesics should be limited and carefully monitored. Their use should be limited to situations wherein a more specific or less potentially problematic agent cannot be used or is ineffective. They may be very effective as backup medications when other migraine medications have failed. For an individual attack, patients should take one or two tablets or capsules, with a maximum of six per attack. The most frequent adverse reactions are drowsiness and dizziness. Drug use should be limited to no more than two to three treatment days per week (Silberstein, 2000b).

Isometheptene and Isometheptene Combination Agents

The combination of acetaminophen, isometheptene (a sympathomimetic) and dichloralphenazone (a chloral hydrate derivative) is used in the treatment of migraine and tension-type headache (Ryan, 1974; Yuill et al., 1972). In two placebo-controlled trials, isometheptene attained borderline significance in relieving headache pain (Diamond and Medina, 1975; Ryan, 1974; Ogden, 1963). Isometheptene mucate plus acetaminophen plus dichloralphenazone was significantly more effective than placebo in two of three trials, although the magnitude of the effect was relatively modest (Diamond, 1976; Diamond and Medina, 1975; Ryan, 1974).

The combination was compared with its constituents (acetaminophen and isometheptene, respectively) and no significant advantages were found (Diamond, 1976; Ryan, 1974). The combination was significantly more effective at reducing headache intensity (Yuill et al., 1972) and associated with significantly less nausea and vomiting than ergotamine plus caffeine. A recent multicenter, double-blind, randomized, parallel trial found no statistically significant difference in efficacy between the isometheptene-containing combination and sumatriptan for mild to moderate migraine with or without aura (Freitag et al., 1999a). Headache recurrence was not significantly different over the 24-hour evaluation period for patients who responded in the first 4 hours. Adverse events associated with isometheptene combinations were not significantly more frequent than with placebo or with the comparator medications described above.

Isometheptene-containing compounds are superior to placebo, with a small but statistically significant effect. Based on clinical evidence and favorable tolerability, they may be a reasonable choice for patients with mild to moderate headache. The initial dose is two capsules, with a maximum of five capsules per attack. Contraindications include glaucoma, renal failure, significant hypertension, heart or liver disease, and use of monoamine oxidase inhibitors (MAOIs). Adverse reactions include transient dizziness and skin rash.

Opioids

Opium is the Greek term for the juice of the poppy plant. Opiates are drugs derived from opium (Ferrante, 1996). "Opioid" is a more inclusive term that applies to all agonists or antagonists with morphine-like activity, such as opiates or endogenous or synthetic opioid peptides (Reisine and Pasternak, 1996). The term "narcotic" is derived from the Greek word for stupor, but because of its legal meaning, it is no longer used pharmacologically. Three families of endogenous opioid peptides, each derived from a different polypeptide precursor, have been identified: the enkephalins (from proenkephalin), the endorphins (from pro-opiomelanocortin), and the dynorphins (from prodynorphin). In addition, there is good evidence for the presence of endogenous morphine and codeine. Morphine- and codeine-like substances have been isolated from the brain of several species, and biosynthetic pathways for morphine production, similar to that used by the opium poppy, have been demonstrated in mammals (Silberstein and McCrory, 1999).

Saper and colleagues (2000) reported the results of a 5-year prospective study using sustained, long-acting opioids in the treatment of over 300 patients with intractable daily or almost-daily headache. Of 160 patients treated for 3 to 5 years, only 23% demonstrated evidence of significant improvement, although a slightly larger group reported feeling better but without corroborative evidence, such as reduction in previous medication usage or an increase in daily activity. Up to 40% of patients showed some evidence of noncompliance (self-adjustment of doses, etc.) in the first year despite the highly structured program, which required monthly or bimonthly visits during the entire course of the study. The authors recommended that only patients who have failed all reasonable methods of treatment, including intense, advanced-care interventions, including full detoxification and hospitalization, should be placed on sustained opioid therapy. Exceptions might include pregnant women and patients with profound medical illnesses or medication requirements that would make the use of standard medications inappropriate. Based upon clinical observations during the period of the study, the authors also suggest that patients with severe Axis I psychiatric illness and those with cluster B personality disorders (borderline, histrionic, antisocial, and narcissistic) not be given sustained opioids.

The AHCPR technical report supports the effectiveness of several opioids for episodic treatment of acute migraine and TTH (Table 9–15). However, opioid drugs are often used as rescue medications after other treatments have failed, and the available trials do not address this situation. All clinical trials of opioid drugs are conducted over short time frames. By focusing on relieving the pain of acute headache attacks, these studies do not address clinically important issues about frequent or prolonged use of opioid analgesics, such as rebound headache, tolerance, and dependence (Silberstein and McCrory, 1999).

Opioids may be considered for patients who have infrequent, moderate to severe headaches that do not respond to standard medication. Opioids are particularly useful for patients who cannot use specific headache medications because of coexisting disease or the lack of a diagnosis (such as a patient who presents to the emergency department with a new headache). They are a safe treatment for the pregnant patient when given in limited amounts. They are useful for severe, middle-of-the-night headache and as a rescue medication. (A self-administered rescue medication should be prescribed for severe migraine since most treatments do not always work. In fact, the triptans may not work at all in as many as 20% to 30% of attacks.) While rescue medications often do not maintain normal function, they relieve pain and suffering without the discomfort and expense of a visit to the physician's office or emergency department. Rescue medications include opioids and neuroleptics (Silberstein and McCrory, 1999).

Opioids can be used in patients who have not overused or abused medication or violated treatment recommendations. They should be avoided or used cautiously and restrictively in patients who have demonstrated severe addictive tendencies and perhaps have a family history of addictive disease. Strict limits (no more than 2 treatment days/week) should be set and small amounts of medication prescribed to avoid the risk of excessive use in treatment-resistant patients (Portenoy et al., 1990; Saper et al., 1999a). In addition, use the lowest dose and least potent agent

Table 9–15 Clinical trials of opioids

Drug	Population	Findings
APAP/codeine	Migraine	Better for HA relief than placebo (2 of 3 trials)
		No better than aspirin (1 trial)
	Tension-type	No better complete relief than Fioricet at 2 hours (1 trial)
		Less complete relief than Fioricet at 4 hours (1 trial)
APAP/codeine/doxylamine	Migraine	No better (HA complete relief, SPID) than placebo (2 of 2 trials)
		No better SPID than APAP/codeine (1 trial)
APAP/codeine/buclizine	Migraine	Better HA relief than placebo (1 of 3 trials)
		No better for HA severity than ergotamine/cyclizine/caffeine (Migril)
Butorphanol (IM)	Migraine	No better for HA relief than meperidine/hydroxyzine (IM) (1 trial)
		No better for HA relief than dihydroergotamine/metoclopramide (IV) (1 trial)
Butorphanol (IN)	Migraine	Better for HA severity than placebo (2 of 2 trials)
Doleron	Migraine	Better for HA relief than aspirin (1 of 1 trial)
		No better for HA relief than ergotamine tartrate
Doleron novum	Migraine	Better for HA relief than aspirin (1 of 1 trial)
		No better for HA relief than ergotamine tartrate
Fiorinal with codeine	Tension-type	Better for PID than placebo (3 of 3 trials)
		Better for PID than Fiorinal (1 of 3 trials)
		Less HA relief than butorphanol (1 trial)
Meperidine (IV)	Migraine	No better than ketorolac (IM) (1 trial)
Meperidine/promethazine (IV)	Migraine	No better than placebo (1 trial)
		No better than ketorolac (IM) (2 of 2 trials)
		No better for HA relief than dihydroergotamine/metoclopramide (IV) (1 trial)
Meperidine/dimenhydrinate (IV)	Migraine	Less reduction in HA severity than chlorpromazine (IV) (1 trial)
		No better for HA severity than methotrimeprazine (IV) (1 trial)
Meperidine/hydroxyzine (IM)	Migraine	No better for HA relief than butorphanol (IM)
		Less HA relief than dihydroergotamine/metoclopramide (IV) (2 trials)
		No better HA relief than ketorolac (IM) (1 trial)

Key to abbreviations: APAP, acetaminophen; IM, intramuscular; IN, intranasal; IV, intravenous; HA, headache; SPID, summed pain intensity difference.

available when possible; carefully review other concurrently used medications to avoid enhanced sedation, respiratory suppression, or other untoward reactions; calculate and prescribe the appropriate number of pills to be used between visits, based on the frequency of attacks and attack requirements (refills are discouraged, as are call-in requests for additional medication); carefully delineate the guidelines for usage, including for which type of headache, how many times per day the drug can be used, and how frequently per week it can be used; and establish a visit pattern that is consistent with the frequency of headaches and the amount and type of medications prescribed (Saper et al., 1999b). The limits can be relaxed in migraincurs who have menstrual headache and in pregnant women. Opioids are often useful in the pregnant patient, and occasional opioid use in the patient who cannot tolerate or does not respond to ergots, triptans, or other symptomatic medications is appropriate.

Opioids should be administered by the most appropriate route for the clinical circumstance. The dosages should be adjusted to account for differences in bioavailability between the oral, parenteral, and rectal routes of administration (Table 9–16). The selection of a specific drug should be based on its route of administration, adverse effect profile, time to peak drug levels, and bioavailability. A nonoral route should be considered when there is severe nausea or vomiting. The agonist–antagonist opioids, such as butorphanol and nalbuphine, have lower abuse potential than the pure agonists. Parenteral butorphanol (2 to 3 mg) produces analgesia

Table 9–16 Doses of opioids equivalent to 10 mg parenteral morphine

Drug	Oral dose (mg)	Oral-to-parenteral dose ratio	Parenteral dose (mg)
Butorphanol	NA	NA	2
Codeine	200	1.5:1	130
Hydromorphone	7.5	5:1	1.5
Meperidine	300	4:1	75
Methadone	20	2:1	10
Morphine			
Single dose	60	6:1	10
Repeated dose	30	3:1	10
Oxycodone	15	2:1	30

and respiratory depression equal to that of 10 mg of morphine (with similar onset, peak, and duration of action) or 80 mg of meperidine. Butorphanol's plasma half-life is about 3 hours; higher values are observed in the elderly. Like other κ-receptor agonists, there is much less of an increase in respiratory depression with higher doses compared to morphine and other μ-receptor agonists. Excessive administration, improper selection, and use for frequent headaches have led to numerous cases of physical and psychologic dependence. Usage patterns exceeding a bottle of butorphanol a day are not uncommon. Recent work suggests that withdrawal from butorphanol results in focal increases in extracellular levels of glutamate within the locus ceruleus that may act through the NMDA glutamate receptor (Hoshi et al., 1996; Saper et al., 1999b).

Butorphanol NS (1 mg followed by an additional 1 mg 1 hour later) was compared to IM methadone 10 mg in a placebo-controlled, double-blind, double-dummy study in 96 patients. Both active agents provided statistically significant pain relief over placebo during the entire course of the study. Butorphanol was statistically superior at the p < 0.05 level in the first 2 hours of the study. Global satisfaction and time to remedication both favored butorphanol NS (transnasal butorphanol, or TNB) in the acute treatment of migraine (Diamond et al., 1991).

Based on the evidence reports, the following recommendations can be made. Butorphanol is a treatment option for migraine and headache patients when other medications cannot be used or as a rescue medication when significant sedation would not jeopardize the patient. As with all opioids and most acute headache treatments, overuse and dependence factors limit the usefulness of butorphanol for acute migraine treatment (Saper et al., 2000).

The major side effects of butorphanol are drowsiness, weakness, sweating, feelings of floating, and nausea. The incidence of psychotomimetic side effects is lower than that with equianalgesic doses of pentazocine but qualitatively similar.

Oral opioid combinations (e.g., aspirin or acetaminophen plus codeine) may be considered for use in acute migraine when sedation side effects will not put the patient at risk and/or the risk for abuse has been addressed. Commonly used combinations include aspirin or acetaminophen plus butalbital, a short-acting barbiturate effective at reducing anxiety (Silberstein, 1984). These combinations, available with or without caffeine, may be prescribed.

For an individual attack, patients should take one to two capsules immediately, with a maximum of six per attack. Although Scholz et al. (1988) found that codeine use did not correlate with the development of chronic daily headache, prudence calls for a smaller monthly use of combination analgesics with codeine.

Parenteral opioids may be considered for rescue therapy in a supervised setting for acute migraine when sedation side effects will not put the patient at risk and/or the risk for abuse has been addressed.

In general, we recommend no more than two to three usage days per week, with strict monthly limits of these agents to prevent overuse. Monthly limits should be established below maximal allowable usage, although individual consideration on a patient-by-patient basis is appropriate.

Ergotamine and Dihydroergotamine

Ergotamine is a choice for moderate to severe migraine if analgesics do not provide headache relief or produce significant side effects (Ziegler, 1987) and cost is a factor. Some patients still respond preferentially to rectal ergotamine. Ergotamine tartrate, originally derived from a rye fungus (*Claviceps purpurea*), is an ergopeptide, which consists of a natural D-lysergic acid linked to a tricyclic peptide moiety by a peptide bond.

Ergotamine has α-adrenergic and serotonergic agonist activity and vasoconstricting actions, stimulating arterial smooth muscle through serotonin receptors. It also constricts venous capacitance vessels. Both ergotamine and DHE are agonists at the serotonin 5-HT_{1A}, 5-HT_{1B}, 5-HT_{1D}, 5-HT_{1E}, and 5-HT_{1F} receptors (Peroutka, 1990a,b). Dihydroergotamine is a derivative of ergotamine which has been reduced at the 9–10 double bond on the D-lysergic acid moiety. Ergotamine and DHE bind avidly to their receptor sites, producing a long k_{off}. This produces a multiphasic metabolism and excretion pattern of drug elimination that may require up to 72 hours for a single dose of ergotamine.

Dihydroergotamine differs from ergotamine (Berde and Stuermer, 1978). While both DHE and ergotamine inhibit the reuptake of noradrenaline at sympathetic nerve endings, DHE is a weaker arterial vasoconstrictor but almost as potent a venoconstrictor as ergotamine, constricting venous capacitance vessels while having a negligible effect on resistance vessels. It is a more potent α-adrenergic blocker than ergotamine and inhibits the baroreceptor circulatory reflex. In both laboratory animals and humans, DHE is much less emetic and has less effect on the uterus than ergotamine. It is very difficult to

induce experimental gangrene in the rat tail with high doses of DHE.

DOSAGE FORMS AND BIOAVAILABILITY

Ergotamine tartrate is available as a sublingual preparation and, in combination with caffeine, as an oral tablet and a suppository. Caffeine may enhance ergotamine's oral absorption (Schmidt and Fanchamps, 1974) and is an analgesic itself (Ward et al., 1991). Oral absorption of ergotamine is erratic. Bioavailability is highly dependent on the route of administration. Ergotamine given by suppository to normal volunteers produced blood levels 20- to 30-fold higher than the same dose given orally (Sanders et al., 1986).

EFFICACY AND SAFETY

The AHCPR reviewed 23 controlled trials of ergotamine tartrate, ergotamine-containing compounds, and ergostine-containing compounds. The results were not consistent and difficult to interpret due to the fact that many of these trials are older and used outdated dosing strategies and outcome measures (Gray et al., 1999c,d). (More recent studies testing the efficacy of ergot alkaloids, specifically DHE, used current headache outcome measures and reported improved efficacy results.)

Five placebo-controlled trials of ergotamine had findings that ranged from no effect to large differences favoring ergotamine (Hakkarainen et al., 1982; Kangasniemi and Kaaja, 1992; Behan, 1978; Ostfeld, 1961; Waters, 1970). Three trials comparing ergotamine plus caffeine with placebo also reported mixed results (Sargent et al., 1988; Friedman et al., 1989; Ryan, 1970). One placebo-controlled trial supported the efficacy of ergostine plus caffeine (Ryan, 1970). A proprietary combination of ergotamine, caffeine, pentobarbital, and Bellafoline was shown, in one trial each, to be superior to placebo and ergotamine plus caffeine (Friedman et al., 1989). Otherwise, no significant differences were shown between ergotamine tartrate, ergotamine plus caffeine, ergotamine plus caffeine plus butalbital plus belladonna alkaloids (Kinnunen et al., 1988), and ergostine (Ryan, 1970; Kinnunen et al., 1988).

Ergotamine was significantly more effective than aspirin in two studies (Hakkarainen et al., 1978, 1979). Ergotamine was not significantly different from ketoprofen PR (Kangasniemi and Kaaja, 1992), naproxen sodium (Treves et al., 1992), tolfenamic acid (Hakkarainen et al., 1979), aspirin plus dextropropoxyphene chloride plus phenazone plus [2-diaminoethyl]phentiazin carboxyl chloride plus caffeine (Hakkarainen et al., 1978), aspirin plus dextropropoxyphene napsylate plus phenazone (Hakkarainen et al., 1980), metoclopramide (Hakkarainen and Allonen, 1982), or an isometheptene combination (Behan, 1978). Ergotamine plus caffeine was less effective than oral sumatriptan (Multinational Oral Sumatriptan and Cafergot Comparative Study Group, 1991) or the combination of isometheptene, dichloralphenazone, and acetaminophen (Yuill et al., 1972) and not significantly different from DHE NS (Hirt et al., 1989) or naproxen sodium (Sargent et al., 1988).

Ergot alkaloids were consistently associated with higher rates of adverse events, especially nausea and vomiting, than were placebo, sumatriptan, isometheptene, NSAIDs, and dextropropoxyphene compounds. Most ergotamine combinations (ergotamine plus caffeine, ergotamine plus caffeine plus pentobarbital plus Bellafoline, and ergotamine plus metoclopramide) had lower rates of nausea and vomiting than ergotamine alone (Gray et al., 1999c).

ERGOTAMINE USAGE

The evidence to support the efficacy of ergotamine for the treatment of migraine is inconsistent. Ergots had more adverse events compared to placebo, sumatriptan, isometheptene, NSAIDs, or dextropropoxyphene compounds. Selected patients with moderate to severe migraine may respond to ergot derivatives. For individual attacks, patients can take up to six (1 mg) tablets or two suppositories over 24 hours. Use should not exceed two dosage days/week (Saper, 1986). In certain circumstances, these limits may be liberalized (e.g., cluster headache, intractable menstrual migraine). Determine the subnauseating dose of ergotamine prior to its initial

use, when the patient is headache-free. This will avoid overdosing, increased headache and nausea, underdosing, and lack of efficacy (Silberstein, 1991). Since the rectal route of administration produces higher blood levels than the oral route, the patient should start with the predetermined subnauseating dose (one-third to one-half of a suppository) at the time of the acute headache attack (Silberstein, 1991).

Patients who cannot tolerate ergotamine because of nausea can be pretreated with metoclopramide (Volans, 1978), prochlorperazine (Kanto et al., 1981), promethazine (Phenergan) (Silberstein, 1991), or a mixture of a barbiturate and a belladonna alkaloid. Oral metoclopramide might also enhance oral absorption of ergotamine. Patients who cannot tolerate ergotamine or obtain no relief from it and still need an ergot should use DHE. Overuse of ergotamine and most acute migraine medications can lead to chronic daily headache and their use must be limited (see Chapter 11).

Dihydroergotamine is available in 1 mg/ml ampules, which can be administered IM, SC, IV, or NS. Bioavailability and blood levels are highest with IV injection (Kanto et al., 1981) and most erratic with SC injection (Schran and Tse, 1985). Patients can be taught to self-administer DHE IM. Bioavailability of the NS is approximately 40%.

Nine placebo-controlled trials reported on the efficacy and safety of DHE NS (Bousser and Loria, 1985; Dihydroergotamine Nasal Spray Multicenter Investigators, 1995; Gallagher, 1996; Krause and Bleicher, 1985; Massiou, 1987; Paiva et al., 1985; Rohr and Dufresne, 1985; Tulunay et al., 1987; Ziegler et al., 1994). These trials demonstrated the superiority of DHE NS, although the magnitude of the benefit was small to moderate. Three comparisons of different doses of DHE NS were inconclusive (Gallagher, 1996; Krause and Bleicher, 1985; Paiva et al., 1985). Two placebo-controlled trials did not clearly establish whether DHE IV (with an added antiemetic) is effective or ineffective for the treatment of acute migraine (Callaham and Raskin, 1986; Klapper and Stanton, 1991b).

Two trials compared DHE NS to other treatments. One found no significant difference between DHE and ergotamine plus caffeine (Hirt et al., 1989). The other trial found that 6 mg of SC sumatriptan was significantly better than 1 mg with the option for a second 1 mg dose of DHE NS 1 hour later (Touchon et al., 1996). One milligram of DHE SC was less effective than 6 mg of sumatriptan SC for headache relief at 1 and 2 hours, but this difference was not seen at 3, 4, and 24 hours following treatment (Winner et al., 1996). Subcutaneous DHE had a significantly lower incidence of headache recurrence than SC sumatriptan. Dihydroergotamine plus metoclopramide IV afforded better headache pain relief at 30 and 60 minutes than did meperidine plus hydroxyzine IM (Belgrade et al., 1989; Klapper and Stanton, 1993). A single trial compared a 50% lower dose of DHE (0.5 mg) plus metoclopramide (1 mg) IV to meperidine (75 mg) plus promethazine (25 mg) IM and found no differences between treatments (Scherl and Wilson, 1995). In a more recent trial (not included in the AHCPR technical report; Gray et al., 1999c), DHE plus hydroxyzine IM was as effective as meperidine plus hydroxyzine IM (Carleton et al., 1998).

The most common adverse event associated with DHE NS was mild to moderate rhinitis, which was clearly related to the route of administration. Compared with ergotamine plus caffeine, DHE NS had a similar incidence of adverse events. Compared with SC sumatriptan, it had a significantly lower rate of adverse events. Nausea and vomiting are the most common adverse events associated with IV DHE treatment (Gray et al., 1999d).

Dihydroergotamine NS is rapidly absorbed, with peak plasma concentrations occurring within 45 minutes. The bioavailability is 40% of the same dose given IM. The side effects of nasal DHE are mild and transient and include nasal stuffiness, nausea, and (rarely) vomiting (Lataste, 1989). It is safe and effective for the treatment of acute migraine attacks. It is an appropriate treatment choice and should be considered a first-line treatment for patients with moderate to severe migraine. Because of their inability to tolerate or take

oral medications, patients with nausea and vomiting may be given DHE NS. Initial treatment with DHE NS is a reasonable choice when the headache is moderate to severe or an adequate trial of NSAIDs or other nonopiate analgesics (including combination NSAIDs such as acetaminophen plus aspirin plus caffeine) has failed to provide adequate relief in the past. After priming the device, the patient delivers one spray (approximately 0.5 mg) into each nostril. This is repeated in 10 to 15 minutes. An additional set of sprays may be used in 2 hours, for a total dose of 3 mg.

Contraindications to the use of ergotamine tartrate or DHE include renal or hepatic failure, pregnancy, hypertension, sepsis, and coronary, cerebral, and peripheral vascular disease.

No placebo-controlled trials in migraine patients have demonstrated the efficacy and safety of DHE SC, IM, or IV as monotherapy. Clinical opinion suggests that DHE SC is relatively safe and effective when compared with other migraine therapies, and DHE SC has fewer adverse events than DHE. Because of their inability to tolerate or take oral medication, patients with nausea and vomiting may be given DHE SC, IV, or IM. Initial treatment with DHE SC is a reasonable choice when the headache is moderate to severe or an adequate trial of NSAIDs or other nonopiate analgesics (including combination NSAIDs such as acetaminophen plus aspirin plus caffeine) has failed to provide adequate relief in the past. DHE IM may be considered in patients with moderate to severe migraine. A trial to determine the subnauseating dose of DHE may be considered when the patient is headache-free. The patient should take up to 1 mg of DHE in a 3 ml syringe with a 1″ 22-gauge needle. Start by instructing the patient to inject DHE 0.25 mg (0.25 cc) IM and then in 0.25 mg increments every 15 minutes until a maximum of 1.0 mg has been injected or nausea has developed. The incidence of nausea is much lower with IM than with IV injection and lower still than with oral or rectal ergotamine tartrate (Tillgren, 1947). Dosage for individual attacks should be limited to 1 mg IM or IV (maximum of 3 mg/day). Monthly limits are 18 ampules or 12 events. Unlike ergotamine, DHE may not produce rebound headache, but this remains uncertain. We recommend limiting its use to prevent overuse of IM injections and the development of refractoriness. Exceptions include cluster headache, menstrual migraine, and use during detoxification.

In the treatment of moderate to severe migraine, DHE IV plus antiemetics has been shown to be effective and moderately safe compared with parenteral opiates. This is an appropriate treatment choice for patients with severe migraine. In some patients, DHE may produce nausea. Pretreatment with metoclopramide, promethazine, or a combination of atropine and a barbiturate, or perhaps ondansetron might counter this side effect and treat the nausea associated with the migraine as well.

The combination of prochlorperazine IV 5 mg followed by DHE IV is a safe and effective means of terminating a migraine attack (Callaham and Raskin, 1986). The combination of metoclopramide IV and DHE IV was more effective at treating an acute migraine attack than meperidine IM (Belgrade et al., 1989). One can mix 10 mg (2 ml) of prochlorperazine and 1 mg (1 ml) of DHE in a syringe and inject 2 cc of this IV. If the headache is not relieved in 15 to 30 minutes, the remainder of the dose can be injected (Raskin, 1990b).

Repetitive IV DHE has become the mainstay of acute symptomatic treatment for intractable headache (Raskin, 1986; Silberstein et al., 1990a; Edmeads, 1988). Repetitive IV DHE was effective at eliminating intractable headache in 89% of patients within 48 hours (Raskin, 1986). Diazepam IV was only partially effective at eliminating such headaches (13% within 3 to 6 days). Silberstein et al. (1990a) also found that repetitive IV DHE was effective at eliminating prolonged migraine, cluster headache, and chronic daily headaches with or without rebound.

Intravenous DHE has a sustained therapeutic effect, but it is uncertain whether this is directly related to the effects of the DHE itself (Silberstein et al., 1990a), the active metabolite 8-OH-DHE (Aellig, 1984; Muller-Schweinitzer, 1984), the termination of drug

"rebound" (Saper, 1986; Diener et al., 1988), or the removal of the patient from a stressful environment (Silberstein et al., 1990a).

Patients treated with DHE should have a heparin lock inserted for medication administration. Patients may be pretreated with an antinauseant, such as metoclopramide 10 mg IV or ondansetron 8 mg IV, which is continued as needed before each infusion of DHE. Initially, DHE is administered at a test dose of 0.5 mg (0.25 in children) given via IV push over 3 to 5 minutes. If the headache persists, another 0.5 mg of DHE is given and 1.0 mg of DHE is administered every 8 hours. If the patient is controlled on 0.5 mg of DHE, the dose is repeated every 8 hours. If nausea persists, the next dose of DHE can be reduced to 0.25 mg. Dihydroergotamine is tapered and discontinued (after 3 to 5 days) if the patient is headache-free or fails to respond to the medication. Alternative delivery methods include an IV drip of DHE diluted in normal saline. There are two methods of doing this. In the first method, DHE is diluted in 50 cc of normal saline and administered over 30 to 60 minutes. In the other method, DHE is infused continuously for up to 3 days (Ford and Ford, 1997). These alternative delivery methods may reduce local venous reactions as well as other adverse events, such as nausea and chest pain.

Selective Serotonin Agonists ("Triptans")

The first selective $5\text{-}HT_{1B/1D}$ agonist to be developed and tested was sumatriptan, followed by zolmitriptan, naratriptan, rizatriptan, eletriptan, almotriptan, and frovatriptan (Table 9–17). (The latter three agents are still in clinical development.) Sumatriptan was first available as an SC injection, then as an oral tablet, and more recently as a NS. Its importance is clearly demonstrated by the large number of copycat "triptans" that followed it. Sumatriptan is the most extensively studied agent in the history of migraine, with over 27,000 patients and over 140,000 attacks treated in clinical trials as of May 1997. Sumatriptan is extensively metabolized in the liver by MAO-A; therefore, its use as an oral

Table 9–17 Selective serotonin (5-HT$_1$) receptor agonists

Drug	Manufacturer	Status
Sumatriptan	Glaxo Smith Kline	Launched
Zolmitriptan	Zeneca	Launched
Rizatriptan	Merck	Launched
Naratriptan	Glaxo Smith Kline	Launched
Eletriptan	Pfizer	Phase III
Frovatriptan	Vanguard/Elan	Phase III
Almotriptan	Almirall/Pharmacia Upjohn	Phase III

or NS formulation is contraindicated in patients who are on MAOIs. The injectable form, however, has been shown to be safe and well tolerated in this setting (Freitag et al., 1998). Substantial drug–drug interaction with other traditional migraine-preventive medications, including β blockers, calcium channel antagonists, selective serotonin reuptake inhibitors (SSRIs), and tricyclic antidepressants, were not found. There was also no difference in the likelihood of improved response with preventive therapies or between preventive therapies. Headache recurrence and adverse events were also similar in the various treatment groups.

Fourteen placebo-controlled trials consistently showed that SC sumatriptan (6 mg) was superior to placebo for headache relief and complete relief at 1 and 2 hours (Brewerton et al., 1988; Cumberbatch et al., 1997; Ferrari and Saxena, 1993a; Fozard and Gray, 1989; Fozard, 1990; Goadsby and Gundlach, 1991; Goadsby and Hoskin, 1996; Gordon et al., 1993; Humphrey and Feniuk, 1991; Kimball et al., 1960; Lance, 1992; Moskowitz, 1990; Silberstein et al., 1992; Somerville, 1976). A second dose of sumatriptan SC, administered 1 hour after the first, provided no added benefit (Moskowitz, 1990; Gordon et al., 1993).

Two trials directly compared SC and oral formulations of sumatriptan. Methodologic differences between the trials complicated their comparison and interpretation, but both studies found SC sumatriptan to be significantly more effective than oral sumatriptan at 2 and 4 hours (Carpay et al., 1997; Gruffydd-Jones et al., 1997).

One trial each compared SC sumatriptan with SC DHE (Winner et al., 1996) and DHE NS (Touchon et al., 1996). In both trials, 1- and 2-hour data on headache relief and complete relief favored sumatriptan, while 2- to 24-hour recurrence rates favored DHE.

Sumatriptan SC was effective for the treatment of recurrent headache after initially successful treatment with sumatriptan (DiGiovanni and Dunbar, 1970), but sumatriptan administered during the migraine aura, before the onset of headache pain, was no more effective than placebo at preventing the development of a moderate to severe headache (Ensink, 1991).

Significantly more patients reported adverse events with SC sumatriptan than with placebo or DHE NS but less than with SC DHE. The most commonly reported adverse effects with sumatriptan SC were injection-site reactions, flushing, dizziness/vertigo, and paresthesia/tingling. Some patients reported transient chest symptoms in many of the trials included in the analysis (Gray et al., 1999c).

Eleven placebo-controlled trials provided consistent evidence that oral sumatriptan 100 mg is significantly more effective than placebo for headache relief and complete relief at 2 and 4 hours (Jackson, 1996; Cutler et al., 1995, 1996; Myllyla et al., 1998; Nappi et al., 1994; Oral Sumatriptan Dose-Defining Study Group, 1991; Oral Sumatriptan International Multiple-Dose Study Group, 1991; Pini et al., 1995; Sargent et al., 1995; Tfelt-Hansen et al., 1995). In the United States sumatriptan is available in 25 and 50 mg doses. Three trials have supported the efficacy of these lower doses (Cutler et al., 1995; Pfaffenrath et al., 1998; Sargent et al., 1995). In the only multidose study reporting 4-hour outcomes, headache relief and complete relief rates with the 50 mg dose were comparable to those reported with the 100 mg dose and superior to the 25 mg dose (Pfaffenrath et al., 1998). In general, the proportions of patients who reported relief with oral sumatriptan were lower than with SC sumatriptan. Two trials directly comparing SC and oral sumatriptan suggested that the SC formulation provides superior relief (Carpay et al., 1997; Gruffydd-Jones et al., 1997).

One trial each compared sumatriptan 100 mg with aspirin plus metoclopramide (Oral Sumatriptan and Aspirin-plus-Metoclopramide Comparative Study Group, 1992), lysine acetylsalicylate plus metoclopramide (Tfelt-Hansen et al., 1995), and a rapid-release formulation of tolfenamic acid (Myllyla et al., 1998). They found no significant differences between the analgesic compounds and sumatriptan for headache relief at 2 hours, and only one of the three trials found sumatriptan to be significantly better for complete relief (Oral Sumatriptan and Aspirin-plus-Metoclopramide Comparative Study Group, 1992). Sumatriptan was significantly more effective than ergotamine plus caffeine for both headache relief and complete relief at 2 hours (Orholm et al., 1986).

A second dose of oral sumatriptan, 2 to 4 hours after the first, did not provide any additional relief of the initial headache (Ferrari et al., 1994; Scott et al., 1996) and did not prevent headache recurrence (Ferrari et al., 1994; Scott et al., 1996; Rapoport et al., 1995). Four trials of sumatriptan showed it was significantly better than placebo at relieving recurrent headache pain (Pini et al., 1995; Ferrari et al., 1994; Cady et al., 1994; Teall et al., 1998).

Six placebo-controlled trials support the efficacy of sumatriptan NS for headache relief at 1 and 2 hours (Finnish Sumatriptan Group and the Cardiovascular Clinical Research Group, 1991; Salonen et al., 1994; Diamond et al., 1998; Ryan et al., 1997). A dose-response relationship was demonstrated, with superiority to placebo at the 10, 20, and 40 mg doses. Results with the 5 mg dose were mixed, and the 1 mg dose was shown to be ineffective. Significantly more patients reported adverse events with sumatriptan NS

than with placebo, the most common symptom being "taste disturbance."

One trial each tested the efficacy of sumatriptan IM (Kelly et al., 1997) and sumatriptan PR (Tepper et al., 1998). Sumatriptan IM 6 mg was as effective as chlorpromazine IV at 1 and 2 hours post-treatment. Sumatriptan PR (12.5 mg or 25 mg) was significantly more effective than placebo at 2 hours, with a stronger clinical benefit observed with the higher dose (Swedish Medical Product Agency, 1997).

Sumatriptan relieves headache pain, nausea, photophobia, and phonophobia and restores the patient's ability to function normally. Sumatriptan (or another triptan) is often prescribed at the initial consultation as a first-line drug for severe attacks and as backup medication for less severe attacks that do not adequately respond to simple or combination analgesics. We prefer SC injection or the NS for patients who need rapid relief or who have severe nausea or vomiting. Oral sumatriptan is used for gradual-onset headache when rapid pain relief is not required. Although 80% of patients get pain relief from an initial SC dose of sumatriptan, headache recurs in about one-third of patients within a day. Recurrences respond well to a second dose of sumatriptan and sometimes to simple and combination analgesics.

Adverse events, most commonly malaise/fatigue, dizziness/vertigo, asthenia, and nausea, were generally more frequent (and in some cases significantly more frequent) with the oral 5-HT$_{1B/1D}$ agonists than with placebo. The incidence of adverse events was dose-dependent with rizatriptan and zolmitriptan. Significantly more patients reported adverse events with sumatriptan than with aspirin/lysine acetylsalicylate plus metoclopramide. For all treatments in this drug class, small numbers of patients reported transient chest symptoms (Gray et al., 1999c,d).

None of the triptans should be used for patients who have clinical ischemic heart disease, Prinzmetal's angina, uncontrolled hypertension, or strictly vertebrobasilar migraine or who are at high risk for these conditions. Sumatriptan's common side effects include pain at the injection site, tingling, flushing, burning, and warm or hot sensations. Dizziness, heaviness, neck pain, and dysphoria can also occur. These side effects generally abate within 45 minutes. Sumatriptan causes noncardiac chest pressure in approximately 4% of patients. We get an electrocardiogram on patients over the age of 40 and those who have risk factors for heart disease before using any of the triptans. We often give the first triptan dose in the office when the patient does not have a headache.

Second-Generation Triptans

Acute migraine treatment advanced significantly with the introduction of sumatriptan, the first specific 5-$HT_{1B/1D}$ agonist; however, there is still room for improvement. After oral administration of the drug, approximately half of patients do not respond at 2 hours and about three-quarters have at least some residual headache pain. About one-third of patients using the oral formulation experience headache recurrence within a day. A number of new 5-$HT_{1B/1D}$ agonists (triptans), whose mechanism of action is similar to sumatriptan but whose pharmacokinetics differ, have been developed. At least three are now in clinical use in North America and Europe. These may produce better migraine response and lower recurrence rates, and they may be better tolerated.

Naratriptan, rizatriptan, and zolmitriptan are full agonists, while eletriptan is a partial agonist. Each compound has been shown in experimental settings to constrict extracerebral intracranial vessels, inhibit activity in peripheral trigeminal neurons, and, since each can penetrate the CNS to some extent, block transmission in the trigeminal nucleus. Each compound can constrict the human coronary artery.

Oral eletriptan is rapidly absorbed, with high bioavailability (50%) and a long half-life (5 hours). There is some concern, however, regarding eletriptan's possible interaction with other compounds that are metabolized at the cytochrome P-450 site. In a dose-ranging comparative trial, 2-hour responses were 67% at 40 mg and 77% at 80 mg with excellent therapeutic gains. In this study, headache recurrences were about one-third, similar to sumatriptan. Two trials of eletriptan provided less information but suggested that this agent may also be effective in some doses (40 mg, 80 mg) (Saxena and Verdouw, 1984; Seibyl et al., 1991). Abstracts not included in the AHCPR technical report have recently become available.

Reches (1999) compared the efficacy, safety, and tolerability of oral eletriptan and Cafergot in the acute treatment of migraine using oral doses (40 and 80 mg) of the 5$HT_{1B/1D}$ agonist in a double-blind, randomized, placebo-controlled, parallel-group trial. Seven hundred thirty-three patients received 40 mg eletriptan, 80 mg eletriptan, Cafergot (2 mg ergotamine tartrate, 200 mg caffeine), and placebo (in the ratio 2:2:2:1). At 2 hours after treatment, a significantly higher proportion of patients in the eletriptan groups had a headache response compared with the cafergot group (54% to 68% vs. 33%, p < 0.0001), and more eletriptan patients were completely pain-free (28% to 38% vs. 10%, p < 0.0001).

Pryse-Phillips (1999) compared oral eletriptan (40 to 80 mg) and oral sumatriptan (50 to 100 mg) for the treatment of acute migraine in a randomized, placebo-controlled trial in sumatriptan-naive patients. Seven hundred seventy-four patients took placebo, 40 mg eletriptan, 80 mg eletriptan, 50 mg sumatriptan, or 100 mg sumatriptan (in the ratio 1:2:2:2:2) as their first dose to treat an acute attack of migraine with or without aura. Headache response rates were higher in the eletriptan than in the sumatriptan group at 1 hour (30% to 37% vs. 24% to 27%, p < 0.05 for eletriptan; 80 mg vs. sumatriptan 50 mg) and 2 hours (64% to 67% vs. sumatriptan dose) after treatment. At 2 hours, significantly more patients in the eletriptan groups were completely pain-free than in the sumatriptan groups (p < 0.01). Eletriptan was also more effective than sumatriptan at providing relief of functional disability, nausea, photophobia, and phonophobia. Headache recurrence rates were low in the eletriptan groups (19% for 40 mg and 16% for 80 mg). In general, treatment-related adverse events were transient and mild or moderate in intensity.

Table 9–18 Pharmacologic characteristics of selected triptans

Parameter	Sumatriptan	Zolmitriptan	Naratriptan	Rizatriptan	Eletriptan
T_{max} (hours)	2	2.5	2–3	1	1
Half-life (hours)	2	3	6	2–3	5
Bioavailability	14	40	60–70	40–45	50
Lipophilicity (log $D_{pH7.4}$)	−1.3	−0.7	−0.2	−0.7	+0.5

Oral naratriptan differs from sumatriptan primarily in its longer half-life, longer T_{max}, higher oral bioavailability (70%), and lipophilicity (Table 9–18). Studies of more than 4,000 patients indicate that the drug has a well-defined dose-response relationship for headache relief, with a mean response of 48% at 2 hours after administration, but therapeutic gains are comparatively modest (21%) (Table 9–19). Two trials tested the efficacy of naratriptan and found a significant clinical benefit over placebo for the 1 and 2.5 mg doses at 4 hours post-treatment (Humphrey et al., 1990; Saxena, 1974). Relief rates with naratriptan were lower than with the other oral 5-$HT_{1B/1D}$ agonists. A direct comparative crossover study of patients prone to headache recurrence showed that about one-third fewer experienced recurrence when they used naratriptan compared with sumatriptan. However, 24-hour comparisons of naratriptan and sumatriptan found relief rates to be similar. The studies showed excellent tolerability for the 2.5 mg dose of naratriptan, with an adverse event rate close to that of placebo.

Rizatriptan has rapid oral absorption and high oral bioavailability at 45% for the 10 mg dose. Four trials found that rizatriptan was significantly better than placebo for headache relief and complete relief at 2 hours; doses tested ranged from 5 to 40 mg, with higher rates of relief reported with the higher doses (doses currently available in the United States: rizatriptan 5 and 10 mg) (Muller, 1992, 1986; Peroutka and Snyder, 1979; Saxena et al., 1971). One study directly compared oral sumatriptan (100 mg) and rizatriptan (10, 20, 40 mg) and found that a high dose of rizatriptan (40 mg) produced significantly better results at 2 hours (Visser et al., 1996). There were no significant differences at 2 hours between sumatriptan and the lower doses of rizatriptan. When directly compared with sumatriptan 100 mg, rizatriptan 10 mg had a cumulative benefit of about 20% in terms of patients who achieved headache response in the first 2 hours and a cumulative advantage of about 15% when compared with sumatriptan 50 mg. Rizatriptan has shown high consistency from attack to attack in for-

Table 9–19 Headache response and therapeutic gain for selected triptans at 2 hours

	Headache response	Therapeutic gain[a] for response
Almotriptan (25 mg)	57%–68%	19%–27%
Eletriptan (40 mg)	54%–65%	22%–41%
Eletriptan (80 mg)	68%–77%	30%–53%
Frovatriptan (2.5 mg)	40%	16%
Naratriptan (2.5 mg)	48% (45%–51%)	21% (18%–24%)
Rizatriptan (10 mg)	73% (69%–73%)	34% (30%–38%)
Sumatriptan (20 mg NS)	60%–86%	28%–55%
Sumatriptan (50 mg)	56% (51%–61%)	33% (29%–36%)
Sumatriptan (6 mg SC)	80%–85%	51%
Zolmitriptan (2.5 mg)	64% (59%–69%)	34% (27%–41%)

[a]Therapeutic gain is the difference between the response to active drug and the response to placebo. It can be used to compare drugs tested in different clinical trials and is presented here with 95% confidence intervals based on published and abstracted studies.

mal blinded consistency studies in a useful wafer formulation that many patients, particularly those with nausea as a prominent feature, find convenient as it dissolves on the tongue and requires no water, although absorption is gastrointestinal and transbuccal (Silberstein et al., 1998). Rizatriptan has a significant interaction with propranolol, which requires that the dose be halved to 5 mg and is contraindicated with MAOIs because of its route of metabolism. Rizatriptan was significantly better than placebo at relieving recurrent headache pain (Teall et al., 1998).

Zolmitriptan was the second selective $5HT_{1B/1D}$ agent marketed in the United States. It has high oral bioavailability (40%), has a T_{max} of about 2.5 hours, and is metabolized by the cytochrome P-450 system to an active metabolite that is degraded by MAO-A. Therefore, patients taking MAOIs are limited to a total zolmitriptan dose of 5 mg/day. Three trials showed zolmitriptan (2.5 or 5 mg) to be significantly more effective than placebo for headache relief and complete relief at 2 and 4 hours (Saxena, 1972; Saxena et al., 1971, 1986). The only trial that directly compared the 2.5 and 5 mg doses of zolmitriptan found no significant difference between them (Saxena, 1972). Zolmitriptan demonstrated a headache response of 64% with a therapeutic gain of 34% for the 2.5 mg dose and a headache response of 65% and a 37% therapeutic gain for the 5 mg dose. The recommended starting dose of 2.5 mg provides the best balance of benefit and side effects, although some patients may benefit from the higher 5 mg dose. In all studies, zolmitriptan reduced the incidence of photophobia, phonophobia, and nausea compared with placebo. In formal comparisons with sumatriptan 100 mg, zolmitriptan 5 mg was no different; and in a recent comparison with zolmitriptan 2.5 mg, no clinically relevant differences were seen. The most frequently reported adverse events include asthenia, nausea, somnolence, dizziness, and paresthesias. A randomized, controlled, parallel trial that compared sumatriptan 25 and 50 mg with zolmitriptan 2.5 and 5 mg over the course of a series of headaches showed that both doses of zolmitriptan were either comparable or statistically superior to

both doses of sumatriptan for headache relief, consistency of response, and 24-hour headache relief rates (Edwards, 1999).

Zolmitriptan (Solomon et al., 1997) was significantly better than placebo at relieving recurrent headache pain. One small study did not support the use of zolmitriptan during the aura phase for the short-term prevention of migraine (Dowson, 1996).

A recent placebo-controlled, randomized trial with the newly developed $5\text{-}HT_{1B/1D}$ agonist almotriptan SC also reported significant headache relief for the acute treatment of migraine (Cabarrocas, 1987). This was recently published as an abstract and not included in the AHCPR technical report. Specifically, placebo-controlled, randomized trials in migraine patients suggest clinically significant migraine relief with oral almotriptan (Cabarrocas and Zayas, 1998). A single oral dose of 6.25 or 12.5 mg of almotriptan or placebo was administered during three different migraine attacks (Robert et al., 1999). The overall percentages of attacks were 38.4%, 59.9%, and 70.3% for placebo, 6.25 mg, and 12.5 mg, respectively. Pain-free values at 2 hours were 15.5%, 29.9%, and 38.8% for placebo, 6.25 mg, and 12.5 mg, respectively.

Frovatriptan is a $5HT_{1B/1D}$ receptor agonist with a high affinity for the $5HT_{1B/1D}$ receptors, potent agonism in isolated human cerebral arteries, functional selectivity for isolated cerebral arteries compared to coronary arteries, and limited coronary constrictor activity relative to sumatriptan. A randomized, double-blind, placebo-controlled, parallel-group, outpatient study of placebo and 2.5, 5, 10, 20, or 40 mg of frovatriptan allocated in a 1:1:1:2:2:2 ratio was performed in 38 U.S. centers. At 2 hours, there was a twofold significant difference in response rates between all doses of frovatriptan (40% to 48%) and placebo (22%) (p ≤ 0.012). More patients had relief of associated migraine symptoms and functional improvement in each of the frovatriptan groups than in the placebo group. Fewer patients took rescue medication in the frovatriptan groups (23% to 36%) than in the placebo group (50%). Lower doses were as effective as higher doses. Low recurrence rates were observed, 9% to 14% for frovatriptan and 18% for placebo; while no dose response for efficacy was observed, a dose relationship for safety was seen. Frovatriptan was effective and well tolerated across a wide range of doses. The initial clinical data suggest that frovatriptan has a promising profile for the acute treatment of migraine. In a follow-up study, a dose response was observed for both efficacy and, to a lesser extent, safety. At 2 hours, headache response to 2.5 mg was statistically significantly superior to placebo. Recurrence rates in this study were consistent with the previous study (Vanguard, personal communication).

Three placebo-controlled, phase III studies were undertaken to confirm the efficacy of a 2.5 mg oral dose of frovatriptan (Goldstein and Keywood, 1998; Ryan and Keywood, 1998; Rapoport, 1998). Patients treated three separate attacks in each study and recorded their response to treatment on diary cards. At 2 hours, primary efficacy parameters for frovatriptan 2.5 mg were significantly (p $\leq$ 0.001) superior to placebo: 39% (placebo 21%), 46% (placebo 27%), and 36% (placebo 23%), respectively. The 4-hour responses were 56% (placebo 31%), 65% (placebo 38%), and 62% (placebo 32%). Median times to first response were 3.75 (placebo 5.57), 2.67 (placebo 6.00), and 3.75 (placebo 8.50) hours (McDaris and Hutchison, 1999). Frovatriptan 2.5 mg was tested in patients with substantial coronary artery disease risk factors, including an active diagnosis of coronary artery disease. No substantial changes in blood pressure, pulse rate, or electrocardiogram were found over a 24-hour continuously monitored patient study. No chest pain was reported by frovatriptan-treated patients and there was a statistically significantly greater incidence of 12-lead electrocardiogram changes among placebo patients compared to the frovatriptan patients at 4 hours (Rosenorm et al., 1988). However, the risk of an adverse cardiovascular event with any triptan is very rare and perhaps idiosyncratic.

Triptans are effective and relatively safe for the acute treatment of migraine headaches. To date, no evidence supports their use during the aura phase of a migraine attack. Triptans are appropriate first-line treatment

choices and may be considered for patients with moderate to severe migraine who have no contraindications to these agents. Because of their inability to take oral medications, patients with nausea and vomiting may be given intranasal or SC sumatriptan. Initial treatment with any triptan is a reasonable choice when the headache is moderate to severe or an adequate trial of NSAIDs or other nonopiate analgesics (including combination NSAIDs such as acetaminophen plus aspirin plus caffeine) has failed to provide adequate relief in the past.

LY334370 is a novel, selective $5HT_{1F}$ receptor agonist that is effective in neurogenic inflammation models and at central inhibition of c-fos expression but lacks vasoconstriction preclinically. A double-blind, parallel, dose-response trial evaluated 131 patients who treated migraine headaches of moderate or severe pain intensity with LY334370 (20, 60, and 200 mg) or placebo. Headache pain intensity of none or mild at 2 hours (2-hour response) was 19% for placebo, 18% for 20 mg, 50% for 60 mg, and 71% for 200 mg. Headache pain intensity of none at 2 hours (2-hour pain-free) was 4%, 0%, 27%, and 38%, respectively. The 2-hour recurrence after response (worsening in headache pain intensity after response at 2 hours) was 19% and 13% for the 60 and 200 mg doses, respectively. These data strongly suggest that nonvasoactive drugs are effective in migraine treatment. Table 9–20 will help with the choice of a triptan.

Neuroleptics and Antiemetics

The associated symptoms of migraine, such as nausea and vomiting, can be as disabling as the headache pain itself. The gastric stasis and delayed gastric emptying that are associated with migraine can decrease the effectiveness of oral medication (Boyle et al., 1990; Volans, 1978; Tfelt-Hansen et al., 1980). The medications used to treat migraine can produce nausea, as can migraine itself. In addition, many of the antiemetics are themselves effective in migraine headache treatment.

Neuroleptics may be used as an adjunct treatment for nausea or as primary ther-

Table 9–20 Clinical stratification of acute specific migraine treatments

Clinical situation	Treatment options
Failed analgesics/NSAIDS	First tier
	Sumatriptan 50 mg PO/NS
	Rizatriptan 10 mg PO
	Zolmitriptan 2.5 mg PO
	Eletriptan 80 mg PO
	DHE 2 mg NS
	Second tier
	Naratriptan 2.5 mg
	Ergotamine 1–2 mg PO or 1–2 mg PR
	(if headache infrequent)
Early nausea or problem taking tablets	DHE 2 mg NS
	DHE 1 mg IM, SC
	Rizatriptan 10 mg MLT wafer
	Sumatriptan 20 mg NS
	Sumatriptan 6 mg SC
Headache recurrence or long-lasting headache	DHE 2 mg NS
	DHE 1 mg IM, SC
	Ergotamine (most effective PR)
	Naratriptan 2.5 mg PO
Tolerating triptans poorly	DHE 2 mg NS
	Naratriptan 2.5 mg
Early vomiting	DHE 2 mg NS
	DHE 1 mg IM, SC Sumatriptan 25 mg
	PR (available in Europe)
	Sumatriptan 6 mg SC
	Sumatriptan 20 mg NS
	DHE 1 mg IM, SC
Very rapidly developing symptoms	Sumatriptan 6 mg SC

Adapted with permission from Silberstein et al. (1998). Migraine: Diagnosis and treatment. In *Headache in Clinical Practice* (S. D. Silberstein, R. B. Lipton, and P. J. Goadsby, eds.), pp. 61–90. Isis Medical Media, Oxford.

Key to abbreviations: NSAID, nonsteroidal anti-inflammatory drug; DHE, dihydroergotamine.

apy. Neuroleptics can be administered orally (PO), rectally (PR), IM, or IV. Monitor for hypotension and sedation. Avoid orthostatic hypotension by maintaining the patient supine for several hours following IV neuroleptics and using supplementary IV fluids if necessary.

Sixteen trials (AHCPR technical report) have compared the efficacy of rectally and parenterally administered medications that are commonly recognized as antiemetics (Coppola et al., 1995; Shrestha et al., 1996; Bell et al., 1990; Lane et al., 1989; Stiell et al., 1991; Jones et al., 1994; Amery and Waelkens, 1983; Cameron et al., 1995; Chappell et al., 1994; Ellis et al., 1993; Jones et al., 1996; Waelkens, 1984; McEwen et al., 1987; Rowat et al., 1991; Tek et al., 1990; Tfelt-Hansen et al., 1980). Prochlorperazine administered IV, IM, or PR (one trial each) (Jones et al., 1994, 1996; Rowat et al., 1991)

was significantly superior to placebo in headache pain relief. In two of three trials, metoclopramide IV was more effective than placebo (Coppola et al., 1995; Ellis et al., 1993; Tek et al., 1990). One study suggested that metoclopramide IV was more effective than oral ibuprofen (Ellis et al., 1993). Metoclopramide IM (Jones et al., 1996) or PR (Tfelt-Hansen et al., 1980) showed a trend toward improvement, but significant differences compared with placebo were not reached. Chlorpromazine IM was not significantly different from placebo (McEwen et al., 1987).

Prochlorperazine IV and IM was significantly superior to metoclopramide in the corresponding forms (Coppola et al., 1995; Jones et al., 1996), but another study found no differences between IV chlorpromazine and metoclopramide (Cameron et al., 1995). Metoclopramide IM was not different from placebo in providing headache relief when administered as add-on therapy to acetamin-ophen plus diazepam (Tfelt-Hansen et al., 1980). Chlorpromazine IV was not signifi-cantly different from DHE IV or ketorolac IM (Bell et al., 1990; Shrestha et al., 1996) but was superior to meperidine IV (Lane et al., 1989) and lidocaine IV (Bell et al., 1990); however, neither of these comparative agents was effective for acute migraine.

Metoclopramide, prochlorperazine, and chlorpromazine had the common adverse event of drowsiness or sedation. Acute dys-tonic reactions and akathisia were rare (Gray et al., 1999c,d).

Studies of specific oral agents, such as domperidone and prochlorperazine, have suggested some clinical benefit but were lim-ited (Gray et al., 1999b,c). No studies were identified for other oral antiemetics as mono-therapy to manage acute migraine attacks for headache relief. Oral antiemetics may be used as an adjunct in the treatment of nausea associated with migraine.

Metoclopramide IM is not effective as monotherapy for acute migraine headache. Metoclopramide IM may be considered an adjunct to control nausea in the treatment of migraine.

Metoclopramide IV was effective for acute migraine in two out of three studies (Gray et al., 1999c). It may be an appropriate choice as adjunct therapy for headache pain or nau-sea in the appropriate setting. It may be used as monotherapy for migraine pain. Metoclo-pramide (Reglan) is available as tablets, syrup, and injectable form (dose 10 to 20 mg) and is useful in the treatment of migraine. It decreases gastric atony and enhances the ab-sorption of coadministered medications (Al-bibi and McCallum, 1983).

Prochlorperazine IM, IV, or PR was rela-tively safe and effective for the treatment of migraine headache and associated nausea and vomiting. Prochlorperazine IV, IM, and PR may be a therapeutic choice for migraine in the appropriate setting. Prochlorperazine PR may be considered an adjunct in the treat-ment of acute migraine with nausea and vom-iting. Prochlorperazine (Compazine) can be administered IV 7.5 to 15 mg over 5 to 10

minutes via a saline drip or "slow push" (Cal-laham and Raskin, 1986; Jones et al., 1989).

Promethazine, available in tablet, liquid, suppository, and injectable forms (dose 25 to 50 mg) is also useful for the control of nausea and vomiting but, unlike metoclopramide, does not enhance gastric emptying. Some pa-tients find promethazine more tolerable than metoclopramide because it has fewer extra-pyramidal side effects.

Hydroxyzine (dose 50 to 100 mg PO, 75 mg IM) may be useful in controlling both nausea and headache. Perphenazine (dose 2 to 4 mg PO, 5 mg IM), chlorpromazine (dose 25 to 50 mg orally, 25 to 100 mg PR), and prochlorperazine (dose 10 mg IM or PR) may be similarly useful and are discussed in more detail below.

Chlorpromazine (Thorazine) can be ad-ministered IV (10 to 25 mg three to four times/day) diluted in 20 to 30 ml of saline by rapid drip or slow push over several minutes. Chlorpromazine can also be administered IM or PR.

Perphenazine (Trilafon, 5 mg IM), halo-peridol (Haldol 5 mg IM), and thiothixene (Navane, 5 mg IM) can also be used as pri-mary or adjunct treatment for intractable mi-graine. Haloperidol was shown to be effective in acute migraine treatment in an open case series (Fisher, 1995).

Droperidol is a parenteral neuroleptic. A pilot study of IV droperidol in 35 patients (32 women and three men, mean age 43) with status migrainosus (n = 25) or refractory mi-graine (n = 10) was conducted in an ambu-latory infusion center. Headache was graded as severe in 21 and moderate in 14 patients. Droperidol (2.5 mg) was given IV every 30 minutes until either three doses were given or the patient was completely or almost head-ache-free (Wang et al., 1997).

The success rate (headache-free or mild headache) was 88% (22/25) in patients with status migrainosus and 100% (10/10) in pa-tients with refractory migraine. The average time to headache improvement was 40 minutes (n = 35), to mild headache 60 minutes (n = 32), and to headache-free 105 minutes (n = 28). Nausea, vomiting, and light and sound sensitivity resolved in all but five patients. Four patients had an asymptomatic systolic blood pressure drop to 20 mm Hg. Sedation was common (34/35), akathisia unusual (5/35), and dystonia rare (1/35). At follow-up 24 hours after discharge, the recurrence rate (headache intensity from none or mild to moderate or severe) was 23% in status migrainosus patients and 10% in refractory migraine patients. Twenty-one patients were still sedated, while 19 had extrapyramidal symptoms, mainly restlessness. Droperidol appears to be safe and effective at treating status migrainosus and refractory migraine. Hypotension was uncommon. Patients should be warned of sedation and akathisia (Wang et al., 1997), which can be treated with diphenhydramine or benzotropine.

Krusz et al. (1999b) treated 45 patients, taken from a population of migraineurs in a headache clinic, with IV droperidol. The average dose per treatment was 3.2 mg, using increments of 0.625 mg per dose. The average reduction in headache severity was 86.1%, using a 0 to 10 Visual Analog Scale rated by each patient. The average time to maximum reduction of headache was about 40 minutes. Droperidol is useful at aborting ongoing migraine headache, acts rapidly, and is devoid of side effects when used in the dosage range employed in this study.

Studies testing the efficacy of the 5-HT$_3$ antagonists granisetron (Rowat et al., 1991) and zatosetron (Chappell et al., 1994) did not demonstrate a statistically significant clinical benefit for headache relief. Sufficient studies have not been done to demonstrate the clinical efficacy of this class of drug. Evidence is insufficient at this time to establish or refute a role for 5-HT$_3$ antagonists as monotherapy in the management of acute attacks. The 5-HT$_3$ antagonists may be considered as adjunct therapy to control nausea in selected patients with migraine attacks. Ondansetron, a selective 5-HT$_3$-receptor antagonist that has no antidopaminergic activity and no effect on gastrointestinal motility, is available IV for the nausea associated with migraine (dose 0.15 mg/kg diluted in 50 ml of 5% dextrose in water or normal saline solution).

Other Acute Treatment

Preventive Medications Used in the Acute Treatment of Migraine

β-ADRENERGIC BLOCKERS

Featherstone (1983) and Tokola and Hokkanan (1978) have suggested that propranolol (40 to 80 mg) can abort an acute attack of migraine with or without aura. However, Fuller and Guiloff (1990) could not demonstrate propranolol's effectiveness in a placebo-controlled, double-blind study. This could be a result of a large placebo effect in the open studies or failure to study a subset of migraineurs who might respond to propranolol.

CALCIUM ANTAGONISTS

Verapamil IV (10 mg) and sublingual nimodipine (40 mg) have not been effective at treating acute attacks of migraine (Andersson and Vinge, 1990). Nifedipine may be useful for treating the aura of migraine but is ineffective at treating the headache (Scholz and Hoffert, 1987). Some recent studies suggest that IV (Soyka et al., 1989; Pfaffenrath et al., 1990) or sublingual (Takeshima et al., 1988) flunarizine is effective in the acute treatment of migraine, perhaps in part due to its dopaminergic blocking effect.

DIVALPROEX

Small open studies have suggested that IV divalproex is effective in acute migraine treatment. Fourteen consecutive patients with moderate to severe headaches of 24 to 72 hours' duration were given 500 mg of valproate IV over 15 to 30 minutes or 10 mg metoclopramide with 1 mg DHE IM. In the IV valproate group, 71.4% of patients improved to a state of mild or no headache at 1 hour, 85.7% at 2 hours, and 71.4% at 4 hours. Migraine-associated symptoms of nausea, photophobia, and phonophobia showed similar improvement. In the DHE group, 42.8% of patients improved to a state of mild or no headache at 1 and 2 hours and 57.1% at 4 hours (Edwards et al., 1999).

Czapinski and Motyl (1999) studied 25 patients (18 women and 7 men) with an acute migraine attack, with or without aura, within 6 hours of onset. They were given either valproate IV 5 minutes at 15 mg/kg of body weight or 0.9% NaCl according to the same protocol. Ten of 13 patients treated with valproate showed a decrease or subsidence of pain, in contrast to 4 of 12 patients in the placebo group. Complete pain relief occurred as soon as 10 minutes, with a range of 10 to 25 minutes (Mathew et al., 1999a).

LIDOCAINE

Lidocaine IV demonstrated limited benefit over placebo in one small study that failed to demonstrate clinically significant benefit or harm (Reutens et al., 1991). In a second trial, lidocaine was significantly less effective than chlorpromazine IV and not more effective than DHE IV (Bell et al., 1990). One study suggested that intranasal lidocaine is effective at relieving headache pain quickly (within 15 minutes), but pronounced local adverse events and a high incidence of recurrence were also reported (Maizels et al., 1996). A recently published abstract (not included in the AHCPR technical report) stated that intranasal lidocaine provided rapid relief; however, the previously reported high incidence of recurrence was not confirmed in this later study (Maizels et al., 1996). Since lidocaine IV is not significantly better than placebo and is less effective than other parenteral therapies for treatment of acute migraine, evidence is insufficient to support a role of lidocaine IV in the management of acute migraine.

CORTICOSTEROIDS

Studies have suggested that corticosteroids are effective in the treatment of headache (Gallagher, 1986). The mechanism by which the corticosteroids exert their effect in migraine is uncertain. They may control neurogenic inflammation or have an effect on the hypothalamic–pituitary axis. One study suggested that inclusion of dexamethasone in an opioid regimen provides added relief (Gallagher, 1986). Two small studies provided insufficient data from which to draw conclu-

sions about the efficacy or safety of either dexamethasone IV or hydrocortisone IV for the acute treatment of migraine (Klapper and Stanton, 1991b; Kozubski, 1992). In one study, dexamethasone IV (6 mg) following pretreatment with metoclopramide IV was effective in the treatment of acute migraine (Klapper and Stanton, 1991a). No good-quality studies support or refute the effectiveness of steroids for acute migraine. Corticosteroids may be considered as a treatment choice for rescue therapy in patients with status migrainosus. Clinical experience also supports the view that oral steroids can assist in terminating an otherwise refractory migraine (Saper, 1989). We believe that high-dose IV steroids, alone or in conjunction with neuroleptics or DHE, can terminate a refractory headache cycle (Saper, 1990; Silberstein et al., 1990a).

Hydrocortisone or methylprednisolone sodium succinate (Solu-Medrol) can be given IV in the following manner: 100 mg via a saline drip over 10 minutes every 6 hours for 24 hours; every 8 hours for 24 hours; every 12 hours for 24 hours; and then a final dose. Dexamethasone (Decadron) can be administered IV or IM, starting at a dose of 8 to 20 mg/day in divided doses, rapidly tapering over 2 to 3 days. Oral dexamethasone 1.5 mg twice daily for 2 days with a taper over 3 more days has also proven useful for less disabled migraineurs with prolonged migraine headache.

MAGNESIUM

The efficacy of IV magnesium sulfate ($MgSO_4$) 1 g was evaluated and the clinical response correlated to the basal serum ionized magnesium (IMg^{2+}) level. In an outpatient headache clinic, a consecutive sample of patients with moderate or severe headache of any type was studied (n = 16 migraine without aura, n = 9 cluster headaches, n = 4 chronic TTHs, and n = 11 chronic migrainous headaches. Total serum magnesium was measured by atomic absorption spectroscopy, and IMg^{2+} was measured with ion-selective electrodes. Complete pain relief was observed in 80% of patients within 15 minutes of $MgSO_4$ infusion. No recurrence or worsening of pain was observed within 24 hours in 56% of patients. Patients treated with $MgSO_4$ also had complete elimination of migraine-associated symptoms such as nausea, photophobia, and phonophobia. Of the 18 patients who did well, 16 (89%) had a low serum IMg^{2+} level. Of the eight patients with no relief, only 37.5% had a low IMg^{2+} level. Intravenous infusion of 1 g of $MgSO_4$ may relieve headache pain in patients with low serum IMg^{2+} levels (Gray et al., 1999b).

NEUROACTIVE STEROIDS

Neuroactive steroids alter the excitability of membrane-bound receptors in the nervous system and thus differ from steroid hormones, which regulate gene transcription through interactions with intracellular receptors. Neuroactive steroids modulate neurotransmission through specific, positive allosteric interaction with a steroid recognition site on the $GABA_A$ receptor ion-channel complex and inhibit voltage-gated Ca^{2+} currents and NMDA receptor function (Gasior et al., 1999).

Ganaxolone is a member of a novel class of neurosteroids called epalons, which modulate $GABA_A$ receptors in the CNS by interacting with the epalon receptor. The epalons, chemically related to progesterone, have no hormonal activity but have potent antiepileptic, anxiolytic, sedative, and hypnotic activity. Ganaxolone chemically is 3-hydroxy-3-methyl-5-pregnan-20-one. It is being developed for the treatment of epilepsy and migraine. In a phase II migraine trial, 252 premenopausal women between the ages of 18 and 55 were given a liquid suspension of one of four doses of ganaxolone or placebo. There was a substantial increase in response as a function of the plasma at 2 and 4 hours postdose. Patients with a plasma drug level of 80 mg/ml or more were more likely to experience pain relief. A tablet formulation, designed to increase the predictability of absorption, will be used for further relevant trials (Kapicioglu et al., 1997).

Octreotide, a long-acting somatostatin analogue, inhibits 5-HT, bradykinin, prostaglandin, substance P, and vasoactive intestinal polypeptide release. In a double-blind, placebo-controlled trial, octreotide 100 μg SC was more effective than placebo at reducing headache at 2 hours.

NITRIC OXIDE SYNTHETASE INHIBITORS

Nitric oxide is formed from the amino acid L-arginine, catalyzed by a family of enzymes known as NO synthases (NOSs). Some of these enzymes are constitutive (cNOS) and calcium/calmodulin-dependent and result in the release of NO from the endothelium and neurons in response to receptor stimulation. Other NOSs are inducible (iNOS) and cause the release of NO from macrophages, astrocytes, and microglia (Thomsen et al., 1994).

Nitric oxide exerts many of its actions by stimulating soluble guanylate cyclase. It is a powerful vasodilator. It is the most important of the so-called endothelium-derived relaxing factors. It is a noxious molecule (Hibbs et al., 1988), and pain, by definition, is a sensation elicited by noxious stimulation. It plays a role in the central processing of pain by interacting with CNS NMDA receptors, resulting in hyperalgesia (Kolesnikov et al., 1992). The NO donors cause CGRP release from perivascular nerve endings in experimental animals.

Nitric oxide may play a pivotal role in migraine pain. Migraineurs are hypersensitive to nitroglycerin, and the NO donor nitroglycerin (glyceryl trinitrate) triggers genuine migraine attacks.

In a double-blind study, 15 patients were randomized to receive the NOS inhibitor L-N^a-methylarginine hydrochloride (546C88) and three patients to receive placebo. The placebo-treated patients were used in the statistical evaluation together with 11 historical controls who had received IV placebo in recent double-blind studies. Patients were treated in hospital with 6 mg/kg 546C88 or placebo (5% dextrose) given IV over 15 minutes for a single spontaneous migraine attack. Of those treated in the trial, 10 of 15 had headache relief at 2 hours compared to 2 of 14 in the control group. Most of these patients were historic (i.e., came from prior trials). It is thus possible that the relief could have been due to a placebo effect (Lassen et al., 1997).

Krusz and Belanger (1999a) reported on the effectiveness of propofol (2,6-diidopropylphenol), an IV anesthetic agent, in treating acute migraine and other headaches in an outpatient headache clinic. Forty-two patients were treated for intractable headaches that were refractory to the usual therapy. Headaches were rated as 7 or higher (out of 10) on VAS. Propofol was administered IV, 20 to 30 mg every 3 to 5 minutes. In no case was the patient asleep during any phase of treatment. The average reduction in headache severity was 94.7%. Time to maximal reduction was 15 to 30 minutes. The average dose of propofol was 95 mg. Propofol has numerous mechanisms of action, including at $GABA_A$ receptors, with reduction in sympathetic neuronal activity, stimulation of NO release, depression of spinal nociceptive neurotransmission, and depression of NMDA receptor excitation.

Civamide, chemically related to capsaicin, a vanniloid receptor agonist that blocks the release of CGRP and substance P, was studied in a multicenter, blinded trial. Both doses (20 and 150 μg) were effective in at least 50% of patients; however, nasal burning also occurred in 88% of subjects (Diamond et al., 1999a).

Failed Drugs

NEUROKININ

Lanepitant, a high-affinity selective neurokinin-1 (NK-1) receptor antagonist effective in the dural inflammation model, was not effective in acute migraine treatment. Lanepitant 30, 80, and 240 mg PO was no more effective than placebo in a controlled, double-blind, crossover trial. However, absorption of the drug during a migraine attack was less than 10% of that of fasted volunteers. This suggests that the negative result was due to inadequate plasma concentration of the drug and says nothing about drug efficacy or the predictive value of the Moskowitz model (Goldstein et al., 1997). RPR100893–201, another NK-1 antagonist, was also not effective in acute migraine treatment at a 20 mg oral dose. Again sufficient plasma concentration

may not have been achieved (Diener et al., 1995).

ENDOTHELIAL ANTAGONISTS

The endothelin family of peptides are potent endogenous vasoconstrictor and pressor agents. Two receptor subtypes, ET_A and ET_B, have been cloned and are found on smooth-muscle cells. The ET_B subtype is also found on endothelial cells and mediates endothelin-dependent vasodilation by the release of NO and prostacyclin (Ferro and Webb, 1996). Bosantan, a mixed endothelin ($ET_{A/B}$) receptor antagonist, was ineffective in the treatment of migraine even when administered IV. In this case, the pharmacokinetics of oral absorption was circumvented (Brandli et al., 1996; Clozel et al., 1994).

PREVENTIVE TREATMENT

Preventive medications are usually taken, whether or not headache is present, to reduce the frequency, duration, or severity of attacks. Preventive treatment can be either episodic, short-term (subacute), or chronic. Episodic preventive treatment is used when there is a known headache trigger, such as exercise or sexual activity. Patients can be instructed to pretreat prior to the exposure or activity. For example, single doses of indomethacin can be used to prevent exercise-induced migraine. Short-term prevention is used in patients undergoing a time-limited exposure to a provoking factor, such as ascent to a high altitude or menstruation. These patients can be treated with daily medication just before and during the exposure (Silberstein et al., 1998). Standard chronic preventive treatment is often maintained for months or even years.

Most current recommendations for migraine prevention focus on the number of attacks that occur each month. These recommendations do not take into account the patient's response to acute medication, the patient's needs or preferences, or the characteristics of the attack. Circumstances that might warrant chronic preventive treatment include (1) recurring migraine that significantly interferes with the patient's daily routine despite acute treatment (e.g., two or more attacks a month that produce disability and last 3 or more days or that are infrequent but produce profound disability); (2) failure of, contraindication to, or troublesome side effects from acute medications; (3) overuse of acute medications; (4) special circumstances, such as hemiplegic migraine or attacks with a risk of permanent neurologic injury; (5) very frequent headaches (more than two per week) with the risk of rebound headache development; and (6) patient preference, i.e., the desire to have as few acute attacks as possible. These rules are stricter during pregnancy, when severe, disabling attacks accompanied by nausea, vomiting, and possibly dehydration are required for chronic treatment to be prescribed (Silberstein, 1997a, 2000b).

The major medication groups (Table 9–21) for preventive migraine treatment include β-adrenergic blockers, antidepressants, calcium channel antagonists, serotonin antagonists, anticonvulsants, NSAIDs, and others (including riboflavin, minerals, and herbs). If preventive medication is indicated, the agent should be preferentially chosen from one of the first-line categories, based on the drug's side effect profile and the patient's coexistent and comorbid conditions (Table 9–10) (Tfelt-Hansen and Lipton, 1993). The following principles will increase the chances of success.

Start the drug at a low dose and increase it slowly until therapeutic effects develop, the

Table 9–21 Preventive prescription drugs

Anticonvulsants
  Valproate, gabapentin, topiramate, tiagabine
Antidepressants
  TCAs, SSRIs, MAOIs
β-Adrenergic blockers
  Propranolol/nadolol/metoprolol/atenolol
Calcium channel antagonists
  Verapamil/nimodipine
Serotonin antagonists
  Methysergide/methergine
Others
  NSAIDs, riboflavin, magnesium, neuroleptics

Key to abbreviations: TCA, tricyclic antidepressant; SSRI, selective serotonin reuptake inhibitor; MAOI, monoamine oxidase inhibitor; NSAID, nonsteroidal anti-inflammatory drug.

ceiling dose for the chosen drug is reached, or side effects become intolerable. Migraineurs often require a lower dose of a preventive medication than is needed for other indications. Tricyclic antidepressants (TCAs) such as amitriptyline are often used in doses of 75 to 200 mg/day for depression, while 10 to 75 mg/day is often effective for migraine. In addition, migraineurs may be more sensitive to a medication's side effect. A starting dose of 25 to 50 mg/day of amitriptyline is common in patients with depression, whereas it can produce intolerable side effects in migraineurs (Silberstein, 1997a). Divalproex is often effective at a dose of 500 to 750 mg/day for migraine, while higher doses may be necessary to effectively treat epilepsy and mania (Silberstein, 1996b). It is important to remember that some patients may respond to lower doses of preventive medications, but it may be necessary to increase the dose to tolerance before assuming that the agent is ineffective.

Give each treatment an adequate trial. A full therapeutic trial may take 2 to 6 months. In controlled clinical trials, efficacy is often first noted at 4 weeks and continues to increase for 3 months. In practice, a common mistake is to treat a patient with a new preventive medication for 1 or 2 weeks without effect and discontinue treatment after a breakthrough headache.

Avoid interfering, overused, and contraindicated drugs. To obtain maximal benefit from preventive medication, the patient should not overuse analgesics, opioids, triptans, or ergot derivatives. In addition, OCs, hormonal replacement therapy, or vasodilating drugs, such as nifedipine or nitroglycerine, may interfere with preventive drugs.

Re-evaluate therapy. Migraine headaches may improve independently of treatment; if the headaches are well controlled, slowly taper and, if possible, discontinue the drug. Many patients experience continued relief with a lower dose of the medication, and others may not require it at all. In all cases, dose reduction frequently provides a better risk-to-benefit ratio.

Be sure that a woman of childbearing potential is aware of any potential risks, and pick the medication that will have the least adverse effect on the fetus (Silberstein, 1997a). Ideally, she should be on adequate contraception before starting migraine medication. However, some women who are pregnant or attempting to become pregnant may still require preventive medications. If this is absolutely necessary, inform the patient and her partner of any potential risks, and pick the medication that will have the least adverse effect on the fetus (Silberstein, 1997a).

Involve patients in their care to maximize compliance. Take patient preferences into account when drugs of relatively equivalent efficacy can be used. Discuss the rationale for a particular treatment, when and how to use it, and what side effects are likely. Address patient expectations. Discuss with the patient the expected benefits of therapy and how long it will take to achieve them (Silberstein, 2000b).

β Adrenergic Blockers

β Blockers, the most widely used class of drugs in prophylactic migraine treatment, are 60% to 80% effective at producing a greater than 50% reduction in attack frequency. Rabkin et al. (1966) serendipitously discovered propranolol's effectiveness in headache treatment in patients who were being treated for angina (Weber and Reinmuth, 1972; Diamond and Medina, 1976).

The AHCPR technical report analyzed 74 controlled trials of β blockers for migraine prevention, including 46 trials of propranolol, 14 trials of metoprolol, and trials of acebutolol, alprenolol, atenolol, bisoprolol, nadolol, oxprenolol, pindolol, practolol, and timolol (Gray et al., 1999a).

Evidence consistently showed propranolol's efficacy in a daily dose of 120 to 240 mg for migraine prevention. Twelve of 21 placebo-controlled trials of propranolol allowed estimation of effect sizes for headache frequency or headache index (Sargent et al., 1985; Pradalier et al., 1989; Ahuja and Verma, 1985; Borgesen et al., 1974; Dahlof, 1987; Forssman et al., 1976; Johnson et al., 1986; Mikkelsen and Falk, 1982; Pita et al., 1977; Stensrud and Sjaastad, 1976a; Tfelt-Hansen et al., 1984; Wideroe and Vigander, 1974). The 12

effect-size estimates were statistically homogeneous and, when combined, indicated a high degree of certainty that propranolol provides moderate reduction in headache frequency or index.

The relative efficacy of the different β blockers has not been clearly established, and most studies show no significant difference between drugs. Direct comparisons have demonstrated few significant differences in efficacy between propranolol and flunarizine (Gawel et al., 1992; Lucking et al., 1988; Ludin, 1989; Shimell et al., 1990), amitriptyline (Ziegler et al., 1987; Mathew, 1981), naproxen sodium (Sargent et al., 1985), mefenamic acid (Johnson et al., 1986), tolfenamic acid (Mikkelsen et al., 1986; Kjaersgaard-Rasmussen et al., 1994), divalproex sodium (Kaniecki, 1997), and methysergide (Behan and Reid, 1980; Steardo et al., 1982). All of these treatments were effective for migraine prevention. One trial comparing propranolol and amitriptyline suggested that propranolol is more efficacious in patients with migraine alone and amitriptyline is superior for patients with mixed migraine and TTH (Mathew, 1981).

Four trials comparing metoprolol with placebo reported mixed results (Langohr et al., 1985; Andersson et al., 1983; Kangasniemi et al., 1987; Steiner et al., 1988). Direct comparisons of metoprolol with propranolol (Steardo et al., 1982; Gerber et al., 1991; Andersson et al., 1983; Olsson et al., 1984), flunarizine (Grotemeyer et al., 1990; Sorensen et al., 1991), and pizotifen (Vilming et al., 1985) demonstrated few significant differences, suggesting that metoprolol is efficacious for the prevention of migraine. Timolol (Stensrud and Sjaastad, 1976b; Briggs and Millac, 1979; Stellar et al., 1984), atenolol (Forssman et al., 1983; Johannsson et al., 1987; Stensrud and Sjaastad, 1974), and nadolol (Tobita et al., 1987; Freitag and Diamond, 1984; Olerud et al., 1986; Ryan and Sudilovsky, 1983; Ryan, 1984; Sudilovsky et al., 1986) are also likely to be beneficial based on comparisons with placebo or with propranolol.

The β blockers with intrinsic sympathomimetic activity (acebutolol, alprenolol, oxprenolol, pindolol) have not been effective at preventing migraine (Ekbom and Lundberg,

1972; Ekbom and Zetterman, 1977; Nanda et al., 1978; Ekbom, 1994; Sjaastad and Stensrud, 1972). These drugs, which are partial agonists, exert intrinsic sympathomimetic activity, and this property may make them ineffective (Fanchamps, 1985). A review of the pharmacological characteristics of the various β blockers suggested that the only factor that correlates with their efficacy is the absence of partial agonist activity (Shanks, 1987). Since all of the negative studies are small and of low power, the possibility that beneficial effects have escaped detection cannot be excluded. In fact, pindolol (Anthony et al., 1972) and practolol (Sales and Bada, 1975) were effective in open-label studies.

A few trials have used long-acting or extended-release preparations of propranolol or metoprolol, but evidence was insufficient to determine whether these preparations were more efficacious and/or better tolerated than regular formulations (Pita et al., 1977; Wideroe and Vigander, 1974; Steardo et al., 1982; Andersson et al., 1983; Kuritzky and Hering, 1987; Solomon, 1986).

No absolute correlation has been found between propranolol's dose and its clinical efficacy (Andersson and Vinge, 1990). One meta-analysis of 53 studies (2,403 treated patients) revealed that, on average, propranolol yielded a 44% reduction in migraine activity compared with a 14% reduction in migraine activity with placebo. Variations in propranolol dose levels across studies were unrelated to the magnitude of the propranolol treatment effect. Overall, one of six patients discontinued propranolol treatment (Holroyd et al., 1991).

The choice of β blocker should be based on specific properties such as β_1 selectivity, convenience of drug formulation, and idiosyncratic drug effectiveness. Before giving up on β blockers as a group, it may be worthwhile to utilize combined or alternate trials. There may be continued improvement after the drug is discontinued. In a 6-month clinical trial of propranolol, approximately 46% of patients who experienced a reduction in migraine frequency maintained their improvement for up to 6 additional months after discontinuation (Diamond et al., 1982).

The mechanism of action of β blockers is not certain, but it appears that their antimigraine effect is due to inhibition of β_1-mediated mechanisms (Ablad and Dahlof, 1986).

β Blockade results in inhibition of norepinephrine (NE) release by blocking prejunctional β receptors. In addition, it results in a delayed reduction in tyrosine hydroxylase activity (the rate-limiting step in NE synthesis) in the superior cervical ganglia. In the rat brain-stem, delayed reduction of the locus ceruleus neuron firing rate has been demonstrated after propranolol administration (Ablad and Dahlof, 1986). This could explain the delay in the prophylactic effect of the β blocker.

The action of β blockers most likely is central and could be mediated by (1) inhibiting central β receptors interfering with the vigilance-enhancing adrenergic pathway, (2) interaction with 5-HT receptors (but not all β blockers bind to the 5-HT receptors), and (3) cross-modulation of the serotonin system (Koella, 1985; Silberstein and Silberstein, 1990b).

Schoenen et al. (1986) have shown that contingent negative variation (CNV), an event-related slow negative scalp potential, is significantly increased and its habituation reduced in patients with untreated common migraine. After treatment with β blockers, CNV normalizes, which is consistent with central adrenergic hyperactivity in migraine. Migraineurs with elevated CNV scores have a much better response to β-blocker therapy (80% effective) than migraineurs with a low or normal score (22% effective), suggesting that the CNV may predict the response to β-blocker treatment (Schoenen et al., 1986). Migraineurs exhibit enhanced centrally mediated secretion of epinephrine after exposure to light (Stoica and Enulescu, 1990); this returns to normal after treatment with propranolol.

The β blockers that are clinically useful in the treatment of migraine consist of both the nonselective blocking agents (propranolol, nadolol, and timolol) and the selective β_1 blockers (metoprolol and atenolol).

All β blockers can produce behavioral side effects, such as drowsiness, fatigue, lethargy, sleep disorders, nightmares, depression, memory disturbance, and hallucinations, indicating that they all affect the CNS. Adverse events most commonly reported in clinical trials with β blockers were fatigue, depression, nausea, dizziness, and insomnia. These symptoms appeared to be fairly well tolerated and were seldom the cause of premature withdrawal from trials (Gray et al., 1999a). In experimental animals, β blockers reduce spontaneous motor activity, counteract amphetamine-induced hyperactivity, and produce slow-wave and paradoxical sleep disturbances. The central effect of β blockers is used to treat anxiety (Koella, 1985). Common side effects include gastrointestinal complaints and decreased exercise tolerance. Less common are orthostatic hypotension, significant bradycardia, impotence, and aggravation of intrinsic muscle disease. Propranolol has been reported to have an adverse effect on the fetus (Featherstone, 1983). Congestive heart failure, asthma, and insulin-dependent diabetes are contraindications to the use of nonselective β blockers.

Case reports (Prendes, 1980; Gilbert, 1982; Bardwell and Trott, 1987; Kumar and Cooney, 1990) have implicated propranolol in the development of migrainous infarction or increasing visual symptoms in patients with migraine with aura. However, Kangasniemi et al. (1987), in a double-blind placebo-controlled study, found that metoprolol was effective in prophylaxis of migraine with aura. Hedman et al. (1988) looked at the modification of aura symptoms by metoprolol. Patients had fewer migraine attacks during metoprolol treatment, and those that occurred were less severe. There was no change in the total visual and nonvisual aura symptoms, but scintillations and paresthesias were more common, while speech disturbances were less frequent.

At this time, it appears that β blockers are not absolutely contraindicated in migraine with aura unless a clear stroke risk is present; the reported adverse reactions to propranolol may be either coincidental or idiosyncratic, but the actual risk is uncertain.

Treatment with β blockers must be individualized following the principles of prophylactic therapy. If the first β blocker is ineffective or has significant side effects, it may be worthwhile to try a second one. Some authors

have commented on continued improvement (Rosen, 1983) and lack of rebound (Diamond et al., 1982) after discontinuing propranolol. However, it seems more reasonable to slowly taper β blockers since stopping them abruptly can cause increased headache (Kangasniemi et al., 1987) and the withdrawal symptoms of tachycardia and tremulousness (Frishman, 1987).

Propranolol (Inderal) is a nonselective β blocker with a half-life of 4 to 6 hours, also available in an effective long-acting formulation (Inderal LA) (Pradalier et al., 1989; Diamond et al., 1987). The therapeutically effective dose of propranolol ranges from 40 to 400 mg/day, with no correlation between propranolol and 4-hydroxypropranolol plasma levels and headache relief (Cortelli et al., 1985). The short-acting form can be given three to four times a day, the long-acting form once or twice a day (we recommend twice a day). Start with 40 mg/day in divided doses and slowly increase to tolerance.

Nadolol (Corgard) is a nonselective β blocker with a long half-life. It is less lipid-soluble than propranolol and has fewer CNS side effects. The dose ranges from 20 to 160 mg/day, given once or in split doses. Some authorities prefer it to propranolol since it has fewer side effects (Sudilovsky et al., 1987).

Timolol (Blocadren) is a nonselective β blocker with a short half-life. The dose ranges from 20 to 60 mg/day in divided doses.

Atenolol (Tenormin) is a selective β_1 blocker with fewer side effects than propranolol. The dose ranges from 50 to 200 mg/day.

Metoprolol (Lopressor) is a selective β_1 blocker with a short half-life. The dose ranges from 100 to 200 mg/day, in divided doses. A long-acting preparation (Toprol XL) may be given once a day.

Antidepressants

The available antidepressants consist of a number of different classes of drugs with different mechanisms of action: (1) the monoamine oxidase inhibitors (MAOIs), including the selective and reversible and the nonselective and irreversible types; (2) the monoamine reuptake inhibitors, including nonselective TCAs, selective serotonin reuptake inhibitors (SSRIs), and selective serotonin and norepinephrine reuptake inhibitors (SNRIs); (3) the monoamine receptor-targeted drugs, including serotonin (trazadone), α_2 antagonist (mirtazapine), and dopamine (bupropion). Future drugs may be based on substance P antagonism.

The TCAs, SSRIs, and SNRIs increase synaptic NE or serotonin (5-HT) by inhibiting high-affinity reuptake. Some are more potent inhibitors of NE, others of 5-HT reuptake. The MAOIs block the degradation of catecholamines. The therapeutic action of antidepressant treatment was initially believed to be a consequence of increased synaptic NE and 5-HT. However, this does not account for the temporal discrepancy between the rapid drug-induced effects on amine uptake, which occur within hours; the antidepressant effects, which take 2 to 3 weeks; and prophylactic headache response, which takes 3 to 10 days or longer (Heninger and Charney, 1987).

The most consistent neurochemical finding with antidepressant treatment (including TCAs, SSRIs, MAOIs and electroconvulsive therapy) is a decrease in β-adrenergic receptor density and NE-stimulated cAMP response. Increased α_1-receptor system sensitivity is not seen as consistently with antidepressant treatment. Long-term antidepressant treatment decreases 5-HT$_2$ receptor-binding and imipramine-binding sites (related to the 5-HT uptake system) but does not change 5-HT$_1$ receptor binding. A strong interaction exists between the NE and 5-HT systems. β-Receptor downregulation in antidepressant treatment is dependent on an intact 5-HT system, while lesions of the NE system block the decrease in 5-HT$_2$ receptor binding (Heninger and Charney, 1987).

The decrease in 5-HT$_2$ receptor-binding sites does not correlate with a decrease in function; in fact, there may be enhanced physiologic responsiveness. If one records the electric activity of neurons following iontophoretic application of 5-HT, one finds that the response is enhanced following antidepressant treatment, suggesting that an enhancement of the second-messenger system has occurred. In addition, antidepressant treatment decreases the sensitivity of the presynaptic 5-HT autoreceptors, thereby enhancing 5-HT release (Heninger and Charney, 1987).

The TCAs upregulate the GABA$_B$ receptor, downregulate the histamine receptor, and enhance the neuronal sensitivity to substance P. Some TCAs are 5-HT$_2$ receptor antagonists. Bupropion is both a dopamine and NE reuptake inhibitor.

The mechanism of headache prophylaxis with antidepressants is uncertain but does not result from treating masked depression. Antidepressants are useful in treating many chronic pain states, including headache, independent of the presence of depression; and the response occurs sooner than the expected antidepressant effect (Couch et al., 1976; Panerai et al., 1990; Kishore-Kumar et al., 1990). (Most clinical studies have concentrated on pain and headache other than migraine.) In animal pain models, antidepressants potentiate the effects of coadministered opioids (Feinmann, 1985). The clinically effective antidepressants in headache prophylaxis either inhibit 5-HT reuptake or are antagonists at the 5-HT$_2$ receptors (Richelson, 1990).

Exogenous delivery of the neurotrophic factors brain-derived neurotrophic factor (BDNF) and neurotrophin-3 (NT-3) promotes the function, sprouting, and regrowth of 5-HT-containing neurons in the brains of adult rats. Similar infusions of BDNF into the dorsal raphe nucleus produce an antidepressant effect, as evaluated by several "learned helplessness" paradigms (Altar, 1999). Also, BDNF accelerated the regrowth of serotonergic nerve fibers following their destruction by a serotonergic neurotoxin, parachloroamphetamine.

Treatment with antidepressants, including specific inhibitors of 5-HT or noradrenaline reuptake, or MAOIs elevated BDNF mRNA levels in the rat hippocampus. Reminiscent of the delay in treating depression in humans, these compounds augmented BDNF mRNA after 3 weeks of chronic treatment but not after 1 day of treatment (Altar, 1999). Brain-derived neurotrophic factor is a large, lipophobic protein and, when given peripherally, does not cross the blood–brain barrier. The 5-HT receptors (including the 5-HT$_{2A}$ subtype), phosphodiesterase inhibition, and β-adrenoreceptors appear to be positively coupled to the production of BDNF mRNA in some brain areas (Altar, 1999).

Further evidence linking BDNF and depression comes from studies in which stress, often a precipitating factor in depression, has decreased BDNF mRNA. The stress of being immobilized (which induces learned helplessness) or system injections of glucocorticoids lower BDNF, but not NT-3, mRNA levels in the hippocampus and other brain areas (Altar, 1999). Thus, a potential new mechanism of action of the antidepressants is an interaction with BDNF.

A total of 16 controlled trials have investigated the efficacy of the TCAs amitriptyline and clomipramine and the SSRIs fluoxetine, and fluvoxamine (Adly et al., 1992; Andersson and Petersen, 1981; Bonuso et al., 1983; Couch and Hassanein, 1976, 1979; Gomersall and Stuart, 1973; Jacobs, 1972; Kangasniemi et al., 1983; Langohr et al., 1985; Mathew, 1981; Monro et al., 1985; Noone, 1980; Saper et al., 1994; Zeeberg et al., 1981; Ziegler et al., 1987; Orholm et al., 1986; Bank, 1999). Amitriptyline has been more frequently studied than the other agents and is the only antidepressant with fairly consistent support for efficacy in migraine prevention. Three placebo-controlled trials found amitriptyline significantly better than placebo at reducing headache index or frequency (Couch and Hassanein, 1976, 1979; Gomersall and Stuart, 1973; Ziegler et al., 1987). One trial conducted in patients with frequent severe or disabling headaches found no significant difference between amitriptyline and propranolol (Ziegler et al., 1987). In another trial, amitriptyline was significantly more efficacious than propranolol for patients with mixed migraine and TTH, while propranolol was significantly better for patients with migraine alone (Mathew, 1981). Amitriptyline was significantly better than timed-released dihydroergotamine (TR-DHE) at reducing headache index in a group of patients with mixed migraine and TTH (Ahuja and Verma, 1985). However, analysis of the data on headache duration, stratified by severity, showed that amitriptyline was significantly better than TR-DHE at reducing the number of hours of moderate and mild TTH-like pain. In contrast, TR-DHE was significantly better than amitriptyline at reducing the number of hours of extremely severe and severe migraine-like pain.

The evidence was insufficient to support the efficacy of clomipramine (Langohr et al., 1985; Noone, 1980) and fluvoxamine (Bank, 1999) for migraine prevention. Fluoxetine was significantly better than placebo in one (Adly et al., 1992), but not a second (Saper et al., 1994), migraine-prevention trial.

Anticholinergic symptoms were frequently reported with the TCAs studied, including amitriptyline. Adverse events were less common with SSRIs, with nausea and sexual dysfunction being the most frequently observed symptoms (Gray et al., 1999a).

The TCAs most commonly used for migraine and TTH prophylaxis include amitriptyline, nortriptyline, doxepin, and protriptyline. Imipramine and desipramine have been used at times. Most have not been vigorously evaluated; their use is based on anecdotal or uncontrolled reports (Silberstein, 2000b).

Pharmacology of Tricyclic Antidepressants

There is wide individual variation in the absorption, distribution, and excretion of the TCAs, with a 10- to 30-fold variation in individuals' drug metabolism. A therapeutic window may exist above which the TCAs are ineffective, but this has been evaluated only for nortriptyline treatment of depression. The presence of a therapeutic window and the wide variation in TCA metabolism necessitate individualized dosing and may prompt monitoring of TCA plasma levels if there are issues of toxicity or compliance. The TCAs are lipid-soluble with a high volume of distribution and avidly bind to plasma proteins. The antihistamine and antimuscarinic activity of the TCAs accounts for many of their side effects (Richardson and Richelson, 1984).

The TCA dose range is wide and must be individualized. With the exception of protrip-

Table 9–22 Tricyclic antidepressants: adverse effects and neurotransmitter receptors

Cholinergic	Blurred vision, dry mouth, sinus tachycardia, constipation, urinary retention, memory disturbances, speech blockage, decreased sweating
Serotonergic	Nausea, increased bowel motility, sweating
Histamine type-1	Sedation, drowsiness, hypotension, weight gain, potentiates other CNS depressants
Histamine type-2	Mental confusion
α_1-Adrenergic	Postural hypotension, dizziness, reflex tachycardia
Dopaminergic	Tremor, increased muscle tonus, myoclonic jerks, tardive dyskinesia

tyline, TCAs are sedating. Start with a low dose of the chosen TCA at bedtime, except when using protriptyline, which should be administered in the morning. If the TCA is too sedating, switch from a tertiary TCA (amitriptyline, doxepin) to a secondary TCA (nortriptyline, protriptyline). If a patient develops insomnia or nightmares, give the TCA in the morning. The SSRIs can be given as a single dose in the morning. They are less sedating than the TCAs, and some patients may require a hypnotic for sleep induction. Bipolar patients can become manic on antidepressants.

Side effects are common with TCA use. Their adverse effects are due to their interaction with multiple neurotransmitters and their receptors. The antimuscarinic adverse effects are most common. Adverse effects related to antihistaminic activity and α-adrenergic mediation (Table 9–22) are from cerebral intoxication, but cardiac toxicity and orthostatic hypotension can occur. Antimuscarinic side effects include dry mouth, a metallic taste, epigastric distress, constipation, dizziness, mental confusion, tachycardia, palpitations, blurred vision, and urinary retention. Antihistaminic activity may be responsible for carbohydrate cravings, which

contributes to weight gain. Adrenergic activity is responsible for the orthostatic hypotension and reflex tachycardia and palpitations that patients may experience. Paradoxically, excess sweating can also occur. Rarely, amitriptyline and others will cause inappropriate secretion of antidiuretic hormone. Any antidepressant treatment may change depression to hypomania or frank mania (particularly in bipolar patients). Ten percent of patients may develop tremors, and confusion or delirium may occur, particularly in older patients, who are more vulnerable to the muscarinic side effects. Antidepressant treatments may also reduce the seizure threshold (Baldessarini, 1990). There are differences among the TCAs and properties that may be useful in selecting an agent and modifying drug regimens to reduce adverse effects (Tables 9–22, 9–23).

TERTIARY AMINES

Amitriptyline (Elavil, Endep) is a tertiary amine tricyclic that is sedating and has antimuscarinic activity. Patients with coexistent depression are more tolerant and require higher doses of amitriptyline. Start at a dose of 10 to 25 mg at bedtime. The dose ranges from 10 to 400 mg/day.

Table 9–23 Relative potency of tricyclic antidepressants on neurotransmitters and other side effects

Drug	Serotonin	Norepinephrine	Dopamine	Sedation	Cholinergic
Amitriptyline	+++	++	++	+++	+++++
Amoxapine	++	++++	+++++	+	++
Desipramine	++++	+++++	+++	+	+++
Doxepin	+++	++	++	+++	+++
Imipramine	++++	++	++++	++	++++
Maprotiline	+	+++	++++	+	++
Nortriptyline	++++	++++	++	+	+++
Protriptyline	++++	+++++	++	0	+++++
Trimipramine	+	+	+++	+/−	++++

Doxepin (Sinequan, Adapin) is a sedating tertiary amine TCA. Start at a dose of 10 mg at bedtime. The dose ranges from 10 to 300 mg/day.

SECONDARY AMINES

Nortriptyline (Pamelor, Aventyl) is a secondary amine that is less sedating than amitriptyline. Nortriptyline is a major metabolite of amitriptyline. If insomnia develops, give the drug earlier in the day or in divided doses. Start at a dose of 10 to 25 mg at bedtime. The dose ranges from 10 to 150 mg/day.

Protriptyline (Vivactil) is a secondary amine similar to nortriptyline. Start at a dose of 5 mg/day. The dose ranges from 5 to 60 mg/day.

Monoamine Reuptake Inhibitors: Selective Serotonin Reuptake Inhibitors

Fluoxetine, fluvoxamine, paroxetine, sertraline, and citalopram are specific serotonergic uptake inhibitors with minimal antihistaminic and antimuscarinic activity. In general, side effects are less than with the TCAs. They produce less weight gain (and even, in some cases, weight loss) and fewer cardiovascular side effects than the TCAs (Abramowicz, 1990). The most common side effects include anxiety, nervousness, insomnia, drowsiness, fatigue, tremor, sweating, anorexia, nausea, vomiting, and dizziness or lightheadedness. Headache was noted in 20.3% of patients on fluoxetine; however, it was also noted in 19.9% of patients on placebo (Barnhart, 1991). The combination of an SSRI and a TCA can be beneficial in treating refractory depression (Weilburg et al., 1989) and, in our experience, resistant cases of migraine.

The efficacy analysis summarized in the AHCPR evidence report (Gray et al., 1999a) did not indicate a clear benefit of the racemic mixture of fluoxetine (Prozac) over placebo. In contrast, a recent randomized, controlled trial of *S*-fluoxetine indicated a possible clinical benefit in migraine prevention, as measured by a reduction in migraine frequency, as early as 1 month after initiation of therapy (Steiner et al., 1998). Anecdotal reports (Markley et al., 1991) and our experience indicate its benefit in migraine prophylaxis. Some researchers have reported that fluoxetine does not improve or may worsen headache (Solomon and Kunkel, 1990).

Start at a dose of 10 mg in the morning. The dose ranges from 10 to 80 mg/day.

Other Antidepressants

SELECTIVE SEROTONIN AND NOREPINEPHRINE REUPTAKE INHIBITORS

Venlafaxine is a potent selective serotonin and norepinephrine reuptake inhibitor. It is occasionally associated with hypertension. The dose ranges from 75 to 275 mg/day, in divided doses or as a long-acting preparation.

Mirtazapine is an antagonist at central α_2 presynaptic NE receptors, resulting in increased NE and 5-HT action. In addition, it is a potent 5-HT$_2$ and 5-HT$_3$ receptor antagonist. The dose ranges from 15 to 45 mg at bedtime.

Pies (1983) found trazodone, an atypical non-TCA that is a highly selective SSRI, to be effective in a patient with features of both migraine and TTH; most investigators, including ourselves, rarely find it effective. Trazodone is metabolized to mCPP, a known migraine precipitant, perhaps by being a 5-HT$_{1C}$ receptor agonist (Brewerton et al., 1988). Plasma levels of mCPP in patients on trazodone are 40% that of the parent drug (Curzon et al., 1990).

Other antidepressants can be tried in resistant cases, particularly those complicated by depression. Bupropion is useful for smoking cessation and neuropsychiatric comorbidity.

MONOAMINE OXIDASE INHIBITORS

Monoamine oxidase exists in two subtypes: MAO-A, which preferentially deaminates NE and 5-HT, and MAO-B, which preferentially deaminates dopamine. Phenelzine is a nonspecific inhibitor of MAO-A and -B. L-Deprenyl is a selective MAO-B inhibitor that may be effective in the treatment of Parkinson's disease.

The MAOI phenelzine (Nardil) at a dose of 15 mg TID was shown (in an open study) to be effective in 80% of 25 patients who were resistant to other forms of treatment (including cyproheptadine and methysergide) (Anthony and Lance, 1969). Many authorities find that phenelzine can be extremely effective in migraine prophylaxis when simpler treatments fail (Raskin, 1988; Saper et al., 1993; Lance, 1986).

The dose of phenylzine ranges from 30 to 90 mg/day, in divided doses. All patients on MAOI-A must be on a restricted diet and avoid the use of certain medications to prevent hypertensive crisis. Meperidine, sympathomimetics (including Midrin), alcohol, and foods with a high tyramine content (cheddar cheese, fava beans, banana peel, tap beers, Marmite and Veggie-Mite concentrated, yeast extract, sauerkraut, soy sauce, and other soybean condiments) must be avoided (Raskin, 1988; Mosniam et al., 1996; Shulman and Walker, 1999; Tollefson, 1983).

The most common side effects of MAOIs include insomnia, orthostatic hypotension, constipation, increased perspiration, weight gain, peripheral edema, and, less commonly, inhibition of ejaculation or reduced libido. Insomnia can be reduced by giving most of the medication early in the day. The risk of hypertensive crisis may be reduced by having the patient take the MAOI 3 to 4 hours before or after eating or taking the entire dose at bedtime as gut MAO activity rapidly returns to normal (Raskin, 1988). Sublingual nifedipine has been used to treat hypertensive crisis when it occurs in MAOI users (Clary and Schweitzer, 1987).

The MAOI and amitriptyline combination has been reported to be relatively safe and effective in the treatment of refractory depression when the two drugs are started concurrently (Lader, 1983; Saper, 1989). Some headache experts have used this combination to treat refractory migraine (Raskin, 1988; Freitag et al., 1987; Saper, 1989). Combination therapy may decrease the risk of hypertensive crisis. A clinical trial demonstrated that administering amitriptyline to patients who were on an MAOI could prevent the occurrence of hypertensive crisis from the ingestion of cheeses or other high-tyramine foods (Pare et al., 1982). However, severe reactions, including hyperthermia, delirium,

and seizures, have been reported (White and Simpson, 1984). The newer atypical antidepressants, such as fluoxetine, must not be combined with an MAOI since fatal outcomes have been reported. One must wait 5 weeks after stopping fluoxetine before starting an MAOI and 2 to 3 weeks after stopping an MAOI before starting fluoxetine.

CALCIUM CHANNEL ANTAGONISTS

Calcium, in combination with a calcium-binding protein such as calmodulin or troponin, regulates many functions, including muscle contraction, neurotransmitter and hormone release, and enzyme activity. Its extracellular concentration is high; its intracellular free concentration is 10,000-fold smaller. The concentration gradient is established by membrane pumps and the intracellular sequestering of free calcium. When stimulated, the cell can open calcium channels in the plasma membrane or release intracellular stores of calcium (Snyder and Reynolds, 1985).

Two types of calcium channels exist: calcium-entry channels, which allow extracellular calcium to enter the cell, and calcium-release channels, which allow intracellular calcium (in storage sites in organelles) to enter the cytoplasm. They include ryanodine and IP_3 receptors (Greenberg, 1997). Calcium-entry channel subtypes include those voltage-gated and opened by depolarization, ligand-gated and opened by chemical messengers such as glutamate, and capacitive and activated by depletion of intracellular calcium stores.

There are six functional subclasses of voltage-gated calcium (Ca^{2+}) channels: T, L, N, P, Q, and R. They fall into two major categories: high-voltage activated channels and the unique low-voltage activated T-type, which is activated at negative potentials (Varadi et al., 1996).

Voltage-gated calcium channels are heteromers containing protein subunits of about 30 to 230 kD that form calcium-selective pores across the cell membrane. These subunits have different functions, and subunit isoforms give rise to distinct channel subtypes. The α_1 subunit, which consists of four homologous domains of six transmembrane segments each, forms the transmembrane pore and contains most of the channel's known drug-binding sites. Molecular cloning has revealed at least six α_1 genes associated with auxiliary subunits, including a membrane-spanning $\alpha_2-\delta$ complex, which increases the amplitude of calcium currents and binds the anticonvulsant gabapentin, and a cytoplasmic β subunit, which modifies the channel's current amplitude, voltage dependence, and activation and inactivation properties (Greenberg, 1997).

The three major classes of L-type Ca^{2+} channel blockers are the dihydropyridines (e.g., nifedipine), the benzothiazepines (e.g., diltiazem), and the phenylalkylamines (e.g., verapamil). Regions of the α_1 subunit contain the binding sites for all of these drugs (Varadi et al., 1996).

Calcium channel subtypes with different electrophysiologic and pharmacologic properties are due to differences in α_1-subunit structure. L-type (long-lasting) calcium channels are expressed in a variety of cardiovascular, endocrine, and neural tissues and are involved in muscle contraction and hormone release. L-type channels contain class S, C, or D α_1 subunits and are sensitive to dihydropyridine drugs like nifedipine and nimodipine, as well as verapamil and diltiazem. α_{1s} subunits are expressed only in skeletal muscle, whereas α_{1c} and α_{1d} subunits are found on neurons. T-type (transient) calcium channels differ from most other channel subtypes since they are activated at low voltages. They are found in cardiac muscle and neurons, where they may be involved in pacemaker activity. The novel calcium channel antagonist mibefradil blocks T-type channels preferentially. N-type (neither L- nor T-type) channels contain α_{1b} subunits and are blocked by peptide toxins from predatory cone snails, ω-toxin GVIA from conus geographus, and ω-toxin MVIIA from conus magus. P- (Purkinje cell) and Q-type channels contain α_{1a} subunits and are closely related. They are blocked by ω-agatoxin IVA (venom of the American funnel well spider *Agelenopsis aperta*). Both N- and P/Q-type channels are located primarily on neurons, especially at presynaptic terminals,

and are involved in neurotransmitter release (Greenberg, 1997).

The mechanism of action of the calcium channel antagonists in migraine prevention is uncertain. They were introduced into the treatment of migraine on the assumption that they prevent hypoxia of cerebral neurons, contraction of vascular smooth muscles, and inhibition of Ca^{2+}-dependent enzymes involved in prostaglandin formation. Perhaps it is their ability to block 5-HT release, interfere with neurovascular inflammation, or interfere with the initiation and propagation of spreading depression that is critical (Wauquier et al., 1985). The discovery that an abnormality in an α_{1a} subunit can produce FHM has led to a search for more fundamental associations (see Chapter 6).

The AHCPR technical report identified 45 controlled trials of calcium antagonists, including flunarizine (25 trials), nimodipine (11 trials), nifedipine (five trials), verapamil (three trials), cyclandelate (three trials), and nicardipine (one trial) (Gray et al., 1999a). Flunarizine was compared with placebo in eight migraine-prevention trials, and effect sizes could be calculated for seven studies (Aldeeb et al., 1992; Diamond and Freitag, 1993; Louis, 1981; Mendenopoulos et al., 1985; Pini et al., 1985; Sorensen et al., 1986; Thomas et al., 1991b) but not the eighth study (Frenken and Nuijten, 1984). A meta-analysis of these seven heterogeneous trials was statistically significant in favor of flunarizine. Flunarizine was not significantly different from propranolol (Gawel et al., 1992; Lucking et al., 1988; Ludin, 1989; Shimell et al., 1990), metoprolol (Sorensen et al., 1991; Grotemeyer et al., 1987), pizotifen (Cerbo et al., 1986; Gabai and Spierings, 1989; Rascol et al., 1986), or methysergide (Steardo et al., 1986).

Nimodipine had mixed results in placebo-controlled trials. Three placebo-controlled studies suggested no significant differences [Ansell et al., 1988; Migraine-Nimodipine European Study Group (MINES), 1989], while two reported relatively large and statistically significant differences in favor of nimodipine (Gelmers, 1983; Ansell et al., 1988). Nimodipine was not different from flunarizine (Bussone et al., 1987), pizotifen (Cerbo et al., 1986; Louis and Spierings, 1982; Rascol et al., 1986), or propranolol (Formisano et al., 1991).

The evidence for nifedipine was difficult to interpret. Two comparisons with placebo yielded similar effect sizes that were statistically insignificant, but the 95% confidence intervals associated with these estimates were large and did not exclude either a clinically important benefit or harm associated with nifedipine (McArthur et al., 1989; Shukla et al., 1995). Similarly ambiguous results were reported in one comparison with flunarizine (Lamsudin and Sadjimin, 1993) and in two comparisons with propranolol (Gerber et al., 1991; Albers et al., 1989). One trial found that metoprolol was significantly better than nifedipine at reducing headache frequency (Gerber et al., 1991).

Verapamil was more effective than placebo in two of three trials, but both positive trials had high dropout rates, rendering the findings uncertain (Solomon, 1986; Markley et al., 1984). The single negative placebo-controlled trial included a propranolol treatment arm. This trial reported no significant difference between verapamil, propranolol, and placebo (Solomon, 1986). The efficacy of nicardipine is supported by a single comparison with placebo in 30 patients with migraine with aura (Leandri et al., 1990). Dotarzine at 50 and 100 mg showed statistically significant efficacy in a multicenter, placebo-controlled, parallel trial. However, long-term studies beyond 3 months of active treatment may be required to attain maximal benefit (Diamond et al., 1999b).

Diltiazem (60 to 90 mg QID) was effective in two small open studies (Riopelle and McCans, 1982; Smith and Schwartz, 1984).

Side effects of the Ca^{2+} antagonists are dependent on the drug and include dizziness and headache (particularly with nifedipine), depression, vasomotor changes, tremor, gastrointestinal complaints (including constipation), peripheral edema, orthostatic hypotension, and bradycardia. Patients frequently report an initial increase in headache. Headache improvement frequently requires weeks of treatment. The AHCPR technical report provided little useful information on the risk of adverse events with these agents. Adverse events most commonly associated with flunarizine were sedation, weight gain, and abdominal pain. Symptoms reported with other calcium channel antagonists included dizziness, edema, flushing, and constipation. Two trials of verapamil and one of nifedipine reported high dropout rates due to adverse events (Gray et al., 1999a). Side effects with nifedipine were frequent (54%) and included dizziness, edema, flushing, headache, and mental symptoms (McArthur et al., 1989).

Verapamil (Calan, Isoptin) is available as a 40, 80, or 120 mg tablet or as a 120, 180, or 240 mg sustained-release preparation. Start at a dose of 80 mg two to three times a day, with a maximum of 640 mg/day in divided doses. The sustained-release preparation of verapamil can be given once or twice a day, but unreliable absorption reduces reliability. The most common side effect is constipation; dizziness, nausea, hypotension, headache, and edema are less common. Bioavailability is 20%. The absorbed drug is tightly protein-bound. Peak plasma levels occur in 5 hours; the half-life ranges from 2.5 to 7.5 hours.

Diltiazem (Cardizem) is available in 30, 60, 90, and 120 mg tablets. Start at a dose of 30 mg two to three times a day, with a maximum of 360 mg/day in divided doses. Side effects are infrequent: hypotension, A-V block, and headaches are occasionally seen. Bioavailability is 50%; the drug is tightly protein-bound.

Nifedipine (Procardia) is available in 10 or 20 mg capsules. Start at a dose of 10 mg/day. This can be increased to a maximum of 120 mg/day in divided doses. Side effects are common and include hypotension, headache, nausea, and vomiting. Bioavailability is 50%; almost all of the drug is protein-bound.

Nimodipine (Nimotop) is available in 30 mg capsules. The dose is 30 to 60 mg QID. Side effects are infrequent. However, the cost of the drug may be prohibitive in the United States.

Flunarizine (Sibellium) is not available in the United States. The dose is 5 to 10 mg/day. The most prominent side effects include weight gain, somnolence, dry mouth, dizziness, hypotension, and occasional extrapyramidal reactions.

Anticonvulsants

Anticonvulsant medication is increasingly recommended for migraine prevention because of placebo-controlled, double-blind trials that prove them effective. Despite earlier researchers' belief that anticonvulsants are more effective in children who have paroxysmal electroencephalograms (Rapoport et al., 1989), they are effective regardless of the electroencephalogram (Prensky, 1987). With the exception of valproic acid and phenobarbital, many anticonvulsants interfere with the efficacy of the OCs (Coulam and Annagers, 1979; Hanston and Horn, 1985).

Nine controlled trials of five different anticonvulsants were included in the AHCPR technical report (Anthony et al., 1972; Hering and Kuritzky, 1992; Jensen et al., 1994b; Klapper, 1994, 1997; Mathew et al., 1995a; Rompel and Bauermeister, 1970; Stensrud and Sjaastad, 1979). The only placebo-controlled trial of carbamazepine suggested a significant benefit, but this trial was inadequately described in several important respects (Rompel and Bauermeister, 1970). Another trial, comparing carbamazepine with clonidine and pindolol, suggested that carbamazepine had a weaker effect on headache frequency than either comparator treatment, although differences from clonidine were not statistically significant (Anthony et al., 1972). A significantly higher percentage of patients reported adverse events with carbamazepine than with placebo or pindolol; there was no significant difference in this respect between carbamazepine and clonidine.

In our experience, carbamazepine (Tegretol), 600 to 1200 mg/day (beginning at 100 mg twice/day) may be effective in the preventive treatment of migraine, particularly in patients who have coexisting mania or hypomania, especially if there is rapid cycling; however, monitoring of plasma levels and white blood count is essential.

Valproic acid possesses anticonvulsant activity in a wide variety of experimental epilepsy models. Valproate at high concentrations increases GABA levels in synaptosomes, perhaps by inhibiting its degradation; it enhances the postsynaptic response to GABA, and at lower concentrations, it increases potassium conductance, producing neuronal hyperpolarization. Valproate turns off the firing of the 5-HT neurons of the dorsal raphe, which are implicated in controlling head pain.

Disordered GABA metabolism during migraine has been reported (Welch et al., 1975). Imbalance in the plasma concentrations of GABA, an inhibitory amino acid, and glutamic acid, an excitatory amino acid, has also been observed (Ferrari et al., 1990; Jensen et al., 1994a; Kaniecki, 1997; Klapper, 1994, 1997; Mathew et al., 1995a; Rompel and Bauermeister, 1970; Stensrud and Sjaastad, 1979). Five studies provided strong and consistent support for the efficacy of divalproex sodium (Behan, 1985; Klapper, 1994, 1997) and sodium valproate (Hering and Kuritzky, 1992; Jensen et al., 1994a). Two placebo-controlled trials of each of these agents showed them to be significantly better than placebo at reducing headache frequency (Klapper, 1997; Mathew et al., 1995a; Hering and Kuritzky, 1992; Jensen et al., 1994a). A single study, reported in abstract form only, compared divalproex sodium with propranolol and found differences favoring divalproex sodium; however, the statistical significance of these results could not be determined (open-label study with high dropout rates) (Klapper, 1994). A more recent study (published after December 1996 and therefore not included in the AHCPR technical report) found divalproex sodium to be more effective compared with placebo but not significantly different compared with propranolol for prevention of migraine in patients without aura (Kaniecki, 1997). An extended-release form of divalproex sodium demonstrated comparable efficacy to the tablet formulation. The adverse effect profile in the clinical trial, however, showed almost identical adverse effect rates for the placebo and active treatment arms (Silbertstein et al., 2000a).

Valproic acid is a simple eight-carbon, two-chain fatty acid with 80% bioavailability after oral administration. It is highly protein-bound, with an elimination half-life of between 8 and 17 hours.

Nausea, vomiting, and gastrointestinal distress are the most common side effects of valproate therapy. These are generally self-limited and slightly less common with divalproex sodium than with sodium valproate. When the therapy is continued, the incidence of gastrointestinal symptoms decreases, particularly after 6 months. In three of four placebo-controlled trials (Gray et al., 1999a), the overall percentage of patients reporting adverse events with divalproex sodium or sodium valproate was not higher than with placebo. The fourth trial found significantly higher rates of nausea, asthenia, somnolence, vomiting, tremor, and alopecia when patients used divalproex sodium.

In an open-label study, Silberstein et al. (1999) evaluated the long-term safety of divalproex sodium in patients who had completed one of two previous double-blind, placebo-controlled studies evaluating the safety and efficacy of divalproex in migraine prophylaxis. Of 163 patients enrolled, 46 had been treated with placebo and 117 had been treated with divalproex. The results, including data from the double-blind study, represented 198 patient-years of divalproex exposure. The average dose was 974 mg/day. Reasons for premature discontinuation (67%) included administrative problems (31%), drug intolerance (21%), and treatment ineffectiveness (15%). The most frequently reported adverse events were nausea (42%), infection (39%), alopecia (31%), tremor (28%), asthenia (25%), dyspepsia (25%), and somnolence (25%). Divalproex was found to be safe, and initial improvements were maintained for periods in excess of 1,080 days. No unexpected adverse events or safety concerns unique to the use of divalproex in the prophylactic treatment of migraine were found.

Valproate has little effect on cognitive functions, and it rarely causes sedation. On rare occasions, valproate administration is associated with severe adverse reactions, such as hepatitis or pancreatitis. The frequency varies with the number of concomitant medications used, the patient's age, the presence of genetic and metabolic disorders, and the patient's general state of health. These idiosyncratic reactions are unpredictable (Pellock and Willmore, 1991).

The risk of valproate hepatotoxicity is highest in children under the age of 2 years, especially those treated with multiple antiepileptic drugs, those with metabolic disorders, and those with severe epilepsy accompanied by mental retardation and organic brain disease (Driefuss et al., 1987). The relative risk of hepatotoxicity from valproate is low in migraineurs. Hepatic failure, however, cannot be predicted by laboratory monitoring since hepatic function tests can be normal until the clinical symptoms are advanced. Some patients progress to fatal hepatotoxicity without ever developing any specific hepatic function abnormalities. Vomiting was the most frequently reported initial symptom in fatal cases of hepatotoxicity. Combined symptoms of nausea, vomiting, and anorexia occurred in 82% of valproate-associated hepatotoxicity cases, whereas lethargy, drowsiness, and coma were described in 40%.

Valproate is potentially teratogenic and should not be used in pregnant women or women considering pregnancy (Silberstein, 1996b). Hyperandrogenism, resulting from elevated testosterone levels, ovarian cysts, and obesity, is of particular concern in young women with epilepsy who use valproate (Vainionpaa et al., 1999). It is uncertain if valproate can cause these symptoms in young women with migraine or mania.

Because of valproate's potential idiosyncratic interactions with barbiturates (severe sedation, coma), migraine patients who are on valproate should not be given barbiturate-containing combination analgesics for symptomatic headache relief. If these drugs are used, they should be given with caution and at a low dose. Absolute contraindications to valproate are pregnancy and a history of pancreatitis or a hepatic disorder such as chronic hepatitis or cirrhosis of the liver. Other important contraindications are hematologic disorders, including thrombocytopenia, pancytopenia and bleeding disorders.

Valproic acid is available as 250 mg capsules and as a syrup (250 mg/5 ml). Divalproex sodium is a stable coordination complex comprised of sodium valproate and valproic acid in a 1:1 molar ratio. Depakote is an enteric-coated form of divalproex sodium available as 125, 250, and 500 mg capsules and a sprinkle formulation. Start with 250 to 500 mg/day in divided doses and slowly increase the dose; monitor serum levels if there is a question of toxicity or compliance. (The usual therapeutic level is from 50 to 100 mg/ml.) The maximum recommended daily dose is 60 mg/kg.

Silberstein (1996b) published the following practical recommendations and clinical guidelines for using valproate in headache prophylaxis. (1) Before initiating divalproex sodium, perform a physical examination and take a thorough medical history, with special attention to hepatic, hematologic, and bleeding abnormalities. Obtain screening baseline laboratory studies to help identify risk factors that could influence drug selection. (2) To minimize gastrointestinal side effects, use the enteric-coated divalproex sodium formulation if available. Begin with a dose of 250 mg at bedtime. If nausea still occurs, use the sprinkle formulation (125 mg) and very slowly increase the dose. Slowly increase the dose to 500 to 750 mg/day. (3) Obtain follow-up divalproex levels to test for compliance, toxicity, and drug reactions as needed. (4) See the patient on a regular basis (every 1 to 2 months) during the first 6 to 9 months of therapy. (5) It is not necessary to monitor blood and urine in otherwise healthy and asymptomatic patients on monotherapy. (6) If mild hepatic transaminase elevation occurs, continue divalproex sodium at the same dose or a lower dose until the enzymes normalize. (7) Tremor may occur in 10% of treated patients. If this is bothersome, decrease the dose of divalproex sodium or use propranolol.

Vigabatrin, an anticonvulsant similar pharmacologically to sodium valproate, was compared with placebo in a double-blind study in drug-resistant migraineurs. Seventeen women and six men between 25 and 60 years of age, who had migraine with or without aura, randomly received either vigabatrin or matched placebo tablets for 12 weeks. After a 4-week washout period, an alternative treatment was given. The dose was increased slowly to 1,000 to 2,000 mg daily, according to the patients' tolerance and response, during the first 6 weeks of each phase; after that, no further dosage adjustment was made. Serum drug levels were monitored at 4-week intervals. There were four dropouts, and three patients were withdrawn for poor compliance. Treated patients had a 40% to 90% reduction in migraine attack frequency. Analysis of variance indicated a significant reduction in migraine attack frequency in women but not in men. Vigabatrin possibly decreased migraine attack frequency in women who previously derived no benefit from any other medication (Ghose et al., 1996).

Gabapentin (600 to 1,800 mg) was effective in episodic migraine and chronic migraine in a 12-week open-label study (Mathew, 1996). Gabapentin was not effective in one placebo-controlled, double-blind study (Wessely et al., 1987); but a more recent trial (not included in the AHCPR technical report and reported in abstract form with limited information on adverse events) reported clinical efficacy for gabapentin in migraine prevention (Mathew et al., 1998). This randomized, placebo-controlled, double-blind trial showed that gabapentin 1,800 to 2,400 mg was superior to placebo at reducing the frequency of migraine attacks. The study consisted of a 1-week screening phase, a 4-week single-blind placebo baseline phase, a 4-week titration phase, and an 8-week stable-dosing phase. Following screening, 145 subjects (81% women) who experienced three to eight migraine episodes a month and had failed no more than two prophylactic antimigraine regimes were randomized 2:1 to gabapentin (n = 99) or placebo (n = 46). During the titration phase, a dose escalation of gabapentin to 2,400 mg daily or matching placebo was administered. During the last 8 weeks of the study, dosages remained fixed. The primary efficacy measurement was the migraine headache rate during the final 4-week stabilization phase. Additional efficacy parameters included the 50% responder rate and the average duration of migraine headaches. Preliminary results indicate that, subjects receiving gabapentin had a median headache rate of 2.7 vs. 3.3 in the placebo group. The responder rate was 36% for gabapentin and 14% for placebo (p = 0.02). The two treatment groups were comparable with respect to treatment-limiting adverse events.

Limited data were reported on adverse events associated with gabapentin. The most common adverse events reported in association with these treatments were dizziness or giddiness and drowsiness. Relatively high patient withdrawal rates due to adverse events were reported in some trials (Gray et al., 1999a).

Topiramate is a structurally unique anticonvulsant that was discovered by serendipity. It was originally synthesized as part of a research project to discover structural analogs of fructose 1,6-diphosphate capable of inhibiting the enzyme fructose-1,6-bisphosphatase, thereby blocking gluconeogenesis, but it has not to date demonstrated clinical evidence of hypoglycemic activity. Topiramate is a derivative of the naturally occurring monosaccharide D-fructose and contains a sulfamate functionality. The structural resemblance of its O-sulfamate moiety to the sulfonamide moiety in acetazolamide prompted an evaluation of possible anticonvulsant effects. Its activity in traditional seizure tests and animal models of epilepsy was predictive of clinical effectiveness, and topiramate is currently marketed for the treatment of epilepsy.

Topiramate is rapidly and almost completely absorbed. The blood plasma concentration increases linearly as a function of dose in humans over the pharmacologically relevant range (Streeter et al., 1994). It is not extensively metabolized in humans and is eliminated predominantly unchanged in the urine. The average elimination half-life is approximately 21 hours (Easterling et al., 1988). Topiramate readily enters the CNS parenchyma; in rats, the concentration in whole brain was approximately one-third that in blood plasma 1 hour after oral dosing.

The anticonvulsant activity of most antiepileptic drugs is thought to be due to a state-dependent blockade of voltage-dependent Na^+ or Ca^{2+} channels or an ability to enhance the activity of GABA at $GABA_A$ receptors (Rogawski and Porter, 1990; MacDonald and McLean, 1986). Topiramate can influence the activity of some types of voltage-activated Na^+ and Ca^{2+} channel, $GABA_A$ receptor, and the α-amino-3-hydroxy-5-methylisoxazole-4-propionic acid (AMPA)/kainate subtype of glutamate receptors. Topiramate also inhibits some isozymes of carbonic anhydrase (CA) and exhibits selectivity for CA II and CA IV (Dodgson et al.; Shank et al., 1994).

Preliminary evidence suggesting that topiramate blocks Na^+ channels in a voltage-sensitive, use-dependent manner was obtained using cultured rat hippocampal neurons (DeLorenzo et al., 2000). Topiramate can reduce the amplitude of tetrodotoxin-sensitive voltage-gated Na^+ currents in rat cerebellar granule cells as measured by whole-cell current-clamp recordings (Zona et al., 1997). Although topiramate was effective at therapeutically relevant concentrations in all reported studies, some studies suggest that topiramate is less effective than phenobarbital, carbamazepine, and lamotrigine at blocking Na^+ channels. Therefore, Na^+ channel blockade may not be a major factor underlying the anticonvulsant activity of topiramate.

Topiramate can directly modulate the action of GABA on $GABA_A$ receptors, and the modulatory effect differs from that of the benzodiazepines or the barbiturates. However, the modulatory effect was always positive (White et al., 1997; 2000); i.e., topiramate always increased GABA-induced Cl currents (Brown et al., 1993).

Topiramate exerts a complex and variable antagonistic or negative modulatory effect on kainate-evoked currents (Gibbs et al., 2000). An initial antagonism (phase I) occurred within 2 to 4 minutes and readily reversed when topiramate was removed from the bathing fluid. When topiramate was applied constantly for more than 10 minutes, the magnitude of the antagonistic effect increased (phase II) and did not reverse during a 2- to 4-hour washout period. The delayed effect (phase II) might reflect an intracellular action, and topiramate might somehow alter the phosphorylation state of the receptor–channel complex. An alteration of the phosphorylation state of kainate-activated channels underlies the delayed (phase II) effect of topiramate.

Topiramate has been tested for inhibitory activity on six isozymes of carbonic anhydrase (CA I, CA II, CA III, CA IV, CA V, and CA VI). These studies revealed that topiramate selectively, but not specifically, inhibits CA II and CA IV. In humans, the K_i is between 1 and 10 μM. At high therapeutic doses (200 mg twice daily), the concentration of topiramate in the blood plasma of humans can be approximately 25 μM (Sachdeo et al., 1996), and based on the brain-to-plasma concentration ratio in rats, the concentration in the CNS parenchyma may be 10 μM. Therefore, CA II and CA IV are likely to be inhibited appreciably in various tissues, including the CNS, in patients receiving high doses of topiramate.

The relevance of the CA inhibitory activity to the anticonvulsant activity of topiramate is not known. Tolerance to the anticonvulsant activity of acetazolamide is well known and is thought to be due to upregulation of CA in the CNS (Anderson et al., 1989). The cross-tolerance study demonstrated that tolerance develops more readily to acetazolamide than to topiramate and that mice who were tolerant to acetazolamide were not tolerant to topiramate (Shank et al., 1994). These findings suggest that the inhibitory effect on CA II and CA IV is not a major factor underlying topiramate's anticonvulsant activity. However, there is now compelling evidence that inhibition of these isozymes could serve as an anticonvulsant mechanism. Research has revealed that the contribution of HCO_3 to the ionic current through dendritic $GABA_A$ receptors is increased during periods of high-frequency receptor activation (Taira et al., 1997; Staley et al., 1995).

Studies indicate that the effects of topiramate on voltage-activated NA^+ channels, voltage-activated calcium channels, $GABA_A$ receptors, and AMPA/kainate receptors are unique. One common characteristic is that they are all regulated by protein phosphorylation (Krebs, 1994; Roche et al., 1996; Wang and Kelly, 1995; Sigel, 1995). One or more subunits of each complex is phosphorylated by PKA, PKC, and possibly CA^{2+}/calmodulin-activated kinases. The consensus peptide sequence at the PKA-mediated phosphorylation

site exhibits homology; e.g., the GluR6 subunit of the AMPA/kainate receptor contains an RRQS, the β subunit of the $GABA_A$ receptor contains RRAS, and some subtypes of the primary subunit of Na^+ and Ca^{2+} channels contain RRNS and RRPT, respectively. If topiramate were to bind selectively to these sites only in the dephosphorylated state, such an interaction could explain the immediate and delayed effects and the variable nature of topiramate's activity. The reasoning is as follows. Immediately upon binding to the site, topiramate could exert either a positive or negative allosteric modulatory effect; secondarily, topiramate would prevent PKA from accessing the serine hydroxyl site, thereby preventing phosphorylation, which, over time, would shift a population of channels toward the dephosphorylated state.

This hypothesis has several predictive and testable elements: a topiramate-induced decrease in the degree of channel phosphorylation, an inverse relationship between the level of topiramate's effect on channel conductance and the degree of channel phosphorylation, a positive effect of PKA (and PKC?) inhibitors on the activity of topiramate, and a negative effect of phosphatase inhibitors on the activity of topiramate.

Electrophysiological and biochemical studies have revealed a combination of pharmacological properties of topiramate. Based on evidence that some of the effects of topiramate on AMPA/kainate receptors are influenced by the phosphorylation state of the receptors, it has been postulated that topiramate may bind to the membrane channel complexes at phosphorylation sites in the inner loop and thereby allosterically modulate ionic conductance through the channels.

Topiramate has been associated with weight loss, not weight gain (a common reason to discontinue preventive medication), with chronic use. Shuaib et al. (1999) studied 37 patients with frequent migraines (more than ten headaches a month) who were treated with topiramate (25 to 100 mg/day). In addition to migraine, most had chronic daily headache and all had failed treatment on a number of preventive drugs. Patients maintained a daily diary to record the frequency and severity of headaches and the amount and type of rescue medication used. Over a 3- to 9-month follow-up, 11 patients (30%) had significant improvement in headache frequency (>60% decrease) and 11 patients had moderate improvement in headache severity (40% to 60% decrease). Three patients discontinued therapy due to side effects (lightheadedness, ringing in the ears, and numbness in the hands), and eight patients did not report any improvement despite having been on therapy for over 12 weeks.

Edwards et al. (1999) enrolled 30 patients with migraine in a placebo-controlled, double-blind prevention trial of topiramate. There was a 4-week baseline screening phase, followed by a 6-week titration of 200 mg QID of topiramate in divided doses or placebo. This was followed by a one-half week steady state. Percentages of responders (patients with ≥ 50% reduction in 28-day migraine headache frequency) during the 18-week double-blind phase were topiramate 46.7% and placebo 6.7% (statistically significant p = 0.035).

Potter et al. (2000) evaluated the efficacy and safety of topiramate in migraine prophylaxis. Forty patients, 18 to 65 years old, having migraine with or without aura were randomized to topiramate or placebo (1:1 ratio). Study duration was 20 weeks (baseline, titration, and maintenance phases of 4, 8, and 8 weeks; 19 patients were randomized to topiramate and 21 to placebo). Thirty-five patients completed the study. The mean topiramate dose was 125 mg (range 25–200 mg). The baseline 28-day headache frequency was 5.14 in topiramate patients and 4.37 in placebo patients. The mean 28-day headache rate over the entire double-blind phase was 3.31 (topiramate) vs. 3.83 (placebo, p = 0.0025). Mean reduction in headache rate was 1.83 (topiramate) vs. 0.55 (placebo, p = 0.0025). The median percent reduction in monthly headache rate was 33% (topiramate) vs. 8% (placebo, p = 0.0061).

Tiagabine was studied by Freitag et al. (1999b) in an open-label clinical trial of 41 patients. All patients had been previously treated with divalproex sodium and discontin-

ued therapy due to adverse events or relative lack of efficacy. Tiagabine was initiated at a dose of 4 mg at bedtime for 1 week and then increased to 4 mg twice a day. Patients were re-evaluated at 1-month intervals and further dosage adjustments made. Five patients experienced a remission, and 33 of 41 patients had at least a 50% reduction in attacks. The mean duration of treatment at final assessment was 3.9 months. The mean dose of tiagabine was 10 mg/day. There were no apparent differences between men and women, age-related responses, or type of migraine. Fourteen adverse events were reported by 12 patients.

Serotonin Antagonists

Methysergide

Methysergide (Sansert) is a semisynthetic ergot alkaloid that is structurally related to methylergonovine. It is a 5-HT$_2$ receptor antagonist and 5-HT$_{1B/D}$ agonist. It was one of the first drugs developed for migraine prevention, but its usefulness is limited by reports of retroperitoneal and retropleural fibrosis associated with long-term, mostly uninterrupted, administration. The AHCPR technical report identified 17 controlled trials of methysergide for migraine prevention (Behan and Reid, 1980; Steardo et al., 1982, 1986; Barrie et al., 1968; Andersson, 1973; Cangi et al., 1989; Forssman et al., 1972; Hudgson et al., 1967; Lance et al., 1963; Pedersen and Moller, 1966; Presthus, 1971; Ryan, 1968; Shekelle and Ostfeld, 1964; Sicuteri, 1973). Four placebo-controlled trials suggested that methysergide was significantly better than placebo at reducing headache frequency (Lance et al., 1963; Pedersen and Moller, 1966; Ryan, 1968; Shekelle and Ostfeld, 1964).

Four comparison trials showed no statistically significant differences between methysergide and pizotifen (Ryan, 1968; Andersson, 1973; Forssman et al., 1972; Presthus, 1971). Two trials directly comparing methysergide and propranolol failed to demonstrate any statistically significant differences between them (Behan and Reid, 1980; Steardo et al.,

1982). The only trial comparing methysergide with metoprolol reported an unusually low response to metoprolol (6%) and, thus, a misleading relative increase in efficacy of methysergide (Behan and Reid, 1980).

Methysergide was compared with flumedroxone (Hudgson et al., 1967), oxitriptan (Sicuteri, 1973; Titus et al., 1986), lisuride (Herman et al., 1977), dihydroergokryptine (Cangi et al., 1989), ergotamine (Barrie et al., 1968), and flunarizine (Steardo et al., 1986). These trials were too small to demonstrate equivalence and failed to show any statistically significant differences.

Methysergide was associated with a higher incidence of adverse events than placebo. Gastrointestinal complaints were most common and included nausea, vomiting, abdominal pain, and diarrhea. Also frequently reported were leg symptoms (restlessness or pain), dizziness, giddiness, drowsiness, lassitude, and paresthesia. Adverse events were no more common with methysergide than with pizotifen. The duration of the trials reviewed here was too short to detect the fibrotic complications sometimes observed with long-term methysergide use.

Side effects of methysergide noted in clinical practice include transient muscle aching, claudication, abdominal distress, nausea, weight gain, and hallucinations. Frightening hallucinatory experiences after the first dose are not uncommon (Curran et al., 1967). Curran and Lance (1964) have treated leg claudication with vasodilators with some enhancement of methysergide's effectiveness, suggesting that its action on headache is not a result of vasoconstriction. The major complication of methysergide is the rare (1/5,000) development of retroperitoneal, pulmonary, or endocardial fibrosis (Graham, 1967; Elkind et al., 1968).

Methysergide is indicated for the treatment of migraine and cluster headache. The dose ranges from 2 to 8 mg/day, with the higher doses being given two or three times a day. Many clinicians use higher doses, up to 14 mg/day, without adverse events and with higher efficacy (Raskin, 1988). To minimize early adverse events, patients can start with a dose of 1 mg/day and increase the dose grad-

ually by 1 mg every 2 to 3 days. (This can be accomplished by breaking the 2 mg tablets.) A trial of at least 2 months should be given with doses up to at least 8 mg/day. Methysergide, in general, should not be taken continuously for long periods since doing so may produce retroperitoneal fibrosis (Graham, 1967; Graham et al., 1966; Bana et al., 1974). Instead, the drug should be given for 6 months, stopped for 1 month, and then restarted. To avoid an increase in headache when methysergide is stopped, the patient should be weaned off the drug over a 1-week period. Some authorities use methysergide on a continuous basis with careful monitoring (Raskin, 1988), which includes auscultation of the heart and yearly echocardiography, chest X-ray, and abdominal MRI. The drug should be discontinued immediately upon suspicion of pulmonary or cardiac retroperitoneal fibrosis (Raskin, 1988; Silberstein, 1998b).

Contraindications to the use of methysergide include pregnancy, peripheral vascular disorders, severe arteriosclerosis, coronary artery disease, severe hypertension, thrombophlebitis or cellulitis of the legs, peptic ulcer disease, fibrotic disorders, lung diseases, collagen disease, liver or renal function impairment, valvular heart disease, debilitation, or serious infection. All patients receiving methysergide should remain under the supervision of the treating physician and be examined regularly for development of the rare pulmonary/cardiac or peritoneal fibrosis or of vascular complications (Silberstein, 1998b).

Methysergide is an effective migraine-preventive medication that is an appropriate consideration in resistant headaches with a high attack frequency. All of the open and controlled studies attest to its efficacy. In addition to being effective at reducing attack frequency, it often acts synergistically with ergotamine for breakthrough attacks. Due to its side effect profile, it should be reserved for severe cases in which other migraine-preventive drugs are not effective.

Ergonovine is an ergot alkaloid 5-HT antagonist which is anecdotally said to be an effective migraine-preventive drug (Raskin, 1988). Gallagher (1989) found it useful in the treatment of menstrual migraine in an open trial. Side effects are uncommon and include nausea, abdominal pain, and aching legs. The dose is 0.2 to 0.4 mg three to four times a day. Contraindications include Prinzmetal's angina, peripheral vascular disease, asthma, and pregnancy.

Ergonovine is no longer commercially available. We have used methylergonovine maleate, a principal metabolite of methysergide and a 5-HT antagonist, in place of ergonovine. The dose is 0.2 to 0.4 mg three to four times a day. Side effects and contraindications are the same as for methysergide.

Cyproheptadine (Periactin), an antagonist at the 5-HT$_2$, histamine H$_1$, and muscarinic cholinergic receptors, is widely used in the prophylactic treatment of migraine in children (Barlow, 1984; Forsythe and Hockaday, 1988; Raskin, 1988). Curran and Lance (1964) found cyproheptadine to be more effective than placebo but less effective than methysergide. Cyproheptadine is available as 4 mg tablets. The total dose ranges from 12 to 36 mg/day (given two to three times or at bedtime). Common side effects are sedation and weight gain; dry mouth, nausea, lightheadedness, ankle edema, aching legs, and diarrhea are less common. Cyproheptadine may inhibit growth in children (Smyth and Lazarus, 1974) and reverse the effects of SSRIs.

Pizotifen (Sandomigran), a 5-HT$_2$ receptor antagonist structurally similar to cyproheptadine, is not available in the United States. Controlled and uncontrolled studies in Europe (Peatfield, 1986) have shown this drug to be of benefit in 40% to 79% of patients. The usual dose is 3.0 mg at bedtime. Side effects include drowsiness and weight gain (Capildeo and Rose, 1982).

Miscellaneous Prophylactic Drugs

Clonidine (Catapres) is an imidazoline that activates α_2-adrenergic receptors. Clonidine inhibits the firing of locus ceruleus neurons (the major source of noradrenergic neurons) induced by opiate withdrawal by activating presynaptic inhibitory α_2 receptors. This is the basis of clonidine's clinical effectiveness in treating opiate (Aghajanian, 1978; Bakris et al., 1982), alcohol, and cigarette withdrawal

(Baumgartner and Rowen, 1987) and in controlling menopausal hot flashes (Nagamani et al., 1987).

The AHCPR technical report included 16 controlled trials of clonidine (Adam et al., 1978; Anthony et al., 1972); Behan, 1985; Boisen et al., 1978; Bredfeldt et al., 1989; Das et al., 1979; Elkind et al., 1989; Kallanranta et al., 1977; Kass and Nestvold, 1980; Louis et al., 1985; Mondrup and Moller, 1977; Ryan and Diamond, 1975; Shafar et al., 1972; Sjaastad and Stensrud, 1971; Stensrud and Sjaastad, 1976a; Wilkinson, 1970). The evidence from these trials suggests that α_2 agonists are minimally, and not conclusively, efficacious. Three of 11 placebo-controlled trials of clonidine found a significant difference in favor of the active agent, but the magnitude of the effect was small (Kallanranta et al., 1977; Sjaastad and Stensrud, 1971; Stensrud and Sjaastad, 1976a).

Two comparative trials comparing clonidine with the β blockers metoprolol (Louis et al., 1985) and propranolol (Kass and Nestvold, 1980) yielded mixed results. Two additional comparative trials showed no significant differences among clonidine, practolol (Kallanranta et al., 1977), and pindolol (Anthony et al., 1972). (The latter two agents are β blockers with intrinsic sympathomimetic activity.) One trial each found no significant differences between clonidine and pizotifen (Behan, 1985) or between clonidine and carbamazepine (Anthony et al., 1972).

The most common adverse events reported with clonidine in clinical trials were drowsiness and tiredness, but these were usually neither serious nor cause for withdrawal from the trials. In studies comparing clonidine with β blockers, adverse events occurred at similar rates for both interventions.

Clonidine (Catapres) is available as 0.1, 0.2, and 0.3 mg tablets and as a patch delivering 0.1 mg (TTS 1), 0.2 mg (TTS 2), or 0.3 mg (TTS 3) a day. The dose ranges from 0.1 to 2 mg/day.

Calcitonin is a single-chain polypeptide hypocalcemic hormone secreted by the thyroid gland. Salmon calcitonin (100 IU/day) is effective at treating pain, perhaps by increasing the circulating levels of β-endorphin, adrenocorticotropin, and cortisol (Ustdal et al., 1989). Salmon calcitonin given IM (Gennari et al., 1986) or NS (Micieli et al., 1988) and an analog of eel calcitonin given IM (Patti et al., 1987) are proposed as effective in migraine prophylaxis.

Captopril (Capoten) is an angiotensin-converting enzyme (ACE) and enkephalinase inhibitor that also inhibits the breakdown of bradykinin. In an open study, Sicuteri (1981) found captopril to be effective in 11 of 11 hypertensive patients and in 12 of 24 normotensive patients, perhaps by inhibiting the degradation of enkephalins. Minervini and Pinto (1987), in a small double-blind study, found captopril to be more effective than placebo.

The total dose ranges from 25 to 150 mg given in divided doses two or three times a day. Side effects are uncommon and include proteinuria, hypotension, angioedema, skin rash, and loss of taste. Cough unresponsive to medication occurs in 5% to 20% of patients treated with ACE inhibitors (Abramowicz, 1991). Birth defects have been reported in children born to women using ACE inhibitors.

Papaverine, a vasodilator chemically related to verapamil, has been shown to be effective in a number of small series of patients (Poser, 1974; Sillanpaa and Koponen, 1978; Vijayan, 1977; Raskin, 1988). The total dose ranges from 300 to 600 mg/day. The drug is rapidly absorbed and well tolerated. Side effects include nausea, drowsiness, vertigo, and constipation. A rare eosinophilic hepatitis has been reported.

Lanepitant is a potent inhibitor of neurogenic dural inflammation. Patients with three to eight migraine headaches during a 1 month placebo lead-in period were randomized to a double-blind, parallel comparison of 200 mg QID lanepitant (n = 42) and placebo (n = 42). Lanepitant was ineffective at preventing or reducing the severity of migraine. Since absorption in this study was not impaired by gastric stasis associated with the migraine attack, the lack of effect may have been due to ineffectiveness of the NK-1 blockade rather than insufficient plasma concentration (Goldstein et al., 1999).

Natural Products

Feverfew (Tanacetum parthenium) is a medicinal herb used in self-treatment of migraine. Four trials were conducted, two in the AHCPR and two after the reports became available. The AHCPR technical report listed two trials, distinctly different in design, that compared feverfew with placebo and no treatment. One trial was conducted in a self-selected group of feverfew users and showed that withdrawing feverfew led to a statistically significant increase in headache frequency (Johnson et al., 1985a). A pilot study of 17 migraineurs who ate fresh feverfew leaves daily was undertaken at the City of London Migraine Clinic. Patients were given capsules of freeze-dried feverfew or placebo. Those receiving placebo had a tripling in the frequency of migraine attacks. Patients on placebo reported increased nervousness, tension headaches, insomnia, or joint stiffness constituting a "post-feverfew syndrome" (perhaps another example of rebound).

The other, more conventional trial was conducted in a larger group of migraineurs, most of whom (71%) had never used feverfew (Murphy et al., 1988). This trial reported a smaller difference between feverfew and the control treatment than did the other trial but still found the difference to be statistically significant in favor of feverfew. Two trials were not included in the AHCPR report. One was a double-blind, randomized, crossover trial that tested the efficacy of feverfew compared with placebo and reported that treatment with feverfew was associated with a significant reduction in pain intensity and nonheadache symptoms (nausea, vomiting, photophobia, and phonophobia) (Palevitch et al., 1997). The other trial reported no significant differences between feverfew given as an alcoholic extract and placebo for reducing migraine frequency (Deweerdt et al., 1996).

Limited information indicates that adverse events were no more common with feverfew than with the control treatment (Gray et al., 1999a). Feverfew has side effects that include mouth ulceration and a more widespread oral inflammation associated with loss of taste. The mechanism of action of feverfew is uncertain. Feverfew is rich in sesquiterpene lactones, especially parthenolide, which may be a nonspecific NE, 5-HT, bradykinin, prostaglandin, and acetylcholine antagonist. The biologic variation in the sesquiterpene lactone content and the long-term safety and effectiveness of feverfew are of concern (Johnson et al., 1985a).

Until recently it was generally assumed that parthenolides represent the active principle of feverfew. This hypothesis was supported by in vitro experiments that emphasized its biological activity. These studies have demonstrated that the plant has inhibitory effects on platelet aggregation and release of serotonin from blood platelets and leukocytes (Heptinstall et al., 1985, 1987). One trial that used feverfew extract with a standardized and constant concentration of parthenolides to treat migraine did not show any beneficial effect (Deweerdt et al., 1996). Thus, the clinical effectiveness of feverfew for migraine prevention has not been established beyond reasonable doubt. More clinical trials are needed, both on a larger scale and with various feverfew extracts, including parthenolide-free sesquiterpene lactone chemotypes (Vogler et al., 1998).

A mitochondrial dysfunction resulting in impaired oxygen metabolism may play a role in migraine pathogenesis (Welch et al., 1989; Montagna et al., 1994; Sangiorgi et al., 1994; Watanabe et al., 1996). Riboflavin (vitamin B_2) is the precursor of flavin mononucleotide and flavin adenine dinucleotide, which are required for the activity of flavoenzymes involved in the electron transport chain. Given to patients with MELAS or mitochondrial myopathies on the assumption that at large doses it might augment activity of mitochondrial complexes I and II, riboflavin improved clinical as well as biochemical parameters (Arts et al., 1983; Penn et al., 1992; Antozzi et al., 1994; Scholte et al., 1995).

Based on the results of an open trial in migraine, a placebo-controlled, double-blind trial of high-dose vitamin B_2 (400 mg) was performed and showed significant benefit (Schoenen et al., 1998). Schoenen et al. (1998) compared riboflavin (400 mg) with placebo in migraineurs in a 3-month randomized trial. Riboflavin was significantly superior to placebo at reducing the attack frequency (p = 0.005), headache days (p = 0.012), and migraine index (0.012). The proportion of patients improved by at least 50% in headache days, i.e., "responders," were 15% for placebo and 59% for riboflavin (p = 0.002), and the number needed to treat for effectiveness was 2.3. Only three adverse events occurred: two in the riboflavin group (diarrhea and polyuria) and one in the placebo group (abdominal cramps). None was serious. Because of its high efficiency, excellent tolerability, and low cost, riboflavin is an interesting option for prophylaxis and a candidate for a comparative trial with an established prophylactic drug.

Lithium is effective in the treatment of cluster headache. Based on the analogy to cluster, Medina (1982) found lithium carbonate to be effective at treating cyclic migraine, a disorder in which patients have bouts of migrainous headaches separated by headache-free periods. Lithium may be a particularly useful adjunctive medication in bipolar or manic patients. Side effects include hand tremor, polyuria, thirst, and ankle edema. Long-term complications include hypothyroidism, oliguric renal failure, and diabetes insipidus. The dose of lithium is 900 to 1,800 mg/day, titrated to give a serum level between 0.6 and 1.2 mEq/l. Combining lithium with verapamil can cause adverse responses (lithium toxicity) at standard doses. The lithium dose must be substantially reduced when it is given with verapamil, even when the blood level is in the therapeutic range (Price and Shalley, 1987; Price and Giannini, 1986).

Magnesium supplementation has been shown to be effective in one of two trials. One study enrolled 81 patients who had IHS migraine. Their mean attack frequency was 3.6/month. After a prospective baseline period of 4 weeks, these patients received 600 mg (24 mmol) of oral magnesium (trimagnesium dicitrate) or placebo daily for 12 weeks. In weeks 9 to 12, the attack frequency was reduced by 41.6% in the magnesium group and by 15.8% in the placebo group compared to the baseline (p < 0.05). The number of days with migraine and symptomatic drug consumption also decreased significantly in the magnesium group. Adverse events were diarrhea (18.6%) and gastric irritation (4.7%) (Peikert et al., 1996).

In another multicenter, prospective, randomized, double-blind, placebo-controlled study, the migraine prophylactic effect of 20 mmol magnesium-L-aspartate-hydrochloride trihydrate given in divided doses was evaluated. Included in this study were patients with a 2-year history of two to six attacks a month of migraine without aura. The efficacy endpoint was a reduction of at least 50% in intensity or duration of migraine attacks at the end of the twelfth week of treatment compared to baseline. With a calculated total sample size of 150 patients, an interim analysis was planned after treatment of at least 60 patients was completed; this analysis, in fact, was performed with 69 patients (64 women, 5 men). Of these, 35 had received magnesium and 34 placebo. There were ten responders in each group (28.6% magnesium and 29.4% placebo). The trial was discontinued for this reason, as determined by the study protocol. There was no benefit from magnesium compared to placebo in the number of migraine days or migraine attacks (Pfaffenrath et al., 1996).

The studies differed in the amount of magnesium (24 vs. 20 mmol) and in the salt (dicitrate vs. aspartate). These differences may produce differences in bioavailability and efficacy and account for the reported difference.

Abortive Agents for Migraine Prophylaxis

Aspirin

O'Neill and Mann (1979) and Masel et al. (1980) found that aspirin (650 mg/day) decreased headache frequency. Two major multicenter trials, however, clearly proved the efficacy of acetylsalicylic acid (ASA) in the prophylaxis of migraine: in 1988 the British Physician Trial showed that a daily dose of 500 mg ASA reduced the frequency of migraine by an average of 30% (Peto et al., 1988). In a double-blind trial of low-dose aspirin (325 mg every other day) in 22,071 U.S. male physicians (Physician Health Study), Buring et al. (1990) found a 20% reduction in headache frequency. Although this is statistically significant, it may not be clinically significant. In a small open trial, Baldratti et al. (1983) compared the efficacy of ASA (13.5 mg/kg) with propranolol (1.8 mg/kg). In this trial, both drugs were equally effective and reduced the frequency, duration, and intensity of the attacks to the same extent. In a double-blind crossover trial, ASA (500 mg daily) was statistically less effective than propranolol (200 mg daily) (Grotemeyer et al., 1990). High-dose aspirin use may lead to overuse and the development of rebound headaches. Aspirin in low doses clearly is indicated for the prophylaxis of myocardial infarction and transient ischemic attacks. We use aspirin only in patients with prolonged or nonvisual aura.

Nonsteroidal Anti-inflammatory Drugs

Some NSAIDs may be effective in migraine prophylaxis. These include sodium naproxen, naproxen, fenoprofen, ketoprofen, and tolfenamic acid (Pradalier et al., 1988). Some headache disorders (chronic paroxysmal hemicrania, hemicrania continua) are defined by their responsiveness to indomethacin (Sjaastad and Spierings, 1984; Sjaastad and Dale, 1976; Bordini et al., 1991). Although NSAIDs are effective, they must be used with caution because of their adverse effects on gastrointestinal and renal function (Feldman and Schlezinger, 1970).

Ergotamine

The prophylactic use of ergotamine is discouraged. The exception is women with primarily menstrual migraine, who can use ergotamine only at the time of headache vulnerability without the danger of developing rebound headache.

Dihydroergotamine

Some studies have shown that an oral programmed-release form of DHE (DHE methanesulfonate, DHE retard) at a dose of

5 mg three times a day is effective in the prophylactic treatment of migraine (Centonze et al., 1983; Fontanari et al., 1983; Martucci et al., 1983; Mastrosimone and Iaccarino, 1987). The DHE retard form is not available in the United States.

Newer Treatments

Silbertstein et al. (2000) evaluated the safety and efficacy of pericranial botulinum toxin type A (Botox) injections as prophylactic treatment of chronic moderate to severe migraine. One hundred twenty-three patients who had chronic IHS-defined migraine and a history of two to eight moderate to severe migraine attacks during a 1-month baseline were randomized to treatment with either 0, 25, or 75 U of botulinum toxin type A injected symmetrically into glabellar, frontalis, and temporalis muscles. Diaries were kept for 3 months postinjection. At 12 centers, 41, 42, and 40 patients were randomized to 0, 25, and 75 U botulinum toxin type A treatment groups and had baseline frequencies of migraine of 4.41, 4.45, and 3.95 attacks per month, respectively. The 25 U botulinum toxin type A treatment group fared significantly better than the placebo group by the following measures: reduction in mean frequency of moderate to severe migraines during days 31 to 60, incidence 50% reduction and incidence two headache decrease in mild to severe migraines at days 61 to 90, reduction in mild to severe migraine during days 61 to 90, reduction of days with phonophobia during days 31 to 90, and improvement by patient global assessment for days 31 to 60 postinjection. The 75 U botulinum toxin type A treatment group was significantly better than the placebo group on patient global assessment for days 31 to 60 but not other parameters. Botulinum toxin type A treatment was well tolerated, but high-dose botulinum toxin type A showed significantly more treatment-related adverse events than placebo. No serious treatment-related adverse events were reported. Pericranial injection of botulinum toxin type A (25 U) showed significant differences compared to vehicle in reducing migraine frequency and associated symptoms during 90 days following injection (Silberstein et al., 2000).

SETTING TREATMENT PRIORITIES

The goals of treatment are to relieve or prevent the pain and associated symptoms of migraine and to optimize the patient's ability to function normally. The medications used to treat migraine can be divided into four major categories: (1) drugs with documented high efficacy and mild to moderate adverse events, which include β blockers, amitriptyline, and divalproex; (2) drugs with lower documented efficacy and mild to moderate adverse events, which include SSRIs, calcium channel antagonists, gabapentin, riboflavin, and NSAIDs; (3) drug use based on opinion, mild to moderate adverse events, major adverse events, or complex management; (4) drugs with documented high efficacy but significant adverse events or drugs that are difficult to use, which include methysergide and MAOIs; and (5) drugs with proven limited or no efficacy, which include cyproheptadine, lithium, and phenytoin. Choose a drug based on its proven efficacy, the patient's preferences and headache profile, side effects, and the presence or absence of coexisting or comorbid disease (Tables 9–10, 9–24). Use the drug with the best risk-to-benefit ratio for the individual patient and take advantage of the drug's side effect profile. An underweight patient would be a candidate for one of the medications that commonly produce weight gain, such as a TCA; in contrast, one should avoid these drugs in the overweight patient. Tertiary TCAs that have a sedating effect would be useful at bedtime for patients with insomnia. The older patient with cardiac disease or patients with significant hypotension may not be able to use TCAs or calcium channel or β blockers but could easily use divalproex. In the athletic patient, β blockers should be used with caution. Medication that can impair cognitive functioning should be avoided in patients who are dependent on their wits (Silberstein et al., 1998; Silberstein, 1997b).

Comorbid and coexistent diseases have important implications for treatment. The pres-

Table 9–24 Preventive drugs

High efficacy: low to moderate AEs
  Propranolol, timolol, amitriptyline, divalproex
Low efficacy: low to moderate AEs
  NSAIDs: aspirin, flurbiprofen, ketoprofen, naproxen
    sodium
  β-blockers: atenolol, metoprolol, nadolol
  Calcium channel blockers: nimodipine, verapamil
  Anticonvulsants: gabapentin, topiramate, tiagabine
  Other: fenoprofen, feverfew, vitamin B$_2$
  Pizotifen
Unproven efficacy: low to moderate AEs
  Antidepressants: doxepin, nortriptyline, imipramine,
    protriptyline venlafaxine, fluvoxamine,
    mirtazepine, paroxetine, protriptyline, sertraline,
    trazodone
Major AEs or complex management
  Methergine, MAOIs
Proven not effective or of low efficacy
  Acebutolol, carbamazepine, clomipramine,
    clonazepam, indomethacin, lamotrigine,
    nabumetone, nicardipine, nifedipine, pindolol

Key to abbreviations: AE, adverse effects; NSAID, nonsteroidal anti-inflammatory drug; MAOI, monoamine oxidase inhibitor.

Drug combinations are commonly used for patients with refractory headache disorders. Some combinations, such as antidepressants and β blockers, are suggested; others, such as β blockers and calcium channel blockers, should be used with caution or avoided altogether; and some, such as MAOIs and SSRIs, are contraindicated because of potentially lethal interactions (Table 9–25). Many clinicians use the combination of an antidepressant (such as a TCA or SSRI) and a β blocker and find that they act synergistically (Silberstein, 1997a). Combining methysergide with a vasodilator, such as a calcium channel blocker, to decrease side effects has been advocated (Silberstein, 1998b). Divalproex in combination with antidepressants is a logical choice to treat refractory migraine that is complicated by depression or bipolar disease.

ence of a second illness provides therapeutic opportunities but also imposes certain therapeutic limitations. In some instances, two or more conditions may be treated with a single drug. When migraine and hypertension and/or angina occur together, β blockers or calcium channel blockers may be effective for all conditions (Solomon, 1989). For the patient with migraine and depression, TCAs or SSRIs may be especially useful. For the patient with migraine and epilepsy (Mathew et al., 1995b; Hering and Kuritzky, 1992) or migraine and bipolar illness (Silberstein, 1996b; Bowden et al., 1994), divalproex sodium is the drug of choice. The pregnant migraineur who has a comorbid condition that needs treatment should be given a medication that is effective for both conditions and has the lowest potential for adverse effects on the fetus. In individuals with more than one disease, certain categories of treatment may be relatively contraindicated. For example, β blockers should be used with caution in the depressed migraineur, while TCAs, neuroleptics, or sumatriptan may lower the seizure threshold and should be used with caution in the epileptic migraineur.

Table 9–25 Drug combinations

Suggested
  Antidepressants
    β-Blocker
    Calcium channel blocker
    Divalproex
    Methysergide
  Methysergide
    Calcium channel blocker
  SSRI
    TCAs
Cautious use
  β-Blocker
    Calcium channel blocker
    Methysergide
  MAOIs
    Amitriptyline or nortriptyline
  Methysergide
    Dihydroergotamine
Contraindications
  MAOIs
    SSRIs
    Most TCAs (except amitriptyline or nortriptyline)
    Doxepin and trazadone
    Carbamazepine
  Midrin
    Most triptans (caution with zolmitriptan and SC
      sumatriptan, safe with naratriptan)
  NSAIDs
    Lithium
  Methysergide
    Ergotamine, triptans (caution with
      dihydroergotamine)

Key to abbreviations: SSRI, selective serotonin reuptake inhibitor; TCA, tricyclic antidepressant; MAOI, monoamine oxidase inhibitor; NSAID, nonsteroidal anti-inflammatory drug.

Some clinicians cautiously use the combination of phenelzine and amitriptyline in refractory headache patients (Silberstein, 1997b; Freitag et al., 1987).

ACUTE MEDICATION FOR PREVENTIVE TREATMENT

Preventive medication is considered to be effective if it decreases the frequency of attacks by more than 50%. Thus, patients treated with preventive medication may continue to have attacks of episodic migraine and TTH. Menstrual migraine attacks often persist to a greater extent than nonmenstrual attacks. Preventive medication may also decrease the intensity and duration of the attacks and may make acute medications more effective. Using preventive and acute medication together presents a new set of complexities.

The amount of acute medication must be limited to prevent the development of drug-induced daily rebound headache and loss of efficacy of the preventive medication. This is one of the causes of secondary failure of preventive medication.

Certain acute medications should be used with caution in the presence of certain preventive medications (Table 9–26). Ergotamine, DHE, and sumatriptan could potentially have enhanced vasospastic properties in the presence of methysergide. However, many authorities have found that the ergots are more effective in patients being treated with methysergide (Curran et al., 1967). The MAOIs decrease first-pass metabolism of the triptans other than naratriptan. This increases the half-life and the area under the curve of these agents. Therefore, the dose of oral zolmitriptan should be reduced and used cautiously, if at all, and none but SC sumatriptan and oral naratriptan should be used in patients taking MAOIs. Meperidine and sympathomimetics are a potentially lethal addition to MAOIs and may result in serotonin syndrome or hypertensive crisis.

Summary

Most patients require acute headache treatment. Some require preventive treatment. Patients on preventive medication still require acute treatment for breakthrough attacks. Many patients find that their acute attacks are more manageable if they are on a preventive medication. The choice of preventive treatment depends on the individual drug's efficacy and side effects; the patient's clinical features, headache frequency, and response to prior treatment; and the presence of any comorbid or coexistent disease.

SPECIAL SITUATIONS

Treatment of Menstrual Migraine

Menstrual migraine (MM) may differ from non-MM in that it is not associated with an aura, is of longer duration, and may be more subject to headache recurrence after treatment. Drugs that are proven effective or commonly used for the acute treatment of MM include NSAIDs, DHE, triptans, and the combination of aspirin, acetaminophen, and caffeine (AAC). The AAC combination was as effective in women with MM as it was

Table 9–26 Cautions in acute medication use

Drug	Caution	Contraindicated
Methysergide	Ergotamine, DHE, 5-HT$_1$ agonists	
Monoamine oxidase inhibitors	Sumatriptan SC, naratriptan, zolmitriptan, and frovatriptan	Meperidine, sympathomimetics (Midrin), dextromethorphan, rizatriptan, sumatriptan (PO, IN), eletriptan
NSAIDs	Other NSAIDs or aspirin-containing compounds	
Divalproex	Overuse of short-acting barbiturates	

Key to abbreviations: DHE, dihydroergotamine; NSAID, nonsteroidal anti-inflammatory drug.

in women with migraine not associated with menses in a placebo-controlled, double-blind trial that used the IHS criteria. The nonselective 5-HT$_1$ agonist DHE, available in parenteral and NS forms, is effective for the treatment of MM (D'Alessandro et al., 1983; Silberstein et al., 1990a; Diamond et al., 1996). Sumatriptan, zolmitriptan, and rizatriptan are as effective for menstrually associated migraine (Solbach and Waymer, 1993) as for nonmenstrually related migraine and, in addition, control the nausea and vomiting associated with attacks (De Lignieres et al., 1986; Sheftel et al., 1992). If severe MM cannot be controlled with NSAIDs, ergots, DHE, or selective 5-HT$_1$ agonists (triptans), then analgesics combined with opioids, opioids alone (Silberstein and Saper, 1993), high-dose corticosteroids, major tranquilizers (chlorpromazine, haloperidol, thiothixene, droperidol), or a course of IV DHE can be tried (Silberstein and Saper, 1993; Silberstein et al., 1990a). Women with frequent, severe MM are candidates for preventive therapy (either continuous or short-term) and often respond better to acute therapy when on preventive treatment.

Women who are using preventive medication but continue to have MM can increase the medication dose prior to their menses. Women who do not use preventive medicine or have migraine exclusively with their menses can just be treated perimenstrually with short-term prophylaxis (Silberstein and Merriam, 1991; Raskin, 1988; Silberstein and Saper, 1993). Regular periods and a predictable relationship between the attacks and the menses are essential for this strategy to succeed. Treating coexistent PMS may help control premenstrual headache. Drugs that have been used perimenstrually for short-term prophylaxis include NSAIDs, ergotamine, DHE, methysergide, methergine, the triptans, and magnesium. In adequate doses, NSAIDs can be used preventively 1 to 2 days before the expected onset of headache and continued for the duration of vulnerability. If the first NSAID fails, a different NSAID from another chemical class should be tried.

Ergotamine and DHE can be used prophylactically at the time of menses without significant risk of developing ergot dependence (Silberstein and Merriam, 1991; Raskin, 1988; Edelson, 1985; Silberstein, 1984). Ergotamine tartrate, at bedtime or twice a day, is an effective prophylactic agent (Raskin, 1988). Ergotamine in combination with belladonna and phenobarbital (Bellergal) may be useful in treating other perimenstrual symptoms in addition to headache (Robinson et al., 1977). Ergonovine maleate, an ergot derivative no longer available, provided a 65% improvement in headache severity and duration when given perimenstrually (Gallagher, 1989). Methylergonovine maleate is sometimes used in its place. As a nasal spray, DHE, given every 8 hours for 6 days beginning 3 days before the expected onset of headache, was used in a placebo-controlled, double-blind, short-term trial for the treatment of MM; the mean pain severity rating for DHE NS was lower than placebo for 67.5% of the 40 evaluable patients (Silberstein, 1996a).

Newman et al. (1998) used oral sumatriptan (25 mg TID) 2 to 3 days before the expected headache onset and continued for a total of 5 days in an open-label study of 20 women with MM. In 126 sumatriptan-treated cycles, headache was absent in 52.4% of subjects and reduced in severity by 50% or greater in 42%. Breakthrough headaches were rare and significantly reduced in severity compared with the baseline headaches. Naratriptan, which has a longer half-life than sumatriptan, is currently in placebo-controlled, double-blind trials for short-term perimenstrual prophylaxis of MM.

A placebo-controlled, double-blind study of 24 women with premenstrual syndrome (PMS) and migraine has shown that oral magnesium (360 mg of magnesium pyrrolidone carboxylic acid) decreases the severity of PMS symptoms and the duration and intensity of MM that occur prior to the onset of menstruation (Facchinetti et al., 1991). Perhaps responders belong to the subset of women with low serum ionized magnesium.

Popular but ineffective treatments for MM include diuretics and vitamins. Diuretics help with fluid retention but not with MM (Lundberg, 1986; Reid and Yen, 1981). The efficacy of pyridoxine to treat both PMS and MM has not been proven in double-blind studies (Williams et al., 1985; Hagen et al., 1985). In fact, high doses of pyridoxine have been reported to cause a sensory neuropathy (Schaumburg et al., 1983).

If severe MM cannot be controlled by these measures, then hormonal therapy may be indicated. Successful hormonal or hormonal modulation therapy of MM has been reported with estrogens (De Lignieres et al., 1986) [alone or combined with progesterone or testosterone (Magos et al., 1986)], combined OCs, synthetic androgens, estrogen modulators and antagonists (Calton and Burnett, 1984), and medical oophorectomy with a gonadotropin-releasing hormone (GnRH) analog with or without add-back therapy and prolactin release inhibitors (Thomas et al., 1991a). Progesterone is not effective in the treatment of headache or the symptoms of PMS (Freeman et al., 1990) despite many favorable anecdotal reports (Dalton, 1973; Bancroft and Backstrom, 1985).

The estradiol cutaneous patch provides a relatively stable plasma-estrogen level over the time of application (Anonymous, 1986; Judd, 1987; Stumpf, 1990). Levels are less stable with higher-dose patches. Serum estrogen levels rise within 4 hours of applying the transdermal patch and are proportional to the dose [patch transdermal therapeutic system (TTS): patch TTS 25 ≈ serum level of 23 pg/ml, TTS 50 ≈ 39 ng/ml, and TTS 100 ≈ 74 pg/ml] (Schwartz et al., 1995).

Pradalier et al. (1994) found that using the TTS 25 patch from 4 days before to 4 days after menstruation was not as effective as using the TTS 100 patch. Dennerstein et al. (1978) suggested that a serum estradiol level of 60 to 80 pg/ml is needed during the crucial week to prevent MM.

Combinations of estrogens and progestogens or progestogens alone in the form of OCs may be a reasonable approach for some patients who have intractable MM, particularly if it is associated with severe dysmenorrhea (Kappius and Goolkasian, 1987). Tamoxifen (Nolvadex) (O'Dea and Davis, 1990; Powles, 1986), a selective estrogen receptor modulator (SERM) that binds to a cytosolic

estrogen receptor, may be effective in resistant MM. A dose of 5 to 15 mg/day for days 7 to 14 of the luteal cycle has provided significant relief of menstrual headache without side effects. The effectiveness on MM of raloxifene, a new SERM with a different profile, is unknown (Delmas et al., 1997).

Neither hysterectomy nor oophorectomy has been proven to be effective in unselected cases of migraine. However, medical ovariectomy using GnRH analogs to suppress ovulation are effective in refractory PMS (Conn and Crowley, 1991; Muse et al., 1984; Hammarback and Backstrom, 1988).

In two placebo-controlled, double-blind studies, GnRH was significantly better than placebo at controlling both the behavioral and the physical symptoms of PMS (headache, breast fullness and tenderness, bloating, and fatigue) (Muse et al., 1984; Hammarback and Backstrom, 1988). Analogs of GnRH may be effective in severe MM. Since GnRH analogs induce hypogonadism, with many of the same short-term and long-term side effects as menopause, treatment is usually limited to 6 months unless replacement estrogens are used (Conn and Crowley, 1991; Pickersgill, 1998).

Add-back therapy can be used to limit these side effects and is not usually detrimental to effective GnRH agonist treatment (Pickersgill, 1998). Add-back treatment prevents bone mineral loss and minimizes the adverse effects of hypoestrogenism. Combined add-back regimens are lipid-neutral (Lemay and Faure, 1994; Howell et al., 1995; Surrey et al., 1995), protect against bone loss (Lemay and Faure, 1994; Maheux and Lemay, 1992; Howell et al., 1995; Simberg et al., 1996; Leather et al., 1993; Moghissi, 1996; Maheux et al., 1991), diminish vasomotor symptoms (Kiiholma et al., 1995; Maheux and Lemay, 1992; Howell et al., 1995; Friedman et al., 1993, 1994; Kiesel et al., 1996), decrease symptoms and blood loss in women with dysfunctional uterine bleeding (Thomas et al., 1991a), and improve symptoms associated with ovarian hyperandrogenism (Lemay and Faure, 1994; Elkind-Hirsch et al., 1995; Azziz et al., 1995; Pickersgill, 1998).

Administration of GnRH agonist, alone or with add-back therapy, may be an effective treatment for carefully selected patients who have severe perimenstrual migraine headaches (Murray and Muse, 1997).

Another strategy is a dopamine receptor agonist, either short-term or continuous. Bromocriptine (Parlodel) (Wentz, 1985; Andersch et al., 1978; Ylostalo et al., 1982; Andersen et al., 1977), a dopamine D2 receptor agonist, is an inhibitor of prolactin release. A dose of 2.5 to 5 mg/day during the luteal phase of the menstrual cycle may decrease the premenstrual symptoms of breast engorgement, irritability, and headache. In an open trial (Herzog, 1995), 24 women with severe, disabling MM (occurring within 3 days of menstruation) were treated with continuous bromocriptine 2.5 mg three times daily. Seventy-five percent of the women had at least a 25% reduction in headache compared to baseline. Overall headache frequency decreased 72%. None of the patients had less than a 10% increase in headache; three could not tolerate bromocriptine, and three did not benefit.

A sequential approach to the treatment of menstrual migraine is outlined in Table 9–27.

Menopausal Migraine

Menopause is the permanent cessation of menstruation. Sex steroid hormone levels are low and gonadotropin levels are elevated. Menopause is associated with both early and late symptoms (Table 9–28) (Utian, 1987a,b). Hot flushes, a vasomotor change, correlate with bursts of activity in hypothalamic pacemaker neurons leading to pulses of GnRH and, thus, luteinizing hormone (Rebar and Spitzer, 1987; Ravnikar, 1990). Hormonal replacement with estrogens (estrogen replacement therapy), alone or in combination with progestins (hormone replacement therapy), is often used to treat symptoms and prevent osteoporosis (Shoemaker et al., 1977; LaRosa, 1995). Estrogen replacement therapy may delay the onset and decrease the risk of Alzheimer's disease (Tang et al., 1996) and improve cognition, but this remains undetermined (Yaffe et al., 1998). Estrogen therapy

Table 9–27 Preventive treatment of menstrual migraine

Perimenstrual use of standard preventive drugs
Perimenstrual use of nonstandard preventive drugs
   Nonsteroidal antiinflammatory drugs
   Ergotamine and its derivatives
   Triptans
   Magnesium
Hormonal therapy
   Estrogens (with or without androgens or progestin)
   Combined oral contraceptives
   Synthetic androgens (danazol)
   Antiestrogen (tamoxifen)
   Medical oophorectomy (gonadotropin-releasing hormone analogues)
Dopamine agonists (bromocriptine)

may decrease the risk for coronary artery disease and hip fracture, but long-term, unopposed estrogen therapy increases the risk for endometrial carcinoma (Grady et al., 1992).

Headache management can be difficult in women who require hormonal replacement therapy for menopausal symptoms but develop headaches as a result of the therapy. Several empirical strategies may be utilized (Table 9–26). Reducing the dose of estrogen or changing the type of estrogen from a conjugated estrogen to pure estradiol, to synthetic ethinyl estradiol, or to a pure estrone may significantly reduce headache. In a controlled double-blind, crossover trial of menopausal women, Aylward et al. (1974) found that oral estropipate decreased the frequency and intensity of headache whereas ethinyl estradiol increased the headache. Changing

Table 9–28 Hormonal replacement treatment of headache

Estrogens
   Reduce estrogen dose
   Change estrogen type from conjugated estrogen to pure estradiol to synthetic estrogen to pure estrone
   Convert from interrupted to continuous dosing
   Convert from oral to parenteral dosing
   Add androgens
   Switch to selective estrogen receptor modulator
Progestin
   Switch from interrupted (cyclic) to continuous lower dose
   Change progestin type
   Change delivery system (PO to vaginal)
   Discontinue progestin (periodic endometrial biopsy or vaginal ultrasound)

from interrupted to continuous administration may be very effective if the headaches are associated with estrogen withdrawal. Techniques may be combined. Kudrow (1975) reported a 58% improvement in headache control with a reduced, continuous dose of estrogen. Parenteral estrogens, with or without adjunct hormones, can be effective. Greenblatt and Bruneteau (1974) studied postmenopausal women with oral estrogen-induced headaches and found that their headaches could be improved by switching from oral to parenteral estrogens (estradiol) and adding androgens (testosterone). The estradiol cutaneous patch, which provides a physiological ratio of estradiol to estrone and a steady-state concentration of estrogen, has been associated anecdotally with fewer headache side effects; however, this has not been proven in any controlled study (Anonymous, 1986; Judd, 1987; Stumpf, 1990). The new SERM raloxifene can also be used if a woman requires, but cannot tolerate, nonselective estrogen.

Progestins, used to prevent endometrial hyperplasia, can cause headache in addition to other symptoms of PMS, particularly if used cyclically. Giving a lower dose of a progestin (medroxyprogesterone, 2.5 vs. 7.5 mg) continuously can often control this. Another strategy is to change the type of progestin. Women who received norethindrone had less depression than those who received medroxyprogesterone acetate (Smith et al., 1994). For women with a uterus who have intolerable mental symptoms with progestins, an estrogen-only regimen may be used in con-

junction with an annual endometrial biopsy or vaginal ultrasonography to measure the endometrial thickness. If the endometrial echo complex is less than 4 mm, it may not be necessary to perform a biopsy since the endometrial cancer risk is very low (Mishell et al., 1997).

Another strategy is to use targeted drug delivery. The new adhesive vaginal gel containing micronized progesterone in an emulsion system was designed to maximize progesterone's therapeutic effect on the uterus while minimizing the potential for systemic side effects. Direct uterine progesterone delivery allows lower systemic progestin levels, providing endometrial protection with fewer progesterone side effects. It is available as a 4% (45 mg) or 8% (90 mg) formulation (Crinone) that can be given every other day (Medical Economics Company, 1999).

Treating Migraine During Pregnancy

Most women with migraine improve during pregnancy. Some women have their first attack during pregnancy. Migraine often recurs postpartum and can begin for the first time in general. Despite drug use, migraineurs do not differ from nonmigraineurs in miscarriages, toxemia, congenital anomalies, or stillbirths.

Death to the conceptus, teratogenicity, fetal growth abnormalities, perinatal effects, postnatal developmental abnormalities, delayed oncogenesis, and functional and behavioral changes can result from drugs or other agents (Table 9–29) (Blake and Niebyl,

Table 9–29 Drug effects and definitions

Effect	Definition
Spontaneous abortion	Death of the conceptus, most due to chromosomal abnormality
Embryotoxicity	The ability of drugs to kill the developing embryo
Congenital anomalies	Deviation from normal morphology or function
Teratogenicity	The ability of an exogenous agent to produce a permanent abnormality of structure or function in an organism exposed during embryogenesis or fetal life
Fetal effects	Growth retardation, abnormal histogenesis (also congenital abnormalities and fetal death), the main outcome of fetal drug toxicity during the second and third trimesters of pregnancy.
Perinatal effects	Effects on uterine contraction, neonatal withdrawal, or hemostasis
Postnatal effects	Drugs may have delayed long-term effects: delayed oncogenesis and functional and behavioral abnormalities

Table 9–30 Food and Drug Administration risk categories

Category A	Controlled human studies show no risk
Category B	No evidence of risk in humans but no controlled human studies
Category C	Risk to humans not ruled out
Category D	Positive evidence of risk to humans from human and/or experimental animal studies
Category X	Contraindicated in pregnancy

1988). According to the Perinatal Collaborative Project, a prospective and concurrent epidemiologic study of more than 50,000 pregnancies, many drugs have little or no human teratogenic risk.

The Food and Drug Administration (FDA) lists five categories of labeling for drug use in pregnancy (Table 9–30) (Medical Economics Company, 1999; Briggs et al., 1994). These categories are intended to provide therapeutic guidance, weighing the risks as well as the benefits of the drug. Although this is an improvement over previous labeling, it is still not ideal. An alternate rating system is TERIS, an automated teratogen information resource wherein ratings for each drug or agent are based on a consensus of expert opinion and the literature (Table 9–31) (Friedman and Polifka, 1994). It was designed to assess the teratogenic risk to the fetus from a drug exposure. A recent study found that the FDA categories have little, if any, correlation to the TERIS teratogenic risk. Friedmann and Polifka (1994) looked at 157 of the most frequently prescribed drugs and found poor correlation between the TERIS rating and the FDA pregnancy categories. This discrepancy results in part from the fact that the FDA categories were designed to provide therapeutic guidance and the TERIS ratings are useful for estimating

Table 9–31 TERIS risk rating

Undetermined (C)
None (A)
None–minimal (A)
Minimal (B)
Minimal–small (D)
High (X)

the teratogenic risks of a drug and not vice versa.

The major concern in managing the pregnant migraineur is the effect of both medication and migraine on the fetus. Because of the possible risk of injury to the fetus, medication use should be limited; however, it is not contraindicated during pregnancy (Silberstein, 1997a). Since migraine usually improves after the first trimester, many women can manage their headaches with this reassurance along with nonpharmacologic means of coping, such as ice, massage, and biofeedback (Silberstein, 1991, 1993b). Some women, however, continue to have severe, intractable headaches, sometimes associated with nausea, vomiting, and possible dehydration. These conditions not only are disruptive to the patient, but they may pose a risk to the fetus that is greater than the potential risk of the medications used to treat the pregnant patient (Silberstein, 1992, 1993b).

Symptomatic treatment, designed to reduce the severity and duration of symptoms, is used for an acute headache attack (Tables 9–30, 9–31). Rest, reassurance, and ice packs should be used to treat individual attacks. Symptomatic drugs are indicated for headaches that do not respond to nonpharmacologic treatment. Acetaminophen (alone or with codeine), NSAIDs, codeine alone, or other narcotics can be used during pregnancy. Aspirin in low, intermittent doses is not a significant teratogenic risk, although large doses, especially near term, may be associated with maternal and fetal bleeding. Aspirin should probably not be used unless there is a definite therapeutic need for it (other than headache). Barbiturates and benzodiazepines, if used at all, should be limited. Ergotamine, DHE, and sumatriptan should be avoided (Silberstein, 1993b).

The associated symptoms of migraine, such as nausea and vomiting, can be as disabling as the headache pain itself. In addition, some medications that are used to treat migraine can produce nausea. Metoclopramide, which decreases the gastric atony seen with migraine and enhances the absorption of coadministered medications, is extremely useful in migraine treatment. Mild nausea can be treated with phosphorylated carbohydrate solution (Emetrol) or doxylamine succinate and vitamin B_6 (pyridoxine). More severe nausea may require the use of injections or suppositories. Trimethobenzamide, chlorpromazine, prochlorperazine, and promethazine are available orally, parenterally, and by suppository; all can be used safely. We frequently use promethazine and prochlorperazine suppositories. Corticosteroids can be utilized occasionally. Some use prednisone in preference to dexamethasone, which crosses the placenta more readily.

Severe attacks of migraine should be treated aggressively (Raskin, 1988; Silberstein and Corbett, 1993). Intravenous fluids should be administered for hydration in conjunction with prochlorperazine 10 mg IV to control both nausea and head pain. Intravenous narcotics or corticosteroids can be added if necessary.

Preventive Treatment

Increased frequency and severity of migraine associated with nausea and vomiting may justify the use of daily prophylactic medication. This treatment option should be used only when absolutely necessary, with the consent of the patient and her partner after the risks have been completely explained. Preventive therapy is designed to reduce the frequency and severity of headache attacks. Consider prophylaxis when patients experience at least three or four prolonged, severe attacks that are relatively frequent and particularly incapacitating or unresponsive to symptomatic therapy and may result in dehydration and fetal distress (Silberstein, 1993b). β-Adrenergic blockers such as propranolol have been used under these circumstances, although adverse effects, including intrauterine growth retardation, have been reported. If the migraine is so severe that drug treatment is essential, the patient should be told of the risks posed by all of the drugs that are used (Tables 9–32, 9–33, 9–34) (Silberstein, 1993b). If the patient has a coexistent illness that requires treatment, select one drug that will treat both disorders. For example, propranolol can be used to treat hypertension and mi-

graine, while fluoxetine can be used to treat comorbid depression.

Drug Exposure

The neurologist should work with the obstetrician to manage the pregnant patient's headaches. If a woman inadvertently takes a medication while she is pregnant or becomes pregnant while taking a medication, determine the dose, timing, and duration of the exposure(s). Ascertain the patient's past and present state of health and the presence of mental retardation or chromosomal abnormalities in the family. Using a reliable source of information (such as TERIS), determine if the drug is a known teratogen (although for many drugs this is not possible) (Blake and Niebyl, 1988; Briggs et al., 1994; Friedman et al., 1990; Gilstrap and Little, 1992; Shepard, 1973).

If the drug is teratogenic or the risk is unknown, have the obstetrician confirm the gestational age by ultrasound. If the exposure occurred during embryogenesis, then high-resolution ultrasound can be performed to determine whether damage to specific organ systems or structures has occurred. If the high-resolution ultrasound is normal, it is reasonable to reassure the patient that the fetal structure is normal (within the 90% sensitivity of the study) (Gilstrap and Little, 1992). Have the obstetrician discuss the results of these studies with the mother and the significant other; formal prenatal counseling may be helpful in uncertain cases (Gilstrap and Little, 1992).

Status Migrainosus

The IHS defines status migrainosus as an attack of migraine, the headache phase of which lasts more than 72 hours whether it is treated or not (Headache Classification Committee of the International Headache Society, 1988). The headache is continuous throughout the attack or is interrupted by headache-free intervals that last less than 4 hours. Relief during periods of sleep is disregarded. No clear distinction is made between transformed migraine and prolonged status mi-

Table 9–32 Some therapeutic medications

	Fetal risk	
	FDA	TERIS
Simple analgesics		
Aspirin	C[a] (D)[b]	None–minimal
Acetaminophen	B[a]	None
Caffeine	B[a]	None–minimal
NSAIDS		
Ibuprofen	B[a] (D)	None–minimal
Indomethacin	B[a] (D)	None
Naproxen	B[a] (D)	Undetermined
Narcotics		
Butorphanol	C_M[c] (D)	
Codeine	C_M (D)	None–minimal
Meperidine	B[a] (D)	None–minimal
Methadone	B[a] (D)	None–minimal
Morphine	B[a] (D)	None–minimal
Ergots and serotonin agonists		
Ergotamine	X_M	Minimal
Dihydroergotamine	X_M	Undetermined
Sumatriptan	C_M	Undetermined
Naratriptan		
Eletriptan		
Rizatriptan		
Zolmitriptan		
Corticosteroids		
Dexamethasone	C[a]	None–minimal
Prednisone	B[a]	None–minimal
Barbiturates		
Butalbital	C[a] (D)	None–minimal
Phenobarbital	D[a]	None–minimal
Benzodiazepam		
Chlordiazepoxide	D[a]	None–minimal
Diazepam	D[a]	None–minimal

[a]Briggs, not manufacturers list.

[b]In parentheses, risk factor if used at end of third trimester.

[c]Subscript M, manufacturers.

Table 9–33 Neuroleptics/antiemetics

	Fetal risk	
	FDA	TERIS
Antihistamines		
Cyclizine (Marezine)	B[a]	
Cyproheptadine	B_M[b]	Undetermined
Dimenhydrinate (Dramamine)	B_M	None–minimal
Meclizine (Antivert)	B_M	None–minimal
Neuroleptics		
Phenothiazines		
Chlorpromazine (Thorazine)	C[a]	None–minimal
Prochlorperazine (Compazine)	C[a]	None
Metoclopramide (Reglan)	B_M	Minimal
Other		
Emetrol	B	
Doxylamine succinate	—	None
Vitamin B_6 (pyridoxine)	B	None

[a]Briggs, not manufacturers list.

[b]Subscript M, manufacturers.

Table 9–34 Guidelines for prophylactic treatment of headache

| | Dose | Fetal risk | |
		FDA	TERIS
β-Blockers			
Propranolol (Inderal, InderalLA)	40–320 mg/day	$C_M{}^b$	Undetermined
Nadolol (Corgard)	40–240 mg/day	C_M	Undetermined
Atenolol (Tenormin)	50–120 mg/day	C_M	Undetermined
Timolol (Blocadren)	10–30 mg/day	C_M	Undetermined
Antidepressants			
Nortriptyline (Pamelor, Aventyl)	10–100 mg/day	D^a	Undetermined
Amitriptyline (Elavil, Endep)	10–250 mg/day	D^a	None–minimal
Doxepin (Sinequan, Adapin)	10–150 mg/day	C^a	Undetermined
Fluoxetine (Prozac)	10–80 mg/day	B_M	None
Calcium channel blockers			
Verapamil (Calan)	240–720 mg/day	C_M	Undetermined
Nifedipine (Procardia)	30–180 mg/day	C_M	Undetermined
Diltiazem (Cardizem)	120–360 mg/day	C_M	Undetermined
Serotonin antagonists			
Methysergide (Sansert)	2–8 mg/day in divided doses up to 14 mg/day	D	Undetermined
Methylergonovine maleate (Methergine)	0.2–0.4 mg qid	C_M	Undetermined
Anticonvulsants			
Phenytoin (Dilantin)	200–400 mg/day	D^a	Small–moderate
Valproic acid (Depakene and Depakote, enteric-coated)	500–3,000 mg/day	D^a	Small–moderate

[a]Briggs, not manufacturers list.

[b]Subscript M, manufacturers.

grainosus because no upper time limit is given to status migrainosus. Factors responsible for triggering status migrainosus include emotional stress, depression, abuse of medications, anxiety, diet, hormonal factors, and multiple nonspecific factors (Couch and Diamond, 1983). Status migrainosus may be secondary to an acute neurologic disorder. However, acute CNS events can trigger an otherwise typical migraine.

There are no large series or double-blind treatment trials on status migrainosus, although reports of the treatment of isolated migraine attacks may include many patients whose attacks approximate the 72-hour criterion mentioned above (Lane and Ross, 1995; Callaham and Raskin, 1986; Jones et al., 1989; Saadah, 1992). Patients with status migrainosus need aggressive treatment. They usually present in the emergency department but can be treated in outpatient infusion centers. The principles of treatment for status migrainosus include the following: (1) fluid and electrolyte replacement (if indicated), (2) drug detoxification, (3) IV pharmacotherapy

to control pain, (4) treatment of associated symptoms of nausea and vomiting, and (5) concurrent implementation of migraine prophylaxis (if indicated).

Detoxification guidelines: (1) Fluid replacement for 24 to 48 hours. (2) Ergotamine tartrate can be discontinued abruptly if DHE is administered. Otherwise, it should be tapered over 2 to 3 days. (3) Analgesics not containing opiates or barbiturates and triptans can be stopped abruptly. (4) Combined analgesics containing barbiturates should be discontinued gradually. Rapid discontinuation can be achieved by giving phenobarbital. (5) Narcotic withdrawal must be carried out slowly or through replacement with methadone and subsequent rapid taper. Side effects can be reduced by giving clonidine hydrochloride and/or phenobarbital or a benzodiazepine derivative (Bakris et al., 1982; Gold et al., 1980).

Patients with severe treatment-resistant headaches benefit from aggressive, acute inpatient management. Criteria for hospitalization include severe, intractable headache accompanied by (1) dehydration, requiring parenteral therapy for pain interruption; (2) dependence on analgesic or ergotamine medication; or (3) significant comorbid neurologic, medical, or psychiatric illnesses (Silberstein and Saper, 1993). An approach to treatment is outlined in Table 9–35.

Oral, rectal, IM, or IV neuroleptics may be used as primary therapy or as adjunct treatment for nausea. Patients who receive neuroleptics must be monitored carefully for hypotension, sedation, and dystonic reactions. Orthostatic hypotension can be avoided by maintaining the patient supine for several hours following neuroleptic administration.

Five milligrams of prochlorperazine IV followed by DHE IV is a safe and effective means of terminating a migraine attack (Callaham and Raskin, 1986). The combination of metoclopramide IV and DHE IV is more effective for an acute migraine attack than is meperidine IM (Belgrade et al., 1989). One can mix 10 mg (2 ml) of prochlorperazine and 1 mg (1 ml) of DHE in a syringe and inject 2 cc IV. If the headache is not relieved in 15 to 30 minutes, the remainder of the dose can be injected. At times, the addition of 5 to 10 mg of diazepam IV will help to terminate the headache attack (Raskin, 1990b). Other choices include haloperidol and droperidol (Wang et al., 1997).

Patients who have truly intractable headaches should be admitted to the hospital and treated with repetitive DHE IV (Raskin, 1986; Silberstein et al., 1990a; Silberstein and Young, 1995b).

Parenteral corticosteroids, either alone or in combination with other symptomatic medications, have been used to treat severe, resistant headaches. Clinical experience also supports the view that steroids, such as a rapidly tapering short course of prednisone (starting with 80 to 100 mg/day) or dexamethasone (Decadron, starting with 8 to 20 mg/day), will assist in terminating an otherwise refractory migraine. Inpatients can be treated with high-dose IV corticosteroids (Solu-Medrol up to 500 mg/day to start), alone or in conjunction with neuroleptics or DHE, to help terminate a headache cycle.

Some clinicians advocate using indomethacin rectal suppositories or ketorolac IM, especially in situations where neuroleptics, narcotics, and DHE are relatively contraindicated.

A maximum of two doses of sumatriptan (6 mg SC) separated by 1 hour can be given within 24 hours. However, sumatriptan should not be given for at least 24 hours following ergotamine or DHE. A repeat injection is not effective if a prior injection failed. Headache recurrence, which occurs in about 40% of patients, may limit sumatriptan's use in status migrainosus and chronic daily headache.

After acute treatment is completed, many patients with status migrainosus require continuing care. This should include a preventive treatment program using standard migraine-preventive drugs.

Table 9–35 Treatment of status migrainosus

Start an IV
Pretreat with prochlorperazine (5–10 mg IV) or metoclopramide (10 mg IV)
Treat with dihydroergotamine (0.6–1.0 mg IV)
If headache persists, in 1 hour give additional dihydroergotamine (0.5 mg IV)
Additions: dexamethasone (4 mg IV), diazepam (5–10 mg IV)
Alternatives: ketorolac (30–60 mg IM), opioids, chlorpromazine (0.1 mg/kg), sumatriptan (6 mg SC)
Consider IV fluids

REFERENCES

Ablad, B. and C. Dahlof (1986). Migraine and β-blockade: Modulation of sympathetic neurotransmission. *Cephalalgia* 6:7–13.

Abramowicz, M. (1990). Fluoxetine (Prozac) revisited. *Med. Lett. Drugs Ther.* 32:83–85.

Abramowicz, M. (1991). Drugs for hypertension. *Med. Lett. Drugs Ther.* 33:33–38.

Adam, E.I., S.M. Gore, and W.H. Price (1978). Double-blind trial of clonidine in the treatment of migraine in a general practice. *J. R. Coll. Gen. Pract.* 28:587–590.

Adham, N., H.T. Kao, and L.E. Schechter (1993). Cloning of another human serotonin receptor (5-HT$_{1F}$): A fifth 5-HT$_1$ receptor subtype coupled to the inhibition of adenylate cyclase. *Neurobiology* 90:408–412.

Adly, C., J. Straumanis, and A. Chesson (1992). Fluoxetine prophylaxis of migraine. *Headache* 32:101–104.

Aellig, W.H. (1984). Investigation of the venoconstrictor effect of 8'hydroxydihydroergotamine, the main metabolite of dihydroergotamine, in man. *Eur. J. Clin. Pharmacol.* 26:239–242.

Aghajanian, G.K. (1978). Tolerance of locus coeruleus neurones to morphine and suppression of withdrawal response by clonidine. *Nature* 276:186–188.

Ahuja, G.K. and A.K. Verma (1985). Propranolol in prophylaxis of migraine. *Indian J. Med. Res.* 82:263–265.

Albers, G.W., L.T. Simon, A. Hamik et al. (1989). Nifedipine versus propranolol for the initial prophylaxis of migraine. *Headache* 29:215–218.

Albibi, R. and R.W. McCallum (1983). Metoclopramide: Pharmacology and clinical application. *Ann. Intern. Med.* 98:86–95.

Aldeeb, S.M., N. Biary, Y. Bahou et al. (1992). Flunarizine in migraine: A double-blind placebo-controlled study (in a Saudi population). *Headache* 32:461–462.

Altar, C.A. (1999). Neurotrophins and depression. *Trends Pharmacol. Sci.* 20:59–61.

Alvarez, W.C. (1934). The present day treatment of migraine. *Mayo Clin. Proc.* 9:22

American Psychiatric Association. (1994). *Diagnostic and Statistical Manual of Mental Disorders.* APA, Washington, D.C.

Amery, W.K. and J. Waelkens (1983). Prevention of the last chance: An alternative pharmacologic treatment of migraine. *Headache* 23:37–38.

Amery, W.K., J. Waelkens, and I. Caers (1986a). Dopaminergic mechanisms in premonitory phenomena. In *The Prelude to the Migraine Attack* (W.K. Amery and A. Wauquier, eds.), pp. 64–77. Bailliere Tindall, London.

Amery, W.K., J. Waelkens, and V. Van den Bergh (1986b). Migraine warnings. *Headache* 26:60–66.

Andersch, B., L. Hahn, C. Wendestam et al. (1978). Treatment of premenstrual syndrome with bromocriptine. *Acta Endocrinol. (Copenh.)* 88:165–174.

Andersen, A.N., J.F. Larsen, O.R. Steenstrup et al. (1977). Effect of bromocriptine on the premenstrual syndrome: A double-blind clinical trial. *Br. J. Obstet. Gynecol.* 84:370–374.

Andersen, A.R., P. Tfelt-Hansen, and N.A. Lassen (1987). The effect of ergotamine and dihydroergotamine on cerebral blood flow in man. *Stroke* 18:120–123.

Anderson, R.E., P. Chiu, and D.M. Woodbury (1989). Mechanisms of tolerance to the anticonvulsant effects of acetazolamide in mice: relation to the activity and amount of carbonic anhydrase in brain. *Epilepsia* 30:208–216.

Andersson, K. and E. Vinge (1990). Beta-adrenoceptor blockers and calcium antagonists in the prophylaxis and treatment of migraine. *Drugs* 39:355–373.

Andersson, P.G. (1973). BC105 and deseril in migraine prophylaxis: A double-blind study. *Headache* 13:68–73.

Andersson, P.G. (1988). Ergotism: The clinical picture. In *Drug-induced Headache* (H.C. Diener and M.S. Wilkinson, eds.), pp. 16–19. Springer, Berlin.

Andersson, P.G., S. Dahl, J.H. Hansen et al. (1983). Prophylactic treatment of classical and nonclassical migraine with metoprolol: A comparison with placebo. *Cephalalgia* 3:207–212.

Andersson, P.G., H.H. Hinge, O. Johansen et al. (1989). Double-blind study of naproxen vs placebo in the treatment of acute migraine attacks. *Cephalalgia* 9:29–32.

Andersson, P.G. and E.N. Petersen (1981). Propranolol and femoxetine, a 5HT-uptake inhibitor, in migraine prophylaxis: A double-blind crossover study. *Acta Neurol. Scand.* 64:280–288.

Anonymous. (1986). Transdermal estrogen. *Med. Lett. Drugs Ther.* 28:119–120.

Ansell, E., T. Fazzone, R. Festenstein et al. (1988). Nimodipine in migraine prophylaxis. *Cephalalgia* 8:269–272.

Anthony, M., H. Hinterberger, and J.W. Lance (1967). Plasma serotonin in migraine and stress. *Arch. Neurol.* 16:544–592.

Anthony, M. and J.W. Lance (1969). Monoamine oxidase inhibition in the treatment of migraine. *Arch. Neurol.* 21:263–268.

Anthony, M., J.W. Lance, and B. Somerville (1972). A comparative trial of prindolol, clonidine and carbamazepine in the interval therapy of migraine. *Med. J. Aust.* 6:1343–1346.

Anthony, M. and B.K. Rasmussen (1993). Migraine without aura. In *The Headaches* (J. Olesen, P. Tfelt-Hansen, and M.A. Welch, eds.), pp. 255–261. Raven Press, New York.

Antozzi, C., B. Garavaglia, M. Mora et al. (1994). Late-onset riboflavin-responsive myopathy with combined multiple acyl coenzyme. A dehydrogenase and respiratory chain deficiency. *Neurology* 44:2153–2158.

Applebaum, R.S. (1984). Diet and migraine. *J. Am. Diet. Assoc.* 84:942

Arts, W.F., H.R. Scholte, J.M. Boggard et al. (1983). NADH-CoQ reductase deficient myopathy: Successful treatment with riboflavin. *Lancet* 2:581–582.

Awidi, A.S. (1982). Efficacy of flurbiprofen in the treatment of acute migraine attacks: A double-blind cross-over study. *Curr. Ther. Res.* 32:492–497.

Aylward, M., F. Holly, and R.J. Parker (1974). An evaluation of clinical response to piperazine estrone sulphate ("Harmogen") in menopausal patients. *Curr. Med. Res. Opin.* 2:417–423.

Azziz, R., T.M. Ochoa, E.L. Bradley et al. (1995). Leuprolide and estrogen versus oral contraceptive pills for the treatment of hirsutism: A prospective randomized study. *J. Clin. Endocrinol. Metab.* 80:3406–3411.

Bakris, G.L., P.D. Cross, and J.E. Hammarstein (1982). The use of clonidine for the management of opiate abstinence in a chronic pain patient. *Mayo Clin. Proc.* 57:657–660.

Baldessarini, R.J. (1990). Drugs and the treatment of psychiatric disorders. In *The Pharmacological Basis of Therapeutics* (A.G. Gilman, T.W. Rall, A.S. Nies et al., eds.) pp. 383–435. Pergamon, New York.

Baldratti, A., P. Cortelli, G. Proccaccianti et al. (1983). Propranolol and acetylsalicylic acid in migraine prophylaxis. Double-blind crossover study. *Acta Neurol. Scand.* 67:181–186.

Bana, D.S., P.S. MacNeal, P.M. LeCompte et al. (1974). Cardiac murmurs and endocardial fibrosis associated with methysergide therapy. *Am. Heart J.* 88:640–655.

Bancroft, J. and T. Backstrom (1985). Premenstrual syndrome. *Clin. Endocrinol. (Oxf.)* 22: 313–336.

Bank, J. (1999). A comparative study of amitriptyline and fluvoxamine in migraine prophylaxis. *Headache* 34:476–478.

Bardwell, A. and J. Trott (1987). Stroke in migraine as a consequence of propranolol. *Headache* 27:381–383.

Barlow, C.F. (1984). *Headaches and Migraine in Children.* JB Lippincott, Philadelphia.

Barnhart, E.R. (1991). *Physicians' desk reference,* Medical Economics, Montvale, NJ.

Barrie, M.A., W.R. Fox, M. Weatherall et al. (1968). Analysis of symptoms of patients with headaches and their response to treatment with ergot derivatives. *Q. J. Med.* 146:319–336.

Baumgartner, C., P. Wessly, C. Bingol et al. (1989). Long-term prognosis of analgesic withdrawal in patients with drug-induced headaches. *Headache* 29:510–514.

Baumgartner, G.R. and R.C. Rowen (1987). Clonidine vs chlordiazepoxide in the management of acute alcohol withdrawal syndrome. *Arch. Intern. Med.* 147:1223–1226.

Baxter, G., G. Kennett, F. Blaney et al. (1995). 5-HT$_2$ receptor subtypes: A family reunited. *Trends Pharmacol. Sci.* 16:105–110.

Bayless, T.M., B. Rothfeld, L. Massa et al. (1975). Lactose and milk intolerance: Clinical implications. *N. Engl. J. Med.* 292:1156–1159.

Beaver, W.T. (1984). Combination analgesics. *Am. J. Med.* 77:38–53.

Beer, M.S., D.N. Middlemiss, and G. McAllister (1993). 5-HT$_1$-like receptors: Six down and still counting. *Trends Pharmacol. Sci.* 14:228–231.

Behan, P.O. (1978). Isometheptene compound in the treatment of vascular headache. *Practitioner* 221:937–939.

Behan, P.O. (1985). Prophylactic treatment for migraine: A comparison of pizotifen and clonidine. *Cephalalgia* 5:524–525.

Behan, P.O. and M. Reid (1980). Propranolol in the treatment of migraine. *Practitioner* 224: 201–204.

Belgrade, M.J., L.J. Ling, M.B. Schleevogt et al. (1989). Comparison of single-dose meperidine, butorphanol, and dihydroergotamine in the treatment of vascular headache. *Neurology* 39: 590–592.

Bell, R., D. Montoya, A. Snualb et al. (1990). A comparative trial of three agents in the treatment of acute migraine headache. *Ann. Emerg. Med.* 19:1079–1082.

Bentley, D., A. Katchbuvian, and J. Brostoff (1984). Abdominal migraine and food sensitivity in children. *Clin. Allergy* 14:499–500.

Berde, B. and E. Stuermer (1978). Introduction to the pharmacology of ergot alkaloids and related compounds as a basis of their therapeutic application. In *Ergot Alkaloids and Related Compounds* (B. Berde and H.O. Schild, eds.), pp. 1–28. Springer-Verlag, Berlin.

Berridge, M.J. (1989). Inositol triphosphate, calcium, lithium, and cell signaling. *JAMA* 262: 1834–1841.

Bickerstaff, E.R. (1987). Migraine variants and complications. In *Migraine: Clinical and Research Aspects* (J.N. Blau, ed.), pp. 55–75. Johns Hopkins University Press, Baltimore.

Bille, B. (1962). Migraine in school children. *Acta Pediatr. Scand.* 51:1–151.

Bix, K.J., D.J. Pearson, and S.J. Bentley (1984). A psychiatric study of patients with supposed food allergy. *Br. J. Psychiatry* 145:121–126.

Blake, D.A. and J.R. Niebyl (1988). Requirements and limitations in reproductive and teratogenic risk assessment. In *Drug Use in Pregnancy* (J.R. Niebyl, ed.), pp. 1–9. Lea & Febiger, Philadelphia.

Blake, P.Y., A.S. Mark, J. Kattah et al. (1995). MR of oculomotor nerve palsy. *Am. J. Neuroradiol.* 16:241–251.

Blau, J.N. (1980). Migraine prodromes separated from the aura: Complete migraine. *BMJ* 281: 658–660.

Blau, J.N. (1982). Resolution of migraine attacks: Sleep and the recovery phase. *J. Neurol. Neurosurg. Psychiatry* 45:223–226.

Blau, J.N. (1984). Migraine pathogenesis: The neural hypothesis reexamined. *J. Neurol. Neurosurg. Psychiatry* 47:437–442.

Blau, J.N. (1987). Adult migraine: The patient observed. In *Clinical and Research Aspects* (J.N. Blau, ed.), pp. 3–30. Johns Hopkins University Press, Baltimore.

Boisen, E., S. Deth, P. Hubbe et al. (1978). Clonidine in the prophylaxis of migraine. *Acta Neurol. Scand.* 58:288–295.

Bom, A.H., J.P. Heiligers, P.R. Saxena et al. (1989). Reduction of cephalic arteriovenous shunting by ergotamine is not mediated by 5-HT$_1$-like or 5-HT$_2$ receptors. *Br. J. Pharmacol.* 97:383–390.

Bonuso, S., E. DiStasio, P. Barone et al. (1983). Timed-release dihydroergotamine in the prophylaxis of mixed headache: A study versus amitriptyline. *Cephalalgia* 3:175–178.

Bordini, C., F. Antonaci, L.J. Stovner et al. (1991). "Hemicrania Continua"—a clinical review. *Headache* 31:20–26.

Borgesen, S.E., J.L. Nielsen, and C.E. Moller (1974). Prophylactic treatment of migraine with propranolol: A clinical trial. *Acta Neurol. Scand.* 50:651–656.

Bouchelet, I., Z. Cohen, W. Yong et al. (1996). Molecular basis for a possible role of 5-hydroxytryptamine (5-HT) 2B receptors in the aetiology of migraine headache. In *Proceedings from the International Business Communications Conference on Serotonin Receptors in the Central Nervous System*, Philadelphia, January 25–26, 1996.

Boureau, F., J.M. Joubert, V. Lasserre et al. (1994). Double-blind comparison of an acetaminophen 400mg–codeine 25mg combination versus aspirin 1000mg and placebo in acute migraine attack. *Cephalalgia* 14:156–161.

Bousser, M.G. and Y. Loria (1985). Efficacy of dihydroergotamine nasal spray in the acute treatment of migraine attacks. *Cephalalgia* 5:554–555.

Bousser, M.G., H. Ratinahirana, and X. Darbois (1990). Migraine and pregnancy [abstract]. *Neurology* 40:437.

Bovill, J.G. (1997). Mechanisms of actions of opioids and nonsteroidal antiinflammatory drugs. *Eur. J. Anesthesiol.* 14:9–15.

Bowden, C.L., A.M. Brugger, and A.C. Swann (1994). Efficacy of divalproex vs lithium and placebo in the treatment of mania. *JAMA* 271:918–924.

Boyle, R., P.O. Behan, and J.A. Sutton (1990). A correlation between severity of migraine and delayed emptying measured by an epigastric impedance method. *Br. J. Clin. Pharmacol.* 30:405–409.

Bradshaw, P. and M. Parsons (1965). Hemiplegic migraine, a clinical study. *Q. J. Med.* 133:65–85.

Branchek, T., J. Zgombick, M. Macchi et al. (1991). Cloning and expression of a human 5-HT$_{1D}$ receptor. In *Serotonin—Molecular Biology, Receptors and Functional Effects* (J.R. Fozard and P.R. Saxena, eds.), pp. 21–32. Birkhauser, Basel.

Brandli, P., B.M. Loffler, V. Breu et al. (1996). Role of endothelin in mediating neurogenic plasma extravasation in rat aura mater. *Pain* 64:315–322.

Bredfeldt, R.C., J.E. Sutherland, and J.E. Kruse (1989). Efficacy of transdermal clonidine for headache prophylaxis and reduction of narcotic

use in migraine patients. A randomized crossover trial. *J. Fam. Pract.* 29:153–156.

Brewerton, T.D., D.L. Murphy, E.A. Mueller et al. (1988). Induction of migraine like headaches by the serotonin agonist *m*-chlorophenylpiperazine. *Clin. Pharmacol. Ther.* 43:605–609.

Briggs, G.G., R.K. Freeman, and S.J. Yaffe (1994). *Drugs in Pregnancy and Lactation*, Williams & Wilkins, Baltimore.

Briggs, R.S. and P.A. Millac (1979). Timolol in migraine prophylaxis. *Headache* 19:379–381.

Brooks, P.M. and R.O. Day (1991). Nonsteroidal antiinflammatory drugs: Differences and similarities. *N. Engl. J. Med.* 324:1716–1725.

Brown, S.D., H.H. Wolf, E.A. Swinyard et al. (1993). The novel anticonvulsant topiramate enhances GABA-mediated chloride flux. *Epilepsia* 34:122.

Buring, J.E., R. Peto, and C.H. Hennekens (1990). Low-dose aspirin for migraine prophylaxis. *JAMA* 264:1711–1713.

Bussone, G., S. Baldini, G. D'Andrea et al. (1987). Nimodipine versus flunarizine in common migraine: A controlled pilot trial. *Headache* 27:76–79.

Cabarrocas, F. (1987). First efficacy data on subcutaneous almotriptan, a novel 5HT$_{1D}$ agonist. For and on behalf of the Almotriptan Subcutaneous Study Group. *Cephalagia* 17:421.

Cabarrocas, X. and J.M. Zayas (1998). Efficacy data on oral almotriptan, a novel 5HT$_{1B/1D}$ agonist. *Headache* 38:377.

Cady, R.K., D. Gutterman, J.A. Saiers et al. (1997). Responsiveness of nonIHS migraine and tension-type headache to sumatriptan. *Cephalalgia* 17:588–590.

Cady, R.K., J. Rubino, D. Crummett et al. (1994). Oral sumatriptan in the treatment of recurrent headache. *Arch. Fam. Med.* 3:766–772.

Cady, R.K., J.K. Wendt, J.R. Kirchner et al. (1991). Treatment of acute migraine with subcutaneous sumatriptan. *JAMA* 265:2831–2835.

Callaham, M. and N. Raskin (1986). A controlled study of dihydroergotamine in the treatment of acute migraine headache. *Headache* 26:168–171.

Calton, G.J. and J.W. Burnett (1984). Danazol and migraine. *N. Engl. J. Med.* 310:721–722.

Cameron, J.D., P.L. Lane, and M. Speechley (1995). Intravenous chlorpromazine vs intravenous metoclopramide in acute migraine headache. *Acad. Emerg. Med.* 2:597–602.

Campbell, W.B. (1990). Lipid-derived autocoids: Eicosanoids and platelet-activating factor. In *The Pharmacological Basis of Therapeutics* (A.G. Gilman, T.W. Rall, and P. Taylor, eds.), pp. 600–617. Pergamon, New York.

Cangi, F., M. Boccuni, A. Zanotti et al. (1989). Dihydroergokryptine (DEK) in migraine prophylaxis in a double-blind study vs methysergide. *Cephalalgia* 9:448–449.

Cao, Y., K.M.A. Welch, and S.K.V.E. Aurora (1997). Functional MRI of visually-triggered headache in migraine patients. Eighth Congress of the International Headache Society [abstract]. *Cephalalgia* 17:254.

Capildeo, R. and F.C. Rose (1982). Single-dose pizotifen, 1.5mg nocte: A new approach in the prophylaxis of migraine. *Headache* 22:272–275.

Carleton, S.C., R.F. Shesser, M.P. Pietrzak et al. (1998). Double-blind, multicenter trial to compare the efficacy of intramuscular dihydroergotamine plus hydroxyzine versus intramuscular meperidine plus hydroxyzine for the emergency department treatment of acute migraine headache. *Ann. Emerg. Med.* 32:129–138.

Carpay, H.A., P. Matthijsse, M. Steinbuch et al. (1997). Oral and subcutaneous sumatriptan in the acute treatment of migraine: An open randomized cross-over study. *Cephalalgia* 17:591–595.

Carter, C.M., J. Egger, and J.F. Soothill (1985). A dietary management of severe childhood migraine. *Hum. Nutr. Appl. Nutr.* 39:294–303.

Casaer, P. (1989). Alternating hemiplegia in childhood. In *Migraine and Other Headaches* (M.D. Ferrari and X. Lataste, eds.), pp. 39–51. Parthenon, Park Ridge, NJ.

Cashman, J. and G. McAnulty (1995). Nonsteroidal antiinflammatory drugs in perisurgical pain management: Mechanisms of action and rationale for optimum use. *Drugs* 49:51–70.

Celentano, D.D., W.F. Stewart, and M.S. Linet (1990). The relationship of headache symptoms with severity and duration of attacks. *J. Clin. Epidemiol.* 43:983–994.

Centonze, V., E. Attolini, L. Santoiemma et al. (1983). DHE retard for prophylactic therapy of migraine: Efficacy and tolerability. *Cephalalgia* 3:179–184.

Cerbo, R., M. Casacchia, R. Formisano et al. (1986). Flunarizine-pizotifen single-dose double-blind cross-over trial in migraine prophylaxis. *Cephalalgia* 6:15–18.

Cernex Pharmaceuticals (1993). *Imitrex (sumatriptan succinate). Subcutaneous Product Monograph.* Cernex, Research Triangle Park, NC.

Chabriat, H., J.E. Joire, J. Danchot et al. (1994). Combined oral lysine acetylsalicylate and metoclopramide in the acute treatment of migraine: A multicenter double-blind placebo-controlled study. *Cephalalgia* 14:297–300.

Chabriat, H., E. Tournier-Lasserve, K. Vahedi et al. (1995a). Autosomal dominant migraine with MRI white-matter abnormalities mapping to the CADASIL locus. *Neurology* 45:1086–1091.

Chabriat, H., K. Vahedi, M.T. Iba-Zizen et al. (1995b). Clinical spectrum of CADASIL: A study of seven families. *Lancet* 346:934–939.

Chappell, A.S., J.J. Bay, G.D. Botzum et al. (1994). Zatosetron, a 5HT₃ receptor antagonist in a multicenter trial for acute migraine. *Neuropharmacology* 33:509–513.

Clary, C. and E. Schweitzer (1987). The treatment of MAOI hypertensive crisis with sublingual nifedipine. *Clin. Psychiatry* 48:249–250.

Clozel, M., V. Breu, A.G. Gray et al. (1994). Pharmacologic characterization of bosentan, a new potent orally active nonpeptide endothelin receptor antagonist. *J. Pharmacol. Exp. Ther.* 270:228–235.

Cohen, G.R., J.W. Harbison, C.J. Blair et al. (1984). Clinical significance of transient visual phenomena in the elderly. *Ophthalmology* 91:436–442.

Conn, P.M. and W.F. Crowley (1991). Gonadotropin-releasing hormone and its analogues. *N. Engl. J. Med.* 324:93–103.

Connor, H.E. and D.T. Beattie (1999). 5-Hydroxytryptamine receptor subtypes: Relation to migraine. In *Migraine and Headache Pathophysiology* (L. Edvinsson, ed.), pp. 43–52. Martin Dunitz, London.

Coppola, M., D.M. Yealy, and R.A. Leibold (1995). Randomized, placebo-controlled evaluation of prochlorperazine versus metoclopramide for emergency department treatment of migraine headache. *Ann. Emerg. Med.* 26:541–546.

Cortelli, P., T. Sacquegna, F. Albani et al. (1985). Propranolol plasma levels and relief of migraine. *Arch. Neurol.* 42:46–48.

Couch, J.R. and S. Diamond (1983). Status migrainosus: Causative and therapeutic aspects. *Headache* 23:94–101.

Couch, J.R. and R.S. Hassanein (1976). Migraine and depression: Effect of amitriptyline prophylaxis. *Trans. Am. Neurol. Assoc.* 101:234–237.

Couch, J.R. and R.S. Hassanein (1979). Amitriptyline in migraine prophylaxis. *Arch. Neurol.* 36:695–699.

Couch, J.R., D. Ziegler, and R. Hassanein (1976). Amitriptyline in the prophylaxis of migraine: Effectivenes and relationship of antimigraine and antidepressant effects. *Neurology* 26:121–127.

Coulam, C.B. and J.R. Annagers (1979). New anticonvulsants reduce the efficacy of oral contraception. *Epilepsia* 20:519–525.

Critchley, M. (1967). Migraine: from cappadocia to queen square. In *Background to Migraine* (R. Smith, ed.). Heinemann, London.

Cumberbatch, M.J., R.G. Hill, and R.J. Hargreaves (1997). Rizatriptan has central antinociceptive effects against durally evoked responses. *Eur. J. Pharmacol.* 328:37–40.

Curran, D.A., H. Hinterberger, and J.W. Lance (1967). Methysergide. *Res. Clin. Stud. Headache* 1:74–122.

Curran, D.A. and J.W. Lance (1964). Clinical trial of methysergide and other preparations in the management of migraine. *J. Neurol. Neurosurg. Psychiatry* 27:463–469.

Curzon, G., G.A. Kennett, K. Shah et al. (1990). Behavioral effects of *m*-chlorophenylpiperazine (m-CPP), a reported migraine precipitant. In *Migraine, A Spectrum of Ideas* (M. Sandler and G. Collins, eds.), pp. 173–181. Oxford University Press, Oxford.

Cutler, N., G.R. Mushet, R. Davis et al. (1995). Oral sumatriptan for the acute treatment of migraine: Evaluation of three dosage strengths. *Neurology* 45:S5–S9.

Cutler, N.R., J. Claghorn, J.J. Sramek et al. (1996). Pilot study of MK462 in migraine. *Cephalalgia* 16:113–116.

Cutrer, F.M. and A. O'Donnell (1999). Recent advances in functional neuroimaging. *Curr. Opin. Neurol.* 12:255–259.

Cutrer, F.M., A.G. Sorenson, R.M. Weisskoff et al. (1998). Perfusion-weighted imaging defects during spontaneous migrainous aura. *Ann. Neurol.* 43:25–31.

Czapinski, P. and R. Motyl (1999). Randomized comparative placebo-controlled assessment of intravenous valproic acid effectiveness and safety in patients with acute migraine [abstract]. *Cephalalgia* 19:372–373.

Dahlof, C. (1987). No clearcut longterm prophylactic effect of one month of treatment with propranolol in migraineurs. *Cephalalgia* 7:459–460.

Dahlof, C. and R. Bjorkman (1993). Diclofenac-K (50 and 100mg) and placebo in the acute treatment of migraine. *Cephalalgia* 13:117–123.

D'Alessandro, R., G. Gamberini, A. Lozito et al. (1983). Menstrual migraine, intermittent prophylaxis with a timed-release pharmacological formulation of dihydroergotamine. *Cephalalgia* 15:158.

Dalessio, D.J. (ed.). (1980). *Wolff's Headache and Other Head Pain*, 4th ed. Oxford University Press, Oxford.

Dalessio, D.J. (ed.). (1987). *Wolff's Headache and Other Head Pain*, 5th ed. Oxford University Press, Oxford.

Dalton, K. (1973). Progesterone suppositories and pessaries in the treatment of menstrual migraine. *Headache* 13:151–159.

Darland, T., M.M. Heinricher, and D.K. Grandy (1998). Orphanin FQ/nociceptin: A role in pain and analgesia, but so much more. *Trends Neurosci.* 21:215–221.

Das, S.M., G.K. Ahuja, and A.S. Narainaswamy (1979). Clonidine in prophylaxis of migraine. *Acta Neurol. Scand.* 60:214–217.

Davis, C.P., P.R. Torre, C. Williams et al. (1995). Ketorolac versus meperidine-plus-promethazine treatment of migraine headache: Evaluations by patients. *Am. J. Emerg. Med.* 13:146–150.

Dawson, T.M., V.L. Dawson, and S.H. Snyder (1992). A novel neuronal messenger molecule in brain: The free radical, nitric oxide. *Ann. Neurol.* 32:297–311.

de Arcaya, A.A., L. Cerezal, A. Canga et al. (1999). Neuroimaging diagnosis of Tolosa-Hunt syndrome: MRI contribution. *Headache* 39:321–325.

Delbene, E., M. Poggioni, U. Garagiola et al. (1987). Intramuscular treatment of migraine attacks using diclofenac sodium: A crossover clinical trial. *J. Int. Med. Res.* 15:44–48.

De Lignieres, B., M. Vincens, P. Mauvais-Jarvis et al. (1986). Prevention of menstrual migraine by percutaneous estradiol. *Br. Med. J. Clin. Res.* 293:1540.

Delmas, P.D., N.H. Bjarnason, B.H. Mitlak et al. (1997). Effects of raloxifene on bone mineral density, serum cholesterol concentrations, and uterine endometrium in postmenopausal women. *N. Engl. J. Med.* 337:1641–1647.

DeLorenzo, R.J., S. Sombati, and D.A. Coulter (2000). Effects of topiramate on sustained repetitive firing and spontaneous recurrent seizure discharges in cultured hippocampal neurons. *Epilepsia* 41:S40–S44.

DenBoer, M.O., C.M. Villalon, J.P. Heiligers et al. (1991a). The role of 5-HT$_1$-like receptors in the reduction of porcine cranial arteriovenous anastomotic shunting by sumatriptan. *Br. J. Pharmacol.* 102:323–330.

DenBoer, M.O., C.M. Villalon, J.P. Heiligers et al. (1991b). The role of 5-HT$_1$-like receptors. *Br. J. Pharmacol.* 104:183–189.

Dennerstein, L., B. Laby, G.D. Burrows et al. (1978). Headache and sex hormone therapy. *Headache* 18:146–153.

Deweerdt, C.J., H.P. Bootsma, and H. Hendriks (1996). Herbal medicines in migraine prevention: Randomized double-blind placebo-controlled crossover trial of feverfew preparation. *Phytomedicine* 3:225–230.

Diamond, S. (1964). Depressive headaches. *Headache* 4:255–259.

Diamond, S. (1976). Treatment of migraine with isometheptene, acetaminophen, and dichloralphenazone combination: A double-blind, crossover trial. *Headache* 15:282–287.

Diamond, S. and D.J. Dalessio (1982). Drug abuse in headache. In *The Practicing Physician's Approach to Headache* (S. Diamond and D.J. Dalessio, eds.), pp. 114–121. Williams & Wilkins, Baltimore.

Diamond, S., A. Elkind, R.T. Jackson et al. (1998). Multiple-attack efficacy and tolerability of sumatriptan nasal spray in the treatment of migraine. *Arch. Fam. Med.* 7:234–240.

Diamond, S. and F.G. Freitag (1993). A double-blind trial of flunarizine in migraine prophylaxis. *Headache Q.* 4:169–172.

Diamond, S., F.G. Freitag, G. Chu et al. (1991). A placebo-controlled comparative study versus intramuscular methadone. In *New Advances in Headache Research* (C. Rose, ed.), pp. 319–324. Smith Gordon, London.

Diamond, S., F.G. Freitag, M.L. Diamond et al. (1996). Subcutaneous dihydroergotamine mesylate (DHE) in the treatment of menstrual migraine. *Headache Q.* 7:145–147.

Diamond, S., F.G. Freitag, J. Prager et al. (1985). Olfactory aura in migraine. *N. Engl. J. Med.* 312:1390–1391.

Diamond, S., L. Kudrow, J. Stevens et al. (1982). Long-term study of propranolol in the treatment of migraine. *Headache* 22:268–271.

Diamond, S., J. Medina, J. Diamond-Falk et al. (1979). The value of biofeedback in the treatment of chronic headache: A five-year retrospective study. *Headache* 19:90–96.

Diamond, S. and J.L. Medina (1975). Isometheptene—a nonergot drug in the treatment of migraine. *Headache* 15:211–213.

Diamond, S. and J.L. Medina (1976). Double-blind study of propranolol for migraine prophylaxis. *Headache* 16:24–27.

Diamond, S. and D. Montrose (1984). The value of biofeedback in the treatment of chronic headache: A four-year retrospective study. *Headache* 24:5–18.

Diamond, S., S.B. Phillips, and J.E. Bernstein (1999a). Intranasal civamide for the acute treatment of migraine headache. *Headache* 39:350.

Diamond, S., R.E. Ryan, J.A. Klapper et al. (1999b). Dotarizine in the prophylaxis of migraine headaches. *Headache* 39:350.

Diamond, S., G.D. Solomon, F.G. Freitag et al. (1987). Long-acting propranolol in the prophylaxis of migraine. *Headache* 27:70–72.

Diener, H.C. (1999). The efficacy and safety of acetylsalicylic acid lysinate compared to subcutaneous sumatriptan and parenteral placebo in the acute treatment of migraine. A double-blind, double-dummy, randomized multicenter, parallel group study. The ASASUMAMIG Study Group. *Cephalagia* 19:581–588.

Diener, H.C., W.D. Gerber, and S. Geiselhart (1988). Short- and long-term effects of withdrawal therapy in drug-induced headache. In *Drug-induced Headache* (H.C. Diener and M. Wilkinson, eds.), pp. 133–142. Springer-Verlag, Berlin.

Diener, H.C., A. Hartung, J.A. Gobel et al. (1995). Substance-P antagonist RPR 100893–201 is not effective in human migraine attacks. In *6th International Headache Research Seminar*, Copenhagen.

DiGiovanni, A.J. and B.S. Dunbar (1970). Epidural injections of autologous blood for postlumbar-puncture headache. *Anesth. Analg.* 49:268–271.

Dihydroergotamine Nasal Spray Multicenter Investigators (1995). Efficacy, safety, and tolerability of dihydroergotamine nasal spray as monotherapy in the treatment of acute migraine. *Headache* 35:177–184.

Diserio, F., J. Patin, and A. Friedman (1989). USA trials of dihydroergotamine nasal spray in the acute treatment of migraine headache. *Cephalalgia* 9:344–345.

Dodgson, S.J., R.P. Shank, and B.E. Maryanoff (2000). Topiramate as an inhibitor of carbonic anhydrase isoenzymes. *Epilepsia* 41:35–39.

Dowson, A. (1996). Can oral 311C90, a novel 5HT$_{1D}$ agonist, prevent migraine headache when taken during an aura? *Eur. Neurol.* 36:28–31.

Driefuss, F.E., N. Santilli, D.H. Langer et al. (1987). Valproic acid hepatic fatalities: A retrospective review. *Neurology* 37:379–385.

Drummond, P.D. (1986). A quantitative assessment of photophobia in migraine and tension headache. *Headache* 26:465–469.

Drummond, P.D. (1987). Scalp tenderness and sensitivity to pain in migraine and tension headache. *Headache* 27:45–50.

Drummond, P.D. and J.W. Lance (1984). Clinical diagnosis and computer analysis of headache symptoms. *J. Neurol. Neurosurg. Psychiatry* 47:128–133.

Dryden, S., H.M. Frankish, A. Kilpatrick et al. (1994). The serotonin agonist mCPP reduces neuropeptide Y concentrations in the paraventricular nucleus of the rat: Could this explain its hypophagic action? *Clin. Sci. (Colch.)* 86:43.

Dryden, S., Q. Wang, H.M. Frankish et al. (1995). The serotonin (5-HT) antagonist methysergide increases neuropeptide Y (NPY) synthesis and secretion in the hypothalamus of the rat. *Brain Res.* 699:12–18.

Duarte, C., F. Dunaway, L. Turner et al. (1992). Ketorolac versus meperidine and hydroxyzine in the treatment of acute migraine headache: A randomized, prospective, double-blind trial. *Ann. Emerg. Med.* 21:1116–1121.

Ducros, A., A. Joutel, and K. Vahedi (1995). Toward the identification of a second locus for familial hemiplegic migraine. *Cephalalgia* 15:9.

Ducros, A., A. Joutel, and K. Vahedi (1997). Mapping of a second locus for familial hemiplegic migraine to 1q21-q23 and evidence of further heterogeneity. *Ann. Neurol.* 42:885–890.

Duke University and Center for Clinical Health Policy Research. (1999). *Behavioral and Physical Treatments for Migraine*. Technical Review 2.2, 290-94-2025, pp. 1–116. Duke University Press, Durham, NC.

Easterling, D.E., T. Zakszewski, and M.D. Moyer (1988). Plasma pharmacokinetics of topiramate, a new anticonvulsant, in humans. *Epilepsia* 29:662.

Edelson, R.N. (1985). Menstrual migraine and other hormonal aspects of migraine. *Headache* 25:376–379.

Edmeads, J. (1988). Emergency management of headache. *Headache* 28:675–679.

Edwards, K., V. Santarcangelo, P. Shea et al. (1999). Intravenous valproate for acute treatment of migraine headaches [abstract]. *Cephalalgia* 19:356.

Edwards, K.R., M.J. Glautz, P. Shea et al. (2000). Topirimate for migraine prophylaxis: A double-blind, randomized, placebo controlled study. *Headache* 40:407.

Egger, J., J. Wilson, C.M. Carter et al. (1983). Is migraine food allergy? *Lancet* ii:865–869.

Eglen, R.M., J.R. Hasper, D.J. Chang et al. (1997). The 5-HT₇ receptor: Orphan found. *Trends. Pharmacol. Sci.* 18:104–107.

Ekbom, K. (1994). Alprenolol for migraine prophylaxis. *Headache* 34:476–478.

Ekbom, K. and P.O. Lundberg (1972). Clinical trial of LB-56 (d-1-4-(2-hydroxy-3-isopropyl-aminopropoxy) indol): An adrenergic beta-receptor blocking agent in migraine prophylaxis. *Headache* 12:15–17.

Ekbom, K. and M. Zetterman (1977). Oxprenolol in the treatment of migraine. *Acta Neurol. Scand.* 56:181–184.

Elkind, A.H., A.P. Friedman, A. Bachman et al. (1968). Silent retroperitoneal fibrosis associated with methysergide therapy. *JAMA* 206:1041–1044.

Elkind, A.H., C. Webster, and R.K. Herbertson (1989). Efficacy of guanfacine in a double-blind parallel study for migraine prophylaxis. *Cephalalgia* 9:369–370.

Elkind-Hirsch, K.E., C. Anania, M. Mack et al. (1995). Combination gonodotrophin-releasing hormone agonist and oral contraceptive therapy improves treatment of hirsute women with ovarian hyperandrogenism. *Fertil. Steril.* 63:970–978.

Ellis, G.L., J. Delaney, D.A. Dehart et al. (1993). The efficacy of metoclopramide in the treatment of migraine headache. *Ann. Emerg. Med.* 22:191–195.

Ensink, F. (1991). Subcutaneous sumatriptan in the acute treatment of migraine. *J. Neurol.* 238:S66–S69.

Epstein, M.T., J.M. Hockaday, and T.D.R. Hockaday (1975). Migraine and reproductive hormones throughout the menstrual cycle. *Lancet* i:543–548.

Facchinetti, F., P. Borella, G. Sances et al. (1991). Oral magnesium successfully relieves premenstrual mood changes. *Obstet. Gynecol.* 78:177.

Fanchamps, A. (1985). Why do not all beta-blockers prevent migraine? *Headache* 25:61–62.

Featherstone, H.J. (1983). Low dose propranolol therapy for aborting acute migraine. *West. J. Med.* 138:416–417.

Feinmann, C. (1985). Pain relief by antidepressants: Possible modes of action. *Pain* 23:1–8.

Ferguson, A. (1990). Food sensitivity or self-deception? *N. Engl. J. Med.* 323:476

Ferrante, F.M. (1996). Principles of opioid pharmacotherapy: Practical implications of basic mechanisms. *J. Pain Symptom Manage.* 11:265–273.

Ferrari, M.D., M.H. James, D. Bates et al. (1994). Oral sumatriptan: Effect of a second dose, and incidence and treatment of headache recurrences. *Cephalalgia* 14:330–338.

Ferrari, M.D., J. Odink, K.D. Bos et al. (1990). Neuroexcitatory plasma amino acids are elevated in migraine. *Neurology* 40:1582–1586.

Ferrari, M.D., J. Odink, C. Tapparelli et al. (1989). Serotonin metabolism in migraine. *Neurology* 39:1239–1242.

Ferrari, M.D. and P.R. Saxena (1993a). Clinical and experimental effects of sumatriptan in humans. *Trends Pharmacol. Sci.* 14:129–133.

Ferrari, M.D. and P.R. Saxena (1993b). On serotonin and migraine: A clinical and pharmacological review. *Cephalalgia* 13:151–165.

Ferro, C.J. and D.J. Webb (1996). The clinical potential of endothelin receptor antagonists in cardiovascular medicine. *Drugs* 51:12–27.

Finnish Sumatriptan Group and Cardiovascular Clinical Research Group. (1991). A placebo-controlled study of intranasal sumatriptan for the acute treatment of migraine. *Eur. Neurol.* 31:332–338.

Fisher, C.M. (1980). Late life migraine accompaniments as a cause of unexplained transient ischemic attacks. *Can. J. Neurol. Sci.* 7:9–17.

Fisher, H. (1995). A new approach to emergency department therapy of migraine headache. *J. Emerg. Med.* 136:119–122.

Fontanari, D., L. Perulli, F. Conte et al. (1983). Planned release dihydroergotamine in common migraine and "tension-vascular headache" multicenter clinical trial. *Cephalalgia* 3:189–191.

Forbes, J.A., W.T. Beaver, K.F. Jones et al. (1991). Effect of caffeine on ibuprofen analgesia in postoperative surgery pain. *Clin. Pharmacol. Ther.* 49:674–684.

Ford, R.G. and K.T. Ford (1997). Continuous intravenous dihydroergotamine in the treatment of intractable headache. *Headache* 37:129–136.

Formisano, R., P. Falaschi, R. Cerbo et al. (1991). Nimodipine in migraine: Clinical efficacy and endocrinological effects. *Eur. J. Clin. Pharmacol.* 41:69–71.

Forssman, B., K.G. Henriksson, V. Johannsson et al. (1976). Propranolol for migraine prophylaxis. *Headache* 16:238–245.

Forssman, B., K.G. Henriksson, and S. Kihlstrand (1972). A comparison between BC105 and methysergide in the prophylaxis of migraine. *Acta Neurol. Scand.* 48:204–212.

Forssman, B., C.J. Lindblad, and V. Zbornikova (1983). Atenolol for migraine prophylaxis. *Headache* 23:188–190.

Forsythe, I. and J.M. Hockaday (1988). Management of childhood migraine. In *Migraine in*

Childhood (J.M. Hockaday, ed.), pp. 63–74. Butterworths, London.

Fozard, J.R. (1982). Serotonin, migraine and platelets. *Progress. Pharmacol.* 414:135–146.

Fozard, J.R. (1990). 5-HT in migraine: Evidence from 5-HT receptor antagonists for a neuronal etiology. In *Migraine: A Spectrum of Ideas* (M. Sandler and G.M. Collins, eds.), pp. 128–146. Oxford University Press, New York.

Fozard, J.R. (1992). Pharmacological relevance of 5-HT$_3$ receptors. In *Serotonin Receptor Subtypes: Pharmacological Significance and Clinical Implications* (S.Z. Langer, N. Brunello, G. Racagni et al. eds.), pp. 44–55. Karger, Basel.

Fozard, J.R. (1995). The 5-hydroxytryptamine–nitric oxide connection: The key link in the initialization of migraine? *Arch. Intern. Pharmacodyn.* 329:111–119.

Fozard, J.R. and J.A. Gray (1989). 5-HT$_{1C}$ receptor activation: A key step in the initiation of migraine? *Trends Pharmacol. Sci.* 10:307–309.

Fozard, J.R. and H.O. Kalkman (1994). 5-Hydroxytryptamine (5-HT) and the initiation of migraine: New perspectives. *Arch. Pharmacol.* 350:225–229.

Freeman, E., K. Rickels, S.J. Sondheimer et al. (1990). Ineffectiveness of progesterone suppository treatment for premenstrual syndrome. *JAMA* 264:349–353.

Freitag, F., S. Diamond, M. Diamond et al. (1998). Subcutaneous sumatriptan in patients treated with monoamine oxidase inhibitors and other prophylactic agents. *Headache Q.* 9:165–171.

Freitag, F.G., R. Cady, A. Elkind et al. (1999a). Comparative study of Midrin and sumatriptan succinate in the treatment of migraine headache [abstract]. *Headache* 19:355.

Freitag, F.G. and S. Diamond (1984). Nadolol and placebo comparison study in the prophylactic treatment of migraine. *J. Am. Osteopath. Assoc.* 84:343–347.

Freitag, F.G., S. Diamond, M.L. Diamond et al. (1999b). The prophylaxis of migraine with the GABA-agonist, tiagabine: A clinical report [abstract]. *Headache* 19:354.

Freitag, F.G., S. Diamond, and G.D. Solomon (1987). Antidepressants in the treatment of mixed headache: MAO inhibitors and combined use of MAO inhibitors and tricyclic antidepressants in the recidivist headache patient. In *Advances in Headache Research* (F.C. Rose, ed.), pp. 271–275. John Libbey, London.

Frenken, C.W. and S.T. Nuijten (1984). Flunarizine, a new preventive approach to migraine: A double-blind comparison with placebo. *Clin. Neurol. Neurosurg.* 86:17–20.

Friedman, A.J., M. Daly, M. Juneau-Norcross et al. (1993). A prospective, randomized trial of gonadotrophin-releasing hormone agonist plus estrogen–progestin or progestin "add-back" re-

gimes for women with leiomyomata uteri. *J. Clin. Endocrinol Metab.* 76:1439–1445.

Friedman, A.J., M. Daly, M. Juneau-Norcross et al. (1994). Long-term medical therapy for leiomyomata uteri: A prospective, randomized study of leuprolide acetate depot plus either estrogen–progestin or progestin add-back for 2 years. *Hum. Reprod.* 9:1618–1625.

Friedman, A.P., F.J. Diserio, and D.S. Hwang (1989). Symptomatic relief of migraine: Multicenter comparison of cafergot pb, cafergot, and placebo. *Clin. Ther.* 11:170–182.

Friedman, A.P., K.H. Finley, and J.R. Graham (1962). Classification of headache. *Arch. Neurol.* 6:173–176.

Friedman, J.M., B.B. Little, R.L. Brent et al. (1990). Potential human teratogenicity of frequently prescribed drugs. *Obstet. Gynecol.* 75:594–599.

Friedman, J.M. and J.E. Polifka (1994). *Teratogenic Effects of Drugs: A Resource for Clinicians (TERIS)*, Johns Hopkins University Press, Baltimore.

Frishman, W.H. (1987). Beta adrenergic blocker withdrawal. *Am. J. Cardiol.* 59:32F.

Frölich, J.C. (1997). A classification of NSAIDs according to the relative inhibition of cyclooxygenase isoenzymes. *Trends Pharmacol. Sci.* 15:34.

Fuller, G.N. and R.J. Guiloff (1990). Propranolol in acute migraine: A controlled study. *Cephalalgia* 10:229–233.

Gabai, I.J. and E.L.H. Spierings (1989). Prophylactic treatment of cluster headache with verapamil. *Headache* 29:167–168.

Gallagher, R.M. (1986). Emergency treatment of intractable migraine. *Headache* 26:74–75.

Gallagher, R.M. (1989). Menstrual migraine and intermittent ergonovine therapy. *Headache* 29:366–367.

Gallagher, R.M. (1996). Acute treatment of migraine with dihydroergotamine nasal spray. Dihydroergotamine Working Group. *Arch. Neurol.* 53:1285–1291.

Gardner, K., M.M. Barmada, L.J. Ptacek et al. (1997). A new locus for hemiplegic migraine maps to chromosome 1q31. *Neurology* 49:1231–1238.

Gasior, M., R.B. Carter, and J.M. Witkin (1999). Neuroactive steroids: Potential therapeutic use in neurological and psychiatric disorders. *Trends Pharmacol. Sci.* 20:107–112.

Gawel, M.J., J. Kreeft, R.F. Nelson et al. (1992). Comparison of the efficacy and safety of flunarizine to propranolol in the prophylaxis of migraine. *Can. J. Neurol. Sci.* 19:340–345.

Gelmers, H.J. (1983). Nimodipine, a new calcium antagonist, in the prophylactic treatment of migraine. *Headache* 23:106–109.

Gennari, C., M.S. Chierichetti, S. Gonnelli et al. (1986). Migraine prophylaxis with salmon calcitonin: A cross-over, double-blind, placebo-controlled study. *Headache* 26:13–16.

Gerber, W.G., H. Diener, E. Scholz et al. (1991). Responders and nonresponders to metoprolol, propranolol and nifedipine treatment in migraine prophylaxis: A dose-range study based on time-series analysis. *Cephalalgia* 11:37–45.

Ghose, K., B. Niven, A. McLeod et al. (1996). Vigabatrin in the prophylaxis of drug resistant migraine: A double-blind crossover comparison with placebo. *Cephalalgia* 16:367.

Gibbs, J.W., S. Sombati, R.J. DeLorenzo, and D.A. Coulter (2000). Cellular actions of topiramate: blockade of kainate-evoked inward currents in cultured hippocampal neurons. *Epilepsia* 41: S10–S16.

Gilbert, G.J. (1982). An occurrence of complicated migraine during propranolol therapy. *Headache* 22:81–83.

Gilman, A.G. (1989). G proteins and regulation of adenylyl cyclase. *JAMA* 262:1819–1825.

Gilstrap, L.C., III and B.B. Little (1992). *Drugs and Pregnancy* (L.C. Gilstrap III and B.B. Little, eds.), pp. 23–29. Elsevier, New York.

Glover, V., J. Littlewood, M. Sandler et al. (1983). Biochemical predisposition to dietary migraine: The role of phenolsulfotransferase. *Headache* 23:53–58.

Goadsby, P.J. and A.L. Gundlach (1991). Localization of [^{3}H]-dihydroergotamine binding sites in the cat central nervous system: Relevance to migraine. *Ann. Neurol.* 29:91–94.

Goadsby, P.J. and K.L. Hoskin (1996). Inhibition of trigeminal neurons by intravenous administration of the serotoinin (5HT)-1-D receptor agonist zolmitriptan (311C90): Are brain stem sites a therapeutic target in migraine? *Pain* 67: 355–359.

Gold, M.S., A.C. Pottash, D.R. Sweeney et al. (1980). Opiate withdrawal using clonidine, a safe, effective, and rapid nonopiate treatment. *JAMA* 243:343–346.

Goldner, J.A. and L.P. Levitt (1987). Treatment of complicated migraine with sublingual nifedipine. *Headache* 27:484–486.

Goldstein, D.J., W.W. Offen, E.G. Klein et al. (1999). Lanepitant, an NK-1 antagonist, in migraine prophylaxis [abstract]. *Cephalalgia* 19: 377.

Goldstein, D.J., O. Wang, J.R. Saper et al. (1997). Ineffectiveness of neurokinin-1 antagonist in acute migraine: A crossover study. *Cephalalgia* 17:785–790.

Goldstein, J., M.J. Gawel, P. Winner et al. (1988). Comparison of butorphanol nasal spray and fiorinal with codeine in the treatment of migraine. *Headache* 38:516–522.

Goldstein, J. and C. Keywood (1998). A study of the efficacy and safety of low doses of frovatriptan (VML251), a potent cerebroselective 5-hydroxytryptamine (5HT)1B/1D agonist in the acute treatment of migraine [abstract]. *Eur. J. Neurol.* 5:S46–S47.

Goldstein, M. and T.C. Chen (1982). The epidemiology of disabling headache. In *Advances in Neurology* (M. Critchley, ed.), pp. 377–390. Raven Press, New York.

Gomersall, J.D. and A. Stuart (1973). Amitriptyline in migraine prophylaxis. Changes in pattern of attacks during a controlled clinical trial. *J. Neurol. Neurosurg. Psychiatry* 36:684–690.

Gordon, M.L., R.B. Lipton, S.L. Brown et al. (1993). Headache and cortical responses to *m*-chlorophenylpiperazine are highly correlated. *Cephalalgia* 13:400–405.

Grady, D., S.M. Rubin, D.B. Petitti et al. (1992). Hormone therapy to prevent disease and prolong life in postmenopausal women. *Ann. Intern. Med.* 117:1016–1037.

Graham, J. (1967). Cardiac and pulmonary fibrosis during methysergide therapy for headache. *Am. J. Med. Sci.* 254:1–12.

Graham, J.R., H.I. Suby, P.R. LeCompte et al. (1966). Fibrotic disorders associated with methysergide therapy for headache. *N. Engl. J. Med.* 274:360–368.

Gray, R.N., R.E. Goslin, D.C. McCrory et al. (1999a). *Drug Treatments for the Prevention of Migraine Headache.* Technical Review 2.3, Agency for Health Care Policy and Research No. 290-94-2025, National Technical Information Service accession 127953.

Gray, R.N., D.C. McCrory, K. Eberlein et al. (1999b). *Drug Treatments for Acute Migraine Headache.* Agency for Health Care Policy and Research 290-94-2025, National Technical Information Service accession 127854.

Gray, R.N., D.C. McCrory, K. Eberlein et al. (1999c). *Parenteral Drug Treatments for Acute Migraine Headache.* Technical Review 2.5, Agency for Health Care Policy and Research 290-94-2025, National Technical Information Service accession 127862.

Gray, R.N., D.C. McCrory, K. Eberlein et al. (1995d). *Self-administered Drug Treatments for Acute Migraine Headache.* Technical Review 2.4, Agency for Health Care Policy and Research 290-94-2025, National Technical Information Service accession 127854.

Greenberg, D.A. (1997). Calcium channels in neurological disease. *Ann. Neurol.* 42:275–282.

Greenblatt, R.B. and D.W. Bruneteau (1974). Menopausal headache—psychogenic or metabolic? *J. Am. Geriatr. Soc.* 283:186–190.

Griffin, M.R., J.M. Piper, J.R. Daugherty et al. (1991). Nonsteroidal antiinflammatory drug use and increased risk for peptic ulcer disease in elderly persons. *Ann. Intern. Med.* 114:257–263.

Grotemeyer, K.H., H.W. Scharafinski, H.P. Schlake et al. (1990). Acetylsalicylic acid vs metoprolol in migraine prophylaxis: A double-blind crossover study. *Headache 30*:639–641.

Grotemeyer, K.H., H.P. Schlake, I.W. Husstedt et al. (1987). Metoprolol versus flunarizine: A double blind crossover study. *Cephalalgia 7*:465–466.

Gruffydd-Jones, K., C.A. Hood, and D.B. Price (1997). A within-patient comparision of subcutaneous and oral sumatriptan in the acute treatment of migraine in general practice. *Cephalalgia 17*:31–36.

Hachinski, V., J.W. Norris, J. Edmeads et al. (1978). Ergotamine and cerebral blood flow. *Stroke 9*:594–596.

Hachinski, V.C., J. Porchawka, and J.C. Steele (1973). Visual symptoms in the migraine syndrome. *Neurology 23*:570–579.

Hagen, I., B. Nesheim, and T. Tuntland (1985). No effect of vitamin B-6 against premenstrual tension: A controlled clinical study. *Acta Obstet. Gynecol. Scand. 64*:667–670.

Hakkarainen, H. and H. Allonen (1982). Ergotamine vs metoclopramide vs their combination in acute migraine attacks. *Headache 22*:10–12.

Hakkarainen, H., B. Gustafsson, and O. Stockman (1978). A comparative trial of ergotamine tartrate acetyl salicylic acid and dextropropoxyphene compound in acute migraine attacks. *Headache 18*:35–39.

Hakkarainen, H., J. Parantainen, G. Gothoni et al. (1982). Tolfenamic acid and caffeine: A useful combination in migraine. *Cephalalgia 2*:173–177.

Hakkarainen, H., H. Quiding, and O. Stockman (1980). Mild analgesics as an alternative to ergotamine in migraine. A comparative trail with acetylsalicylic acid, ergotamine tartrate, and dextropropoxyphene compound. *J. Clin. Pharmacol. 20*:590–595.

Hakkarainen, H., H. Vapaatalo, G. Gothoni et al. (1979). Tolfenamic acid is as effective as ergotamine during migraine attacks. *Lancet 2*:326–328.

Hammarback, S. and T. Backstrom (1988). Induced anovulation as a treatment of premenstrual tension syndrome: A double-blind crossover study with GnRH-agonist versus placebo. *Acta Obstet. Gynecol. Scand. 67*:159–166.

Hansen, S.L., L. Borelli-Miller, P. Strange et al. (1990). Opthalmoplegic migraine: Diagnostic criteria, incidence of hospitalization and possible etiology. *Acta Neurol. Scand. 81*:54–60.

Hansten, P.D. and J.R. Horn (1985). Drug interaction. *Newsletter 5*:7–10.

Hasselmark, L., R. Malingren, and J. Hanneiz (1987). Effect of carbohydrate-rich low in protein tryptophan in classic and common migraine. *Cephalalgia 7*:87–92.

Havanka-Kanniainen, H. (1989). Treatment of acute migraine attack: Ibuprofen and placebo compared. *Headache 29*:507–509.

Headache Classification Committee of the International Headache Society. (1988). Classification and diagnostic criteria for headache disorders, cranial neuralgia, and facial pain. *Cephalalgia 8*:1–96.

Hedman, C., A.R. Andersen, P.G. Andersson et al. (1988). Symptoms of classic migraine attacks: Modifications brought about by metoprolol. *Cephalalgia 8*:279–284.

Hemler, M., W.E. Lands, and W.L. Smith (1976). Purification of the cyclooxygenase that forms prostaglandins. Demonstration of two forms of iron in the holoenzyme. *J. Biol. Chem. 251*: 2629–2636.

Heninger, G.R. and D.S. Charney (1987). Mechanism of action of antidepressant treatments: Implications for the etiology and treatment of depressive disorders. In *Psychopharmacology: The Third Generation of Progress* (H.Y. Meltzer, ed.), pp. 535–544. Raven Press, New York.

Henry, P., J.F. Dartigues, M.P. Benetier et al. (1985). Ergotamine- and analgesic-induced headaches. In *Migraine. Proceedings of the 5th International Migraine Symposium, London* (C. Rose, ed.), pp. 197–205.

Heptinstall, S., W.A. Groenewegen, P. Spangenberg et al. (1987). Extracts of feverfew may inhibit platelet behavior via neutralization of sulphydryl groups. *J. Pharm. Pharmacol. 39*:459–465.

Heptinstall, S., A. White, L. Williamson et al. (1985). Extracts of feverfew inhibit granule secretion in blood platelets and polymorphonuclear leukocytes. *Lancet i*:1071–1074.

Hering, R. and A. Kuritzky (1992). Sodium valproate has a prophylactic effect in migraine: A double-blind study vs placebo. *Cephalalgia 12*: 81–84.

Herman, W.M., R. Horowski, K. Dannehl et al. (1977). Clinical effectiveness of lisuride hydrogen maleate: A double-blind trail versus methysergide. *Headache 17*:54–60.

Herzog, A.G. (1995). Continuous bromocriptine therapy in menstrual migraine [Abstract]. *Neurology 45*:465.

Hibbs, J.B., R.R. Taintor, Z. Vavrin et al. (1988). Nitric oxide: A cytotoxic activated macrophage effector molecule. *Biochem. Biophys. Res. Commun. 157*:87–94.

Hirt, D., X. Lataste, and P. Taylor (1989). A comparison of DHE nasal spray and cafergot in acute migraine. *Cephalalgia 9*:410–411.

Hoffert, M.J., M.J. Scholz, R. Kauter (1992). A double-blind controlled study of nifedipine as an abortive treatment in acute attacks of migraine with aura. *Cephalalgia 12*:323–324.

Holroyd, K.A., D.B. Penzien, and G.E. Coordingley (1991). Propranolol in the management of recurrent migraine: A meta-analytic review. *Headache 31*:333–340.

Hoshi, K., T. Ma, and I.K. Ho (1996). Precipitated kappa-opioid receptor agonist withdrawal increases glutamate in rat locus coeruleus. *Eur. J. Pharmacol.* 314:301–306.

Hosking, G. (1988). Special forms: Variants of migraine in childhood. In *Migraine in Childhood* (J.M. Hockaday, ed.), pp. 35–53. Butterworths, Boston.

Howell, R., D. Crook, D.K. Edmonds et al. (1995). Gondotrophin-releasing hormone analogue (goserelin) plus hormone replacement therapy for the treatment of endometriosis: A randomized control trial. *Fertil. Steril.* 64:474–481.

Hoyer, D., D.E. Clarke, J.R. Fozard et al. (1994). International Union of Pharmacology classification of receptors for 5-hydroxytryptamine (serotonin). *Pharmacol. Rev.* 46:157–203.

Hoyer, D. and G.R. Martin (1997). 5-HT receptor classification and nomenclature: Towards a harmonization with the human genome. *Neuropharmacology* 36:419–428.

Hudgson, P., J.B. Foster, and D.J. Newell (1967). Controlled trial of demigran in the prophylaxis of migraine. *BMJ* 2:91–93.

Humphrey, P.P., E. Apperley, W. Feniuk et al. (1990). A rational approach to identifying a fundamentally new drug for the treatment of migraine. In *Cardiovascular Pharmacology of 5-Hydroxytryptamine: Prospective Therapeutic Applications* (P.R. Saxena, D.I. Wallis, W. Wouters et al., eds.), pp. 416–431. Kluwer, Dordrecht.

Humphrey, P.P. and W. Feniuk (1991). Mode of action of the antimigraine drug sumatriptan. *Trends Pharmacol. Sci.* 12:444–446.

Humphrey, P.P., P. Hartig, and D. Hoyer (1993). A proposed new momenclature for 5-HT receptors. *Trends Pharmacol. Sci.* 14:233–238.

Hupp, S.L., L.B. Kline, and J.J. Corbett (1989). Visual disturbances of migraine. *Surv. Ophthalmol.* 33:221–236.

Hutchinson, M., J. O'Riordan, M. Javed et al. (1995). Familial hemiplegic migraine and autosomal dominant arteriopathy with leukoencephalopathy. *Ann. Neurol.* 38:817–824.

Isler, H. (1986). Frequency and time course of premonitory phenomena. In *The Prelude to the Migraine Attack* (W.K. Amery and A. Wauquier, eds.), pp. 44–53. Bailliere Tindall, London.

Jackson, N.C. (1996). A comparison of oral eletriptan (UK-116,044) (20–80 mg) and oral sumatriptan (100 mg) in the acute treatment of migraine, for the Eletriptan Steering Committee [Abstract]. *Cephalalgia* 16:368–369.

Jacobs, H. (1972). A trial of opipramol in the treatment of migraine. *J. Neurol. Neurosurg. Psychiatry* 35:500–504.

Jen, J., Q. Yue, S.F. Nelson et al. (1999). A novel nonsense mutation in CACNA1A causes episodic ataxia and hemiplegia. *Neurology* 53:34–37.

Jensen, K., P. Tfelt-Hansen, M. Lauritzen et al. (1986). Classic migraine, a prospective recording of symptoms. *Acta Neurol. Scand.* 73:359–362.

Jensen, R., T. Brinck, and J. Olesen (1994a). Sodium valproate has a prophylactic effect in migraine without aura. *Neurology* 44:647–651.

Jensen, R., T. Brinck, and J. Olesen (1994b). Sodium valproate has prophylactic effect in migraine without aura: A triple-blind, placebo-controlled crossover study. *Neurology* 44:241–244.

Jewett, D.L., G. Fein, and M.H. Greenberg (1990). A double-blind study of symptom provocation to determine food sensitivity. *N. Engl. J. Med.* 323:429–433.

Johannsson, V., L.R. Nilsson, T. Widelius et al. (1987). Atenolol in migraine prophylaxis: A double-blind crossover multicenter study. *Headache* 27:372–374.

Johnson, E.S., N.P. Kadam, D.M. Hylands et al. (1985a). Efficacy of feverfew as prophylactic treatment of migraine. *BMJ* 291:569–573.

Johnson, E.S., D.M. Ratcliffe, and M. Wilkinson (1985b). Naproxen sodium in the treatment of migraine. *Cephalalgia* 5:5–10.

Johnson, K.W., J.M. Schaus, M.M. Durkin et al. (1997). $5HT_{1F}$ receptor agonists inhibit neurogenic dural inflammation in guinea pigs. *Neuroreport* 8:2237–2240.

Johnson, R.H., R.W. Hornabrook, and D.G. Lambie (1986). Comparison of mefenamic acid and propranolol with placebo in migraine prophylaxis. *Acta Neurol. Scand.* 73:490–492.

Jones, E.B., E.R. Gonzales, J.G. Boggs et al. (1994). Safety and efficacy of rectal prochlorperazine for the treatment of migraine in the emergency department. *Ann. Emerg. Med.* 24:237–241.

Jones, J., S. Pack, and E. Chun (1996). Intramuscular prochlorperazine versus metoclopramide as single-agent therapy for the treatment of acute migraine headache. *Am. J. Emerg. Med.* 14:262–264.

Jones, J., D. Sklar, J. Dougherty et al. (1989). Randomized double-blind trial of intravenous prochlorperazine for the treatment of acute headache. *JAMA* 261:1174–1185.

Joutel, A., C. Corpechot, A. Ducros et al. (1996). Notch3 mutations in CADASIL, a hereditary adult-onset condition causing stroke and dementia. *Nature* 383:707–710.

Joutel, A., K. Vahedi, C. Corpechot et al. (1997). Strong clustering and sterotyped nature of Notch3 mutations in CADASIL patients. *Lancet* 350:1511–1515.

Judd, H. (1987). Efficacy of transdermal estradiol. *Obstet. Gynecol.* 156:1326–1331.

Kahn, R.S., O. Kalus, S. Wetzler et al. (1990). Effects of serotonin antagonists on *m*-chlorophenylpiperazine–mediated responses in normal subjects. *Psychiatry Res.* 33:189–198.

Kalkman, H.O. (1999). Minireview: Is migraine prophylactic activity caused by 5-HT$_{2B}$ or 5-HT$_{2C}$ receptor blockade? *Life Sci.* 54:641–644.

Kallanranta, T., H. Hakkarainen, E. Hokkanen et al. (1977). Clonidine in migraine prophylaxis. *Headache* 17:169–172.

Kangasniemi, P., A.R. Andersen, P.G. Andersson et al. (1987). Classic migraine: Effective prophylaxis with metoprolol. *Cephalalgia* 7:231–238.

Kangasniemi, P. and R. Kaaja (1992). Ketoprofen and ergotamine in acute migraine. *J. Intern. Med.* 231:551–554.

Kangasniemi, P.J., T. Nyrke, A.H. Lang et al. (1983). Femoxetine—a new 5HT uptake inhibitor—and propranolol in the prophylactic treatment of migraine. *Acta Neurol. Scand.* 68:262–267.

Kaniecki, R.G. (1997). A comparison of divalproex with propranolol and placebo for the prophylaxis of migraine without aura. *Arch. Neurol. 54:* 1141–1145.

Kanto, J., H. Allonen, and K. Koski (1981). Pharmacokinetics of dihydroergotamine in healthy volunteers and in neurological patients after a single intravenous injection. *Int. J. Clin. Pharmacol. Ther. Toxicol.* 19:127–130.

Kapicioglu, S., E. Gokce, Z. Kapicioglu et al. (1997). Treatment of migraine attacks with a long-acting somatostatin analogue (octreotide, SMS 201-995). *Cephalalgia* 17:27–30.

Kappius, R.E.K. and P. Goolkasian (1987). Group and menstrual phase effect in reported headaches among college students. *Headache* 27: 491–494.

Karachalios, G.N., A. Fotiadou, N. Chrisikos et al. (1992). Treatment of acute migraine attack with diclofenan sodium: A double-blind study. *Headache* 32:98–100.

Kass, B. and K. Nestvold (1980). Propranolol (Inderal) and clonidine (Catapressan) in the prophylactic treatment of migraine: A comparative trial. *Acta Neurol. Scand.* 61:351–356.

Kaufman, H.S. and D. Starr (1991). Prevention of red wine headache (RWH): A blind controlled study. In *Advances in Headache Research* (F.C. Rose, ed.), pp. 369–373. Smith Gordon, London.

Kelly, A.M., M. Ardagh, C. Curry et al. (1997). Intravenous chlorpromazine versus intramuscular sumatriptan for acute migraine. *J. Accid. Emerg. Med.* 14:209–211.

Kiesel, L., K.W. Schweppe, M. Sillem et al. (1996). Should add-back therapy for endometriosis be deferred for optimal results? *Br. J. Obstet. Gynaecol.* 103:15–17.

Kiiholma, P., R. Tuimala, S. Kivinen et al. (1995). Comparison of the gonadotrophin-releasing hormone agonist goserelin acetate along verus goserelin combined with estrogen-progestogen add-back therapy in the treatment of endometriosis. *Fertil. Steril.* 64:903–908.

Kimball, R.W., A.P. Friedman, and E. Vallejo (1960). Effect of serotonin in migraine patients. *Neurology* 10:107–111.

Kinnunen, E., T. Erkinjuntti, and M. Färkkilä (1988). Placebo controlled double-blind trial of pirprofen and an ergotamine tartrate compound in migraine attacks. *Cephalalgia* 8:175–179.

Kishore-Kumar, R., M.B. Max, S.C. Schafer et al. (1990). Desipramine relieves post-herpetic neuralgia. *Clin. Pharmacol. Ther.* 47:305–312.

Kjaersgaard-Rasmussen, M.J., B. Holt-Larsen, L. Borg et al. (1994). Tolfenamic acid versus propranolol in the prophylactic treatment of migraine. *Acta Neurol. Scand.* 89:446–450.

Klapper, J.A. (1994). An open label crossover comparison of divalproex sodium and propranolol HCl in the prevention of migraine headaches. *Headache Q.* 5:50–53.

Klapper, J.A. (1997). Divalproex sodium in migraine prophylaxis: A dose-controlled study. *Cephalalgia* 17:103–108.

Klapper, J.A. and J. Stanton (1993). Current emergency treatment of severe migraine headaches. *Headache* 33:560–562.

Klapper, J.A. and J.S. Stanton (1991a). Kertrolac versus DHE and metoclopramide in the treatment of migraine headaches. *Headache* 31:523–524.

Klapper, J.A. and J.S. Stanton (1991b). The emergency treatment of acute migraine headache: A comparison of intravenous dihydroergotamine, dexamethasone, and placebo. *Cephalalgia* 11: 159–160.

Kloster, R., K. Nestvold, and S.T. Vilming (1992). A double-blind study of ibuprofen versus placebo in the treatment of acute migraine attacks. *Cephalalgia* 12:169–171.

Koehler, S.M. and A. Glaros (1988). The effect of aspartame on migraine headache. *Headache* 28: 10–13.

Koella, W.P. (1985). CNS-related (side-)effects of β-blockers with special reference to mechanisms of action. *Eur. J. Clin. Pharmacol.* 28:55–63.

Kolesnikov, Y., C.G. Pick, and G.W. Pasternack (1992). N^G-Nitro-1-arginine prevents morphine tolerance. *Eur. J. Pharmacol.* 221:399–400.

Kozubski, W. (1992). Metamizole and hydrocortisone for the interruption of a migraine attack—preliminary study. *Headache Q.* 3:326–328.

Krause, K.H. and M.A. Bleicher (1985). Dihydroergotamine nasal spray in the treatment of migraine attacks. *Cephalalgia* 5:138–139.

Krebs, E.G. (1989). Role of the cyclic AMP–dependent protein kinase in signal transduction. *JAMA* 262:1815–1818.

Krebs, E.G. (1994). The growth of research on protein phosphorylation. *Trends. Biochem. Sci.* 19:439.

Krootila, K., O. Oksala, A. Zschauer et al. (1992). Inhibitory effect of methysergide on calcium gene–related peptide–induced vasodilatation and ocular irritative changes in the rabbit. *Br. J. Pharmacol.* 106:404–408.

Krusz, J.C. and J. Belanger (1999a). Propofol—a highly effective treatment for acute headaches [Abstract]. *Cephalalgia* 19:358.

Krusz, J.C., V. Scott, and J. Belanger (1999b). IV droperidol as a treatment for acute migraine headaches [Abstract]. *Cephalalgia* 19:356.

Kudrow, L. (1975). The relationship of headache frequency to hormone use in migraine. *Headache* 15:36–49.

Kudrow, L. (1982). Paradoxical effects of frequent analgesic use. *Adv. Neurol.* 33:335–341.

Kumar, K.L. and T.G. Cooney (1990). Visual symptoms after atenolol therapy for migraine. *Ann. Intern. Med.* 112:712–713.

Kunkle, E.C., S.R. Bronson, and H.G. Wolff (1942). Studies on headache: The mechanisms and significance of the headache associated with brain tumor. *Bull. N. Y. Acad. Med.* 18:400–422.

Kupersmith, M.J., W.K. Hass, and N.E. Chase (1987). Isoproterenol treatment of visual symptoms in migraine. *Stroke* 27:484–486.

Kuritzky, A. and R. Hering (1987). Prophylactic treatment of migraine with long acting propranolol: A comparison with placebo. *Cephalalgia* 7:457–458.

Kuritzky, A., K.E. Ziegler, and R. Hassanein (1981). Vertigo, motion sickness and migraine. *Headache* 21:227–231.

Ladecola, C. (1993). Regulation of the cerebral microcirculation during neural activity: Is nitric oxide the missing link? *Trends Pharmacol. Sci.* 16:206–214.

Lader, M. (1983). Combined use of tricyclic antidepressants and monoamine oxidase inhibitors. *J. Clin. Psychiatry* 44:20–24.

Lampl, C., A. Buzath, D. Klinger et al. (1999). Lamotrigine in the prophylactic treatment of migraine aura—a pilot study. *Cephalalgia* 19:58–63.

Lamsudin, R. and T. Sadjimin (1993). Comparison of the efficacy between flunarizine and nifedipine in the prophylaxis of migraine. *Headache* 33:335–338.

Lance, J.W. (1982). *Mechanisms and Management of Headache*. Butterworth Scientific, London.

Lance, J.W. (1986). The pharmacotherapy of migraine. *Med. J. Aust.* 144:85–88.

Lance, J.W. (1992). History of involvement of 5-HT in primary headaches. In *5-Hydroxytryptamine Mechanisms in Primary Headaches* (J. Olesen and P.R. Saxena, eds.), pp. 19–28. Raven Press, New York.

Lance, J.W. and M. Anthony (1966). Some clinical aspects of migraine. *Arch. Neurol.* 15:356–361.

Lance, J.W., R.D. Fine, and D.A. Curran (1963). An evaluation of methysergide in the prevention of migraine and other vascular headaches. *Med. J. Aust.* 1:814–818.

Lane, P.L., B.A. McLellan, and C.J. Boggoley (1989). Comparative efficacy of chlorpromazine and meperidine with dimenhydrinate in migraine headache. *Ann. Emerg. Med.* 18:360–365.

Lane, P.L. and R. Ross (1995). Intravenous chlorpromazine—preliminary results in acute migraine. *Headache* 25:302–304.

Langohr, H.D., W.D. Gerber, E. Koletzki et al. (1985). Clomipramine and metoprolol in migraine prophylaxis: A double-blind crossover study. *Headache* 25:107–113.

Larkin, G.L. and J.E. Prescott (1992). A randomized, double-blind, comparative study of the efficacy of ketorolac tromethamine versus meperidine in the treatment of severe migraine. *Ann. Emerg. Med.* 21:919–924.

LaRosa, J.C. (1995). Has HRT come of age? *Lancet* 345:76–77.

Larsen, B.H., L.V. Christiansen, B. Andersen et al. (1990). Randomized double-blind comparison of tolfenamic acid and paracetamol in migraine. *Acta Neurol. Scand.* 81:464–467.

Lassen, L.H., M. Ashina, I. Christiansen et al. (1997). Nitric oxide synthase inhibition in migraine. *Lancet* 349:401–402.

Lataste, X. (1989). Dihydroergotamine nasal spray. In *Migraine and Other Headaches* (M.D. Ferrari and X. Lataste, eds.), pp. 249–260. Parthenon, Park Ridge, NJ.

Lauritzen, M. (1986). Spreading cortical depression as a mechanism of the aura in classic migraine. In *The Prelude to the Migraine Attack* (W.K. Amery and A. Wauquier, eds.), pp. 134–141. Bailliere Tindall, London.

Leandri, M., S. Rigardo, R. Schizzi et al. (1990). Migraine treatment with nicardipine. *Cephalalgia* 10:111–116.

Leao, A.A.P. (1944). Spreading depression of activity in cerebral cortex. *J. Neurophysiol.* 7:359–390.

Leather, A.T., J.W.W. Studd, N.R. Watson et al. (1993). The prevention of bone loss in young treated with GnRH analogues with add-back estrogen therapy. *Obstet. Gynecol.* 81:104–107.

Lemay, A. and N. Faure (1994). Sequential estrogen–progestin addition to gonadotrophin-releasing hormone agonist suppression for the chronic treatment of ovarian hyperandrogenism: A pilot study. *J. Clin. Endocrinol. Metab.* 79:1716–1722.

Levy, D.E. (1988). Transient CNS deficits: A common, benign sydrome in young adults. *Neurology* 38:831–836.

Limmroth, V., D. Wermelskirchen, F. Tegtmeier et al. (1997). Alniditan blocks neurogenic edema by activation of $5HT_{1B/1D}$ receptors in anesthetized rats more effectively than sumatriptan. *Cephalalgia* 17:402.

Lipton, R.B., J.G. Baggish, W.F. Stewart et al. (2000a). Efficacy and safety of acetaminophen in the non-prescription treatment of migraine. *Arch. Intern. Med.* 160:3486–3492.

Lipton, R.B., R.K. Cady, S. O'Quinn et al. (1999). Sumatriptan treats the full spectrum of headache in individuals with disabling IHS migraine [Abstract]. *Neurology* 52:A256.

Lipton, R.B. and S.D. Silberstein (1994). Why study the comorbidity of migraine? *Neurology* 44:4–5.

Lipton, R.B., W.F. Stewart, R.E. Ryan et al. (1998). Efficacy and safety of the nonprescription combination of acetaminophen, aspirin, and caffeine in alleviating headache pain of an acute migraine attack: Three double-blind, randomized, placebo-controlled trials. *Arch. Neurol.* 55:210–217.

Lipton, R.B., W.F. Stewart, A.M. Stone et al. (2000). Stratified care vs. step care strategies for migraine. The disability in strategies of care (DISC) study a randomized trial. *JAMA* 284:2499–2505.

Littlewood, J.T., C. Gibb, V. Glover et al. (1987). Red wine as a migraine trigger. In *Advances in Headache Research*,(F.C. Rose, ed.), pp. 123–127. John Libbey, London.

Littlewood, J.T., V. Glover, P.T. Davies et al. (1988). Red wine as a cause of migraine. *Lancet* i:558–559.

Longmore, J., D. Shaw, D. Smith et al. (1997). Differential distribution of 5HT(1D)- and 5HT(1B)-immunoreactivity within the human trigeminocerebrovascular system: Implications for the discovery of new antimigraine drugs. *Cephalalgia* 17:833–842.

Louis, P. (1981). A double-blind placebo-controlled prophylactic study of flunarizine (Sibelium) in migraine. *Headache* 21:235–239.

Louis, P., J. Schoenen, and C. Hedman (1985). Metoprolol vs clonidine in the prophylactic treatment of migraine. *Cephalalgia* 5:159–165.

Louis, P. and E.L. Spierings (1982). Comparison of flunarizine (Sibelium) and pizotifen (Sandomigran) in migraine treatment: A double-blind study. *Cephalalgia* 2:197–203.

Luciani, R., D. Carter, L. Mannix et al. (2000). Prevention of migraine during prodrome with naratriptan. *Cephalalgia* 20:122–126.

Lucking, C.H., W. Oestreich, R. Schmidt et al. (1988). Flunarizine vs propranolol in the prophylaxis of migraine: Two double-blind comparative studies in more than 400 patients. *Cephalalgia* 8:21–26.

Ludin, H.P. (1989). Flunarizine and propranolol in the treatment of migraine. *Headache* 29:219–224.

Lundberg, P.O. (1986). Endocrine headaches. In *Handbook of Clinical Neurology* (F.C. Rose, ed.), pp. 431–440. Elsevier, New York.

MacDonald, A., I. Forsythe, and C. Wall (1989). Dietary treatment of migraine. In *Headache in Children and Adolescents* (G. Lanzi, U. Balottin, and A. Cernibori, eds.), pp. 333–338. Elsevier, New York.

MacDonald, R.L. and M.J. McLean (1986). Anticonvulsant drugs: Mechanisms of action. In *Advances in Neurology* (A.D. Escueta, A.A. Ward, D.M. Woodbury et al., eds.), pp. 713–736. Raven Press, New York.

MacLennan, S.J. and G.R. Martin (1990). Comparison of the effects of methysergide and methylergometrine with GR 43175 on feline carotid blood flow distribution. *Br. J. Pharmacol.* 99:221.

Magos, A.L., M. Brincat, and J.W.W. Studd (1986). Treatment of the premenstrual syndrome by subcutaneous estradiol implants and cyclical oral noresthisterone: Placebo controlled study. *Br. Med. J. Clin. Res.* 292:1629–1633.

Maheux, R. and A. Lemay (1992). Treatment of perimenopausal women: Potential long-term therapy with a depot GnRH agonist combined with hormone replacement therapy. *Br. J. Obstet. Gynecol.* 99:13–17.

Maheux, R., A. Lemay, P. Blanchet et al. (1991). Maintained reduction of uterine leiomyoma following addition of hormonal replacement therapy to a monthly luteinizing hormone-releasing hormone agonist implant: A pilot study. *Hum. Reprod.* 6:500–505.

Maizels, M., B. Scott, W. Cohen et al. (1996). Intranasal lidocaine for treatment of migraine: A randomized, double-blind, controlled trial. *JAMA* 276:319–321.

Mamounas, L.A., M.A. Wilson, K.J. Axt et al. (1992). Morphological aspects of serotonergic innervation. In *Serotonin, CNS Receptors and Brain Function* (P.B. Bradley, S.L. Handley, S.J. Cooper et al., eds.), pp. 97–118. Pergamon Press, New York.

Manzoni, G., S. Farina, M. Lanfranchi et al. (1985). Classic migraine—clinical findings in 164 patients. *Eur. Neurol.* 24:163–169.

Marcus, D.A., L. Scharff, D. Turk et al. (1997). A double-blind provocative study of chocolate as a trigger of headache. *Cephalalgia* 17:855–862.

Mark, A.S., J. Casselman, D. Brown et al. (1998). Ophthalmoplegic migraine: Reversible enhancement and thickening of the cisternal segment of the oculomotor nerve on contrast-enhanced MR images. *Am. J. Neuroradiol.* 19:1887–1891.

Markley, H.G., J.C.D. Cleronis, and R.W. Piepko (1984). Verapamil prophylactic therapy of migraine. *Neurology* 34:973–976.

Markley, H.G., P.A. Gasser, M.E. Markley et al. (1991). Fluoxetine in prophylaxis of migraine: Clinical experience. *Cephalalgia* 11:164–165.

Martucci, N., V. Manna, P. Mattesi et al. (1983). Ergot derivatives in the prophylaxis of migraine: A multicentric study with a timed-release dihydroergotamine formulation. *Cephalalgia* 3: 151–155.

Masel, B.E., A.L. Chesson, B.H. Peters et al. (1980). Platelet antagonists in migraine prophylaxis: A clinical trial using aspirin and dipyridamole. *Headache* 20:13–18.

Massiou, H. (1987). Dihydroergotamine nasal spray in prevention and treatment of migraine attacks: Two controlled trials versus placebo. *Cephalalgia* 7:440–441.

Massiou, H., C. Tzourio, and M.G. Bousser (1997). Methodology of treatment trials for migraine prophylaxis. In *Headache Treatment. Trial Methodology and New Treatment* (J. Olesen and P. Tfelf-Hansen, eds.), pp. 125–133. Lippincott-Raven, Philadelphia.

Mastrosimone, F. and C. Iaccarino (1987). Progress in migraine: Treatment with dihydroergotamine-retard. *Cephalalgia* 7:168–170.

Masyczek, R. and C.S. Pugh (1983). The "red wine" reaction. *Ann. J. Enol. Vitic.* 34:260–264.

Mathew, N., J. Saper, and L. Magnus-Miller (1998). Efficacy and safety of gabapentin (Neurontin®) in migraine prophylaxis [abstract]. In *17th Annual Meeting of the American Pain Society Program*, San Diego, CA.

Mathew, N.T. (1981). Prophylaxis of migraine and mixed headache. A randomized controlled study. *Headache* 21:105–109.

Mathew, N.T. (1990). Drug induced headache. *Neurol. Clin.* 8:903–912.

Mathew, N.T. (1996). Gabapentin in migraine prophylaxis. *Cephalalgia* 16:367

Mathew, N.T., J. Kailasam, L. Meadors et al. (1999a). Intravenous valproate sodium (Depacon®) aborts migraine rapidly: A preliminary report [abstract]. *Cephalalgia* 19:373.

Mathew, N.T., J.R. Saper, S.D. Silberstein et al. (1995a). Migraine prophylaxis with divalproex. *Arch. Neurol.* 52:281–286.

Mathew, N.T., J.R. Saper, S.D. Silberstein et al. (1995b). Prophylaxis of migraine headaches with divalproex sodium. *Arch. Neurol.* 52:281–286.

Mattsson, P. and P.O. Lundberg (1999). Characteristics and prevalence of transient visual disturbances indicative of migraine visual aura. *Cephalalgia* 19:479–484.

May, M. (1986). Idiopathic (Bell's) palsy, herpes zoster and other facial nerve disorders of viral origin. In *The Facial Nerve* (M. May, ed.), pp. 365–399. Thieme Medical, New York.

McAllister, G., A. Charlesworth, C. Snodin et al. (1992). Molecular cloning of a serotonin receptor from human brain (5HT1E): A fifth 5HT1-like subtype. *Neurobiology* 89:5517–5521.

McArthur, J.C., K. Marek, A. Pestronk et al. (1989). Nifedipine in the prophylaxis of classic migraine: A crossover, double-masked, placebo-controlled study of headache frequency and side effects. *Neurology* 39:284–286.

McCall, R.B. (1999). Preclinical and clinical studies in migraine using the selective $5HT_{1D}$ receptor agonist PNU-142633. In *IBC Third Annual Conference on Migraine: Novel Drug and Therapeutic Development Program, Philadelphia, May 20, 1999*.

McCormack, K. (1994). Nonsteroidal antiinflammatory drugs and spinal nociceptive processing. *Pain* 59:9–43.

McCrory, D.C., R.E. Goslin, and R.N. Gray (1998). *Evidence Report: Butalbital-containing compounds for the Treatment of Tension-Type and Migraine Headache*. Duke University Center for Health Policy Research, Raleigh, NC.

McCroy, D., D.B. Matchar, J.H. Rosenberg et al. (1999). Evidenced-based guidelines for migraine hadache: overview of program description and methodology, Neurology [serial on line]. Available at http://www.neurology.org. Accessed April 25, 2000.

McDaris, H.L. and J. Hutchison (1999). A review of overall clinical efficacy [abstract]. *Cephalalgia* 19:363–364.

McEwen, J.I., H.M. O'Connor, and H.B. Dinsdale (1987). Treatment of migraine with intramuscular chlorpromazine. *Ann. Emerg. Med.* 16: 758–763.

McQuay, H.J., D. Carroll, P.G. Watts et al. (1999). Codeine 20mg increases relief from ibuprofen 400mg after third molar surgery. Repeat dose comparison in an ibuprofen-codeine combination. *Pain* 37:7–13.

McQueen, J., R.H. Loblay, A.R. Savain et al. (1989). A controlled trial of dietary modification in migraine. In *New Advances in Headache Research* (F.C. Rose, ed.), pp. 235–242. Smith Gordon, London.

Medical Economics Company. (1999). *Physicians' Desk Reference*. Medical Economics Company, Montvale, NJ.

Medina, J.L. and S. Diamond (1978). The role of diet in migraine. *Headache* 18:31–34.

Medina, J.L. (1982). Cyclic migraine: A disorder responsive to lithium carbonate. *Psychosomatics* 23:625–637.

Medina, J.L. and S. Diamond (1977). The clinical link between migraine and cluster headaches. *Arch. Neurol.* 34:470–472.

Mendenopoulos, G., T. Manafi, I. Logothetis et al. (1985). Flunarizine in the prevention of classical migraine: A placebo-controlled evaluation. *Cephalalgia* 5:31–37.

Micieli, G., A. Cavallini, E. Martignoni et al. (1988). Effectiveness of salmon calcitonin nasal spray preparation in migraine treatment. *Headache* 28:196–200.

Migraine-Nimodipine European Study Group (MINES). (1989). European multicenter trial of nimodipine in the prophylaxis of common migraine (migraine without aura). *Headache* 29: 633–638.

Miguel, M.D. and M. Hamon (1992). 5-HT$_1$ receptor subtypes: Pharmacological heterogeneity. In *Serotonin Receptor Subtypes: Pharmacological Significance and Clinical Implications* (S.Z. Langer, N. Brunello, G. Racagni et al., eds.), pp. 13–30, Karger, Basel.

Mikkelsen, B., K.K. Pedersen, and L.V. Christiansen (1986). Prophylactic treatment of migraine with tolfenamic acid, propranolol, and placebo. *Acta Neurol. Scand.* 73:423–427.

Mikkelsen, B.M. and J.V. Falk (1982). Prophylactic treatment of migraine with tolfenamic acid: A comparative double-blind crossover study betwen tolfenamic acid and placebo. *Acta Neurol. Scand.* 66:105–111.

Mikoshiba, K. (1993). Inositol 1,4,5-triphosphate receptor. *Trends Pharmacol. Sci.* 14:86–89.

Miller, F.W. and T.J. Santoro (1985). Nifedipine in the treatment of migraine headache and amaurosis fugax in patients with systemic lupus erythematosus. *N. Engl. J. Med.* 311:921.

Minervini, M.G. and K. Pinto (1987). Catopril relieves pain and improves mood depression in depressed patients with classical migraine. *Cephalalgia* 7:485–486.

Mishell, D.R., M.A. Stenchever, W. Droegemueller et al. (1997). Menopause: Endocrinology, consequences of estrogen deficiency, effects of hormonal replacement therapy, treatment regimens. In *Comprehensive Gynecology* (D.R. Mishell, M.A. Stenchever, W. Droegemueller et al., eds.), pp. 1159–1198. Mosby, St. Louis.

Moffett, A.M., M. Swash, and D.F. Scott (1974). Effect of chocolate: A double-blind study. *J. Neurol. Neurosurg. Psychiatry* 37:445–448.

Moghissi, K.S. (1996). Add-back therapy in the treatment of endometriosis: The North America experience. *Br. J. Obstet. Gynaecol.* 103:14.

Mondrup, K. and C.E. Moller (1977). Prophylactic treatment of migraine with clonidine: A controlled clinical trial. *Acta Neurol. Scand.* 56: 405–412.

Monro, P., C. Swade, and A. Coppen (1985). Mianserin in the prophylaxis of migraine: A double-blind study. *Acta Psychiatr. Scand.* 72: 98–103.

Monsma, F.J., Y. Shen, R.P. Ward et al. (1992). Cloning and expression of a novel serotonin receptor with high affinity for tricyclic psychotropic drugs. *Mol. Pharmacol.* 43:320–327.

Montagna, P., P. Cortelli, L. Monari et al. (1994). ^{31}P-Magnetic resonance spectroscopy in migraine without aura. *Neurology* 44:666–669.

Morrison, B.W., S. Christensen, W. Yuan et al. (1999). Analgesic efficacy of the cyclooxygenase-2-specific inhibitor rofecoxib in postdental surgery pain: A randomized, controlled trial. *Clin. Ther.* 21:943–953.

Moskowitz, M.A. (1990). Basic mechanisms in vascular headache. *Neurol. Clin.* 8:801–815.

Moskowitz, M.A. (1992a). Interpreting vessel diameter changes in vascular headaches. *Cephalalgia* 12:5–7.

Moskowitz, M.A. (1992b). Neurogenic versus vascular mechanisms of sumatriptan and ergot alkaloids in migraine. *Trends Pharmacol. Sci.* 13: 307–311.

Mosniam, A., F.G. Freitag, R. Ignacio et al. (1996). Apparent lack of correlation between tyramine and phenylethylamines content and the occurrence of food precipitated migraine. *Headache Q.* 7:239–249.

Mueller, E.A., D.L. Murphy, and T. Sunderland (1986). Further studies of the putative serotonin agonist, *m*-chlorophenylpiperazine: Evidence for a serotonin receptor mediated mechanism of action in humans. *Psychopharmacology* 89: 388–391.

Muller, S.E. (1986). Serotonergic receptors in brain vessels. In *Neural Regulation of Brain Circulation* (C. Owman and J.E. Hardebo, eds.), pp. 219–234. Elsevier, Amsterdam.

Muller, S.E. (1992). Ergot alkaloids in migraine: Is the effect via 5-HT receptors. In *5-Hydroxytryptamine Mechanisms in Primary Headaches* (J. Olesen and P.R. Saxena, eds.), pp. 297–304. Raven Press, New York.

Muller-Schweinitzer, E. (1984). Pharmacological actions of the main metabolites of dihydroergotamine. *Eur J. Clin. Pharmacol.* 26:699–705.

Multinational Oral Sumatriptan and Cafergot Comparative Study Group. (1991). A randomized, double-blind comparison of sumatriptan and cafergot in the acute treatment of migraine. *Eur. Neurol.* 31:314–322.

Murphy, J.J., S. Heptinstall, and J.R. Mitchell (1988). Randomized double-blind placebo controlled trial of feverfew in migraine prevention. *Lancet* 2:189–192.

Murray, S.C. and K.N. Muse (1997). Effective treatment of severe menstrual migraine headaches with gonadotropin-releasing hormone agonist and "add-back" therapy [abstract]. *Fertil. Steril.* 67:390–393.

Murray, W.J. (1964). Evaluation of aspirin in treatment of headache. *Clin. Pharmacol. Ther.* 5:21–25.

Muse, K.N., N.S. Cetel, L.A. Fitterman et al. (1984). The premenstrual syndrome: Effects of "medical ovariectomy." *N. Engl. J. Med. 311*: 1345–1349.

Myllyla, V.V., H. Havanka, L. Herrala et al. (1998). Tolfenamic acid rapid release versus sumatriptan in the acute treatment of migraine: Comparable effect in a double-blind, randomized, controlled, parallel-group study. *Headache 38*: 201–207.

Nagamani, M., M.E. Kelver, and E.R. Smith (1987). Treatment of menopausal hot flashes with transdermal administration of clonidine. *Am. J. Obstet. Gynecol. 156*:561–565.

Nanda, R.N., R.H. Johnson, J. Gray et al. (1978). A double-blind trial of acebutolol for migraine prophylaxis. *Headache 18*:379–381.

Nappi, G., G. Micieli, C. Tassorelli et al. (1993). Effectiveness of a piroxicam fast dissolving formulation sublingually administered in the symptomatic treatment of migraine without aura. *Headache 33*:296–300.

Nappi, G., F. Sicuteri, M. Byrne et al. (1994). Oral sumatriptan compared with placebo in the acute treatment of migraine. *J. Neurol. 241*:138–144.

Nattero, G., I. Savi, G. Cadario et al. (1991). Food and headache: Adverse reaction or psychic suggestion? In *New Advances in Headache Research* (F.C. Rose, ed.), pp. 199–203. Smith Gordon, London.

Nelson, D.L. (1996). *Proceedings from the International Business Communications conference on serotonin receptors in the central nervous system, Philadelphia, January 25–26, 1996.*

Nelson, J.A., M.D. Wolfe, W.T. Yuh et al. (1992). Cranial nerve involvement with Lyme borreliosis demonstrated by magnetic resonance imaging. *Neurology 42*:671–673.

Neri, I., F. Granella, R.M.G.C. Nappi et al. (1993). Characteristics of headache at menopause: A clinico-epidemiologic study. *Maturitas 17*:31–37.

Newman, L.C., R.B. Lipton, C.L. Lay et al. (1998). A pilot study of oral sumatriptan as intermittent prophylaxis of menstruation-related migraine. *Neurology 51*:307–309.

Nishizuka, Y. (1989). The family of protein kinase C for signal transduction. *JAMA 262*:1833.

Noone, J.F. (1980). Clomipramine in the prevention of migraine. *J. Int. Med. Res. 8*:49–52.

O'Connor, P.S. and T.J. Tredici (1981). Acephalgic migraine: Fifteen years experience. *Ophthalmology 88*:999–1003.

O'Dea, P.K. and E.H. Davis (1990). Tamoxifen in the treatment of menstrual migraine. *Neurology 40*:1471.

Ogden, H.D. (1963). Controlled studies of a new agent in vascular headache. *Headache 3*:29–31.

Olerud, B., C.L. Gustavsson, and B. Furberg (1986). Nadolol and propranolol in migraine management. *Headache 26*:490–493.

Olesen, J. (1978). Some clinical features of the acute migraine attack. An analysis of 750 patients. *Headache 18*:268–271.

Olesen, J. (1984). The significance of trigger factors in migraine. In *Progress in Migraine Research* (F.C. Rose, ed.), pp. 21–22. Pitman, London.

Olesen, J., A. Aebelholt, and B. Veilis (1979). The Copenhagen Acute Headache Clinic: Organization, patient material and treatment results. *Headache 19*:223–227.

Olesen, J. and L. Edvinsson (1988). *Basic Mechanisms of Headache.* Elsevier, New York.

Olsson, J.E., H.C. Behring, B. Forssman et al. (1984). Metoprolol and propranolol in migraine prophylaxis: A double-blind multicenter study. *Acta Neurol. Scand. 70*:160–180.

O'Neill, B.P. and J.D. Mann (1979). Aspirin prophylaxis in migraine. *Lancet 2*:1179–1181.

Ophoff, R.A., G.M. Terwindt, and M.N. Vergouwe (1996). Familial hemiplegic migraine and episodic ataxia type-2 are caused by mutations in the Ca^{2+} channel gene *CACNLA4*. *Cell Tissue Res. 87*:543–552.

Oral Sumatriptan and Aspirin-plus-Metoclopramide Comparative Study Group. (1992). A study to compare oral sumatriptan with oral aspirin plus oral metoclopramide in the acute treatment of migraine. *Eur. Neurol. 32*:177–184.

Oral Sumatriptan Dose-Defining Study Group. (1991). Sumatriptan—an oral dose-defining study. *Eur. Neurol. 31*:300–305.

Oral Sumatriptan International Multiple-Dose Study Group. (1991). Evaluation of a multiple-dose regimen of oral sumatriptan for the acute treatment of migraine. *Eur. Neurol. 31*:306–313.

Orholm, M., P.F. Honor, and I. Zeeberg (1986). A randomized general practice group-comparative study of femoxetine and placebo in the prophylaxis of migraine. *Acta Neurol. Scand. 74*:235–239.

Ostfeld, A.M. (1961). A study of migraine pharmacotherapy. *Am. J. Med. Sci. 241*:192–198.

Pachner, A.R., P. Duray, and A.C. Steere (1989). Central nervous system manifestations of Lyme disease. *Arch. Neurol. 46*:790–795.

Packard, R.C. (1979). What does the headache patient want? *Headache 19*:370–374.

Paiva, T., P. Esperanca, L. Marcelino et al. (1985). A double-blind trial with dihydroergotamine nasal spray in migraine crisis. *Cephalalgia 5*:140–141.

Palacios, J.M., C. Waeber, G. Mengod et al. (1991). Molecular neuroanatomy of 5-HT receptors. In *Serotonin—Molecular Biology, Receptors and Functional Effects* (J.R. Fozard and P.R. Saxena, eds.), pp. 5–20. Birkhauser, Basel.

Palevitch, D., G. Earon, and R. Carusso (1997). Feverfew (*Tanacetum parthenium*) as a prophylactic treatment for migraine: A double-blind placebo-controlled study. *Phytother. Res. 11*: 508–511.

Panerai, A.E., G. Monza, P. Movilia et al. (1990). A randomized, within-patient, cross-over, placebo-controlled trial on the efficacy and tolerability of the tricyclic antidepressants chlorimipramine and nortriptyline in central pain. *Acta Neurol. Scand.* 82:34–38.

Pare, C.M., N. Kline, C. Hallstrom et al. (1982). Will amitriptyline prevent the "cheese" reaction of monoamine-oxidase inhibitors? *Lancet* 9: 183–186.

Pasternak, G.W. (1993). Review: Pharmacological mechanisms of opioid analgesics. *Clin. Neuropharmacol.* 16:1–18.

Patti, F., U. Scapagnini, F. Nicoletti et al. (1987). A short-term trial of an analogue of eel-calcitonin in headache. *Headache* 27:334–339.

Pearce, I., G.J. Frank, and J.M. Pearce (1983). Ibuprofen compared with paracetamol in migraine. *Practitioner* 227:465–467.

Pearce, J.M.S. (1984). Migraine: A cerebral disorder. *Lancet* ii:86–89.

Peatfield, R. (1986). Drugs acting by modification of serotonin function. *Headache* 26:129–131.

Pedersen, E. and C.E. Moller (1966). Methysergide in migraine prophylaxis. *Pharmacol. Ther.* 7:520–526.

Peikert, A., C. Wilimzig, and R. Kohne-Volland (1996). Prophylaxis of migraine with oral magnesium: Results from a prospective, multicenter, placebo-controlled and double-blind randomized study. *Cephalalgia* 16:257–263.

Pellock, J.M. and L.J. Willmore (1991). A rational guide to routine blood monitoring in patients receiving antiepileptic drugs. *Neurology* 41: 961–964.

Penn, A.M., J.W. Lee, P. Thuillier et al. (1992). MELAS syndrome with mitochondrial tRNA$^{LEU(UUR)}$ mutation: Correlation of clinical state, nerve conduction, and muscle^{31}P magnetic resonance spectroscopy during treatment with nicotinamide and riboflavin. *Neurology* 42: 2147–2152.

Peroutka, S.J. (1990a). Developments in 5-hydroxytryptamine receptor pharmacology in migraine. *Neurol. Clin.* 8:829–838.

Peroutka, S.J. (1990b). The pharmacology of current antimigraine drugs. *Headache* 30:12.

Peroutka, S.J. (1993). 5-Hydroxytryptamine receptors. International Society for Neurochemistry. *J. Neurochem.* 60:408–416.

Peroutka, S.J. and S.H. Snyder (1979). Multiple serotonin receptors: Differential binding of ^{3}H-5-hydroxytryptamine, ^{3}H-lysergic acid diethylamide and 3H-spiroperidol. *Mol. Pharmacol.* 16:687–689.

Peto, R., R. Gray, R. Collins et al. (1988). Randomized trial of prophylactic daily aspirin in British male doctors. *BMJ* 296:313–316.

Pfaffenrath, V., G. Cunin, G. Sjonell et al. (1998). Efficacy and safety of sumatriptan tablets (25mg, 50mg, and 100mg) in the acute treatment of migraine: Defining the optimum doses of oral sumatriptan. *Headache* 38:184–190.

Pfaffenrath, V., W. Oestreich, and W. Haase (1990). Flunarizine (10 and 20mg) i.v. versus placebo in the treatment of acute migraine attacks: A multicenter double-blind study. *Cephalalgia* 10:77–81.

Pfaffenrath, V., P. Wessely, C. Meyer et al. (1996). Magnesium in the prophylaxis of migraine—a double-blind, placebo-controlled study. *Cephalalgia* 16:436–440.

Pfeiffer, A., V. Brantl, A. Herz et al. (1986). Psychotomimesis mediated by κ opiate receptors. *Science* 233:774–776.

Pickersgill, A. (1998). GnRH agonists and add-back therapy: Is there a perfect combination? *Br. J. Obstet. Gynaecol.* 105:475–485.

Pies, R. (1983). Trazodone and intractable headaches. *J. Clin. Psychiatry* 44:317.

Pigott, T.A., J. Zohar, J.L. Hill et al. (1991). Metergoline blocks the behavioral and neuroendocrine effects of orally administered *m*-chlorophenylpiperazine in patients with obsessive-compulsive disorder. *Biol. Psychiatry* 29:418–426.

Pini, L.A., A. Ferrari, G. Guidetti et al. (1985). Influence of flunarizine on the altered electronystagmographic (ENG) recordings in migraine. *Cephalalgia* 5:173–175.

Pini, L.A., E. Sternieri, L. Fabbri et al. (1995). High efficacy and low frequency of headache recurrence after oral sumatriptan. The Oral Sumatriptan Italian Study Group. *J. Int. Med. Res.* 23:96–105.

Piros, E.T., T.G. Hales, and C.J. Evans (1996). Functional analysis of cloned opioid receptors in transfected cell lines. *Neurochem. Res.* 21: 1277–1285.

Pita, E., A. Higueras, J. Bolanos et al. (1977). Propranolol and migraine: A clinical trial. *Arch. Farmacol. Toxicol.* 3:273–278.

Podell, R.N. (1984). Is migraine a manifestation of food allergy? *Postgrad. Med.* 75:221–224.

Portenoy, R.K., K.M. Foley, and C.E. Inturrisi (1990). The nature of opioid responsiveness and its implications for neuropathic pain: New hypotheses derived from studies of opioid infusions. *Pain* 43:273–286.

Poser, C.M. (1974). Papaverine in prophylactic treatment of migraine. *Lancet* i:1290.

Potter, D.L., D.E. Hart, C.S. Calder et al. (2000). A double-blind, randomized, placebo-controlled, parallel study to determine the efficacy of Topamax® (topiramate) in the prophylactic treatment of migraine [abstract]. *Neurology* 52(7, Suppl. 3):A15.

Powles, T.J. (1986). Prevention of migrainous headaches by tamoxifen. *Lancet* ii:1344.

Pradalier, A., A. Clapin, and J. Dry (1988). Treatment review: Nonsteroid antiinflammatory drugs in the treatment and long-term prevention of migraine attacks. *Headache* 28:550–557.

Pradalier, A., G. Rancurel, G. Dordain et al. (1985). Acute migraine attack therapy: Comparison of naproxen sodium and an ergotamine tartrate compound. *Cephalalgia* 5:107–113.

Pradalier, A., G. Serratrice, M. Colard et al. (1989). Long-acting propranolol on migraine prophylaxis: Results of a double-blind, placebo-controlled study. *Cephalalgia* 9:247–253.

Pradalier, A., D. Vincent, P.H. Beaulieu et al. (1994). Correlation between estradiol plasma level and therapeutic effect on menstrual migraine. In *New Advances in Headache Research* (F.C. Rose, ed.), pp. 129–132. Smith-Gordon, London.

Prendes, J.L. (1980). Consideration on use of propranolol in complicated migraine. *Headache* 20: 93–95.

Prensky, A.L. (1987). Migraine in children. In *Migraine: Clinical and Research Aspects* (J.N. Blau, ed.), pp. 31–53. Johns Hopkins University Press, Baltimore.

Presthus, J. (1971). BC105 and methysergide (Deseril) in migraine prophylaxis. *Acta Neurol. Scand.* 47:514–518.

Price, W.A. and A.J. Giannini (1986). Neurotoxicity caused by lithium–verapamil synergism. *J. Clin. Pharmacol.* 26:717–719.

Price, W.A. and J.E. Shalley (1987). Lithium–verapamil toxicity in the elderly. *J. Am. Geriatr. Soc.* 35:177–179.

Pryse-Phillips, W. (1999). Comparison of oral eletriptan (40–80mg) and oral sumatriptan (50–100mg) for the treatment of acute migraine: A randomized, placebo-controlled trial in sumatriptan-naive patients [abstract]. *Cephalalgia* 19:355.

Rabkin, R., D.P. Stables, N.W. Levin et al. (1966). The prophylactic value of propranolol in angina pectoris. *Am. J. Cardiol.* 18:370–383.

Rapoport, A. (1998). The dose range characteristics of frovatriptan (VML251) a potent cerebroselective 5-hydroxytryptamine (5-HT$_{1B/1D}$ agonist in the acute treatment of migraine [abstract]. *Cephalalgia* 18:384.

Rapoport, A.M. (1992). The diagnosis of migraine and tension-type headache, then and now. *Neurology* 42:11–15.

Rapoport, A.M., F.D. Sheftell, and B. Gordon (1989). The successful treatment of migraine with anticonvulsant medication in patients with abnormal EEGs. *Headache* 29:309.

Rapoport, A.M., W.H. Visser, N.R. Cutler et al. (1995). Oral sumatriptan in preventing headache recurrence after treatment of migraine attacks with subcutaneous sumatriptan. *Neurology* 45:1505–1509.

Rapoport, A.M. and R.E. Weeks (1988). Characteristics and treatment of analgesic rebound headache. In *Drug-induced Headache* (H.C. Diener and M. Wilkinson, eds.), pp. 162–167. Springer-Verlag, Berlin.

Rascol, A., J.L. Montastruc, and O. Rascol (1986). Flunarizine versus pizotifen: A double-blind study in the prophylaxis of migraine. *Headache* 26:83–85.

Raskin, N.H. (1981). Chemical headaches. *Annu. Rev. Med.* 32:63–71.

Raskin, N.H. (1986). Repetitive intravenous dihydroergotamine as therapy for intractable migraine. *Neurology* 36:995–997.

Raskin, N.H. (1988). Migraine treatment. In *Headache* (N.H. Raskin, ed.), pp. 229–230. Churchill-Livingstone, New York.

Raskin, N.H. (1990a). Conclusions. *Headache* 30: 24.

Raskin, N.H. (1990b). Modern pharmacotherapy of migraine. *Neurol. Clin.* 8:857–865.

Raskin, N.H. and R.K. Schwartz (1980). Icepick-like pain. *Neurology* 30:203–205.

Rasmussen, B.K., R. Jensen, and J. Olesen (1991a). A population-based analysis of the diagnostic criteria of the International Headache Society. *Cephalalgia* 11:129–134.

Rasmussen, B.K., R. Jensen, M. Schroll et al. (1991b). Epidemiology of headache in a general population—a prevalence study. *J. Clin. Epidemiol.* 44:1147–1157.

Ratinahirana, H., Y. Darbois, and M.G. Bousser (1990). Migraine and pregnancy: A prospective study in 703 women after delivery. *Neurology* 40:437.

Ravnikar, V. (1990). Physiology and treatment of hot flushes. *Obstet. Gynecol.* 75:S3–S8.

Rebar, R.W. and I.B. Spitzer (1987). The physiology and measurement of hot flushes. *Am. J. Obstet. Gynecol.* 156:1284–1288.

Reches, A. (1999). Comparison of the efficacy, safety and tolerability of oral eletriptan and Cafergot® for the acute treatment of migraine. On behalf of the Eletriptan Steering Committee [abstract]. *Cephalalgia* 19:355.

Reid, R.L. and S.S.C. Yen (1981). Premenstrual syndrome. *Am. J. Obstet. Gynecol.* 139:85–104.

Reisine, T. and G. Pasternak (1996). Opioid analgesics and antagonists. In *Goodman & Gilman's The Pharmacological Basis of Therapeutics* (J.G. Hardman, L.E. Limbird, P.B. Molinoff et al., eds.), pp. 521–556. McGraw-Hill, New York.

Reutens, D.C., D.M. Fatovich, E.G. Stewart-Wynne et al. (1991). Is intravenous lidocaine clinically effective in acute migraine? *Cephalalgia* 11:245–247.

Richardson, J.W. and E. Richelson (1984). Antidepressants: A clinical update for medical practitioners. *Mayo Clin. Proc.* 59:330–337.

Richelson, E. (1990). Antidepressants and brain neurochemistry. *Mayo Clin. Proc.* 65:1227–1236.

Riopelle, R. and J.L. McCans (1982). A pilot study of the calcium channel antagonist diltiazem in migraine syndrome prophylaxis. *Can. J. Neurol. Sci.* 9:269.

Robert, M., X. Cabarrocas, J.M. Zayas et al. (1999). Overall response of oral almotriptan in the treatment of three migraine attacks. On behalf of the Almotriptan Multiple Attacks Study Group [abstract]. *Cephalalgia* 19:363.

Robinson, K., K.M. Huntington, and M.G. Wallace (1977). Treatment of the premenstrual syndrome. *Br. J. Obstet. Gynaecol.* 84:784–788.

Roche, K.W., R.J. O'Brien, A.L. Mammen, and R.L. Huganir (1996). Characterization of multiple phosphorylation sites on the AMP receptor GluR1 subunit. *Neuron* 16:1179–1188.

Rogawski, M.A. and R.J. Porter (1990). Antiepileptic drugs: pharmacological mechanisms and clinical efficacy with consideration of promising development stage compounds. *Pharmacol. Rev.* 42:223–286.

Rohr, J. and J.J. Dufresne (1985). Dihydroergotamine nasal spray for the treatment of migraine attacks: A comparative double-blind crossover study with placebo. *Cephalalgia* 5:142–143.

Rompel, H. and P.W. Bauermeister (1970). Aetiology of migraine and prevention with carbamazepine (Tegretol). *S. Afr. Med. J.* 44:75–80.

Rosen, J.A. (1983). Observations on the efficacy of propranolol for the prophylaxis of migraine. *Ann. Neurol.* 13:92–93.

Rosenorm, J., V. Eskesen, and K. Schmidt (1988). Unruptured intracranial aneurysms: An assessment of the annual risk of rupture based on epidemiological and clinical data. *J. Neurosurg.* 2:369–377.

Roth, B.L., S.C. Craigo, M.S. Choudhary et al (1994). Binding of typical and atypical antipsychotic agents to 5-hydroxytryptamine-6 and 5-hydroxytryptamine-7 receptors. *J. Pharmacol. Exp. Ther.* 268:1403–1410.

Rowat, B.M., C.F. Merrill, A. Davis et al. (1991). A double-blind comparison of granisetron and placebo for the treatment of acute migraine in the emergency department. *Cephalalgia* 11:207–213.

Rozen, T.D. (1999). Successful treatment of a prolonged migrainous aura with intravenous furosemide: Does this help prove the existence of cortical spreading depression in humans [abstract]? *Headache* 39:378.

Ruat, M., E. Traiffort, J.M. Arrang et al. (1993). A novel rat serotonin (5-HT$_6$) receptor: Molecular cloning, localization, and stimulation of cAMP accumulation. *Biochem. Biophys. Res. Commun.* 193:268–276.

Russell, M.B. and J. Olesen (1995). Increased familial risk and evidence of genetic factor in migraine. *BMJ* 311:541–544.

Russell, M.B. and J. Olesen (1996). A nosographic analysis of the migraine aura in a general population. *Brain* 119:355–361.

Russell, M.B., B.K. Rasmussen, J. Brennum et al. (1992). Presentation of a new instrument: The diagnostic headache diary. *Cephalalgia* 12:369–374.

Ryan, R., A. Elkind, C.C. Baker et al. (1997). Sumatriptan nasal spray for the acute treatment of migraine: Results of two clinical studies. *Neurology* 49:1225–1230.

Ryan, R. and C. Keywood (1998). A preliminary study of frovatriptan (VML251), a potent cerebroselective 5-hydroxytryptamine (5-HT)$_{1B/1D}$ agonist for the acute treatment of migraine [abstract]. *Eur. J. Neurol.* 5:S46.

Ryan, R.E. (1968). Double-blind crossover comparison of BC105, methysergide, and placebo in the prophylaxis of migraine headache. *Headache* 8:118–126.

Ryan, R.E. (1970). Double-blind clinical evaluation of the efficacy and safety of ergostine—caffeine and placebo in migraine headache. *Headache* 9:212–220.

Ryan, R.E. (1974). A study of Midrin® in the symptomatic relief of migraine headache. *Headache* 14:33–42.

Ryan, R.E. (1984). Comparative study of nadolol and propranolol in prophylactic treatment of migraine. *Am. Heart J.* 108:1156–1159.

Ryan, R.E. and S. Diamond (1975). Double-blind study of clonidine and placebo for the prophylactic treatment of migraine. *Headache* 15:202–210.

Ryan, R.E. and A. Sudilovsky (1983). Nadolol: Its use in the prophylactic treatment of migraine. *Headache* 23:26–31.

Saadah, H.A. (1992). Abortive headache therapy in the office with intravenous dihydroergotamine plus prochlorperazine. *Headache* 32:143–146.

Sachdeo, R.C., S.K. Sachdeo, S.A. Walker et al. (1996). Steady-state pharmacokinetics of topiramate and carbamazepine in patients with epilepsy during monotherapy and concomitant therapy. *Epilepsia* 37:774–780.

Sacks, O. (1985). *Migraine: Understanding a Common Disorder*. University of California Press, Berkeley.

Saito, K., S. Markowtiz, and M.A. Moskowitz (1988a). Ergot alkaloids block neurogenic extravasation in dura mater: Proposed action in vascular headaches. *Ann. Neurol.* 24:732–737.

Saito, K., S. Markowtiz, and M.A. Moskowitz (1988b). Ergot alkaloids specifically block the development of neurogenic inflammation within the dura mater induced by chemical or electrical stimulation. *Ann. Neurol.* 24:732–737.

Sales, F. and J.L. Bada (1975). Practolol and migraine. *Lancet* i:742.

Salfield, S.A., B.L. Waywardly, and W.T. Houlsby (1987). Controlled study of exclusion of dietary vasoactive amines in migraine. *Arch. Dis. Child.* 62:458–460.

Salonen, R., E. Ashford, C. Dahlof et al. (1994). Intranasal sumatriptan for the acute treatment of migraine. International Intranasal Sumatriptan Study Group [Abstract]. *J. Neurol. 241*:463–469.

Sanders, S.W., N. Haering, H. Mosberg et al. (1986). Pharmacokinetics of ergotamine in healthy volunteers following oral and rectal dosing. *Eur. J. Clin. Pharmacol. 30*:331–334.

Sangiorgi, S., M. Mochi, R. Riva et al. (1994). Abnormal platelet mitochondrial function in patients affected by migraine with and without aura. *Cephalalgia 14*:21–23.

Saper, J.R. (1983). *Headache Disorders: Current Concepts in Treatment Strategies*. Wright-PSG, Littleton, MA.

Saper, J.R. (1986). Changing perspectives of chronic headache. *Clin. J. Pain 2*:19–28.

Saper, J.R. (1987). Egotamine dependency–a review. *Headache 27*:435–438.

Saper, J.R. (1989). Chronic headache syndromes. *Neurol. Clin. 7*:387–412.

Saper, J.R. (1990). Chronic headache syndromes. *Neurol. Clin. 8*:891–901.

Saper, J.R. and J.M. Jones (1986). Ergotamine tartrate dependency: Features and possible mechanisms. *Clin. Neuropharmacol. 9*:244–256.

Saper, J.R., A.E. Lake, R.H. Hamel et al. (2000). Sustained, scheduled opioid therapy for patients with intractable headache: A 5-year prospective study. Presented to the American Headache Society, ACHE Award Lecture, Montreal, Quebec, June.

Saper, J.R. and J.H. Lossing (1974). Prolonged trance-like stupor in epilepsy. Petit mal status-wave stupor, spaced-out status. *Arch. Intern. Med. 134*:1079–1082.

Saper, J.R., S.D. Silberstein, C.D. Gordon et al. (1993). *Handbook of Headache Management*. Williams & Wilkins, Baltimore.

Saper, J.R., S.D. Silberstein, C.D. Gordon et al. (1999a). *Handbook of Headache Management: A Practical Guide to Diagnosis and Treatment of Head, Neck, and Facial Pain*. Lippincott-Williams & Wilkins, Baltimore.

Saper, J.R., S.D. Silberstein, C.D. Gordon et al. (1999b). Medications used in the pharmacotherapy of headache. In *Handbook of Headache Management: A Practical Guide to Diagnosis and Treatment of Head, Neck, and Facial Pain* (J.R. Saper, S.D. Silberstein, C.D. Gordon et al., eds.), pp. 61–145. Lippincott-Williams & Wilkins, Baltimore.

Saper, J.R., S.D. Silberstein, A.E. Lake et al. (1994). Double-blind trial of fluoxetine: Chronic daily headache and migraine. *Headache 34*:497–502.

Sargent, J., J.R. Kirchner, R. Davis et al. (1995). Oral sumatriptan is effective and well tolerated for the acute treatment of migraine: Results of a multicenter study. *Neurology 45*:S10–S14.

Sargent, J., P. Solbach, H. Damasio et al. (1985). A comparison of naproxen sodium to propranolol hydrochloride and a placebo control for the prophylaxis of migraine headache. *Headache 25*:320–324.

Sargent, J.D., B. Baumel, K. Peters et al. (1988). Aborting a migraine attack: Naproxen sodium versus ergotamine plus caffeine. *Headache 28*:263–266.

Saxena, P.R. (1972). The effects of antimigraine drugs on the vascular responses evoked by 5-hydroxytryptamine and related biogenic substances on the external carotid bed of dogs: Possible pharmacologic implications to their antimigraine action. *Headache 12*:44–54.

Saxena, P.R. (1974). Selective vasoconstriction in carotid vascular bed by methysergide: Possible relevance to its antimigraine effect. *Eur. J. Pharmacol. 27*:99–105.

Saxena, P.R. and S.G. DeVlaam (1974). Role of some biogenic substances in migraine and relevant mechanism in antimigraine action of ergotamine. Studies in an animal experimental model for migraine. *Headache 13*:142–163.

Saxena, P.R., D.J. Duncker, A.H. Bom et al. (1986). Effects of MDL72222 and methiothepin on carotid vascular responses to 5-hydroxytryptamine in the pig: Evidence for the presence of vascular 5-hydroxytryptamine1-like receptors. *Arch. Pharmacol. 333*:198–204.

Saxena, P.R., P. VanHouwelingen, and I.L. Bonta. (1971). The effect of mianserin hydrochloride on the vascular responses to 5-hydroxytryptamine and related substances. *Eur. J. Pharmacol. 13*:295–305.

Saxena, P.R. and P.D. Verdouw (1984). Effects of methysergide and 5-hydroxytryptamine on carotid blood flow distribution in pigs: Further evidence for the presence of atypical 5-HT receptors. *Br. J. Pharmacol. 82*:817–826.

Scharff, L. and D.A. Marcus (1999). The association between chocolate and migraine: A review. *Headache Q. 10*:199–205.

Schaumburg, H.H., R. Byck, R. Gerstl et al. (1969). Monosodium L-glutamate: Its pharmacology and role in the Chinese restaurant syndrome. *Science 163*:826–828.

Schaumburg, H., J. Kaplan, A. Windebank et al. (1983). Sensory neuropathy from pyridoxine abuse. *N. Engl. J. Med. 309*:445–448.

Scherl, E.R. and J.F. Wilson (1995). Comparison of dihydroergotamine with metoclopramide versus meperidine with promethazine in the treatment of acute migraine. *Headache 35*:256–259.

Schiffman, S.S., C.E. Buckley III, H.A. Sampson et al. (1987). Aspartame and susceptibility to headache. *N. Engl. J. Med. 317*:1181.

Schmidt, R. and A. Fanchamps (1974). Effect of caffeine on intestinal absorption of ergotamine in man. *Eur. J. Clin. Pharmacol. 7*:213–216.

Schmitt, T., F. Erbguth, and A. Taghavy (1993). Oculomotor paralysis as the leading symptom of meningovascular syphilis: Report of two patients and review of the literature. *Nervenarzt 64*: 668–672.

Schoenen, J., J. Jacquy, and M. Lenaerts (1998). Effectiveness of high-dose riboflavin in migraine prophylaxis. A randomized controlled trial. *Neurology 50*:466–470.

Schoenen, J., A. Maertens de Noordout, M. Timsit-Bertheir et al. (1986). Contingent negative variation and efficacy of β-blocking agents in migraine. *Cephalalgia 6*:231–233.

Scholte, H.R., H.F. Busch, H.D. Bakker et al. (1995). Riboflavin-responsive complex I deficiency. *Biochim. Biophys. Acta 1271*:75–83.

Scholz, E., H.C. Diener, S. Geiselhart et al. (1988). Drug-induced headache: Does a critical dosage exist? In *Drug-induced Headache* (H.C. Diener, ed.), pp. 29–43. Springer-Verlag, Berlin.

Schran, H.F. and F.L.S. Tse (1985). Pharmacokinetics of dihydroergotamine following subcutaneous administration in humans. *Int. J. Clin. Pharmacol. Ther. Toxicol. 23*:1–4.

Schwartz, J., R. Freeman, and W. Frishman (1995). Clinical pharmacology of estrogens: Cardiovascular actions and cardioprotective benefits of replacement therapy in postmenopausal women. *J. Clin. Pharmacol. 35*:1–16.

Scott, R.J., W.R. Aitchison, P.R. Barker et al. (1996). Oral sumatriptan in the acute treatment of migraine and migraine recurrence in general practice. *QJM 89*:613–622.

Seibyl, J.P., J.H. Krystal, L.H. Price et al. (1991). Effects of ritanserin on the behavioral, neuroendocrine, and cardiovascular responses to metachlorophenylpiperazine in healthy human subjects. *Psychiatry Res. 38*:227–236.

Selby, G. and J.W. Lance (1960). Observation on 500 cases of migraine and allied vascular headaches. *J. Neurol. Neurosurg. Psychiatry 23*:23–32.

Shafar, J., E.R. Tallett, and P.A. Knowlson (1972). Evaluation of clonidine in prophylaxis of migraine. Double-blind trial and followup. *Lancet i*:403–407.

Shank, R.P., J.F. Gardocki, J.L. Vaught et al. (1994). Topiramate: preclinical evaluation of structurally novel anticonvulsant. *Epilepsia 35*: 450–460.

Shanks, R.G. (1987). A review of the relationship between beta-adrenoreceptor antagonists and their action in migraine. In *Advances in Headache Research* (F.C. Rose, ed.), pp. 161–166. John Libbey, London.

Sheftel, F., S.D. Silberstein, and A. Rapoport. (1992). Pharmacological treatment of chronic headache. *Drug Ther. 22*:47–59.

Shekelle, R.B. and A.M. Ostfeld (1964). Methysergide in the migraine syndrome. *Clin. Pharmacol. Ther. 5*:201–204.

Shepard, T.H. (1973). *Catalog of Teratogenic Agents*. Johns Hopkins University Press, Baltimore.

Shimell, C.J., V.U. Fritz, and S.L. Levien (1990). A comparative trial of flunarizine and propranolol in the prevention of migraine. *S. Afr. Med. J. 77*:75–77.

Shoemaker, E.S., J.P. Forney, and P.C. MacDonald (1977). Estrogen treatment of postmenopausal women. *JAMA 238*:1524–1530.

Shrestha, M., R. Singh, J. Moreden et al. (1996). Ketorolac vs chlorpromazine in the treatment of acute migraine without aura. A prospective, randomized, double-blind trial. *Arch. Intern. Med. 156*:1725–1728.

Shuaib, A., F. Ahmed, M. Muratoglu et al. (1999). Topiramate in migraine prophylaxis: A pilot study [Abstract]. *Cephalalgia 19*:379–380.

Shukla, R., R.K. Garg, D. Nag et al. (1995). Nifedipine in migraine and tension headache: A randomized double-blind crossover study. *J. Assoc. Physicians India 43*:770–772.

Shulman, K.I. and S.E. Walker (1999). Refining the MAOI diet. Tyramine content of pizzas and soy products. *J. Clin. Psychiatry 60*:191–193.

Sicuteri, F. (1973). The ingestion of serotonin precursors (L-5-hydroxytryptophan and L-tryptophan) improves migraine headache. *Headache 13*:19–22.

Sicuteri, F. (1981). Enkephalinase inhibition relieves pain syndromes of central dysnociception (migraine and related headache). *Cephalalgia 1*: 229–232.

Sigel, E. (1995). Functional modulation of ligand-gated $GABA_A$ and NMDA receptor channels by phosphorylation. *J. Receptor Signal Transduct. Res. 15*:325.

Silberstein, S.D. (1984). Treatment of headache in primary care practice. *Am. J. Med. 77*:65–72.

Silberstein, S.D. (1990). Twenty questions about headaches in children and adolescents. *Headache 30*:716–727.

Silberstein, S.D. (1991). Appropriate use of abortive medication in headache treatment. *Pain Manage. 4*:22–28.

Silberstein, S.D. (1992). Evaluation and emergency treatment of headache. *Headache 32*: 396–407.

Silberstein, S.D. (1993a). Chronic daily headache and tension-type headache. *Neurology 43*: 1644–1649.

Silberstein, S.D. (1993b). Headaches and women: Treatment of the pregnant and lactating migraineur. *Headache 33*:533–540.

Silberstein, S.D. (1994). Serotonin (5-HT) and migraine. *Headache 34*:408–417.

Silberstein, S.D. (1995). Migraine symptoms: Results of a survey of self-reported migraineurs. *Headache* 35:387–396.

Silberstein, S.D. (1996a). DHE-45 in the prophylaxis of menstrually related migraine. *Cephalalgia* 16:371.

Silberstein, S.D. (1996b). Divalproex sodium in headache—literature review and clinical guidelines. *Headache* 36:547–555.

Silberstein, S.D. (1997a). Migraine and pregnancy. *Neurol. Clin.* 15:209–231.

Silberstein, S.D. (1997b). Preventive treatment of migraine: An overview. *Cephalalgia* 17:67–72.

Silberstein, S.D. (1998a). Drug-induced headache. *Neurol. Clin. N. Am.* 16:107–123.

Silberstein, S.D. (1998b). Methysergide. *Cephalalgia* 18:421–435.

Silberstein, S.D. and J.J. Corbett (1993). The forgotten lumbar puncture. *Cephalalgia* 13:212–213.

Silberstein, S.D. and S.D. Collins (1999). Safety of divalproex sodium in migraine prophylaxis: An open label Long-term study. *Headache* 39:633–643.

Silberstein, S.D., J.R. Fozard, and L. Murphy (1992). More on mCPP and migraine (letter). *Headache* 32:242–243.

Silberstein, S.D. and R.B. Lipton (1994). Overview of diagnosis and treatment of migraine. *Neurology* 44:6–16.

Silberstein, S.D. and R.B. Lipton (1996). Migraine epidemiology. *Neurol. Clin.* 14:421–434.

Silberstein, S.D. and R.B. Lipton (1997). Chronic daily headache. In *Headache* (P.J. Goadsby and S.D. Silberstein, eds.), pp. 201–225. Butterworth-Heinemann, Woburn, MA.

Silberstein, S.D., R.B. Lipton, and P.J. Goadsby (1998). Migraine: Diagnosis and treatment. In *Headache in Clinical Practice* (S.D. Silberstein, R.B. Lipton, and P.J. Goadsby, eds.), pp. 61–90. Isis Medical Media, Oxford.

Silberstein, S.D., R.B. Lipton, and M. Sliwinski (1996). Classification of daily and near-daily headaches: Field trial of revised IHS criteria. *Neurology* 47:871–875.

Silberstein, S.D., N. Mathew, J. Saper et al. (2000). Migraine Clinical Research Group: Botulinum toxin type A as a migraine preventive treatment. *Headache* 40:445–450.

Silberstein, S.D. and D.C. McCrory (1999). Opioids. In *Monographs in Clinical Neuroscience. Drug Treatment of Migraine and Other Frequent Headaches.* (H.C. Diener, ed.). Karger, Basel.

Silberstein, S.D. and G.R. Merriam (1991). Estrogens, progestins, and headache. *Neurology* 41:775–793.

Silberstein, S.D. and G.R. Merriam (1997). Sex hormones and headache. In *Headache* (P.J.

Goadsby and S.D. Silberstein, eds.), pp. 143–173. Butterworth-Heinemann, Woburn, MA.

Silberstein, S.D. and J.R. Saper (1993). Migraine: Diagnosis and treatment. In *Wolff's Headache and Other Head Pain* (D.J. Dalessio and S.D. Silberstein, eds.), pp. 96–170. Oxford University Press, New York.

Silberstein, S.D., E.A. Schulman, and M.M. Hopkins (1990a). Repetitive intravenous DHE in the treatment of refractory headache. *Headache* 30:334–339.

Silberstein, S.D. and M.M. Silberstein (1990b). New concepts in the pathogenesis of headache. Part II. *Pain Manage.* 3:334–342.

Silberstein, S.D. and W.B. Young (1995a). Migraine aura and prodrome. *Semin. Neurol.* 45:175–182.

Silberstein, S.D. and W.B. Young (1995b). Safety and efficacy of ergotamine tartrate and DHE in the treatment of migraine and status migrainosus. *Neurology* 45:577–584.

Sillanpaa, M. and M. Koponen (1978). Papaverine in the prophylaxis of migraine and other vascular headache in children. *Acta Paediatr. Scand.* 67:209–212.

Simberg, N., A. Titinen, A. Silfvast et al. (1996). High bone density in hyperandrogenic women: Effect of gonadotrophin-releasing hormone agonist alone or in conjunction with estrogen-progestin replacement. *J. Clin. Endocrinol. Metab.* 81:646–651.

Simkins, R.T., N. Tepley, G.L. Barkley et al. (1989). Spontaneous neuromagnetic fields in migraine: Possible link to spreading cortical depression. *Neurology* 39:325.

Simon, M.I., M.P. Strathmann, and N. Gautam (1991). Diversity of G proteins in signal transduction. *Science* 252:802–909.

Sjaastad, O. and I. Dale (1976). A new (?) clinical headache entity: Chronic paroxysmal hemicrania 2. *Acta Neurol. Scand.* 54:140–159.

Sjaastad, O. and E.L. Spierings (1984). Hemicrania continua: Another headache absolutely responsive to indomethacin. *Cephalalgia* 4:65–70.

Sjaastad, O. and P. Stensrud (1971). 2-(2,6-Dichlorophenylamino)-2-imidazoline hydrochloride (ST 155 or Catapresan) as a prophylactic remedy against migraine. *Acta Neurol. Scand.* 47:120–122.

Sjaastad, O. and P. Stensrud (1972). Clinical trial of a beta-receptor blocking agent (LB46) in migraine prophylaxis. *Acta Neurol. Scand.* 48:124–128.

Smith, R. and A. Schwartz (1984). Diltiazem prophylaxis in refractory migraine. *N. Engl. J. Med.* 310:1327–1328.

Smith, R.N.J., E.F.N. Holland, and J.W.W. Studd (1994). The symptomatology of progestogen intolerance. *Maturitas* 18:87.

Smyth, G.A. and L. Lazarus (1974). Suppression of growth hormone secretion by melatonin and cyproheptadine. *J. Clin. Invest.* 54:116–121.

Snyder, S.H. and I.J. Reynolds (1985). Calcium-antagonist drugs: Receptor interactions that clarify therapeutic effects. *N. Engl. J. Med.* 313: 995–1002.

Solbach, M.P. and R.S. Waymer (1993). Treatment of menstruation-associated migraine headache with subcutaneous sumatriptan. *Obstet. Gynecol.* 82:769–772.

Solomon, G. and R. Kunkel (1990). Effects of fluoxetine on premenstrual syndrome in chronic headache sufferers. *Headache* 30:301.

Solomon, G.D. (1986). Verapamil and propranolol in migraine prophylaxis: A double-blind cross-over study. *Headache* 26:325.

Solomon, G.D. (1989). Management of the headache patient with medical illness. *Clin. J. Pain* 5:95–99.

Solomon, G.D., R.K. Cady, J.A. Klapper et al. (1997). Clinical efficacy and tolerability of 2.5mg zolmitriptan for the acute treatment of migraine. *Neurology* 49:1219–1225.

Solomon, S. and R.B. Lipton (1991). Criteria for the diagnosis of migraine in clinical practice. *Headache* 31:384–387.

Somerville, B.W. (1971). The role of progesterone in menstrual migraine. *Neurology* 21:853–859.

Somerville, B.W. (1972). A study of migraine in pregnancy. *Neurology* 22:824–828.

Somerville, B.W. (1976). Platelet-bound and free serotonin levels in jugular and forearm venous blood during migraine. *Neurology* 26:41–45.

Sorensen, P.S., K. Hansen, and J. Olesen (1986). A placebo-controlled, double-blind, cross-over trial of flunarizine in common migraine. *Cephalalgia* 6:7–14.

Sorensen, P.S., B.H. Larsen, M.J. Rasmussen et al. (1991). Flunarizine versus metoprolol in migraine prophylaxis: A double-blind, randomized parallel group study of efficacy and tolerability. *Headache* 31:650–657.

Soyka, D., Z. Taneri, W. Oestreich et al. (1989). Flunarizine IV in the acute treatment of common or classical migraine attacks—a placebo-controlled double-blind trial. *Headache* 29:21–27.

Speed, W.G. (1989). Closed head injury sequelae: Changing concepts. *Headache* 29:643–647.

Spierings, E.L. (1984). The role of arteriovenous shunting in migraine. In *The Pharmacological Basis of Migraine Therapy* (W.K. Amery, J.V. Van Nueten, and A. Wauquier, eds.), pp. 36–49. Pitman, London.

Spierings, E.L. (1989). Treatment of the migraine attack. In *Migraine and Other Headaches* (M.D. Ferrari and X. Lataste, eds.), pp. 241–248. Parthenon, Park Ridge, NJ.

Spierings, E.L. (1996). *Management of Migraine.* Butterworth Heinemann, Boston.

Staley, K.J. and B.L. Soldo (1995). Ionic mechanisms of neuronal excitation by inhibitory GABA$_A$ receptors. *Science* 269:977–981.

Steardo, L., S. Bonuso, E. DiStasio et al. (1982). Selective and nonselective beta-blockers: Are both effective in prophylaxis of migraine? A clinical trial versus methysergide. *Acta Neurol.* 4:196–204.

Steardo, L., E. Marano, P. Barone et al. (1986). Prophylaxis of migraine attacks with a calcium-channel blocker; flunarizine versus methysergide. *J. Clin. Pharmacol* 26:524–528.

Steiner, T.J. (1997). Ethical aspects of headache treatment trials. In *Headache Treatment. Trial Methodology and New Treatment* (J. Olesen and P. Tfelt-Hansen, eds.), pp. 71–78. Lippincott-Raven, Philadelphia.

Steiner, T.J., F. Ahmed, L.J. Findley et al. (1998). S-Fluoxetine in the prophylaxis of migraine: A phase II double-blind randomized placebo-controlled study. *Cephalalgia* 18:283–286.

Steiner, T.J., R. Joseph, C. Hedman et al. (1988). Metoprolol in the prophylaxis of migraine: Parallel-groups comparison with placebo and dose-ranging followup. *Headache* 28:15–23.

Stellar, S., S.P. Ahrens, A.R. Meibohm et al. (1984). Migraine prevention with timolol: A double-blind crossover study. *JAMA* 252:2576–2580.

Stensrud, P. and O. Sjaastad (1974). Clinical trial of a new antibradykinin, antiinflammatory drug, ketoprofen (19.583 r.p.) in migraine prophylaxis. *Headache* 14:96–100.

Stensrud, P. and O. Sjaastad (1976a). Clonidine (Catapresan)—double-blind study after long-term treatment with the drug in migraine. *Acta Neurol. Scand.* 53:233–236.

Stensrud, P. and O. Sjaastad (1976b). Short-term trial of propranolol in racemic form (Inderal), D-propranolol and placebo in migraine. *Acta Neurol. Scand.* 53:229–232.

Stensrud, P. and O. Sjaastad (1979). Clonazepam (Rivotril) in migraine prophylaxis. *Headache* 19: 333–334.

Stewart, W.F., A. Schechter, and R.B. Lipton (1994a). Migraine heterogeneity: Disability, pain intensity, attack frequency, and duration. *Neurology* 44:S24–S39.

Stewart, W.F., A.L. Shechter, and R.B. Lipton (1994b). Migraine heterogeneity: Disability, pain intensity, attack frequency, and duration. *Neurology* 44:S24–S39.

Stiell, I.G., D.G. Dufour, D. Moher et al. (1991). Methotrimeprazine versus meperidine and dimenhydrinate in the treatment of severe migraine: A randomized, controlled trial. *Ann. Emerg. Med.* 20:1201–1205.

Stoica, E. and O. Enulescu (1990). Propranolol corrects the abnormal catecholamine response to light during migraine. *Eur. Neurol.* 30:19–22.

Streeter, A.J., P.L. Stahle, J.F. Hills et al. (1994).

Pharmacokinetics of topiramate in the rat. *Pharm. Res. 11*:372.

Stumpf, P.G. (1990). Pharmacokinetics of estrogen. *Obstet. Gynecol. 75*:9–17.

Sudilovsky, A., A.H. Elkind, R.E. Ryan et al. (1987). Comparative efficacy of nadolol and propranolol in the management of migraine. *Headache 27*:421–426.

Sudilovsky, A., M.A. Stern, and J.H. Meyer (1986). Nadolol: The benefits of an adequate trial duration in the prophylaxis of migraine. *Headache 26*:325.

Surrey, E.S., B. Voigt, N. Fournet et al. (1995). Prolonged gonadotrophin-releasing hormone agonist treatment of symptomatic endometriosis: The role of cyclic sodium etidronate and low-dose norethindrone add-back therapy. *Fertil. Steril. 63*:747–755.

Swedish Medical Product Agency. (1997). http://www.mpa.se/sve/mono/imig.sht (Monograph in Swedish on sumatriptan suppositories published on the internet by Swedish Medical Product Agency).

Taira, T., K. Lamsa, and K. Kaila (1997). Posttetanic excitation mediated by GABA(A) receptors in rat CA1 pyramidal neurons. *J. Neurophysiol. 77*:2213–2218.

Takeshima, T., S. Nishikawa, and K. Takashashi (1988). Sublingual administration of flunarizine for acute migraine: Will flunarizine take the place of ergotamine? *Headache 28*:602–606.

Tang, M.X., D. Jacobs, Y. Stern et al. (1996). Effect of oestrogen during menopause on risk and age at onset of Alzheimer's disease. *Lancet 348*:429–432.

Teall, J., M. Tuchman, N. Cutler et al. (1998). Rizatriptan (MAXALT) for the acute treatment of migraine and migraine recurrence. A placebo-controlled, outpatient study (Rizatriptan 022 Study Group). *Headache 38*:281–287.

Tek, D.S., D.S. McClellan, J.S. Olshaker et al. (1990). A prospective, double-blind study of metoclopramide hydrochloride for the control of migraine in the emergency department. *Ann. Emerg. Med. 19*:1083–1087.

Tepper, S.J., A. Cochran, S. Hobbs et al. (1998). Sumatriptan suppositories for the acute treatment of migraine. S2B351 Study Group. *Int. J. Clin. Pract. 52*:31–35.

Tfelt-Hansen, P. (1993). Sumatriptan for the treatment of migraine attacks—a review of controlled clinical trials. *Cephalalgia 13*:238–244.

Tfelt-Hansen, P., P. Henry, L.J. Mulder et al. (1995). The effectiveness of combined oral lysine acetylsalicylate and metoclopramide compared with oral sumatriptan for migraine. *Lancet 346*:923–926.

Tfelt-Hansen, P. and R.B. Lipton (1993). Prioritizing treatment. In *The Headaches* (J. Olesen, P. Tfelt-Hansen, and K.M.A. Welch, eds.), pp. 359–362. Raven Press, New York.

Tfelt-Hansen, P. and J. Olesen (1984). Effervescent metoclopramide and aspirin (Migravess) versus effervescent aspirin or placebo for migraine attacks: A double-blind study. *Cephalalgia 4*:107–111.

Tfelt-Hansen, P., J. Olesen, A. Aebelholt-Krabbe et al. (1980). A double blind study of metoclopramide in the treatment of migraine attacks. *J. Neurol. Neurosurg. Psychiatry 43*:369–371.

Tfelt-Hansen, P., B. Standnes, P. Kangasniemi et al. (1984). Timolol vs propranolol vs placebo in common migraine prophylaxis: A double-blind multicenter trial. *Acta Neurol. Scand. 69*:1–8.

Thomas, E.J., K.J. Okuda, and N.M. Thomas (1991a). The combination of depot gonadotrophin releasing hormone agonist and cyclical hormone replacement therapy for dysfunctional uterine bleeding. *Br. J. Obstet. Gynaecol. 98*:1155–1159.

Thomas, M., M. Behari, and G.K. Ahuja (1991b). Flunarizine in migraine prophylaxis: An Indian trial. *Headache 31*:613–615.

Thomsen, L.L., H.K. Iversen, L.H. Lassen et al. (1994). The role of nitric oxide in migraine pain: Therapeutic implications. *CNS Drugs 2*:417–422.

Tillgren, N. (1947). Treatment of headache with dihydroergotamine tartrate. *Acta Med. Scand. 196*:222–228.

Titus, F., A. Davalos, J. Alom et al. (1986). 5-Hydroxytryptophan versus methysergide in the prophylaxis of migraine. Randomized clinical trial. *Eur. Neurol. 25*:327–329.

Tobita, M., M. Hino, N. Ichikawa et al. (1987). A case of hemiplegic migraine treated with flunarizine. *Headache 27*:487–488.

Tokola, R. and E. Hokkanen (1978). Propranolol for acute migraine. *BMJ 2*:1089.

Tokola, R.A., P. Kangasniemi, P.J. Neuvonen et al. (1984). Tolfenamic acid, metoclopramide, caffeine and their combinations in the treatment of migraine attacks. *Cephalalgia 4*:253–263.

Tollefson, G.D. (1983). Monoamine oxidase inhibitors: A review. *J. Clin. Psychiatry 44*:280–288.

Touchon, J., L. Bertin, A.J. Pilgrim et al. (1996). A comparison of subcutaneous sumatriptan and dihydroergotamine nasal spray in the acute treatment of migraine. *Neurology 47*:361–365.

Tournier-Lasserve, E. (1999). Hemiplegic migraine, episodic ataxia type 2, and the others. *Neurology 53*:3–4.

Tournier-Lasserve, E., A. Joutel, and J. Melki (1993). Cerebral autosomal arteriopathy with subcortical infarcts and leukoencephalopathy maps to chromosomes. *Nat. Genet. 3*:256–259.

Treves, T.A., M. Streiffler, and A.D. Korczyn (1992). Naproxen sodium versus ergotamine tartrate in the treatment of acute migraine attacks. *Headache 32*:280–282.

Tulunay, F.C., O. Karan, N. Aydin et al. (1987). Dihydroergotamine nasal spray during migraine attacks. A double-blind crossover study with placebo. *Cephalalgia* 7:131–133.

Ustdal, M., P. Dogan, A. Soyeur et al. (1989). Treatment of migraine with salmon calcitonin: Effects on plasma beta-endorphin, ACTH, and cortisol levels. *Biomed. Pharmacother.* 43:687–691.

Utian, W.H. (1987a). Overview on menopause. *Am. J. Obstet. Gynecol.* 156:1280–1283.

Utian, W.H. (1987b). The fate of the untreated menopause. *Obstet. Gynecol. Clin. North Am.* 14:1–11.

Vainionpaa, L.K., J. Rattya, M. Knip et al. (1999). Valproate-induced hyperandrogenism during pubertal maturation in girls with epilepsy. *Ann. Neurol.* 45:444–450.

Van den Bergh, V., W.K. Amery, and J. Waelkens (1987). Trigger factors in migraine: A study conducted by the Belgian migraine society. *Headache* 27:191–196.

Varadi, G., Y. Mori, G. Mikala et al. (1996). Molecular determinants of Ca^{2+} channel function and drug action. *Trends Pharmacol. Sci.* 16:43–49.

Vijayan, N. (1977). Brief therapeutic report: Papaverine prophylaxis of complicated migraine. *Headache* 17:159–162.

Vilming, S., B. Standnes, and C. Hedman (1985). Metoprolol and pizotifen in the prophylactic treatment of classical and common migraine: A double-blind investigation. *Cephalalgia* 5:17–23.

Visser, W.H., G.M. Terwindt, S.A. Reines et al. (1996). Rizatriptan vs sumatriptan in the acute treatment of migraine. A placebo-controlled, dose-ranging study. Dutch/United States Rizatriptan Study Group [Abstract]. *Arch. Neurol.* 53:1132–1137.

Vogler, B.K., M.H. Pittler, and E. Ernst (1998). Feverfew as a preventive treatment for migraine: A systematic review. *Cephalalgia* 18:704–708.

Volans, G.N. (1978). Research review: Migraine and drug absorption. *Pharmacokinetics* 3:313–318.

Von Euler, U.S. (1937). On the specific vasodilating and plain muscle stimulating substance from accessory genital glands in man and certain animals (prostaglandin and vesiglandin). *J. Physiol.* 88:213–234.

Waeber, C. and J.M. Palacios (1991). 5-HT_{1C}, 5-HT_{1D} and 5-HT_2 receptors in mammalian brain: Multiple affinity states with a different regional distribution. In *Serotonin—Molecular Biology, Receptors and Functional Effects* (J.R. Fozard and P.R. Saxena, eds.), pp. 107–131. Birkhauser, Basel.

Waelkens, J. (1984). Dopamine blockade with domperidone: Bridge between prophylactic and abortive treatment of migraine? A dose-finding study. *Cephalalgia* 4:85–90.

Wallace, J.L. and G. Cirino (1994). The development of gastrointestinal-sparing nonsteroidal antiinflammatory drugs. *Trends Pharmacol. Sci.* 15:405–406.

Wang, J.H. and P.T. Kelly (1995). Postsynaptic injection of CA2+/CaM induces synaptic potentiation requiring CaMKII and PKC activity. *Neuron* 15:443–452.

Wang, S.J., S.D. Silberstein, and W.B. Young (1997). Droperidol treatment of status migrainosus and refractory migraine. *Headache* 37:377–382.

Ward, N.C., C. Whitney, D. Avery et al. (1991). The analgesic effects of caffeine in headache. *Pain* 44:141–155.

Watanabe, H., T. Kuwabara, M. Ohkubo et al. (1996). Elevation of cerebral lactate detected by localized ^{1}H-magnetic resonance spectroscopy in migraine during the interictal period. *Neurology* 47:1093–1095.

Waters, W.E. (1970). A randomized controlled trial of ergotamine tartrate. *Br. J. Prev. Soc. Med.* 24:65.

Waters, W.E. (1986). *Headache*. Wright-PSG, Littleton, MA.

Watson, S. and D. Girdlestone (1995). TiPS on nomenclature. *Trends Pharmacol. Sci.* 16(1):15–16.

Wauquier, A., D. Ashton, and R. Marranes (1985). The effects of flunarizine in experimental models related to the pathogenesis of migraine. *Cephalalgia* 5:119–120.

Weber, R.B. and O.M. Reinmuth (1972). The treatment of migraine with propranolol. *Neurology* 22:366–369.

Wei, E.P., M.A. Moskowitz, P. Boccalini et al. (1992). Calcitonin gene–related peptide mediates nitroglycerine and sodium nitroprusside–induced vasodilation in feline cerebral arterioles. *Circ. Res.* 70:1313–1319.

Weilburg, J.B., J.F. Rosenbaum, J. Biederman et al. (1989). Fluoxetine added to nonMAOI antidepressants converts nonresponders to responders: A preliminary report. *J. Clin. Psychiatry* 50:447–449.

Weinshank, R.L., N. Adham, J. Zgombick et al. (1992). Molecular analysis of serotonin receptor subtypes. In *Serotonin Receptor Subtypes: Pharmacological Significance and Clinical Implications* (S.Z. Langer, N. Brunello, G. Racagni et al., eds.), pp. 1–12. Karger, Basel.

Welch, K.M.A., E. Chabi, K. Bartosh et al. (1975). Cerebrospinal fluid gamma aminobutyric acid levels in migraine. *BMJ* 3:516–517.

Welch, K.M.A., G. D'Andrea, N. Tepley et al. (1990). The concept of migraine as a state of central neuronal hyperexcitability. *Neurol. Clin.* 8:817–828.

Welch, K.M.A., S.R.D.G. Levine, L. Schultz et al. (1989). Preliminary observations on brain energy metabolism in migraine studied by in vivo [31]phosphorus NMR spectroscopy. *Neurology 39*: 538–541.

Wentz, A.C. (1985). Management of the menopause. In *Novak's Textbook of Gynecology* (H.W. Jones, A.C. Wentz, and L.S. Burnett, eds.), pp. 397–442. Williams and Wilkins, Baltimore.

Wessely, P., C. Baumgartner, D. Klinger et al. (1987). Preliminary results of a double-blind study with the new migraine prophylactic drug gabapentin. *Cephalalgia 7*:477–478.

White, H.S., S.D. Brown, J.H. Woodhead et al. (1997). Topiramate enhances GABA-mediated chloride flux and GABA-evoked chloride currents in murine brain neurons and increase seizure threshold. *Epilepsy Res. 28*:167–179.

White, H.S., S.D. Brown, J.H. Woodhead et al. (2000). Topiramate modulates GABA-evoked currents in murine cortical neurons by a non-benzodiazepine mechanism. *Epilepsia 41*:S17–S20.

White, K. and G. Simpson (1984). The combined use of MAOIs and tricyclics. *J. Clin. Psychiatry 45*:67–69.

Whitty, C.W.M. (1967). Migraine without headache. *Lancet ii*:283–285.

Whitty, C.W.M. (1986). Familial hemiplegic migraine. In *Handbook of Clinical Neurology* (F.C. Rose, ed.), pp. 141–153. Elsevier, New York.

Wideroe, T.E. and T. Vigander (1974). Propranolol in the treatment of migraine. *BMJ 2*:699–701.

Wijman, C., P.A. Wolf, C.S. Kase et al. (1998). Migrainous visual accompaniments are not rare in late life: The Framingham Study. *Stroke 29*: 1539–1543.

Wilkinson, M. (1970). Preliminary report on the use of clonidine (Boehringer Ingelheim) in the treatment of migraine. *Res. Clin. Stud. Headache 3*:315–320.

Wilkinson, M. (1986). Clinical features of migraine. In *Handbook of Clinical Neurology*, (F.C. Rose, ed.), pp. 117–133. Elsevier, New York.

Wilkinson, M. (1988a). Introduction. In *Drug-induced headache* (H.C. Diener and M. Wilkinson, eds.), pp. 1–2. Springer-Verlag, Berlin.

Wilkinson, M. (1988b). Treatment of migraine. *Headache 28*:659–661.

Williams, M.J., R.I. Harris, and B.C. Dean (1985). Controlled trial of pyridoxine in the premenstrual syndrome. *J. Int. Med. Res. 1*:174–179.

Winner, P., O. Ricalde, B. Leforce et al. (1996). A double-blind study of subcutaneous dihydroergotamine vs subcutaneous sumatriptan in the treatment of acute migraine. *Arch. Neurol. 53*: 180–184.

Winther, K. (1995). Ketanserin: A selective serotonin antagonist in relation to platelet aggregation and migraine attack rate. *Cephalalgia 5*: 402–403.

Woods, R.P., M. Iacoboni, and J.C. Mazziotta (1994). Bilateral spreading cerebral hypoperfusion during spontaneous migraine headaches. *N. Engl. J. Med. 331*:1689–1692.

Yaffe, K., G. Sawaya, I. Lieberburg et al. (1998). Estrogen therapy in postmenopausal women: Effects on cognitive function and dementia. *JAMA 279*:688–695.

Ylostalo, P., A. Kauppila, J. Puolakka et al. (1982). Bromocriptine and noresthisterone in the treatment of premenstrual syndrome. *Obstet. Gynecol. 58*:292–298.

Youdim, M.B.H., S.M. Bonham-Carter, M. Sandler et al. (1971). Conjugation defect in tyramine sensitive migraine. *Nature 230*:127–128.

Yuill, G.M., W.R. Swinburn, and L.A. Liversedge (1972). A double-blind crossover trial of isometheptene mucate compound and ergotamine in migraine. *Br. J. Clin. Pract. 26*:76–79.

Zeeberg, I., M. Orholm, J.D. Nielsen et al. (1981). Femoxetine in the prophylaxis of migraine: A randomized comparison with placebo. *Acta Neurol. Scand. 64*:452–459.

Zgombick, J.M., L.E. Schechter, M. Macchi et al. (1992). Human gene *S31* encodes the pharmacologically defined serotonin 5-hydroxytryptamine1E receptor. *Mol. Pharmacol. 42*:180–185.

Ziegler, D., R. Ford, J. Kriegler et al. (1994). Dihydroergotamine nasal spray for the acute treatment of migraine. *Neurology 44*:447–453.

Ziegler, D.K. (1987). The treatment of migraine. In *Wolff's Headache and Other Head Pain* (D.J. Dalessio, ed.), pp. 87–111. Oxford University Press, New York.

Ziegler, D.K. and R.S. Hassanein (1990). Specific headache phenomena: Their frequency and coincidence. *Headache 30*:152–156.

Ziegler, D.K., A. Hurwitz, R.S. Hassanein et al. (1987). Migraine prophylaxis. A comparison of propranolol and amitriptyline. *Arch. Neurol. 44*: 486–489.

Zona, C., M.T. Ciotti, and M. Avoli (1997). Topiramate attenuates voltage-gated sodium currents in rat cerebellar granule cells. *Neurosci. Lett. 231*:123–126.

10

Episodic Tension-Type Headaches

SEYMOUR SOLOMON
LAWRENCE C. NEWMAN

In the past, the term "tension headache" was used to denote a common headache, but what did "tension" mean? Was it muscle tension or psychological tension? Because the mechanisms of this headache were not well understood, the International Headache Society (IHS) adopted the term "tension-type headache" (TTH) in 1988 (Headache Classification Committee of the International Headache Society, 1988).

Epidemiological studies of the general population have shown that TTH is the most common type of headache, with a lifetime prevalence of 78% and a yearly prevalence of 38% (Rasmussen et al., 1991b; Schwartz et al., 1998). Almost one-third of TTH sufferers have headaches on more than 14 days a year.

DIAGNOSIS

In 1988, the IHS published a classification system for headache, outlining the criteria that must be present to diagnose episodic TTH (Table 10–1) (Headache Classification Committee of the International Headache Society, 1988). The criteria distinguish TTH from migraine. Neither premonitory symptoms nor neurological aura symptoms occur with TTH. In contrast to migraine, the typical

pain characteristics of TTH are not pulsating, not unilateral, not severe in intensity, and not aggravated by routine physical activity; rather, the pain is a dull ache, pressure, or tight sensation. The location is usually bilateral but may be scattered. (The so-called typical band-like sensation around the head is the exception rather than the rule). The pain may extend from the cranium down the back of the neck or, less commonly, to the temporomandibular joints (TMJ) (the IHS classification places TMJ dysfunction/oromandibular dysfunction under the heading of TTH) (Headache Classification Committee of the International Headache Society, 1988).

There is often overlap of TTH and migraine features. In a major epidemiological study, TTHs were nonpulsating in 78% of patients, but pulsation occurred when the headaches increased in intensity (Rasmussen et al., 1991a). Headaches were not aggravated by physical activity in 72% of patients. Ninety percent of patients reported their headaches to be bilateral. Unilateral headache was reported in 10% to 20% of TTH patients, and a pulsating quality was noted in 14% (Rasmussen, 1992; Iversen et al., 1990). Typically, nausea is not associated with TTH, nor are photophobia and phonophobia; however, one or the other may occur, usually mild in de-

Table 10–1 Diagnostic criteria: episodic tension-type headache

A. At least ten previous headache episodes fulfilling criteria B–D listed below, number of days with such headache <180/year (<15/month).
B. Headache lasting from 30 minutes to 7 days
C. At least two of the following pain characteristics:
  1. Pressing/tightening (non-pulsating) quality
  2. Mild or moderate intensity (may inhibit, but does not prohibit activities)
  3. Bilateral location
  4. No aggravation by walking stairs or similar routine physical activity
D. Both of the following:
  1. No nausea or vomiting (anorexia may occur)
  2. Photophobia and phonophobia are absent, or one but not the other is present
E. No evidence of temporally related structural or metabolic disease

gree. Nausea, phonophobia, and photophobia were noted in 4%, 11%, and 13% of patients, respectively (Rasmussen et al., 1991a). Episodic TTH is arbitrarily characterized as lasting from 30 minutes to 7 days and, to distinguish episodic from chronic TTH, the frequency of episodic TTH is less than 15 headaches a month. The median frequency of TTH was 6 days a month, ranging from 2 to 12 days, and mean headache duration was 12 hours, ranging from 30 minutes to 72 hours. Virtually all patients report that the intensity of their pain was mild to moderate, but intensity increases with increased headache frequency (Ziegler et al., 1972). To avoid confusing this benign headache with one that may have identical characteristics but is due to structural or metabolic disease, the IHS criteria require at least ten previous headaches in the past and no temporally related organic disease (Headache Classification Committee of the International Headache Society, 1988).

In summary, the associated features of migraine, such as nausea, vomiting, photophobia and phonophobia, and aggravation by routine physical activity are usually absent during TTH; but their exclusion is not absolute. When these symptoms occur with TTH, they are much less prominent and much less consistent than with migraine (Iversen et al., 1990). Other symptoms often reported by patients with TTH include tiredness

(81%), sleep disturbances (53%), and light-headedness (51%) (Chun, 1985; Rasmussen, 1993).

Triggering factors are less common or less obvious in patients with TTH than in migraineurs. Lack of sleep is a common triggering factor. Sleep deprivation evoked TTH in 39% of a healthy population (Blau, 1990). Emotional stress may precipitate or aggravate migraine and TTH, just as relaxation may ameliorate both headache types. Similarly, menstruation may trigger or exaggerate both TTH and migraine.

Not only may some features of migraine occur with TTH, but a bout of TTH may evolve into an attack of typical migraine as the intensity of pain increases (Saper, 1986). Moreover, many people experience an episode of TTH at one time and a bout of migraine at another time. Sixty-two percent of migraineurs have TTH and 25% of people with TTH also have migraine (Ziegler and Hassanein, 1990).

The course of TTH is variable. Frequent bouts of episodic TTH may evolve into chronic TTH, with headaches occurring daily or almost every day. Overuse of analgesics or other medications designed for episodic use is a major factor in the evolution of migraine or TTH to chronic TTH (Mathew et al., 1987, 1990).

DIFFERENTIAL DIAGNOSIS

Headaches that are secondary to underlying disease may mimic either migraine or TTH. Because there is no laboratory test that will make the diagnosis of TTH (or any of the other primary headaches), one must always consider underlying structural or metabolic disease when evaluating a patient who fulfills the diagnostic criteria of TTH.

The differential diagnosis of TTH is extensive because the clinical features are not specific. The diagnostic criteria differentiate TTH from the other primary headaches, but virtually all structural and metabolic diseases may cause a symptom complex identical to that of episodic TTH. On the one hand, a patient with a primary headache such as episodic TTH may be misdiagnosed as having a "sinus headache" because he or she has a postnasal drip with thickening of the sinus mucosa or a "cervicogenic headache" because of neck stiffness and cervical spondylosis on x-ray. On the other hand, one should not be falsely reassured that the patient has a benign primary headache just because routine physical and neurologic examinations are normal. Examples include increased intracranial pressure without papilledema, as might occur with any mass such as a chronic subdural hematoma or pseudotumor cerebri, or metabolic changes, such as those associated with subtle carbon monoxide poisoning.

Other disorders may have symptoms very similar to episodic TTH. The pain of TMJ/oromandibular dysfunction or disease may radiate to the temple and beyond and may be misdiagnosed as TTH. However, other features of the TMJ syndrome should distinguish it from TTH. Pain arising from disease or dysfunction of the cervical structures may radiate to the occipital areas and sometimes to other parts of the head, but neck movement is an almost invariable triggering factor that distinguishes this site of pain from episodic TTH. Fibromyalgia is a label applied to scattered pains throughout the body with 11 or more tender sites without evidence of underlying disease. The unknown mechanism of this condition may be operative in some people with episodic TTH. Underlying disease of the head and neck may trigger a TTH. Look for and treat dental disease and sinusitis, as well as less common disorders.

The index of suspicion must be raised and further evaluation pursued if the headaches are of recent onset, if the qualities of the headache change, if there are important symptoms other than those associated with the primary headaches, and, of course, if there are positive neurologic signs.

PATHOPHYSIOLOGY

The term "TTH" includes headaches of diverse pathophysiology. Some believe that TTHs are fragments of migraine or are one end of a primary headache spectrum with mi-

graine at the other end (Raskin, 1988). The response to sumatriptan suggests that TTH has a pathogenesis akin to migraine in some people but an independent mechanism in others. Sumatriptan effectively treated TTH only in patients who also had attacks of migraine (Lipton et al., 2000). As years pass and migraine increases in frequency, the features of migraine tend to fade and the qualities of TTH evolve (Drummond and Lance, 1984).

The IHS classification lists eight possible etiologic factors for TTH: oromandibular dysfunction, psychosocial stress, anxiety, depression, delusional phenomena, muscle stress, drug overuse, and structural or metabolic diseases (Headache Classification Committee of the International Headache Society, 1988). There have been few scientific studies documenting these relationships, and some of the factors may be manifestations of coping strategies, reactions to the headache, or comorbid or coexistent conditions associated with the headache. Of these conditions, oromandibular/TMJ dysfunction is often overdiagnosed. People with TTH often have tenderness of pericranial muscles, including those in the area of the TMJ, but these findings are independent of TMJ dysfunction (Jensen et al., 1993).

In some people, TTH is associated with excessive scalp or neck muscle contraction. The IHS classification, recognizing that concept, divides TTHs into those associated with disorders of pericranial muscles and those without (Headache Classification Committee of the International Headache Society, 1988). Pericranial muscle disorder is based on the finding of increased tenderness of these muscles or increased level of electromyographic (EMG) activity. Most agree that TTH is a heterogeneous disorder. Peripheral factors in muscles and joints, as well as central biochemical factors and the psyche, may all play a part.

TENDERNESS

Unless there is associated pericranial muscle disorder, patients with TTH have normal examinations. Palpation may reveal tender points or nodules that evoke localized pain or trigger points where sustained pressure induces referred pain (Jensen and Paiva, 1993). Pericranial tenderness can be assessed by palpating the frontalis, temporalis, lateral and medial pterygoid, masseter, sternocleidomastoid, and trapezius muscles. Evaluation of tenderness is dependent on the reaction of the patient to the force of the examiner. The response will vary with the examiner (Jensen, 1995). However, during episodic TTH, muscle tenderness is increased but, curiously, pressure-pain thresholds tested by algometry are not affected (Jensen, 1995; Bove and Nilsson, 1999). Increased tenderness is often noted over the site of the headache and may persist for several days after cessation of the headache (Drummond, 1987; Lous and Olesen, 1982).

Scalp tenderness is not specific. In a random population-based study, 66% of people with episodic TTH had a pericranial muscular factor, predominantly tenderness (Jensen and Rasmussen, 1996). Because muscle tenderness can also be elicited in migraineurs, this finding in patients with TTH cannot be considered diagnostic (Drummond, 1987; Lous and Olesen, 1982). However, people with a history of TTH were more tender than migraineurs (Sandrini et al., 1994). Tenderness scores increased with increasing frequency and intensity of headache and during the headache. In one study, pressure-pain thresholds did not differentiate people with TTH, migraine, or the control population (Jensen and Rasmussen, 1996). Another group, however, found that the pressure-pain threshold over the frontalis was lower in TTH sufferers than in controls and migraineurs (Sandrini et al., 1994). An electronic pressure algometer showed that patients with chronic TTH had lower pain thresholds over both cephalic and extracephalic locations when muscle tenderness was present (Jensen et al., 1998). This was not true of patients with episodic TTH.

ELECTROMYOGRAPHY

Increased activity of pericranial muscles on EMG is not specific for TTH or migraine

(Sandrini et al., 1994; Lichstein et al., 1991). There have been many EMG studies in people with tension headache, but the results have not been consistent (Sandrini et al., 1994; Jensen et al., 1998; Lichstein et al., 1991; Arena et al., 1991; Hatch et al., 1991; Murphy and Lehrer, 1990; Schoenen et al., 1991). A meta-analysis concluded that people with TTH do not have significantly higher frontalis EMG levels at rest than control populations (Wittrock, 1997). Moreover, neither the degree of pain nor muscle tenderness was related to EMG levels (Sandrini et al., 1994; Peterson et al., 1995). During periods of stress, EMG levels of activity were higher in TTH patients and controls, but there was no statistical difference between the 2 groups (Rugh et al., 1990). In chronic TTH patients who had a muscular disorder, EMG levels were significantly greater than in those who did not have a muscular disorder (Jensen et al., 1998). The authors suggested that prolonged nociceptive stimuli from pericranial muscles sensitize the central nervous system, leading to increased pain sensitivity; this may be a factor in the conversion of episodic TTH to chronic TTH (Jensen et al., 1998).

OTHER TESTS

Many tests in people with TTH have shown differences when compared to control subjects or migraineurs. Unfortunately, the findings are not sufficiently specific to be diagnostic. There is as yet no biological marker for TTH.

The exteroceptive suppression test measures the early and late suppression of reflex temporal muscle activity after electrical stimuli to the labial commissure; it reflects the excitability of inhibitory interneurons in the brain stem (Godaux and Desmedt, 1975). Patients with TTH have a reduction in the duration or absence of the late exteroceptive suppression (ES2) of temporal muscle activity; this is more prominent in patients with chronic TTH than in those with the episodic form (Schoenen, 1993). Unfortunately, values of the ES2 duration for controls, migraineurs, and patients with TTH overlap and the sensitivity of this study has not been fully assessed.

Cerebrovascular changes in patients with TTH have been detected by transcranial Doppler ultrasound (Wallasch, 1993). The mean flow velocities in a group of patients with episodic TTH during the headache-free period were increased in the anterior, middle, and posterior cerebral arteries compared with a control group and a group of patients with chronic TTH. However, similar increases in mean flow velocities have been noted in migraine sufferers both during attacks and while headache-free (Thie et al., 1990a,b; Abernathy et al., 1990).

Another similarity between TTH and migraine is the finding of white matter abnormalities on magnetic resonance imaging in about one-third of patients (DeBenedittis et al., 1995). With computed tomography (CT), 22% of patients with TTH had single or multiple lacunar infarcts without clinical signs, but this group was older than patients with normal CT examinations (Nagata et al., 1993). Platelet activation has been reported during migraine and episodic TTH but not during chronic TTH or in controls (Kitano et al., 1994; Oishi and Mochizuki, 1998).

Some biochemical changes are common to both migraine and TTH. Ionized serum magnesium levels are low in both conditions (Mauskop et al., 1993). Some biochemical differences are noted between migraine and TTH, particularly with regard to serotonin and methionine enkephalin; but studies of platelet serotonin have not provided consistent results (Ferrari, 1993). In any case, these tests are not readily available and not specific.

When contingent negative variations were studied, patients with TTH showed a decrease in the interstimulus interval amplitude and a decrease in the late-wave component compared with controls and migraineurs (Wallasch et al., 1993).

PSYCHOLOGICAL FACTORS

The role of psychological factors in people who have TTH is uncertain. There is no doubt that pain intensity is increased by emo-

tional stress and that stress can trigger a headache (Donias et al., 1991). Somatization of anxiety or depression is an accepted mechanism but is probably more applicable to chronic TTH than the episodic form. There is no consistent factor, and the etiological relationship of psychological factors in people with TTH has been challenged by some investigations (Featherstone, 1985; Bakal, 1982). In most studies, episodic TTH was not clearly differentiated from chronic TTH.

Psychological evaluations of patients with TTH do not reveal consistent findings. The Minnesota Multiphasic Personality Inventory (MMPI) did not reveal significant differences between TTH patients and migraineurs (Pfaffenrath et al., 1991). Psychometric tests in patients with TTH and controls revealed significantly higher levels of anxiety, depression, and suppressed anger in TTH patients (Hatch et al., 1991). Those with TTH associated negative emotions such as anger and anxiety with attacks of headache significantly more than migraineurs (Donias et al., 1991). The frequency of TTH rose with increasing frequency of daily annoyances, and at least one psychosocial stress event or psychiatric disorder was noted in 85% of patients with TTH (DeBenedittis and Lorenzetti, 1992; Puca et al., 1999). Increased emotional tension levels were higher in patients with TTH, both during and between bouts of headache, than in control subjects (Cathcart and Pritchard, 1998). In one study, TTH sufferers had higher levels of depression and trait anxiety than a control group (Ficek and Wittrock, 1995). However, in a prospective longitudinal epidemiological study of a cohort of 19- and 20-year-olds, neither anxiety nor affective disorders was more prevalent in people with TTH than in controls (Merikangas, 1994).

THERAPY

Episodic TTH is the most common type of headache, and the vast majority of people who experience these headaches take simple analgesics or no medicine at all and do not consult a health-care professional for this almost inevitable human experience. People may seek help if episodic TTHs occur with unusual frequency or intensity. The main categories of treatment for TTH are pharmacological therapy and nondrug modalities. Medications for acute attacks of TTH start with simple analgesics [aspirin, acetaminophen, or nonsteroidal anti-inflammatory drugs (NSAIDs)] that do not require a doctor's prescription. Caffeine, an analgesic adjuvant, is often added to these agents (Solomon, 1994).

Failure of the simple drugs may be due to inadequate dosage. As a general rule, medications used for an acute headache should be taken at a relatively high dose and as early as possible. One thousand milligrams of aspirin or acetaminophen; 660 or 750 mg of naproxen; two tablets of the combination 250 mg of aspirin, 250 mg of acetaminophen, and 65 mg of caffeine will usually abort a TTH of moderate intensity. A 25 mg dose of ketoprofen was more effective than the 12.5 mg dose, and both were more effective than 1,000 mg of acetaminophen and significantly more effective than placebo in a study of 703 subjects with TTH (Mehlisch et al., 1998). Fifty milligrams of ketoprofen, but not acetaminophen (paracetamol), was more effective than placebo at ameliorating TTH (Dahlof and Jacobs, 1996).

If over-the-counter analgesics fail, then prescription medications are appropriate. High-dose NSAIDs may be prescribed. A combination of 325 mg of aspirin or acetaminophen with 40 mg of caffeine and 50 mg of butalbital is very effective. In rare instances, codeine may need to be added to the above combination to achieve pain relief; however, stronger opioids are almost never necessary for an attack of TTH (Solomon, 1994).

The most troublesome side effect of nonopioid analgesics, other than acetaminophen, is upper gastrointestinal irritation. Addition of a barbiturate or codeine may cause drowsiness. Prolonged use of aspirin and NSAIDs may cause renal disease, and acetaminophen may exacerbate hepatic disease. Aspirin and NSAIDs may impair platelet function with associated bleeding tendencies. In addition to the cautious use of analgesics in people with renal or liver disease, the main contraindications are hypersensitivity to aspirin and gastrointestinal disease.

An often overlooked danger in using medications for acute attacks of headache is the possibility of evoking a paradoxical effect. When an agent designed for episodic acute headache is taken daily or almost every day, a rebounding of the headache mechanism, leading to daily or almost-daily headaches, may result (Mathew et al., 1990). The medication appears harmless. It transiently relieves the pain, but when the analgesic effect wears off and some degree of headache returns, the natural tendency is to take more medication. This is a common reason for episodic TTH or migraine to evolving to chronic TTH or daily headache (Mathew et al., 1990). As a rule of thumb, acute medication should be taken no more than 2 days a week.

Except when episodic TTH frequency exceeds 15 days a month, prophylactic medication is not required. These measures are discussed in Chapter 9. Muscle relaxants appear to be logical medications for TTH associated with disorders of the pericranial muscles, but there have been few well-controlled studies using only muscle relaxants for episodic TTH. In some studies of tension headache, prior to the subclassifications of episodic and chronic TTH, a muscle relaxant or an antianxiety agent was combined with analgesics (Atkinson, 1979; Glassman and Soyka, 1980).

Depression, anxiety, or both may coexist with, aggravate, or cause TTH (Diamond, 1987; DeBenedittis et al., 1990), and the patient must be evaluated for these conditions and appropriately treated. However, these factors apply more to chronic TTH and migraine than to episodic TTH.

Nonpharmacological treatment modalities should always be considered in the management of TTH and migraine. These psychological and behavioral techniques are discussed in Chapter 9. They include teaching healthy habits with regard to sleep, meals, and exercise and eliminating unhealthy habits, such as smoking and drinking.

Studies that alter EMG activity by biofeedback have revealed conflicting results. Clinical improvement after biofeedback and reduction of EMG activity of pericranial muscles were noted in some studies but not in others (Budzynski et al., 1973; Cram, 1980; Hoffman, 1979; Andrasik and Holroyd, 1980). Indeed, the same lack of improvement in headache efficacy was noted when patients were taught to increase or decrease pericranial EMG activity (Philips and Hunter, 1981). Biofeedback-assisted relaxation has been used for juveniles with TTH (Bussone et al., 1998). Over a period of 1 year, there was an 86% reduction in headache intensity and duration, in contrast to placebo, which was associated with a 50% reduction. Self-help relaxation in adolescents with episodic TTH reduced headache frequency and intensity to a modest degree, although significantly better than in a control group (Larsson et al., 1990). Biofeedback techniques are commonly used to evoke a relaxation response. Other cognitive pain-coping methods, such as behavior modification and stress management, may be helpful.

Physical measures, such as needling or anesthetic injections of trigger points, may be useful (Davidoff, 1998). Physical therapy may be warranted for patients who have TTH associated with pericranial muscle disorders (Hammell et al., 1996). These modalities include ergonomic instruction, posture and positioning training, massage and other manual therapies, ultrasound, heat or cold application, and cold spray and stretch techniques. The use of transcutaneous electrical stimulations and acupuncture may also be considered in this broad category.

Attention to psychological factors is always appropriate. Many patients are concerned about an underlying brain tumor or other serious disease. Reassurance in this regard is important. Learning of the patients' interactions with family, friends, teachers, or employers may give the physician clues to some of the headache mechanisms and their management. Discussion of the term "TTH" is advisable. Explain that muscle tension and emotional tension are as likely to be consequences as causes of the headache and that anxiety and depression may coexist and aggravate the headache because of common biological dysfunctions. Asserting that the condition is psychosomatic is often counterproductive.

REFERENCES

Abernathy, M., J. Wieneke, M. Ramos et al. (1990). Transcranial Doppler: Intracranial blood flow velocities in headache-free migraineurs and non-headache-prone volunteers. *Neurology 40* (Suppl. 1):213.

Andrasik, F. and K.A. Holroyd (1980). A test of specific and nonspecific effects in the biofeedback treatment of tension headache. *J. Consult. Clin. Psychol. 48*:575–586.

Arena, J.G., S.L. Hannah, G.M. Bruno et al. (1991). Effect of movement and position of muscle activity in tension headache sufferers during and between headaches. *J. Psychosom. Res. 35*:187–195.

Atkinson, D. (1979). A single dose placebo-controlled study to assess the effectiveness of adding a muscle relaxant to a compound analgesic in the treatment of tension headaches. *J. Intern. Med. 7*:560–565.

Bakal, D.A. (1982). *The Psychobiology of Chronic Headache*. Springer, New York.

Blau, J.N. (1990). Sleep deprivation headache. *Cephalalgia 10*:157–160.

Bove, G.M. and N. Nilsson (1999). Pressure pain threshold and pain tolerance in episodic tension-type headache do not depend on the presence of headache. *Cephalalgia 19*:174–178.

Budzynski, T.H., J.M. Stoyva, S. Adler et al. (1973). EMG biofeedback and tension headache: A controlled outcome study. *Psychosom. Med. 35*:484–496.

Bussone, G., L. Grazzi, D. D'Amico et al. (1998). Biofeedback-assisted relaxation training for young adolescents with tension-type headache: A controlled study. *Cephalalgia 18*:463–467.

Cathcart, S. and D. Pritchard (1998). Relationships between arousal-related moods and episodic tension-type headache: A biopsychological study. *Headache 38*:214–221.

Chun, W.X. (1985). An approach to the nature of tension headache. *Headache 25*:188–189.

Cram, J.R. (1980). EMG biofeedback and the treatment of tension headaches: A systematic analysis of treatment components. *Behav. Ther. 11*:699–710.

Dahlof, C.G.H. and L.D. Jacobs (1996). Ketoprofen, paracetamol and placebo in the treatment of episodic tension-type headache. *Cephalalgia 16*:117–123.

Davidoff, R.A. (1998). Trigger points and myofascial pain: Toward understanding how they affect headaches. *Cephalalgia 18*:436–448.

De Benedittis, G. and A. Lorenzetti (1992). Minor stressful life events (daily hassles) in chronic primary headache: Relationship with MMPI personality patterns. *Headache* 32:330–332.

De Benedittis, G., A. Lorenzetti, and A. Pieri (1990). The role of stressful life events in the onset of chronic primary headache. *Pain 40*:65–75.

DeBenedittis, G., A. Lorenzetti, C. Sina et al. (1995). Magnetic resonance imaging in migraine and tension-type headache. *Headache* 35:264–268.

Diamond, S. (1987). Muscle contraction headache. In *Wolff's Headache and Other Head Pain*, 5th ed. (D.J. Dalessio, ed.), pp. 172–189. Oxford University Press, New York.

Donias, S.H., S. Peioglou-Harmoussi, G. Georgiadis et al. (1991). Differential emotional precipitation of migraine and tension-type headache attacks. *Cephalalgia 11*:47–52.

Drummond P.D. (1987). Scalp tenderness and sensitivity to pain in migraine and tension headache. *Headache 27*:45–50.

Drummond, P.D. and J.W. Lance (1984). Clinical diagnoses and computer analyses of headache symptoms. *J. Neurol. Neurosurg. Psychiatry 47*: 128–133.

Featherstone, H.J. (1985). Migraine and muscle contraction headaches: A continuum. *Headache* 25:194–198.

Ferrari, M.D. (1993). Biochemistry of tension-type headache. In *Tension-type Headache: Classification, Mechanisms, and Treatment* (J. Olesen and J. Schoenen eds.), pp. 117–126. Raven Press, New York.

Ficek, S.K. and D.A. Wittrock (1995). Subjective stress and coping in recurrent tension-type headache. *Headache* 35:455–460.

Glassman, J.M. and J.P. Soyka (1980). Muscle contraction (tension) headache; a double blind study comparing the efficacy and safety of meprobamate–aspirin with butalbital–aspirin–phenacetin–caffeine. *Curr. Ther. Res. 28*:904–909.

Godaux, E. and J.E. Desmedt (1975). Exteroceptive suppression and motor control of the masseter and temporalis muscles in normal man. *Brain Res. 85*:447–458.

Hammell, J.M., T.M. Cook, and J.C. Rosecrance (1996). Effectiveness of a physical therapy regimen in the treatment of tension-type headache. *Headache 36*:149–153.

Hatch, J.P., T.J. Prihoda, P.J. Moore et al. (1991). A naturalistic study of the relationships among electromyographic activity, psychological stress, and pain in ambulatory tension-type headache patients and headache-free controls. *Psychosom. Med.* 53:576–584.

Hatch, J.P., L.S. Schoenfeld, N.N. Boutros et al. (1991). Anger and hostility in tension-type headache. *Headache 31*:302–304.

Headache Classification Committee of the International Headache Society. (1988). Classification and diagnostic criteria for headache disorders, cranial neuralgias, and facial pain. *Cephalalgia* 8(Suppl. 7):1–96.

Hoffmann, E. (1979). Autonomic, EEG and clinical changes in neurotic patients during EMG biofeedback training. *Res. Commun. Psychol. Psych. Behav. 4*:209–239.

Iversen, H.K., Langemark, M., Andersson, P.G. et al. (1990). Clinical characteristics of migraine and episodic tension-type headache in relation to old and new diagnostic criteria. *Headache 30*: 514–519.

Jensen, R. (1995). Mechanisms of spontaneous tension-type headaches: An analysis of tenderness, pain thresholds and EMG. *Pain 64*:251–256.

Jensen, R., L. Bendtsen, and J. Olesen (1998). Muscular factors are of importance in tension-type headache. *Headache 38*:10–17.

Jensen, R. and T. Paiva (1993). Episodic tension-type headache. In *The Headaches* (J. Olesen, P. Tfelt-Hansen and K.M.A. Welch, eds.), pp. 497–502. Raven Press, New York.

Jensen, R. and B.K. Rasmussen (1996). Muscular disorders in tension-type headache. *Cephalalgia 16*:97–103.

Jensen, R., B.K. Rasmussen, and J. Olesen (1993). Cephalic muscle tenderness and pressure pain threshold in headache. *Pain 52*:193–199.

Kitano, A., T. Shimomura, T. Takeshima et al. (1994). Increased 11-dehydrothromboxane B_2 in migraine: Platelet hyperfunction in patients with migraine during headache-free period. *Headache 34*:515–518.

Larsson, B., L. Melin, and A. Doberl (1990). Recurrent tension headache in adolescents treated with self-help relaxation training and a muscle relaxant drug. *Headache 30*:665–671.

Lichstein, K.L., S.M. Fischer, T.L. Eakin et al. (1991). Psycho-physiological parameters of migraine and muscle-contraction headaches. *Headache 31*:27–34.

Lipton, R.B., W.F. Stewart, R. Cady et al. (2000). Sumatriptan for the range of headaches in migraine sufferers: Results of the spectrum study. *Headache 40*:783–791.

Lous, I. and J. Olesen (1982). Evaluation of pericranial tenderness and oral function in patients with common migraine, muscle contraction headache and combination headache. *Pain 12*: 385–393.

Mathew, N.T., R. Kurman, and F. Perez (1990). Drug-induced refractory headache: Clinical features and management. *Headache 30*:634–638.

Mathew, N.T., U. Reuveni, and F. Perez (1987). Transformed or evolutive migraine. *Headache* 27:102–106.

Mauskop, A., B.T. Altura, R.Q. Cracco et al. (1993). Serum ionized magnesium levels in patients with tension-type headaches. In *Tension-type Headache: Classification, Mechanisms, and Treatment* (J. Olesen and J. Schoenen, eds.), pp. 137–140. Raven Press, New York.

Mehlisch, D.R., M. Weaver, and B. Fladung (1998). Ketoprofen, acetaminophen and placebo in the treatment of tension headache. *Headache* 38:579–589.

Merikangas, K.R. (1994). Psychopathology and headache syndromes in the community. *Headache* 34:S17–S26.

Murphy, A.I. and P.M. Lehrer (1990). Headache versus nonheadache state: A study of electrophysiological and affective changes during muscle contraction headaches. *Behav. Med.* 16:23–30.

Nagata, K., Y. Hirata, Y. Satoh et al. (1993). Neurologic and radiologic profiles of tension-type headache. In *Tension-type Headache: Classification, Mechanisms, and Treatment* (J. Olesen and J. Schoenen, eds.), pp. 131–136. Raven Press, New York.

Oishi, M. and Y. Mochizuki (1998). B-Thromboglobulin and 11-dehydrothromboxane B_2 in tension-type headache. *Headache* 38:676–678.

Peterson, A.L., G.W. Talcott, W.J. Kelleher et al. (1995). Site specificity of pain and tension in tension-type headaches. *Headache* 35:89–92.

Pfaffenrath, V., J. Hummelsberger, W. Pollmann et al. (1991). MMPI personality profiles in patients with primary headache syndromes. *Cephalalgia* 11:263–268.

Philips, C. and M. Hunter (1981). The treatment of tension headache—I. Muscular abnormality and biofeedback. *Behav. Res. Ther.* 19:485–498.

Puca, F., S. Genco, M.P. Prudenzano et al. (1999). The Italian Collaborative Group for the Study of Psychopathological Factors in Primary Headaches. Psychiatric comorbidity and psychosocial stress in patients with tension-type headache from headache centers in Italy. *Cephalalgia* 19:159–164.

Raskin, N.H. (1988). *Headache*, 2nd ed., pp. 215–224. Churchill Livingstone, New York.

Rasmussen, B.K. (1992). Migraine and tension-type headache in a general population: Psychosocial factors. *Int. J. Epidemiol.* 21:1138–1143.

Rasmussen, B.K. (1993). Migraine and tension-type headache in a general population: Precipitating factors, female hormones, sleep pattern and relation to life-style. *Pain* 53:65–72.

Rasmussen, B.K., R. Jensen, and J. Olesen (1991a). A population-based analysis of the diagnostic criteria of the International Headache Society. *Cephalalgia* 11:129–134.

Rasmussen, B.K., R. Jensen, M. Schroll et al. (1991b). Epidemiology of headache in a general population—a prevalence study. *J. Clin. Epidemiol.* 44:1147–1157.

Rugh, J.D., J.P. Hatch, P.J. Moore et al. (1990). The effects of psychological stress on electro-myographic activity and negative affect in ambulatory tension-type headache patients. *Headache* 30:216–219.

Sandrini, G., F. Antonaci, E. Pucci et al. (1994). Comparative study with EMG, pressure algometry and manual palpation in tension-type headache and migraine. *Cephalalgia* 14:451–457.

Saper, J.R. (1986). Changing perspectives of chronic headache. *Clin. J. Pain* 2:19–28.

Schoenen, J. (1993). Central mechanisms in tension-type headache: Assessment by neurophysiologic methods, in particular exteroceptive suppression of temporalis muscle activity. In *Tension-type Headache: Classification, Mechanisms, and Treatment* (J. Olesen and J. Schoenen, eds.), pp. 147–160. Raven Press, New York.

Schoenen, J., P. Gerard, V. DePasqua et al. (1991). EMG activity in pericranial muscles during postural variation and mental activity in healthy volunteers and patients with chronic tension-type headache. *Headache* 31:321–324.

Schwartz, B.S., W.F. Stewart, D. Simon et al. (1998). Epidemiology of tension-type headache. *JAMA* 279:381–383.

Solomon, S. (1994). OTC analgesics in treating common primary headaches: A review of safety and efficacy. *Headache* 34(Suppl 1):13–21.

Thie, A., A. Fuhlendorf, K. Spitzer et al. (1990a). Transcranial Doppler evaluation of common and classic migraine. Part I. Ultrasonic features during the headache-free period. *Headache* 30:201–208.

Thie, A., A. Fuhlendorf, K. Spitzer et al. (1990b). Transcranial Doppler evaluation of common and classic migraine. Part II. Ultrasonic features during attacks. *Headache* 30:209–215.

Wallasch, T.M. (1993). Transcranial Doppler ultrasonic findings in episodic and chronic tension-type headache. In *Tension-type Headache: Classification, Mechanisms, and Treatment* (J. Olesen and J. Schoenen, eds.), pp. 127–130. Raven Press, New York.

Wallasch, T.M., P. Kropp, T. Weinschutz et al. (1993). Contingent negative variation in tension-type headache. In *Tension-type Headache: Classification, Mechanisms, and Treatment* (J. Olesen and J. Schoenen, eds.), pp. 173–175. Raven Press, New York.

Wittrock, D.A. (1997). The comparison of individuals with tension-type headache and headache-free controls on frontal EMG levels: A meta-analysis. *Headache* 37:424–432.

Ziegler, D.K. and R.S. Hassanein (1990). Specific headache phenomena: Their frequency and coincidence. *Headache* 30:152–156.

Ziegler, D.K., R. Hassanein, and K. Hassanein (1972). Headache syndromes suggested by factor analysis of symptom variables in a headache prone population. *J. Chron. Dis.* 25:353–363.

11

Chronic Daily Headache, Including Transformed Migraine, Chronic Tension-Type Headache, and Medication Overuse

STEPHEN D. SILBERSTEIN
RICHARD B. LIPTON

There is no consensus on the classification of very frequent headache disorders, sometimes referred to as chronic daily headache (CDH). Some authors use CDH to refer to chronic or transformed migraine; others use it for any headache disorder that occurs on a daily or near-daily basis, regardless of cause. The International Headache Society (IHS) has not addressed the classification of very frequent primary headache disorders. In this chapter, we use CDH to refer to the broad group of people with very frequent headaches (15 or more days/month), including those headaches associated with medication overuse. We divide CDH into primary and secondary varieties.

Primary CDH sufferers have headaches not related to a structural or systemic illness, more than 15 days/month. Population-based studies in the United States, Europe, and Asia suggest that 4% to 5% of the general population have primary CDH (Scher et al., 1998; Castillo et al., 1999; Wang et al., 2000) and that 0.5% have severe headaches on a daily basis (Newman et al., 1994). In population samples, chronic tension-type headache

(CTTH) is the leading cause of primary CDH (Rasmussen, 1992). Patients with frequent headaches account for the majority of consultations in headache subspecialty practices (Silberstein et al., 1994a). These patients often overuse medication, which may play a role in initiating or sustaining the pattern of pain. Anxiety, depression, and other psychologic disturbances may accompany the headaches (Silberstein et al., 1994a). These disorders require treatment. They are also less common causes of primary CDH of short duration (Table 11–1).

Secondary CDH occurs 15 or more times a month and has some identifiable underlying cause. Secondary causes of frequent headache are reviewed in Table 11–1. These include post-traumatic headache, cervical spine disorders, headache associated with vascular disorders, headache associated with nonvascular intracranial disorders, and other disorders (i.e., temporomandibular joint disorder or sinus infection).

Patients with primary CDH are difficult to classify using the IHS system as it is currently framed (Solomon et al., 1992b; Sanin et al.,

Table 11–1 Chronic daily headache

Primary chronic daily headache
  Headache duration ≥4 hours
    Chronic migraine (previously transformed
      migraine)
    Chronic tension-type headache
    New daily persistent headache
    Hemicrania continua
  Headache duration <4 hours
    Cluster headache
    Paroxysmal hemicranias
    Hypnic headache
    Idiopathic stabbing headache
Secondary chronic daily headache
  Post-traumatic headache
  Cervical spine disorders
    Headache associated with vascular disorders
      (arteriovenous malformation; arteritis, including
      giant cell arteritis; dissection; and subdural
      hematoma)
    Headache associated with nonvascular intracranial
      disorders [intracranial hypertension, infection
      (EBV, HIV), neoplasm]
    Other (temporomandibular joint disorder, sinus
      infection)

Key to abbreviations: EBV, Epstein-Barr virus; HIV, human immunodeficiency virus.

1994; Messinger et al., 1991; Pfaffenrath and Isler, 1993). When they can be classified, many of these individuals meet criteria for two or three distinct disorders, including CTTH, migraine headache, and medication-withdrawal headache in various combinations. Several lines of evidence (outlined below) suggest that many patients with primary CDH begin with episodic migraine and develop a chronic form of migraine. It seems inappropriate to classify their headaches, without regard to natural history, as a form of TTH (Silberstein et al., 1994a).

An approach to classifying frequent headache is presented in Table 11–1. We first define a primary or secondary CDH syndrome. We subclassify primary CDH on the basis of average headache duration a day (≥4 hours or <4 hours). Chronic migraine (formerly transformed migraine), new daily persistent headache (NDPH), and hemicrania continua are primary CDH disorders not yet included in the IHS classification (Table 11–2).

Primary CDH of shorter duration (<4 hours) includes chronic cluster headache, chronic paroxysmal hemicrania, hypnic headache, idiopathic stabbing headache, and the

cranial neuralgias. Both the short- and long-duration primary and secondary disorders can be associated with medication-overuse syndromes.

Causes of secondary CDH include post-traumatic headache and headache associated with cervical spine disorders, including cervical disc lesions (discussed in Chapters 14, 16, and 19) (Edmeads, 1988; Brain, 1963; Mathew, 1991; Lake et al., 1993). Other secondary causes of frequent headache include chronic meningitis and idiopathic intracranial hypertension (Mathew, 1982; Mathew et al., 1982, 1987; Olesen et al., 1993; Saper, 1983). Cervicogenic headache (Sjaastad et al., 1983) is a unilateral pain disorder that does not switch sides (Sjaastad, 1990), occurs mainly in women, and may be associated with ipsilateral blurred vision, tinnitus, lacrimation, tingling, difficulty swallowing, photophobia, arm pain, and, when more severe, nausea and anorexia. "Neck triggers" and reduced cervical range of motion are characteristic. It is uncertain whether cervicogenic headache is an independent entity or migraine or TTH with a cervical trigger (Pfaffenrath and Kaube, 1990). This makes its classification uncertain.

Patients with CDH can have idiopathic intracranial hypertension and are easily diagnosed when papilledema is present. Some patients do not have papilledema; this condition can mimic primary CDH (see Chapter 16). This issue is further complicated by the ob-

Table 11–2 Proposed headache classification for chronic daily headache

Daily or near-daily headache lasting >4 hours for >15
  days/month
  1.8 Chronic migraine (previously transformed
    migraine)
    1.8.1 with medication overuse
    1.8.2 without medication overuse
  2.2 Chronic tension-type headache
    2.2.1 with medication overuse
    2.2.2 without medication overuse
  4.7 New daily persistent headache
    4.7.1 with medication overuse
    4.7.2 without medication overuse
  4.8 Hemicrania continua
    4.8.1 with medication overuse
    4.8.2 without medication overuse

Modified from Silberstein, S.D., R.B. Lipton, S. Solomon et al. (1994a). Classification of daily and near daily headaches: Proposed revisions to the IHS classification. *Headache* 34:1–7.

servation of Mosek et al. (1999), who prospectively measured cerebrospinal fluid opening pressure in 24 patients who had CDH without papilledema. The average cerebrospinal fluid opening pressure was 170 ± 41 mm of cerebrospinal fluid, and five patients (21%) had an opening pressure of greater than 200 mm of cerebrospinal fluid. Chronic daily headache patients had a mean cerebrospinal fluid opening pressure that was 13 mm higher than nonheadache patients (p = 0.05) after adjusting for body mass index, age, sex, and various nonheadache disorders. The odds of having a cerebrospinal fluid opening pressure greater than 200 mm cerebrospinal fluid were five times greater for CDH patients than nonheadache patients.

Several authors have examined the relative frequency of some of these conditions in CDH patients in clinic-based studies. Mathew et al. (1987) found that 77% of patients with CDH had what they labeled "transformed migraine." Solomon et al. (1992a) found that most of their CDH patients had transformed migraine. Sandrini et al. (1993) classified 90 consecutive CDH patients who attended an outpatient clinic in Italy. Most had CDH evolving from migraine (75.0%), 16.7% had CDH that had begun de novo, and 7.7% had CDH that had evolved from episodic tension-type headache (ETTH). They differentiated two subsets of patients with CDH evolving from migraine: "transformed migraine" referred to those patients who had distinct bouts of migraine that evolved into CDH with the disappearance of typical migraine attacks and "migraine with interparoxysmal headache" was defined as recurrent bouts of migraine with a constant, low-severity headache between attacks. This can also be described as coexistent migraine and CTTH.

Silberstein et al. (1990) studied 300 patients who were admitted to an inpatient unit with chronic refractory headache. Most patients (72%) had CDH associated with medication overuse. Fifty patients who overused medication were followed for 2 years (Silberstein and Silberstein, 1992). Most had transformed migraine (74%), some had NDPH (24%), and only 2% had CTTH with a diag-

nosis of prior ETTH. Most patients (80%) reverted to episodic headache following detoxification, suggesting that both transformed migraine and NDPH associated with medication overuse are perpetuated by drug overuse. This will be validated only after long-term follow-up.

In this chapter, we discuss the classification and treatment of primary CDH of long duration, highlighting the four categories outlined above. At present, the IHS provides criteria for only one of these disorders. We propose revisions to the IHS system and offer criteria for chronic migraine, CTTH, NDPH, and hemicrania continua (Silberstein et al., 1994a). We also discuss the role of medication overuse in the development and treatment of these disorders as well as their mechanisms and treatment (Table 11–2).

CHRONIC MIGRAINE

Many studies have described the process and associated features of chronic migraine (CM) (Silberstein et al., 1995; Mathew, 1982; Mathew et al., 1982, 1987; Olesen et al., 1993; Saper, 1983). This disorder has been variously called transformed or evolutive migraine or mixed headache. Patients with CM often have a past history of episodic migraine that typically began in their teens or twenties (Silberstein et al., 1995). Most patients with this disorder are women, 90% of whom have a history of migraine without aura. Patients often report a process of transformation characterized by headaches that become more frequent over months to years, with the associated symptoms of photophobia, phonophobia, and nausea becoming less severe and less frequent (Mathew, 1982, 1987; Mathew et al., 1982, Saper, 1983). Patients often develop (or transform into) a pattern of daily or nearly-daily headaches that phenomenologically resemble CTTH; i.e., the pain is often mild to moderate and is not always associated with photophobia, phonophobia, or gastrointestinal features. Other features of migraine, including aggravation by menstruation and other trigger factors, as well as unilaterality and gastrointestinal symptoms, may persist.

Attacks of full-blown migraine superimposed on a background of less severe headaches occur in many patients. The term "transformed migraine" (TM) has been used to refer to this process. We prefer the term "CM" because a history of transformation is often missing (see below).

About 80% of CDH patients seen in subspecialty clinics overuse symptomatic medication (Mathew, 1993; Mathew et al., 1982, 1987; Saper, 1983). Headaches often increase in frequency during a period of increasing medication use. Stopping the overused medication frequently results in distinct headache improvement, although improvement may take days to weeks. Many patients have significant long-term improvement after detoxification.

In clinic-based studies, 80% of patients with CM have depression (Mathew, 1993; Saper, 1983). The depression often lifts when the pattern of medication overuse and daily headache is interrupted. Although CM is recognized as a clinical entity, widely accepted formal diagnostic criteria are lacking. We proposed and then revised criteria for CM (Table 11–3). We believe that CM is a form of migraine and that the diagnosis is best made in patients with a past history of IHS migraine who describe a process of transformation, as noted above. The period of transformation is characterized by increasing headache frequency and decreasing prominence of associated migrainous features.

In our initial proposal ("1994 criteria") (Silberstein et al., 1994a), the diagnosis of CM (then called TM) depended on a past history of IHS migraine and a process of transformation leading to headaches that last more than 4 hours/day and at least 15 days/month. The period of transformation was characterized by increasing headache frequency and decreasing prominence of associated migrainous features. We elected not to require particular characteristics for the daily or near-daily headaches, in part because these headaches are pleomorphic. Patients with CM often continue to have episodic superimposed bouts of full-blown migraine. Some patients find that their migraine headaches disappear completely (Sandrini et al., 1993; Silberstein, 1993). For this reason, we did not originally utilize the continuing occurrence of superimposed migraine attacks as part of our definition.

We tested our 1994 criteria for CM in 150 consecutive patients who presented to a headache subspecialty clinic with more than 15 headaches/month (Silberstein et al., 1995). Our objective was to develop a comprehensive classification system with appropriate categories for patients who were difficult to classify using the IHS system. We wanted to be able to assign a clinically useful diagnosis to every patient with CDH. Despite our revisions, we were unable to classify 29% of patients. A review of our classification failures revealed that 41% of the patients were not

Table 11–3 Revised criteria for chronic migraine

1.8 Chronic migraine
  A. Daily or almost daily (>15 days/month) head pain for >1 month
  B. Average headache duration of >4 hours/day (if untreated)
  C. At least one of the following:
    1. History of episodic migraine meeting any IHS criteria 1.1 to 1.6
    2. History of increasing headache frequency with decreasing severity of migrainous features over at least 3 months
    3. Headache at some time meets IHS criteria for migraine 1.1 to 1.6 other than duration
  D. Does not meet criteria for new daily persistent headache (4.7) or hemicrania continua (4.8)
  E. At least one of the following:
    1. There is no suggestion of one of the disorders listed in groups 5–11
    2. Such a disorder is suggested, but it is ruled out by appropriate investigations
    3. Such a disorder is present, but first migraine attacks do not occur in close temporal relation to the disorder

Modified from Silberstein, S.D., R.B. Lipton, S. Solomon et al. (1994a). Classification of daily and near daily headaches: Proposed revisions to the IHS classification. *Headache* 34:1–7.

able to provide an accurate history of prior headaches, while 55% could not describe a period of escalation, often because consultation occurred many years after the daily or near-daily headaches developed (Silberstein et al., 1995). As most of these patients had a clinical diagnosis of CM, we reasoned that our criteria, as originally proposed, might have been too restrictive. Patients simply could not recall their history.

Based on these data, we developed our revised criteria for TM (Table 11–3), now CM. Our criteria provide three alternative diagnostic links to migraine: (1) a prior history of IHS migraine, (2) a clear period of escalating headache frequency with decreasing severity of migrainous features (which were both required in the 1994 criteria), and (3) current superimposed attacks of headaches that meet all of the IHS criteria for migraine except duration.

To avoid undue diagnostic overlap, we proposed hierarchical rules. If a patient meets the criteria for two disorders, the rules establish which diagnosis should be used. Thus, the diagnosis of CM precludes a diagnosis of either episodic migraine (IHS 1.1 to 1.7) or CTTH. If a patient has episodic migraine and independent, coincidental CTTH, there is a risk that he or she may be misclassified as TM or CM. With these revisions, we were able to classify virtually all of our primary CDH patients. The number of CM patients increased dramatically. Using our revisions, virtually every patient not classified as CM or CTTH met the criteria for NDPH or hemicrania continua. Thus, the objective of comprehensiveness was met. Reliability and validity still need to be studied.

Krymchantowski et al. (1999) retrospectively evaluated 215 CM headache clinic patients with clear-cut prior IHS episodic migraine with or without aura. All patients had daily moderate pain, and some had intermittent attacks of severe headache: 46.5% had bilateral pain, 37.1% had hemicranial pain, 12.1% had diffuse pain, and 26.5% had pain in other locations. Throbbing pain occurred in 40.9% of patients; 36.2% had tightening pain, 17.2% had a combination of throbbing

and dull pain, 4.2% had burning pain, and 7.4% had other types of headache.

Migraine transformation most often develops when there is medication overuse, but transformation may occur without overuse (Mathew et al., 1982, 1990). Using the IHS criteria, a firm diagnosis of "headache induced by substance use or exposure" requires that the headaches remit after the overused medication is discontinued. This criterion is difficult to apply reliably, and diagnosis is impossible until the overused medication is discontinued. As an alternative, we provide definitions for medication overuse based on a review of published reports and clinical experience (see below) (Silberstein et al., 1994b).

CHRONIC TENSION-TYPE HEADACHE

Daily headaches may also develop in patients with a history of ETTH. These headaches are usually diffuse or bilateral and frequently involve the posterior aspect of the head and neck. In patients with CTTH, in contrast to those with CM, prior or coexistent episodic migraine is absent, as are most features of migraine. We proposed several modifications to the current classification of CTTH (Table 11–4). Chronic tension-type headache (2.2) requires head pain on at least 15 days/month for at least 6 months. Although the pain criteria are identical to those for ETTH, the IHS classification allows nausea but not vomiting. There is a need for operational rules regarding nausea, photophobia, and phonophobia and for their prominence (Pfaffenrath and Isler, 1993). It is possible that mild nausea or mild photophobia and phonophobia may prove to be compatible with the diagnosis of CTTH if better measures of symptom severity are developed (Pfaffenrath and Isler, 1993; Mathew et al., 1982). However, the need to include any of these migrainous features in the IHS definition of CTTH may result from including CM under the rubric of CTTH. If CM is classified separately, there may not be a need to include migrainous features in the diagnostic criteria for CTTH. For

Table 11–4 Proposed criteria for chronic tension-type headache

2.2 Chronic tension-type headache
 A. Average headache frequency >15 days/month (180 days/year) with average duration of ≥4 hours/day (if
    untreated) for 6 months fulfilling criteria B–D listed below
 B. At least 2 of the following pain characteristics:
    1. Pressing/tightening quality
    2. Mild or moderate severity (may inhibit, but does not prohibit, activities)
    3. Bilateral location
    4. No aggravation by walking stairs or similar routine physical activity
 C. History of episodic tension-type headache in the past (needs to be tested)
 D. History of evolutive headaches which gradually increased in frequency over at least a 3-month period
    (needs to be tested)
 E. Both of the following:
    1. No vomiting
    2. No more than one of nausea, photophobia, or phonophobia (needs to be tested)
 F. Does not meet criteria for hemicrania continua (4.8), new daily persistent headache (4.7), or chronic
    migraine (1.8)
 G. At least one of the following:
    1. There is no suggestion of one of the disorders listed in groups 5–11
    2. Such a disorder is suggested, but it is ruled out by appropriate investigations
    3. Such a disorder is present, but first headache attacks do not occur in close temporal relation to the
       disorder

Modified from Silberstein, S.D., R.B. Lipton, S. Solomon et al. (1994a). Classification of daily and near daily headaches: Proposed revisions to the IHS classification. *Headache* 34:1–7.

the present, the criteria we propose continue to permit only one of the symptom criteria (nausea, photophobia, and phonophobia). Migraine and CTTH might coexist with the proviso that the nonmigrainous headaches have no migrainous features. Guitera et al. (1999) have suggested, based on population-based epidemiologic data, that CTTH and migraine can coexist if and only if the current headache has no migrainous features and there is a remote history of migraine.

Chronic tension-type headache that has evolved from ETTH presupposes prior evidence of ETTH. Diagnostic confidence increases if ETTH frequency increases to meet the criteria of CTTH. Although there is no explicit headache duration in the IHS definition of CTTH, available evidence does not support a critical value. (We arbitrarily chose 4 hours to separate out cluster headache and the other shorter-duration daily headaches.) One could argue that CTTH could begin without preceding ETTH, analogous to chronic cluster (i.e., unremitting from onset). However, cluster headache includes a series of episodic attacks, not a constant headache. Does CTTH, unremitting from onset, differ from NDPH? We believe that there is a bi-

ologic difference between them, but this has not been proven. It is likely that CTTH and NDPH are themselves etiologically and biologically heterogeneous. We also distinguish between CTTH associated with medication overuse (2.2.01) and CTTH not associated with medication overuse (2.2.0.2).

Pfaffenrath and Isler (1993) proposed alternative modifications of the CTTH criteria to allow some migrainous features, such as pulsatile pain, predominantly one-sided pain location, photophobia and phonophobia, mild nausea, and anorexia but not severe nausea or vomiting. They recognized that some primary CDH patients could not be classified within the current IHS system. They advocated expanding the CTTH group instead of expanding the migraine group. We prefer to expand the migraine group because of the arguments outlined above that tie TM to migraine. In the absence of a definitive biologic marker or gold standard for migraine diagnosis, it is difficult to argue absolutely for either position. Classification rules for patients with current migraine or current ETTH and the hierarchy that relates these disorders require further definition. As genetic markers emerge, biologically homogeneous subgroups of primary CDH may well be defined. The IHS is now revising their criteria and may elect to expand migraine and add CM.

Russell et al. (1999) evaluated CTTH in a family study of 122 probands and 377 first-degree relatives. Sensitivity, specificity, predictive values, and chance-corrected agreement rate for the diagnosis of CTTH were 68%, 86%, 53% (PVpos), 92% (PVneg), and 0.48, respectively. The low sensitivity of CTTH assessed by proband report indicates that a clinical interview of family members is necessary. Clinically interviewed parents, siblings, and children had a 2.1- to 3.9-fold increased risk of CTTH compared with the general population. The proband's gender did not influence the risk of CTTH among first-degree relatives. The significantly increased familial risk, with no increased risk found in spouses, suggests that a genetic factor is involved in CTTH.

We elected not to classify NDPH as a type of de novo CTTH, for it is not clear whether or not this condition is etiologically related to TTH. Since NDPH and CTTH have similar characteristics, the absence or presence of a past history of headache distinguishes the disorders. New daily persistent headache requires the absence of a history of evolution from migraine or ETTH. Excluding all patients with a history of ETTH is problematic as almost 70% of men and 90% of women have had a TTH in the past. We allow a diagnosis of NDPH in patients with migraine or ETTH if these disorders do not increase in frequency to give rise to NDPH. The constancy of location is uncertain and needs to be field-tested. New daily persistent headache may or may not be associated with medication overuse (4.7.1, 4.7.2). A diagnosis of NDPH takes precedence over TM and CTTH.

NEW DAILY PERSISTENT HEADACHE

New daily persistent headache (Vanast, 1986) is characterized by the relatively abrupt onset of an unremitting primary CDH; i.e., a patient develops a headache that does not remit (Table 11–5). It is likely to be a heterogeneous disorder. Some cases may reflect a postviral syndrome (Vanast, 1986). The daily headache develops abruptly, over less than 3 days. Patients with NDPH are generally younger than those with TM (Vanast, 1986).

HEMICRANIA CONTINUA

Hemicrania continua (HC) is a rare, indomethacin-responsive headache disorder characterized by a continuous, moderately severe, unilateral headache that varies in intensity, waxing and waning without disappearing completely (Newman et al., 1993). It may alternate sides, although this is rare (Bordini et al., 1991). Hemicrania continua is frequently associated with jabs and jolts (idiopathic stabbing headache). Exacerbations of pain are of-

Table 11–5 Proposed criteria for new daily persistent headache

4.7 New daily persistent headache
  A. Average headache frequency >15 days/month for >1 month
  B. Average headache duration >4 hours/day (if untreated). Frequently constant without medication but may fluctuate
  C. No history of tension-type headache or migraine which increases in frequency and decreases in severity in association with the onset of new daily persistent headache (over 3 months)
  D. Acute onset (developing over <3 days) of constant unremitting headache
  E. Headache is constant in location? (Needs to be tested)
  F. Does not meet criteria for hemicrania continua (4.8)
  G. At least one of the following:
    1. There is no suggestion of one of the disorders listed in groups 5–11
    2. Such a disorder is suggested, but it is ruled out by appropriate investigations
    3. Such a disorder is present, but first headache attacks do not occur in close temporal relation to the disorder

Modified from Silberstein, S.D., R.B. Lipton, S. Solomon et al. (1994a). Classification of daily and near daily headaches: Proposed revisions to the IHS classification. *Headache* 34:1–7.

ten associated with autonomic disturbances, such as ptosis, miosis, tearing, and sweating. Hemicrania continua is not triggered by neck movements, but tender spots in the neck may be present (Table 11–6). Some patients may have photophobia, phonophobia, and nausea.

Although the disorder almost invariably has a prompt and enduring response to indomethacin, the requirement of a therapeutic response as a diagnostic criterion is problematic. It effectively excludes the diagnosis of HC in patients who were never treated with indomethacin (perhaps because another agent helped) and patients who failed to respond to indomethacin. Treatment response is generally not part of IHS case definitions of headache disorders. Cases have been described that did not respond to indomethacin but meet the phenotype; for this reason, we have provided an alternate means of diagnosis (Table 11–6). A case responding to the piroxicam-β-cyclodextrin further suggests that while the nonsteroidal anti-inflammatory

drug (NSAID) response is of great interest, it points to, rather than expresses, the pathophysiology.

Hemicrania continua exists in continuous and remitting forms. In the remitting variety, distinct headache phases last weeks to months, with prolonged pain-free remissions (Newman et al., 1993; Iordanidis and Sjaastad, 1989; Pareja et al., 1990). In the continuous variety, headaches occur on a daily, continuous basis, sometimes for years. The continuous variety can be subclassified into (1) an evolutive, unremitting form that arises from the remitting form (Sjaastad and Tjorstad, 1987; Sjaastad and Antonaci, 1993) and (2) an unremitting form characterized by continuous headache from the onset (Zukerman et al., 1987). Both forms meet the criteria in Table 11–6. Fifteen percent of patients have the remitting form, 32% have the evolutive form, and 53% have the unremitting form. A chronic form evolving to a remitting form (Pareja, 1995), a bilateral case, and a patient whose attacks alternated sides (Newman et al., 1993) have been described. Hemicrania continua takes precedence over the diagnosis of other types of primary CDH. Many patients with HC overuse acute medication; it must be differentiated from TM.

Hemicrania continua is differentiated from cluster headache and chronic paroxysmal hemicrania primarily by its continuous, moderate pain and the lack of autonomic features between painful exacerbations. Although there are no reports of secondary HC, it can be aggravated by a C7 root irritation due to a disc herniation (Sjaastad et al., 1985). A case of a mesenchymal tumor in the sphenoid bone in which the response to indomethacin faded after 2 months has also been reported (Antonaci and Sjaastad, 1992). These cases suggest that escalating doses or loss of indomethacin's efficacy should be treated with suspicion and the patient re-evaluated. Hemicrania continua is seen in non-Caucasian populations (Joubert, 1991).

The relative rarity of HC has made it difficult to study its pathophysiology. Pain pressure thresholds are reduced in patients with HC as they are in chronic paroxysmal hemicrania patients (Antonaci et al., 1994). In con-

Table 11–6 Proposed criteria for hemicrania continua

4.8 Hemicrania continua[a]
  A. Headache present for at least 1 month
  B. Strictly unilateral headache
  C. Pain has all 3 of the following present:
    1. Continuous but fluctuating
    2. Moderate severity, at least some of the time
    3. Lack of precipitating mechanisms
  D. 1. Absolute response to indomethacin or
     2. One of the following autonomic features with severe pain exacerbation
        (a) Conjunctival infection
        (b) Lacrimation
        (c) Nasal congestion
        (d) Rhinorrhea
        (e) Ptosis
        (f) Eyelid edema
  E. May have associated stabbing headaches
  F. At least one of the following:
     1. There is no suggestion of one of the disorders listed in groups 5–11
     2. Such a disorder is suggested, but it is ruled out by appropriate investigations
     3. Such a disorder is present, but first headache attacks do not occur in close temporal relation to the disorder

[a]Hemicrania continua is usually nonremitting, but rare cases of remission have been reported.

Modified from Goadsby, P.J. and R.B. Lipton (1997). A review of paroxysmal hemicranias, SUNCT syndrome and other short-lasting headaches with autonomic features, including new cases. *Brain* 120:193–209.

trast, orbital phlebography is relatively normal compared to patients with chronic paroxysmal hemicrania (Antonaci, 1994), although this area is controversial (Bovim et al., 1992). Pupillometric studies have shown no clear abnormality in HC (Antonaci et al., 1992), and studies of facial sweating have shown modest changes, similar to those seen in chronic paroxysmal hemicrania (Antonaci, 1991).

Espada et al. (1999) reported five men and four women who had HC diagnosed using Goadsby and Lipton's (1997) draft diagnostic criteria (eight continuous and one remitting, with a mean age at onset of 53.3 years, range 29–69). All nine patients had initial relief with indomethacin (mean daily dose 94.4 mg, range 50–150). Follow-up was possible in eight patients. Indomethacin could be discontinued after 3, 7, and 15 months, respectively, and patients remained pain-free. Three patients discontinued treatment because of side effects and had headache recurrence; two had relief with aspirin. Two other patients continue to take indomethacin with partial relief.

DRUG OVERUSE AND REBOUND HEADACHE

Patients with frequent headaches often overuse analgesics, opioids, ergotamine, and triptans (Katsarava et al., 1999). Medication overuse may be both a response to chronic pain and a consequence of chronic pain, or in headache-prone patients, medication overuse may produce drug-induced "rebound headache" accompanied by dependence on symptomatic medication. In addition, medication overuse can make headaches refractory to prophylactic medication (Mathew et al., 1990; Mathew, 1990; Diamond and Dalessio, 1982; Wilkinson, 1988; Saper, 1987, 1989). Although stopping the acute medication may result in the development of withdrawal symptoms and a period of increased headache, there is generally subsequent headache improvement (Saper, 1989; Andersson, 1988; Baumgartner et al., 1989; Rapoport et al., 1986; Saper and Jones, 1986). Many primary CDH patients withdrawn from ergotamine

and analgesics and given no further therapy no longer had daily headaches, although about 40% still had episodic migraine attacks (Dichgans et al., 1984; Rapoport, 1988).

In subspecialty centers, most patients with drug-induced headache have a history of episodic migraine that has been converted into CM as a result of medication overuse (Mathew et al., 1987, 1990; Mathew, 1990; Rapoport, 1988; Kudrow, 1982; Diener et al., 1989; Rasmussen et al., 1989). Patients with TTH, HC, and NDPH may also overuse symptomatic medications. Drug-induced primary CDH or, as Isler (1988) has termed it, "painkiller headache" has been reported since the 17th century, with occurrences reaching epidemic proportions in Switzerland after World War II.

The epidemiology of chronic drug-induced headache is uncertain since some cases are drug-induced and some are just associated with drug overuse. In European headache centers, 5% to 10% of patients have drug-induced headache. One series of 3,000 consecutive headache patients reported that 4.3% had drug-induced headaches (Micieli et al., 1988). Experiences in the United Kingdom (P. Goadsby, personal communication) suggest that drug-associated headache is more common than the literature suggests. In American specialty headache clinics, as many as 80% of patients who presented with primary CDH used analgesics on a daily or near-daily basis (Rapoport, 1988). Other headache clinics report a smaller percentage but a majority nonetheless (Solomon et al., 1992a). In India, in contrast, medication overuse is less common (Ravishankar, 1997).

Diener and Tfelt-Hansen (1993) summarized 29 studies including 2,612 patients with chronic drug-induced headache. Migraine was the primary headache in 65% of patients, TTH in 27%, and mixed or other headaches (i.e., cluster headache) in 8%. Women had more drug-induced headaches than men (3.5:1; 1,533 women, 442 men). The mean duration of primary headache was 20.4 years. The mean admitted time of frequent drug intake was 10.3 years in one study, and the mean duration of daily headache was 5.9 years. Results from headache diaries show that the number of tablets or suppositories taken daily averaged 4.9 (range 0.25–25). Patients averaged 2.5 to 5.8 different pharmacologic components simultaneously (range 1–14) (Diener and Tfelt-Hansen, 1993).

Patients attending an outpatient neurology clinic in Austria reported taking, on average, 6.3 different headache pain drugs (Schnider et al., 1994). Of these patients, 26.5% reported using both prescription and over-the-counter medications, 31.3% used over-the-counter medications only, and 27.7% used prescription drugs only. Acetaminophen (average dose 500 mg) was the most frequently used analgesic. Most patients attending a London migraine clinic used multiple medications (Silberstein and Saper, 1993). Acetaminophen, again, was the most commonly used analgesic (34.9%), followed by aspirin (22.9%).

In a cross-sectional survey carried out in Tromsø in 1986–87, 19,137 men and women (aged 12 to 56 years) from the general population were asked about their drug use over the preceding 14 days. On average, 28% of the women and 13% of the men had used analgesics. The most significant predictor of analgesic use was headache; a lesser association was found with infections. Drug use in women was associated with symptoms of depression. Drug use in men was associated with sleeplessness. Higher drug use was associated with smoking and high coffee consumption but not with frequent alcohol intake (Eggen, 1993).

In a representative sample of the Swiss population, 4.4% of men and 6.8% of women took analgesics at least once a week; 2.3% took them daily (Gutzwiller and Zemp, 1986). Analgesic dependence was more frequent than dependence on tranquilizers, hypnotics, and stimulating drugs in psychiatric inpatients in Switzerland (Kieholz and Ladewig, 1981). In Germany, possibly 1% of the population take up to ten pain tablets every day (Schwarz et al., 1985).

In the United States, 20.2% of a national sample survey of 20,468 individuals reported "severe headache;" 62.6% of the women and 74.6% of the men used over-the-counter medications, while prescription drugs were used by 34.5% of the women and 21.3% of the men. Over-the-counter analgesic use was greater than prescription medication use among migraineurs as well as among those suffering from undefined severe headache (Celentano et al., 1992). This could be either a cause or a result of the severe headache.

A random telephone survey of 24,159 households in Canada produced a sample of 1,573 households with one or more eligible headache sufferers. Ninety percent of the IHS-diagnosed migraineurs reported using over-the-counter drugs and 44% reported using prescription drugs. In this sample, 1.5% of migraineurs had rebound headache resulting from ergotamine tartrate or analgesic overuse. Drug-induced rebound headache is a major public health problem in both the clinic and the community (Robinson, 1993).

CLINICAL FEATURES OF REBOUND HEADACHE

Analgesic rebound headache has not been demonstrated in placebo-controlled trials. However, stopping daily low-dose caffeine frequently results in withdrawal headache (Silverman et al., 1992). In a controlled study of caffeine withdrawal, 64 normal adults (71% women) with low to moderate caffeine intake (the equivalent of about 2.5 cups of coffee/day) were given a 2-day caffeine-free diet and either placebo or replacement caffeine. Under double-blind conditions, 50% of the patients who were given placebo had a headache by day 2 compared to 6% of those given caffeine. Nausea, depression, and flu-like symptoms were common in the placebo group. This study is relevant since caffeine is frequently used by headache sufferers for pain relief, often in combination with analgesics or ergotamine. The study is a model for short-term caffeine withdrawal but does not demonstrate the long-term consequences of detoxification. In a community-based telephone survey of 11,112 subjects in Lincoln and Omaha, Nebraska, 61% reported daily caffeine consumption and 11% of the caffeine consumers reported symptoms upon stopping coffee (Potter et al., 2000). A group of those who reported withdrawal were assigned to one of three regimes: abrupt caffeine withdrawal, gradual withdrawal, and no change. One-third of the abrupt-withdrawal group and an occasional member of the gradual-withdrawal group had symptoms that included headache and tiredness.

The actual dose limits and the time needed to develop rebound headaches have not been defined in rigorous studies, nor is the relationship of drug half-life to rebound development known. Our clinical knowledge is derived from observing patterns of medication use in patients who present with rebound headaches. Because there may be large individual differences in susceptibility to rebound headaches, anecdotal data must be generalized cautiously. It is believed that overuse occurs when patients take three or more simple analgesics a day more often than 5 days a week, triptans or combination analgesics containing barbiturates, sedative, or caffeine more often than 3 days a week, or opioids or ergotamine tartrate more often than 2 days a week (Mathew et al., 1990; Diamond and Dalessio, 1982; Mathew, 1990; Saper, 1987; Wilkinson, 1988).

Specific limits are necessary to prevent analgesic, ergotamine, and triptan overuse. Wilkinson (1988), Saper and Jones (1986), Mathew et al. (1987), and Scholz et al. (1988) compared ergotamine intake in patients with and without primary CDH. In the groups without primary CDH, the maximum ergotamine intake was 24 mg/month. However, one patient with primary CDH consumed only 7 mg/month. The frequency of days of ergotamine use (treatment days, events) is as important as, if not more important than, the total monthly dose (Saper, 1983; Saper and Jones, 1986). Rebound headache can develop in patients taking as little as 0.5 to 1 mg of ergotamine three times a week (Silberstein, 1993; Wilkinson, 1988; Saper, 1987; Baumgartner et al., 1989).

Scholz et al. (1988) studied simple analgesic consumption in patients with and without rebound headache. Patients with rebound headache consumed between 1,200 and 1,500 mg of analgesics a day. Increased caffeine, but not codeine, consumption was correlated with the development of primary CDH. Barbiturate consumption was significantly higher in patients with primary CDH (60 to 500 mg/day, mean 160 mg/day) than in those without primary CDH (mean <60 mg/day). All of the triptans (sumatriptan, rizatriptan, naratriptan, and zolmitriptan), selective 5-HT$_1$ agonists that are effective in acute migraine treatment, have been reported to induce rebound headache (Catarci et al., 1994; Diener et al., 1991; Gaist et al., 1996). Katsarava et al. (1999) reported the first cases and the specific clinical features of drug-induced headache following the frequent use of zolmitriptan and naratriptan. All patients remained responsive to triptans. Six patients had never previously used triptans or ergotamine derivatives but developed drug-induced headache within 6 months of taking the drug. Four patients consumed 7.5 to 10 mg of zolmitriptan or 10 to 12 mg of naratriptan weekly. The weekly dosages necessary to initiate drug-induced headache with the centrally penetrant triptans may be lower than with ergotamines or sumatriptan and the time of onset might be shorter. Increasing attack frequency can be the first sign that drug-induced headache is developing. We recommend limiting the use of triptans to 3 days/week.

Most daily headache patients overuse symptomatic medication and may develop psychologic dependence, tolerance, and abstinence syndromes (Mathew et al., 1990). Medication overuse may be responsible, in part, for the transformation of episodic migraine or ETTH into daily headache and for the perpetuation of the syndrome. However, medication overuse is not the *sine qua non* of CM or CTTH. Some patients develop CM or CTTH without overusing medication, and others continue to have daily headaches long after the overused medication has been discontinued. Medication overuse is usually motivated by a patient's desire to treat the headaches (Kaiser, 1999). However, some headache patients may overuse combination analgesics to treat a mood disturbance. Medication overuse rarely represents a form of primary substance abuse.

There are those who doubt the existence of drug-induced headache (Fisher, 1988). When Fisher (1988) failed to find analgesic rebound headache in patients who were using analgesics for arthritis, he attempted to refute the concept. His work has been reinterpreted to suggest that headache-prone patients are especially vulnerable to the rebound phenomenon. Headache-prone patients often develop daily headaches if they are put on analgesics for a nonheadache indication (Bowdler et al., 1990; Lance et al., 1988).

In addition to exacerbating the headache disorder, drug overuse has other serious effects. The overuse of acute drugs may interfere with the effectiveness of preventive headache medications. Prolonged use of large amounts of medication may cause renal or hepatic toxicity in addition to tolerance, habituation, or dependence. (*Tolerance* refers to the decreased effectiveness of the same dose of an analgesic, often leading to the use of higher doses to achieve the same degree of effectiveness. *Habituation* and *dependence* are, respectively, the psychologic and physical need to repeatedly use drugs.)

PSYCHIATRIC COMORBIDITY

Anxiety, depression, panic disorder, and bipolar disease are more frequent in migraineurs than in nonmigraine control subjects (Merikangas et al., 1990; Breslau and Davis, 1993). Since CM evolves from migraine, one would expect to find psychiatric comorbidity in CM. In fact, depression occurs in 80% of CM patients. The Minnesota Multiphasic Personality Inventory (MMPI) was abnormal in 61% of primary CDH patients compared with 12.2% of patients with episodic migraine. Zung and Beck Depression Scale scores were significantly higher in primary CDH patients than in migraine controls (Mathew, 1990, 1991; Mathew et al., 1990; Saper, 1987). Comorbid depression often improves when the cycle of daily head pain is broken. Mongini et al. (1997) found that several MMPI and State and Trait anxiety index 2 scores decreased after headache improvement occurred, but 12 of 20 patients continued to have a conversion V configuration on the MMPI.

Mitsikostas and Thomas (1999) found that the average Hamilton rating scores for anxiety and depression were significantly higher in headache sufferers (17.4 and 14.2, respectively) than in healthy controls (6.8 and 5.7, respectively). High headache attack frequency, a long history of headaches, and female gender correlated with the Hamilton rating elevation for both anxiety and depression. Patients with CTTH, mixed headache, or drug-abuse headache had the highest Hamilton rating scores for depression and anxiety.

Verri et al. (1998) found current psychiatric comorbidity in 90% of primary CDH patients, 81% of migraineurs, and 83% of chronic low back pain patients (no significant differences). Generalized anxiety disorders were the most common in each group (primary CDH 69.3%, $p \leq 0.001$; migraine 59.5%, $p \leq 0.05$; chronic low back pain 65.7%, $p \leq 0.001$). The most common mood disorder in primary CDH was major depressive disorder (25%). This was significantly more frequent than dysthymia ($p \leq 0.001$) and significantly more frequent ($p \leq 0.05$) in primary CDH than in chronic low back pain patients. Somatoform disorders (including somatization, conversion disorder, and hypochondriasis) were found in 5.7% of primary CDH patients, always concomitant with anxiety and mood disorders.

Psychiatric comorbidity is a predictor of intractability. The MMPI was abnormal in 100% of patients with primary CDH who failed to respond to aggressive management (31% of the primary CDH group) compared with 48% of the responders. Physical, emotional, or sexual abuse, parental alcohol abuse, and a positive dexamethasone suppression test also correlated highly with a poor response to aggressive management. Curioso et al. (1999) found that 31 of 69 (45%) primary CDH patients had an adjustment disorder, 16 (23%) had major depression, 12 (17%) were dysthymic, 6 (9%) had generalized anxiety disorder, 1 (2%) was bipolar, and 3 (4%) were normal. The risk of a bad outcome after treatment was significantly greater for patients with major depression compared to those without. Primary CDH patients who have major depression or abnormal Beck Depression Inventory scores have worse outcomes at 3 to 6 months compared with patients who are not depressed.

Monzon and Lainez (1998), using the Medical Outcomes Study Short Form (SF-36) questionnaire, found that patients with primary CDH had significantly worse scores in physical functioning, role functioning (physical), bodily pain, general health perceptions, and mental health than migraineurs (Solomon et al., 1993).

Guitera et al. (1999) analyzed the impact of CDH on health-related quality of life using the SF-36 in a population sample, 4.7% of whom met the criteria for CDH of Silberstein et al. (1996). Controls consisted of 89 healthy subjects and 89 episodic migraineurs. All SF-36 scores were significantly reduced in the CDH patients compared with the healthy subjects. Transformed migraine patients did not differ from TTH patients. Transformed migraine patients had a general reduction in quality of life compared with episodic migraine patients. Chronic daily headache patients who overused analgesics scored significantly lower in physical role and bodily pain than those who did not overuse. The impact that CDH has on quality of life depends more on the chronicity of the headache disorder than on individual attack severity. Analgesic overuse worsens the impact.

Puca et al. (1999) evaluated 234 adult CDH patients using a structured clinical interview, the Structured Clinical Interview for the Diagnostic and Statistical Manual of Mental Disorders-IV edition and the Symptom Check List 90R. At least one psychiatric disorder was detected in 66% of the CDH patients (anxiety disorders 45%, mood disorders 33%). The prevalence of psychopathologic symptoms was more than 78%. At least one psychosocial stress factor was found in 42% of cases. Sixty-four percent of patients overused symptomatic drugs.

EPIDEMIOLOGY

In population-based surveys, primary CDH occurs in 4.1% of Americans, 4.45% of Greeks, 3.9% of elderly Chinese, and 4.7% of Spaniards. Population-based estimates for the 1-year period prevalence of CTTH are 1.7% in Ethiopia (Tekle Haimanot et al., 1995), 3% in Denmark (Rasmussen, 1995), 2.2% in Spain (Castillo et al., 1999), 2.7% in China (Wang et al., 2000), and 2.2% in the United States (Scher et al., 1998).

Using a validated, computer-assisted telephone interview, Scher et al. (1998) ascertained the prevalence of primary CDH in 13,343 individuals aged 18 to 65 years in Baltimore County, Maryland. Subjects were selected by random-digit dialing and interviewed by telephone about their headaches. Those reporting 180 or more headaches a year were classified as having frequent headache. Three mutually exclusive subtypes of frequent headache were identified: TM, CTTH, and unclassified frequent headache. The overall prevalence of primary CDH was 4.1% (5.0% women, 2.8% men; 1.8:1 women-to-men ratio). Frequent headache was 33% more common in Caucasians (4.4%) than in African-Americans (3.3%). In both men and women, prevalence was highest in the lowest educational category. More than half (52% women, 56% men) met the criteria for CTTH (2.2%), almost one-third (33% women, 25% men) met the criteria for CM (1.3%), and the remainder (15% women, 19% men) were unclassified (0.6%). Overall, 30% of women and 25% of men who were frequent headache sufferers met IHS criteria for migraine (with or without aura). On the basis of chance, migraine and CTTH would co-occur in 0.22% of the population; CM occurring in 1.3% of this population would suggest that their co-occurrence is more than random (Lipton et al., 2001a).

Castillo et al. (1999) sampled 2,252 subjects older than 14 years in Cantalucia, Spain. Subjects who had headaches more than 10 days a month were interviewed, examined, given a diary, and followed up. The response rate was 83.5%. Overall, 4.7% had CDH. Using the criteria of Silberstein et al. (1994a), none had HC, 0.1% had NDPH, 2.2% had CTTH, and 2.4% had CM. Overuse of symptomatic medication occurred in 19% of CTTH patients and 31.1% of CM patients.

Eight patients had a previous history of migraine without aura and now had primary CDH with only the characteristics of TTH. These headaches met the criteria of CM but could have been migraine and coincidental CTTH.

Wang et al. (2000) looked at the characteristics of primary CDH in a population of elderly Chinese (over 65 years of age) in two townships on Kinmen Island in August 1993. Chronic daily headache was diagnosed by a neurologist via a structured questionnaire and clinical interview. Primary CDH was diagnosed as a headache that occurred more than 15 days a month for at least 6 months in the previous year; it was subclassified into CTTH, CM, and other primary CDH. Person-to-person biannual follow-up of the primary CDH patients was done in June 1995 and August 1997. Seventy-seven percent of the eligible population (1,533/2,003) participated. Sixty patients (3.9%) had CDH. Significantly more women than men had primary CDH (5.6% and 1.8%, p < 0.001). Of the primary CDH patients, 42 (70%) had CTTH (2.7%), 15 (25%) had CM (1%), and 3 (5%) had other CDH. Only 23% of patients had consulted a physician for headache in the previous year. By multivariate logistic regression, the significant risk factors of primary CDH included analgesic overuse [odds ratio (OR) = 79], a history of migraine (OR = 6.6), and Geriatric Depression Scale-Short Form score of 8 or above (OR = 2.6). At follow-up in 1995 and 1997, approximately two-thirds of patients still had CDH. Compared with patients in remission, patients with persistent primary CDH in 1997 had a significantly higher frequency of analgesic overuse (33% vs. 0%, p = 0.03) and major depression (38% vs. 0%, p = 0.04).

PATHOPHYSIOLOGY OF CHRONIC DAILY HEADACHE

The nucleus caudalis (NC) of the trigeminal complex, the major relay nucleus for head and face pain, receives nociceptive input from cephalic blood vessels and pericranial muscles, as well as inhibitory and facilitatory supraspinal input. Recent evidence suggests that central pain facilitatory neurons (on-cells) are present in the ventromedial medulla. In addition, neurons in the trigeminal NC can be sensitized as a result of intense neuronal stimulation. Usually, the pain from intensive stimulation or injury diminishes as healing progresses. However, another type of pain occurs when the peripheral or central nervous system malfunctions. Three spatio-temporal characteristics of pain can be seen during both normal and pathophysiologic pain: (1) as pain intensity increases, the area in which it is experienced often enlarges (*radiation*); (2) the pain may outlast the evoking stimulus; and (3) repeated nociceptive stimuli may increase the perceived pain intensity, even without increased input (*sensitization*).

Chronic pain may be due to ongoing peripheral activation of nociceptors (i.e., chronic inflammation), although it may occur in the absence of painful stimuli. Although the source of pain in primary CDH is unknown and may be dependent on the subtype of CDH, recent work suggests several mechanisms that could contribute to the process: (1) abnormal excitation of peripheral nociceptive afferent fibers (perhaps due to chronic neurogenic inflammation), (2) enhanced responsiveness of NC neurons (central sensitization), (3) decreased pain modulation, (4) spontaneous central pain, or (5) a combination of these.

Peripheral Mechanisms

In migraine, trigeminal nerve activation is accompanied by the release of vasoactive neuropeptides, including calcitonin gene–related peptides (CGRP), substance P, and neurokinin A from the nerve terminals. These mediators produce mast cell activation, sensitization of the nerve terminals, and extravasation of fluid into the perivascular space around the dural blood vessels. Intense neuronal stimulation causes induction of c-fos (an immediate-early gene product) in the trigeminal NC of the brain stem. Substance P and CGRP further amplify the trigeminal terminal sensitivity by stimulating the release of bradykinin and other inflammatory mediators from non-neuronal cells (Moskowitz, 1992). Inflammatory mediators increase the responsiveness of and turn on silent, or sleeping, nociceptors. Neurotropins, such as nerve growth factor, are synthesized locally and can also activate mast cells and sensitize nerve terminals (Montalcini et al., 1995). Bradykinin and kallidin, both acting through the B_1 and B_2 receptors, can activate primary afferent nociceptors (Rang and Urban, 1995). Prostaglandins and nitric oxide (a diffusible gas that acts as a neurotransmitter) (Edelman and Gally, 1992) are endogenous mediators that can be produced locally and can sensitize nociceptors. Repeated episodes of neurogenic inflammation may chronically sensitize nociceptors and thus contribute to the development of daily headache.

Central sensitization is manifested by increased spontaneous impulse discharges, increased responsiveness to noxious and nonnoxious peripheral stimuli, and expanded receptive fields of nociceptive neurons. In animal models, conditioning stimuli that activate unmyelinated C fibers result in a marked and prolonged increase in the flexion–withdrawal reflex in rats. Repetitive C-fiber stimulation at constant intensity induces the phenomenon of *windup*, which is the increase in dorsal horn nociceptive neuron responsiveness in both magnitude and duration with each subsequent stimulus above a certain frequency (Mendell, 1966).

Morphine pretreatment and N-methyl-D-aspartate (NMDA) receptor antagonists block windup, which is mediated by NMDA and tachykinin receptors. It may be the trigger to long-lasting neuronal sensitization. Neurons that exhibit windup are less sensitive to opioids than those that do not (Post and Silberstein, 1994). Windup is accompanied by calcium entry via NMDA channels. The increased intracellular calcium induces translocation (from the cytosolic to the membrane-bound form) and activation of protein kinase C and phosphorylation of the NMDA channel, which relieves the Mg^{2+} block on the ion channel (Price et al., 1994). The increased calcium may also be responsible for the induction of the two early gene products, c-fos and c-jun, which can alter other peptides,

proteins, and receptors (Price et al., 1994). This results in increased glutamate sensitivity. Nerve growth factor and inflammatory cytokines may change the phenotype of sensory neurons, making them more sensitive to nociception (Woolf, 1995). Nerve growth factor increases the synthesis, transport, and neuronal content of substance P and CGRP. It also regulates two ion channels in sensory neurons: the capsaicin receptor ion channel and the tetrodotoxin-resistant Na^+ channel (Dray et al., 1994).

Does central sensitization play a role in headache? In animal models of head pain, there is good evidence for c-fos activation in the trigeminal NC. In the NC superior dorsal horn, c-fos is a marker for nociceptive stimulation and may be one signal for the adaptive responses of the nervous system to insult (Mungliani and Hunt, 1995). This may produce long-lasting neuronal sensitization with increased activation of the trigeminal vascular system.

Brief chemical irritation of the dura with a cocktail of four inflammatory mediators (histamine, serotonin, bradykinin, and prostaglandin E_2) made meningeal perivascular neurons pain-sensitive for a period of 1 to 2 hours, becoming more sensitive to mechanical forces (>2 g) (Strassman et al., 1996). This can explain the intracranial hypersensitivity (i.e., the worsening pain during coughing, bending over, or any head movement) and the throbbing pain of migraine (Anthony and Rasmussen, 1993).

Brief dural chemical irritation also results in temporary changes in central trigeminal neurons that receive convergent input from the dura and the skin. Their threshold decreased and their excitability increased in response to brushing and heating (<42°C) of the periorbital skin, stimuli to which they showed only minimal or no response prior to chemical stimulation (Burstein et al., 1998). Sensitization may be the basis of the extracranial tenderness that accompanies migraine. In addition, the threshold of cardiovascular responses to facial and intracranial stimuli is reduced (Yamamura et al., 1999). The enhanced neuronal responses represent a state of central sensitization, and the enhanced cardiovascular responses represent a state of intracranial hypersensitivity and cutaneous allodynia.

Burstein et al. (1998) predicted that cutaneous allodynia is present in migraine patients during attacks. They examined the pain thresholds of patients during and between migraine attacks. Many patients had periorbital cutaneous allodynia ipsilateral to the headache. Patients with allodynia were significantly older than those without cutaneous allodynia, hinting at a possible correlation between age and sensitization. These findings provide a neural basis for the pathophysiology of migraine pain and suggest a basis for continued head pain.

Bendtsen et al. (1996) found evidence for sensitization in patients with CTTH. Pericranial myofascial tenderness, evaluated by manual palpation, was considerably higher in patients than in controls ($p < 0.00001$). The stimulus–response function from highly tender muscle was qualitatively different from normal muscle, suggesting that myofascial pain may be mediated by low-threshold mechanosensitive afferents projecting to sensitized dorsal horn neurons.

Lassen et al. (1997) discovered that nitroglycerin, a nitric oxide donor, can induce headache in CTTH patients. In a randomized, double-blind, crossover trial, 16 CTTH patients (who never had migraine) and 16 healthy volunteers received an IV infusion of nitroglycerin (0.5 $\mu g \cdot kg^{-1} \cdot min^{-1}$ for 20 minutes) or placebo on nonheadache days. The primary end point was the difference between the area under the headache curve (AUC, duration times intensity) recorded on an active day and on a placebo day. In patients, the median AUC on a nitroglycerin day, 2,221, was significantly higher than on a placebo day, 730 ($p = 0.008$). Peak pain intensity occurred 8 hours after nitroglycerin infusion. On a nitroglycerin day, the median AUC in patients, 2,221, was also significantly higher than in controls, 43 ($p = 0.0001$). This study suggests that nitric oxide may play an important role in the pathophysiology of CTTH.

Ashina et al. (1999a) randomized 16 CTTH patients in a double-blind, crossover-designed

trial to either IV infusions of 6 mg/kg L-N^6 methyl arginine hydrochloride (L-NMMA) or placebo on 2 days, separated by at least 1 week. Trapezius muscle hardness (measured with a meter) and pericranial myofascial tenderness (evaluated by a standardized validated manual palpation) were recorded at baseline and at 60 and 120 minutes after beginning the infusion. Compared with baseline, muscle hardness and tenderness were significantly reduced at 60 and 120 minutes. Placebo had no significant effect. Compared with placebo, the summary score of muscle hardness was significantly reduced, while tenderness showed a nonsignificant reduction following treatment with L-NMMA. Increased muscle hardness in CTTH patients may reflect sensitization of second-order neurons due to prolonged nociceptive input from myofascial tissues. The decrease in muscle hardness following treatment with L-NMMA may be caused by decreased central sensitization.

Pain Modulation

The mammalian nervous system contains networks that modulate nociceptive transmission. In the rostroventromedial medulla are so-called off-cells, which inhibit, and on-cells, which facilitate nociception (Fields et al., 1991). These cells are believed to modulate the activity of the trigeminal NC and dorsal horn neurons. Increased on-cell activity in the brain stem's pain-modulation system could enhance the response to both painful and nonpainful stimuli. Opiate withdrawal results in increased firing of on-cells, decreased firing of off-cells, and enhanced nociception (Fields et al., 1991). A similar mechanism may occur during drug-induced headaches. Primary CDH may result, in part, from enhanced neuronal activity in the NC as a result of enhanced on-cell or decreased off-cell activity. Other conditioned stimuli associated with pain and stress can also turn on the system and may account for some of the association between pain and stress.

Jensen and Olesen (1996) used sustained teeth clenching to trigger TTH in 58 patients with frequent, but not daily, CTTH or ETTH and 58 matched controls. Within 24 hours, 69% of patients (more than expected) and 17% of controls developed TTH. Shortly after clenching, electromyographic (EMG) amplitude was significantly increased in the trapezius, but not in the temporal, muscle and tenderness (which was increased at baseline in the headache patients) further increased only in patients who subsequently developed headache. Mechanical pain thresholds remained unchanged in the group that developed headache but increased in the group that did not develop headache. Pain tolerance decreased in patients who developed headache, was unchanged in the remaining patients, and increased in controls, suggesting that headache patients do not effectively activate their antinociceptive system. This study clearly shows that peripheral mechanisms alone cannot explain TTH, but they could act as a trigger for a central process. Tenderness, not muscle contraction, correlates with headache development.

Changes of the second suppressive period of the exteroceptive suppression (ES) of the temporalis muscle activity have been found in patients with CTTH and may reflect an abnormal endogenous pain control system. *Exteroceptive suppression* is the inhibition of voluntary EMG activity of the temporalis muscle induced by trigeminal nerve stimulation (Schoenen et al., 1987). There are two successive periods of ES (ES1 and ES2) (silent periods) (Fig. 11–1). It was originally reported that ES2, a multisynaptic reflex subject to limbic and other modulation, was absent in 40% of patients with CTTH and reduced in duration in 87%. The oligosynaptic reflex, ES1, was normal. It may be that ES2 is absent in more headache-prone patients (Paulus et al., 1992; Nakashima and Takahashi, 1991).

Schoenen et al. (1987) measured the ES2, pain threshold, EMG activity, anxiety scores, and response to biofeedback in 32 women with CTTH and found an abnormal EMG in 62.5% of the patients if three different muscles and three states were tested. The EMG was abnormal in only 40% if only one muscle and one state were tested. A decreased pain threshold was found in half the patients

tested in one of three muscles but in only 34% if only one muscle was tested. Duration of ES2 was reduced in 87% of patients.

Schepelmann et al. (1998) compared ES2 values in patients with the fibromyalgia syndrome to patients with CTTH and controls. The duration of ES2 ($\pm$SD) in fibromyalgia syndrome patients was 30.6 $\pm$ 7.5 ms and was not significantly different from the control group (33.1 $\pm$ 7.8 ms), whereas it was significantly shortened in CTTH patients (22.9 $\pm$ 11.5 ms).

Lipchik et al. (1996) evaluated masseter ES2 suppression and tenderness in the pericranial muscles of young adults with CTTH, ETTH, migraine without aura, migraine with aura, and controls. Pericranial muscle tenderness better distinguished diagnostic subgroups and better distinguished recurrent headache sufferers from controls than did masseter ES2. Chronic TTH sufferers had the highest pericranial muscle tenderness, and controls exhibited the lowest tenderness (p < 0.01). The association between pericranial muscle tenderness and CTTH was independent of the intensity, frequency, and chronicity of headaches. Pericranial muscle tenderness may be present early in the development of tension headache, while ES2 suppression may emerge only later.

An adequate pain stimulus induces two pain sensations: the first is acute, short-lasting, and well localized and the second longer-lasting and less localized. The second pain intensity increases with repeat stimulation and is enhanced in chronic headaches (Fusco et al., 1997). Fusco et al. (1997) examined second pain in subjects with ETTH, CDH, migraine without aura, and controls using percutaneous electrical shock. Second pain intensity was significantly greater in the group of patients with CDH compared with the other groups.

Fusco et al. (1999) evaluated the effect of dextromethorphan and Mg^{2+} on temporal summation of second pain in seven patients with CM and five with other chronic headaches, using a sequence of four electrical shocks delivered on the medial forearm at 3-second intervals. Pain intensity was measured with a visual analog scale. The stimulus was repeated 1 hour after a 100 mg oral dose of dextromethorphan, 10 minutes after the end of a slow IV infusion of Mg^{2+}, or both. First pain intensity did not change. The exaggerated temporal summation of second pain in chronic headache was confirmed. Dextromethorphan significantly decreased this; Mg^{2+} alone had no effect, but it did increase dextromethorphan's effect. Pharmacologic modulation of NMDA receptors may improve chronic headaches.

Ashina et al. (1999b) measured trapezius muscle hardness in 20 CTTH patients and 20 healthy controls. The patients were examined on 2 days, one with headache and one without headache. Pericranial myofascial tenderness (manual palpation) and muscle hardness (using a meter) were measured in 30 healthy controls and five patients outside of headache. In patients, muscle hardness on days with headache did not differ significantly from muscle hardness on days without headache. Muscle hardness positively correlated with the local tenderness score recorded from the trapezius muscle on days both with and without headache. The total tenderness score on days with headache was significantly higher than the total tenderness score on days without headache. There was a significant difference between the total tenderness score recorded in patients without headache, 15 ± 11, and controls, 4 ± 4 (p = 0.002). Muscle hardness was significantly higher in patients on days without headache than in controls. The authors found that muscle hardness and tenderness are permanently altered in CTTH and not only a consequence of actual pain. The positive correlation between muscle hardness and tenderness supports the clinical observation that tender muscles are harder than normal muscles.

Sakai et al. (1995) found that pericranial muscle hardness was significantly greater in women than in men. In TTH patients, the trapezius muscles were significantly harder in patients than they were in normal subjects. Posterior neck muscle hardness was also significantly greater in patients than in normal subjects. There was no significant difference in muscle hardness between ETTH and CTTH. Muscle hardness was reduced in patients who displayed clinical improvement.

Reduced Achilles tendon pain thresholds were found in half of CTTH patients when compared with headache-free controls (Schoenen et al., 1991). Biofeedback moderately but significantly increased the pain threshold, perhaps by normalizing limbic input to the brain-stem pain-modulating system. Increased EMG activity or decreased pain thresholds were found in 72% of patients (Schoenen et al., 1991), consistent with a diagnosis of "CTTH associated with disorder of pericranial muscles," but these findings were not present in the remaining 28% of patients, consistent with a diagnosis of "CTTH unassociated with such disorder." Headache severity, anxiety, ES2, and response to biofeedback did not differ between these two groups, suggesting that their separation may be artificial or a consequence of the headache.

Welch et al. (1999) used magnetic resonance imaging (MRI) to evaluate CM patients. Seven CM patients and nine normal adults were imaged with a 3-Tesla MRI system. The CM group had a significant decrease in R2 of the red nucleus and substantia nigra compared with the normal group. In addition, a significant decrease in R2* left and a marginally significant decrease in R2* right was observed in the red nucleus of the CM group. There was a moderately significant decrease in the left side and a significant decrease in the right side of R2* of the substantia nigra. There was no significant difference in the R2 values between the two groups, in either the red nucleus or the substantia nigra of the midbrain hemispheres. Decreased R2 and R2* indicate reduced non-heme iron or reduced deoxyhemoglobin. Chronic migraine appears to be associated with persistently altered function in the red nucleus and substantia nigra.

Spontaneous Central Pain Activation

Post and Silberstein (1994) suggested the kindling model for epilepsy as a model for nonepileptic, progressive disorders such as mania. In kindling, low-level electrical stimulation induces a complex series of neurochemical and anatomic changes, including C-fos activation. Post and Silberstein (1994) suggested that in the process of headache transformation, spontaneous recurrent migraine headaches might be analogous to the low levels of electrical stimulation in the kindling model. Preventive migraine treatment could provide a dual benefit by preventing the occurrence of episodes and blocking the sensitization process that could lead to syndrome progression.

In primary CDH, hypersensitivity of neurons in the trigeminal NC may exist as a result of supraspinal facilitation. The vascular nociceptor may be hypersensitive in CM; in CTTH associated with a disorder of the pericranial muscles, the myofascial nociceptor may be hypersensitive. In CTTH not associated with a disorder of the pericranial muscles, there may be less myofascial nociceptor hypersensitivity and a general increase in nociception. Chronic TTH and CM may result from a defective interaction between endogenous nociceptive brain-stem activity and peripheral input. Physical or psychologic stress or nonphysiologic working positions can increase nociception from strained muscles that could trigger or sustain an attack in an individual with altered pain modulation and could produce CTTH. Emotional mechanisms may also reduce endogenous antinociception. Long-term potentiation of nociceptive neurons and decreased activity in the antinociceptive system could cause primary CDH. Sensitization of the trigeminal NC neurons can result in normally nonpainful stimuli becoming painful, producing trigger spots, an overlap in the symptoms of migraine and TTH, and activation of the trigeminal vascular system.

Drug-Induced Headache Mechanisms

Overuse of analgesics, opioids, barbiturates, ergotamine-containing compounds, or triptans may contribute to the transformation of episodic into chronic migraine. Some believe that drug-induced primary CDH is due to a rebound effect wherein medication withdrawal triggers the next headache, which in turn leads to the consumption of more drug. This may produce a vicious cycle, resulting in more frequent drug use and drug-induced primary CDH. Formulations of drugs that maintain sustained, nonfluctuating levels might avoid the development of drug-induced headache (Post and Silberstein, 1994).

In the headache-prone individual, primary CDH may be a result of enhanced nociception. Continued high fluctuating doses of ergots, analgesics, opioids, or triptans could result in resetting of the pain-control mechanisms in susceptible individuals, perhaps by enhancing on-cell activity, enhancing central sensitization through NMDA receptors, or blocking adaptive antinociceptive changes. The consequences of drug discontinuation depend on the type of therapeutic response the drug engenders. Different drugs are effective in different phases of migraine. Some drugs are effective only acutely, others are effective only preventively, and some are effective only for infrequent episodic headache and not for frequent intractable migraine. Compensatory adaptive changes associated with frequent headaches (if they occur) may not be enough to allow continued drug effectiveness. If tolerance has decreased drug effectiveness, a drug holiday could renew the response (Post and Silberstein, 1994). Drug overuse may, in part, prevent the occurrence of antinociceptive adaptive changes. The analgesic washout period could be a result of the time required for the system to reset. The failure of preventive drugs could result from the lack of endogenous antinociceptive agents. A similar phenomenon occurs in contingent tolerance in the seizure kindling model (described below).

Cerebral blood flow increases in the brain stem and cortex of patients with migraine without aura. During the headache, the increased cerebral blood flow in the cortex, but not the brain stem, is reversed by sumatriptan, as is the headache. This area of the brain stem is rich in opioids and includes the pain-control centers. Dihydroergotamine (DHE) and centrally penetrant triptans selectively bind to this area of the brain stem, while sumatriptan may not. Perhaps this area of the brain stem integrates the phenomenon we call migraine, or it could be activated as a result of the migraine attack. If the first explanation is correct, ongoing activity in this area of the brain stem could produce recurrent or daily headache. If this area is responsible for controlling pain, then its failure to activate could explain ongoing headache activity. Acute migraine medications may induce daily headache by preventing the development of adaptive changes and perhaps by maintaining brain-stem activation (Weiller et al., 1995).

Contingent Tolerance Phenomena

The long-term effectiveness of anticonvulsants can be studied in amygdala-kindled animals. Repeated pretreatment with carbamazepine before kindling results in a loss of drug efficacy and constitutes a unique form of associative or contingent tolerance. Animals treated with carbamazepine after seizures occur do not show tolerance. Giving the drug after seizures occur can reverse tolerance once it has developed (Pazzaglia and Post, 1992). Some neurobiologic alterations following seizures may thus be adaptive, or anticonvulsant, in contrast to more enduring changes related to the primary pathophysiology of the kindled process (Post and Silberstein, 1994).

Clinical strategies based on these concepts might be used to reverse tolerance in the long-term treatment of migraine or CM. Switching a patient to a drug that has a different mechanism of action and does not show cross-tolerance or discontinuing the ineffective drug and reintroducing it later may be effective in some migraine or CM patients.

TREATMENT

Overview

Patients suffering from long-duration CM can be difficult to treat, especially when the disorder is complicated by medication overuse, comorbid psychiatric disease, low frustration tolerance, and physical and emotional dependence (Mathew et al., 1987; Saper, 1987). We recommend the following steps: first, exclude secondary headache disorders; second, diagnose the specific primary headache disorder

(i.e., CM, HC); and third, identify comorbid medical and psychiatric conditions, as well as exacerbating factors, especially medication overuse. Limit all symptomatic medications (with the possible exception of the long-acting NSAIDs). Patients should be started on a program of preventive medication (to decrease reliance on symptomatic medication), with the explicit understanding that the drugs may not become fully effective until medication overuse has been eliminated and detoxification (the washout period) completed (Silberstein and Saper, 1993). Patients need education and continuous support during this process.

Patients who overuse medication may not become fully responsive to acute and preventive treatments for 2 to 10 weeks after medication overuse is eliminated. Withdrawal symptoms include severely exacerbated headaches accompanied by nausea, vomiting, agitation, restlessness, sleep disorder, and (rarely) seizures. Barbiturates and benzodiazepine must be tapered gradually to avoid a serious withdrawal syndrome. The washout period may last 3 to 8 weeks; once it is over, there is frequently considerable headache improvement (Silberstein et al., 1990; Mathew et al., 1990; Baumgartner et al., 1989; Raskin, 1986).

Inpatient infusion (in an ambulatory infusion unit) and outpatient detoxification options are available. If outpatient detoxification proves difficult or dangerous, hospitalization may be required. Diener et al. (1988) were able to detoxify only 1.5% of 200 patients on an outpatient basis. Hering and Steiner (1991), in contrast, successfully used outpatient detoxification in 37 of 46 patients who were taking simple analgesics or ergotamine. A recent consensus paper by the German Migraine Society (Diener et al., 1992) recommends outpatient withdrawal for highly motivated patients who do not take barbiturates or tranquilizers with their analgesics. Inpatient treatment is recommended for patients who fail outpatient treatment, have high depression scores, or take tranquilizers, codeine, or barbiturates (Diener et al., 1992). The Standards of Care of the National Headache Foundation suggest that hospitalization may be necessary for severe dehydration, for which inpatient parenteral therapy may be necessary; diagnostic suspicion (confirmed by appropriate diagnostic testing) of organic etiology; prolonged, unrelenting headache with associated symptoms, such as nausea and vomiting, which, if allowed to continue, would pose a further threat to the patient's welfare; status migrainosus; dependence on analgesics, ergots, opiates, barbiturates, or tranquilizers; pain that is accompanied by serious adverse reactions or complications from therapy wherein continued use of such therapy aggravates or induces further illness; pain that occurs in the presence of significant medical disease but appropriate treatment of headache symptom aggravates or induces further illness; failed outpatient detoxification, for which inpatient pain and psychiatric management may be necessary; or treatment requiring copharmacy with drugs that may cause a drug interaction, thus necessitating careful observation (monoamine oxidase inhibitors and β-blockers). We have proposed guidelines for hospitalization (Table 11–7).

Disturbances in mood and function are common and require management with behavioral methods of pain management and supportive psychotherapy (including biofeedback, stress management, and cognitive behavioral therapy). Treatment of the comorbid psychiatric illness is often necessary before the primary CDH comes under control. "Chronobiologic interventions," such as encouraging regular habits of sleep, exercise, and meals, are often useful (Silberstein and Saper, 1993).

Psychophysiologic therapy involves reassurance, counseling, stress management, relaxation therapy, and biofeedback. The use of traditional acupuncture is controversial and has not proved more effective than placebo (Tavola et al., 1992). Physical therapy consists of modality treatments (heat, cold packs, ultrasound, and electrical stimulation); improvement of posture through stretching, exercise, and traction; trigger point injections; occipital nerve blocks; and a program of regular exercise, stretching, balanced meals, and adequate sleep (Silberstein, 1984). It has been our experience that treating painful trigger areas in the neck can result in the improvement of intractable primary CDH.

Acute Pharmacotherapy

Choice of acute pharmacotherapy depends on the diagnosis. Chronic migraine patients who do not overuse symptomatic medication can treat acute migrainous headache exacerbations with antimigraine drugs including triptans, DHE, and NSAIDs. These drugs must be strictly limited to prevent superimposed rebound headache that will complicate treatment and require detoxification. The risk of rebound is much lower for DHE and triptans than for analgesics, opioids, and ergotamine. Chronic TTH and NPDH can be treated with nonspecific headache medications, and HC can be treated with supplemental doses of indomethacin.

Preventive Pharmacotherapy

Patients with very frequent headaches should be treated primarily with preventive medications, with the explicit understanding that their medications may not become fully effective until the overused medication has been eliminated. It may take 3 to 6 weeks for treatment effects to develop.

The following principles guide the use of preventive treatment: (1) from among the first-line drugs, choose preventive agents based on their side effect profiles, comorbid conditions, and specific indications (e.g., indomethacin for HC); (2) start at a low dose; (3) gradually increase the dose until efficacy is achieved, until the patient develops side effects, or until the ceiling dose for the drug in question is reached; (4) treatment effects develop over weeks, and treatment may not become fully effective until rebound is eliminated; (5) if one agent fails and all other things are equal, choose an agent from another therapeutic class; (6) prefer monotherapy, but be willing to use combination therapy; (7) communicate realistic expectations (Silberstein and Lipton, 1994).

Most preventive agents used for primary CDH have not been examined in well-designed double-blind studies. Table 11–8 sum-

Table 11–7 Criteria for hospitalization

I. Emergency or urgent admission
  A. Certain migraine variants (e.g., hemiplegic migraine, suspected migrainous infarction, basilar migraine with serious neurologic symptoms such as syncope, confusional migraine, etc.)
    1. When a diagnosis has not been established during a previous similar occurrence
    2. When established outpatient treatment plan has failed
  B. Diagnostic suspicion of infectious disorder involving CNS (e.g., brain abscess, meningitis) with initiation of appropriate diagnostic testing
  C. Diagnostic suspicion of acute vascular compromise (e.g., aneurysm, subarachnoid hemorrhage, carotid dissection) with initiation of appropriate diagnostic testing
  D. Diagnostic suspicion of a structural disorder causing symptoms requiring an acute setting (e.g., brain tumor, increased intracranial pressure) with initiation of appropriate diagnostic testing
  E. Low cerebrospinal fluid headache when an outpatient blood patch has failed and an outpatient treatment plan has failed or no obvious cause
  F. Medical emergency presenting with a severe headache
  G. Severe headache associated with intractable nausea and vomiting producing dehydration or postural hypotension or unable to retain oral medication and unable to be controlled in an outpatient setting or with admission to observation status
  H. Failed outpatient treatment of an exacerbation of episodic headache disorder with
    1. Failure to respond to "rescue" or backup medications or
    2. Failure to respond to outpatient treatment with IV dihydroergotamine on a schedule of a minimum of twice daily
II. Nonemergent admission
  A. Coexistent psychiatric disease documented by psychologic or psychiatric evaluation with sufficient severity of illness such that a failure to admit could pose a health risk to the patient or impair the implementation of outpatient treatment
  B. Coexistent or risk of disease (e.g., unstable angina, unstable diabetes, recent transient ischemic attack, myocardial infarction in the past 6 months, renal failure, hypertension, age >65) necessitating monitoring for treatment of headache significant enough to warrant admission
  C. Severe chronic daily headaches involving chronic medication overuse when there is
    1. Daily use of potent opioids and/or barbiturates
    2. Daily use of triptans, simple analgesics, or ergotamine in a patient with a documented failed trial of withdrawal of these medications
  D. Impaired daily functioning (e.g., threatened relationships, many lost days at work or school due to headache), with a failure to respond to 2 days of outpatient treatment with IV dihydroergotamine, IV neuroleptics, or IV corticosteroids on a schedule of a minimum of twice daily or equivalent treatment

marizes the efficacy, safety, and evidence for a number of agents (Silberstein and Saper, 1993).

Antidepressants are attractive agents for use in primary CDH (CM, CTTH, and NDPH) since many patients have comorbid depression and anxiety. The most widely used tricyclic antidepressants are nortriptyline (Aventyl, Pamelor); amitriptyline (Elavil), which has been effective in many, but not all, studies (Bussone et al., 1991; Couch et al., 1976; Diamond and Baltes, 1971; Lance and Curran, 1964; Pluvinage, 1994; Pfaffenrath et al., 1986, 1994; Holroyd et al., 1991; Gobel et al., 1994; Cerbo et al., 1998; Mitsikostas et al., 1997; Bonuccelli et al., 1996); and doxepin (Sinequan) (Morland et al., 1979). In an open–label study in 82 nondepressed pa-

tients with either ETTH or CTTH, Cerbo et al. (1998) found that amitriptyline (25 mg/day) significantly reduced (p < 0.05) analgesic consumption and the frequency and duration of headache in CTTH but not in ETTH.

Fluoxetine (Prozac), a selective serotonin reuptake inhibitor, is coming into wider use for daily headaches; evidence from a double-blind study demonstrates its efficacy in primary CDH (Bussone et al., 1991; Saper et al., 1994). Fluvoxamine appears to be effective (Manna et al., 1994) and may have analgesic properties (Palmer and Benfield, 1994). Other selective serotonin reuptake inhibitors, including paroxetine (Foster and Bafaloukos, 1994), and monoamine oxidase inhibitors may have a therapeutic role; but this has not been proven (Langemark and Olesen, 1994).

Table 11–8 Summary of prophylactic drugs for use in chronic migraine[a]

Drug	Clinical efficacy	Side effects	Clinical evidence[b]
Antidepressants			
Amitriptyline	+++	++	+++
Doxepin	+++	++	++
Fluoxetine	++	+	+++
Anticonvulsants			
Divalproex	+++	++	++
Topiramate	+++	++	++
β Blockers			
Propranolol, nadolol, etc.	++	+	+
Calcium channel blockers			
Verapamil	++	+	+
Miscellaneous			
Methysergide	+++	+++	+

[a]All categories are rated from + to ++++ based on a combination of published literature and clinical experience.

[b]Ratings of +++ for clinical evidence indicate at least one double-blind, placebo-controlled study. A rating of ++ indicates well-designed open studies and + indicates ratings based on clinical experience. A rating of ++++ requires at least two double-blind, placebo-controlled trials.

Modified from Tfelt-Hansen, P. and R.B. Lipton (1993). Prioritizing treatment. In *The Headaches* (J. Olesen, P. Tfelt-Hansen, and K.M.A. Welch, eds.), pp. 359–362. Raven Press, New York.

β Blockers (propranolol, nadolol) remain a mainstay of therapy for migraine (Silberstein and Saper, 1993) and are used for primary CDH (Pfaffenrath et al., 1986; Mathew, 1981). Clinicians fear that β blockers may exacerbate depression; however, this issue is controversial (Bright and Everitt, 1992). β blockers are relatively contraindicated in patients who have asthma and Raynaud's disease.

Calcium channel blockers are very well tolerated (Silberstein and Saper, 1993); anecdotal evidence supports their use for CM. Verapamil (Calan) is the most widely prescribed agent in this family. Diltiazem (Cardizem) and nifedipine (Procardia) may also be considered. Flunarizine (Silberstein and Saper, 1993; Lake et al., 1993) is widely used in Canada and Europe but is not available in the United States.

The anticonvulsant divalproex sodium (Depakote) (Jensen et al., 1994) is an important drug in migraine prophylaxis, even in patients who have failed other agents. Four double-blind, placebo-controlled studies have demonstrated its efficacy in migraine (Jensen et al., 1994; Mathew et al., 1995; Hering and Kuritzky, 1998; Klapper, 1995). Smaller open studies support its utility in CM (Mathew and Ali, 1991). Doses lower than those used in epilepsy (250 mg twice/day) may be sufficient. Divalproex sodium is an especially useful agent in patients with comorbid epilepsy and manic-depressive illness and, possibly, anxiety disorders. In an open-label study, Edwards et al. (1999) assessed the possible benefit of sodium valproate in 20 consecutive CDH patients who were refractory to multiple standard treatments. Eleven (55%) had a response (mild or no headaches within 1 to 4 weeks). The doses ranged from 375 to 1,500 mg/day. Two patients (10%) discontinued medication due to side effects (nausea and difficulty thinking).

Topiramate is a new antiepileptic agent that has GABA-agonist properties and few side effects when used in low doses. Its chronic use has been associated with weight loss, not weight gain. Shuaib et al. (1999) treated 37 patients who had more than ten migraine headaches a month with topiramate (25 to 100 mg/day) in an open-label study. Most patients had CDH in addition to migraine; all had failed previous preventive treatment. Over a 3- to 9-month follow-up, 11 patients (30%) had an excellent result (headache frequency decreased by over 60%), 11 patients had a good result (headache frequency decreased 40% to 60%), three patients discontinued therapy due to side effects, and eight patients had no improvement. This uncontrolled study suggests that topiramate may be useful for CM.

The ergot derivative methysergide (Silberstein, 1998) is the first Food and Drug Administration–approved migraine prophylactic drug and one that is sometimes unreasonably feared. It is an effective migraine-preventive agent and can be safely combined with tricyclic antidepressants, selective serotonin reuptake inhibitors, or calcium channel blockers. The usual initial dose of methysergide is 2 mg twice/day. It can be increased to a maximum of 8 mg/day (2 mg four times/day); higher doses, although not recommended by the *Physicians' Desk Reference*, are sometimes useful.

Fontes-Ribeiro et al. (1999) treated 78 CTTH patients (65 evaluable) with L-5-hydroxytryptophan (100 mg) or placebo three times a day for 8 weeks, after a washout period of 2 weeks and with a follow-up period of 2 more weeks. Only analgesic drugs were permitted. There was a trend toward reduction in the number of headache days and headache intensity, but this was not statistically significant due to the high placebo effect (about 30%). The decrease in analgesic consumption was statistically significant. During the 2 weeks of follow-up, there was a significant decrease in the number of headache days (a postdrug effect).

The NSAIDs can be used for both symptomatic and preventive headache treatment. Naproxen sodium is effective at prevention at a dose of one or two 275 mg tablets twice/day (Miller et al., 1997). Other NSAIDs found to be effective include tolfenamic acid, ketoprofen, mefenamic acid, fenoprofen, and ibuprofen (Johnson and Tfelt-Hansen, 1993; Mylecharane and Tfelt-Hansen, 1993). Aspirin was effective in one study (Kangasniemi et al., 1983) and equal to placebo in another (Scholz et al., 1987). We believe that the short-acting NSAIDs, such as ibuprofen and aspirin, cause rebound headache and that their use should be limited. Rebound poten-

tial of the other NSAIDs is uncertain. Indomethacin is the drug of choice for HC, and the response to this medication defines the disorder. We give indomethacin a therapeutic trial to rule out HC but otherwise limit the use of NSAIDs.

Although monotherapy is preferred, it is sometimes necessary to combine preventive medications. Antidepressants are often used with β blockers or calcium channel blockers, and divalproex sodium may be used in combination with any of these medications.

Other Treatments

Open and small placebo-controlled trials have suggested that CTTH may improve following injection with botulinum toxin A (Botox); whether this is due to paralysis of muscles or to unknown mechanisms is uncertain. Botulinum toxin has been shown to be effective at decreasing the frequency of migraine attacks (Silberstein et al., 2000).

Mauskop (1999) used botulinum toxin to treat 12 refractory CDH patients (five men, seven women), who overused acute medications almost daily. Injections were given into the frontalis, temporalis, glabellar, and, when occipital pain was present, rectus muscles. Six to 11 points were injected with 50 to 100 U of botulinum toxin. Only one patient obtained good relief; she has had repeated injections. The most likely potential cause of the low efficacy of botulinum toxin in this group of patients is rebound from acute medication overuse.

Porta et al. (1999), in a randomized, single-blind trial, compared botulinum toxin A to methylprednisolone. Injections were given in tender points of the cranial muscles, which were determined using pressure pain threshold measurements obtained via an electronic algometer. Inclusion criteria included a diagnosis of IHS ETTH or CTTH, age between 18 and 70 years, and no preventive treatment. At 30 and 60 days postinjection, both treatment groups had a significant reduction in pain scores (using a visual analog scale) compared with baseline. At 60 days postinjection, the reduction in pain scores was statistically significantly greater in botulinum toxin A–

treated patients compared with steroid-treated patients.

Smuts et al. (1999) conducted a double-blind, placebo-controlled, randomized study of 40 CTTH patients (29 women, 11 men) who were previously unsuccessfully treated with either amitriptyline or sodium valproate. Patients received intramuscular injections of either botulinum toxin A (100 U in 2 ml saline) or placebo (2 ml saline) at predefined areas in the neck and temporal muscles. The number of headache-free days was significantly increased in the botulinum toxin A group compared with controls 3 months following treatment. A clear shift toward the lower headache scores for the botulinum toxin A group was retained throughout the study period. A statistically significant reduction in the average pain score was achieved for the botulinum toxin A group compared with the placebo group over the 3-month period. No serious adverse events were reported.

Gobel et al. (1999) treated ten CTTH patients in a double-blind trial with either 10 IU botulinum toxin (Botox) injected into the frontal and auricular muscles on each side and 20 IU injected into the splenius capitis muscle on each side or the corresponding quantity of NaCl as placebo. No significant change in headache intensity, headache hours a day, or frequency of analgesic intake was observed between the treatment groups. Standardized bilateral injection of botulinum toxin A into muscles with increased tension or pain sensitivity was not effective in this study.

Ashina et al. (1999c) treated 16 CTTH patients in a randomized, double-blind, crossover trial. Patients received IV infusion of 6 mg/kg L-NMMA or placebo on 2 days, separated by at least 1 week, in a randomized order. Headache intensity was measured on a 100 mm visual analog scale and on a verbal rating scale at baseline and at 30 minutes, 60 minutes, and 120 minutes after the start of treatment. The primary end point was reduction of pain intensity on the visual analog scale by the active treatment compared with placebo. Compared with placebo L-NMMA reduced pain intensity significantly more.

Treatment of Medication Overuse

Outpatient

There are two general outpatient strategies. One approach is to taper the overused medication, gradually substituting a long-acting NSAID as effective preventive therapy is established. The alternative strategy is to abruptly discontinue the overused drug, substitute a transitional medication to replace the overused drug, and subsequently taper the transitional drug. Drugs used for this purpose include NSAIDs, DHE, corticosteroids, and triptans (Diener et al., 1991; Bonuccelli et al., 1996; Drucker and Tepper, 1998). Serious withdrawal syndromes that can be produced by the overused drug must be prevented. For example, if high doses of a butalbital-containing analgesic combination are abruptly discontinued, phenobarbital should be used to prevent barbiturate-withdrawal syndrome. Similarly, benzodiazepines must be gradually tapered. Outpatient treatment is preferred for motivated patients but is not always safe or effective.

Patients who do not need hospital-level care but cannot be safely or adequately treated as outpatients can be considered for ambulatory infusion treatment. Outpatient ambulatory infusion treatment is effective for migraine status and uncomplicated primary CDH with and without rebound. It must be done in a hospital or a supervised medical setting, where the patient can be monitored frequently (every 15 minutes). Under these circumstances, repetitive IV treatment can be given twice a day for several days in a row. Although ambulatory infusion treatment is better for many patients than outpatient treatment, major concerns still exist. Contraindications to outpatient ambulatory infusion treatment include the likelihood of withdrawal symptoms occurring at night when patients are withdrawn from long-acting or potent drugs; psychiatric disorders that interfere with treatment (these patients cannot be treated aggressively as outpatients); and comorbid medical illness that requires prolonged monitoring. No long-term observation is available, and many problems manifest themselves in an intensely monitored, interactive environment.

Inpatient

If outpatient treatment fails or is not safe or if there is significant medical or psychiatric comorbidity present, inpatient treatment may be needed (Silberstein and Saper, 1993). The goals of inpatient headache treatment include the following: (1) medication withdrawal and rehydration, (2) pain control with parenteral therapy, (3) establishment of effective preventive treatment, (4) interruption of the pain cycle, (5) patient education, and (6) establishment of outpatient methods of pain control. The detoxification process can be enhanced and shortened and the patient's symptoms made more tolerable by the use of repetitive IV DHE coadministered with metoclopramide (Fig. 11–1) (Raskin, 1986), which helps to control nausea and is an effective antimigraine drug in its own right. Following 10 mg

of IV metoclopramide, DHE 0.5 mg is administered IV. Subsequent doses are adjusted based on pain relief and side effects. Patients who are not candidates for DHE or do not respond can use repetitive IV neuroleptics, such as chlorpromazine, droperidol, and prochlorperazine, and/or corticosteroids. These agents may also supplement repetitive IV DHE in refractory patients (Silberstein et al., 1990). Hospitalization is also used as a time for patient education, for introducing behavioral methods of pain control, and for adjusting an outpatient program of preventive and acute therapy.

Our (Silberstein et al., 1990) experience with more than 300 patients has shown that repetitive IV DHE is a safe and effective means of rapidly controlling intractable headache. Of 214 patients suffering from daily headache with rebound, 92% became headache-free, usually within 2 to 3 days, with an average hospital stay of 7.3 days. With more aggressive treatment, average length of

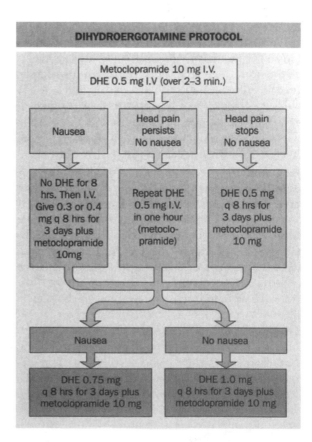

Figure 11–1 Dihydroergotamine treatment protocol. After Raskin.[51]

stay is now 3 days. Pringsheim and Howse (1998) reported similar but less robust results (see below).

PROGNOSIS

The "natural history" of primary CDH, and rebound headache in particular, has never been studied and probably never will be for ethical and technical reasons. Recognition of the rebound process is probably therapeutic in and of itself and could affect the patient's behavior or the physician's approach. Retrospective analysis suggests that there may be periods of stable drug consumption and periods of accelerated medication use. Patients treated aggressively generally improve. There are no reports of spontaneous improvement of rebound headache, although this may happen. We (Silberstein and Silberstein, 1992) performed follow-up evaluations on 50 hospitalized primary CDH drug-overuse patients who were treated with repetitive IV DHE and became headache-free. Once detoxified, treated, and discharged, most patients did not resume daily analgesic or ergotamine use.

Seventy-two percent continued to show significant improvement at 3 months, and 87% continued to show significant improvement after 2 years. This suggests at least a 70% improvement at 2 years in the initial group (35/50), allowing for patients lost to follow-up.

Our (Silberstein and Silberstein, 1992) 2-year success rate of 87% is consistent with the long-term success rates reported in the literature (Table 11–9). In a series of 23 papers (Hering and Steiner, 1991; Andersson, 1988; Tfelt-Hansen and Krabbe, 1981; Schoenen et al., 1989; Isler, 1982; Dichgans et al., 1984; Granella et al., 1998; Baumgartner et al., 1989; Diener et al., 1988, 1989, 1992; Mathew, 1990; Mathew et al., 1990; Rapoport et al., 1986; Lake et al., 1990; Henry et al., 1984; Andersson, 1975; Silberstein and Silberstein, 1992; Pini et al., 1996; Schnider et al., 1996; Pringsheim and Howse, 1998; Monzon and Lainez, 1998; Suhr et al., 1999) published between 1975 and 1999, the success rate of withdrawal therapy (often accompanied by pharmacologic and/or behavioral intervention) in patients overusing analgesics, ergotamine, or both was between 48% and 91%,

Table 11–9 Drug-induced headache: long-term follow-up

Year	Author	Drug[a]	Number of patients	Follow-up (months)	Positive results (%)	Released rate (%)
1975	Andersson	E	44	6	91	9
1981	Tfelt-Hansen and Krabbe	E	40	12	47.6	29
1982	Ala-Hurula	E	23	3–6	78	19
1982	Isler	A	104	1–30	77.9	58.6
1984	Dichgans et al.	E/A	52	16	77	9
1984	Henry et al.	E/A	22	3	78	33
1986	Rapoport et al.	A	90	4	82	?
1988	Diener et al.	E/A	85	35	69	?
1988	Andersson	E	32	6	50	?
1989	Baumgartner et al.	E/A	38	16	60.5	24
1989	Diener et al.	A	139	34		
1989	Schoenen et al.	A	121	6	50	20
1990	Lake et al.	E/A	100	3–12	87	
1990	Mathew et al.	E/A	200	3	86	?
1991	Hering and Steiner	E/A	46	6	80.4	4
1992	Silberstein and Silberstein	E/A	50	24	87	13
1996	Pini et al.	E/A/T	104	4	72	28
1996	Schnider et al.	E/A	38	60	50	39.5
1998	Pringsheim and Howse	E/A/T	132	3	56	
1998	Granella et al.	A	95	6	?	22
1999	Monzon et al.	E/A	104	12	66	?
1999	Suhr et al.	E/A/T	101	72 ± 48		20.8
1999	Lorenzatto et al.	E/A/T	140	12	84.6	

[a]E, ergotamine tartrate; A, analgesics; T, triptans.

with the rate being reported as 77% or higher in ten papers (Table 11–9).

Henry et al. (1984) hospitalized, detoxified, and followed 22 primary CDH drug-overuse patients for 4 to 24 months. Nine of 15 patients showed marked improvement, one showed slight improvement, and five did not improve. Rapoport et al. (1986) studied 90 patients with primary CDH who discontinued analgesics. After 1 month, 30% were significantly improved, and 67% were significantly improved within 2 months, 80% after 3 months, and 82% after 4 months. The authors suggested that an "analgesic washout period" exists that may be as long as 3 months for some patients.

Diener et al. (1988) hospitalized 85 patients who were overusing analgesics or various migraine drugs (including ergotamine). The length of admission was 14 days. They detoxified these patients and followed them for 10 to 75 months (mean 35 months) after discharge. Sixty-nine percent had at least 50% improvement, 29.4% were unchanged, and one had deteriorated. Fifty-four patients with drug-induced headache were hospitalized by Baumgartner et al. (1989) for 2 weeks. They were detoxified and started on a prophylactic drug. At an average of 16.8 months (13.6 months) after treatment and discharge, 38 patients were evaluated: 76.3% had reduced their analgesic intake and 60.5% had experienced a significant relief in headache intensity and frequency.

Lake et al. (1990) reported on 100 patients who had been hospitalized with severe refractory primary CDH frequently complicated by symptomatic medication overuse. At follow-up between 3 months and 1 year after discharge, the mean number of severe headaches was reduced 64% and the mean number of dysfunctional days was reduced 70%. Overall, 87% of patients reported at least a 50% headache reduction.

Hering and Steiner (1991) followed 46 migraineurs who developed primary CDH as a result of analgesic overuse. Six months after analgesic and ergotamine withdrawal, 80.4% (n = 37) were no longer overusing the agents and no longer had primary CDH.

Mathew et al. (1990; Mathew, 1990) stud-ied 200 patients who were overusing daily symptomatic medication, 58% of whom were taking prophylactic medication without achieving benefit. At the 3-month follow-up, if the analgesics had been discontinued and prophylactic medication started or modified, a reduction of approximately 86% in the weekly headache index was achieved, with a dropout rate of 10.3%. If symptomatic medication had been continued, only 21% improvement was achieved. It is interesting to note that merely discontinuing symptomatic medication resulted in 58% improvement.

Schnider et al. (1996) followed 38 primary CDH inpatients who had overused ergotamine and/or analgesics and were detoxified. After 5 years, 19 patients had headache 8 or fewer days a month and 18 had no or only mild headaches. Outcome was related to headache frequency and duration of drug use. Fifteen patients (39.5%) had relapsed and were again overusing acute drugs.

Pini et al. (1996) evaluated 102 primary CDH patients who were overusing ergotamine, analgesics (including butalbital combinations), and/or sumatriptan. Patients were treated as either outpatients or inpatients based on the therapeutic schedule to be followed. Both groups showed equal improvement at 1 and 4 months in the headache index, but there was a higher relapse rate in the outpatients (38%) compared with the inpatients (25%). This suggests that the more complicated and refractory patients were admitted to the hospital.

Granella et al. (1998) looked for factors associated with the evolution of migraine without aura into chronic migraine. Risk factors included head trauma (OR = 3.3), analgesic use with every attack (OR = 2.8), and long duration of oral contraceptive use.

Pringsheim and Howse (1998) detoxified 174 inpatients who were overusing ergotamine, analgesics, and triptans and treated them with repetitive IV DHE; 132 patients were followed after 3 months by telephone. Sixty-one percent had an immediate good result. Of these, 56% continued to do well at 3 months and 5% relapsed.

Suhr et al. (1999) conducted a prospective study of 257 primary CDH patients allocated to inpatient (n = 147) or outpatient (n = 110) treatment depending on the personal situation of the patient. Only 5% of the patients were headache-free at follow-up, which was up to 5 years after treatment. Total relapse to drug overuse was 20.8%, occurring in 14.0% of outpatients and 25.0% of inpatients. No baseline analysis of headache days a month or mean pain intensity was given, but there was no significant difference in these outcomes between groups.

Monzon et al. (1999) prospectively studied the long-term (6 and 12 months) outcome of 164 consecutive primary CDH patients and analyzed various etiologic causal factors. One hundred eighteen (72%) patients had CM, 33 (20%) patients had CTTH, and 13 (8%) patients had NDPH. One hundred forty-nine patients were treated with outpatient therapy, and 15 refractory patients were admitted to a comprehensive inpatient treatment facility. At 6 months, 54 patients had an excellent result, 64 had a good result, and 41 had a fair result; five patients continued to have CM. At 12 months, 104 patients were analyzed: 23 had an excellent result, 46 had a good result, and 28 had a fair result; seven patients continued to have CM. There were no statistically significant differences in evolution when transformation factors were analyzed. Although differences were not statistically significant, treatment was less efficacious when inpatient therapy was necessary and when patients had a history of analgesic abuse or traumatic life events. This, again, suggests that the more severe and intractable cases were admitted to the hospital.

Lorenzatto et al. (1999), using the criteria proposed by Silberstein et al. (1996), retrospectively studied 140 patients (101 women and 39 men aged 17 to 83) who had CDH, i.e., their overused acute drugs. The patients were taken off and treated with preventive medications and education. After 1 month, 23.6% of patients had more than a 50% improvement in headache intensity and frequency and 56.4% had a similar improvement. Fifty percent improvement after 3 months was observed after 6 months in 70.2% of patients, after 9 months in 82.6%, and after 12 months in 84.6%.

WHY TREATMENT FAILS

When patients fail to respond to therapy or announce at the first consultation that they have already tried everything and nothing will work, it is important to try to identify the reason or reasons that treatment has failed (Lipton et al., 2001b) (Table 11–10). The cause of treatment failure may be an incomplete or incorrect diagnosis: e.g., (1) an undiagnosed secondary headache disorder is the major source of the head pain; (2) a misdiagnosed primary headache disorder is present (i.e., HC is mistaken for CM, episodic paroxysmal hemicrania or hypnic headache is mistaken for cluster); or (3) two or more different headache disorders are present. In addition, pharmacotherapy may have been inadequate or important exacerbating factors, such as medication overuse, may have been missed.

PREVENTION

Headache sufferers often do not realize that excessive or frequent self-treatment may perpetuate or exacerbate their headaches. Since most headache sufferers do not seek medical

Table 11–10 Why treatment fails

Diagnosis is incomplete or incorrect
- An undiagnosed secondary headache disorder is present
- A primary headache disorder is misdiagnosed
- Two or more different headache disorders are present

Important exacerbating factors may have been missed
- Medication overuse (including over-the-counter)
- Caffeine overuse
- Dietary or lifestyle triggers
- Hormonal triggers
- Psychosocial factors
- Other medications that trigger headaches

Pharmacotherapy has been inadequate
- Ineffective drug
- Excessive initial doses
- Inadequate final doses
- Inadequate duration of treatment

Other factors
- Unrealistic expectations
- Comorbid conditions complicate therapy
- Inpatient treatment required

Modified from Lipton, R.B., S.D. Silberstein, P.J. Goodsby et al. (2001b). Why headache treatment fails? Submitted for publication.

advice until and unless the pain becomes frequent or intense, the opportunity for diagnosis and physician intervention to halt the cycle is often missed. Physicians need to screen CDH patients for analgesic overuse. Headache patients must be informed about the risks of analgesic overuse and rebound headache. Yet, even when patients are aware of the risks, they may still overmedicate. This requires continued vigilance on the part of the treating physician.

Because patients who overuse medication may feel ashamed and out of control, an accurate history may be difficult to obtain. To facilitate this process, the condition of medication rebound should be explained as part of the natural history of migraine. Even if the patient is not rebounding at the time, all symptomatic headache medications, with the possible exception of the long-acting NSAIDs, should be limited to prevent rebound headache.

Patients with drug-induced CDH, while difficult to treat, often return to a state of intermittent episodic headache after detoxification and treatment with a preventive medication.

REFERENCES

Ala-Hurula, V., V. Myllyla, and E. Hokkanen (1982). Ergotamine abuse: results of ergotamine discontinuation, with special reference to the plasma concentrations. *Cephalagia* 2:189.

Andersson, P.G. (1975). Ergotamine headache. *Headache* 15:118–121.

Andersson, P.G. (1988). Ergotism: The clinical picture. In *Drug-induced Headache* (H.C. Diener and M.S. Wilkinson, eds.), pp. 16–19. Springer, Berlin.

Anthony, M. and B.K. Rasmussen (1993). Migraine without aura. In *The Headaches* (J. Olesen, P. Tfelt-Hansen, and M.A. Welch, eds.), pp. 255–261. Raven Press, New York.

Antonaci, F. (1991). The sweating pattern in hemicrania continua. A comparison with chronic paroxysmal hemicrania. *Funct. Neurol.* 6:371–375.

Antonaci, F. (1994). Chronic paroxysmal hemicrania and hemicrania continua: Orbital phlebography and MRI studies. *Headache* 34:32–34.

Antonaci, F., T. Sand, and O. Sjaastad (1992). Hemicrania continua and chronic paroxysmal hemicrania: A comparison of pupillometric findings. *Funct. Neurol.* 7:385–389.

Antonaci, F., G. Sandrini, A. Danilov et al. (1994). Neurophysiological studies in chronic paroxysmal hemicrania and hemicrania continua. *Headache* 34:479–483.

Antonaci, F. and O. Sjaastad (1992). Hemicrania continua: A possible symptomatic case, due to mesenchymal tumor. *Funct. Neurol.* 7:471–474.

Ashina, M., L. Bendtsen, R. Jensen et al. (1999a). Possible mechanisms of action of nitric oxide synthase inhibitors in chronic tension-type headache. *Brain* 122:1629–1635.

Ashina, M., L. Bendtsen, R. Jensen et al. (1999b). Muscle hardness in patients with chronic tension-type headache: Relation to actual headache state. *Pain* 79:201–205.

Ashina, M., L.H. Lassen, L. Bendtsen et al. (1999c). Effect of inhibition of nitric oxide synthase on chronic tension-type headache: A randomized crossover trial. *Lancet* 353:287–289.

Baumgartner, C., P. Wessly, C. Bingol et al. (1989). Long-term prognosis of analgesic withdrawal in patients with drug-induced headaches. *Headache* 29:510–514.

Bendtsen, L., R. Jensen, and J. Olesen (1996). Qualitatively altered nociception in chronic myofascial pain. *Pain* 65:259–264.

Bonuccelli, U., A. Nuti, C. Lucetti et al. (1996). Amitriptyline and dexamethasone combined treatment in drug-induced headache. *Cephalalgia* 16:197–200.

Bordini, C., F. Antonaci, L.J. Stovner et al. (1991). "Hemicrania continua"—a clinical review. *Headache* 31:20–26.

Bovim, G., G. Jenssen, and K. Ericson (1992). Orbital phlebography: A comparison between cluster headache and other headaches. *Headache* 32:408–412.

Bowdler, I., J. Killian, and S. Gänsslen-Blumberg (1990). The association between analgesic abuse and headache—coincidental or causal. *Headache* 30:494.

Brain, W.R. (1963). Some unsolved problems of cervical spondylosis. *BMJ* 1:771–777.

Breslau, N. and G.C. Davis (1993). Migraine, physical health and psychiatric disorders: A prospective epidemiologic study of young adults. *J. Psychiatr. Res.* 27:211–221.

Bright, R.A. and D.E. Everitt (1992). Beta-blockers and depression: Evidence against association. *JAMA* 267:1783–1787.

Burstein, R., H. Yamamura, A. Malick et al. (1998). Chemical stimulation of the intracranial dura induces enhanced responses to facial stimulation in brainstem trigeminal neurons. *J. Neurophysiol.* 79:964–982.

Bussone, G., G. Sandrini, G. Patruno et al. (1991). Effectiveness of fluoxetine on pain and depression in chronic headache disorders. In *Head-*

ache and Depression: Serotonin Pathways as a Common Clue (G. Nappi, G. Bono, G. Sandrini et al., eds.), pp. 265–272. Raven Press, New York.

Castillo, J., P. Munoz, V. Guitera et al. (1999). Epidemiology of chronic daily headache in the general population. *Headache* 39:190–196.

Catarci, T., F. Fiacco, and C. Argentino (1994). Ergotamine-induced headache can be sustained by sumatriptan daily intake. *Cephalalgia* 14:374–375.

Celentano, D.D., W.F. Stewart, and R.B. Lipton (1992). Medication use and disability among migraineurs: A national probability sample. *Headache* 32:223–228.

Cerbo, R., P. Barbanti, G. Fabbrini et al. (1998). Amitriptyline is effective in chronic but not in episodic tension-type headache: Pathogenetic implications. *Headache* 38:453–457.

Couch, J.R., D.K. Ziegler, and R. Hassainein (1976). Amitriptyline in the prophylaxis of migraine. *Arch. Neurol.* 26:121–127.

Curioso, E.P., W.B. Young, A.L. Shechter et al. (1999). Psychiatric comorbidity predicts outcome in chronic daily headache patients [Abstract]. *Neurology* 52:A471.

Diamond, S. and B. Baltes (1971). Chronic tension headache treated with amitriptyline: A double blind study. *Headache* 11:110–116.

Diamond, S. and D.J. Dalessio (1982). Drug abuse in headache. In *The Practicing Physician's Approach to Headache* (S. Diamond and D.J. Dalessio, eds.), pp. 114–121. Williams and Wilkins, Baltimore.

Dichgans, J., H.D. Diener, W.D. Gerber et al. (1984). Analgetika-induzierter dauerkopfschmerz. *Dtsch. Med. Wochenschr* 109:369.

Diener, H.C., J. Dichgans, E. Scholz et al. (1989). Analgesic-induced chronic headache: Long-term results of withdrawal therapy. *J. Neurol.* 236:9–14.

Diener, H.C., W.D. Gerber, and S. Geiselhart (1988). Short- and long-term effects of withdrawal therapy in drug-induced headache. In *Drug-induced Headache* (H.C. Diener and M. Wilkinson, eds.), pp. 133–142. Springer-Verlag, Berlin.

Diener, H.C., J. Haab, C. Peters et al. (1991). Subcutaneous sumatriptan in the treatment of headache during withdrawal from drug-induced headache. *Headache* 31:205–209.

Diener, H.C., V. Pfaffenrath, D. Soyka et al. (1992). Therapie des medikamenten-induzierten dauerkopfschmerzes. *Dtsch. Med. Wochenschr.* 134:159–162.

Diener, H.C. and P. Tfelt-Hansen (1993). Headache associated with chronic use of substances. In *The Headaches* (J. Olesen, P. Tfelt-Hansen, and K.M.A. Welch, eds.), pp. 721–727. Raven Press, New York.

Dray, A., L. Urban, and A. Dickenson (1994). Pharmacology of chronic pain. *Trends Pharmacol. Sci.* 15:190–197.

Drucker, P. and S. Tepper (1998). Daily sumatriptan for detoxification from rebound. *Headache* 38:687–690.

Edelman, G.M. and J.A. Gally (1992). Nitric oxide: Linking space and time in the brain. *Proc. Natl. Acad. Sci. USA* 89:11651–11652.

Edmeads, J. (1988). The cervical spine and headache. *Neurology* 38:1874–1878.

Edwards, K., V. Santarcangelo, P. Shea et al. (1999). Intravenous valproate for acute treatment of migraine headaches [Abstract]. *Cephalalgia* 19:356.

Eggen, A.E. (1993). The Tromsø study: Frequency and predicting factors of analgesic drug use in a free-living population (12–56 years). *J. Clin. Epidemiol.* 46:1297–1304.

Espada, F., F. Morales-Asín, I. Escalza et al. (1999). Hemicrania continua: Nine new cases [Abstract]. *Cephalalgia* 19:442.

Fields, H.L., M.M. Heinricher, and P. Mason (1991). Neurotransmitters as nociceptive modulatory circuits. *Annu. Rev. Neurosci.* 14:219–245.

Fisher, C.M. (1988). Analgesic rebound headache refuted. *Headache* 28:666.

Fontes-Ribeiro, C.A. (1999). L-5-Hydroxytryptophan in the prophylaxis of chronic tension-type headache: A double-blind randomized placebo-controlled study [Abstract]. *Cephalalgia* 19:453.

Foster, C.A. and J. Bafaloukos (1994). Paroxetine in the treatment of chronic daily headache. *Headache* 34:587–589.

Fusco, B.M., O. Colantoni, and M. Giavovazzo (1997). Alteration of central excitation circuits in chronic headache and analgesic misuse. *Headache* 37:486–491.

Fusco, B.M., O. Colantoni, C. Saturnino et al. (1999). Altered "second pain" in chronic headaches: Pharmacological modulation [Abstract]. *Cephalalgia* 19:399–400.

Gaist, D., J. Hallas, S.H. Sindrup et al. (1996). Is overuse of sumatriptan a problem? A population-based study. *Eur. J. Clin. Pharmacol.* 50:161–165.

Goadsby, P.J. and R.B. Lipton (1997). A review of paroxysmal hemicranias, SUNCT syndrome and other short-lasting headaches with autonomic features, including new cases. *Brain* 120:193–209.

Gobel, H., V. Hamouz, C. Hansen et al. (1994). Chronic tension-type headache: Amitriptyline reduces clinical headache-duration and experimental pain sensitivity but does not alter pericranial muscle activity readings. *Pain* 59:241–249.

Gobel, H., V. Lindner, P. Krack et al. (1999). Treatment of chronic tension-type headache with botulinum toxin [Abstract]. *Cephalalgia 19*: 455.

Granella, F., A. Cavallini, G. Sandrini et al. (1998). Long-term outcome of migraine. *Cephalalgia 18*:30–33.

Guitera, V., P. Muñoz, J. Castillo et al. (1999). Impact of chronic daily headache in the quality of life: A study in the general population [Abstract]. *Cephalalgia 19*:412–413.

Gutzwiller, F. and E. Zemp (1986). Der analgetikakonsum in der bevölkerung und socioökonomische aspekte des analgetikaabusus. In *Das Analgetikasyndrom* (M.J. Mihatsch, ed.), pp. 197–205. Thieme, Stuttgart.

Henry, P., J.F. Dartigues, M.P. Benetier et al. (1984). Ergotamine- and analgesic-induced headache. In C. Rose (ed.), Migraine: Proceedings from the Fifth International Migraine Symposium, London, 1984:197.

Hering, R. and A. Kuritzky (1998). Sodium valproate in the prophylactic treatment of migraine: A double-blind study versus placebo. *Cephalalgia 12*:81–84.

Hering, R. and T.J. Steiner (1991). Abrupt outpatient withdrawal from medication in analgesic-abusing migraineurs. *Lancet 337*:1442–1443.

Holroyd, K.A., J.M. Nash, and J.D. Pingel (1991). A comparison of pharmacologic (amitriptyline HCl) and nonpharmacologic (cognitive-behavioral) therapies for chronic tension headaches. *J. Consult. Clin. Psychol. 59*:387–393.

Iordanidis, T. and O. Sjaastad (1989). Hemicrania continua: A case report. *Cephalalgia 9*:301–303.

Isler, H. (1982). Migraine treatment as a cause of chronic migraine. In *Advances in Migraine Research and Therapy* (F.C. Rose, ed.), pp. 159–164. Raven Press, New York.

Isler, H. (1988). Headache drugs provoking chronic headache: Historical aspects and common misunderstandings. In *Drug-induced Headache* (H.C. Diener and M. Wilkinson, eds.), pp. 87–94. Springer-Verlag, Berlin.

Jensen, R., T. Brinck, and J. Olesen (1994). Sodium valproate has a prophylactic effect in migraine without aura. *Neurology 44*:647–651.

Jensen, R. and J. Olesen (1996). Initiating mechanisms of experimentally induced tension-type headache. *Cephalalgia 16*:175–182.

Johnson, E.S. and P. Tfelt-Hansen (1993). Nonsteroidal antiinflammatory drugs. In *The Headaches* (J. Olesen, P. Tfelt-Hansen, and K.M.A. Welch, eds.), pp. 391–395. Raven Press, New York.

Joubert, J. (1991). Hemicrania continua in black patient—the importance of the non-continuous stage. *Headache 31*:480–482.

Kaiser, R.S. (1999). Substance abuse and headache. In *41st Annual Scientific Meeting*. American Association for the Study of Headache, Boston, MA.

Kangasniemi, P.J., T. Nyrke, A.H. Lang et al. (1983). Femoxetine—a new 5HT uptake inhibitor—and propranolol in the prophylactic treatment of migraine. *Acta Neurol. Scand. 68*:262–267.

Katsarava, Z., V. Limmroth, G. Fritsche et al. (1999). Drug-induced headache following the use of zolmitriptan or naratriptan [Abstract]. *Cephalalgia 19*:414.

Kieholz, P. and D. Ladewig (1981). Probleme des medikamentenmissbrauches. *Schweis. Arztezeitung. 62*:2866–2869.

Klapper, J. (1995). Divalproex sodium in the prophylactic treatment of migraine [Abstract]. *Headache 35*:290.

Krymchantowski, A.V., J.S. Barbosa, W.S. Lorenzatto et al. (1999). Clinical features of transformed migraine [Abstract]. *Cephalalgia 19*: 336–337.

Kudrow, L. (1982). Paradoxical effects of frequent analgesic use. *Adv. Neurol. 33*:335–341.

Lake, A., J. Saper, S. Madden et al. (1990). Inpatient treatment for chronic daily headache: A prospective long-term outcome [Abstract]. *Headache 30*:299–300.

Lake, A.E., J.R. Saper, S.F. Madden et al. (1993). Comprehensive inpatient treatment for intractable migraine: A prospective long-term outcome study. *Headache 33*:55–62.

Lance, F., C. Parkes, and M. Wilkinson (1988). Does analgesic abuse cause headache de novo? *Headache 28*:61–62.

Lance, J.W. and D.A. Curran (1964). Treatment of chronic tension headache. *Lancet 1*:1236–1239.

Langemark, M. and J. Olesen (1994). Sulpiride and paroxetine in the treatment of chronic tension-type headache. *Headache 34*:20–24.

Lassen, L.H., M. Ashina, I. Christiansen et al. (1997). Nitric oxide synthase inhibition in migraine. *Lancet 349*:401–402.

Lipchik, G.L., K.A. Holroyd, C.R. France et al. (1996). Central and peripheral mechanisms in chronic tension-type headache. *Pain 64*:475.

Lipton, R.B., A.I. Scher, W.F. Stewart et al. (2001a). Frequent headache: A far too common problem. Advanced Studies in Medicine, in press.

Lipton, R.B., S.D. Silberstein, P.J. Goodsby et al. (2001b). Why headache treatment fails? Submitted for publication.

Lorenzatto, W.S., C.F. Cheim, M. Adriano et al. (1999). Long-term outcome in chronic daily headache [Abstract]. *Cephalalgia 19*:413.

Manna, V., F. Bolino, and L. DiCicco (1994). Chronic tension-type headache, mood depression and serotonin. *Headache 34*:44–49.

Mathew, N.T. (1981). Prophylaxis of migraine and mixed headache. A randomized controlled study. *Headache 21*:105–109.

Mathew, N.T. (1982). Transformed migraine. *Cephalalgia 13*:78–83.

Mathew, N.T. (1987). Transformed or evolutional migraine. *Headache* 27:305–306.

Mathew, N.T. (1990). Drug induced headache. *Neurol. Clin.* 8:903–912.

Mathew, N.T. (1991). Chronic daily headache: Clinical features and natural history. In *Headache and Depression: Serotonin Pathways as a Common Clue* (G. Nappi, G. Bono, G. Sandrini et al., eds.), pp. 49–58. Raven Press, New York.

Mathew, N.T. (1993). Transformed migraine. *Cephalalgia* 13:78–83.

Mathew, N.T. and S. Ali (1991). Valproate in the treatment of persistent chronic daily headache. An open label study. *Headache* 31:71–74.

Mathew, N.T., R. Kurman, and F. Perez (1990). Drug induced refractory headache—clinical features and management. *Headache* 30:634–638.

Mathew, N.T., U. Reuveni, and F. Perez (1987). Transformed or evolutive migraine. *Headache* 27:102–106.

Mathew, N.T., J.R. Saper, S.D. Silberstein et al. (1995). Migraine prophylaxis with divalproex. *Arch. Neurol.* 52:281–286.

Mathew, N.T., E. Stubits, and M.R. Nigam (1982). Transformation of migraine into daily headache: Analysis of factors. *Headache* 22:66–68.

Mauskop, A. (1999). Botulinum toxin in the treatment of chronic daily headaches [Abstract]. *Cephalalgia* 19:453.

Mendell, L.M. (1966). Physiologic properties of unmyelinated fibre projection to the spinal chord. *Exp. Neurol.* 16:316–332.

Merikangas, K.R., J. Angst, and H. Isler (1990). Migraine and psychopathology: Results of the Zurich cohort study of young adults. *Arch. Gen. Psychiatry* 47:849–853.

Messinger, H.B., E.L.H. Spierings, and A.J.P. Vincent (1991). Overlap of migraine and tension-type headache in the International Headache Society classification. *Cephalalgia* 11:233–237.

Micieli, G., G.C. Manzoni, F. Granella et al. (1988). Clinical and epidemiological observations on drug abuse in headache patients. In *Drug-induced Headache* (H.C. Diener and M. Wilkinson, eds.), pp. 20–28. Springer-Verlag, Berlin.

Miller, D.S., C.A. Talbot, W. Simpson et al. (1997). A comparison of naproxen sodium, acetaminophen and placebo in the treatment of muscle contraction headache. *Headache* 27:392–396.

Mitsikostas, D.D., S. Gatzonis, A. Thomas et al. (1997). Buspirone vs. amitriptyline in the treatment of chronic tension-type headache. *J. Neurol. Scand.* 96:247–251.

Mitsikostas, D.D. and A.M. Thomas (1999). Comorbidity of headache and depressive disorders. *Cephalalgia* 19:211–217.

Mongini, F., N. Defilippi, and C. Negro (1997). Chronic daily headache. A clinical and psycho-logic profile before and after treatment. *Headache* 37:83–87.

Montalcini, R.L., R. Daltos, F. Dellavalle et al. (1995). Update of the NGF saga. *J. Neurol. Sci.* 130:119–127.

Monzon, M.J. and M.J. Lainez (1998). Quality of life in migraine and chronic daily headache patients. *Cephalalgia* 18:638–643.

Monzon, M.J., M.J.A. Lainez, F. Morales et al. (1999). Long-term prognosis of chronic daily headache [Abstract]. *Cephalalgia* 19:410.

Morland, T.J., O.V. Storli, and T.E. Mogstad (1979). Doxepin in the prophylactic treatment of mixed "vascular" and tension headache. *Headache* 19:382–383.

Mosek, A., J.W. Swanson, W.M. O'Fallon et al. (1999). CSF opening pressure in patients with chronic daily headache [Abstract]. *Cephalalgia* 19:323.

Moskowitz, M.A. (1992). Neurogenic versus vascular mechanisms of sumatriptan and ergot alkaloids in migraine. *Trends Pharmacol. Sci.* 13:307–311.

Mungliani, R. and S.P. Hunt (1995). Molecular biology of pain. *Br. J. Anaesth.* 75:186–192.

Mylecharane, E.J. and P. Tfelt-Hansen (1993). Miscellaneous drugs. In *The Headaches* (J. Olesen, P. Tfelt-Hansen, and K.M.A. Welch, eds.), pp. 397–402. Raven Press, New York.

Nakashima, K. and K. Takahashi (1991). Exteroceptive suppression of the masseter, temporalis and trapezius muscles produced by mental nerve stimulation in patients with chronic headaches. *Cephalalgia* 11:23–28.

Newman, L.C., R.B. Lipton, and S. Solomon (1993). Hemicrania continua: 7 new cases and a literature review. *Headache* 32:267.

Newman, L.C., R.B. Lipton, S. Solomon et al. (1994). Daily headache in a population sample: Results from the American Migraine Study. *Headache* 34:295.

Olesen, J., P. Tfelt-Hansen, and K.M.A. Welch (eds.) (1993). *The Headaches*. Raven Press, New York.

Palmer, K.J. and P. Benfield (1994). Fluvoxamine: An overview of its pharmacologic properties and a review of its use in nondepressive disorders. *CNS Drugs* 1:57–87.

Pareja, J.A. (1995). Chronic paroxysmal hemicrania: Dissociation of the pain and autonomic features. *Headache* 35:111–113.

Pareja, J.A., T. Palomo, M.A. Gorriti et al. (1990). Hemicrania episodica—a new type of headache or pre-chronic stage of hemicrania continua. *Headache* 30:344–346.

Paulus, W., J. Schoenen, and A. Straube (1992). Exteroceptive suppression of temporalis muscle activity in various types of headache. *Headache* 32:41–44.

Pazzaglia, P.J. and R.M. Post (1992). Contingent tolerance and reresponse to carbamazepine: A case study in a patient with trigeminal neuralgia and bipolar disorder. *J. Neuropsychiatry Clin. Neurosci.* 4:76–81.

Pfaffenrath, V., H.C. Diener, H. Isler et al. (1994). Efficacy and tolerability of amitriptylinoxide in the treatment of chronic tension-type headache: A multicentre controlled study. *Cephalalgia* 14:149–155.

Pfaffenrath, V. and H. Isler (1993). Evaluation of the nosology of chronic tension-type headache. *Cephalalgia* 13:60–62.

Pfaffenrath, V. and H. Kaube (1990). Diagnostics of cervicogenic headache. *Funct. Neurol.* 5:159–164.

Pfaffenrath, V., U. Kellhammer, and W. Pollmann (1986). Combination headache: Practical experience with a combination of beta-blocker and an antidepressive. *Cephalalgia* 6:25–32.

Pini, L.A., M. Bigarelli, G. Vitale et al. (1996). Headaches associated with chronic use of analgesics: A therapeutic approach. *Headache* 36:433–439.

Pluvinage, R. (1994). Le traitement des migraines et des cephalees psychogenes par l'amitriptyline. *Semin. Hop. Paris* 54:713–716.

Porta, M., M. Loiero, and M. Gamba (1999). Treatment of tension-type headache by botulinum toxin in pericranial muscles [Abstract]. *Cephalalgia* 19:453–454.

Post, R.M. and S.D. Silberstein (1994). Shared mechanisms in affective illness, epilepsy, and migraine. *Neurology* 44:S37–S47.

Potter, D.L., D.E. Hart, C.S. Calder et al. (2000). A double-blind, randomized, placebo-controlled, parallel study to determine the efficacy of Topamax® (topiramate) in the prophylactic treatment of migraine [Abstract]. *Neurology* 57(7, Suppl 3):A15.

Price, D.D., J. Mao, and D.J. Mayer (1994). Central neural mechanisms of normal and abnormal pain states. In *Progress in Pain Research and Management* (H.L. Fields and J.C. Liebeskind, eds.), pp. 61–84. IASP Press, Seattle.

Pringsheim, T. and D. Howse (1998). Inpatient treatment of chronic daily headache using dihydroergotamine: A long-term followup study. *Can. J. Neurol. Sci.* 25:146–150.

Puca, F., S. Genco, M.P. Prudenzano et al. (1999). Psychiatric comorbidity and psychosocial stress in patients with tension-type headache from headache centers in Italy. The Italian Collaborative Group for the Study of Psychopathological Factors in Primary Headaches. *Cephalalgia* 19:159–164.

Rang, H.P. and L. Urban (1995). New molecules in analgesia. *Br. J. Anaesth.* 75:145–156.

Rapoport, A.M. (1988). Analgesic rebound headache. *Headache* 28:662–665.

Rapoport, A.M., R.E. Weeks, F.D. Sheftell et al. (1986). The "analgesic washout period": A crit-

ical variable in the evaluation of headache treatment efficacy. *Neurology* 36:100–101.

Raskin, N.H. (1986). Repetitive intravenous dihydroergotamine as therapy for intractable migraine. *Neurology* 36:995–997.

Rasmussen, B.K. (1992). Migraine and tension-type headache in a general population: Psychosocial factors. *Int. J. Epidemiol.* 21:1138–1143.

Rasmussen, B.K. (1995). Epidemiology of headache. *Cephalalgia* 15:45–68.

Rasmussen, B.K., R. Jensen, and J. Olesen (1989). Impact of headache on sickness absence and utilization of medical services. *J. Epidemiol. Community Health* 46:443–446.

Ravishankar, K. (1997). Headache pattern in India: A headache clinic analysis of 1000 patients. *Cephalalgia* 17:143–144.

Robinson, R.G. (1993). Pain relief for headaches. *Can. Fam. Physician* 39:867–872.

Russell, M.B., S. Stergaard, L. Endtsen et al. (1999). Familial occurrence of chronic tension-type headache. *Cephalalgia* 19:207–210.

Sakai, F., S. Ebihara, M. Akiyama et al. (1995). Pericranial muscle hardness in tension-type headache: A noninvasive measurement method and its clinical application. *Brain* 118:523–531.

Sandrini, G., G.C. Manzoni, C. Zanferrari et al. (1993). An epidemiologic approach to nosography of chronic daily headache. *Cephalalgia* 13:72–77.

Sanin, L.C., N.T. Mathew, L.R. Bellmyer et al. (1994). The International Headache Society (IHS) headache classification as applied to a headache clinic population. *Cephalalgia* 14:443–446.

Saper, J.R. (1983). *Headache Disorders: Current Concepts in Treatment Strategies*. Wright-PSG, Littleton, MA.

Saper, J.R. (1987). Egotamine dependency—a review. *Headache* 27:435–438.

Saper, J.R. (1989). Chronic headache syndromes. *Neurol. Clin.* 7:387–412.

Saper, J.R. and J.M. Jones (1986). Ergotamine tartrate dependency: Features and possible mechanisms. *Clin. Neuropharmacol.* 9:244–256.

Saper, J.R., S.D. Silberstein, A.E. Lake et al. (1994). Double-blind trial of fluoxetine: Chronic daily headache and migraine. *Headache* 34:497–502.

Schepelmann, K., M. Dannhausen, I. Kotter et al. (1998). Exteroceptive suppression of temporalis muscle activity in patients with fibromyalgia, tension-type headache, and normal controls. *Electroencephalog. Clin. Neurophysiol.* 107:196–199.

Scher, A.I., W.F. Stewart, J. Liberman et al. (1998). Prevalence of frequent headache in a population sample. *Headache* 38:497–506.

Schnider, P., S. Aull, C. Baumgartner et al. (1996). Long-term outcome of patients with headache and drug abuse after inpatient withdrawal: Five-year follow-up. *Cephalalgia* 16:481–485.

Schnider, P., S. Aull, and M. Feucht (1994). Use and abuse of analgesics in tension-type headache. *Cephalalgia* 14:162–167.

Schoenen, J., D. Bottin, F. Hardy et al. (1991). Cephalic and extracephalic pressure pain threshold in chronic tension-type headache. *Pain* 47:145–149.

Schoenen, J., B. Jamart, P. Gerard et al. (1987). Exteroceptive suppression of temporalis muscle activity in chronic headache. *Neurology* 37: 1834–1836.

Schoenen, J., P. Lenarduzzi, and J. Sianard-Gainko (1989). Chronic headaches associated with analgesics and/or ergotamine abuse: A clinical survey of 434 consecutive outpatients. In *New Advances in Headache Research* (F.D. Rose, ed.), pp. 29–43. Smith-Gordon, London.

Scholz, E., H.C. Diener, S. Geiselhart et al. (1988). Drug-induced headache: Does a critical dosage exist? In *Drug-induced Headache* (H.C. Diener, ed.), pp. 29–43. Springer-Verlag, Berlin.

Scholz, E., W.D. Gerber, H.C. Diener et al. (1987). Dihydroergotamine vs. flunarizine vs. nifedipine vs. metoprolol vs. propranolol in migraine prophylaxis: A comparative study based on time series analysis. In *Advances in Headache Research* (E. Scholz, W.D. Gerber, H.C. Diener et al., eds.), pp. 139–145. John Libbey, London.

Schwarz, A., U. Farber, and G. Glaeske (1985). Daten zu analgetikakonsum and analgetikanephropathie in der bundesrepublik. *Offentliche Gesundheitswesen* 47:298–300.

Shuaib, A., F. Ahmed, M. Muratoglu et al. (1999). Topiramate in migraine prophylaxis: A pilot study [Abstract]. *Cephalalgia* 19:379–380.

Silberstein, S.D. (1993). Chronic daily headache and tension-type headache. *Neurology* 43: 1644–1649.

Silberstein, S.D. (1984). Treatment of headache in primary care practice. *Am. J. Med.* 77:65–72.

Silberstein, S.D. (1998). Methysergide. *Cephalalgia* 18:421–435.

Silberstein, S.D. and R.B. Lipton (1994). Overview of diagnosis and treatment of migraine. *Neurology* 44:6–16.

Silberstein, S.D., R.B. Lipton, and M. Sliwinski (1995). Assessment for revised criteria of chronic daily headache. *Neurology* 45:A394.

Silberstein, S.D., R.B. Lipton, and M. Sliwinski (1996). Classification of daily and near-daily headaches: Field trial of revised IHS criteria. *Neurology* 47:871–875.

Silberstein, S.D., R.B. Lipton, S. Solomon et al. (1994a). Classification of daily and near daily headaches: Proposed revisions to the IHS classification. *Headache* 34:1–7.

Silberstein, S.D. and J.R. Saper (1993). Migraine: Diagnosis and treatment. In *Wolff's Headache and Other Head Pain* (D.J. Dalessio and S.D. Silberstein, eds.), pp. 96–170. Oxford University Press, New York.

Silberstein, S.D., E.A. Schulman, and M.M. Hopkins (1990). Repetitive intravenous DHE in the treatment of refractory headache. *Headache* 30: 334–339.

Silberstein, S.D. and J.R. Silberstein (1992). Chronic daily headache: Prognosis following inpatient treatment with repetitive IV DHE. *Headache* 32:439–445.

Silberstein, S.D., N.Mathew, J. Saper, and S. Jenkins for the Botox Migraine Clinical Research Group (2000). Botulinum toxin type A as a migraine preventive treatment. *Headache* 40:445–450.

Silverman, K., S.M. Evans, E.C. Strain et al. (1992). Withdrawal syndrome after the double-blind cessation of caffeine consumption. *N. Eng. J. Med.* 327:1109–1114.

Sjaastad, O. (1990). The headache challenge in our time: Cervicogenic headache. *Funct. Neurol.* 5:155–158.

Sjaastad, O. and F. Antonaci (1993). Chronic paroxysmal hemicrania (CPH) and hemicrania continua: Transition from one stage to another. *Headache* 33:551–554.

Sjaastad, O., C. Saunte, and T.A. Fredriksen (1985). Bilaterality of cluster headache. *Cephalalgia* 5:55–58.

Sjaastad, O., C. Saunte, and H. Hovdahl (1983). "Cervicogenic headache." An hypothesis. *Cephalalgia* 3:249–256.

Sjaastad, O. and K. Tjorstad (1987). Hemicrania continua: A third Norwegian case. *Cephalalgia* 7:175–177.

Smuts, J.A., M.K. Baker, H.M. Smuts et al. (1999). Botulinum toxin type A as prophylactic treatment in chronic tension-type headache [Abstract]. *Cephalalgia* 19:454.

Solomon, G.D., F.G. Skobieranda, and L.A. Gragg (1993). Quality of life and well-being of headache patients: Measurement by the Medical Outcomes Study instrument. *Headache* 33:351–358.

Solomon, S., R.B. Lipton, and L.C. Newman (1992a). Clinical features of chronic daily headache. *Headache* 32:325–329.

Solomon, S., R.B. Lipton, and L.C. Newman (1992b). Evaluation of chronic daily headache —comparison to criteria for chronic tension-type headache. *Cephalalgia* 12:365–368.

Strassman, A.M., S.A. Raymond, and R. Burstein (1996). Sensitization of meningeal sensory neurons and the origin of headaches. *Nature* 384: 560–564.

Suhr, B., S. Evers, B. Bauer et al. (1999). Drug-induced headache: Long-term results of stationary versus ambulatory withdrawal therapy. *Cephalalgia* 19:44–49.

Tavola, T., C. Gala, G. Conte et al. (1992). Traditional Chinese acupuncture in tension-type headache: A controlled study. *Pain* 48:325–329.

Tekle Haimanot, R., B. Seraw, L. Forsgren et al. (1995). Migraine, chronic tension-type headache, and cluster headache in an Ethiopian rural community. *Cephalalgia* 15:482–488.

Tfelt-Hansen, P. and A.A. Krabbe (1981). Ergotamine. Do patients benefit from withdrawal? *Cephalalgia* 1:29–32.

Tfelt-Hansen, P. and R.B. Lipton (1993). Prioritizing treatment. In *The Headaches* (J. Olesen, P. Tfelt-Hansen, and K.M.A. Welch, eds.), pp. 359–362. Raven Press, New York.

Vanast, W.J. (1986). New daily persistent headaches: Definition of a benign syndrome. *Headache* 26:317.

Verri, A.P., P. Cecchini, C. Galli et al. (1998). Psychiatric comorbidity in chronic daily headache. *Cephalalgia* 18:45–49.

Wang, S.J., J.L. Fuh, S.R. Lu et al. (2000). Chronic daily headache in Chinese elderly: prevalence, risk factors and biannual follow-up. *Neurology* 54:314–319.

Weiller, C., A. May, V. Limroth et al. (1995). Brainstem activation in spontaneous human migraine attacks. *Nat. Med.* 1:658–660.

Welch, K.M.A., V. Nagesh, K. Rozell et al. (1999). Functional MRI of chronic daily headache [Abstract]. *Cephalalgia* 19:462–463.

Wilkinson, M. (1988). Introduction. In *Drug-induced Headache* (H.C. Diener and M. Wilkinson, eds.), pp. 1–2. Springer-Verlag, Berlin.

Woolf, C.J. (1995). Somatic pain: Pathogenesis and prevention. *Br. J. Anaesth.* 75:169–176.

Yamamura, H., A. Malick, N.L. Chamberlin et al. (1999). Cardiovascular and neuronal responses to head stimulation reflect central sensitization and cutaneous allodynia in a rat model of migraine. *J. Neurophysiol.* 81:479–493.

Zukerman, E., S.N. Hannuch, S. de Carvalho et al. (1987). Hemicrania continua: A case report. *Cephalalgia* 7:171–173.

12

Cluster Headache: Diagnosis, Management, and Treatment

DAVID W. DODICK
J. KEITH CAMPBELL

Cluster headache, the most painful of the primary headaches, has been known in the past by a confusing variety of names. Although "cluster headache" is now the generally accepted name for this severe unilateral headache of brief duration, it is still sometimes referred to as "migrainous neuralgia" (Harris, 1936), especially in Europe. "Erythroprosopalgia," "histaminic cephalgia," "petrosal neuralgia," "sphenopalatine neuralgia," "Sluder's neuralgia," "vidian neuralgia," and "erythromelalgia of the head" are just some of the older terms for the condition.

Horton et al. (1939) described many of the features of cluster headache and reported their experience in treating this "new syndrome of vascular headache" with histamine. Later, the condition became known as "Horton's headache" or "histaminic cephalgia" (Horton, 1952). The connection to histamine arose from the observation that injections of it would provoke a severe but brief unilateral headache with associated autonomic symptoms in those prone to such attacks.

Symonds (1956) provided a careful description of cluster headache under the term "a particular variety of headache." This paper brought the condition to the attention of many neurologists and internists. Noting the tendency for the headache attacks to cluster

in time, Kunkle et al. (1952) used the term "cluster pattern" to convey the periodicity of the groups of attacks.

CLASSIFICATION

Long classified as a primary headache, cluster headache was considered to be a variant of migraine. This is no longer a tenable view; therefore, in 1988, the Headache Classification Committee of the International Headache Society (IHS) classified cluster headache as distinct from migraine but placed it in the same group as the much less common, but in some respects similar, chronic paroxysmal hemicrania (CPH) (Table 12–1) (Sjaastad and Dale, 1974) (see Chapter 14).

DEFINITIONS

Several of the terms relating to cluster headache can be confusing and require defining. An individual attack, lasting on average 60 to 90 minutes, is called a *cluster headache* or *cluster attack*. The time during which recurrent attacks are occurring, usually weeks but at times months or years, is referred to as the *cluster period* or sometimes, especially by pa-

Table 12–1 International Headache Society classification of cluster headache and chronic paroxysmal hemicrania

---

3. Cluster headache and chronic paroxysmal hemicrania
  3.1 Cluster headache
    3.1.1 Cluster headache periodicity undetermined
    3.1.2 Episodic cluster headache
    3.1.3 Chronic cluster headache
      3.1.3.1 Unremitting from onset
      3.1.3.2 Evolved from episodic
  3.2 Chronic paroxysmal hemicrania
  3.3 Cluster headache-like disorder not fulfilling above criteria

---

tients, simply as a *cluster* (of attacks). When attacks cease, the individual is in remission. This may last from a few days to years.

Episodic cluster headache infers that remissions or periods of freedom from pain characterize the course of the disorder. The IHS description of episodic cluster headache states that attacks "occur in periods lasting 7 days to 1 year separated by pain-free periods lasting 14 days or more."

Chronic cluster headache refers to attacks that occur for more than 1 year without remission or have remissions that last less than 14 days. The chronic form of the disease can evolve from the episodic form (secondary chronic form) (Ekbom and Olivarius, 1971) or may develop de novo as primary chronic cluster headache. The rarest variety is the secondary episodic pattern, which begins as the chronic form and then becomes episodic.

Although not accepted by the IHS Classification Committee, several cluster-like conditions have been described in which cluster headaches and trigeminal neuralgia appear to be blended together so that both types of pain occur. The term "cluster-tic" has been used in relation to this combination of symptoms (Green and Apfelbaum, 1978). In some individuals, cluster headache and migraine coexist. This combination has been termed "cluster-migraine" (Medina and Diamond, 1977), but the term should be avoided as it has also been applied to episodes of migraine that occur in clusters without any of the features of cluster headache. "Cluster-vertigo" (Gilbert, 1965, 1970) is not sufficiently sub-

stantiated to warrant inclusion in the IHS classification.

CLINICAL MANIFESTATIONS

In its commonest form, episodic cluster headache occurs at least once every 24 hours for weeks at a time. A period of freedom from attacks, a remission, usually follows and may last from weeks to years (Ekbom, 1970a; Kudrow, 1980). Most often, the remission is followed by a further period of attacks, but any cluster period may be an individual's last. A common pattern, especially in the first few years of cluster headache, is for exacerbations (periods at risk) to occur seasonally, e.g., every spring or every fall for a few years (Ekbom, 1970b). This periodicity generally becomes less evident after a few years, and periods of cluster activity become much less predictable, occurring at almost any time of the year. Periodicity was studied in a large series of patients (Kudrow, 1987; Kudrow and Kudrow, 1990); the most likely times for a cluster to start were apparently associated with the number of hours of daylight, more exacerbations within the two weeks following the summer and winter solstices and fewer exacerbations starting within 2 weeks of the onset and offset of daylight-saving time. Approximately 85% of individuals afflicted by cluster headache have the episodic form (Rasmussen, 1999).

On average, a cluster period lasts 6 to 12 weeks, while remissions last for an average of 12 months (Ekbom, 1970a; Kudrow, 1980). Considerable variations of these average durations between patients and in the individual are characteristic, especially after the disorder has persisted for a few years. Despite this variability, many individuals describe the onset of their yearly cluster in relation to the same season for a number of years. Such patients are always pleasantly surprised by the nonappearance of a cluster in any particular year and unpleasantly surprised by the unexplained appearance of a cluster at a different time of year.

When exacerbations lengthen, remissions shorten, or more clusters occur than usual, an individual may be switching from the episodic form of the disease to the chronic form. In chronic cluster headache, attacks occur daily or almost daily for more than a year with no more than a 2-week remission. Once chronic cluster headache has developed, whether de novo or by transformation from the episodic form, it tends to persist for years, even into old age, although long-term follow-up has shown that as many as 50% of affected individuals eventually revert or switch to an episodic form (Manzoni et al., 1991; Krabbe, 1986). Chronic cluster headache occurs in approximately 15% of those affected by cluster headache. The chronic form is unremitting from onset (primary chronic cluster) in 10% of sufferers and evolves from the episodic form in 5%.

During a cluster period, or in the chronic phase, individual attacks of headache occur daily or almost daily. When only one attack occurs in 24 hours, it is not uncommon for each attack to occur at the same time each day or each night for days or weeks on end. Unlike migraine or trigeminal neuralgia, nocturnal attacks of cluster headache are more frequent than daytime attacks. Onset of the first attack about 90 minutes after falling asleep has been related to the onset of rapid eye movement (REM) sleep (Dexter and Riley, 1975; Kudrow et al., 1984). There is little doubt that sleep disturbances rapidly compound when several attacks of headaches occur each night. Sleep deprivation results in early-onset REM sleep, which may trigger a further attack. As this seemingly vicious cycle persists, even a daytime nap can induce REM sleep and a further attack of headache.

THE INDIVIDUAL ATTACK

An attack of cluster headache lasts an average of 45 to 90 minutes, with shorter and longer attacks contributing to a bell-shaped curve of duration distribution. Almost without exception, attacks are strictly unilateral in any cluster period and may remain unilateral on the same side throughout the individual's history. Less frequently, the pain occurs on the opposite side of the head and face in a subse-

quent cluster, and even less frequently, attacks will switch sides from one attack to another.

Cluster headache is usually described as coming on without warning. Some observers have described a vague premonitory warning sensation prior to an attack (Blau and Engel, 1998), but in general, the onset of pain is unheralded, rapidly escalates in intensity, and is recognized as a pain of great intensity, the so-called suicide headache. Until recently, cluster headache was not considered to be associated with aura symptoms seen in migraine, but Silberstein et al. (2000) reported on a group of six cluster headache patients who had stereotyped aura (visual aura in five of six patients) preceding their individual cluster attacks.

Gastrointestinal symptoms are not typical of cluster headache attacks. Nausea has been described in as many as 40% of patients, but vomiting is rare. In some patients, nausea may be secondary to drug ingestion. The reported frequency of photophobia in patients with cluster headache has varied between 5% and 72%, while phonophobia was reported only occasionally, in 12% to 39% of cluster headache cases (Ekbom, 1970a; Nappi et al., 1992). However, recent quantitative data suggest that cluster headache patients resemble migraine patients, who in general are markedly more sensitive to light and sound than controls (Vingen et al., 1999)

Quality and Intensity of the Pain

The pain of cluster headache is often described in such graphic terms as "boring," "tearing," or "burning" and with such descriptive analogies as "a hot poker in the eye" or as if "the eye is being pushed out." The intensity is arguably the most severe of the primary headache syndromes, comparable to the pain intensity associated with trigeminal neuralgia and the syndrome of short-lasting unilateral neuraligiform pain with conjunctival injection and tearing (SUNCT).

Behavior During an Attack

In contrast to migraine, it is common for those suffering a cluster headache to be restless and occasionally even violent. Most are unwilling to lie down but prefer to pace about or sit and rock back and forth. Some sufferers exert pressure on the painful area with a hand or place either an ice pack or a hot pack over the affected eye and temple. Many individuals isolate themselves from family members or leave the house to get into cold or fresh air for the duration of the attack. Violent, destructive behaviors that result in self-inflicted injuries occur rarely. Many contemplate suicide during an attack, while others beg a family member to end their suffering.

As attacks appear to be triggered by REM sleep, desperate individuals will attempt to remain awake for as long as possible. The resulting sleep deprivation shortens the REM latency time so that when sleep occurs, as it inevitably does, an attack occurs shortly thereafter. The resulting vicious cycle of pain and lack of sleep can rapidly demoralize the unfortunate individual and lead to depression and suicidal ideation.

Location

The pain of cluster headache is most frequently maximal around the eye and orbits on the affected side. It may radiate into the ipsilateral temple, forehead, cheek, and even the jaw. Ekbom (1970a) described an upper and a lower syndrome based on the distribution of the pain radiating out from the affected eye/orbit. In the upper syndrome, the pain, which is maximal around the eye, radiates to the forehead and/or temple and/or parietal region. In the lower syndrome, the pain radiates infraorbitally to the upper and lower teeth and jaw and even into the ipsilateral neck.

Temporal Profile

After starting without warning or after a mild pain in the temple, cluster headache pain rapidly worsens and reaches a peak intensity within 5 to 10 minutes. The pain may stay at maximal intensity or fluctuate slightly for 45 to 90 minutes and then decrease in a stepwise manner. In some patients, a period of repetitive peaks of pain separated by brief valleys

of lesser pain characterizes the attack profile. The end of the attack usually comes quite suddenly, with rapidly decreasing intensity and finally freedom from pain.

The most articulate description of an attack of cluster headache was written by Kudrow (1980), himself a cluster headache sufferer.

Following a period of perhaps several hours of feeling quite elated and energetic, I experienced a fullness in my ears, somewhat more on the right side than the left, having a character similar to that which occurs during rapid descent in an airplane or elevator. I then became aware of a dull discomfort, an extension of ear fullness at the base of my skull—further extending over the entire head, on both sides, though somewhat more on the right. At this point, two or three minutes have elapsed; seemingly short but long enough for me to know that a "cluster" has indeed begun and will ultimately get worse. Such anticipation causes me considerable consternation regarding any decision to continue my activities, or cancel plans and find a place to be alone; giving way to a slowly increasing anxiety, fear, panic and withdrawal. I become aware of myself "listening" for changes in my head. Is the cluster prematurely aborting itself, progressing further, or unchanging? A sudden stab, only fleeting, strikes my temple, then again —somewhere near the apex of my skull and upper molars in my face, always on the right side. It strikes me again, deep into the skull base, and as quickly, changes location to a small area above my eyebrow. My nose is stuffed and yet runs simultaneously. If I could sneeze, I feel the attack would end. Yet in spite of all tricks, I find myself unable to induce sneezing. While the sharp stabs continue in this fashion, a slow crescendo of dull pain presents itself in an area of hand's length and breadth over the eye and temporal region. The pain area narrows into a smaller area, and yet, as if magnified, enlarges in intensity. I find myself bending my neck downward, though slightly, as if my head is being gently pushed from behind. My neck, up to the base of my skull, is tight and feels as if I was wearing a neck collar. I feel compelled to remove my tie and loosen my shirt collar even though I know that it will not offer me even a modicum of relief.

In an effort to alter this persistent discomfort, I drop my head between my legs while seated. My face and eyes seem to fill with fluid, but the pain persists and remains unchanged. Despite my suntan, as I look into the mirror, a gaunt, sickly, pale face peers back. My right lid is only slightly drooping and the white of my eye is charted with many red vessels, giving the eye an overall color of pink. Right and left pupils appear equal and constricted, as is usual for light-eyed people. Having difficulty standing in one place too long, I leave the mirror to continue alternating my pacing and sitting.

As usual, I am struck with the additional fear that the pain will never end, but dismiss it as impossible, since even if that were the case, I would surely kill myself.

The pain, now located somewhere behind my eye and slightly above it, worsens. The pain is best described as a "force" pushing with such incredible power through my eye that my head appears to be moving backward, yielding to its resistance. The "force" wanes and waxes, but the duration of successive exacerbations seems to increase. The cluster attack is at its peak which is celebrated by an outpouring of tears from only my right eye. I have now been in cluster for thirty-five minutes—ten minutes at its peak.

My wife peeks into the room which I hold forth. I look up and see her expression of pity, frustration, and helplessness. She sees my tortured face as I have seen it in the mirror at this stage before; a drooling mouth, agape, gray face wet on one side, an almost closed eyelid; and smelling of pain and anguish. She closes the door and leaves, feeling hurt for me, anger for the stupidity of medical science, and guilt—since deep within her mind is the suspicion that she is the cause for my suffering.

I cry for her, but cry more for myself. The pain is so incredible. Suddenly I am overwhelmed by a fury. I lift a chair high over my head and crash it to the floor. With a doubled fist I strike the wall. The pain persists.

Waning periods soon become longer in duration and I allow myself to suspect that the peak is behind me—but cautiously, since I have been too often disappointed.

Indeed, the pain is ending. The descent from the mountain is rapid. The "force" is gone. Only severe pain remains. My nose and eye continue to run. The road back, as with all travel, covers the same territory, but faster. Stabbing, easily tolerated pain is felt. Then gone. Dull, aching fullness, neck stiffness, all disappear, replaced in turn by a welcome sensation of pins and needles over the right scalp area—similar to the way one's leg feels after it has been "asleep." Thus my head has awakened after a nightmare of torment.

Eye and nose dry, I let out a sigh. I collect my pile of wet tissues that are strewn all over the floor and deposit them in a wastepaper basket. The in-

nocent chair, now uprighted, I rub my slightly bruised fist.

Thus, having ended the battle and cleaned up its field, I open the door and enter my pain-free world . . . until tomorrow.

AUTONOMIC FEATURES

All of the autonomic features (Table 12–2) are transient, lasting only for the duration of the attack, with the exception of a partial Horner's syndrome (57% to 69%) with ptosis or meiosis, both of which may persist after many acute attacks, although this is rare (Lance and Anthony, 1971b). Lacrimation and conjunctival injection are the most common local signs of autonomic involvement, being present in more than 80% of patients. Nasal stuffiness or rhinorrhea is experienced by 68% to 76% of patients during attacks. It is usually ipsilateral to the pain but may, on rare occasions, occur on both sides. Forehead sweating, facial flushing, and edema are rare. Fluctuations in heart rate, blood pressure, and cardiac rhythm, including premature ventricular beats, transient episodes of atrial fibrillation, and first-degree atrioventricular or sinoatrial block, can occur (Russell and Storstein, 1983). Autonomic symptoms may not be clinically evident in up to 3% of cluster headache sufferers (Nappi et al., 1992).

Table 12–2 Autonomic features of cluster headache

Ipsilateral to the pain
  Partial Horner's syndrome with sparing of facial sweating
  Nasal obstruction
  Tearing due to temporary blockage of nasolacrimal duct
  Conjunctival injection
  Increased sweating (rare)
  Flushing (rare)
  Edema of facial tissues including the gums and palate (very rare)
  "Cold spot" supraorbitally as detected by thermography (Kudrow, 1979a)
Systemic
  Bradycardia (may be severe enough to induce syncope)
  Hypertension
  Increased gastric acid production

PHYSICAL CHARACTERISTICS

The typical heavy facial features common to many cluster headache sufferers were noted by Graham (1969). Deep nasolabial furrows, *peau d'orange* skin, and telangiectasia led to the description of "leonine facies." Women with cluster headache often have a masculine appearance, according to Kudrow (1993). Many of the characteristic facial features are most likely due to heavy tobacco and alcohol use, which are also characteristics of this population. Kudrow (1979b) reported that two-thirds of the patients in his large series had hazel-colored eyes. He also noted that many of those subject to cluster headache are tall, about 3 inches above average.

High gastric acid production and an increased incidence of peptic ulceration are also typical of those with cluster headache, but this could be due to the tendency to overuse alcohol often noted in those who have cluster headache.

PSYCHOLOGICAL CHARACTERISTICS

Graham (1969) claimed that men with cluster headaches looked lion-like but inwardly were like mice. He also reported a high incidence of emotional trauma prior to the onset of headaches. Neither observation is accepted as valid.

The personality type characteristically associated with cluster headache, particularly in men, is type A, hard-driving, energetic, and ambitious; but there are many exceptions. Cigarette smoking is almost universal in men with cluster headache and almost as frequent in women with cluster headache. Similar, but somewhat less consistent, is the heavy use of alcohol. However, there are exceptions to these characteristic behaviors. While several Minnesota Multiphasic Personality Inventory (MMPI) studies (Kudrow and Sutkus, 1979; Andrasik et al., 1982; Cuypers et al., 1981) failed to show a higher than normal incidence of neuroses or other psychopathology in cluster headache populations, patients with the chronic form of the disorder can become despondent and, according to Onofrio and

Campbell (1986), "fill the (consulting) room with emotional electricity."

TRIGGER FACTORS

Once a cluster period begins, individual headaches can, in many patients, be triggered or precipitated by alcohol and other vasodilators, notably nitroglycerin (Ekbom, 1968) and histamine. When in remission, i.e., between clusters, alcohol rarely precipitates an attack; thus, most sufferers will avoid alcohol as soon as a drink triggers an attack and will remain abstinent until the cluster is over. The mechanism whereby alcohol induces an attack is not understood. Nitroglycerin acts through its role as a source of nitric oxide, which leads to vasodilation.

Allergies, food sensitivities, hormonal changes, and stress appear to play little part in the pathogenesis of cluster headache. Trauma to the head has been recognized (legally) as a cause of cluster headache (Reik, 1987; Turkewitz et al., 1992), but it is hard to prove a cause-and-effect relationship.

DIFFERENTIAL DIAGNOSIS

Although the history of a cluster headache is often unmistakable, other possibilities should be considered in the differential diagnosis. Migraine may present with recurrent unilateral headache even with ipsilateral autonomic symptoms, particularly during severe attacks. However, the periodicity of cluster headache is often very stereotyped for a given patient, and the attacks of cluster headache are short-lived (45 to 90 minutes) compared to migraine (4 to 72 hours). Furthermore, cluster attacks are almost always unilateral, frequently nocturnal, can occur several times per day, and usually are not associated with aura, nausea, or vomiting.

Temporal arteritis pain is usually continuous but may wax and wane, and systemic symptoms (fever, polymyalgia, weight loss) are often associated with this disorder. Trigeminal neuralgia is characterized by paroxysmal shock-like electric jabs of unilateral pain, most commonly limited to the distribution of the second and/or third divisions of the trigeminal nerve. The pain can be triggered by stimulation of limited areas of facial skin or oral mucosa. Other disorders to be considered are dissection of the cervicocephalic cerebral blood vessels (carotid or vertebral), sinusitis, glaucoma, intracranial aneurysms, tumors or arteriovenous malformations, and even cervical cord lesions (meningioma) or infarction. In many of these instances, however, the history and examination disclose features that are worrisome for a secondary cause, the history lacks the stereotypical periodicity of attack and remission phases, or the response to conventional medications is lacking.

Finally, a number of primary headache syndromes may closely resemble cluster headache, such as chronic and episodic paroxysmal hemicrania, SUNCT syndrome, and hemicrania continua (Table 12–3). Collectively, these disorders have been referred to as "trigeminal-autonomic cephalgias" because of the trigeminal distribution of pain and the associated autonomic signs (Goadsby and Lipton, 1997). They are characterized by discrete, short-lasting, episodic attacks of intense, unilateral, orbital-temporal headache associated with robust ipsilateral autonomic signs. These syndromes may be associated with nocturnal attacks and may be precipitated by alcohol. The SUNCT syndrome appears to be the only other headache disorder that predominates in men. These disorders differ from cluster headache mainly in the higher frequency and shorter duration of individual attacks, with an almost inverse relationship across these disorders; as attack frequency increases, duration tends to decrease

(Table 12–3). The distinction between cluster headache and other paroxysmal hemicranias is important because of the different responses to therapy. The paroxysmal hemicranias and hemicrania continua often respond in a dramatic fashion to indomethacin, whereas patients with SUNCT syndrome derive no benefit from indomethacin or drugs typically used to treat cluster headache.

GENETICS AND FAMILY HISTORY

In contrast to migraine, cluster headache has not previously been considered an inherited condition. However, between 1947 and 1985, a total of 12 studies collectively revealed a family history in 4% (47/1,182) of patients with cluster headache (Russell 1997). In addition, cluster headache occurs in approximately 1 in 1,500 (D'Alessandro et al., 1986), which suggests an increased familial risk. Since that time, a number of studies have found a positive family history in approximately 7% of cluster sufferers, which represents a 14-fold increased risk of cluster headache in first-degree relatives of probands with cluster headache (Kudrow and Kudrow, 1994; Russell, 1997; Russell et al., 1994) and a twofold increased risk in second-degree relatives. The importance of genetics in cluster headache is also underscored by twin studies that demonstrate 100% concordance in five pairs of monozygotic twins (Eadie and Sutherland, 1966; Couturier et al., 1991; Roberge et al., 1992; Sjaastad et al., 1993). Complex segregation analysis suggests that an autosomal dominant gene has a role in the inheritance of cluster headache in some families (Russell, 1997).

Table 12–3 Cluster headache: comparison with other trigeminal autonomic cephalgias

Feature	Cluster	CPH	EPH	SUNCT
Gender (M:F)	4:1	1:3	1:1	4:1
Attack duration	15–180 min	2–45 min	1–30 min	5–250 s
Attack frequency	1–8/day	1–40/day	3–30/day	1/day–30/h
Autonomic features	++	++	++	++
Alcohol	++	+	+	+
Indomethacin effect	+/−	++	++	−

Key to abbreviations: CPH, chronic paroxysmal hemicrania; EPH, episodic paroxysmal hemicrania; SUNCT, short-lasting unilateral neuralgiform pain with conjunctival injection and tearing.

EPIDEMIOLOGY

Cluster headache is rare, but the exact prevalence is still a matter of debate because of the paucity of epidemiologic surveys. A large survey of 9,803 Swedish army recruits, all 18-year-old men, revealed a prevalence of 92/100,000 (confidence interval 42–174) (Ekbom et al., 1978), while the prevalence in a large population-based survey from the republic of San Marino was 69/100,000 (confidence interval 39–114) (D'Alessandro et al., 1986). Since cluster headache predominates in men, the difference in prevalence between these two studies may be explained by the difference in study populations. The Swedish data were extrapolated by Kudrow (1980) to the distribution of age at onset from headache clinic data to yield a prevalence rate of approximately 0.4%. The Swedish data was extrapolated by Kudrow to the distribution of age of onset from headache clinic data to yield a prevalence rate of approximately 0.4% (Kudrow, 1980). A population-based incidence study from Rochester, Minnesota, based on a retrospective review of more than 6,400 patient medical records, revealed an age-adjusted incidence of cluster headache of 15.6/100,000 person-years for men and 4.0/100,000 person-years for women (Swanson, 1994). As the authors pointed out, data derived from incidence studies provide a better basis for the generation of hypotheses regarding disease etiology since prevalence rates may vary as a function of patient survival and migration.

DEMOGRAPHICS

Cluster headache has long been recognized to predominate in men. The gender ratio has varied between 5.0:1 and 6.7:1 in the larger case series, which have included at least 200 patients (Horton, 1956; Lovshin, 1961; Ekbom, 1981; Kudrow, 1980; Krabbe, 1986; Manzoni et al., 1988). The largest case series, including 1,176 patients (Horton, 1956) and 425 patients (Kudrow, 1980), have reported male-to-female ratios of 6.7:1 and 5:1, respectively. However, recent evidence suggests a progressively decreasing male preponderance. In a study of 482 patients from Parma, Italy, Manzoni (1997) reported a male-to-female ratio of 3.5:1. The male-to-female ratio based on the year of onset decreased from 6.2:1 in the 1960s to 2.1:1 in the 1990s (Manzoni, 1998). It is unclear whether this represents a true rise in the incidence of cluster headache in women or whether the disorder is becoming better recognized in women. Several authors have stressed the importance of changing lifestyles, such as the changing role of women in society and in the workplace. However, the importance of these changes in altering the sex predilection of cluster headache is unclear.

Although cluster headache has been reported to begin in childhood, the mean age at onset is 27 to 31 years in both men and women, approximately 10 years later than that of migraine (Ekbom, 1970b; Kudrow, 1980). Several authors have reported a higher prevalence of cluster headaches among African-Americans than Caucasians, particularly among black women, where the male-to-female ratio is only 3:1 (Lovshin, 1961; Kudrow, 1980). Data from the North American and European continents suggest that there is little ethnic difference in the occurrence of cluster headache.

PATHOGENESIS

A unifying pathophysiologic explanation of cluster headache is not available. A complete hypothesis must account for the three major features of the syndrome, which include the trigeminal distribution of the pain, the ipsilateral autonomic features, and the tendency for attacks to cluster with striking circadian and circannual consistency, which is the signature feature of cluster headache.

Based on the clinical features of the disorder, three conclusions can be drawn. First, because the pain of cluster headache is invariably centered around the eye and forehead, it is probable that the ipsilateral trigeminal nociceptive pathways are integrally involved. Second, the ipsilateral autonomic features suggest activation of the cranial parasympathetic system (lacrimation and rhinorrhea) and the ipsilateral sympathetic nerves (ptosis and meiosis). The cavernous carotid artery has been suggested as a likely site of involvement since it is here that the trigeminal, parasympathetic, and sympathetic fibers converge. Finally, the remarkable and often clockwork consistency and seasonal prediliction of attacks strongly suggest that a central pacemaker is integrally involved in the genesis of this disorder.

PAIN AND AUTONOMIC FEATURES

Blood Flow/Cavernous Sinus Hypothesis

Cluster headache has traditionally been thought of as a "vascular" headache disorder. A number of observations have indicated that there is vasodilation of the ipsilateral ophthalmic artery during an attack of cluster headache. These include findings of increased corneal indentation, pulse amplitude, intraocular pressure, and skin temperature around the eye, as well as decreased blood flow velocities at ultrasonography (Lance and Anthony, 1971a; Friedman and Wood, 1976; Sjaastad and Dale, 1974; Kudrow, 1979a; Sjaastad, 1992). Magnetic resonance angiography performed during spontaneous attacks of cluster headache revealed marked dilation of the ophthalmic artery ipsilateral to the pain (Waldenlind et al., 1993). This confirmed the original observation of marked dilation of the ipsilateral ophthalmic artery during catheter in a patient undergoing angiography during a spontaneous cluster headache (Ekbom and Greitz, 1970). Recently, positron emission tomographic (PET) studies during precipitated attacks of cluster headache have demonstrated bilateral activation (more marked on the side of the headache) in the region of the cavernous sinus, thought to be indicative of increased flow in the cavernous portion of the internal carotid arteries (May et al., 1998b). From a clinical standpoint, involvement of the cavernous carotid artery would be consistent with the location of the pain and the third-order neuron postganglionic Horner's syndrome often seen during attacks.

Indeed, an inflammatory process in the cavernous sinus and tributary veins has been proposed as the mechanism of cluster headache (Hardebo, 1994). This theory is based principally on abnormal orbital phlebography in patients during cluster headache attacks (Hannerz et al., 1987; Sjaastad, 1992), the fact that nitroglycerin and other vasodilators can induce an attack of cluster headache (Ekbom, 1968), and the finding that cluster headache patients have a narrower anterior/middle cranial fossa and possibly a narrower cavernous sinus loggia, which might favor disturbances in local venous drainage from the cavernous sinus region (Afra et al., 1998). An inflammatory "venous vasculitis" was thought to obliterate the venous outflow from the cavernous sinus, leading to vascular congestion. The vascular congestion within the arterial and venous circulation in the cavernous sinus may lead not only to pain but also to injury of the traversing sympathetic fibers that richly invest the carotid artery. The active period ends when the inflammation is suppressed and the sympathetic fibers partially or fully recover.

However, a magnetic resonance imaging (MRI) study of cluster patients showed no definite pathologic changes in the area of the cavernous sinus (Sjaastad and Rinck, 1990). Furthermore, parasellar hyperactivity using single photon emission computed tomography (SPECT) was seen in 50% to 80% of cluster headache patients and in more than 70% of migraine patients, indicating that activation in this region is not specific to cluster headache (Sianard-Gainko et al., 1994). In addition, identical orbital phlebography findings have been demonstrated in patients with Tolosa-Hunt syndrome (Hannerz et al., 1986), hemicrania continua (Antonaci, 1994), SUNCT syndrome (Hannerz et al., 1992; Kruszewski, 1992), chronic paroxysmal hemicrania (Antonaci, 1994), cervicogenic headache, migraine, and tension-type headache (Bovin et al., 1992). The same pattern of activation using PET has also been shown in migraine as well as in healthy controls with experimentally induced first-division trigeminal pain elicited with capsaicin (May et al., 1998b). These data strongly suggest that the flow changes seen during cluster headache attacks are an epiphenomenon of trigeminal activation and do not play a causal role in the genesis of cluster headache.

Furthermore, nitroglycerin induces attacks of cluster headache that are indistinguishable from spontaneous attacks but does so after a latency of approximately 30 to 40 minutes following administration. The headache occurs well after the vasodilatory effect of the drug has resolved, and there is evidence that the provocative action of this compound may be related, at least in part, to activation of the trigeminovascular system (Faniullacci et al., 1997).

Trigeminovascular and Cranial-Parasympathetic Pathways

The pain-sensitive innervation of intracranial structures has its cell bodies of origin in the trigeminal ganglion and is predominantly served by the first, or ophthalmic, division (Feindel et al., 1960; McNaughton, 1966). Animal studies have shown that the cerebral blood vessels and dura mater are innervated by cell bodies from the trigeminal ganglion marked by neuropeptides such as substance P, calcitonin gene–related peptide (CGRP), and neurokinin A (Mayberg et al., 1984; Uddman et al., 1985). Furthermore, both parasympathetic and sympathetic nerves innervate these vessels, and these fibers are distinguished by specific neuropeptide populations (Figure 12–1).

The cranial parasympathetic innervation of the intracranial vessels arises from primary-order neurons located in the superior salivatory nucleus. The efferent fibers exit the brain stem via the seventh cranial nerve (Spencer et al., 1990), traverse the geniculate ganglion, and synapse in the sphenopalatine, otic, and carotid miniganglia (Suzuki et al., 1988). Parasympathetic vasomotor efferents then travel via the ethmoidal nerve to innervate the cerebral blood vessels. In addition, secretomotor efferents innervate both the lacrimal and nasal mucosal glands, which provides the anatomic basis for the cranial autonomic symptoms (lacrimation, nasal congestion, rhinorrhea) seen in patients with cluster headache and other trigeminal-autonomic cephalgias (Goadsby and Lipton,

1997). Cranial parasympathetic fibers contain vasoactive intestinal polypeptide (VIP) and nitric oxide, which colocalize within sphenopalatine ganglion neurons and cerebrovascular parasympathetic nerve fibers (Goadsby et al., 1996).

The physiology of the trigeminal and parasympathetic neurons is reasonably well described in experimental animals. Stimulation of the trigeminal ganglion causes a cerebral vasodilator response with an increase in brain blood flow. This effect is mediated by antidromic activation of trigeminal afferents with release of CGRP, as well as through stimulation of parasympathetic outflow, which is accomplished through a functional reflex between the corresponding nuclei of the trigeminovascular (nucleus caudalis) and cranial parasympathetic (superior salivatory nucleus) systems (Lambert et al., 1984; Goadsby and Duckworth, 1987). In animal models, stimulation of either the superior saggital sinus, a C fiber–innervated pain-sensitive structure (Zagami et al., 1990), or the trigeminal ganglion (Goadsby and Edvinsson, 1994) results in the release of CGRP and VIP into the cranial circulation.

In humans, evidence for activation of the trigeminovascular system in primary headache disorders has been highlighted by a marked increase in the level of CGRP in the cranial venous circulation during attacks of migraine (Goadsby et al. 1997), cluster headache (Goadsby and Edvinsson 1994), and CPH (Goadsby and Edvinsson, 1996). In addition, evidence of parasympathetic activation in humans has been corroborated by the finding of dramatically elevated levels of VIP during attacks of cluster headache (Goadsby and Edvinsson, 1994) and CPH (Goadsby and Edvinsson, 1996), where ipsilateral autonomic features are robust. In patients with migraine, levels of VIP remain relatively unchanged unless there are accompanying signs of autonomic activation, such as tearing or nasal congestion (Goadsby and Lipton, 1997).

These findings support the integral involvement of the trigeminovascular and cranial parasympathetic systems in cluster headache (Goadsby and Edvinsson, 1994). Activation of these pathways provides the anatomic basis

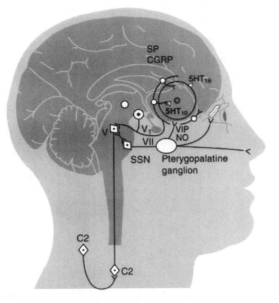

Figure 12–1 Cephalic nociceptive information from pain-sensitive intracranial structures (dura and intracranial blood vessels) arrives in the nervous system via the ophthalmic branch of cranial nerve V with a synapse in the caudal trigeminal nucleus (V). Antidromic activation of the trigeminovascular system leads to release of calcitonin gene–related peptide (*CGRP*) and substance P (*SP*), leading to vasodilation and plasma protein extravasation (neurogenic inflammation). Both peptides are markedly elevated in the cranial venous blood during a cluster attack, indicating activation of this system. A functional brain-stem connection exists between the nucleus of V and the superior salivatory nucleus (*SSN*). The SSN contains the preganglionic parasympathetic neurons, which give rise to fibers that travel with cranial nerve VII and synapse in the pteropalatine ganglion. Postganglionic vasomotor efferents innervate the cerebral blood vessels, and secretomotor efferents innervate the secretory glands of the nasal mucosa and lacrimal glands. Vasomotor efferents contain vasoactive intestinal polyptide (*VIP*), which is released in large amounts during cluster attacks, reflecting activation of the cranial parasympathetic system. The blood vessel in the diagram depicts the cavernous portion of the internal carotid artery, the anatomic location where the trigeminal sensory, parasympathetic, and sympathetic fibers converge. The caudal extent of the trigeminal sensory nucleus descends to C2–3 within the dorsal horn of the spinal cord and converges with nociceptive fibers from this root level. *NO*, nitric oxide; *5-HT*, 5-hydroxytryptamine.

for the expression of first-division trigeminal pain and ipsilateral autonomic symptoms that occur during cluster attacks (Fig. 12–2).

Periodicity

The signature feature of cluster headache is its unmistakable circadian and circannual periodicity. This clock-like rhythmicity is difficult to reconcile or explain on the basis of hemodynamic mechanisms. Indeed, this feature has led several authorities to suggest that cluster headache must be central in origin (Ekbom, 1970a; Kudrow, 1987; Raskin, 1988).

Attacks of cluster headache occur one to eight times a day, often with clockwork regularity, during a permissive time known as cluster periods. Cluster periods last for several weeks to months and are intervened by relatively longer-lasting remission periods, which last 6 months to 2 years. Cluster periods are frequently observed to occur cyclically, often during the same time each year. The frequency of cluster period onset has been related to photoperiod duration, increased in July and January, shortly after the longest and shortest days of the year, respectively. Conversely, cluster period onset decreases following resetting of clocks 1 hour for daylight-saving and standard times in April and October, respectively (Kudrow, 1987).

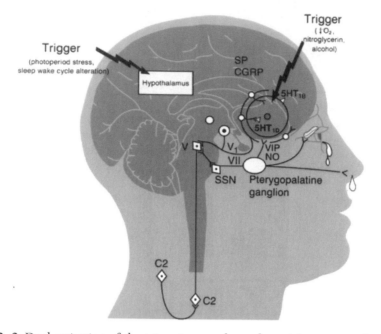

Figure 12–2 Dual activation of the trigeminovascular and cranial parasympathetic systems from centrally or peripherally acting triggers occurs at permissive times known as cluster periods. This period is determined by a dysfunctional hypothalamic pacemaker. Activation of these pathways leads to neurogenic inflammation and vascular dilation of the cavernous carotid artery and congestion within the cavernous sinus, as well as secretion from lacrimal and nasal mucosal glands, thus accounting for the pulsatile periorbital pain and the cranial autonomic symptoms that characterize the clinical profile of a cluster headache. The sympathetic fibers that invest the carotid artery are secondarily involved, leading to a partial third-order neuron Horner's syndrome. *SP*, substance P; *CGRP*, calcitonin gene–related peptide; *5-HT*, 5-hydroxytryptamine; *VIP*, vasoactive intestinal polypeptide; *NO*, nitric oxide; *SSN*, superior salivatory nucleus.

This distinctive periodicity has strongly implicated a disturbance in the biologic clock or pacemaker, which in humans is located in the hypothalamic gray in an area known as the suprachiasmatic nucleus.

Hypothalamic regulation of the endocrine system involves rhythmic and phasic modulation of the hypophyseal hormones and melatonin to maintain homeostasis. Substantially lowered concentrations of plasma testosterone during the cluster headache period in men provided the first evidence of hypothalamic involvement in cluster headache pathogenesis (Kudrow, 1996). This finding was followed by reports of alterations in the production of a wide range of secretory circadian rhythms involving luteinizing hormone (LH), cortisol, and prolactin (PRL), as well as altered responses in the production of cortisol, LH, follicle-stimulating hormone (FSH), PRL, growth hormone (GH), and thyroid-stimulating hormone (TSH) to diverse challenges in cluster headache (Leone and Bussone, 1993).

Melatonin is the most sensitive surrogate marker of circadian function in humans, and its rhythmic secretion is under the control of the suprachiasmatic nucleus (Brzezinski, 1997). The principal environmental stimulus for the entrainment and rhythmic secretion of melatonin is light intensity. Photic information reaches the suprachiasmatic nucleus from a direct retinal–hypophyseal pathway. In humans, the circadian rhythm for the release of melatonin from the pineal gland is closely synchronized with the habitual hours of sleep. Therefore, melatonin levels are normally low during the day and increase during the hours of darkness and sleep. In patients with cluster headache, the 24-hour production of melatonin is reduced, the nocturnal peak in melatonin concentration is blunted during cluster periods, and the *acrophase* (the time from midnight to the moment of peak hormone level) is moved forward (Leone et al., 1995). Pain-induced stress cannot explain this decrease because stress causes a release in endogenous norepinephrine, which increases melatonin production.

Low melatonin may be due to reduced metabolism and reduced availability of serotonin for its synthesis. Evidence of impaired function of the serotonergic system in cluster headache has been supported by recent studies that demonstrate an increase in plasma serotonergic metabolism with low platelet 5-hyfroxytryptamine (5-HT) and increased 5-hydroxyindoleacetic acid (5-HIAA) (D'Andrea et al., 1998). Leone et al. (1997) challenged hypothalamic function in patients with cluster headache using metachlorophenylpiperazine (m-CPP), a central serotonergic agonist that stimulates several 5-HT receptor subtypes, and found an altered cortisol secretion pattern during the active period suggesting impaired central serotonergic function.

The most direct and convincing evidence for the role of the hypothalamus in cluster headache pathogenesis has come from functional and morphometric neuroimaging. Using PET imaging to detect areas of functional activation, May et al. (1998a) demonstrated marked activation in the ipsilateral ventral hypothalamic gray matter during nitroglycerin-induced acute cluster headache attacks. This finding appears to be specific for cluster headache and perhaps other related trigeminal autonomic cephalgias as the same pattern of activation in this region of the hypothalamus was recently demonstrated in a patient with SUNCT syndrome (May et al., 1999b). This pattern of activation has not been seen during attacks of migraine or experimentally induced ophthalmic (first-division) pain induced by capsaicin injection into the forehead of control subjects (May et al., 1998a).

In addition, a voxel-based morphometric analysis of the structural T1-weighted MRI scans of 25 right-handed patients with cluster headache revealed a significant difference in hypothalamic gray matter density between these patients and 29 right-handed healthy male volunteers (May et al., 1999a). This difference consisted of an increase in volume and was present for the entire cohort. This structural difference was bilateral in the diencephalon, coinciding with the inferior posterior hypothalamus. In terms of the stereotaxic coordinates, it was almost identical to the area of activation seen during an acute cluster headache attack with PET imaging. The colocalization of morphologic and functional changes within a discrete hypothalamic region that appears specific to cluster headache may identify the precise anatomic location for the central nervous lesion of cluster headache and explain the profound circadian rhythmicity of this syndrome. However, the nature of the hypothalamic disturbance is as yet unclear.

Mitochondrial Dysfunction

Phosphorus magnetic resonance spectroscopy has shown defective brain and muscle energy metabolism in patients with migraine with and without aura during and between attacks (Welch, 1989; Barbiroli, 1992; Montagna, 1994). A defect of brain and muscle mitochondrial respiration has also been demonstrated in cluster headache patients both during and after the cluster periods (Montagna, 1997). Two cases of cluster headache occurring in conjunction with large-scale mitochondrial deletions and a point mutation in platelet mitochondrial tRNA[Leu(UUR)] have been reported (Shimomura, 1994; Odawara, 1997). One patient had a therapeutic response to ubidecarenone (Odawara, 1997). However, genomic analysis of mitochondrial DNA from cluster sufferers has yielded conflicting results. In a study which examined the mitochondrial genomes of 22 patients with cluster headache, none harbored the reported tRNA[Leu(UUR)] mutation or any other length variations of the ntDNA (Seibel, 1996). Although the data is conflicting, abnormal energy metabolism of excitable cells (brain and muscle) may represent a characteristic of migraine and cluster headache and suggests a shared pathogenesis. Reports on the presence of premonitory symptoms (Blau amd Engel, 1998), photophobia and phonophobia (Vanagaite Vingen et al., 1998), nausea, and visual aura (Silberstein et al., 2000) in patients with cluster headache appear to underscore the potential for a shared pathogenesis between these two disorders. Cluster headache, none harboured the reported tRNA$^{Leu(UUR)}$ mutation or any other length variations of one mtDNA (Seibel, 1996) although the data is conflicting.

Management

Successful cluster headache treatment is governed by the same principles that apply to most medical disorders. Patient education, prophylactic medication, and symptomatic treatment are paramount.

Patient Education

For many patients, the painful experience of the cluster headache attack and the anticipation of future attacks are enough to provoke a state of anxiety and anguish that persists throughout the cluster period. Patients should be told that most attacks may now be prevented within the cluster period by prophylactic measures and that breakthrough attacks can be quickly terminated with acute therapies. However, the cluster period itself can be neither prevented nor shortened.

In all cases, patients should be instructed to avoid afternoon naps and alcoholic beverages, including wine and beer. Alcohol, in most instances, induces acute attacks during active cluster periods but not during remission periods. Patients should be cautioned about prolonged exposure to volatile substances, such as solvents, gasoline, or oil-based paints, during cluster periods. Dietary influences, with the exception of alcohol, appear to have little importance in cluster headache.

Bursts of anger, prolonged anticipatory anxiety, and excessive physical activity should be avoided because cluster attacks are apt to occur during the relaxation period that follows. Prolonged anger, hurt, rage, or frustration during a cluster period is often associated with a new onset of a cluster period.

Altitude hypoxemia at levels above 5,000 feet may induce attacks during cluster periods. Attacks frequently occur during airplane travel because the pressurization in most planes is equilibrated to approximately 5,000 feet. Patients who know a cluster attack will be precipitated by high altitude may prevent it by taking acetazolamide, 250 mg twice a day for 4 days, starting 2 days before the altitude is reached.

Finally, patients may be advised that the onset of cluster periods often follows a long period of sleep alteration, i.e., changes in the sleep–wake cycle. Such changes may result from vacation trips, work-shift changes, new occupations, postsurgical periods, or completion of university studies. Although many variables are associated with changes in lifestyle, the altered sleep–wake patterns that often accompany these changes may be the most important.

Acute (Symptomatic) Therapy

Because of the rapid onset and short time to peak intensity of the pain of cluster headache, fast-acting symptomatic therapy is imperative. Oxygen and subcutaneous sumatriptan provide the most rapid, effective, and reliable relief for attacks of cluster headache.

OXYGEN

Oxygen inhalation has been the standard of care for the symptomatic relief of cluster since it was introduced as an effective therapy by Horton (1956). If oxygen is delivered at the onset of an attack via a non-rebreathing facial mask at a flow rate of 7 l/minute for 15 minutes, approximately 70% of patients will obtain relief within 15 minutes (Kudrow, 1981; Fogan, 1985). Some patients find oxygen to be completely effective if taken when the pain is at maximal intensity, while others note that the attack is delayed for minutes to hours rather than completely aborted. A small placebo-controlled study of hyperbaric oxygen (2 atm) delivered over 30 minutes demonstrated efficacy in six of seven patients within 5 to 13 minutes, with complete or partial interruption of the cluster period (Di Sabato et al., 1993). These therapies have obvious practical limitations since treatment is not always readily available, and although small portable cylinders are available for use at work or when out of the house, some patients find this to be cumbersome and inconvenient.

SUMATRIPTAN

Subcutaneous sumatriptan is the most effective self-administered medication for the symptomatic relief of cluster headache. In a placebo-controlled study, 6 mg of sumatriptan delivered subcutaneously was significantly more effective than placebo, with 74% of patients having complete relief by 15 minutes compared with 26% of placebo-treated patients (Ekbom 1991). In long-term open-label studies, sumatriptan is effective in 76% to 100% of all attacks within 15 minutes, with no evidence of tachyphylaxis or rebound even after repetitive daily use for several months (Ekbom et al., 1995; Gobel et al., 1998). However, sumatriptan is not effective when used before an expected attack in an attempt to prevent an oncoming attack, nor is it useful as a prophylactic agent. The overall efficacy of sumatriptan has been reported to be approximately 8% less in patients with chronic cluster headache than in patients with episodic cluster headache (Gobel et al., 1998). Patients with chronic cluster headache respond very well but to a somewhat lesser extent and more slowly than patients with episodic cluster headache. Although generally well tolerated, sumatriptan is contraindicated in patients with ischemic heart disease or uncontrolled hypertension. Caution must be exercised in patients with cluster headache since the disorder predominates in middle-aged men, who often have risk factors for cardiovascular disease, particularly tobacco abuse, which is present in up to 88% of cluster headache sufferers (Manzoni, 1999).

Sumatriptan nasal spray 20 mg is less effective than subcutaneous injection at relieving pain in the great majority of cluster headache sufferers. In an open randomized study comparing the effectiveness and satisfaction of subcutaneous sumatriptan 6 mg vs. intranasal sumatriptan 20 mg, 49 of 52 treatments with injection resulted in complete relief of pain within 15 minutes, with a mean time-to-pain relief of 9.6 minutes (Hardebo and Dahlof, 1998). The remaining three attacks were reduced by a mean of 87% at 15 minutes. By comparison, only 7 of 52 treatments with nasal spray in the nostril ipsilateral to the pain resulted in complete relief within 15 minutes, with a mean of 13 minutes. No pain relief was obtained in 27 attacks at 15 minutes.

DIHYDROERGOTAMINE

Dihydroergotamine (DHE) is available in the United States in injectable and intranasal formulations. Intravenous DHE-45 provides prompt and effective relief of cluster headache within 15 minutes. The intramuscular and subcutaneous routes of administration provide slower relief because of the lower bioavailability and time to maximal concentration. Because of the rapid peak intensity and relatively short duration of each cluster headache attack, DHE is a less attractive and feasible option than sumatriptan because of the necessity of having to get to an emergency department or physician's office to have an intravenous line placed. In addition, it is not a feasible long-term solution as the attacks are often daily and multiple during a cluster period, which may last months, particularly if prophylactic therapy is not optimal or effective.

A double-blind crossover trial compared intranasal DHE 1 mg with placebo and found no effect on headache frequency or duration, but the pain intensity was significantly reduced with DHE compared to placebo (Andersson and Jespersen, 1986). The effect, however, was not dramatic. It has been suggested that the dosage used (1 mg) was lower than the recommended dosage for migraine and less than what is available in commercial preparations of DHE nasal spray (2 mg). Therefore, DHE at a dose of 2 mg may be more effective than 1 mg, but this has not been studied in a controlled fashion.

ZOLMITRIPTAN

Zolmitriptan is an effective oral agent for the acute treatment of migraine. A double-blind, controlled trial compared the efficacy of 5 and 10 mg oral zolmitriptan to placebo for the treatment of acute cluster headache attacks (Bahra et al., 2000). With headache response defined as a two-point reduction on a five-point pain-intensity scale, 30-minute response rates were 29%, 40%, and 47% following placebo, 5 mg, and 10 mg of zolmitriptan, respectively. The difference reached statistical significance for 10 mg zolmitriptan compared with placebo. In addition, significantly more patients reported mild or no pain 30 minutes after treatment with 5 and 10 mg zolmitriptan (57% and 60%, respectively) than following placebo (42%). Although these efficacy rates do not approach those of oxygen or subcutaneous sumatriptan, zolmitriptan is the first orally administered triptan to demonstrate efficacy in the treatment of cluster headache and remains a therapeutic option for patients who cannot tolerate oxygen or subcutaneous sumatriptan or those who desire oral medication.

LIDOCAINE

Because cocainization of the sphenopalatine ganglion has been helpful in aborting cluster headache attacks (Barre, 1982), intranasal lidocaine has been utilized as an adjunctive therapy since the study of Kittelle et al. (1985). However, in general, whether applied via a spray bottle or by dropping 4% viscous lidocaine in the nostril ipsilateral to the pain, this therapy does not render the patient pain-free and achieves only a moderate reduction in pain in less than one-third of patients (Robbins, 1995). Therefore, it may be useful as adjunctive but not as "stand-alone" therapy for relief of acute cluster attacks.

Preventive Pharmacotherapy

The importance of an effective preventive regimen during cluster periods cannot be overstated. During cluster periods, individual cluster attacks often occur daily for several weeks to months. Furthermore, many patients have more than one attack per day (up to eight), and the attacks are severe, are short-lived, and peak rapidly, making repeated attempts at abortive therapy exhaustive. Furthermore, abortive therapies may be contraindicated, ineffective, or not tolerated or they may simply delay the attack. Treating frequent daily attacks may result in overmedication or toxicity, and finally, repeated attacks of severe pain may unnecessarily prolong suffering.

The primary goals of preventive therapy are to produce a rapid suppression of attacks and to maintain that remission over the expected duration of the cluster period. Secondary objectives are to reduce the headache frequency, as well as attack severity and duration. To achieve these primary goals, preventive therapy can best be thought of in terms of transitional and maintenance prophylaxis (Fig. 12–3).

Transitional Prophylaxis

ERGOTAMINE DERIVATIVES

Both ergotamine tartrate (2 mg) and DHE-45 (1 mg) are effective agents for rapid attack suppression when administered daily for a short period of time. Patients often tolerate these medications for a period of 2 to 3 weeks, and there does not appear to be a risk of rebound in this group of patients. Ergotamine tartrate is more convenient because of its oral route of administration and may be particularly useful when given 1 to 2 hours prior to bedtime for attacks that occur predominantly or exclusively during sleep (Ek-

---

Figure 12–3 Three approaches for the initial prophylaxis of cluster headache incorporating combinations of transitional and maintenance preventive medications. Because the effect of verapamil may be delayed for up to 3 weeks, it is often combined with a transitional medication such as ergotamine or prednisone to suppress attacks during this interval and to limit the need for repeated administration of acute therapy, particularly in patients with multiple attacks in a 24-hour period. Options 2 and 3 are somewhat restrictive because sumatriptan as an acute therapy cannot be used in conjunction with ergotamine or ergotamine-like medications (e.g., methysergide). Melatonin can be used in combination with any medication as an adjunctive therapy. Combination therapy refers to the use of two or more maintenance preventive medications in patients for whom monotherapy is not optimal. Trigeminal root section is considered a last resort in patients who have failed all feasible medical and surgical modalities.

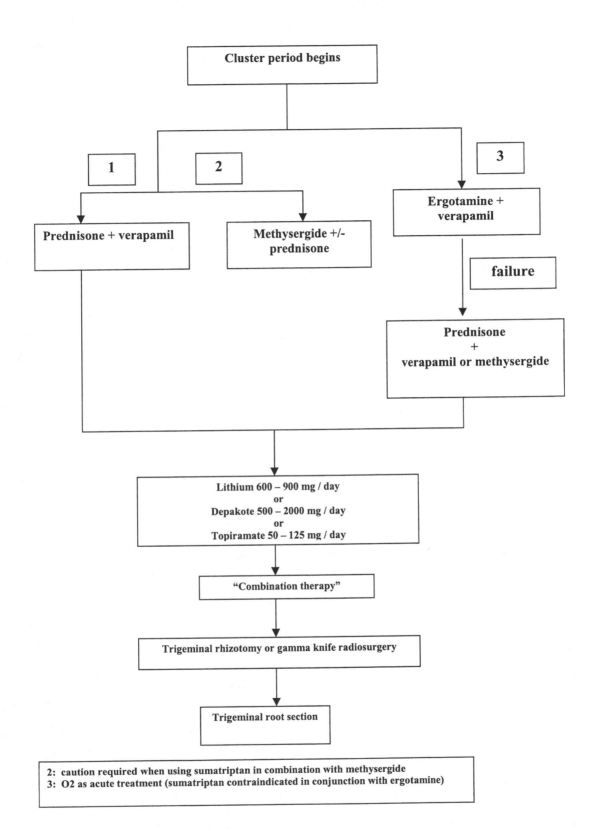

Cluster period begins

1

2

3

Prednisone + verapamil

Methysergide +/- prednisone

Ergotamine + verapamil

failure

Prednisone + verapamil or methysergide

Lithium 600 – 900 mg / day
or
Depakote 500 – 2000 mg / day
or
Topiramate 50 – 125 mg / day

"Combination therapy"

Trigeminal rhizotomy or gamma knife radiosurgery

Trigeminal root section

2: caution required when using sumatriptan in combination with methysergide
3: O2 as acute treatment (sumatriptan contraindicated in conjunction with ergotamine)

bom, 1947; Horton, 1952; Kudrow, 1993). Both agents may also be administered in divided daily dosages (not to exceed 4 mg ergotamine tartrate or 3 mg DHE) when attacks are multiple or occur throughout the day. Both of these agents are contraindicated in patients who are pregnant or have peripheral vascular disease, coronary artery disease, or uncontrolled hypertension. They should not be used for the duration of the cluster period and are not intended for long-term preventive use. They also limit the long-term preventive and abortive options since their use is contraindicated within 24 hours of using sumatriptan, and they are generally not administered concomitantly with methysergide because of the risk of potentiating the vasoconstrictive effects of this drug.

CORTICOSTEROIDS

Corticosteroids (prednisone and dexamethasone) are the most rapid-acting of the prophylactic agents. They represent a very effective initial prophylactic option to rapidly suppress attacks during the time required for the longer-acting maintenance prophylactic agents to take effect since the maximum benefit from other preventive drugs may not be realized until 2 weeks after treatment is begun. Although the data are limited and uncontrolled, the largest open-label study reported marked relief of cluster headache in 77% of 77 episodic cluster headache patients and partial relief in another 12% of patients treated with prednisone (Kudrow, 1980). Prednisone was also found to provide marked relief in 40% of patients with chronic cluster headache and was more effective than methysergide in this patient group. Treatment is usually initiated with 60 mg/day for 3 days, followed by 10 mg decrements every 3 days over an 18-day period.

Dexamethasone at a dose of 4 mg BID for 2 weeks followed by 4 mg/day for 1 week has also been shown to be effective (Anthony and Daher, 1992). However, when dexamethasone or prednisone is tapered, the cluster attacks almost invariably recur. Therefore, corticosteroids are useful primarily for inducing rapid remission in patients with episodic cluster headache, although they may provide a brief respite for patients with chronic cluster headache. Its long-term use in these patients is generally discouraged.

Maintenance Prophylaxis

Maintenance prophylaxis refers to the use of preventive medications throughout the anticipated duration of the cluster period. They are started at the very onset of the cluster period in conjunction with either corticosteroids or ergotamine derivatives but are continued after these initial suppressive agents are discontinued.

VERAPAMIL

Verapamil is considered by many to be the preventive therapy of choice for both episodic and chronic cluster headache. It is generally well tolerated and can be used safely in conjunction with sumatriptan, ergotamine, corticosteroids, and other preventive agents. In an open-label trial involving 48 patients, 69% of patients improved by more than 75% during treatment with verapamil (Gabai and Spierings, 1989). A double-blind, placebo-controlled trial evaluated the efficacy of verapamil 360 mg (three divided dosages) over a 14-day period. A statistically significant reduction in headache frequency and analgesic consumption was seen in the verapamil-treated patients, with a greater reduction in the second week of treatment (Leone et al., 1999).

The initial daily dosage is usually 80 mg TID or 240 mg sustained-release. Dosages employed range from 240 to 720 mg/day in divided doses. Both the regular and extended-released preparations have been shown to be useful, but no direct comparative trials are available. Delayed-release verapamil at dosages up to 720 mg may be effective in cases of refractory cluster headache (Gobel et al., 1999). Because of this apparent dose-response relationship, a total daily dosage of between 480 and 720 mg is recommended before the medication is deemed a failure. Constipation is the most common side effect, but dizziness, edema, nausea, fatigue, hypotension, and bradycardia may also occur.

LITHIUM CARBONATE

Although the beneficial results of lithium carbonate therapy for cluster headache prevention have been derived mainly from open clinical trials, this drug has been and continues to be an effective agent for cluster headache prophylaxis. Collectively, in over 28 clinical trials involving 468 patients, good to excellent results were found in 78% of 304 patients with chronic cluster headache (Ekbom, 1981). The efficacy of lithium in patients with chronic cluster also appears to be durable up to 4 years after treatment (Manzoni et al., 1983). Upon interruption or cessation of lithium therapy in this group, a transition from chronic to episodic cluster headache has been recognized (Ekbom, 1981).

Although somewhat less robust than the response in patients with chronic cluster headache, lithium has induced remission in 63% of 164 patients with episodic cluster (Ekbom, 1981). A double-blind crossover study comparing verapamil (360 mg daily) and lithium (900 mg daily) in 30 patients claimed equal efficacy for the two drugs (Bussone et al., 1990). On the other hand, a single double-blind, placebo-controlled trial failed to show superiority of lithium (800 mg sustained-release) over placebo. However, this study was terminated 1 week after treatment began, and there was an unexpectedly high placebo response rate of 31% (Steiner et al., 1997). The treatment period was therefore too short to be conclusive.

The initial starting daily dosage of lithium carbonate is either 300 mg TID or 450 mg sustained-release. Again, data comparing the two formulations are not available, but a long half-life affords the option of a once-daily dosage regimen, which is simpler and may enhance compliance.

Lithium is often effective at serum concentrations (0.4 to 0.8 mEq/l), less than that usually required for the treatment of bipolar disorder. Most patients will benefit from dosages between 600 and 900 mg/day.

Lithium has the potential for many side effects and has a narrow therapeutic window. The serum concentration should be measured 12 hours after the last dose and should not exceed 1.0 mEq/l. Renal and thyroid function must be measured prior to and during treatment; side effects such as tremor, diarrhea and polyuria must be monitored; and caution must be exercised when other drugs, such as diuretics and nonsteroidal anti-inflammatory drugs, are prescribed.

METHYSERGIDE

Methysergide is a potent prophylactic drug for the treatment of cluster headache, but because of the potential for fibrotic complications, it is not commonly employed for more than 3 months in patients with chronic cluster headache. Good to excellent results have been demonstrated in 70% of patients with episodic cluster headache (Curran et al., 1967; Kudrow, 1980), but the drug appears to lose its effectiveness with repeated use in up to 20% of patients (Kudrow, 1980).

Methysergide is a prodrug of methylergometrine and, thus, should be used with caution in patients receiving other ergotamine derivatives or vasoconstrictive agents. The short-term side effects include nausea, muscle cramps, abdominal pain, and pedal edema. Long-term side effects include fibrosis of the retroperitoneum or pleural and pericardial lining. The daily dose employed is usually 2 mg in three divided doses, but up to 12 mg may be used if tolerated.

VALPROIC ACID

An open-label study in 15 patients with cluster headache demonstrated efficacy of valproic acid (600 to 2,000 mg), with a 73% favorable response rate (Hering and Kuritzky, 1989). Nine of 15 patients had complete suppression of attacks, and the time to pain relief was brief, ranging from 1 to 4 days. Treatment was well tolerated, with only nausea reported; but weight gain, hair loss, tremor, and lethargy are other potential side effects. It has been suggested that patients whose cluster headaches are accompanied by migrainous features, such as nausea, vomiting, photophobia, and phonophobia, may preferentially respond to valproic acid (Wheeler, 1998).

The medication is usually started in divided dosages of 250 mg BID, and 250 mg increments per dose are recommended to find the lowest effective dose and minimize side effects. Pancreatitis, platelet dysfunction, thrombocytopenia, and hepatic dysfunction have been described with this medication, thereby necessitating baseline and follow-up complete blood counts and liver function testing.

TOPIRAMATE

In an open-label study, treatment with topiramate was associated with rapid improvement in ten cluster headache patients (Wheeler and Carrazana, 1999). Cluster period remission occurred in 1 to 3 weeks in nine patients, two of whom had chronic cluster headache. All patients responded to relatively small dosages, ranging between 50 and 125 mg/day in two divided doses; therefore, the drug was well tolerated. Starting at low dosages and making small increments can minimize both the total daily dosage and the potential for side effects. Somnolence, dizziness, ataxia, and cognitive symptoms are the most common side effects reported by patients. Additionally, because of the weak carbonic anhydrase inhibition of this drug, renal calculi and paresthesias have been reported. This favorable preliminary experience must be followed up by further corroborative data.

MELATONIN

Melatonin is the most sensitive surrogate marker of circadian rhythm in humans and is under the control of the suprachiasmatic nucleus (Brzezinski, 1997). Serum melatonin levels are reduced in patients with cluster headache, particularly during a cluster period (Waldenlind et al., 1987; Leone et al., 1995). Based on these observations, the striking circadian rhythmicity of cluster headache, and the importance of the hypothalamus in the pathogenesis of this disorder, the efficacy of 10 mg oral melatonin has been evaluated in a double-blind, placebo-controlled trial (Leone et al., 1996). Cluster headache remission within 3 to 5 days was achieved in five of ten patients who received melatonin compared to zero of ten patients who received placebo.

CAPSAICIN

Capsaicin has been shown to be superior to placebo at reducing attack frequency and severity in a double-blind study when delivered at a dose of 0.025% BID via a cotton-tipped applicator in the ipsilateral nostril for 7 days (Marks et al., 1993). However, because there are more easily administered and effective agents available, this medication does not enjoy widespread use in the treatment of cluster headache.

INDOMETHACIN

Although several other trigeminal-autonomic cephalgias, such as chronic and episodic paroxysmal hemicrania, respond in an absolute way to indomethacin, this medication has not been evaluated in a systematic fashion for the prophylaxis of cluster headache. There is anecdotal evidence to suggest that some cluster headache patients respond to indomethacin, but the response rate appears to be far less than that seen with the other disorders.

OTHERS

A number of other agents have been reported in small open-label studies or within case reports to have demonstrated efficacy in patients with cluster headache. These include methylphenidate, antispasticity drugs (tizanidine and baclofen), clonidine, diltiazem, flunarizine, histamine, somatostatin, and pizotifen. These is a paucity of experience with these drugs, and because of the lack of data, further evidence is needed before recommendations can be made to support their routine use in cluster headache. However, all medical options should be considered in patients with treatment-resistant cluster headache before an ablative surgical procedure is attempted.

REFRACTORY PATIENTS

Medical Therapy

Approximately 10% of patients develop chronic cluster headache which does not respond to monotherapy. In addition, patients with episodic cluster headache with frequent cluster periods may develop resistance, intolerance, or contraindications to prophylactic and/or abortive medications and may require a more definitive surgical procedure for pain control.

Before considering surgery, it is important to realize that some patients may do best with drugs used in combination rather than maximal dosages of one in isolation. For example, lithium or methysergide may be combined with verapamil. Melatonin may also be a useful adjunct in these circumstances as there are few side effects and its long-term use appears to be associated with few adverse events. Alternatively, three medications may be used in combination, such as ergotamine, verapamil, and lithium. This is usually not a feasible long-term therapeutic option as the toxicity of these medications may accumulate and the side effects may become intolerable. In addition, ergotamine is not recommended for long-term use and the use of lithium, ergotamine, or methysergide may restrict the usage of sumatriptan as an abortive agent.

Repetitive IV DHE administered in an inpatient setting over a period of 3 days may be very useful in some patients with both episodic and chronic cluster headache. In one study of 54 intractable cluster headache patients (31 of whom had chronic cluster headache), after a median hospital stay of 6 days, all patients were headache-free after repetitive IV DHE and at 12 months follow-up, 83% and 39% of episodic and chronic cluster headache patients, respectively, remained free of headache (Mather et al., 1991).

Histamine "desensitization" has been used to treat patients with intractable cluster headache with mixed results. This therapy usually entails a prolonged hospital stay of at least 1 week with repetitive administration of IV histamine (Diamond et al., 1986). This treatment modality does not enjoy widespread use at this time.

Surgery

For the most intractable patients who have failed outpatient and inpatient therapy or for whom contraindications or intolerance limits the use of effective medications, surgery may be a feasible option. Only patients whose headaches have been exclusively unilateral should be considered for surgery as patients whose attacks have alternated sides are at risk for a contralateral recurrence after surgery. In addition, only patients with a stable personality and psychologic profile with low addiction proneness should be considered for an ablative procedure.

Although a wide variety of surgical procedures have been utilized, those which are directed toward the sensory trigeminal nerve have been the most successful. The procedure of choice is radiofrequency thermocoagulation of the trigeminal ganglion. This is generally preferred over glycerol gangliorhizolysis as the extent and precision of the lesion can be better controlled with the former and the risk of aseptic meningitis or subarachnoid hemorrhage is higher with the latter.

The overall results of radiofrequency rhizotomies are encouraging, with approximately 75% of patients showing good to excellent results (Onofrio and Campbell, 1986; Mathew and Hurt, 1988). The durability of the procedure is also quite favorable, with only a 20% long-term recurrence rate, while some patients remain pain-free even after 20 years (Taha and Tew, 1995). The best results may require complete analgesia or dense hypalgesia. If the pain is primarily orbital in location, V1 and V2 lesions appear to be adequate; but if the pain also involves the temporal or auricular region, a V3 lesion may be necessary for optimal results. Indeed, in patients whose pain is primarily located around the ear, temple, or cheek, an ablative trigeminal procedure may not be curative or as successful (Taha and Tew, 1995). Transient complications may include diplopia, hyperacusis, ice-pick pain, and jaw deviation, while longer-term complications include corneal anesthesia and, in <4% of cases, anesthesia dolorosa. Aggressive long-term ophthalmic follow-up and eye care are critically important.

Efficacy with gamma knife radiosurgery in six medically recalcitrant cluster headache patients has been reported (Ford et al., 1998). The time to effective relief was either immediate or within 1 week. Four patients were pain-free at more than 8 months follow-up. This study has not been duplicated, and the overall efficacy, safety, and durability of this procedure is as yet unknown. However, it is a noninvasive procedure with a better side-effect profile than the ablative surgeries and may represent a viable alternative in some patients prior to a destructive procedure.

Microvascular decompression (MVD) of the trigeminal nerve with or without MVD or section of the nervus intermedius for chronic cluster headache was reported to be efficacious (Lovely et al., 1998). In their series, 28 patients, two of whom had bilateral cluster headache, underwent 39 operations for MVD of the trigeminal nerve, alone or combined with MVD or section of the nervus intermedius. Twenty-two of the 30 first-time procedures resulted in 50% relief or better, but long-term follow-up (average 5.3 years) showed a fall in the good to excellent relief to 46%. Repeat procedures were ineffective. Three patients who responded with a reduction in pain by more than 50% after MVD of the trigeminal nerve improved to better than 90% after a MVD or section of the nervus intermedius. These procedures require the skill of a very experienced surgical team, and further experience with this combined approach is needed.

Finally, a number of authors have reported satisfactory results in patients with refractory chronic cluster headache after section of the sensory trigeminal nerve at the root exit zone (Watson et al., 1983; Onofrio and Campbell, 1986; Kirkpatrick et al., 1993). Trigeminal sensory rhizotomy via a posterior fossa approach was employed by Onofrio and Campbell (1986) in ten patients, with relief of pain in six and failure of relief in four. In the largest series, Kirkpatrick and colleagues (1993) reported complete or near-complete relief of pain in 12 of 14 patients who underwent a sensory trigeminal rhizotomy using a similar approach. The mean duration of follow-up was 5.6 years. Only one patient developed a contralateral recurrence of attacks. Seven patients who had a partial nerve root section required a second procedure for complete resection. They concluded that a complete sec-

tion was more likely to provide relief than a partial section but agreed with the findings of others that total loss of sensation of all three divisions of the trigeminal nerve did not guarantee relief from the attacks.

Natural History

There is a relative paucity of information regarding the natural history of cluster headache. Manzoni et al. (1991) evaluated 189 consecutive patients who had a disease duration of over 10 years. Approximately 13% of patients with episodic cluster headache converted to a chronic pattern, while another 6% evolved into an intermediate pattern. The remaining 80% continued to have episodic cluster headache. On the contrary, chronic cluster headache evolved into an episodic or intermediate pattern in 33% and 14%, respectively. The prognosis in patients with chronic cluster headache appears to be favorable, with over one-third reverting to an episodic pattern of attacks. It is unclear whether pharmacotherapy contributes to this conversion, but some authors feel that lithium carbonate in particular may play a role in this transformation.

In another study, approximately one-third of patients who had been subject to cluster headache for 20 years or longer reported complete remission (Kudrow, 1982); in another third, the attacks were attenuated in severity so as to obviate the need for medication; in the final third, the pattern of attacks remained unchanged. A Japanese study of 68 cluster headache patients with a mean cluster headache history of 18.9 years who were followed over an 18-year period revealed no change in headache attack severity, frequency, duration, or associated symptoms (Igarashi and Sakai, 1996). There was no change in cluster period onset or duration. However, in all but five patients, the remission periods lengthened from a mean of 1.1 years to a mean of 3.3 years. This change appeared to occur most commonly around the age of 42 years.

The balance of evidence therefore indicates that cluster headache is a durable and often lifelong disorder in the majority of patients. However, in a substantial proportion of patients, complete remission or lengthening of remission phases may occur, while in one-third of patients, chronic cluster may evolve into an episodic pattern.

REFERENCES

Afra, J., A. Proietti Cecchini, and J. Schoenen (1998). Craniometric measures in cluster headache patients. *Cephalalgia* 18:143–145.

Andersson, P.G. and L.T. Jespersen (1986). Dihydroergotamine nasal spray in the treatment of attacks of cluster headache. *Cephalalgia* 6: 51–54.

Andrasik, F., E.B. Blanchard, J.G. Arena et al. (1982). Cross-validation of the Kudrow-Sutkus MMPI classification system for diagnosing headache type. *Headache* 22:2–5.

Anthony M. and B.N. Daher (1992). Mechanism of action of steroids in cluster headache. In: *New Advances in Headache Research*, Vol. 2. (F.C. Rose, ed.), pp. 271–274. Smith Gordon, London.

Antonaci, F. (1994). Chronic paroxysmal hemicrania and hemicrania continua: Orbital phlebography and MRI studies. *Headache* 34:32–34.

Bahra, A., M.J. Gawel, J.E. Hardebo et al. (2000). Oral zolmitriptan is effective in the acute treatment of cluster headache. *Neurology* 54:1832–1839.

Barbiroli, B., P. Montagna, P. Cortelli et al. (1992). Abnormal brain and muscle energy metabolism shown by 31P magnetic resonance spectroscopy in patients affected by migraine with aura. *Neurology* 42:1209–1214.

Barre, F. (1982). Cocaine as an abortive agent in cluster headache. *Headache* 22:69–73.

Blau, J.N. and H.O. Engel (1998). Premonitory and prodromal symptoms in cluster headache. *Cephalalgia* 18:91–93.

Bovin, G., G. Jenssen, and K. Ericson (1992). Orbital phlebography: A comparison between cluster headache and other headaches. *Headache* 32:408–412.

Brzezinski, A. (1997). Melatonin in humans. *N. Engl. J. Med.* 336:186–195.

Bussone, G., M. Leone, and C. Peccarisi (1990). Double blind comparison of lithium and verapamil in cluster headache prophylaxis. *Headache* 30:411–417.

Couturier, E.G., R. Hering, and T.J. Steiner (1991). The first report of cluster headache in identical twins. *Neurology* 41:761.

Cremer, P.D., G.M. Halmagyi, and P.J. Goadsby (1995). Secondary cluster headache responsive to sumatriptan. *J. Neurol. Neurosurg. Psychiatry* 59:633–634.

Curran, D.A., H. Hinterburger, and J.W. Lance (1967). Methysergide. *Res. Clin. Stud. Headache* 1:74–122.

Cuypers, J., H. Altenkirch, and S. Bunge (1981). Personality profiles in cluster headache and migraine. *Headache* 21:21–24.

D'Alessandro, R., G. Gamberini, and G. Benassi (1986). Cluster headache in the Republic of San Marino. *Cephalalgia* 6:159–162.

Diamond, S., F.G. Freitag, and J. Prager (1986). Treatment of intractable cluster headache. *Headache* 26:42–46.

Di Sabato, F., B.M. Fusco, P. Pelaia et al. (1993). Hyperbaric oxygen therapy in cluster headache. *Pain* 52:243–245.

Dexter, J.D. and T.L. Riley (1975). Studies in nocturnal migraine. *Headache* 15:51–62.

Eadie, M.J. and J.M. Sutherland (1966). Migainous neuralgia. *Med. J. Aust.* 1:1053–1057.

Ekbom, K. (1968). Nitroglycerin as a provocative agent in cluster headache. *Arch. Neurol.* 19: 487–493.

Ekbom, K. (1970a). A clinical comparison of cluster headache and migraine. *Acta Neurol. Scand. Suppl.* 41:1–48.

Ekbom, K. (1970b). Patterns of cluster headache with a note on the relations to angina pectoris and peptide ulcer. *Acta Neurol. Scand.* 46:225–237.

Ekbom, K. (1981). Lithium for cluster headache: Review of the literature and preliminary results of long-term treatment. *Headache* 21:132–139.

Ekbom, K. (1990). Evaluation of clinical criteria for cluster headache with special reference to the classification of the International Headache Society. *Cephalalgia* 10:195–197.

Ekbom, K. (1991) Treatment of acute cluster headache with sumatriptan. *N. Engl. J. Med.* 325:322–326.

Ekbom, K.A. (1947). Ergotamine tartrate orally in Horton's "histaminic cephalgia" (also called Harris's "ciliary neuralgia"). *Acta Psychiatr. Scand. Suppl.* 46:106–113.

Ekbom, K., B. Ahlborg, and R. Schele (1978). Prevalence of migraine and cluster headache in Swedish men of 18. *Headache* 18:9–19.

Ekbom, K. and B. de F. Olivarius (1971). Chronic migrainous neuralgia—diagnostic and therapeutic aspects. *Headache* 11:97–101.

Ekbom, K. and T. Greitz (1970). Carotid angiography in cluster headache. *Acta Radiol.* 19:177–186.

Ekbom, K., A. Krabbe, G. Micieli et al. (1995). Sumatriptan Long-Term Study Group. Cluster headache attacks treated for up to three months with subcutaneous sumatriptan (6mg). *Cephalalgia* 15:230–236.

Ekbom, K. and E. Waldenlind (1981). Cluster headache in women: Evidence of hypofertility(?): headaches in relation to menstruation and pregnancy. *Cephalalgia* 1:167–174.

Faniullacci, M., M. Alessandri, R. Sicuteri et al. (1997). Responsiveness of the trigeminovascular system to nitroglycerin in cluster headache patients. *Brain 120*:283–288.

Feindel, W., W. Penfield, and F. McNaughton (1960). The tentorial nerves and localization of intracranial pain in man. *Neurology 10*:555–563.

Fogan, L. (1985). Treatment of cluster headache: A double-blind comparison of oxygen vs. air inhalation. *Arch. Neurol. 42*:362–363.

Ford, R.G., K.T. Ford, S. Swaid et al. (1998). Gamma knife treatment of refractory cluster headache. *Headache 38*:1–9.

Friedman, A.P. and E.H. Wood (1976). Thermography in vascular headache. In *Medical Thermography* (S. Uema, ed.), pp. 80–84. Brentwood, Los Angeles.

Gabai, I.J. and E.H.L. Spierings (1989). Prophylactic treatment of cluster headache with verapamil. *Headache 29*:167–168.

Gilbert, G.J. (1965). Meniere's syndrome and cluster headaches: Recurrent paroxysmal vasodilatation. *JAMA 191*:691–694.

Gilbert, G.J. (1970). Cluster headache and cluster vertigo. *Headache 9*:195–200.

Goadsby, P.J and J.W. Duckworth (1987). Effect of stimulation of trigeminal ganglion on regional cerebral blood flow in cats. *Am. J. Physiol. 253*: R270–R274.

Goadsby, P.J. and L. Edvinsson (1994). Human in vivo evidence for trigeminovascular activation in cluster headache. *Brain 117*:427–434.

Goadsby, P.J. and L. Edvinsson (1996). Neuropeptide changes in a case of chronic paroxysmal hemicrania—evidence for trigemino-parasympathetic activation. *Cephalalgia 16*:448–450.

Goadsby, P.J. and R.B. Lipton (1997). A review of paroxysmal hemicranias, SUNCT syndrome and other short-lasting headaches with autonomic features, including new cases. *Brain 120*:193–209.

Goadsby, P.J., R. Uddman, and L. Edvinsson (1996). Cerebral vasodilation in the cat involves nitric oxide from parasympathetic nerves. *Brain Res. 707*:110–118.

Gobel H., H. Holzgreve, A. Heinze A. et al. (1999). Retarded verapamil for cluster headache prophylaxis [abstract]. *Cephalalgia 19*: 458–459.

Gobel, H., V. Lindner, A. Heinze et al. (1998). Acute therapy for cluster headache with sumatriptan: Findings of a one-year long-term study. *Neurology 51*:908–911.

Graham, J.R. (1969). Cluster headache. Presentation at the International Symposium on Headache, Chicago.

Green, M. and R.I. Apfelbaum (1978). Cluster-tic syndrome [abstract]. *Headache 18*:112.

Hannerz, J., K. Ericson, and G. Bergstrand (1986). A new etiology for visual impairment and chronic headache. The Tolosa Hunt syndrome may be only one manifestation of venous vasculitis. *Cephalalgia 6*: 59–63.

Hannerz, J., K. Ericson, and G. Bergstrand (1987). Orbital phlebography in patients with cluster headache. *Cephalalgia 7*:207–211.

Hannerz, J.E., D. Greitz, P. Hansson et al. (1992). SUNCT may be another manifestation of orbital venous vasculitis. *Headache 32*: 384–389.

Hardebo, J.E. (1994). How cluster headache is explained as an intracavernous inflammatory process lesioning sympathetic fibers. *Headache 34*: 125–131.

Hardebo, J.E. and C. Dahlof (1998). Sumatriptan nasal spray (20 mg/dose) in the acute treatment of cluster headache. *Cephalalgia 18*:487–489.

Harris, W. (1936). Ciliary (migrainous) neuralgia and its treatment. *BMJ 1*:457–460.

Headache Classification Committee of the International Headache Society (1988). Classification and diagnostic criteria for headache disorders, cranial neuralgias and facial pain. *Cephalalgia 8*(Suppl. 7):35–38.

Hering, R. and A. Kuritzky (1989). Sodium valproate in the treatment of cluster headache: An open trial. *Cephalalgia 9*:195–198.

Horton, B.T. (1952). Histaminic cephalgia. *Lancet 2*:92–98.

Horton, B.T. (1956). Histaminic cephalgia. Differential diagnosis and treatment: 1176 patients 1937–1955. *Proc. Staff Meet. Mayo Clin. 31*: 325–333.

Horton, B.T., A.R. MacLean, and W.M. Craig (1939). A new syndrome of vascular headache: Results of treatment with histamine. Preliminary report. *Mayo Clin. Proc. 14*:257–260.

Igarashi, H. and F. Sakai (1996). Natural history of cluster headache [abstract]. *Cephalalgia 16*: 390–391.

Kirkpatrick, P.J., M.D. O'Brien, and J.J. MacCabe (1993). Trigeminal nerve section for chronic migrainous neuralgia. *Br. J. Neurosurg. 7*:483–490.

Kitelle, J.P., D.S. Grouse, and M.E. Seyboro (1985). Cluster headache: Local anesthetic abortive agents. *Arch. Neurol. 42*:496–498.

Krabbe, A.A. (1986). Cluster headache: A review. *Acta Neurol. Scand. 74*:1–9.

Kruszewski, P. (1992). Short-lasting, unilateral, neuralgiform headache attacks with conjunctival injection and tearing (SUNCT syndrome): V. Orbital phlebography. *Cephalalgia 12*:387–389.

Kudrow, L. (1979a). Thermographic and Doppler flow asymmetry in cluster headache. *Headache 19*:204–208.

Kudrow, L. (1979b). Cluster headache: Diagnosis and management. *Headache 19*:142–150.

Kudrow, L. (1980). *Cluster Headache: Mechanisms and Management*, pp. 10–150. Oxford University Press, London.

Kudrow, L. (1981). Response of cluster headache attacks to oxygen inhalation. *Headache 21*:1–4.

Kudrow, L. (1982). Natural history of cluster headache. Part I. Outcome of dropout patients. *Headache* 22:203–206.

Kudrow, L. (1987). The cyclic relationship of natural illumination to cluster period frequency [abstract]. *Cephalalgia* 7(Suppl. 6):76–77.

Kudrow, L. (1993). Cluster headache: Diagnosis, management, and treatment. In *Wolff's Headache and Other Head Pain*, 6th ed., (D.J. Dalessio and S.D. Silberstein, eds.), pp. 171–197. Oxford University Press, New York.

Kudrow, L. and D.B. Kudrow (1990). Association of sustained oxyhemoglobin desaturation and onset of cluster headache attacks. *Headache* 30:474–480.

Kudrow, L. and D.B. Kudrow (1994). Inheritance of cluster headache and its possible link to migraine. *Headache* 34: 400–407.

Kudrow, L., D.J. McGinty, E.R. Phillips et al. (1984). Sleep apnea in cluster headache. *Proceedings of the 12th Scandinavian Migraine Society Meeting, Helsinki, June 17–18*, p. 56.

Kudrow, L. and B.J. Sutkus (1979). MMPI pattern specificity in primary headache disorders. *Headache* 19:18–24.

Kunkle, E.C., J.R. Pfeiffer, W.M. Wilhoit et al. (1952). Recurrent brief headaches in "cluster" pattern. *Trans. Am. Neurol. Assoc.* 77:240–243.

Krabbe, A. (1991). The prognosis in cluster headache. In *New Advances in Headache Research*, Vol. 2 (F.C. Rose, ed.), Smith-Gordon, London.

Lambert, G.A., N. Bogduk, P.J. Goadsby et al. (1984). Decreased carotid arterial resistance in cats in response to trigeminal stimulation. *J Neurosurg* 61:307–315.

Lance, J.W. and M. Anthony (1971a). Thermographic studies in vascular headache. *Med. J. Aust.* 1:240.

Lance, J.W. and M. Anthony (1971b). Migrainous neuralgia or cluster headache? *J. Neurol. Sci.* 13:401–414.

Leone, M., D. D'Amico, A. Attanasio et al. (1999). Verapamil is an effective prophylactic for cluster headache: Results of a double-blind multicenter study versus placebo. In *Cluster Headache and Related Conditions* (J. Olesen and P.J. Goadsby, eds.), pp. 296–299. Oxford University Press, Oxford.

Leone, M., D. D'Amico, F. Moschiano et al. (1996). Melatonin versus placebo in the prophylaxis of cluster headache: A double-blind pilot study with parallel groups. *Cephalalgia* 16:494–496.

Leone, M., V. Lucini, D. D'Amico et al. (1995). Twenty-four hour melatonin and cortisol plasma levels in relation to timing of cluster headache. *Cephalalgia* 15:224–229.

Lovely, T.J., X. Kotsiakis, and P.J. Jannetta (1998). The surgical management of chronic cluster headache. *Headache* 38:590–594.

Lovshin, L.L. (1961). Clinical caprices of histaminic cephalgia. *Headache* 1:3–6.

Manzoni, G.C. (1997). Male preponderance of cluster headache is progressively decreasing over the years. *Headache* 37:588–589.

Manzoni, G.C. (1998). Gender ratio of cluster headache over the years: A possible role of changes in lifestyle. *Cephalalgia* 18:138–142.

Manzoni, G.C. (1999). Cluster headache and lifestyle: Remarks on a population of 374 male patients. *Cephalalgia* 19:88–94.

Manzoni, G.C., G. Bono, M. Lanfranchi et al. (1983). Lithium carbonate in cluster headache: Assessment of its short and long-term therapeutic efficacy. *Cephalalgia* 3:109–114.

Manzoni, G.C., G. Micieli, F. Granella et al. (1991). Cluster headache: Course over ten years in 189 patients. *Cephalalgia* 11:169–174.

Manzoni, G.C., G. Micieli, F. Ganella et al. (1988). Cluster headache in women: Clinical findings and relationship with reproductive life. *Cephalalgia* 8:37–44.

Marks, D.R., A. Rapoport, and D. Padla (1993). A double-blind placebo-controlled trial of intranasal capsaicin for cluster headache. *Cephalalgia* 13:114–116.

Mather, P.J., S.D. Silberstein, E.A. Schulman et al. (1991). The treatment of cluster headache with repetitive intravenous dihydroergotamine. *Headache* 31:525–532.

Mathew, N.T. and W.H. Hurt (1988). Percutaneous radiofrequency trigeminal gangliorhizolysis in intractable cluster headache. *Headache* 28:328–331.

May, A., J. Ashburner, C. Buchel et al. (1999a). Correlation between structural and functional changes in an idiopathic headache syndrome. *Nat. Med.* 5:836–838.

May, A., A. Bahra, C. Buchel et al. (1998a). Hypothalamic activation in cluster headache attacks. *Lancet* 352:275–278.

May, A., A. Bahra, C. Buchel et al. (1999b). Functional magnetic resonance imaging in spontaneous attacks of SUNCT: short-lasting neuralgiform headache with conjunctival injection and tearing. *Ann. Neurol.* 46:787–790.

May, A., H. Kaube, C. Buchel et al. (1998b). Experimental cranial pain elicited by capsaicin: A PET study. *Pain* 74:61–66.

Mayberg, M.R., N.T. Zervas, and M.A. Moskowitz (1984). Trigeminal projections to supratentorial pial and dural blood vessels in cats demonstrated by horseradish peroxidase histochemistry. *J. Comp. Neurol.* 223:46–56.

McNaughton, F.L. (1966). The innervation of the intracranial blood vessels and the dural sinuses. In *The Circulation of the Brain and Spinal Cord* (S. Cobb, A.M. Frantz, W. Penfield et al., eds.), pp. 178–200. Hafner, New York.

Medina, J.L. and S. Diamond (1977). The clinical

link between migraine and cluster headaches. *Arch. Neurol.* 34:470–472.

Montagna, P., P. Cortelli, and B. Barbiroli (1994). Magnetic resonance spectroscopy studies on migraine. *Cephalalgia* 14:184–193.

Montagna, P., R. Lodi, P. Cortelli et al. (1997). Phosphorus magnetic resonance spectroscopy in cluster headache. *Neurology* 48:113–118.

Nappi, G., G. Micieli, A. Cavallini et al. (1992). Accompanying symptoms of cluster attacks: Their relevance to the diagnostic criteria. *Cephalalgia* 3:165–168.

Nattero, G., L. Savi, and G. Pisanti (1980). Doppler flow velocity in cluster headache. Presented at the International Congress, Headache, Florence, Italy.

Odawara, M., A. Tamaeka, H. Mizusawa et al. (1997). A case of cluster headache associated with mitochondrial DNA deletions. *Muscle and Nerve* 20:394–395.

Onofrio, B.M. and J.K. Campbell (1986). Surgical treatment of chronic cluster headache. *Mayo Clin. Proc.* 61:537–544.

Raskin, N.H. (1988). *Headache*, 2nd ed., pp. 229–254. Churchill Livingstone, London.

Rasmussen, B.K. (1999). Epidemiology of cluster headache. In *Cluster Headache and Related Conditions* (J. Olesen and P.J. Goadsby, eds.), pp. 23–26. Oxford University Press, Oxford.

Reik, L., Jr. (1987). Cluster headache after head injury. *Headache* 27:509–510.

Robbins, L. (1995). Intranasal lidocaine for cluster headache. *Headache* 35:83–84.

Roberge, C., J.P. Bouchard, D. Simard et al. (1992). Cluster headache in twins. *Neurology* 42:1255–1256.

Russell, D. and L. Storstein (1983). Cluster headache: A computerized analysis of 24 Holter ECG recordings and description of ECG rhythm disturbances. *Cephalalgia* 3:83–107.

Russell, M.B. (1997). Genetic epidemiology of migraine and cluster headache. *Cephalalgia* 17:683–701.

Russell, M.B., P.G. Andersson, and L.L. Thomsen (1994). Familial occurrence of cluster headache [abstract]. *Genet. Epidemiol.* 11:305–306.

Shimomura, T., A. Kitano, H. Marukawa et al. (1994). Point mutation in platelet mitochondrial tRNA (Leu(UUR)) on a patient with cluster headache. *Lancet* 344:625.

Sianard-Gainko, J., J. Milet, V. Ghuysen et al. (1994). Increased parasellar activity on gallium SPECT is not specific for active cluster headache. *Cephalalgia* 14: 132–133.

Seibel, P., T. Grünewaldt, A. Gundolla et al. (1996). Investigation on the mitochondrial transfer RNA[Leu(UUR)] in blood cells from patients with cluster headache. *J Neurol* 243:305–307.

Silberstein, S.D., R. Nikham, T.D. Rozen et al. (2000). Cluster headache with aura. *Neurology* 54:219–220.

Sjaastad, O. (1992). *Cluster Headache Syndrome*. W.B. Saunders, London.

Sjaastad, O. and I. Dale (1974). Evidence for a new(?), treatable headache entity. *Headache* 14: 105–108.

Sjaastad, O. and P. Rinck (1990). Cluster headache: MRI studies of the cavernous sinus and the base of the brain. *Headache* 30:350–351.

Sjaastad, O., K. Rootwelt, and I. Horven (1975). Cutaneous blood flow in cluster headache. *Headache* 13:173–175.

Sjaastad, O., J.M. Shen, L.J. Stovner et al. (1993). Cluster headache in identical twins. *Headache* 33:214–217.

Spencer, S.E., W.B. Sawyer, H. Wada et al. (1990). CNS projections to the pteropalatine parasympathetic preganglionic neurons in the rat: A retrograde transneuronal viral cell body labeling study. *Brain Res.* 534:149–169.

Steiner, T.J., R. Hering, E.G.M. Couturier et al. (1997). Double-blind placebo-controlled trial of lithium in episodic cluster headache. *Cephalalgia* 17:673–675.

Suzuki, N., J.E. Hardebo, and C. Owman (1988). Origins and pathways of cerebrovascular vasoactive intestinal polypeptide-positive nerves in rat. *J. Cereb. Blood Flow Metab.* 8:697–712.

Swanson, J.W., T. Yanigahara, P.E. Stang et al. (1994). Incidence of cluster headaches: A population-based study in Olmstead County, Minnesota. *Neurology* 44:433–437.

Symonds, C.P. (1956). A particular variety of headache. *Brain* 79:217–232.

Taha, J.M. and J.M. Tew (1995). Long-term results of radiofrequency rhizotomy in the treatment of cluster headache. *Headache* 35:193–196.

Turkewitz, L.J., O. Wirth, G.A. Dawson et al. (1992). Cluster headache following head injury: A case report and review of the literature. *Headache* 32:504–506.

Uddman, R., L. Edvinsson, R. Ekman et al. (1985). Innervation of the feline cerebral vasculature by nerve fibers containing calcitonin gene–related peptide: Trigeminal origin and coexistence with substance P. *Neurosci. Lett.* 62: 131–136.

Vanagaite Vingen, J., J.A. Pareja, and L.J. Stovner (1998). Quantitative evaluation of photophobia and phonophobia in cluster headache. *Cephalalgia* 18:250–256.

Vingen, J.V., J. Pareja, and L.J. Stovner (1999). Increased sensitivity to light and sound during cluster headache bout. In *Cluster Headache and Related Conditions*. (J. Olesen and P.J. Goadsby, eds.), pp. 207–211. Oxford University Press, Oxford.

Waldenlind, E., K. Ekbom, and J. Torhall (1993).

MR-angiography during spontaneous attacks of cluster headache: A case report. *Headache 33*: 291–295.

Waldenlind, E., S.A. Gustafsson, K. Ekbom et al. (1987). Circadian secretion of cortisol and melatonin in cluster headache during active cluster period and remission. *J. Neurol. Neurosurg. Psychiatry 50*:207–213.

Watson, C.P., T.P. Morley, J.C. Richardson et al. (1983). The surgical treatment of chronic cluster headache. *Headache 23*:289–295.

Welch, K.M., S.R. Levine, G. D'Andrea et al. (1989). Preliminary observations on brain en-ergy metabolism in migraine studied by in vivo phosphorus 31NMR spectroscopy. *Neurology 39*:538–541.

Wheeler, S. (1998). Significance of migrainous features in cluster headache: Divalproex responsiveness. *Headache 38*:547–551.

Wheeler, S. and E.J. Carrazana (1999). Topiramate-treated cluster headache. *Neurology 53*: 234–236.

Zagami, A.S., P.J. Goadsby, and L. Edvinsson (1990). Simulation of the superior sagittal sinus in the cat causes release of vasoactive peptides. *Neuropeptides 16*:69–75.

13

Unusual Primary Headache Disorders

LAWRENCE C. NEWMAN
PETER J. GOADSBY

This chapter focuses on a group of uncommon primary headache disorders that are often unrecognized in primary care and general neurologic practice. Although these disorders are less prevalent than other primary headaches, such as migraine and tension-type headaches, it is important to recognize them as they differ in their treatment response and early diagnosis and treatment will prevent needless suffering and disability in affected patients.

PAROXYSMAL HEMICRANIAS

Chronic paroxysmal hemicrania (CPH) was first described in 1974 (Sjaastad and Dale, 1974) but was not officially named until 1976 (Sjaastad and Dale, 1976); it appears in the International Headache Society (IHS) classification (Headache Classification Committee of the International Headache Society, 1988). Chronic paroxysmal hemicrania was originally described as multiple, short-lived, unilateral attacks that occurred on a daily basis, sometimes for years, without remission (Sjaastad and Dale, 1974, 1976; Russell, 1984; Antonaci and Sjaastad, 1989; Sjaastad and Shen, 1991; Sjaastad, 1992; Spierings, 1992). It eventually became clear that not all patients experienced this chronic unremitting course; some patients reported a remitting pattern with discrete headache phases separated by prolonged periods of pain-free remissions (Gearney, 1983; Bogucki and Niewodnicy, 1984; Kudrow et al., 1987; Blau and Engel, 1990; Alberca et al., 1991; Cummings, 1991; Newman et al., 1992a; Spierings, 1988, 1992; Newman et al., 1993; Goadsby and Lipton, 1997). Kudrow et al. (1987) named this pattern episodic paroxysmal hemicrania (EPH). Other patients have experienced an initially episodic course that evolved into the chronic nonrelenting phase (Antonaci and Sjaastad, 1989; Dodick, 1998).

The nomenclature for the various forms of the paroxysmal hemicranias has been controversial. The IHS recognizes only CPH. One nomenclature system uses the term CPH for the entire category and subclassifies the following forms: (1) chronic from onset; (2) chronic evolved from the remitting form; (3) nonchronic/remitting (Antonaci and Sjaastad, 1989). We prefer the terms CPH, EPH, and CPH evolved from EPH to describe these various syndromes (Kudrow et al., 1987; Blau and Engel, 1990; Newman et al., 1992a; Newman and Lipton 1997). These terms are useful in that they are analogous to the IHS nomenclature of cluster headache. Proposed changes to the IHS classification system regarding the paroxysmal hemicranias are listed in Table 13–1 (Goadsby and Lipton, 1997).

Epidemiology

There are more than 100 published case reports of paroxysmal hemicranias; and although these disorders were initially believed to be uncommon, the number of diagnosed cases is surely much higher as these disorders are no longer considered rare. Clinically, it appears that CPH is more common than EPH; only 19 well-documented cases of EPH appear in English publications (Goadsby and Lipton, 1997; Newman et al., 1993; Dodick, 1998). Paroxysmal hemicranias have been re-

ported in different countries throughout the world and across racial boundaries (Rapoport et al., 1981; Petty and Rose, 1983; Haggag and Russell, 1993; Joubert et al., 1987; Joubert, 1988).

Unlike cluster headache, CPH demonstrates a female preponderance, with a sex ratio of approximately 2:1, whereas there is no gender preference for EPH. The disorder usually begins in adulthood. The age at onset ranges from 3 to 81 years, with a mean of approximately 33 years (Sjaastad et al., 1980; Antonaci and Sjaastad, 1989; Kudrow and Kudrow, 1989; Haggag and Russell, 1993; Broeske et al., 1993). A family history of CPH or EPH was not found in any of the reported cases. A documented family history of mi-

Table 13–1 Suggested criteria for the paroxysmal hemicranias

3.2 Paroxysmal hemicrania
   3.2.1 Chronic paroxysmal hemicrania (CPH)
     A. At least 30 attacks fulfilling B–E
     B. Attacks of severe unilateral orbital, supraorbital, and/or temporal pain always on the same side lasting 2–45 minutes
     C. Attack frequency above 5 a day for more than half the time (periods with lower frequency may occur)
     D. Pain is associated with at least one of the following signs/symptoms on the pain side:
       1. Conjunctival injection
       2. Lacrimation
       3. Nasal congestion
       4. Rhinorrhea
       5. Ptosis
       6. Eyelid edema
     E. At least one of the following:
       1. There is no suggestion of one of the disorders listed in groups 5–11
       2. Such a disorder is suggested but excluded by appropriate investigations
       3. Such a disorder is present, but the first headache attacks do not occur in close temporal relation to the disorder
    Note: Most cases respond rapidly and absolutely to indomethacin (usually in doses of 150 mg/day or less)
   3.2.2 Episodic paroxysmal hemicrania (EPH)
     A. At least 30 attacks fulfilling B–F
     B. Attacks of severe unilateral orbital or temporal pain, or both, that is always unilateral and lasts from 1–30 minutes
     C. An attack frequency of 3 or more a day
     D. Clear intervals between bouts of attacks that may last from months to years
     E. Pain is associated with at least one of the following signs/symptoms on the pain side:
       1. Conjunctival injection
       2. Lacrimation
       3. Nasal congestion
       4. Rhinorrhea
       5. Ptosis
       6. Eyelid edema
     F. At least one of the following:
       1. There is no suggestion of one of the disorders listed in groups 5–11
       2. Such a disorder is suggested but excluded by appropriate investigations
       3. Such a disorder is present, but the first headache attacks do not occur in close temporal relation to the disorder
    Note: Most cases respond rapidly and absolutely to indomethacin (usually in doses of 150 mg/day or less)

Reproduced with permission from Goadsby, P.J. and R.B. Lipton (1997). A review of paroxysmal hemicranias, SUNCT syndrome and other short-lasting headaches with autonomic features, including new cases. *Brain 120*:193–209.

graine was evident in 21% of reported cases (Newman and Lipton, 1997). Only one patient reported a positive family history of cluster headaches (Antonaci and Sjaastad, 1989).

Clinical Features

As the clinical profiles of both EPH and CPH are quite similar, we will discuss these entities together.

The pain is strictly unilateral and without side-shift in the vast majority of sufferers. In one report, the pain was bilateral (Pollmann and Pfaffenrath, 1986); and in three patients, the headache demonstrated side-shift (Antonaci and Sjaastad, 1989). Maximal pain is experienced in the ocular, temporal, maxillary, and frontal regions; nuchal and retro-orbital pain have less often been described. The pain may occasionally radiate into the ipsilateral shoulder and arm. Strictly occipital pain has been noted in single reports of CPH (Sjaastad, 1986) and EPH (Dodick, 1998). On rare occasions, toothache or otalgia is the presenting symptom (Delcanho and Graff-Radford, 1993; Boes et al., 1998).

The pain is described as a throbbing, boring, pulsatile, or stabbing sensation that ranges from moderate to excruciating in severity. On occasion, a mild discomfort at the usual site of pain is present interictally (Antonaci and Sjaastad, 1989). During acute attacks, sufferers usually prefer to sit quietly or lie in bed in the fetal position (Stein and Rogado, 1980); rarely, however, some sufferers assume the pacing activity usually seen in cluster.

Attacks of CPH recur one to 40 times daily. There is, however, a marked variability in attack frequency: the frequency of mild attacks ranges from two to 14 daily, and severe attacks recur six to 40 times a day (Newman and Lipton, 1997). The majority of patients report 15 or more attacks a day (Sjaastad et al., 1980; Haggag and Russell, 1993; Newman and Lipton, 1997). Individual headaches usually last between 2 and 25 minutes, with a range of 2 to 120 minutes (Bogucki et al., 1984; Russell, 1984; Sjaastad, 1992; Haggag and Russell, 1993; Newman and Lipton,

1997). In EPH, the daily attack frequency ranges from two to 30, with attacks lasting 3 to 30 minutes each. The headache phase lasts from 2 weeks to 4.5 months; remissions range from 1 to 36 months (Newman et al., 1992a, 1993; Newman and Lipton, 1997; Dodick, 1998). Attacks recur throughout the day and night; nocturnal attacks have been reported to occur in association with REM sleep (Sjaastad and Dale, 1976; Kayed et al., 1978; Sjaastad et al., 1980; Newman et al., 1993; Russell, 1984).

Approximately 19% of patients report the ability to trigger attacks by bending or rotating their head (Antonaci and Sjaastad, 1989; Sjaastad et al., 1984). Pressure on the C_2 root, the greater occipital nerve, or the transverse process of C_4-C_5 may also induce an attack (Sjaastad et al., 1982, 1984).

During acute attacks, one or more ipsilateral autonomic symptoms are usually present. Approximately 60% of sufferers report ipsilateral lacrimation. Homolateral ptosis (33%), conjunctival injection (36%), nasal congestion (42%), and rhinorrhea (36%) also may accompany the headaches (Antonaci and Sjaastad, 1989; Sjaastad, 1992; Haggag and Russell, 1993), and ipsilateral miosis has occasionally been reported (Drummond, 1985; Petty and Rose, 1983). Increased forehead sweating has been reported to occur in some patients on the symptomatic side during acute headache episodes, as has generalized sweating (Sjaastad et al., 1981, 1986). Unlike cluster headache, Horner's syndrome does not appear to accompany attacks of CPH or EPH (de Souza Caralho et al., 1988; Sjaastad, 1986; Sjaastad, 1988). Although the IHS criteria require at least one ipsilateral autonomic feature during attacks, patients with otherwise typical CPH without autonomic symptoms have been described (Bogucki et al., 1984; Pareja, 1995).

Secondary causes of the paroxysmal hemicranias have been reported. Disorders that mimic the paroxysmal hemicranias include circle of Willis aneurysms (Medina, 1992), arteriovenous malformations and cerebrovascular accidents (Newman et al., 1992b; Broeske et al., 1993), collagen vascular disease (Medina, 1992), Pancoast's tumor (Delreux et al., 1989), tumor of the frontal lobe

(Medina, 1992), tumor of the sella turcica (Vijayan, 1992; Gawel and Rothbart, 1992), tumor of the cavernous sinus (Sjaastad et al., 1995), intracranial hypertension (Hannerz and Jogestrand, 1993), and thrombocythemia (MacMillan and Nukada, 1989).

Chronic paroxysmal hemicrania has been reported to occur in association with migraine (Pareja and Pareja, 1992), cluster headache (Jotkowitz, 1978; Pearce et al., 1987; Tehindrazanarivelo et al., 1992; Centonzone et al., 2000), and trigeminal neuralgia (Hannerz, 1993; Caminero et al., 1998; Zukerman et al, 2000).

Laboratory Studies

Excluding the secondary mimics, magnetic resonance imaging (MRI) studies of patients with CPH have been normal (Antonaci, 1994). Segmental narrowing of the ophthalmic veins, similar to the changes seen in cluster headache, have been reported (Antonaci, 1994), although the relevance is uncertain. Ocular blood flow changes, measured by dynamic tonometry, reveal significant attack-related increases in corneal indentation pulse amplitudes, ocular blood flow, and intraocular pressure that are more pronounced on the symptomatic side (Horven et al., 1989; Haggag and Russell, 1993). Increased corneal temperatures have also been reported to occur on the symptomatic side and may reflect the increased ocular blood flow (Drummond, 1985). Pupillometric studies show a consistently smaller pupil on the affected side (de Souza Carvalho et al., 1988). Electrophysiological studies in patients with CPH have revealed reduced pain thresholds, reduced corneal reflex thresholds, and normal blink reflexes (Antonaci et al., 1994). Autonomic studies have yielded inconsistent results, although increased lacrimation and nasal secretion on the symptomatic side and decreased salivation have been reported (Saunte, 1984). Cardiac conduction abnormalities, including bradycardia and sinoatrial block, bundle branch block with runs of atrial fibrillation, extrasystoles, and bradycardia have occurred in patients with CPH (Sjaastad and Dale,

1974; Petty and Rose, 1983; Russell and Storstein, 1984).

Facial thermograms in CPH are similar to those of patients with cluster headache. Interictally, cold spots are observed over the supraorbital margin or inner canthus (Mongini et al., 1990). During attacks of CPH, increases in temperature over the affected region have been reported (Drummond, 1985). Abnormalities in cerebral blood flow, measured by transcranial Doppler, were abnormal in three patients (Shen, 1993).

Abnormalities in the cyclic release of catecholamines and β-endorphin have been observed (Micieli et al., 1989; Goadsby and Lipton, 1997). Increased levels of calcitonin gene–related peptide (CGRP) and vasoactive intestinal peptide (VIP) in the cranial venous blood of a CPH sufferer were also documented. These levels returned to normal following treatment with indomethacin (Goadsby and Edvinsson, 1996).

Treatment

Indomethacin is the treatment of choice for the paroxysmal hemicranias and has been deemed the *sine qua non* for establishing the diagnosis. Therapy is usually initiated at a dose of 25 mg TID and increased to 50 mg TID in 1 week if there is no response or only partial benefit. Headache resolution is usually prompt, occurring 1 to 2 days after the effective dose has been established. Maintenance with doses ranging from 25 to 100 mg daily usually suffices; however, doses up to 300 mg/day may be required. Injectable indomethacin may be used to test this response (Antonaci et al., 1998).

Dosage adjustments are occasionally necessary to treat the clinical fluctuations that are sometimes seen in these disorders; night-time dosing with sustained-release indomethacin often prevents nocturnal exacerbations. During the active headache cycle, patients report that skipping or even delaying doses of indomethacin may result in the prompt reemergence of headaches. In patients suffering from EPH, indomethacin is given for slightly longer than the usual headache period and then gradually tapered. In patients with CPH, chronic treatment is usually required, although long-lasting remissions have been reported following cessation of indomethacin in rare patients with CPH (Sjaastad and Antonaci, 1987).

When patients are refractory to indomethacin therapy, the diagnosis should be reconsidered. Patients requiring continuous, high dosages of indomethacin may have underlying pathology and need careful diagnostic evaluation (Sjaastad et al., 1995). Gastrointestinal side effects secondary to indomethacin may be treated with antacids, misoprostol, or histamine H_2 receptor antagonists and should always be considered for patients who require long-term treatment.

Although the IHS requires indomethacin response as a diagnostic criteria, other agents have also been reported to be of some benefit (Evers and Husstedt, 1996). Acetylsalicylic acid has been efficacious during the early phases of CPH in some patients (Antonaci and Sjaastad, 1989) and possibly during the childhood phase of the disorder (Kudrow and Kudrow, 1989). Partial success has also been reported with verapamil (Coria et al., 1992; Shabbir and McAbee, 1994), steroids (Hannerz et al., 1987), and naproxen (Antonaci and Sjaastad, 1989). A piroxicam derivative was reported to be efficacious in some patients with CPH who were also responsive to indomethacin therapy (Sjaastad and Antonaci, 1995), and acetazolamide therapy successfully treated a patient previously unresponsive to indomethacin (Warner et al., 1994). Sumatriptan has been reported to be beneficial in a patient suffering from bilateral CPH (Hannerz and Jogestrand, 1993), although its usefulness in typical unilateral cases has not been demonstrated (Dahlof, 1990; Goadsby and Lipton, 1997).

SHORT-LASTING UNILATERAL NEURALGIFORM HEADACHES WITH CONJUNCTIVAL INJECTION AND TEARING (SUNCT SYNDROME)

The SUNCT syndrome is one of the rarest of the unusual primary headache disorders and has the most dramatic and variable clinical presentation. The syndrome was first described in 1978 and more fully characterized in 1989 (Sjaastad et al., 1978, 1989). At the time of this writing, 26 sufferers have been reported. The disorder has a male predominance (18 men, 8 women) with a sex ratio of 2.25:1 (Pareja and Sjaastad, 1994, 1997; Bouhassira et al., 1994; Goadsby and Lipton, 1997; Benoliel and Sharav, 1998; Raimondi and Gardella, 1998; May et al., 1999). Suggested clinical criteria for the diagnosis of SUNCT are listed in Table 13–2 (Goadsby and Lipton, 1997).

Clinical Features

The SUNCT syndrome is characterized by very brief headache episodes recurring multiple times per day. The age at onset ranges from 23 to 77 years (mean 51) (Pareja and Sjaastad, 1997). The pain is usually maximal in and around the eye and may radiate to the ipsilateral forehead, temple, nose, cheek, and palate (Pareja and Sjaastad, 1997). Attacks are typically unilateral; in three patients, however, pain was simultaneously experienced on the opposite side (Pareja and Sjaastad, 1997). The pain is usually burning, stabbing, or electric in nature. Paroxysms begin and end

Table 13–2 Criteria for SUNCT

A. At least 30 attacks fulfilling B–E
B. Attacks of unilateral moderately severe orbital or temporal stabbing or throbbing pain lasting 15–120 seconds
C. Attack frequency 3–100/day
D. Pain is associated with at least one of the following signs or symptoms on the affected side, with feature 1 being most often present and very prominent:
   1. Conjunctival injection
   2. Lacrimation
   3. Nasal congestion
   4. Rhinorrhea
   5. Ptosis
   6. Eyelid edema
E. At least one of the following:
   1. There is no suggestion of one of the disorders listed in groups 5–11
   2. Such a disorder is suggested but excluded by appropriate investigations
   3. Such a disorder is present, but the first headache attacks do not occur in close temporal relation to the disorder

abruptly, reaching maximum intensity within 2 to 3 seconds (Pareja and Sjaastad, 1997). Individual headache attacks last between 5 and 250 seconds (mean 49) (Pareja et al., 1996c), although attacks lasting 2 hours each have been described (Pareja et al., 1996b). Some patients experience a dull interictal discomfort that persists between acute episodes (Pareja et al., 1996b), although most patients report being totally pain-free between attacks. Four patients experienced a status-like pattern in which painful paroxysms persisted from 1 to 3 days (Pareja et al., 1996a).

The temporal pattern is also quite variable, with symptomatic periods alternating with periods of pain-free remission in an erratic fashion. Symptomatic periods generally last from a few days to several months and occur once or twice yearly. Remissions range from 1 week to 7 years but usually are of a few months' duration (Pareja and Sjaastad, 1997). During the symptomatic phase, daily attacks recur from 6 to 77 times (mean 28) (Pareja et al., 1996c); however, tremendous variability occurs between patients and within the same patient. Attacks may be as infrequent as once a day or less to more than 30 attacks an hour (Pareja et al., 1996c; Pareja and Sjaastad, 1997). One patient reported attacks that would recur in a repetitive and overlapping fashion for 1 to 3 hours at a time, twice daily (Pareja et al., 1994). Although attacks recur throughout the day, a bimodal distribution with increased attack frequency occurring in the morning and afternoon/evening hours has been described (Pareja et al., 1996c). Nocturnal attacks were experienced by 12 patients (Pareja and Sjaastad, 1997).

Acute attacks of headache in the SUNCT syndrome are accompanied by a variety of associated symptoms, the most prominent of which are ipsilateral conjunctival injection and lacrimation. Ipsilateral nasal congestion, rhinorrhea, and eyelid edema are less commonly reported. Some patients reported that the accompanying autonomic phenomena were bilateral, although more pronounced on the side of the headache (Pareja and Sjaastad, 1997). The associated tearing and conjunctival injection usually begin 1 to 2 seconds following the acute episodes of pain and may persist for a few seconds longer than the painful episodes (Pareja and Sjaastad, 1997). Two patients had associated symptoms that remained for 30 to 60 seconds following headache resolution (Sjaastad et al., 1989; Becser and Berky, 1995), and one patient had eyelid edema that persisted for 5 to 10 minutes (Hannerz et al., 1992). Rhinorrhea, when present, is delayed, occurring relatively late in the course of the headache (Pareja and Sjaastad, 1997).

Many patients can precipitate acute attacks by touching certain trigger zones within the territory of V_1–V_3. Precipitants include touching the hair, forehead, face, nose, and lip on the symptomatic side. Washing, shaving, eating, chewing, tooth-brushing, talking, and coughing were also reported as headache triggers (Pareja and Sjaastad, 1997). Mechanical movements of the neck can also precipitate attacks, although some patients could lessen or abort attacks by continuously rotating their neck (Sjaastad et al., 1989; Pareja and Sjaastad, 1997). Unlike patients with trigeminal neuralgia, most patients have no refractory period.

Secondary causes of SUNCT have been reported in three patients and include homolateral cerebellopontine angle arteriovenous malformations (Bussone et al., 1991; De Benedittis, 1995) and brain-stem cavernous hemangioma (Morales et al., 1994).

Laboratory Studies

Excluding symptomatic cases, computed tomography (CT), MRI, and angiography, when performed, were essentially normal. Orbital phlebography was abnormal, revealing a narrowed superior ophthalmic vein ipsilateral to the headache (Kruszewski, 1992). Intraocular pressure and corneal temperatures are increased, as is forehead sweating, during attacks (Sjaastad et al., 1992; Kruszewski, 1992), but pupillometry and pharmacologic studies of the pupil are normal (Zhao and Sjaastad, 1993). Systolic blood pressure is occasionally increased (Kruszewski et al., 1991), and bradycardia has been reported in association with acute attacks (Kruszewski et al., 1991), although ventilatory function is normal

(Kruszewski et al., 1995). Single photon emission CT and transcranial Doppler studies are normal during attacks (Shen and Johnsen, 1994; Poughias and Aasly, 1995); functional MRI revealed significant activation in the region of the ipsilateral posterior hypothalamus in one patient (May et al., 1999).

Treatment

The SUNCT syndrome has proven to be refractory to a variety of therapeutic approaches. Medications typically employed in the treatment of migraine, cluster, and other short-lived headache syndromes are ineffectual, as are anesthetic blockades (Pareja et al., 1995). Carbamazepine was reported to be of possible benefit in 5 of 18 patients (Pareja and Sjaastad, 1997). Azathiaprine, oral sumatriptan, prednisone, valproate, nifedipine, and lamotrigine were mildly efficacious in single reports (Hannerz et al., 1992; Ghose, 1995; Pareja et al., 1995; D'Andrea et al., 1999). Verapamil and omeprazole were reported to worsen the condition (Pareja et al., 1995).

HYPNIC HEADACHE SYNDROME

The hypnic headache syndrome is a rare primary headache disorder that was first described by Raskin (1988) and Newman et al. (1990). The initial description of the syndrome was a bilateral, throbbing headache without associated autonomic features that lasted from 15 to 60 minutes and recurred once to three times nightly, often during rapid-eye-movement (REM) sleep. At the time of this writing, a total of 37 patients with the disorder have been described. The disorder has a female predominance (26 women, 11 men), with a sex ratio of 2.36:1 (Raskin, 1988; Newman et al., 1990, 1991; Goadsby and Lipton, 1997; Gould and Silberstein, 1997; Morales-Asin et al., 1998; Dodick et al., 1998; Ivanez et al., 1998; Perez-Martinez et al., 1999). Although most patients are elderly, the age at onset ranges from 40 to 82 years (mean 66 years, median 66 years). Headaches occur at a consistent time each night, usually

between 1:00 and 3:00 A.M., and may on rare instances occur during a daytime nap (Dodick et al., 1998). The headaches begin abruptly, are diffuse and throbbing, and spontaneously resolve in 15 to 180 minutes. In ten patients (27%), the headache was hemicranial (Gould and Silberstein, 1997; Dodick et al., 1998; Ivanez et al., 1998; Morales-Asin et al., 1998). No associated autonomic symptoms accompany the pain, but nausea, photophobia, and phonophobia may rarely be present.

All patients have been successfully treated with bedtime doses of lithium carbonate, 300 to 600 mg, although many patients could not tolerate the side effects. Bedtime doses of caffeine (five patients), flunarizine (two patients), indomethacin (one patient), atenolol (one patient), and a combination of ergotamine tartrate, belladonna, and caffeine (one patient) have also been reported to treat this syndrome (Morales-Asin et al., 1998; Dodick et al., 1998; Ivanez et al., 1998). One patient who was treated with prednisone, vincristine, and cyclophosphamide for an unrelated illness experienced headache resolution (Newman et al., 1991). Table 13–3 lists suggested criteria for hypnic headache (Goadsby and Lipton, 1997).

The disorders described in this chapter are relatively rare but probably are more com-

---

Table 13–3 Suggested criteria for hypnic headache

A. Headaches occur at least 15 times per month for at least 1 month
B. Headaches awaken patients from sleep
C. Attack duration of 5–60 minutes
D. Pain is generalized or unilateral[a]
E. Pain is not associated with autonomic features
F. At least one of the following:
　1. There is no suggestion of one of the disorders listed in groups 5–11
　2. Such a disorder is suggested but excluded by appropriate investigations
　3. Such a disorder is present, but the first headache attacks do not occur in temporal relation to the disorder

---

A rapid clinical response to lithium at bedtime is usually expected.

[a]These criteria were modified following reports of ten patients with unilateral hypnic headaches.

Reproduced with permission from Goadsby, P.J. and R.B. Lipton (1997). A review of paroxysmal hemicranias, SUNCT syndrome and other short-lasting headaches with autonomic features, including new cases. *Brain 120*:193–209.

Table 13–4 Clinical features

	CPH	EPH	SUNCT	Hypnic	Cluster
Sex F:M	2:1	1:1	1:2	2:1	1:8
Pain quality	Throbbing, boring, stabbing	Throbbing, boring, stabbing	Burning, stabbing, electric	Throbbing	Stabbing, boring
Pain severity	Very severe	Very severe	Moderate	Moderate	Very severe
Site of maximal pain	Orbit, temple	Orbit, temple	Periorbital	Diffuse, rarely hemicranial	Orbit, temple
Attacks per day	1–40	2–30	6–77	1–3	1 every 2nd day to 8/day
Attack duration	2–25 minutes	3–30 minutes	5–250 seconds	30–60 minutes	15–180 minutes
Autonomic features	Present	Present	Present	Absent	Present
Triggers	Alcohol, bending head, pressing C_4–C_5, C_2, occipital nerve	Alcohol, bending head, pressing C_4–C_5, C_2, occipital nerve	V_1–V_3 trigger points, neck movements	Sleep	Alcohol
Nocturnal attacks	Yes	Yes	Yes	Yes	Yes
Treatment	Indomethacin	Indomethacin	None known	Lithium, caffeine	Verapamil, lithium, methysergide

Key to abbreviations: CPH, chronic paroxysmal hemicrania; EPH, episodic paroxysmal hemicrania; SUNCT, short-lasting unilateral neuralgiform with conjunctival injection and tearing.

mon than previously thought. As these disorders cause significant pain and disability, recognition is essential as treatment response differs from that of migraine, tension-type, and cluster headaches. Table 13–4 reviews the important clinical features of these syndromes and contrasts them with cluster headache, the disorder with which they are often confused.

REFERENCES

Alberca, R. and J.J. Ochoa (1994). Cluster tic syndrome. *Neurology* 44:996–999.

Alberca, R., B. Sureda, C. Narquez et al. (1991). Episodic paroxysmal hemicrania or chronic paroxysmal hemicrania in prechronic state? *Neurologia* 6:219–221.

Antonaci, F. (1994). Chronic paroxysmal hemicrania and hemicrania continua: Orbital phlebography and MRI studies. *Headache* 34:32–34.

Antonaci, F., J.A. Pareja, A.B. Caminero et al. (1998). Chronic paroxysmal hemicrania and hemicrania continua. Parenteral indomethacin: the Indotest. *Headache* 38:122–128.

Antonaci, F., G. Sandrini, A. Danilov et al. (1994). Neurophysiological studies in chronic paroxysmal hemicrania and hemicrania continua. *Headache* 34:479–483.

Antonaci, F. and O. Sjaastad (1989). Chronic paroxysmal hemicrania (CPH): A review of the clinical manifestations. *Headache* 29:648–656.

Becser, N. and M. Berky (1995). SUNCT Syndrome: A Hungarian Case. *Headache* 35:158–160.

Benoliel, R. and Y. Sharav (1998). SUNCT syndrome: Case report and literature review. *Oral Surg. Oral Med. Oral Pathol. Oral Radiol. Endod.* 85:158–161.

Blau, J.N. and H. Engel (1990). Episodic paroxysmal hemicrania: A further case and review of the literature. *J. Neurol. Neurosurg. Psychiatry* 53:343–344.

Boes, C.J., J.W. Swanson, and D.W. Dodick (1998). Chronic paroxysmal hemicrania presenting as otalgia with a sensation of external acoustic meatus obstruction: Two cases and a pathophysiologic hypothesis. *Headache* 38:787–791.

Bogucki, A. and A. Niewodniczy (1984). Chronic cluster with unusual high frequency of attacks: Differential diagnosis with CPH. *Headache* 24:150–151.

Bogucki, A., R. Szymanska, and W. Braciak (1984). Chronic paroxysmal hemicrania: Lack of a prechronic stage. *Cephalalgia* 4:187–189.

Bouhassira, D., N. Attal, M. Esteve et al. (1994)

SUNCT syndrome. A case of transformation from trigeminal neuralgia? *Cephalalgia* 14:168–170.

Broeske, D., N.J. Lenn, and E. Cantos (1993). Chronic paroxysmal hemicrania in a young child: Possible relation to ipsilateral occipital infarction. *J. Child Neurol.* 8:235–236.

Bussone, G., M. Leone, G. Dalla Volta et al. (1991). Short-lasting unilateral neuralgiform headache attacks with tearing and conjunctival injection: The first symptomatic case? *Cephalalgia* 11:123–127.

Caminero, A.B., J.A. Pareja, and J.L. Dobato (1998). Chronic paroxysmal hemicrania-tic syndrome. *Cephalalgia* 18:159–161.

Centonze, V., A. Bassi, V. Causarano V et al. (2000). Simultaneous occurrence of ipsilateral cluster headache and chronic paroxysmal hemicrania: A case report. *Headache* 40:54–56.

Coria, F., L.E. Claveria, F.J. Jimenez-Jimenez et al. (1992). Episodic paroxysmal hemicrania responsive to calcium channel blockers. *J. Neurol. Neurosurg. Psychiatry* 55:166.

Cummings, W.J.K. (1991). Episodic paroxysmal hemicrania. *J. Neurol. Neurosurg. Psychiatry* 54:666.

Dahlof, C. (1993). Subcutaneous sumatriptan does not abort attacks of chronic paroxysmal hemicrania (CPH). *Headache* 33:201–202.

D'Andrea, G., F. Granella, and M. Cadaldini (1999). Possible usefulness of lamotrigine in the treatment of SUNCT syndrome. *Neurology* 22:1609.

De Benedittis, G. (1995). SUNCT syndrome associated with cavernous angioma of the brain stem. *Cephalalgia* 15(Suppl. 14):28.

Delcanho, R.E. and S.B. Graff-Radford (1993). Chronic paroxysmal hemicrania presenting as a toothache. *J. Orofac. Pain* 7:300–306.

Delreux, V., L. Kevers, and A. Callewaert (1989). Hemicranie paroxysitique inaugurant un syndrome de Pancoast. *Rev. Neurol.* 145:151–152.

de Souza Caralho, S., R. Salvesen, T. Sand et al. (1988). Chronic paroxysmal hemicrania. XIII. The pupillometric pattern. *Cephalalgia* 8:219–226.

Dodick, D.W. (1998). Extratrigeminal episodic paroxysmal hemicrania. Further clinical evidence of functionally relevant brain stem connections. *Headache* 38:794–798.

Dodick, D.W., A.C. Mosek, and J.K. Campbell (1998). The hypnic (alarm clock) headache syndrome. *Cephalalgia* 18:152–156.

Drummond, P.D. (1985). Thermographic and pupillary asymmetry in chronic paroxysmal hemicrania. A case study. *Cephalalgia* 5:133–136.

Evers, S. and I.W. Husstedt (1996). Alternatives in drug treatment of chronic paroxysmal hemicrania. *Headache* 36:429–432.

Gawel, M.J. and P. Rothbart (1992). Chronic paroxysmal hemicrania which appears to arise from either third ventricle pathology or internal carotid artery pathology. *Cephalalgia 12*:327.

Gearney, D.P. (1983). Indomethacin-responsive episodic cluster headache. *J. Neurol. Neurosurg. Psychiatry 46*:860–861.

Ghose, R.R. (1995). SUNCT syndrome. *Med. J. Aust. 162*:667–668.

Goadsby, P.J. and L. Edvinsson (1996). Neuropeptide changes in a case of chronic paroxysmal hemicrania—evidence trigemino-parasympathetic activation. *Cephalalgia 16*:448–450.

Goadsby, P.J. and R.B. Lipton (1997). A review of paroxysmal hemicranias, SUNCT syndrome and other short-lasting headaches with autonomic feature, including new cases. *Brain 120*:193–209.

Gould, J.D. and S.D. Silberstein (1997). Unilateral hypnic headache: A case study. *Neurology 49*: 1749–1751.

Haggag, K.J. and D. Russell (1993). Chronic paroxysmal hemicrania. In *The Headaches* (J. Olesen, P. Tfelt-Hansen, and K.M.A. Welch, eds.), pp. 601–608. Raven Press, New York.

Hannerz, J. (1993). Trigeminal neuralgia with chronic paroxysmal hemicrania: The CPH-tic syndrome. *Cephalalgia 13*:361–364.

Hannerz, J., K. Ericson, and G. Bergstrand (1987). Chronic paroxysmal hemicrania: Orbital phlebography and steroid treatment. A case report. *Cephalalgia 7*:189–192.

Hannerz, J., D. Greitz, P. Hansson et al. (1992). SUNCT may be another manifestation of orbital venous vasculitis. *Headache 32*:384–389.

Hannerz, J. and T. Jogestrand (1993). Intracranial hypertension and sumatriptan efficacy on a case of chronic paroxysmal hemicrania which became bilateral (the mechanism of indomethacin in CPH). *Headache 33*:320–323.

Headache Classification Committee of the International Headache Society (1988). Classification and diagnostic criteria for headache disorders, cranial neuralgias and facial pain. *Cephalalgia* 8(Suppl. 7):1–96.

Horven, J., D. Russell, and O. Sjaastad (1989). Ocular blood flow changes in cluster headache and chronic paroxysmal hemicrania. *Headache 29*: 373–376.

Ivanez, V., R. Soler, and P. Barreiro (1998). Hypnic headache syndrome: A case with good response to indomethacin. *Cephalalgia 18*:225–226.

Jotkowitz, S. (1978). Chronic paroxysmal hemicrania and cluster. *Ann. Neurol. 4*:389.

Joubert, J. (1988). Cluster headaches in black patients. A report of 7 cases. *S. Afr. Med. J. 73*: 552–554.

Joubert, J., D. Powell, and J. Djikowski (1987). Chronic paroxysmal hemicrania in a South African black. A case report. *Cephalalgia 7*:193–196.

Kayed, K., O.B. Godtilibsen, and O. Sjaastad (1978). Chronic paroxysmal hemicrania. 4.

AREM sleep locked nocturnal headache attacks. *Sleep 1*:91–95.

Kruszewski, P. (1992). Short-lasting, unilateral, neuralgiform headache attacks with conjunctival injection and tearing (SUNCT syndrome): V. Orbital phlebography. *Cephalalgia 12*:387–389.

Kruszewski, P., M.L. Fasano, A.O. Beubakk et al. (1991). Shortlasting, unilateral, neuralgiform headache attacks with conjunctival injection, tearing and subclinical forehead sweating ("SUNCT" syndrome): II. Changes in heart rate and aterial blood pressure during pain paroxysms. *Headache 31*:399–405.

Kruszewski, P., L.R. White, J.M. Shen et al. (1995). Respiratory studies in SUNCT syndrome. *Headache 35*:344–388.

Kudrow, D.B. and L. Kudrow (1989). Successful aspirin prophylaxis in a child with chronic paroxysmal hemicrania. *Headache 29*:280–281.

Kudrow, L., P. Esperanca, and N. Vijayan (1987). Episodic paroxysmal hemicrania? *Cephalalgia 7*: 197–201

Macmillan, J.C. and H. Nukada (1989). Chronic paroxysmal hemicrania. *N. Z. Med. J. 102*:251–252.

May, A., A. Bahra, C. Buchel et al. (1999). Functional magnetic resonance imaging in spontaneous attacks of SUNCT: Short-lasting neuralgiform headache with conjunctival injection and tearing. *Ann. Neurol. 46*:791–794.

Medina, J.L. (1992). Organic headaches mimicking chronic paroxysmal hemicrania. *Headache 32*:73–74.

Micieli, G., A. Cavallini, F. Facchinetti et al. (1989). Chronic paroxysmal hemicrania: A chronobiological study (case report). *Cephalalgia 9*:281–286.

Mongini, F., C. Caselli, V. Macri et al. (1990). Thermographic findings in cranio-facial pain. *Headache 30*:497–504.

Morales, F., E. Mostacero, J. Marta et al. (1994). Vascular malformation of the cerebellopontine angle associated with SUNCT syndrome. *Cephalalgia 14*:301–302.

Morales-Asin, F., J.A. Mayri, C. Inniguez et al. (1998). The hypnic headache syndrome: Report of three new cases. *Cephalalgia 18*:157–158.

Newman, L.C., M.L. Gordon, R.B. Lipton et al. (1992a). Episodic paroxysmal hemicrania: Two new cases and a literature review. *Neurology 42*: 964–966.

Newman, L.C., S. Herskovitz, R.B. Lipton et al. (1992b). Chronic paroxysmal headache: Two cases with cerebrovascular disease. *Headache 32*:75–76.

Newman, L.C. and R.B. Lipton (1997). Paroxysmal hemicranias. In *Headache. Blue Books of Practical Neurology 17* (P.J. Goadsby and S.D. Silberstein, eds.), pp. 243–250. Butterworth-Heinemann, Boston.

Newman, L.C., R.B. Lipton, and S. Solomon

(1990). The hypnic headache syndrome: A benign headache disorder of the elderly. *Neurology 40*:1904–1905.

Newman, L.C., R.B. Lipton, and S. Solomon (1991). The hypnic headache syndrome. In *New Advances in Headache Research* (F.C. Rose, ed.), pp. 31–34. Smith-Gordon, London.

Newman, L.C., R.B. Lipton, and S. Solomon (1993). Episodic paroxysmal hemicrania: 3 new cases and a review of the literature. *Headache 33*:195–197.

Pareja, J. and J. Pareja (1992). Chronic paroxysmal hemicrania coexisting with migraine. Differential response to pharmacological treatment. *Headache 32*:77–78.

Pareja, J.A. (1995). Chronic paroxysmal hemicrania: Dissociation of the pain and autonomic features. *Headache 35*:111–113.

Pareja, J.A., V. Caballero, and O. Sjaastad (1996a). SUNCT syndrome. Status-like pattern. *Headache 36*:622–624.

Pareja, J.A., J. Joubert, and O. Sjaastad (1996b). SUNCT syndrome. Atypical temporal patterns. *Headache 36*:108–110.

Pareja, J.A., P. Kruszewski, and O. Sjaastad (1995). SUNCT syndrome: Trials of drugs and anesthetic blockades. *Headache 35*:138–142.

Pareja, J.A., J. Pareja, T. Palomo et al. (1994). SUNCT syndrome: Repetitive and overlapping attacks. *Headache 34*:114–116.

Pareja, J.A., J.M. Shen, P. Kruszewski et al. (1996c). SUNCT syndrome: Duration, frequency, and temporal distribution of attacks. *Headache 36*:161–165.

Pareja, J.A. and O. Sjaastad (1994). SUNCT syndrome in the female. *Headache 34*:217–220.

Pareja, J.A. and O. Sjaastad (1997). SUNCT syndrome. A clinical review. *Headache 37*:195–202.

Pearce, S.H.S., J.G.C. Cox, and J.M.S. Pearce (1987). Chronic paroxysmal hemicrania, episodic cluster headache and classic migraine in one patient. *J. Neurol. Neurosurg. Psychiatry 50*:1599.

Perez-Martinez, D.A., A. Berbel-Garcia, A.I. Puente-Munoz et al. (1999). Hypnic headache: A new case. *Rev. Neurol. 28*:883–884.

Petty, R.G. and F.C. Rose (1983). Chronic paroxysmal hemicrania: First reported British case. *BMJ 286*:438.

Pollmann, W. and V. Pfaffenrath (1986). Chronic paroxysmal hemicrania: The first possible bilateral case. *Cephalalgia 6*:55–57.

Poughias, L. and J. Aasly (1995). SUNCT syndrome: Cerebral SPECT images during attacks. *Headache 35*:143–145.

Raimondi, E. and L. Gardella (1998). SUNCT syndrome. Two cases in Argentina. *Headache 38*:369–371.

Rapoport, A.M., F.D. Sheftell, and S.M. Baskin (1981). Chronic paroxysmal hemicrania: Case report of the second known definite occurrence in a male. *Cephalalgia 1*:67–69.

Raskin, N.H. (1988). The hypnic headache syndrome. *Headache 28*:534–536.

Russell, D. (1984). Chronic paroxysmal hemicrania: Severity, duration and time of occurrence of attacks. *Cephalalgia 4*:53–56.

Russell, D. and L. Storstein (1984). Chronic paroxysmal hemicrania: Heart rate changes and ECG rhythm disturbances. A computerized analysis of 24h ambulatory ECG recordings. *Cephalalgia 4*:135–144.

Saunte, C. (1984). Chronic paroxysmal hemicrania: Salivation, tearing and nasal secretion. *Cephalalgia 4*:25–32.

Shabbir, N. and G. McAbee (1994). Adolescent chronic paroxysmal hemicrania responsive to verapamil monotherapy. *Headache 34*:209–210.

Shen, J.M. (1993). Transcranial Doppler sonography in chronic paroxysmal hemicrania. *Headache 33*:493–496.

Shen, J.M. and H.J. Johnsen (1994). SUNCT syndrome: Estimation of cerebral blood flow velocity with transcranial Doppler ultrasonography. *Headache 34*:25–31.

Sjaastad, O. (1986). Chronic paroxysmal hemicrania (CPH). In *Handbook of Clinical Neurology*, Vol. 48 (P.J. Vinken, G.W. Bruyn, H.L. Klawans et al., eds.), pp. 257–266. Elsevier, Amsterdam.

Sjaastad, O. (1988). Cluster headache and its variants. *Headache 28*:667–668.

Sjaastad, O. (1992). *Cluster Headache Syndrome*. W.B. Saunders, London.

Sjaastad, O., J. Aasly, T. Fredriksen et al. (1986). Chronic paroxysmal hemicrania. 10. On the autonomic involvement. *Cephalalgia 6*:113–124.

Sjaastad, O. and F. Antonaci (1987). Chronic paroxysmal hemicrania: A case report. Long-lasting remission in the chronic stage. *Cephalalgia 7*: 203–205.

Sjaastad, O. and F. Antonaci (1995). A piroxicam derivative partially effective in chronic paroxysmal hemicrania and hemicrania continua. *Headache 35*:549–550.

Sjaastad, O., R. Apfelbaum, W. Caskey et al. (1980). Chronic paroxysmal hemicrania (CPH): The clinical manifestations—a review. *Ups. J. Med. Sci. 31*:27–33.

Sjaastad, O. and I. Dale (1974). Evidence for a new (?) treatable headache entity. *Headache 14*: 105–108.

Sjaastad, O. and I. Dale (1976). A new (?) clinical headache entity "chronic paroxysmal hemicrania" 2. *Acta Neurol. Scand. 54*:140–159.

Sjaastad, O., P. Kruszewski, K. Fostad et al. (1992). SUNCT syndrome: VII. Ocular and related variables. *Headache 32*:489–495.

Sjaastad, O., D. Russell, I. Horven et al. (1978). Multiple neuralgiform unilateral headache attacks associated with conjunctival injection and appearing in clusters. A nosological problem. *Proc. Scand. Migraine Soc. 31*.

Sjaastad, O., D. Russell, C. Saunte et al. (1982). Chronic paroxysmal hemicrania. 6. Precipitation of attacks. Further studies on the precipitation mechanism. *Cephalalgia* 2:211–214.

Sjaastad, O., C. Saunte, and J.R. Graham (1984). Chronic paroxysmal hemicrania. VII. Mechanical precipitation of attacks. New cases and localization of trigger points. *Cephalalgia* 4:113–118.

Sjaastad, O., C. Saunte, D. Russell et al. (1981). Cluster headache. The sweating pattern during spontaneous attacks. *Cephalalgia* 1:233–244.

Sjaastad, O., C. Saunte, R. Salvesen et al. (1989). Short-lasting unilateral neuralgiform headache attacks with conjunctival injection, tearing, sweating, and rhinorrhea. *Cephalalgia* 9:147–156.

Sjaastad, O. and J.M. Shen (1991). Cluster headache. Our current concepts. *Acta Neurol.* 13:500–505.

Sjaastad, O., L.J. Stovner, A. Stolt-Nielsen et al. (1995). CPH and hemicrania continua: Requirements of high indomethacin dosages—an ominous sign? *Headache* 35:363–367.

Spierings, E.L. (1988). The chronic paroxysmal hemicrania concept expanded. *Headache* 28:597–598.

Spierings, E.L. (1992). Episodic and chronic paroxysmal hemicrania. *Clin. J. Pain* 8:44–48.

Stein, H.J. and A.Z. Rogado (1980). Headache rounds. Chronic paroxysmal hemicrania: Two new patients. *Headache* 20:72–76.

Tehindrazanarivelo, A.D., J.M. Visy, and M.G. Bousser (1992). Ipsilateral cluster headache and chronic paroxysmal hemicrania: Two case reports. *Cephalalgia* 12:318–320.

Vijayan, N. (1992). Symptomatic chronic paroxysmal hemicrania. *Cephalalgia* 12:111–113.

Warner, J.S., A.W. Wanul, and M.J. McLean (1994). Acetazolamide for the treatment of chronic paroxysmal hemicrania. *Headache* 34:597–599.

Zhao, J.M. and O. Sjaastad (1993). SUNCT syndrome: VIII. Pupillary reaction and corneal sensitivity. *Funct. Neurol.* 8:409–414.

Zukerman, E., M.F.P. Peres, A.O. Kaup et al. (2000). Chronic paroxysmal hemicrania-tic syndrome. *Neurology* 54:1524–1526.

Diagnosis and Treatment of Secondary Headache Disorders

Headaches Associated with Head Trauma

WILLIAM B. YOUNG
RUSSELL C. PACKARD
NABIH RAMADAN

Post-traumatic headache (PTH) is a new headache that follows a blunt or open injury to the head or brain (Headache Classification Committee of the International Headache Society, 1988). *Post-traumatic* (or *postconcussion) syndrome* is a constellation of symptoms that may follow a mild to moderate closed head injury. Symptoms of postconcussion syndrome include headache, depression, irritability, memory impairment, alcohol intolerance, dizziness or vertigo, attention and concentration difficulties, and loss of libido.

DEFINITIONS

Headache is a symptom that may occur after injury to the head, neck, or brain. Minor head injury and minor traumatic brain injury are difficult to define compared with moderate or severe injury, in which structural damage is evident. Recent definitions have used the Glasgow Coma Scale (Table 14–1) (Teasdale and Jennett, 1984) to determine the severity of a traumatic brain injury. Minor head injury was defined by Rimel (1981). His criteria for minor head injury required (1) a period of unconsciousness lasting less than 20 minutes, (2) a Glasgow Coma Scale score of 14 or

greater without subsequent deterioration, and (3) post-traumatic amnesia lasting less than 48 hours. More recently, the American Congress of Rehabilitation Medicine (1993) defined minor traumatic brain injury as "a traumatically induced physiological disruption of brain function" with at least one of the following: (1) any period of loss of consciousness; (2) any memory loss for events just before or after the accident; (3) any alteration in mental state at the time of the accident, and (4) focal neurologic deficits that may or may not be transient (Packard, 1999). The injury should not result in a loss of consciousness of greater than 30 minutes, an initial Glascow Coma Scale score of less than 13 (after 30 minutes), or post-traumatic amnesia exceeding 24 hours (American Congress of Rehabilitation Medicine, 1993).

Concussion has also been variously defined. For many years a concussion was considered to be a brief, reversible brain injury with transient loss of consciousness. We now know that loss of consciousness is not required (Rizzo and Tranel, 1996; Evans, 1996). In this chapter, we consider concussion to be a minor traumatic brain injury. These definitions are evolving. Cantu (1988) defines three grades of sports concussion: (1) grade 1, no

Table 14–1 Glasgow Coma Scale

Eye opening (E)
- Spontaneous   4
- To sound   3
- To pain   2
- None   1

Best motor response (M)
- Obeys   6
- Localizes   5
- Withdraws   4
- Abnormal flexion   3
- Extends   2
- None   1

Verbal response (V)
- Oriented   5
- Confused   4
- Inappropriate   3
- Incomprehensible   2
- None   1

Score equals sum (of) E + M + V and ranges between 3 and 15.

loss of consciousness and post-traumatic amnesia lasts less than 30 minutes; (2) grade 2, loss of consciousness lasts less than 5 minutes and post-traumatic amnesia lasts more than 30 minutes but less than 24 hours; (3) grade 3, prolonged loss of consciousness and prolonged post-traumatic amnesia (Packard, 1999). A recent practice parameter of the American Academy of Neurology modified the Cantu (1988) criteria in the following way: (1) grade 1, confusion with no amnesia and no loss of consciousness; (2) grade 2, confusion with amnesia and no loss of consciousness; (3) grade 3, loss of consciousness (Packard, 1999). *Concussion* is defined as a "trauma-induced alteration in mental status that may or may not involve loss of consciousness." These definitions allow a range of severity and treatment protocols to be considered when evaluating patients and athletes with concussion (Packard, 1999).

The diagnostic criteria established by the International Headache Society (IHS) (Headache Classification Committee of the International Headache Society, 1988) for acute PTH with significant head trauma or confirmatory signs include the following: (1) significance of head trauma documented by at least one of the following: (a) loss of consciousness, (b) post-traumatic amnesia lasting more than 10 minutes, (c) at least two of the following showing relevant abnormality: clinical neuro

logic examination, radiographs of skull, neuroimaging, evoked potentials, cerebrospinal fluid examination, vestibular function test, and neuropsychologic testing; (2) headache occurs less than 14 days after regaining consciousness (or after trauma if there has been no loss of consciousness); and (3) headache disappears within 8 weeks after regaining consciousness (or after trauma if there has been no loss of consciousness) (Headache Classification Committee of the International Headache Society, 1988).

The IHS diagnostic criteria for acute PTH with minor head trauma and no confirmatory signs include the following: (1) head trauma that does not satisfy criterion 1 for "significant" head trauma, as noted above; (2) headache occurring less than 14 days after injury; and (3) headache disappearing within 8 weeks after injury (Headache Classification Committee of the International Headache Society, 1988).

The IHS criteria require the headache to continue for more than 8 weeks after injury to be considered chronic PTH. The new International Classification of Diseases (ICD-10) criteria for PTH have basically adopted the IHS criteria. The IHS definitions of chronicity are variable and somewhat arbitrary. Since the majority of patients with PTH improve in the first 6 months after the injury, it has been suggested that 6 months or more should define chronicity in PTH, which would be in line with the definition of chronic pain (Packard and Ham, 1993).

EPIDEMIOLOGY

Motor vehicle accidents are the most frequent cause of head injury (42%), and men between 15 and 24 years of age are at the highest risk. Other causes of head injury include falls (23%), assaults (14%), and sports injuries (6%) (Kraus et al., 1994). Jennett and Frankowski (1990) found similar figures: motor vehicle accidents, 45%; falls, 30%; and occupational and recreational accidents, 20%. Many of these patients suffer from post-traumatic syndrome and have additional somatic and neuropsychologic symptoms. Since many patients with mild head injuries who subsequently develop PTH are never hospitalized, it is difficult to estimate the true burden of the disorder. Patients with mild head injury, defined as a Glasgow Coma Scale score of 13 to 15 (Table 14–1), are hospitalized at a rate of approximately 200/100,000 each year (Kraus et al., 1994). Post-traumatic headache develops in 30% to 80% of these patients (Evans, 1992; Raskin, 1988; Brenner and Friedman, 1944; Elkind, 1992; Speed, 1987). Of patients who have postconcussion symptoms, 79% to 90% also have headache (Gfeller et al., 1994; Rimel et al., 1981).

The term "whiplash" refers to the sequence of extension, flexion, and lateral motions of the neck that follows impact, with or without direct trauma to the head. Ninety-seven percent of patients who seek help from a physician after whiplash have headaches (Machado et al., 1988). The symptomatology that follows whiplash is remarkably similar to that experienced by patients following head injury. In addition to neck pain, headaches, dizziness, paresthesias, and cognitive and psychologic sequelae are extremely common. Since whiplash injuries usually do not lead to hospitalization, its incidence is even more difficult to calculate than that of head injury or PTH; however, it has been estimated to be approximately one million cases per year in the United States (O'Neill et al., 1972; Foreman and Croft, 1995).

Table 14–2 Sequelae of mild head injury

Headaches
- Tension-type
- Migraine
- Cluster
- Low cerebrospinal pressure
- Occipital neuralgia
- Idiopathic intracranial hypotension
- Supraorbital and infraorbital neuralgia
- Cervicogenic
- Temporomandibular joint syndrome or dysfunction
- Local neuroma
- Mixed

Cranial nerve symptoms and signs
- Dizziness
- Vertigo
- Tinnitus
- Hearing loss
- Blurred vision
- Diplopia
- Convergence insufficiency
- Light and noise sensitivity
- Diminished taste and smell

Psychologic and somatic complaints
- Irritability
- Anxiety
- Depression
- Personality change
- Fatigue
- Sleep disturbance
- Decreased libido
- Decreased appetite

Rare sequelae
- Subdural and epidural hematoma
- Seizures
- Transient global amnesia
- Tremor
- Dystonia

Other
  Seizure-like spells

CLINICAL FEATURES

Symptoms of post-traumatic syndrome (Table 14–2) may develop immediately or be delayed (or not initially recognized) following trauma. Head, neck, and shoulder pain usually begins within 24 to 48 hours of the injury, while local occipital tenderness occurs immediately. Neuralgic symptoms can develop in the frontal or occipital region months after the injury. The IHS criteria for PTH (Table 14–3) require headache onset within 2 weeks of head injury or of regaining consciousness. However, in clinical practice, it is often difficult to determine when the headache actually started since head pain may be mild and

other pains (particularly neck pain) more prominent. Furthermore, patients may develop chronic headaches as long as 24 months after the trauma. These late-onset headaches are similar clinically to chronic PTH. Brenner and Friedman (1944) found that 6% of patients who had mild head injury had headaches that began within 16 months after discharge, while Cartlidge and Shaw (1981) found that 12% had late-acquired headache, at both 6 and 24 months after discharge. These late-onset headaches (which do not meet IHS criteria for PTH) are more prevalent than would be expected by chance. Why these headaches begin late is uncertain. Their relationship to the preceding injury is highly controversial and difficult to establish with

Table 14–3 Acute and chronic post-traumatic headache

5.1.1 With significant head trauma and/or confirmatory signs
Diagnostic criteria
   A. Significance of head trauma documented by at least 1 of the following:
      1. Loss of consciousness
      2. Post-traumatic amnesia lasting more than 10 minutes
      3. At least 2 of the following exhibit relevant abnormality: clinical neurologic examination, x-ray of skull,
         neuroimaging, evoked potentials, spinal fluid examination, vestibular function test, neuropsychologic
         testing
   B. Headache occurs less than 14 days after regaining consciousness (or after trauma if there has been no loss
      of consciousness)
   C. Headache disappears within 8 weeks after regaining consciousness (or after trauma if there has been no
      loss of consciousness), acute, or continues more than 8 weeks (chronic)

5.1.2 With minor head trauma and no confirmatory signs
Diagnostic criteria
   A. Head trauma that does not satisfy 5.1.1A
   B. Headache occurs less than 14 days after injury
   C. Headache disappears within 8 weeks after injury

Reproduced with permission from Headache Classification Committee of the International Headache Society (1988). Classification and diagnostic criteria for headache disorders, cranial neuralgia, and facial pain. *Cephalalgia* 8:1–96.

certainty. Some late-onset headaches may be due to a traumatically lowered headache susceptibility that is not manifest until other factors ultimately push the patient over a headache threshold. The IHS criteria that state that PTH must begin within 2 weeks following injury or regaining consciousness may not have physiologic validity but, instead, may represent an arbitrary compromise to establish causality for disability, compensation, litigation, and insurance purposes.

A variety of pain patterns that resemble the primary headache disorders may develop after head injury (Table 14–2). The most frequently seen pattern resembles tension-type headache (TTH) and occurs in 85% of patients. It is characterized by generalized, persistent, bilateral, mild to moderate pain (Mandel, 1989). The headaches may be exacerbated by very mild physical or mental activity (Kelly, 1988). In one study (De-Benedittis and DeSantis, 1983), headaches were mild in 30% of patients, moderate in 52%, and severe in 18% and the pain was occipital in 51% of patients, frontal in 44%, and generalized in 11% of patients. The studies do not make clear the frequency of the headaches, their tempo, and their associated symptoms. Haas (1995) used the IHS criteria for primary headache disorders to categorize 30 PTH patients. Eight patients' headaches were classified as migraine, 12 as chronic

TTH, two as analgesic-abuse headache, seven as "probable analgesic-abuse headache," and one was unclassifiable.

An otherwise typical migraine with or without aura may be triggered by impact (Haas and Lourie, 1988). Alternatively, a pattern of recurring migraine-like headaches may begin some time after a head injury (Evans, 1992; Mandel, 1989; Packard and Ham, 1996; Binder, 1986; Winston, 1987). In one study (Weiss et al., 1991), 35 patients (27 women and 8 men) had newly acquired migraine with or without aura, beginning within a few days of mild head injury or whiplash injury. Most patients experienced two or three attacks per week. Amitriptyline or propranolol was dramatically effective in 71% of patients. Some patients have PTH with features of migraine and TTH that closely resembles chronic (transformed) migraine (Saper, 1983).

Neuralgic pain that occurs in the frontal or occipitocervical region may be associated with other headache types. Cluster headache-like syndrome has been found in up to 10% of patients (Evans, 1992; Mandel, 1989; Saper, 1983; Gfeller et al., 1994). These headaches may not undergo remissions. Packard and Ham (1996) found them to be quite rare.

The symptoms of post-traumatic syndrome may be unreported. Only 59% of patients who were hospitalized with head injury complained spontaneously of headache; the rest required prompting or direct questioning. At 6 months, only 33% of patients with headache after head injury volunteered this information. Similar percentages of spontaneous complaints of dizziness were noted, while the percentages of patients reporting symptoms of depression, anxiety, and irritability were much smaller (Cartlidge and Shaw, 1981).

In the past, PTH was considered acute if it lasted less than 2 months and chronic if it lasted more than 2 months (Table 14–3). Packard and Ham (1993) suggested that PTH that persists for more than 6 months should be considered chronic since improvement is less likely to occur after this time.

RARE TYPES OF POST-TRAUMATIC HEADACHE

A cerebrospinal fluid (CSF) leak through a dural root sleeve tear or a cribriform plate fracture may cause orthostatic headache. Idiopathic intracranial hypertension (pseudotumor) with and without papilledema has been reported as a consequence of head injury (Silberstein and Marcelis, 1990).

Dysautonomic cephalalgia, a rare type of PTH that occurs following injury to the anterior area of the carotid sheath, was described by Vijayan (1977). This severe, unilateral headache is localized to the frontotemporal area and is associated with ipsilateral pupillary dilation and increased facial sweating.

Temporomandibular joint injury may occur in conjunction with mild head injury. Symptoms include jaw pain with mastication or prolonged talking, incomplete jaw opening, clicking or lateral movements (which by themselves are not clinically relevant), and pain on palpation of the jaw joint or the muscles of mastication. Many experts believe that actual temporomandibular joint injury at the time of head injury or whiplash injury is rare. Temporomandibular joint dysfunction is thought to be a trigger for headache.

Trauma may also cause a fracture of the styloid process and symptoms that resemble Eagle's syndrome: unilateral pain in the throat or neck or referred pain in the shoulder, chest, tongue, eye, cheek, temporomandibular joint, or ear. The pain is usually dull and continuous, but it may be neuralgic. There may be a foreign body sensation in the throat. Symptoms of carotid artery insufficiency may also occur. The fracture should be visualized radiographically (Montalbetti et al., 1995; Wong et al., 1995).

NONHEADACHE SYMPTOMS

Most patients who have post-traumatic syndrome have impaired memory and difficulty concentrating (Rimel et al., 1981). A survey of high school and university students demonstrated that those with self-reported head injury had more cognitive and emotional symptoms than those without such injury (Segalowitz and Lawson, 1995). Some patients have neurocognitive deficits and an inability to process information (Gronwall and Wrightson, 1974). Many have difficulty processing different stimuli simultaneously and appear absentminded because they must devote full concentration to the task at hand. If the information processing capacity is overtaxed, the patient will appear forgetful (Andrasik and Wincze, 1994). Patients with head injury often appear distracted due to their inability to disregard irrelevant stimuli. Other frequently reported symptoms include anger, depression, and personality changes. Irritability, which may be immediate or delayed, is commonly reported after traumatic brain injury (Kim et al., 1999). Constitutional abnormalities include changes in appetite, alterations in sexual drive, weight loss or gain, and menstrual irregularities. Patients may meet the criteria for post-traumatic stress disorder (Hickling et al., 1992) (Table 14–4) with uncertain frequency (Sbordone and Liter, 1995; Jensen and Nielson, 1990b). Post-traumatic stress disorder often requires aggressive intervention (Sbordone and Liter, 1995).

Nonspecific dizziness and episodic and positional vertigo are common among patients with post-traumatic syndrome (Lidvall et al., 1974). Sleep disturbances, including insomnia and daytime drowsiness, are frequent. Nonrestorative sleep and hypersomnolence are

Table 14–4 Post-traumatic Stress Disorder

- Person exposed to traumatic event
- Traumatic event persistently re-experienced
- Persistent avoidance of stimuli associated with trauma and numbing of general responsiveness
- Persistent symptoms of increased arousal
- Duration of the disturbance is more than 1 month
- Disturbance causes clinically significant distress or impairment in social, occupational, or other important areas of functioning

From *American Psychiatric Association: Diagnostic and Statistical Manual of Mental Disorders, 4th edition.* Washington, D.C., American Psychiatric Association, 1994.

common complaints, with polysomnographic studies showing increased fragmentation of nocturnal sleep (Prigatano et al., 1982). Seizure-like events may occur, although few events appear to be epileptic and the electroencephalograph is usually normal. Nonspecific staring episodes, nonvestibular dizziness, and periodic loss of consciousness have been reported. Epilepsy or true syncope is rare. Narcolepsy- or cataplexy-like spells, episodic disorientation, and fugue-like states can occur (Silberstein et al., 1995; Lankford et al., 1994). The attacks are more common when there has been a loss of consciousness at the time of the initial injury (Lake et al., 1995).

CONTROVERSIES SURROUNDING THE DIAGNOSIS OF POST-TRAUMATIC HEADACHE AND POST-TRAUMATIC SYNDROME

Patients with post-traumatic syndrome are often told, either by physicians, insurers, or employers, that they are embellishing or malingering, that they have a primary psychiatric disorder, or that their condition is not related to their injury. This belief is not substantiated, however, since (1) patients with chronic PTH rarely engage in such behavior, (2) the presence of litigation does not appear to influence outcome, (3) patients are not cured by a verdict (Rimel et al., 1981; Mendelson, 1982; Packard, 1992), and (4) symptoms of litigants are similar to those of nonlitigants (Davis and Luxon, 1995). Nonetheless, physicians are often placed in a position of justifying an accurate diagnosis of post-traumatic syndrome.

Miller (1961b) published a series of lectures in the *British Medical Journal* in which he ascribed chronic post-traumatic syndrome to a desire for compensation or a desire not to work. These arguments continue to be used today, to the detriment of the patient. Lidvall et al. (1974), however, conducted a prospective study that demonstrated that poor work adjustment did not predict post-traumatic syndrome but that patients with post-traumatic syndrome subsequently demonstrated poor work adjustment.

Arguing for nonorganicity, Mittenberg et al. (1992) demonstrated that a control population identified the symptoms of post-traumatic syndrome from a checklist in a similar manner to patients who complained of post-traumatic syndrome. He concluded that the symptoms of post-traumatic syndrome are due to the fact that patients expect to experience these symptoms. He suggested that education and reassurance of a favorable prognosis are adequate treatments and that some patients should be treated for anxiety. The findings of Mittenberg et al. (1992) suggest that post-traumatic syndrome is a common syndrome with which most people are familiar, perhaps because they have experienced the symptoms following a minimal concussion or because they have heard about head injuries in sports figures. The crux of post-traumatic syndrome may be the organic magnification or persistence of symptoms commonly experienced by normal individuals, thus accounting for the easy recognizability of these symptoms by controls.

The fact that sports injuries rarely cause post-traumatic syndrome leads to the suggestion that post-traumatic syndrome occurs because of the opportunity for gain. However, the velocities and forces experienced during most sports injuries are much less than those that result from motor vehicle accidents and falls, which are the injuries that commonly cause post-traumatic syndrome. In sports injuries, the head is often fixed, whereas in automobile accidents the head is freely mobile, which results in more severe damage.

Similarly, the observation that seemingly trivial injuries can cause severe disability has led some to conclude that the disability does not have a physiologic basis. There are other disease states in which minor injuries cause severe pain. For example, incomplete peripheral nerve injuries are often excruciatingly painful, whereas nerve transections are usually painless. In some cases, a skull fracture may dissipate the energy of impact and protect the brain from an injury that could lead to post-traumatic syndrome, producing fewer symptoms in a population that superficially appears more injured.

One of the arguments used against the organicity of post-traumatic syndrome is that patients do not have abnormal study results and there are no abnormal signs on examination. "Failure to understand the problem is no proof of psychogenicity" (Strauss and Savitsky, 1934). Many neurologic diseases, such as migraine with aura, have no abnormal signs on examination. Several paraclinical studies show group differences between uninjured mild head injury patients without chronic post-traumatic syndrome and post-traumatic syndrome patients (see below). They do not yet have the sensitivity to distinguish individuals with "organic" PTH from those with psychological or other causes of PTH.

Work factors have been hypothesized to cause prolonged disability. Miller (1961a,b) stated that unskilled workers and less intelligent persons suffer more prolonged disability due to post-traumatic syndrome. The group studied consisted of patients sent by an insurance company; hence, a significant referral bias is likely. Furthermore, jobs that require certain cognitive skills are particularly difficult for patients suffering from post-traumatic syndrome. Laborers whose jobs depend on sustained physical effort and mental vigilance have particular difficulty performing their jobs, whereas patients whose jobs allow more flexibility and do not require physical activity may be better able to cope with the disability. Another author observed that patients who blamed their employer as a large impersonal body had more symptoms than those who did not. This has been attributed to be "clear evidence of nervous and emotional factors at work in the production of symptoms" (Rutherford et al., 1977). The other possibility, that patients who are anxious, depressed, and ir-

ritable and have more symptoms due to their post-traumatic syndrome are more likely to blame others, was not addressed.

Some physicians argue that a patient who has psychiatric symptoms has an illness that does not have an organic cause. Many kinds of brain injury, including stroke and neurodegenerative disease, produce psychiatric symptoms. Chronic pain by itself can induce depression and abnormal behavior; this does not mean that organic pathology does not exist. Having a disabling illness that is not accepted by medical professionals, employers, and family is a legitimate cause of anxiety, depression, and abnormal behaviors.

A recent study (Obelieniene et al., 1998) of Lithuanian automobile accident victims failed to show an increased incidence of headache or neck pain years after injury. This finding was attributed to the fact that insurance was not available to compensate Lithuanian accident victims for lost work and to the general lack of recognition of postconcussion headache/postconcussion syndrome in the community. The methodology behind this study has been criticized. In contrast to Lithuania, postconcussion headache/postconcussion syndrome is recognized across many cultures in the Americas, Europe, and East Asia.

RISK FACTORS

Age, gender, and certain mechanical factors are risks for a poor outcome after head injury or whiplash injury. Compared to men, women have a 1.9-fold increased risk of PTH (Jensen et al., 1990a) and post-traumatic syndrome (Fenton, 1996). Increasing age is associated with a less rapid and less complete recovery (Cartlidge and Shaw, 1981; Bohnen et al., 1992; McClelland et al., 1994; Fenton, 1996). One study found that children under 15 years of age may develop acute, but not chronic, PTH (Keshavan et al., 1981). Jensen and Nielson (1990), however, found that the risk of PTH did not vary with age. Mechanical factors, in addition to the force of impact, are important. If the head is rotated, increased stress is put on the cervical structures and more rotational forces are applied to the brain; thus, PTH is more likely if the head is inclined or rotated prior to impact. A rear-end collision and an unprepared occupant are other factors that increase the likelihood of post-traumatic syndrome (Mendelson, 1982).

The relationship between the severity of the injury and the severity of post-traumatic syndrome has not been conclusively established. In general, the persistence of headache does not correlate with the duration of unconsciousness or the presence of post-traumatic amnesia, skull fracture, electroencephalographic (EEG) abnormalities, or bloody CSF (DeBenedittis and DeSantis, 1983; Lidvall et al., 1974). Yamaguchi (1992) found an inverse relationship between the severity of the injury and the severity of the PTH. Since this study included patients with both moderate and severe head injury, this finding may not apply within the mild head injury group (Yamaguchi, 1992). In one study, the initially hospitalized mild head injury patients had similar symptoms to patients who were discharged from the emergency room. However, *hospitalized* patients recovered more quickly. These findings could support the concept that more severe mild head injury causes less PTH and post-traumatic syndrome, although other explanations are possible (Barrett et al., 1994). Similarly, Wilkinson and Gilchrist (1980) found that severe head injury may, in fact, reduce the incidence of PTH.

Another study found that patients who had lost consciousness had more depression and anger-control problems than patients who did not lose consciousness (Lake et al., 1995). The fact that diplopia, anosmia, and the presence of central nervous system abnormality at 24 hours correlate with the persistence of symptoms 6 weeks after injury suggests that a subset of patients with more severe injury have worse outcomes (Rutherford, 1989). This difference suggests that more research using prospectively followed, stratified patient samples is needed before definitive conclusions can be reached.

Radanov et al. (1995) studied patients 7 days and again 2 years after whiplash injury. Patients who had high multiple-symptom scores shortly after their injury had a significantly greater chance of having symptoms 2 years after the injury. Patients who were still disabled 2 years after their injury had higher multiple-symptom scores at the initial examination compared with patients who were symptomatic but not disabled after 2 years. Radanov et al. (1995) believe that patients with more severe injuries have higher initial-symptom scores and worse outcomes. Alternatively, individual vulnerability could lead to a greater number of initial symptoms and a poorer long-term outcome, regardless of the severity of the initial injury.

There has been speculation that a history of prior headache increases the risk for PTH. Pretraumatic migraine was not a risk factor for developing PTH after hospitalization for cerebral concussion (Jensen and Nielson, 1990; Lidvall et al., 1974). These studies suffered from recall bias since the patients were interviewed 9 to 12 months after the injury. Weiss et al. (1991) reported that 31% of patients who developed migraine-like attacks following mild head or neck trauma had a history of migraine in first-degree relatives. The authors suggested that head or neck trauma triggers the migraine process in susceptible individuals. In another study, in which patients were interviewed immediately following whiplash injury, pretraumatic headache was a significant risk factor for developing PTH (Radanov et al., 1995). Early headache, occurring within 24 hours of injury, is a strong risk factor for post-traumatic syndrome at 6 weeks (Wilkinson and Gilchrist, 1980).

Lidvall et al. (1974) found that while lack of education was not a risk factor for acute post-traumatic syndrome, unskilled laborers were more likely to develop symptoms. Likewise, socioeconomic status may predict employment 3 months after minor head injury. Business managers and executives in the study of Rimel et al. (1981) were employed 3 months after injury, but only 57% of the unskilled laborers were still employed. Higher education also predicted continued employment. These studies do not differentiate between the premorbid effect of lack of education, poor motivation to return to a menial job, poor resources to adjust to the effects of the injury, or employer intolerance (Rimel et al., 1981).

Pre-existing psychopathology may influence the clinical evolution of post-traumatic syndrome. Ross and McNaughton (1944) found that patients with localized PTH did not have pre-existing psychopathology, whereas those with "bizarre" generalized or bilateral headaches had prior "unstable personalities." In another study, patients were assessed for premorbid psychopathology by interviewing them and their relatives within 1 month of head injury. The patient's psychologic state prior to the injury correlated with the subjective symptomatology. However, physical and social dysfunction correlated with the severity of the injury, not with pre-existing factors (Keshavan et al., 1981). In another study, patients with pretraumatic emotional problems had higher scores on scales of cognitive and emotional-vegetative dysfunction after mild head injury (Bohnen et al., 1992). Disability was not measured. These studies suggested that pre-existing psychopathology influenced how symptoms are reported rather than impacting on disability.

Three studies do not support these conclusions. McClelland et al. (1994) found no difference in premorbid personality adjustment between chronic post-traumatic syndrome sufferers and patients whose symptoms resolved. Likewise, Lidvall et al. (1974) found no differences in pretraumatic neuroticism or adjustment to work between similarly injured patients who developed post-traumatic syndrome and those who did not. Fenton (1996) found no differences between premorbid social adjustment, life events, and chronicity of symptoms. These studies have methodologic problems: their psychologic assessments were retrospective, and the methods used to ascertain pre-existing psychopathology were often not well described.

Using the Freiburg Personality Inventory, Radanov et al. (1995) assessed patients shortly after whiplash injury. Scores on the nervousness, depression, openness, neuroticism, and masculinity scales did not correlate with outcome 2 years after injury. In contrast, poor well-being scale scores correlated with the persistence of symptoms but not with disability among patients who were symptomatic 2 years after injury (Sturzenegger, 1991).

PATHOPHYSIOLOGY

Post-traumatic syndrome is probably not a single pathologic entity but a group of traumatically induced disorders with overlapping symptoms. The cognitive, sleep, and psychologic deficits of these patients are manifestations of brain injury. Headache is mainly a manifestation of brain dysfunction, with occasional contributions from persistent musculoskeletal injuries.

Neck, jaw, and scalp tissue injuries may contribute to acute PTH; pain originating from these areas can be referred to the head. Most of these injuries heal completely and cannot, by themselves, account for chronic PTH or the associated neurocognitive symptoms of PTH. However, soft tissue or skeletal injuries may initiate or trigger a transformation process in headache-prone patients similar to the process by which daily intermittent migraine or TTH evolves into chronic daily headache. Postconcussion headache patients have more upper cervical segment joint dysfunction, less endurance of neck flexor muscle, and a higher incidence of moderately tight neck musculature, yet the neck range of motion is normal (Treleaven et al., 1994). These findings could be due to adaptive, and sometimes maladaptive, phenotypic central nervous system changes similar to the phenomenon of central sensitization that is observed in experimental models of chronic pain. One model, based on the kindling phenomenon in experimental epilepsy (Post and Silberstein, 1994), could explain the evolution of peripheral injuries into chronic centrally maintained pain. Nerve or musculoskeletal injuries could induce wind-up and sensitization, which could ultimately result in permanently altered neuronal function. Because these changes occur postsynaptically as well as presynaptically, neuronal function may be altered at distant brain sites involved in the production or experience of pain (Post and Silberstein, 1994).

As a result of head injury or whiplash, shear forces are applied to the brain; this can result in diffuse axonal injury that can be elicited histologically. In experimental models, direct impact is not necessary to produce significant diffuse axonal injury (Gennarelli, 1993). Diffuse axonal injury is most common in the corpus callosum, internal capsule, fornices, dorsolateral midbrain, and pons (Blumbergs et al., 1989). Gennarelli et al. (1975) suggested that there is a continuum of diffuse axonal injury that varies from functional abnormalities alone to structural lesions that become increasingly severe and result in widespread injury. Immunohistochemical studies demonstrate similar, although less severe, histologic findings in the rat fluid percussion model in mild head injury compared with moderate head injury. These changes are delayed in mild injury (Saatman et al., 1998). The relevance and extent of diffuse axonal injury in human mild head injury is not fully elucidated. One report indicates that diffuse axonal injury occurs in concussive mild head injury (Blumbergs et al., 1994).

Because of unsynchronized rotations that may develop between the cerebral hemispheres and the cerebellum (Elson and Ward, 1994), axons in the upper brain stem may be particularly vulnerable to diffuse axonal injury. Evidence of brain-stem vulnerability in humans comes from a demonstration of midbrain hemorrhage on magnetic resonance imaging (MRI) in a patient with mild head injury (Servadei et al., 1994). Brain-stem axons that are sheared in diffuse axonal injury are responsible for control of arousal, vigilance, and sleep (Goodman, 1994). Serotonergic and adrenergic projection fibers are postulated to play a central role in pain modulation (Weiller et al., 1995); when both are injured, head pain results. Reactive *synaptogenesis*, a process of axonal sprouting that restores synaptic contact on denuded dendrites, has been demonstrated in at least one model of head injury (Erb and Povlishock, 1991). This could account for both physiologic improvement through appropriate healing and new or worsening symptoms as aberrant connections are made. Evidence for synaptogenesis in human head injury is awaited.

Head injury usually involves a combination of translational and rotational forces. Restricted rotation makes it more difficult to produce a concussion in animals (Elson and Ward, 1994). Rotational forces occur even

when movement is primarily translational (see below). In studies using windows in cadaver skulls, the brain has been demonstrated to lag behind the skull, due to inertia, when the head is accelerated. As a result of the translational force, the brain is compressed near the point of impact, while negative pressures develop opposite to the site of impact.

Experimental models of head injury have advanced several observations. The angular acceleration model, using subhuman primates, demonstrates axonal changes in the brain stem (Jane et al., 1985) similar to the human autopsy cases of minor head injury (Povlishock and Coburn, 1989). In this model, diffuse axonal injury is a major finding of severe head injury and is probably the cause of coma (Gennarelli et al., 1975). In the cat fluid percussion model of experimental brain injury, a hydraulic pressure pulse, lasting milliseconds, creates a physiologic response similar to that seen in human moderate or mild head injury. Based on microscopic changes observed after this type of head injury, Povlishock and Coburn (1989) speculated that stretching or compression, not shearing, is the cause of axonal injury in this model and possibly in human head injury. Finally, a fluid percussion pulse injury in rats causes loss of cholinergic neurons in the forebrain but not in the brain stem (Schmidt and Grady, 1995). The relevance of these findings to human head injury is unknown.

Finite element modeling is a computerized structural analysis technique used to study the effect of various acceleration forces on the brain. By introducing an adjustment for brain tissue compressibility, Ward and Nahum (1979) created a model that fits with the experimental data. Finite element modeling has shown that rotational brain movements occur even when the motion of the head is primarily translational. It has also shown that various brain compartments have different rotations (Fig. 14–1). Shear stress in the brain stem is influenced by a number of factors, including pressure release at the foramen magnum, motion of the medulla due to neck motion, the influence of individually rotating cerebral hemispheres and the cerebellum, the proximity of the brain stem to the

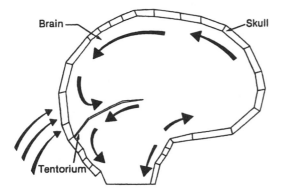

Figure 14–1 Brain motion. From Ward, C. (1981). *Status of Head Injury Modeling. Head and Neck Injury Criteria*, U.S. Department of Transportation, Washington, D.C.

skull, and restraint provided by the tentorium (Elson and Ward, 1994; Ward, 1982).

Ischemic brain injury is common following severe head injury (Goodman, 1994). Posttraumatic vasospasm, which can occur in moderate or severe head injury, correlates with a lower Glasgow Coma Scale score (Zubkov et al., 1999). Abnormal cerebrovascular autoregulation may also occur (Junger et al., 1997). Forty-eight hours after minor head injury, 28% of patients and no controls had poorly functioning or absent autoregulation. There was no correlation with the Glasgow Coma Scale score. Since long-term clinical

outcomes were not studied, the role of this observation in chronic PTH or post-traumatic syndrome is unknown.

A series of neurochemical changes occur with experimental head injury (Table 14–5) (Packard and Ham, 1997). The relevance of these alternatives to human head injury and the role of such changes in the evolution of post-traumatic syndrome are unknown. However, an altered chemical or electrical environment could account for immediate-impact headache or aura. It could result in cellular injury and in post-traumatic syndrome. The similarity between the biochemical changes of migraine headaches and those seen after head injury suggest a shared physiology and possibly a role for similar treatment strategies (Packard, 1999).

The effectiveness of treatments such as repetitive intravenous dihydroergotamine (IV DHE) in PTH suggests a similar or shared mechanism with the primary headache disorders. This could be due to a "final common pathway" of symptom expression, perhaps with central serotonergic dysfunction and trigeminovascular activation (McBeath and Nanda, 1994; Young et al., 1994).

Many authors uphold the "psychogenesis" of chronic PTH and post-traumatic syndrome, but few point out specific mechanisms to account for it. Duckro et al. (1995) used a "path analysis," a directional multiple

Table 14–5 Comparison of biochemical changes in mild head injury and migraine headache

Mild head injury	Migraine
Increased extracellular K^+ and intracellular Na^+, Ca^{2+} and Cl^-	Increased extracellular K^+ and intracellular Na^+, Ca^{2+} and Cl^-
Excessive release of EAAs (primarily glutamate)	Excessive release of EAAs (glutamate and aspartate)
Accumulation of platelet-derived 5-HT in CNS	Excessive firing of dorsal raphe leads to increased 5-HT release and depletion of available 5-HT pool
Increased levels of endogenous opioids (findings mixed)	β-Endorphin content may be reduced in headache-free periods; high met-enkephalin levels during attacks
Decline in intracellular and total brain Mg	Deficiency of Mg levels between and during attacks
Influx of extracellular Ca^{2+} in compromised axolemmas	Increase in intracellular Ca^{2+}/Mg^{2+} ratio
Nitric oxide may be converted to free oxygen radical, potentially leading to tissue injury	Nitric oxide may be involved in migraine pathogenesis; at the vascular endothelium, it is a potent vasodilator; in the spinal cord, it is pronociceptive

Key to abbreviations: EAA, excitatory amino acid; 5-HT, 5-hydroxytryptamine; CNS, central nervous system.

regression analysis, to examine the relationship between post-traumatic pain, disability, depression, and anger. They concluded that depression might cause disability and that expressed and unexpressed anger contribute to depression. However, this statistical technique cannot prove causal relationship, and other explanations for the correlation between depression and disability could be equally valid.

Kelly (1988) posits that nonvalidation of cognitive and physically painful symptoms by medical, legal, and employment authorities leads to an anxiety/depressive reaction that results in the persistence of originally organic symptoms. He relies on the now outdated concept that emotional tension is a principal cause of persistent headache. Recent positron emission tomographic (PET) scan studies have shown a neurobiologic basis for many "psychologic" phenomena, including anxiety, pain, and even hallucinations.

It is likely that at least two processes occur in patients with PTH or post-traumatic syndrome. The first is likely due to diffuse axonal injury and correlates with the acceleration/deceleration forces. When more severe, it is associated with abnormalities on MRI, PET, single photon emission computed tomography, and certain neuropsychologic tests. A challenge to this hypothesis is the observation that patients with severe closed head injury do not report as many symptoms as those with less severe injuries. It could be argued, however, that symptoms of post-traumatic syndrome and PTH are only masked by co-existing illnesses and manifestations of the sequelae of severe head injury. Clinical improvement of diffuse axonal injury may occur over several months, with normalization or amelioration of radiologic tests. Also, neuropsychologic testing may indicate full recovery, but tests for attention may still be abnormal. A second process may be responsible for many of the symptoms that persist after minor head injury. A pre-existing vulnerability may be necessary for the chronic post-traumatic symptoms to manifest since pre-existing headache is a risk factor in some patients. A mechanism similar to the kindling model of epilepsy or, perhaps, aberrant con-nections made by injured axons may underlie this mechanism and explain most of the symptoms of chronic post-traumatic syndrome and PTH. Additional factors, perhaps psychologic, may magnify the expression of symptoms caused by the second process.

For most patients with post-traumatic syndrome, the clinical history of new-onset or changed headache after an injury associated with new cognitive, emotional, and sleep disturbances is so characteristic that, once intracranial pathology is excluded, confirmatory tests are not required before proceeding with treatment. Unfortunately, tests are often conducted for medicolegal reasons, increasing patients' anxiety and self-doubt when they are negative. Negative test results are often used to indicate no abnormality. However, no test has the specificity or sensitivity to make or exclude a diagnosis in a particular individual. Similarly, if post-traumatic syndrome is not a single entity but a syndrome derived from several pathologic processes initiated by head trauma, no single test would be expected to diagnose all patients.

TESTING

Although many studies have been performed in an attempt to establish the extent of the head injury and the diagnosis of post-traumatic syndrome, there is no test that reliably distinguishes patients with post-traumatic syndrome from normal controls or from patients with primary headache disorders.

Computed Tomography and Magnetic Resonance Imaging

Few studies have specifically evaluated brain imaging in post-traumatic syndrome. Most series have included patients with head injury who might have required neurosurgical intervention. Kelly et al. (1986) looked at a group of head injury patients and found no MRI abnormalities among the subgroup of patients with post-traumatic syndrome. Levin et al. (1987) found MRI abnormalities within several weeks of injury in 17 of 20 hospitalized patients with mild or moderate head injury. Magnetic resonance imaging was clearly superior to computed tomography (CT) at identifying these abnormalities, which were located in the white matter or at the gray–white matter junction. Levin et al. (1987, 1992) studied patients who were admitted with mild to moderate head injury and found that a reduction of the mean parenchymal lesion size occurred with the passage of time. Most of the resolutions occurred within the first month, and lesions that were present at 1 month remained at 3 months. Patients who had abnormal MRI had more cognitive deficits than patients who had normal MRI. In the absence of pathologic confirmation, one cannot be certain that these lesions represent diffuse axonal injury with resolving edema. We speculate that the MRI changes resolve with resolution of the edema when the diffuse axonal injury is less severe, whereas the changes are permanent when the diffuse axonal injury is more severe.

Mittle et al. (1994) obtained MRI on 20 consecutively hospitalized head injury patients. These studies were reviewed by two blinded readers, who concurred that diffuse axonal injury was present in 30% of patients. One radiologist diagnosed diffuse axonal injury in 20% of patients, indicating that even MRI may not always provide an unequivocal diagnosis. These MRI findings may not be characteristic of head injury patients who were not hospitalized. Nevertheless, diffuse axonal injury of lesser severity (i.e., not producing MRI abnormalities) could still be present.

There are no prospective studies that establish the value of brain imaging in patients with PTH or post-traumatic syndrome. In the acute setting, it is prudent to image all patients with mild behavioral abnormalities, abnormal findings on clinical examination, or a Glasgow Coma Scale score of less than 15 because of the risk of subsequent deterioration. With subacute or chronic post-traumatic syndrome, there is little information to guide the clinician. Neuroimaging should be guided by findings on clinical examination, the medical history, and the history of symptom evolution or resolution.

Functional Imaging

Single photon emission CT (SPECT) observes the physiologic behavior of the brain. It can contribute information about the spatial distribution of radiolabeled ligands and the time course of ligand uptake and washout. It is analyzed by CT and has been used to study head injury patients but not specifically in PTH or post-traumatic syndrome. In the acute phase of head injury, technetium-99m hexamethylpropyleneamineoxine SPECT is more useful than CT at identifying brain lesions and demonstrating abnormalities of function. It shows more lesions than CT and is helpful in predicting outcome (Abdel-Dayem et al., 1987, 1994; Reid et al., 1990). One study of 20 patients with head injury revealed technetium-99m hexamethylpropyleneamineoxine SPECT abnormalities in 60% of patients, whereas only 25% had abnormalities on CT (Gray et al., 1992). Another study examined 12 patients with mild to moderate head injury 1 to 9 years after the injury. In this study, ten patients had abnormal technetium-99m hexamethylpropyleneamineoxine SPECT, while CT was abnormal in only six (Krelina et al., 1989). Another study showed that the number of lesions on SPECT correlates with the extent of disability (Newton et al., 1992).

Abnormal sites on imaging studies include the basal ganglia and thalamus in 55.2% of patients, the frontal lobes in 23.8%, the temporal lobes in 13%, the parietal lobes in 3.7%, and the insular and occipital regions together in 4.8% (Abdel-Dayem et al., 1998). Another study has shown significant orbitofrontal hypoperfusion in 67% of patients with post-traumatic anosmia; by contrast, there were no group differences in other brain regions and individual abnormalities were infrequent (Varney and Bushnell, 1998). Anosmia may be a marker for orbitofrontal brain injury.

Masdeu et al. (1995) suggested that two types of lesion may be seen on SPECT: circumscribed areas of hypoperfusion that represent contusion and diffuse occipitotemporal hypoperfusion that represents multiple small contusions or diffuse axonal injury. The Academy of Neurology's Therapeutics and Technology Assessment Subcommittee has determined the use of SPECT for the evaluation of head trauma to be "investigational" based on class II evidence (one or more well-designed clinical studies) (American Academy of Neurology, 1996).

Using xenon-inhalation cerebral blood flow, Ramadan et al. (1995) studied the correlation between headache disability and cerebral blood flow. Both the emotional subscale score and the function subscale score of a headache disability inventory correlated with the mean asymmetry score. The same investigators reported that patients with chronic PTH have lower mean initial slope indices, significant regional interhemispheric flow differences, and more interhemispheric asymmetries compared with migraineurs and nonheadache controls (Gilkey et al., 1997). The authors concluded that the cerebral blood flow findings indicate neurovascular instability that persists months to years after the initial head injury.

Like SPECT, PET examines physiologic activity within the brain. In head trauma, PET has revealed widespread abnormalities in cerebral glucose metabolism (Alavi et al., 1987; George et al., 1989) and areas of diminished perfusion that tend to improve with clinical recovery (George et al., 1989). In one study, these areas of perfusion abnormality corresponded with areas of abnormality that had been identified by neuropsychologic testing (Rao et al., 1984).

One month after head injury, patients with minor traumatic brain injury and control subjects showed different brain activation patterns in response to increasing working memory processing loads. Patients with minor traumatic brain injury had significantly more cognitive symptoms but performed as well as controls on a neuropsychologic battery, differing only in response speed, sample reaction time, and distractability tasks of the continuous performance test. The presence of headache was not reported.

Electroencephalography

Electroencephalography is usually of little value in evaluating post-traumatic syndrome in patients with head injury. While it may be abnormal immediately after injury, it often normalizes within minutes to weeks. Persistent findings that were once considered abnormal are now considered normal variants, having the same incidence as in the general population (Schoenhuber and Gentilini, 1989).

Quantitative EEG may or may not be useful in head injury. In one small study (Hughes and Robbins, 1990), quantitative EEG showed a statistically significant increase in both slow and fast activities over the temporal region of the skull. However, the authors concluded that this test offers little benefit to the patient with PTH since there is a great deal of variability within the PTH group and these findings are common in both PTH and control patients. Another study examined the ability of power spectrum analysis to discriminate between 608 head injury patients and 108 age-matched controls and found that head injury could be discriminated from age-matched controls with more than 90% accuracy (Thatcher et al., 1989). No correlation was made between the symptoms of PTH or post-traumatic syndrome and abnormal test results. Therefore, the predictive value of this study is uncertain at this time. In general, these studies indicate that PTH patients, as a group, differ from nonheadache controls; but unlike the study of Ramadan et al. (1995), they cannot reliably differentiate an individual PTH patient from a patient with an idiopathic headache.

Magnetic Source Imaging

Magnetic source imaging combines MRI and magnetoencephalography (Lewine et al., 1999). One study showed abnormalities in 5% of a normal control group, 10% of an asymptomatic mild head injury group, and 65% of a group of patients with persistent symptoms (p < 0.01). These abnormal findings improve as the patient improves. Like the xenon cerebral blood flow studies of Ramadan et al. (1997), this study demonstrates an organic abnormality in patients with postconcussion syndrome.

Evoked Potentials and Electronystagmography

Short-latency somatosensory evoked potentials have not been shown to be of value in testing patients with head injury or post-traumatic syndrome (Bricolo and Turella, 1990). Brain-stem auditory evoked potentials have been found to be abnormal in 10% to 20% of patients with head injury and postconcussion syndrome. The more prolonged the unconsciousness, the greater the incidence of abnormalities (Schoenhuber and Gentilini, 1989). Brain-stem auditory evoked potentials can either improve or deteriorate from 2 days to 1 month after injury (Geets and Louette, 1983). Symptomatic dizziness does not correlate with brain-stem auditory evoked potential abnormalities. While the brain-stem auditory evoked potential separates groups of post-traumatic syndrome patients from groups of controls, it is of no value in distinguishing an individual with post-traumatic syndrome from one without it.

The P300 is an event-related potential manifested by a positive cortical potential that occurs after an infrequent stimulation to which the patient is attending, such as a loud sound in a train of soft sounds. It has been correlated with cognitive functions, such as memory information delivery and decision making, and decreases in amplitude with drowsiness or inattention. Studies of P300 in head injury have yielded mixed results. One study demonstrated significant abnormalities of P300 amplitude and latency in 20 head injury patients compared with 20 control subjects (Pratap-Chand et al., 1988). Werner and Vanderzant (1991) found an abnormal response in only one of 18 patients. Kobylare and colleagues (1995) found a correlation between an abnormal P300 and an abnormal MRI. An interesting study demonstrated that hearing accident-related words (i.e., "stressful") produced a significantly larger P300 than hearing neutral words in patients with mild head injury but not in non-head injury controls. The P300 amplitude difference correlated with the patient's two-way state anxiety score (Granovsky et al., 1998). The role that P300 may play in evaluating head injury is uncertain.

Electronystagmogram is abnormal in 40% to 50% of patients with head injury or "whiplash" in clinic-based studies. Toglia (1969) examined 150 patients who complained of vestibular symptoms following either head injury or whiplash injury, searching for spontaneous, latent, and positional nystagmus. Bithermal caloric tests and rotational tests were performed when possible. Abnormal caloric tests (including both canal paresis and directional preponderance) were found in 63% of whiplash patients and 68% of head injury patients. Abnormal rotatory tests were found in 9 of 16 whiplash patients (56%) and 20 of 24 head injury patients (83%). Rowe and Carlson (1980) studied 19 patients with postconcussive dizziness following head injury and found that 11 patients (58%) had abnormalities consisting of latent or positional nystagmus or calorie-induced nystagmus. None of these patients who had abnormal brain-stem auditory evoked potentials (3 standard deviations) had normal electronystagmograms. Conversely, most patients with abnormal electronystagmograms had normal brain-stem auditory evoked potentials. This suggests that the electronystagmogram may be more sensitive than the brain-stem auditory evoked potential. Mallinson and Longridge (1998) found electronystagmogram abnormalities in patients with whiplash injury and mild head injury but not in whiplash injury alone, although symptoms of dizziness were similar in both groups.

Computerized dynamic posturography was studied in a referral population of dizzy patients after whiplash injury, alone or with mild head injury. Both groups had positive findings, although the type of posturography abnormality was different between groups (Mallinson and Longridge, 1998).

Blood Testing: S-100

The S-100 is a marker of brain injury in head trauma and correlates with the Glasgow Coma Scale score on admission (Herrmann et al., 1999). In hospitalized mild head injury patients, S-100 was detectable in 28% of patients, 36% of whom had contusions on MRI. In patients with detectable S-100 levels, there was a trend toward impaired neuropsycho-logic functioning on measures of attention, memory, and information processing speed (Ingebrigtsen et al., 1999).

Neuropsychologic Testing

Neuropsychologic testing in head injury often shows marked early abnormalities that im-prove or resolve with time. These include in-formation processing, auditory vigilance, re-action time, sustained divided and distributed attention, visual and verbal memory, design fluency imagination, and analytic capacity. Ei-senberg (1989) reported that tests of design fluency and verbal memory improved and normalized over 1 to 3 months in parallel with MRI findings. The paced auditory serial addition test is a widely used test of infor-mation processing that is often abnormal shortly after head injury. Patients are pre-sented with a random series of digits at in-tervals of either 1 to 2 or 2 to 4 seconds (same interval for entire test) and are asked to add the most recently presented number to the one before. The score is expressed as the per-centage correct at each rate or as the mean correct response per second. It has been given serially over 8 weeks postinjury and demonstrates cognitive recovery to normal. Paced auditory serial addition test recovery, however, was delayed in head injury patients with post-traumatic syndrome compared with a non-post-traumatic syndrome control group (Gronwall and Wrightson, 1974).

Within 8 weeks of head injury, a test of auditory vigilance in which patients had to detect the rare instances in which the interval between elements in a string of numbers was longer than in the others showed normaliza-tion (McCarthy, 1977). However, "recovered" head injury patients performed more poorly than normal controls at simulated high alti-tude (Ewing et al., 1980), demonstrating that deficits may reappear under physiologic stress. Several measures of reaction time, which are believed to be indicators of atten-tion deficits, are also impaired in patients with head injury at various times after in-jury, although recovery was demonstrated in one study of mild head injury patients 10

years after injury compared to twin controls (Dencker and Lofving, 1958). In a test of se-lective attention devised by Gentilini et al. (1989), head injury patients were significantly slower but not less accurate than controls 3 months after injury. Tests of sustained and di-vided attention, again devised by Gentilini et al. (1989), showed significant differences from controls at 1 month but were inconclu-sive 3 months after injury. Bohnen et al. (1995) demonstrated that patients with mild head injury and post-traumatic syndrome per-formed less well on a test of sustained atten-tion than mild head injury controls (without post-traumatic syndrome) 12 to 34 months af-ter injury. Gentilini et al. (1989) demon-strated that tests of distributed attention showed deficits 1 and 3 months after head injury. The authors pointed out that the most sensitive tools for revealing cerebral dysfunc-tion test the function of the greatest number of cortical and subcortical areas simultane-ously (Gentilini et al., 1989). Only one study (Bohnen et al., 1995) has been shown to dis-tinguish PTH or post-traumatic syndrome from mild head injury alone (Gentilini et al., 1989).

Keidel et al. (1992) performed repeated neuropsychologic tests on 30 patients with post-traumatic syndrome after whiplash in-jury. Attention and concentration deficits re-covered within 6 weeks. Visual memory, imagination, and analytic capacity recovered within the next 6 weeks. Verbal memory ab-straction, cognitive selectivity, and informa-tion processing speed took more than 12 weeks to recover. These findings demonstrate a hierarchy of functional recovery occurring over a period of greater than 12 weeks after apparently mild injury.

Ham et al. (1994) studied patients with PTH and compared them with patients with chronic "combination headache" and low-back pain and with pain-free controls. Pa-tients with PTH had the highest scale eleva-tions on the Symptom Checklist 90-Revised, a brief screen for somatic and psychologic symptoms that are broken down into nine pri-mary "dimensions," or scales. Elevations were significant on all scales except the hostility and phobic anxiety scales. Patients with PTH scored significantly higher than pain-free controls on the Beck Depression Inventory but did not differ significantly from other pain groups. State anxiety, a measure of acute anxiety, was significantly higher in PTH patients than controls or those with other pain states, but trait anxiety, a measure of anxious personality structure, differed significantly only from controls. Mean headache severity was higher (but not significantly) in the PTH group than in the control headache group. These findings suggest that PTH patients exhibit more psychopathology than individuals with other headache types and normal controls. On some tests, patients with PTH had more psychopathology than patients with low-back pain. In general, these tests do not demonstrate any specific pattern to the psychopathology (Ham et al., 1994).

DIAGNOSIS

The diagnosis of PTH and post-traumatic syndrome is established by symptoms consistent with this syndrome and trauma-related onset. The IHS criteria for PTH require the headache to occur within 14 days after regaining consciousness (or after the trauma if there is no loss of consciousness). There are no IHS criteria for late-onset PTH. The IHS differentiates between acute PTH, which lasts less than 8 weeks, and chronic PTH, which lasts longer (Table 14–3). A worsening of a pre-existing headache disorder does not qualify as PTH. A substantial difference between headache features before and after injury must be present for the designation of PTH.

Other physiologic or psychologic disorders must be meticulously excluded. The differential diagnosis includes, among others, subdural or epidural hematoma, CSF hypotension, cerebral vein thrombosis, cavernous sinus thrombosis, cervical or carotid artery dissection, cerebral hemorrhage, epilepsy, and hydrocephalus.

Many patients diagnosed with post-traumatic syndrome are portrayed as malingerers or are thought to profoundly embellish their symptoms. Most experts believe this is rare.

Binder (1986) suggests that the diagnosis of malingering should be actively made by surreptitiously observing a patient performing a task he or she stated could not be accomplished. Simulators have been shown to perform worse on sensorimotor tests (Heaton et al., 1978) and memory tests (Benton and Spreen, 1961) than would be expected. Performance that is significantly worse than chance on a forced-choice memory test can be interpreted as the deliberate production of wrong answers. Binder (1990) noted that such a result may not distinguish between malingering and conversion reactions. If a patient is suspected of malingering, the clinician should actively search for other clues, such as antisocial or borderline personality, poor work record, prior claims for injury, random test performance, and excessive endorsement of symptoms (Ruff and Willie, 1993).

TREATMENT

Patients with post-traumatic syndrome are often distressed and misunderstood, and they require an objective and comprehensive treatment approach. Treating them inappropriately may create pathologic resentment and disability that is refractory to treatment. The comprehensive approach to treatment utilizes medications, physical modalities, and biofeedback or counseling. Medina (1992) found that 85% of patients had returned to work after being treated aggressively in individualized programs that included medication, biofeedback, stress management, exercise, and neuromuscular relaxation.

In the absence of any known remediable mechanism, treatment should be directed at the identifiable components of post-traumatic syndrome. Headache is treated as if it had arisen as a primary headache disorder. Cervical and soft tissue injury should be identified and treated. Anxiety and depression should be meticulously identified and addressed. Cognitive dysfunction should also be addressed.

Few studies have evaluated specific drug treatments for PTH or looked at which headache responds to which drugs. Most have in-

volved use of the antidepressant amitriptyline. In an uncontrolled study, Tyler et al.
(1980) found amitriptyline to be effective in
90% of PTH patients, not distinguishing between various headache patterns of PTH.
The dose of amitriptyline varied from 75 to
250 mg. Saran (1988) used amitriptyline in
two groups of psychiatric hospital patients
with depression, one with PTH and the other
with idiopathic headaches. Outcome was
based on average daily headache intensity calculated from a headache calendar. Amitriptyline, at an average dose of 175 mg/day,
was effective for the uninjured patients
but not for the post-traumatic syndrome patients. This study is likely to have selected
a particularly intractable subgroup of post-
traumatic syndrome patients and may not apply to all patients with PTH. Depression in
patients with postconcussion syndrome is relatively resistent to tricyclic antidepressant
treatment.

Other antidepressants, including imipramine, doxepin, nortriptyline, selective serotonin reuptake inhibitors, venlafaxine, and
mirtazapine, may be effective in PTH. Done-
pezil is used for the cognitive symptoms of
major head injury, but it has not been studied
after minor head injury or postconcussion
syndrome.

Abortive medications are widely used for
patients with post-traumatic syndrome. One
must be on the lookout for analgesic and ergotamine overuse. Sumatriptan is effective
for the migrainous exacerbation of PTH but
not for the baseline headache (Gawel et al.,
1993). Repetitive IV DHE was effective for
PTH that met the criteria of chronic daily
headache (McBeath and Nanda, 1994; Young
et al., 1994) and appeared to improve cognitive function in one study (Young et al.,
1994). Chlorpromazine IV has been effective
in acute PTH (Herd and Ludwig, 1994). In
patients with daily or near-daily headache,
preventive medications should be used preferentially and the use of abortive medications
should be limited.

In the presence of true epilepsy, anticonvulsant therapy is indicated. Divalproex sodium is our drug of first choice if the patient
has PTH and a seizure disorder. The many

other spells seen in this population rarely respond to anticonvulsant treatment.

Biofeedback and psychotherapy or behavior modification may be helpful for many patients. Biofeedback enables the patient to
recognize muscle tension and bring it under
voluntary control. Ham and Packard (1996)
found that biofeedback enabled 53% of patients to moderately increase their ability to
relax and cope with pain, and 80% of patients
felt it was at least moderately helpful.

If a whiplash type of injury has occurred or
there is significant persistent neck pain suggesting a physical examination, cervical zygoapophyseal joint pain should be searched
for and treated if identified. Lord et al. (1996)
found the prevalence of zygoapophyseal joint
pain in patients with chronic neck pain after
whiplash injury to be 60%. Among patients
with whiplash injury who rated their headaches more severe than their neck pain, the
incidence of C2–3 zygoapophyseal joint pain
(based on diagnostic blocks) was 50% (Lord
et al., 1996). When initially successful, the
benefits of radiofrequency neurotomy last an
average of 422 days, and repeat procedures
are successful (McDonald et al., 1999).

Physical modalities, such as physical therapy and exercise, chiropractic treatment, and
massage, have been beneficial for some patients, particularly when headache is related
to or occurs in association with cervical
trauma. Cold, heat, electrotherapy, and cervical orthoses have been used successfully,
particularly in the acute stage, to improve
functioning. In one open study, manual therapy was more successful than cold packs at
relieving chronic post-traumatic syndrome
(Jensen et al., 1990). After the initial, acute
phase, exercise programs are important to
prevent deconditioning with a decrease in the
overall level of functioning.

Behavior modification or cognitive therapy
is often helpful in providing support and education and improving the patient's ability to
cope. For patients with more severe psychopathology, long-term psychotherapy may be
needed. Medication may be valuable to treat
anxiety and depression.

Cognitive retraining exercises, counseling,
adaptive strategy programs, and vocational re-

habilitation are useful treatments for neuro-cognitive dysfunction. Alexander (1995) suggested that programs that claim to treat attention and memory problems are of uncertain value in head injury in general and are inappropriate for mild head injury. Levin et al. (1990) demonstrated greater improvement in neuropsychologic function in patients with mild head injury who were treated with cytidine diphosphate-choline for the month after injury than in placebo-treated controls. The role for this treatment in the long-term management of postconcussion syndrome is uncertain.

OUTCOME

Prognostic studies have used various definitions of head injury, different study designs, and varying subject characteristics. Results have varied, making it difficult to accurately ascertain the prognosis of patients presenting at various stages of post-traumatic syndrome. At 1 month after mild head injury, 31% (Munderhoud et al., 1980) to 90% (Denker, 1944) of patients had headache. At 2 to 3 months postinjury, 32% (Denny-Brown, 1945) to 78% (Rimel et al., 1981) of patients had headache. One year after injury, the range was 8% (Rutherford et al., 1978) to 35% (Dencker and Lofving, 1958). Two to 4 years after injury, three studies show that 20% to 24% of patients have persistent headache (Cartlidge, 1978; Danker, 1944; Edna and Ceppelen, 1987). Dizziness, memory problems, and irritability are less likely to be noted within the first few months of injury but are more likely to persist (Evans, 1994).

Approximately one-third of patients are unable to return to work after head injury (Rutherford et al., 1978). In one study (Rimel et al., 1981), 34% of previously employed patients who were admitted to a hospital had not returned to work 3 months after injury. Older patients with higher levels of education and employment, greater income, and higher socioeconomic status were more likely to return to work.

Patients with mild traumatic brain injury have 1.8 times the risk of behavioral discharge from the armed services compared to the total discharge population. Mild and moderate head injury patients have 2.6 and 5.4 times the risk of discharge for alcohol and drug abuse, respectively, compared with the total population (Ommaya et al., 1996). An alternate explanation for these findings could be that the behavioral abnormalities are the risk factor for mild head injury (although previous studies, see Risk Factors, in other populations have failed to show that behavioral abnormalities have such a strong effect on outcome).

CONCLUSION

Chronic PTH and post-traumatic syndrome are common and frequently disabling conditions. There is no specific symptom cluster or reliable diagnostic test to unequivocally establish a diagnosis. The diagnosis is thus most reliably made by establishing the onset of symptoms soon after injury. The absence of a generally accepted mechanism for the genesis of chronic symptoms has led to an unfortunate skepticism about the validity of these symptoms, which has hindered the development of more effective treatments. The search for better treatment should continue; if new treatments can be based on interfering with a putative mechanism of symptom genesis (i.e., wind-up, kindling, aberrant reinnervation, neurochemical cascade), they may provide insight into the causes of post-traumatic syndrome. Relying on "psychogenesis" as the sole explanation of the syndrome feeds into a culture that could be harmful to individuals who have already been injured.

REFERENCES

Abdel-Dayem, H.M., H. Abu-Judeh, M. Kumar et al. (1998). SPECT brain perfusion abnormalities in mild or moderate traumatic brain injury. *Clin. Nucl. Med.* 23:309–317.

Abdel-Dayem, H.M., J. Masdeu, and R. O'Connell (1994). Brain perfusion abnormalities following minor/moderate closed head injury: Comparison between early and late imaging in two groups of patients. *Eur. J. Nucl. Med.* 21:750.

Abdel-Dayem, H.M., S.A. Sadek, and K. Kouris (1987). Changes in cerebral perfusion after acute head injury: Comparison of CT with Tc-99m-PAO SPECT. *Radiology* 165:221–226.

Alavi, A., T. Fazekas, W. Alves et al. (1987). Positron emission tomography in the evaluation of head injury. *J. Cereb. Blood Flow Metab.* 7:646.

Alexander, M.P. (1995). Mild traumatic brain injury: Pathophysiology, natural history, and clinical management. *Neurology* 45:1253.

American Academy of Neurology (1996). Assessment of brain SPECT. Report of the Therapeutics and Technology Assessment Subcommittee of the American Academy of Neurology. *Neurology* 46:278.

American Psychiatric Association (1994). *Diagnostic and Statistical Manual of Mental Disorders*, 4th edition. American Psychiatric Association, WAshington, D.C.

Mild Traumatic Brain Injury Committee of the Head Injury Interdisciplinary Special Interests Group of the American Congress of Rehabilitation Medicine. (1993). Definition of mild traumatic brain injury. *J. Head Trauma Rehabil.* 8:86–87.

Andrasik, F. and J.P. Wincze (1994). Emotional and psychologic aspects of mild head injury. *Semin. Neurol.* 14:60.

Barrett, K., A.B. Ward, A. Boughey et al. (1994). Sequelae of minor head injury: The natural consciousness and followup. *J. Accid. Emerg. Med.* 11:79.

Benton, A.L. and O. Spreen (1961). Visual memory test: The simulation of mental incompetence. *Arch. Gen. Psychiatry* 4:79.

Binder, L.M. (1986). Persisting symptoms after mild head injury: A review of the postconcussive syndrome. *J. Clin. Exp. Neuropsychol.* 8:323–346.

Binder, L.M. (1990). Malingering following minor head trauma. *Clin. Neuropsychol.* 4:25.

Blumbergs, P.C., N.R. Jones, and J.B. North (1989). Diffuse axonal injury in head trauma. *J. Neurol. Neurosurg. Psychiatry* 52:838–841.

Blumbergs, P.C., G. Scott, J. Manavis et al. (1994). Staining of amyloid precursor protein to study axonal damage in mild head injury. *Lancet* 344:1055.

Bohnen, N., A. Twinjnstra, and J. Jolles (1992). Posttraumatic and emotional symptoms in different subgroups of patients with mild head injury. *Brain Inj.* 6:481–487.

Bohnen, N.I., J. Jolles, A. Twijnstra et al. (1995). Late neurobehavioral symptoms after mild head injury. *Brain Inj.* 9:27.

Brenner, C. and A.P. Friedman (1944). Posttraumatic headache. *J. Neurosurg.* 1:379–391.

Bricolo, A.P. and G.S. Turella (1990). Electrophysiology of head injury. In *Handbook of Clinical Neurology* (R. Braakman, ed.), pp. 181–206. Elsevier, New York.

Cantu, B.C. (1988). Head and spine injuries in the young athlete. *Clin. Sports Med.* 7:459–472.

Cartlidge, N. E. F. (1978). Post-concussional syndrome. *Scot. Med.* 23:103.

Cartlidge, N. and D. Shaw (1981). *Head Injury* (N. Cartlidge and D. Shaw, eds.), pp. 95–154. W.B. Saunders, Philadelphia.

Davis, R.A. and L.M. Luxon (1995). Dizziness following head injury: A neurotologic study. *J. Neurol.* 242:222.

DeBenedittis, G. and A. DeSantis (1983). Chronic posttraumatic headache: Clinical, psychopathologic features and outcome determinants. *J. Neurosurg. Sci.* 27:177.

Denker, P.G. (1944). The postconcussion syndrome: Prognosis and evaluation of the organic factors. *N.Y. State J. Med.* 44:379–384.

Dencker, S.J. and B.A. Lofving (1958). A psychometric study of identical twins discordant for closed head injury. *Acta Psychiatr. Neurol. Scand.* 122(Suppl):119–126.

Denny-Brown, D. (1945). Disability arising from closed head injury. *JAMA* 127:429–436.

Duckro, P.N., J.T. Chibnall, and T.J. Tomazic (1995). Anger, depression, and disability: A path analysis of relationships in a sample of chronic posttraumatic headache patients. *Headache* 35:7.

Edna T-H and J. Coppelen (1987). Late post concussional symptoms in traumatic head injury. An analysis of frequency and risk factors. *Acta. Neurochir. (Wien)* 86:12–17.

Eisenberg, H.M. (1989). CT and MRI finding in mild to moderate head injury. In *Mild Head Injury* (H.L. Levin, H.M. Eisenberg, and A.L. Benton, eds.), p. 133. Oxford University Press, New York.

Elkind, A.H. (1992). Posttraumatic headache. In *The Practicing Physician's Approach to Headache* (S. Diamond and D.J. Dalessio, eds.), pp. 146–161. Williams and Wilkins, Baltimore.

Elson, L.M. and C.C. Ward (1994). Mechanisms and pathophysiology of mild head injury. *Semin. Neurol.* 14:8–18.

Erb, D.E. and J.T. Povlishock (1991). Neuroplasticity following traumatic brain injury: A study of GABAergic terminal loss and recovery in the cat dorsal lateral vestibular nucleus. *Exp. Brain Res.* 83:253.

Evans, R.W. (1992). The postconcussion syndrome and the sequelae of mild head injury. *Neurol. Clin.* 10:815–847.

Evans, R.W. (1994). The postconcussion syndrome: 130 years of controversy. *Semin. Neurol.* 14:32.

Evans, R.W. (1996). The postconcussion syndrome and the sequelae of mild head injury. In *Neurology and Trauma* (R.W. Evans, ed.). pp. 91–116. W.B. Saunders, Philadelphia.

Ewing, R., D. McCarthy, D. Gronwall et al. (1980). Persisting effects of minor head injury observable during hypoxic stress. *J. Clin. Neuropsychol.* 2:147.

Fenton, G.W. (1996). The postconcussional syndrome reappraised. *Clin. Electroencephalogr.* 27:174–182.

Foreman, S. and A. Croft (1995). *Whiplash Injuries: The Cervical Acceleration/Deceleration Syndrome.* Williams and Wilkins, Baltimore.

Gawel, M.J., P. Rothbart, and H. Jacobs (1993). Subcutaneous sumatriptan in the treatment of acute episodes of posttraumatic headache. *Headache* 33:96–97.

Geets, W. and N. Louette (1983). EEG et potentials évoqués du tronc cérébral dans 125 commotions récentes. *Electroencephalogr. Neurophysiol. Clin.* 13:253.

Gennarelli, T.A. (1993). Mechanisms of brain injury. *J. Emerg. Med.* 1:5–11.

Gennarelli, T.A., L.E. Thibault, J.H. Adams et al. (1975). Diffuse axonal injury and traumatic coma in the primate. In *Trauma of the Central Nervous System* (R.G. Dacey, H.R. Winr, R.W. Rimel et al., eds.), p. 169. Raven Press, New York.

Gentilini, T.M., P. Michelli, and R. Schoenhuber (1989). Assessment of attention in mild head injury. In *Mild Head Injury* (H.S. Levin, H.M. Eisenberg, and A.L. Benton, eds.), p. 163. Oxford University Press, New York.

George, J.K., Z. Alavi, R.A. Zimmerman, et al. (1989). Metabolic (PET) correlates of anatomic leads (CT/MRI) produced by head trauma [abstract]. *J. Nucl. Med.* 30:802.

Gfeller, J.D., J.T. Chibnall, and P.N. Duckro (1994). Postconcussion symptoms and cognitive functioning in posttraumatic headache patients. *Headache* 34:503–507.

Gilkey, S.J., N.M. Ramadan, T.K. Aurora et al. (1997). Cerebral blood flow in chronic posttraumatic headache. *Headache* 37:583–587.

Goodman, J.C. (1994). Pathologic changes in mild head injury. *Semin. Neurol.* 14:19.

Granovsky, Y., E. Sprecher, J. Hemli et al. (1998). P300 and stress in mild head injury patients. *Electroencephalogr. Clin. Neurophysiol.* 108: 554–559.

Gray, B.G., M. Ichise, and D. Chung (1992). Technetium-99m-HMPAO SPECT in the evaluation of patients with remote history of traumatic brain injury: A comparison with x-ray computed tomography. *J. Nucl. Med.* 33:52–58.

Gronwall, D. and P. Wrightson (1974). Delayed recovery of intellectual function after minor head injury. *Lancet* 2:605–609.

Haas, D.C. (1995). Classification of chronic posttraumatic headache. *Cephalalgia* 15:162.

Haas, D.C. and H. Lourie (1988). Trauma-triggered migraine: An explanation for common neurologic attacks after mild head injury. *J. Neurosurg.* 68:181–188.

Ham, L.P., F. Andrasik, R.C. Packard et al. (1994). Psychopathology in individuals with posttraumatic headaches and other pain types. *Cephalalgia* 14:118.

Ham, L.P. and R.C. Packard (1996). A retrospective, followup study of biofeedback-assisted relaxation therapy in patients with posttraumatic headache. *Biofeedback Self Regul.* 21:93–104.

Headache Classification Committee of the International Headache Society (1988). Classification and diagnostic criteria for headache disorders, cranial neuralgia, and facial pain. *Cephalalgia* 8: 1–96.

Heaton, R.K., H.H. Smith, R.A. Lehman et al. (1978). Prospects for faking believable deficits on neuropsychologic testing. *J. Consult. Clin. Psychol.* 46:892.

Herd, A. and L. Ludwig (1994). Relief of posttraumatic headache by intravenous chlorpromazine. *J. Emerg. Med.* 12:849–851.

Herrmann, M., N. Curio, S. Jost et al. (1999). Protein S-100B and neuron specific enolase as early neurobiochemical markers of the severity of traumatic brain injury. *Restor. Neurol. Neurosci.* 14:109–114.

Hickling, E.J., E.B. Blanchard, D.J. Silverman et al. (1992). Motor vehicle accidents, headaches, and posttraumatic stress disorder. *Headache* 32: 147.

Hughes, J.R. and L.D. Robbins (1990). Brain mapping in migraine. *Clin. Electroencephalogr.* 21:14.

Ingebrigtsen, T., K. Waterloo, E.A. Jacobsen et al. (1999). Traumatic brain damage in minor head injury: Relation of serum S-100 protein measurements to magnetic resonance imaging and neurobehavioral outcome. *Neurosurgery* 45: 468–475.

Jane, J.A., O. Steward, and T.A. Gennarelli (1985). Axonal degeneration induced by experimental noninvasive minor head injury. *J. Neurosurg.* 62: 96.

Jennett, B. and R.F. Frankowski (1990). The epidemiology of head injury. In *Handbook of Clinical Neurology* (R. Braakman, ed.), pp. 1–7. Elsevier, New York.

Jensen, O.K. and F.F. Nielson (1990). The influence of sex and pretraumatic headache on the incidence and severity of headache after injury. *Cephalalgia* 10:285–293.

Jensen, O.K., F.F. Nielsen, and L. Vosmar (1990). An open study comparing manual therapy with the use of cold packs in the treatment of posttraumatic headache. *Cephalalgia* 10:241–250.

Junger, E.C., D.W. Newell, G.A. Grant et al. (1997). Cerebral autoregulation following minor head injury. *J. Neurosurg.* 86:425–432.

Keidel, M., L. Yaguez, H. Wilhelm et al. (1992). Prospective followup of neuropsychologic deficits after cervicocephalic acceleration trauma. *Nervenarzt* 63:731.

Kelly, A.B., R.D. Zimmerman, S.E. Gandy et al. (1986). Comparison of magnetic resonance imaging and computed tomography in the evaluation of head injury. *Neurosurgery* 18:45.

Kelly, R. (1988). Headache after cranial trauma. In *Headache: Problems in Diagnosis and Management* (A. Hopkins, ed.), p. 219. W.B. Saunders, London.

Keshavan, M.S., S.M. Channabasavanna, and G.N. Reddy (1981). Posttraumatic psychiatric disturbances: Patterns and predictors of outcome. *Br. J. Psychiatry* 131:157.

Kim, S.H., F. Manes, T. Kosier, et al. (1999). Irritability following traumatic brain injury. *J. Nerv. Ment. Dis.* 187:327–335.

Kobylare, E.J., J. Dunford, B. Jabbari et al. (1995). Auditory event-related potentials in head injury patients. *Neurology* 45:358P.

Kraus, J.F., D.L. McArthur, and T.A. Silberman (1994). Epidemiology of mild brain injury. *Semin. Neurol.* 14:1–7.

Krelina, M., R. Reid, and J. Ballinger (1989). Regional cerebral blood flow in patients with remote close-head injuries [abstract]. *Can. J. Neurol. Sci.* 2:279.

Lake, A.E., B. Branca, T. Lutz et al. (1995). Comorbid symptoms in chronic posttraumatic headache. I: Comparison to intractable migraine. II: Relationship to severity of injury and litigation [abstract]. *Headache* 35:302.

Lankford, D.A., J.J. Wellman, and C. O'Hara (1994). Posttraumatic narcolepsy in mild to moderate closed head injury. *Sleep* 17:S25–S28.

Levin, H.S., E. Amparo, and H.M. Eisenberg (1987). Magnetic resonance imaging and computerized tomography in relation to the neurobehavioral sequelae of mild and moderate head injuries. *J. Neurosurg.* 66:706–713.

Levin, H.S., D. Williams, and H.M. Eisenberg (1990). Treatment of postconcussional symptoms with CDP-choline. *Neurology* 40:326.

Levin, H.S., D.H. Williams, H.M. Eisenberg et al. (1992). Serial MRI and neurobehavioral findings after mild to moderate head injuries. *J. Neurol. Neurosurg. Psychiatry* 55:255.

Lewine, J.D., J.T. Davis, J.H. Sloan et al. (1999). Neuromagnetic assessment of pathophysiologic brain activity induced by minor head trauma. *A.J.N.R.* 20:857–866.

Lidvall, H.F., B. Linderoth, and B. Norlin (1974). Causes of the postconcussional syndrome. *Acta Neurol. Scand.* 40:1–143.

Lord, S.M., L. Barnsley, B.J. Wallis et al. (1996). Chronic cervical zygoapophyseal joint pain after whiplash: A placebo-controlled prevalence study. *Spine* 21:1737–1744.

Machado, E.B., C.J. Michet, D.J. Ballard et al. (1988). Trends in incidence and clinical presentation of temporal arteritis in Olmsted County, Minnesota, 1958–1985. *Arthritis Rheum.* 31: 745–749.

Mallinson, A.I. and N.S. Longridge (1998). Diz-

ziness from whiplash and head injury: Differences between whiplash and head injury. *Am. J. Otol.* 19:814–818.

Mandel, S. (1989). Minor head injury may not be "minor." *Postgrad. Med. J.* 85:213–215.

Masdeu, J.C., H. Abdel-Dayhem, and R.L. VanHeertum (1995). Head trauma: Use of SPECT. *J. Neuroimaging* 5:53.

McBeath, J.G. and A. Nanda (1994). Use of dihydroergotamine in patients with postconcussion syndrome. *Headache* 34:148–151.

McCarthy, D. (1977). Memory and vigilance after concussion. University of Auckland, Auckland. Dissertation.

McClelland, R.J., G.W. Fenton, and W. Rutherford (1994). The postconcussional syndrome revisited. *J. R. Soc. Med.* 87:508–510.

McDonald, G.J., S.M. Lord, and N. Bogduk (1999). Long-term followup of patients treated with cervical radiofrequency neurotomy for chronic neck pain. *Neurosurgery* 45:61.

Medina, J.L. (1992). Efficacy of an individualized outpatient program in the treatment of chronic posttraumatic headache. *Headache* 32:180–183.

Mendelson, G. (1982). Not "cured by a verdict." *Med. J. Aust.* 2:132–134.

Miller, H. (1961a). Accident neurosis: Lecture I. *BMJ* 1:918.

Miller, H. (1961b). Accident neurosis: Lecture II. *BMJ* 1:992.

Mittenberg, W., D. DiGiulio, S. Perrin et al. (1992). Symptoms following mild head injury: expectation as etiology. *J. Neurol. Neurosurg. Psychiatry* 55:200.

Mittle, R.L., R.I. Grossman, J.F. Hiehl et al. (1994). Prevalence of MR evidence of diffuse axonal injury in patients with mild head injury and normal head CT findings. *Am. J. Neuroradiol.* 15:1583.

Montalbetti, L., D. Ferrandi, P. Pergami et al. (1995). Elongated styloid process and Eagle's syndrome. *Cephalalgia* 15:80.

Munderhoud, J.M., M.E. Boclens, and J. Huizenga (1980). Treatment of minor head injuries. *Clin. Neurol. Neurosurg.* 82:127–140.

Newton, M.R., R.J. Greenwood, K.F. Britton et al. (1992). A study comparing SPECT with CT and MRI after closed head injury. *J. Neurol. Neurosurg. Psychiatry* 55:92.

Obelieniene, D., G. Bovim, H. Schrader et al. (1998). Headache after whiplash: A historical cohort study outside the medicolegal context. *Cephalalgia* 18:559–564.

Ommaya, A.K., A.M. Salazar, A.L. Dannenberg et al. (1996). Outcome after traumatic brain injury in the U.S. military medical system. *J. Trauma* 41:972–975.

O'Neill, B., W. Haddon, A.B. Kelley et al. (1972). Automobile head restraints: Frequency of neck claims in relation to the presence of head restraints. *Am. J. Public Health* 62:403.

Packard, R.C. (1992). Posttraumatic headache: Permanency and relationship to legal settlement. *Headache* 32:496–500.

Packard, R.C. (1999). Epidemiology and pathogenesis of posttraumatic headache. *J. Head Trauma Rehabil.* 14:9–21.

Packard, R.C. and L.P. Ham (1993). Posttraumatic headache: Determining chronicity. *Headache* 33:133–134.

Packard, R.C. and L.P. Ham (1996). Incidence of cluster-like posttraumatic headache: An inconsistency. *Headache Q.* 7:139.

Packard, R.C. and L.P. Ham (1997). Pathogenesis of posttraumatic headaches and migraine: A common headache pathway? *Headache* 37:142–152.

Post, R.M. and S.D. Silberstein (1994). Shared mechanisms in affective illness, epilepsy, and migraine. *Neurology* 44:S37–S47.

Povlishock, J.T. and T.H. Coburn (1989). Morphopathologic change associated with mild head injury. In *Mild Head Injury* (H.S. Levin, H.M. Eisenberg, and A.L. Benton, eds.). Oxford University Press, New York. pp. 37–53.

Pratap-Chand, R., M. Sinniah, and F.A. Salem (1988). Cognitive evoked potential (P300): A metric for cerebral concussion. *Acta Neurol. Scand.* 78:185.

Prigatano, G.P., M.L. Stahl, W.C. Orr et al. (1982). Sleep and dreaming disturbances in closed head injury patients. *J. Neurol. Neurosurg. Psychiatry* 45:78.

Radanov, B.P., M. Sturzeneger, and G. DiStefano (1995). Long-term outcome after whiplash injury: A 2-year followup considering features of injury mechanism and somatic, radiologic, and psychosocial findings. *Medicine* 74:281.

Ramadan, N.M., L.L. Norris, and L.R. Shultz (1995). Abnormal cerebral flood flow correlates with disability to chronic posttraumatic headache [abstract]. *J. Neuroimaging* 5:68.

Ramadan, N.M., L.L. Schultz, and S.J. Gilkey (1997). Migraine prophylactic drugs: Proof of efficacy, utilization, and cost. *Cephalalgia* 17:73–80.

Rao, N., P.A. Turski, R.E. Polcyn et al. (1984). ^{18}F Positron emission computed tomography in closed head injury. *Arch. Phys. Med. Rehabil.* 65:780.

Raskin, N.H. (1988). Posttraumatic headache: The postconcussion syndrome. In *Headache* (N.H. Raskin, ed.). Churchill Livingstone, New York. pp. 269–282.

Reid, R.H., K. Gulenchyn, and J.R. Ballinger (1990). Cerebral perfusion imaging with Tc-HM-PAO following cerebral trauma. *Clin. Nucl. Med.* 15:383–388.

Rimel, R.W. (1981). Disability caused by minor head injury. *J. Head Trauma Rehabil.* 6:86–87.

Rimel, R.W., B. Giordani, J.T. Barth et al. (1981). Disability caused by minor head injury. *Neurosurgery* 9:221–228.

Rizzo, M. and D. Tranel (1996). *Head Injury and Postconcussion Syndrome*. Churchill Livingstone, New York.

Ross, W.D. and F.L. McNaughton (1944). Head injury: A study of patients with chronic posttraumatic complaints. *Arch. Neurol. Psychiatry* 52:255.

Rowe, M.J. and C. Carlson (1980). Brainstem auditory evoked potentials in postconcussion dizziness. *Arch. Neurol.* 37:679.

Ruff, M.R. and T. Willie (1993). Malingering and malingering-like aspects of mild closed head injury. *J. Head Trauma Rehabil.* 8:60.

Rutherford, W.H. (1989). Postconcussion symptoms. In *Mild Head Injury* (H.S. Levin, H.M. Eisenberg, and A.Z. Beriton, eds.), p. 217. Oxford University Press, New York.

Rutherford, W.H., J.D. Merrett, and J.R. McDonald (1977). Sequelae of concussion caused by minor head injuries. *Lancet* 1:1–4.

Rutherford, W.H., J.D. Merrett, and J.R. McDonald (1978). Symptoms of one year following concussion from minor head injuries. *Injury* 10:225–230.

Saatman, K.E., D.I. Graham, and T.K. McIntosh (1998). The neuronal cytoskeleton is at risk after mild and moderate brain injury. *J. Neurotrauma* 15:1047–1058.

Saper, J.R. (1983). *Headache Disorders: Current Concepts in Treatment Strategies*. Wright-PSG, Littleton, MA.

Saran, A. (1988). Antidepressants not effective in headache associated with minor closed head injury. *Int. J. Psychiatry Med.* 18:75.

Sbordone, R.J. and J.C. Liter (1995). Mild traumatic brain injury does not produce posttraumatic stress disorder. *Brain Inj.* 9:405.

Schmidt, R.H. and M.S. Grady (1995). Loss of forebrain cholinergic neurons following fluid-percussion injury: Implications for cognitive impairment in closed head injury. *J. Neurosurg.* 83:496.

Schoenhuber, R. and M. Gentilini (1989). Neurophysiologic assessment of mild head injury. In *Mild Head Injury* (H.S. Levin, H.M. Eisenberg, and A.L. Benton, eds.), pp. 142–150. Oxford University Press, New York.

Segalowitz, S.J. and S. Lawson (1995). Subtle symptoms associated with self-reported mild head injury. *J. Learn. Disabil.* 28:309.

Servadei, P., G. Vergoni, A. Pasini et al. (1994). Diffuse axonal injury with brainstem localization: Report of a case in a mild head injured patient. *J. Neurosurg. Sci.* 38:129.

Silberstein, S.D., R.B. Lipton, J.R. Saper et al. (1995). Headache and facial pain: Part A. *Continuum* 1:8.

Silberstein, S.D. and J. Marcelis (1990). Pseudo-tumor cerebri without papilledema. *Headache* 30:304.

Speed, W.G. (1987). Psychiatric aspects of post-traumatic headaches. In *Psychiatric Aspects of Headache* (C. Adler, S. Adler, and R. Packard, eds.), pp. 210–217. Williams and Wilkins, Baltimore.

Strauss, I. and N. Savitsky (1934). Head injury. *Arch. Neurol. Psychiatry* 31:893.

Sturzenegger, M. (1991). Ultrasound findings in spontaneous carotid artery dissection. *Arch. Neurol.* 48:1057–1063.

Teasdale, G. and B. Jennett (1984). Assessment of coma and impaired consciousness: A practical scale. *Lancet* 2:81–84.

Thatcher, R.W., R.A. Walker, I. Gerson et al. (1989). EEG discriminant analyses of mild head trauma. *Electroencephalogr. Clin. Neurophysiol.* 73:1989.

Toglia, J.U. (1969). Dizziness after whiplash injury of the neck and closed head injury. In *The Late Effects of Head Injury* (W.F. Walker, W.F. Caveness, and M. Critchley, eds.), p. 72. Thomas, Springfield, IL.

Treleaven, J., G. Jull, and L. Atkinson (1994). Cervical musculoskeletal dysfunction in postconcussional headache. *Cephalalgia* 14:273–279.

Tyler, G.S., H.E. McNeely, and M.L. Dick (1980). Treatment of posttraumatic headache with amitriptyline. *Headache* 20:213.

Varney, N.R. and D. Bushnell (1998). Neuro-SPECT findings in patients with posttraumatic anosmia: A quantitative analysis. *J. Head Trauma Rehabil.* 13:63–72.

Vijayan, N. (1977). A new posttraumatic headache syndrome. *Headache* 17:19–22.

Ward, C.C. (1982). Finite element modeling of the head and neck. In *Impact injury of the Head and Spine* (C.L. Ewing, ed.), p. 421. Thomas, Springfield, IL.

Ward, C.C. and A.M. Nahum (1979). Correlation between brain injury and intracranial pressures in experimental head impacts. In *Proceedings of the 4th International Conference on the Biomechanics of Trauma*, Goteborg, Sweden, 133.

Weiller, C., A. May, V. Limroth et al. (1995). Brainstem activation in spontaneous human migraine attacks. *Nat. Med.* 1:658–660.

Weiss, H.D., B.J. Stern, and J. Goldbert (1991). Posttraumatic migraine: Chronic migraine precipitated by minor head or neck trauma. *Headache* 31:451–456.

Werner, R.A. and C.W. Vanderzant (1991). Multimodality evoked potential testing in acute mild closed head injury. *Arch. Phys. Med. Rehabil.* 72:31.

Wilkinson, M. and E. Gilchrist (1980). Posttraumatic headache. *Ups. J. Med. Sci.* 31:48.

Winston, K.R. (1987). Whiplash and its relationship to migraine. *Headache* 27:452–457.

Wong, E., G. Lee, and D.T. Mason (1995). Temporal headaches and associated symptoms relating to the styloid process and its attachments. *Ann. Acad. Med.* 24:124.

Yamaguchi, M. (1992). Incidence of headache and severity of head injury. *Headache* 32:422.

Young, W.B., M.M. Hopkins, B. Janyszek et al. (1994). Repetitive intravenous DHE in the treatment of refractory posttraumatic headache [abstract]. *Headache* 34:297.

Zubkov, A.Y., A.S. Pilkington, D.H. Bernanke et al. (1999). Posttraumatic cerebral vasospasm: Clinical and morphological presentations. *J. Neurotrauma* 16:763–770.

15

Headache Associated with Vascular Disorders

MARIE GERMAINE BOUSSER
JANINE GOOD
STEVEN J. KITTNER
STEPHEN D. SILBERSTEIN

Headache can be a manifestation of vascular disease, but it is often unrecognized because its frequency is so much lower than that of migraine or tension-type headache. In this chapter, we will discuss cerebral venous thrombosis, intracerebral and subarachnoid hemorrhage, unruptured vascular malformations, and arterial vascular disease, including ischemic stroke. This will be followed by a discussion of dissection and other causes of carotid or vertebral artery pain, central nervous system angiitis and angiopathy, migraine and stroke, and arterial hypertension.

CEREBRAL VENOUS THROMBOSIS

In the past, cerebral venous thrombosis (CVT) was considered a rare, devastating disease characterized by headache, papilledema, seizures, bilateral focal deficits, and coma that almost invariably led to death. The widespread use of angiography, computerized tomography (CT) of the brain, magnetic resonance imaging (MRI), and magnetic resonance angiography (MRA) in the last 20 years has made early diagnosis of CVT possible and has completely changed our perception of this condition. For example, CVT is much more common than previously thought. It has multiple causes, a wide spectrum of clinical presentations, and an unpredictable but usually favorable outcome. Headache is the most frequent and, at times, the only symptom of CVT, in contrast to arterial stroke. The best diagnostic tools are MRI and MRA, and the treatment of choice is heparin (Bousser and Russell, 1997; Einhaupl et al., 1991).

Pathophysiology

The cause of headache in CVT is multifactorial; it can be due to the causes or the consequences of the venous occlusion. Headache is a prominent symptom in some of the conditions that can cause CVT. They can be focal (such as head trauma, intracranial tumor, cerebral abscess, meningitis, or an infection of the face, ear, nose, or sinuses) or general (such as primary or secondary polycythemia or any infection or febrile disease). These conditions should be systematically searched for in patients with CVT. If one or more is diagnosed first, care must be taken not to overlook the concurrent CVT as the cause of headache.

Headache is often due to the consequences of venous occlusion, particularly intracranial hypertension (ICH) secondary to impaired cerebrospinal fluid (CSF) absorption, either from blockage of arachnoid granulations by a thrombus or from chronic raised venous pressure. The presence of ICH usually indicates thrombosis of the superior sagittal sinus or of both lateral sinuses. Unilateral lateral sinus and jugular vein thromboses cause ICH only if the thrombus extends back to involve the torcular or if the other lateral sinus is hypoplastic. Another potential mechanism for headache in CVT is venous infarction, which is characterized by distended and thrombosed sinuses and cortical veins, often associated with perivenous subarachnoid hemorrhage (SAH) and sometimes with large subdural hemorrhages (Bousser and Russell, 1997).

Headache Characteristics

Headache is the most frequent symptom of CVT, present in 80% to 90% of cases, and it is often the initial symptom (Ameri and Bousser, 1992; Bousser et al., 1985b; Cantu and Barinagarrementeria, 1993; Daif et al., 1995). It has no specific characteristics. It is often diffuse, but it can be unilateral, localized to any region of the head, or even limited to the neck. It varies in severity, ranging from a mild sensation of heaviness to excruciating pain. The mode of onset is usually subacute (more than 48 hours but less than 30 days) but can be sudden. Headache is usually constant, but it can be intermittent, particularly initially, and can even occur in attacks.

While the headache of CVT has no specific clinical characteristic or temporal profile, in over 95% of cases it is associated with neurologic signs that point to an organic intracranial disorder.

Main Patterns of Presentation

Headache in CVT can be associated with any of the signs in Table 15–1, in isolation or in combination. Four main patterns and some unusual presentations exist (Bousser and Russell, 1997).

Table 15–1 Cerebral venous thrombosis: main neurological symptoms and signs (personal series of M.G. Bousser)

Sign/symptom	Incidence (n = 160)
Headache	131 (81.9%)
Papilledema	81 (50.6%)
Seizures	67 (41.8%)
Focal deficits (motor, sensory, aphasia)	62 (38.7%)
Drowsiness, mental changes, confusion, or coma	49 (30.6%)
Multiple cranial nerve palsies	17 (10.6%)
Bilateral cortical signs	7 (4.3%)
Cerebellar signs	4 (2.5%)

Headache with Isolated Intracranial Hypertension

The most homogeneous pattern of presentation is headache with isolated ICH. Headache, progressive over days or weeks, is associated with bilateral papilledema and, less frequently, with sixth-nerve palsy, tinnitus, and transient visual obscurations. This presentation mimics so-called benign or idiopathic ICH (pseudotumor cerebri) and accounts for 40% of our 160 patients. Benign ICH has often been diagnosed in case reports without ruling out CVT despite the fact that superior sagittal and lateral sinus thromboses can cause ICH. In two different series, one prospective and one retrospective, of 24 and 46 patients who had the clinical, CT, and CSF characteristics of benign ICH, sinus thrombosis was present in 25% and 26% of cases, respectively (Tehindrazanarivelo et al., 1992; Leker and Steiner, 1999). In a series of 160 consecutive patients with CVT, 59 had isolated ICH, and of these, 54% had a normal CT scan and 75% had normal CSF contents (Biousse et al., 1999). Since sinus thrombosis is a mimic of idiopathic ICH and since CT scan and CSF can be normal in CVT, we think that a normal MRI/MRA should be added to the traditional diagnostic criteria of idiopathic ICH.

Headache with Focal Signs

The most frequent heterogeneous presentation of CVT is headache with focal signs, which accounts for roughly 75% of published cases. The mode of onset of focal signs, their nature (deficits, seizures, or both), and their possible association with altered consciousness and signs of raised intracranial pressure vary. Acute cases mimic arterial strokes, chronic cases mimic tumors, and subacute cases mimic abscesses.

Subacute Encephalopathy

Subacute encephalopathy is characterized by diffuse headache and a depressed level of consciousness with occasional deficits or seizures but without recognizable features of raised intracranial pressure. The differential diagnosis includes encephalitis, disseminated intravascular coagulation, and cerebral vasculitis.

Cavernous Sinus Thrombosis

Frontal headache is a major symptom of cavernous sinus thrombosis. In acute cases, its distinctive clinical picture usually includes chemosis, proptosis, and ophthalmoplegia, initially unilateral but frequently becoming bilateral. Cavernous sinus thrombosis can also take a more indolent and atypical form, with only mild frontal headache, chemosis, and proptosis (Levine et al., 1988). This can occur by itself or because of the masking effect of an inadequate antibiotic regimen.

Unusual Presentations

The four main pattern groups do not account for all cases of CVT. Isolated headache can be the only symptom (7/160 in our series). Also, CVT can simulate other conditions, including a postural headache occurring after lumbar puncture (LP), particularly in patients with suspected or definite multiple sclerosis. It also occurs after epidural anesthesia. This is of particular concern during the postpartum period (Hubbert, 1987). A persistent headache after a dural puncture, especially when a blood patch is ineffective or when the postdural puncture headache loses its typical postural component and becomes permanent should suggest coexistent pathology, including CVT (Aidi et al., 1999).

Cerebral venous thrombosis can present with a sudden, severe headache with CT scan or LP evidence of SAH. This mimics a ruptured intracranial aneurysm and indicates a need to study the cerebral venous system in patients with SAH without arterial causes (Bousser and Russell, 1997). Benign thunderclap headache (de Bruijn et al., 1996) and migraine attacks (with our without aura) (Newman et al., 1989) can be the presenting symptoms of CVT. Other headache varieties, particularly in patients with lateral sinus thrombosis, are unclassifiable. One patient presented with unilateral hearing loss and diffuse headache (Crassard et al., 1997), and another presented with an isolated, sharp monocular pain as the only signs of ipsilateral lateral sinus thrombosis.

Any new headache, whatever its severity, location, and associated signs, should raise suspicion of organic disease, which may require investigations including CT scan, CSF study, and MRI/MRA.

Investigations

In the above clinical context, CVT must be considered, particularly when an underlying condition that is known to increase the risk of venous thrombosis (e.g., puerperium, postoperative or post-traumatic state, cardiac failure, Behcet's disease) is present.

The best current diagnostic tool is MRI. It is the only study that visualizes the thrombus itself, which appears as an increased signal on both TI and T2 images and is usually obvious between day 5 and day 30 after the onset of symptoms (Dormont et al., 1994; Mattle et al., 1990; Padayachee et al., 1991; Rippe et al., 1990; Tsai et al., 1995). Magnetic resonance venography, helical CT venography, or conventional angiography is indicated for very early (before day 5) or late (after 6 weeks) stages when false-negatives may occur or if the MRI shows equivocal signs. Computed tomographic scanning is performed on an emergency basis to rule out the other conditions that CVT can mimic, such as arterial stroke, abscess, tumor, or SAH. It is diagnostic in about 20% of cases, visualizing the hyperdensity of the thrombosed sinus on plain images and the empty triangle (or delta) sign typical of superior sagittal sinus thrombosis after contrast (Buonanno et al., 1982; Virapongse et al., 1987). A CSF examination is needed when meningitis or encephalitis is suspected and to measure CSF pressure in a patient with isolated ICH. Once the diagnosis is established, it is important to identify causative or predisposing conditions.

Treatment

Treatment should be started as soon as the diagnosis is firmly established. Symptomatic treatment (anticonvulsants and reduction of raised intracranial pressure) and intravenous heparin (dose-adjusted activated partial thromboplastin time) are used, even if a hemorrhagic lesion is present on CT or MRI (Bousser and Russell, 1997; Einhaupl et al., 1991; Villringer et al., 1994; Bousser, 1999c; de Bruijn and Starn, 1999). Whenever possible, the underlying cause should be treated, e.g., antibiotics in septic cases or steroids in Behcet's disease and systemic lupus. As soon as clinical improvement starts, warfarin should be added; when levels are therapeutic, heparin can be discontinued.

Headache treatment usually consists of high doses of oral or intravenous (IV) paracetamol (acetaminophen). Aspirin should be avoided because of its interaction with anticoagulants. Sedatives should be avoided so that the patient's state of consciousness can be monitored. Headache due to ICH often improves rapidly after LP. Improvement is usually rapid, and sometimes spectacular, once heparin is begun. In some cases, the headache remains severe for a week or two, requiring major analgesics or opioids. Look for an underlying condition if headache persists.

The headache and the other neurologic signs may worsen despite optimal symptomatic treatment and adequate heparin treatment. If the deterioration is proven to be due to thrombosis extension, local thrombolysis with urokinase or recombinant tissue-type plasminogen activator can be tried (Smith et al., 1994; Frey et al., 1999). These cases are extremely rare (none in the last 30 cases seen

over 2 years by one of us), and the benefit/risk ratio of thrombolysis in CVT has not been properly assessed (Bousser, 1999c).

Outcome

The prognosis of CVT is better than previously thought, but it remains unpredictable (Barinagarrementeria et al., 1992a). In recent large series, mortality ranged from 33% (Cantu and Barinagarrementeria, 1993) to 4% (6/160 in our series), with three main causes of death: the brain lesion itself, particularly with massive hemorrhagic infarct; intercurrent complications, such as sepsis, uncontrolled seizures, or pulmonary embolism; or the underlying condition (carcinoma, leukemia, septicemia, paroxysmal nocturnal hemoglobinuria, or heart failure). Headache is not reported to be a sequelae of CVT; in contrast, focal deficits or seizures persist in 10% to 30% of cases (Preter et al., 1996). Most patients survive and have excellent recovery of function. In the most recent series (Preter et al., 1996), over 70% of subjects recovered completely.

SUBARACHNOID HEMORRHAGE

Subarachnoid hemorrhage (SAH) from a ruptured aneurysm occurs in 28,000 people a year in North America (Leblanc, 1987). The classical presentation of an aneurysmal SAH is an acute-onset, severe headache associated with a stiff neck, photophobia, nausea, vomiting, and perhaps obtundation or coma; it is easily differentiated from migraine. This catastrophic presentation is often preceded by a more minor hemorrhage that can signal the likelihood of a major rupture within hours, days, or weeks and may be more difficult to diagnose (Leblanc, 1987; Waga et al., 1975; Fontanarosa, 1989; Duffy, 1983; King and Saba, 1974; Bartleson et al., 1981). In most series of patients with "minor leaks" related to SAH, headache, nausea and vomiting are common; loss of consciousness is less common; and seizures or cranial nerve findings are rare. In one study, nonexertional activities preceding the SAH were more frequent than exertional activities (Fontanarosa, 1989). Harling et al. (1989) could not clinically differentiate between SAH and other benign headaches in patients presenting with the sudden onset of their worst headache ever. Both the SAH and non-SAH groups had neck stiffness and photophobia, but the SAH group had significantly more vomiting.

The most common secondary cause of intense and incapacitating abrupt-onset headache is SAH. Since focal neurologic deficits can be absent at presentation, the headache is often misdiagnosed as migraine, particularly if a triptan is given and the patient responds. Of patients presenting to emergency departments with headache, 1% to 4% had SAH (Ramirez-Lassepas et al., 1997). Approximately 80% of nontraumatic SAHs result from ruptured saccular aneurysms, which occur in 30,000 patients annually in the United States (Mayberg et al., 1994) and result in the death of approximately 18,000 individuals (Kassell et al., 1990). Approximately 10% of nontraumatic SAHs are due to nonaneurysmal perimesencephalic hemorrhages (Vermeulen, 1996; Vermeulen and Van Gijn, 1990).

Most intracranial aneurysms (80% to 85%) are located in the anterior circulation, often at the junction of the internal carotid artery and the posterior communicating artery, the anterior communicating artery complex, or the trifurcation of the middle cerebral artery. Posterior circulation aneurysms are usually located at the bifurcation of the basilar artery or the junction of the vertebral artery and the ipsilateral posterior inferior cerebellar artery. Multiple intracranial aneurysms occur in 20% to 30% of patients (Kassell et al., 1990).

Pathophysiology

Pain that follows SAH results from local distention and stretching of the cerebral vessel and the adjacent arachnoid and chemical irritation of the intracranial sensory nerves by the blood. Pain is carried by the fifth, ninth, and tenth cranial nerves and the upper cervical spinal nerves. Headache may also be due to increased intracranial pressure or delayed cerebral ischemia.

Headache Characteristics

The typical headache of SAH is of sudden-onset and severe (thunderclap headache). The headache is usually bilateral but can be unilateral and accompanied by nausea and vomiting and possible loss of consciousness (Schievink, 1997). The physical examination may show nuchal rigidity, retinal hemorrhages (prehyaloid hemorrhage), restlessness, or focal neurologic signs. The International Headache Society (IHS) diagnostic criteria (Headache Classification Committee of the International Headache Society, 1988) for headache associated with SAH include present or past subarachnoid bleeding demonstrated by CSF examination or CT, headache of sudden onset (<60 minutes if it is an aneurysm, <12 hours if it is an arteriovenous malformation), and at least one of the following: severe headache intensity, bilateral headache location, stiff neck, increased body temperature. These criteria have not been validated, and the time limit and elevated temperature criteria are of particular concern.

The Problem of Misdiagnosis

Misdiagnosis can result from three correctable patterns of diagnostic error: (1) failure to appreciate the spectrum of clinical presentations; (2) failure to understand the limitations of CT; and (3) failure to perform and correctly interpret the results of LP (Edlow and Caplan, 2000) (Table 15–2).

Spectrum of Presentation

Between 20% and 50% of patients with documented SAH report a distinct, unusually severe, premonitory headache (thunderclap headache) a few days or weeks before a major aneurysmal rupture (Bassi et al., 1991; Verweij et al., 1988; Linn et al., 1994; Ogawa et al., 1993). Thunderclap headaches develop in seconds, achieve maximal intensity in minutes, and last hours to days. The differential diagnosis includes SAH, aneurysm, thrombosis, localized meningeal inflammation (Raps et al., 1993b), leakage into the aneurysm wall (Day and Raskin, 1986), cerebral

Table 15-2 Reasons for misdiagnosis of subarachnoid hemorrhage

Failure to appreciate the spectrum of presentations of subarachnoid hemorrhage
    Failure to evaluate patients with "warning headaches" (severe, abrupt, unusual headaches)
    Failure to recognize that headache can improve spontaneously or with non-narcotic analgesic drugs
    Over-reliance on the classic presentation, leading to the following incorrect diagnoses:
        Viral syndrome, viral meningitis, or gastroenteritis
        Migraine or tension-type headache
        Sinus-related headache
        Neck pain (rarely back pain)
        Psychiatric disorders
    Focus on secondary head injury (resulting from syncope)
    Focus on electrocardiographic abnormalities
    Focus on high blood pressure
    Lack of knowledge of presentations of unruptured aneurysm
Failure to understand the limitations of computed tomography
    Loss of sensitivity with increasing time between onset of headache and scanning
    False-negative results in cases of small-volume bleeding (spectrum bias)
    Interpretation factors (e.g., variations in expertise of physician reading the scan)
    Technical factors (e.g., variations in thickness of slices taken at the base of the brain, motion artifact)
    False-negative results for blood with a hematocrit of <30%
Failure to perform lumbar puncture and correctly interpret cerebrospinal fluid findings
    Failure to perform lumbar puncture in patients with negative, equivocal, or suboptimal results on computed
        tomography
    Failure to recognize that xanthochromia may be absent very early (<12 hours after hemorrhage) and very late
        (>2 weeks after hemorrhage)
    Failure to realize that visual inspection for the presence of xanthochromia is less sensitive than
        spectrophotometry
    Failure to distinguish properly between "traumatic tap" and true subarachnoid hemorrhage

Reproduced with permission from Edlow, J.A. and L.R. Caplan. (2000). Avoiding pitfalls in the diagnosis of subarachnoid hemorrhage. *N. Engl. J. Med.* 342:29–36.

venous thrombosis (de Bruijn et al., 1996), benign exertional headache, nonaneurysmal perimesencephalic hemorrhage, and benign thunderclap headache (Wijdicks et al., 1988; Linn et al., 1998). Since early recognition and surgery might lead to improved outcome, all patients with thunderclap headache should be evaluated for SAH (Edlow and Caplan, 2000).

Less severe headache can be mistaken for a migraine or tension-type headache. The SAH headache may be in any location, may be localized or generalized, may resolve spontaneously (Weir, 1998), and may be relieved by analgesics and triptans (Seymour et al., 1995). Neck stiffness may take hours to develop and, in some cases, may never appear. The absence of neck stiffness does not exclude SAH (Vermeulen, 1996).

Subarachnoid hemorrhage may be mistaken for other medical conditions. Patients with fever, vomiting, sweating, and tachycardia may be misdiagnosed as having a viral syndrome; some may have severely elevated blood pressure (Kawamura and Meyer, 1991;

Schievink, 1997; Kassell et al., 1990) and be misdiagnosed as a hypertensive emergency. Cardiac arrhythmias occur in 91% of patients with SAH (Andreoli et al., 1987) and electrocardiographic changes consistent with myocardial ischemia can occur, suggesting a primary cardiac disorder (Adams et al., 1980). Subarachnoid blood may be inappropriately attributed to minor head trauma, particularly if the patient fell after the ictus and has a superficial hematoma or laceration.

Computed Tomographic Scanning and Its Limitations

A CT scan without contrast, with 3 mm cuts, is the neuroimaging study of choice; it provides high initial sensitivity that decreases over time (Evans, 1996; Edlow and Caplan, 2000). Thicker cuts (<3 mm) may miss small collections of blood. In the International Cooperative Study of the Timing of Aneurysm Surgery (1980–1983), 3,521 patients had older-generation CT scan; the sensitivity of CT in detecting subarachnoid blood was 92%

during the first 24 hours, decreasing to 58% on day 5 (Kassell et al., 1990). Modern third-generation CT scanners have 98% sensitivity in the first 12 hours (van der Wee et al., 1995) and 93% sensitivity within the first 20 hours (Sames et al., 1996; Morgenstern et al., 1998). The pattern of hemorrhage can predict the presence and location of an aneurysm (Vermeulen, 1996). A ruptured aneurysm should be suspected if the subarachnoid clots are most dense at one of the classical aneurysm sites: the frontal interhemispheric fissure (ACA aneurysm), the chiasmatic cistern on one side (ICA aneurysm), or the most lateral part of the Sylvian fissure (MCA aneurysm) (Vermeulen and Van Gijn, 1990). Blood may be isodense on CT, and the diagnosis of SAH may be missed if the hematocrit is <30%.

Lumbar Puncture and Interpretation of Findings

Lumbar puncture (LP) following SAH may rarely be associated with neurologic deterioration (Hillman, 1986). It should be performed immediately in a patient whose clinical presentation suggests SAH and whose CT scan is negative, equivocal, or technically inadequate (Mayberg et al., 1994; Edlow and Caplan, 2000). The CSF pressure should be measured (high pressure can suggest CVT); it can help distinguish SAH from a traumatic tap. Clear CSF in a second LP at the interspace above the first tap suggests a traumatic tap; use of the three-tube method and the finding of crenated red blood cells are not reliable (Edlow and Caplan, 2000).

Xanthochromia appears by 12 hours after SAH and lasts for weeks. Its presence after 12 hours diagnoses SAH with a high degree of sensitivity (the sensitivity of CT for detecting SAH decreases after the first 12 hours.) The CSF should be immediately centrifuged to avoid contamination by blood from a traumatic tap and, if possible, tested for xanthochomia by spectrophotometry, which is more sensitive than visual inspection. In a study by Vermeulen et al. (1989), all 111 patients with SAH who underwent LP between 12 hours and 2 weeks after the onset of symptoms had xantho-chromic CSF, as determined by spectrophotometry.

If SAH is diagnosed, neurologic and neurosurgical consultation and conventional catheter angiography are indicated.

Complications

Rebleeding can occur within 48 hours of the initial bleed (Kawamura and Meyer, 1991). Hydrocephalus may be immediate or delayed. Acute hydrocephalus occurs in approximately 20% of cases (Mayberg et al., 1994). Vasospasm is a prevalent, often devastating complication that develops several days after the hemorrhage (Greenberg, 1994). Cardiac, pulmonary, and infectious complications frequently occur in patients recovering from SAH. Diabetes insipidus or the syndrome of inappropriate antidiuretic hormones may also occur (Findlay, 1997).

Treatment

Headache and restlessness should be controlled with appropriate analgesics and moderate sedation. Aspirin, while previously considered to be contraindicated because of the potential for rebleeding, may have potential value in preventing vasospasm after aneurysm clipping (Juvela, 1995; Hop et al., 2000). Acetaminophen and opioids are recommended.

Proper timing of aneurysm surgery (early vs. late aneurysm surgery) is still debatable. The advantages of early surgery are eliminating the risks of rebleeding and facilitating the management of vasospasm. Early surgery removes subarachnoid blood and allows safe treatment with induced hypertension, which may reduce the risk of vasospasm. Disadvantages of early surgery include brain swelling, which makes exposure of the aneurysm more difficult and the risk of intraoperative complications greater (Findlay, 1997). Early surgery is recommended for the patient who is in good condition and has an uncomplicated aneurysm. For other clinical situations, the decision depends on the circumstances of the particular case (Mayberg et al., 1994). Surgery during days 4–10 following SAH, the period of highest risk for vasospasm, should be undertaken with caution (Findlay, 1997).

Acute therapy is directed at preventing rebleeding and managing vasospasm. All patients with aneurysmal SAH should be treated with the calcium antagonist nimodipine for neuroprotection (Pickard et al., 1989), and in certain circumstances patients should receive anticonvulsants. Induced arterial hypertension, hypervolemia, and in some instances percutaneous balloon angioplasty are recommended to reverse vasospasm (Findlay, 1997). Pharmacologic treatment is directed at controlling pain, blood pressure, and intracranial pressure (Findlay, 1997).

Outcome

The morbidity and mortality figures of patients with SAH have not changed in recent decades. Approximately 50% of patients die following SAH, and 50% of the survivors are left more or less disabled (Ausman et al., 1989; Bonita and Thomson, 1985; Rasmussen et al., 1981). Disabling headache may occur in one of four survivors (Rasmussen et al., 1981).

THUNDERCLAP HEADACHE AND UNRUPTURED ANEURYSM

Thunderclap headache is the sudden onset of a severe headache that reaches maximum intensity within 1 minute. Benign thunderclap headache is further defined by the absence of SAH. An acute neurologic event must be ruled out in all patients who present with severe, acute-onset headache, although migraine can present in this manner (Silberstein, 1992).

The first or worst attack of migraine may be very difficult to differentiate from SAH, particularly if the pain is of acute onset (thunderclap headache).

Day and Raskin (1986) have stated that all patients presenting with severe, sudden-onset headache should, in addition, be evaluated with angiography for an aneurysm, even if CT, MRI, and LP do not show evidence of SAH. They reported a case of thunderclap headache in which angiography showed an aneurysm and arterial spasm, but the CT scan was normal and the CSF bloodless. Several prospective studies had suggested that thunderclap headache is usually benign and angiography probably not necessary if neurologic examination, CT or MRI, and CSF examination performed at the time of the ictus are normal (Harling et al., 1989; Wijdicks et al., 1988).

Wijdicks et al. (1988) prospectively followed 71 patients with severe, sudden-onset thunderclap headaches who had normal CT and CSF findings. All but two were admitted to the hospital within 2 days of the headache; only seven (10%) reported a previous similar headache. Neurologic examination was normal except for questionable meningismus in ten (14%). Four patients underwent angiography, which was normal. The patients were followed for a mean of 3.3 years; none developed evidence of subsequent SAH. Recurrent headaches developed in 12 patients, beginning as early as 1 day and as long as 4 years after the initial one. Four patients were readmitted and still had normal CT and CSF studies; two of them had normal angiography. A total of 31 patients (44%) developed tension-type headaches or migraine without aura during the follow-up period.

Harling et al. (1989) prospectively followed 14 patients who presented to a regional neurosurgical unit with sudden headache suggestive of SAH but with normal CSF and CT scan. It was not possible, on clinical grounds alone, to distinguish these patients from those who had bled. These patients were followed for a minimum of 18 months. One had no further headache, four had musculoskeletal pain, five had psychogenic pain, and four had migraine-type headaches. None developed an unequivocal SAH, and the investigators concluded that angiography cannot be justified in patients with thunderclap headache.

Markus (1992) compared the clinical features of thunderclap headache to SAH in a prospective series of 55 patients who presented to a district general hospital with a provisional diagnosis of SAH. Criteria for thunderclap headache included a headache starting within seconds and reaching maximum intensity within 1 minute and a normal CSF examination within 48 hours of the onset of headache. The clinical features were compared to those of patients who presented to a regional neurosurgical unit with SAH without focal neurologic symptoms or impairment of consciousness. The thunderclap headache was described as the worst headache they had ever experienced. Most common locations were occipital (50%) and frontal (38%). Three patients had previously experienced a similar thunderclap headache. No patient in the thunderclap group (n = 18) had developed SAH at 24 months of follow-up. This was the evidence for the absence of an unruptured aneurysm.

Hughes (1992) reported two cases of thunderclap headache due to unruptured aneurysms. Case 1 was a healthy 32-year-old man who presented with a severe, abrupt-onset, left-sided headache. When evaluated 12 days after the ictus, the headache was gone, CT was negative, and LP showed nine red blood cells (RBCs). A left middle cerebral artery trifurcation aneurysm was found; no evidence of recent hemorrhage was found at surgery. Case 2 was a 48-year-old woman who presented with a severe, abrupt-onset headache that was different from her usual migraine. She had a large left posterior cerebral artery aneurysm that showed no evidence of rupture at surgery.

Ng and Pulst (1992) reported a 53-year-old woman who presented with the acute onset of the worst headache of her life. Examination, CT, and LP were normal. She was discharged after 36 hours of observation, but she was readmitted 2 days later due to recurring persistent headaches. The next day she was found unresponsive. An angiogram showed a distal right internal carotid artery aneurysm. She died shortly thereafter.

Raps et al. (1993b) looked at the clinical spectrum of unruptured intracranial aneurysms, performing a retrospective study of 111 patients (with 132 unruptured aneurysms) who presented to a tertiary referral center. Aneurysms were defined as unruptured by the absence of visible hemorrhage on CT scan, lack of xanthochromia or RBCs

on CSF examination, and visual inspection at the time of surgery. The study included 85 women and 26 men with a mean age of 51.2 years. Fifty-four symptomatic patients were identified; 19 had acute symptoms: ischemia (n = 7), headache (n = 7), seizures (n = 3), and cranial neuropathy (n = 23). Thirty-five had chronic symptoms attributed to mass effect, including headache (n = 18) and visual loss (n = 10).

Acute severe thunderclap headache comparable to SAH but without nuchal rigidity was seen in 6.3% (7/111) of patients with unruptured aneurysms, most of which were located in the anterior circle of Willis (Raps et al., 1993b). Thus, cataclysmic headache may serve as the symptom of both a ruptured and an unruptured aneurysm. The mechanism for acute headache is likely to involve the vessel wall and may include acute expansion, intraluminal bleeding, or occult hemorrhage. While this study shows conclusively that an unruptured aneurysm can cause thunderclap headache, it does not allow an estimate of the prevalence of this phenomenon in the population due to selection bias.

Intracranial berry aneurysm occurs in 1% to 2% of the adult population (Raps et al., 1993b). If less than 7% of these in a selected series present with thunderclap headache, the prevalence of this headache type in the general population is no more than 0.1%. The age range is 10 to 70 years, and frequency of recurrence is uncertain. Migraine is an episodic disorder with a 1-year prevalence of about 12%. If 5% of migraineurs had an attack of acute-onset headache, prevalence would be about 0.6%, which is approximately an order of magnitude higher than that of thunderclap headache from unruptured aneurysm. This could, in part, account for the failure of clinical prospective series of thunderclap headache to detect large numbers of unruptured aneurysms. In addition, the criterion for detection is rupture, not angiography. Thus, patients followed for 3 years still could have an unruptured aneurysm (the risk for rupture is only 1% annually).

In summary, unruptured aneurysm can cause thunderclap headache. The true frequency of unruptured aneurysms among patients with thunderclap headache is unknown. All patients with a possible unruptured aneurysm should have MRA. The routine use of cerebral angiography is proscribed by the risk of permanent (0.1%) and transient (1.2%) deficits in this low-yield population, but the issue can be a difficult clinical judgment (Leow and Murie, 1988). Increasing risk factors include patients with a particularly high likelihood of aneurysmal SAH, such as those with retinal or subhyloid hemorrhage, nuchal rigidity, seizure, diploplia, loss of consciousness, or focal neurologic signs, and those with a personal or family history of SAH, polycystic kidney disease, or fibromuscular dysplasia (Edlow and Caplan, 2000).

OTHER VASCULAR MALFORMATIONS

Headache in Encephalotrigeminal Angiomatosis (Sturge-Weber Syndrome)

Sturge-Weber syndrome is defined as a facial angioma associated with an ipsilateral meningeal angioma. Neurologic manifestations include seizures (in 80% to 90% of cases), mental retardation (in 40% to 50%) and focal signs, such as hemiplegia, aphasia, or hemianopia, that are often fluctuating (in 25% of cases).

A survey of headache in Sturge-Weber syndrome was performed by Klapper (1994). A questionnaire based on IHS criteria was sent to 500 members of the Sturge-Weber Foundation. Unfortunately, only 71 replies could be evaluated, and no detailed description is given either of the questionnaire or of the varieties of headache. In this population of young subjects (mean age 15 years) with a sex ratio of 1, the prevalence of recurrent headache was 44%, including migraine (28%), glaucoma headache (8%), chronic tension-type headache (4%), episodic tension-type headache (1%), and unclassifiable headache (3%). Ninety-three percent of patients had seizures, and half of them experienced postictal headache. Neurologic symptoms (focal weakness, visual loss, and paresthesias) occurred in association with headache in 58%

of cases, but in the absence of further description, it is impossible to know whether these symptoms correspond to migraine with aura.

A few cases suggest that Sturge-Weber syndrome might be responsible for symptomatic migraine. In one of these (Cambon et al., 1987), a young man experienced typical attacks of migraine with aura with scintillating scotoma, right sensory motor disturbances, and dysphasia that lasted for 30 minutes and was usually followed by left-sided headache. Oxygen[15] positron emission tomography (PET) showed a typical and persisting misery perfusion syndrome. Similar PET abnormalities were found in a young woman with a history of migraine attacks since puberty (first without aura and later with aura) who, while pregnant, suffered a stroke-like episode with a severe right hemiplegia, hemianopia, dysphasia, and seizures. These symptoms cleared completely in 3 months without any sign of infarction on MRI.

These observations suggest that chronic focal oligemia and ensuing tissue hypoxia might precipitate severe, prolonged deficits without cerebral infarction, bearing striking similarities to those reported in some varieties of familial hemiplegic migraine (Fitzsimons and Wolfenden, 1985).

In summary, it is impossible to precisely assess the frequency and characteristics of migraine and other varieties of headache in Sturge-Weber syndrome. Isolated case reports suggest that Sturge-Weber syndrome might be one of the many causes of symptomatic migraine, particularly with prolonged aura, possibly related to chronic oligemia.

INTRACEREBRAL HEMORRHAGE

Headache in intracerebral (intraparenchymal) hemorrhage is accompanied by the rapid development of focal neurologic signs and/or alterations in consciousness; this allows them to be immediately differentiated from the primary headaches.

Pathophysiology

Headache accompanies intracerebral hemorrhage in about 60% of cases and is more common in cerebellar and lobar hemorrhages than in thalamic, caudate, capsuloputaminal, or brain-stem hemorrhages (Melo et al., 1996). The headache of intraparenchymal hemorrhage has been attributed to traction on pain-sensitive intracranial structures (Gorelick et al., 1986). Multivariate analyses of a cohort of 289 patients found that meningeal signs, hematoma location, and female gender were more predictive of headache than hematoma volume, suggesting that headache is more often related to subarachnoid blood and to local anatomic effects in susceptible individuals than to intracranial hypertension (Melo et al., 1996).

Headache Characteristics and Pattern of Presentation

In contrast to SAH, the headache of intracerebral hemorrhage is often unilateral and of mild or moderate severity (Gorelick, 1993). Nausea, vomiting, and severe hypertension are often associated features. Headache laterality predicts the side of the hemorrhage with an 80% predictive value (Melo et al., 1996) but otherwise has limited value for predicting hemorrhage location (Gorelick et al., 1986; Melo et al., 1996).

Cerebellar hemorrhage deserves special discussion (Kase et al., 1998). The headache is often acute and can be maximal at onset and severe, mimicking SAH (Fisher et al., 1965). Occipital location and associated neck stiffness are common (Ott et al., 1974; Melo et al., 1996). Orthostatic headache with aggravation by the upright position and alleviation by lying down has been reported as the presenting symptom in two cases (in addition to early nausea and vomiting, inability to stand or walk without help is a frequent and important symptom) (Fisher et al., 1965). Associated brain-stem compression (Heros, 1982) is indicated most importantly by impaired level of consciousness but also by gaze paresis, peripheral facial weakness, decreased corneal response, Horner's syndrome, unilateral Babinski's sign, and mild hemiparesis. Obtundation, pinpoint pupils, ataxic respirations, and decerebrate posture are late signs of brain-stem compression. Although cere-

bellar hemorrhage often progresses to brainstem compression within hours, it is unpredictable and can occur days to weeks later (Brillman, 1979).

Investigations and Treatment

Diagnosis is by CT scan. Due to risk of herniation, LP is contraindicated. Investigation of the etiology of the intracerebral hemorrhage (Caplan, 1988) may require MRI, MRA, or conventional catheter angiography. Management consists of blood pressure control, correction of any coagulopathy, and neurosurgical intervention, particularly with a cerebellar hemorrhage, wherein surgical evacuation can be lifesaving if accomplished before brain-stem compression. Although cerebellar hematomas of <3 cm diameter, in the absence of hydrocephalus and obliteration of the quadrigeminal cistern, may not require surgery, close clinical monitoring is required in all cases (Little et al., 1978; Heros, 1982). The role of neurosurgical intervention in other locations is being addressed in clinical trials. Persistent neurologic disability is common. Female gender and a history of prehemorrhage headache and post-stroke depression are independent predictors of posthemorrhage headache (Ferro et al., 1998).

ISCHEMIC STROKE

The headache of ischemic stroke, like that of intracerebral hemorrhage, is accompanied by focal neurologic signs and/or alterations in consciousness, usually allowing differentiation from the primary headaches. The headache due to carotid or vertebral artery dissection, with or without stroke, and the complex interrelationship between migraine and stroke will be discussed later in this chapter. The headaches that accompany temporal arteritis are discussed elsewhere in this volume.

Pathophysiology

Headache accompanies ischemic stroke in from 17% (Gorelick et al., 1986) to 34% (Ferro et al., 1995) of cases, depending on the series. It may be more frequent in vertebrobasilar than in carotid territory strokes and infrequent in subcortical infarcts and lacunae due to single perforator disease (Gorelick, 1993; Ferro et al., 1995). The cause of headache in ischemic stroke is not well understood, but it may be due to activation of the trigeminovascular system (Moskowitz, 1984; Moskowitz et al., 1989). Multivariate analyses of a cohort of 182 patients found that the probability of headache onset was directly related to vertebrobasilar stroke and a past history of migraine and inversely related to lacunar stroke (Ferro et al., 1995). Stroke location and predisposition to headache are the most important determinants of headache onset in ischemic stroke.

Headache Characteristics and Pattern of Presentation

The headache of ischemic stroke is usually unilateral and less likely to be severe or associated with vomiting than the headache of SAH or intracerebral hemorrhage (Gorelick et al., 1986). There is no consistent relationship between the headache location and the vascular distribution of the stroke (Gorelick, 1993). A *sentinel* headache, defined as an unusual headache noted by the patient in the days to weeks before stroke onset, has been noted in about 10% of 160 ischemic stroke cases (Gorelick et al., 1986). Other series using slightly different definitions of premonitory headache have noted similar rates: 10% of a mixed group consisting of 90% ischemic strokes and 10% intracerebral hemorrhage or other (Vestergaard et al., 1993) and 11% of an ischemic stroke group (Arboix et al., 1994). There is little information on headache onset in ischemic stroke; in a series of 135 stroke patients comprised clinically of two-thirds ischemic strokes and one-third intracerebral hemorrhages (Portenoy et al., 1984), gradual headache onset and abrupt headache onset were equally likely.

Investigations and Treatment

The diagnosis of ischemic stroke is based on the clinical syndrome with exclusion of extracranial causes. Newer imaging studies, such as diffusion-weighted MRI, have a high sensitivity for the diagnosis of acute stroke (Kidwell et al., 1999; Albers et al., 2000). Thrombolytic therapy given to appropriately selected acute stroke patients within the first 3 hours improves outcome and has revolutionized stroke care (Adams et al., 1996). The immediate use of aspirin post-stroke, in those not undergoing thrombolytic therapy, improves outcome (Chen et al., 2000). The aim of acute stroke investigation is to determine the pathophysiologic mechanism and etiology, which determines subsequent management (Caplan, 1993; Adams et al., 1994). The presentation and management of cerebellar infarction are similar to those of cerebellar hemorrhage (discussed above); timely surgery may be lifesaving. Symptomatic extracranial carotid disease or a cardioembolic source should be excluded and the possibility of vasculitis considered before starting antiplatelet medication. General preventive measures include blood pressure management and aggressive lipid-lowering therapy (Hess et al., 2000; National Cholesterol Education Program 1988) as well as angiotensin-converting enzyme inhibitors (Yusuf et al., 2000).

CAROTID OR VERTEBRAL ARTERY PAIN

In the IHS classification, "carotid or vertebral artery pain" is a subchapter of "headache associated with vascular disorders" that includes artificially grouped headaches directly or indirectly related to proven or presumed lesions of the walls of the internal carotid or vertebral arteries. This includes arterial dissections, vascular surgery, angioplasty with or without stenting, and intracranial endovascular procedures. Pain is not a feature of other arterial lesions, such as fibromuscular dysplasia, moya-moya, postradiotherapy stenosis, arterial kinks, or atheromatous stenosis or occlusion.

"Acute idiopathic carotidynia" is included as a variety of carotid pain and is recognized as a separate entity in the IHS classification with the following four diagnostic criteria: at least one of the following overlying the carotid artery: tenderness, swelling, increased pulsations; appropriate investigations do not reveal structural abnormality; pain over the affected side of the neck that may project to the ipsilateral side of the head; a self-limited syndrome of less than 2 weeks' duration.

The term "carotidynia" was first used by Fay (1927) to refer to tenderness of the bifurcation of the carotid artery sometimes observed in patients with "atypical facial neuralgia." Over the years, carotidynia has come to refer to a distinct syndrome characterized by two cardinal signs: unilateral neck pain and carotid artery tenderness. In the 1960s and 1970s, hundreds of cases of acute or chronic carotidynia were reported. However, a critical review on carotidynia (Biousse and Bousser, 1994) found that the unilateral neck pain had no specific clinical characteristics or temporal pattern and that the physical signs (i.e., local tenderness, swelling, and increased pulsations) are neither constant nor specific. Very few cases were appropriately investigated to rule out structural abnormalities, such as carotid dissections, which have all the characteristics of acute carotidynia. In the literature of idiopathic carotidynia, as defined by the IHS, there is not a single case report in which there has been a normal carotid investigation (Biousse and Bousser, 1994; Biousse et al., 1992).

Carotidynia is not a validated entity but rather a symptom (unilateral neck pain with local tenderness) that can be the result of vascular and nonvascular conditions. Recurring attacks of carotidynia with headache that last a few days are probably related to migraine, attacks that last a few minutes suggest chronic paroxysmal hemicrania, and regular daily attacks of 1 or 2 hours' duration suggest cluster headache. Acute varieties with a self-limited course may be viral in origin, but carotid dissection must be excluded. Chronic varieties with continuous background pain have an important psychologic component. Other causes include carotid artery diseases (occlusion, fibromuscular dysplasia, giant cell arteritis, or carotid endarterectomy), carotid body tumors, lymphadenitis, pharyngitis, dental infection, local aphthous ulcers, and malignant infiltration (Biousse and Bousser, 1994;

Biousse et al., 1992; Vijayan and Watson, 1986). Carotidynia is not a distinct entity but a symptom complex of unilateral neck pain with local tenderness that has multiple causes.

Headache in Carotid and Vertebral Artery Dissections

Cervical and cerebral artery dissections are important causes of ischemic stroke (Fisher, 1982; Mokri et al., 1986; Mitsias and Ramadan, 1992a,b; Biousse et al., 1995; Silbert et al., 1995; Guillon et al., 1998b), accounting for up to 20% of cases in recent series of ischemic strokes in the young. They affect the internal carotid artery (ICA) more frequently than the vertebral artery (VA) and are more common extracranially than intracranially (Guillon et al., 1998b; Mokri et al., 1986). Their cause is unknown, although neck trauma is frequently implicated. So-called spontaneous cases often have an associated underlying disorder, such as fibromuscular dysplasia, elastic tissue disease, arterial hypertension, or migraine. The most typical clinical presentation is sudden-onset cephalic pain followed hours or days later by signs of cerebral or retinal ischemia (Mokri et al., 1986; d'Anglejan-Chatillon et al., 1989; Guillon et al., 1998b).

Pathophysiology

The pathophysiology of head pain in ICA and VA dissections is still poorly understood. No good correlation exists between the characteristics of the pain and those of the dissection (site, presence of stenosis, occlusion, or aneurysm). The pain is most likely referred from dilation or distention of the artery, which stimulates pain-sensitive receptors in the vessel well. Electrical stimulation of the wall of the carotid bifurcation (Fay, 1927) or balloon inflation in the distal carotid artery (Nichols et al., 1990) produces ipsilateral pain in various parts of the face and head depending on the area stimulated (Mitsias and Ramadan, 1992a,b; Nichols et al., 1990). The predominantly occipital distribution of headache in VA dissection can be explained by the upper cervical innervation of the vasculature of the posterior fossa. Why some dissections are painful and others are painless remains a mystery.

Headache Characteristics

Cephalic pain (headache, facial and neck pain) is a crucial symptom in carotid and vertebral artery dissections. It is the most frequent symptom, the most frequent inaugural symptom, and can be the only symptom of dissection. In all series of carotid or vertebral artery dissections, cephalic pain is present in 55% to 100% of cases (Table 15–3). The frequency is underestimated because headache cannot be properly assessed in cases associated with aphasia or disorders of consciousness. Since cephalic pain is the most frequent inaugural symptom in this condition (33% to 86% of cases), early diagnosis and treatment are possible. The mode of onset is variable. In the Mayo Clinic series, the onset of pain was gradual, over a few hours or days in 85% of ICA dissections and in 72% of VA dissections (Silbert et al., 1995), whereas in other series, a sudden onset was the rule (Biousse et al., 1994; Sturzenegger, 1994). The risk of cerebral or retinal ischemia is highest in the first week after headache onset, but it persists up to 1 month (Biousse et al., 1995). Cephalic pain as the only manifestation of dissection is rare: in the Mayo Clinic series, it occurred in 3/135 patients with ICA dissection and in 4/26 patients with VA dissection (Silbert et al.,

1995). In VA dissections, isolated pain is usually due to SAH, which can be the only manifestation of intracranial VA dissection. In ICA dissections, various isolated pain patterns have been reported, including thunderclap headache, lateral cervical pain, and orbital pain (Biousse et al., 1992; Guillon et al., 1998a).

There are no specific characteristics of cephalic pain in ICA/VA dissections. The pain is usually unilateral, severe, and persistent. Pain location is variable and it can involve, in isolation or in combination, any part of the head (70%), neck (20%), or face (10%) (Biousse et al., 1994; Silbert et al., 1995). In 80% of cases, the pain is unilateral and ipsilateral to the dissection; however, bilateral and diffuse headache can occur, even when the dissection is unilateral. The pain is more frequently localized than diffuse, with a predilection for the frontal, orbital, temporal, and upper lateral cervical regions. Cervical pain often radiates toward the ipsilateral mandible, eye, or ear. With VA dissections, the pain is usually located in the occiput and/or posterior neck and more frequently felt medially than laterally, even when dissection is unilateral (Mitsias and Ramadan, 1992a,b; Biousse et al., 1994; Silbert et al., 1995). It can be mistaken for pain of musculoskeletal origin despite the usual absence of cervical spine movement restriction (Sturzenegger, 1994), with potentially dramatic consequences if chiropractic manipulations are performed (Mas et al., 1989).

Table 15–3 Cephalic pain in series of carotid or vertebral artery dissection

Study	Number of patients	Artery involved	Cephalic pain Inaugural (%)	At any time (%)
Fisher (1982)	26	ICA	—	88
Biousse et al. (1994b)	65	ICA	58	74
Sturzenegger (1995)	44	ICA	74	91
Silbert et al. (1989)	135	ICA	47	68
Mas et al. (1987)	15	VA (EC)	80	92
Greselle et al. (1987)	15	VA (EC/IC)	—	100
Sturzenegger (1994)	14	VA (EC/IC)	86	86
Silbert et al. (1995)	26	VA	33	88
De Bray et al. (1997)	16	VA (EC/IC)	65	65
Hosoya et al. (1999)	31	VA (IC)	35	55

Key to abbreviations: ICA, internal carotid artery; VA, vertebral artery; EC, extracranial; IC, intracranial.

The pain is severe in 75% of cases, sometimes excruciating, described as a thunderclap headache, with or without SAH (Biousse et al., 1994; Silbert et al., 1995). It can also be very mild and ignored, particularly when more prominent signs are present. The pain has no specific quality. It is as frequently aching, pressing or sharp in quality, and throbbing (Biousse et al., 1994; Silbert et al., 1995). Most patients who have had prior headaches recognize this pain as being different. However, up to one-third of migraine subjects reported that the pain that accompanied their dissection was indistinguishable from that of their usual migraine attack (Biousse et al., 1994). The dissection, in such cases, can be mistaken for a migraine attack, either without aura when the headache is isolated or with aura when visual symptoms (frequent in ICA and VA dissections) are present (Biousse et al., 1994; Ramadan et al., 1991; Duyff et al., 1997). If a stroke ensues, the dissection will be misinterpreted as a migrainous infarct (Sinclair, 1959; Shuaib, 1991; Ganesan and Kirkham, 1997). This distinction is particularly important since migraine may be a risk factor for dissection (d'Anglejan-Chatillon et al., 1989).

The pain usually lasts several days, but the duration can be 1 hour to several days. In two large series of ICA dissections, the median durations were 3 and 5 days, respectively (Silbert et al., 1995; Biousse et al., 1994); the median duration was 3 days (range 2 to 35 days) in VA dissections (Silbert et al., 1995). In over 90% of cases, the pain resolves in less than 10 days, but cases of long-lasting pain have been reported (Fisher, 1982; Mokri et al., 1986; Silbert et al., 1995), particularly in patients with residual aneurysms (Mokri et al., 1986). Long-lasting pain is uncommon, however, even in patients with residual aneurysms. No cases of persisting headache were observed in a prospective follow-up of 16 patients with aneurysms that developed during extracranial ICA dissection (Guillon et al., 1999).

Severe, unilateral head pain of sudden or rapid onset, particularly when associated with cervical pain, suggests ICA (when the pain is anterior) or VA (when occipital) dissection.

Dissection frequently presents with other varieties of head and neck pain, mimicking migraine, cluster headache, carotidynia, SAH, or Raeder's syndrome. Dissection not only mimics SAH but can cause SAH. In one series of 648 angiographically investigated SAH patients, 14 had intracranial vertebrobasilar dissecting aneurysms; six others were found among patients who initially had stenotic or occlusive lesions (Nakatomi et al., 1997).

Main Patterns of Presentation

Head pain is rarely the only sign of dissection; in most cases, ischemic and/or local signs are present. The most frequently associated sign is retinal or cerebral ischemia. Unilateral head or neck pain in a patient presenting with amaurosis fugax, anterior circulation transient ischemic attacks, or stroke is highly suspicious of ICA dissection (Fisher, 1982; Mokri et al., 1986; Biousse et al., 1994; Silbert et al., 1995; Guillon et al., 1998a,b; Radanov et al., 1995). Similarly, occipital or posterior neck pain with vertebrobasilar symptoms suggests VA dissection (Mas et al., 1987; Greselle et al., 1987; Mitsias and Ramadan, 1992a,b; Sturzenegger, 1994; de Bray et al., 1997; Hosoya et al., 1999). Atypical presentations include cervical cord and dorsal medullary infarction due to VA dissection in a patient presenting with an excruciating retro-orbital paroxysmal headache (de la Sayette et al., 1999). Ischemic signs, if present, typically follow the head pain, usually within a few days to a month (Biousse et al., 1995). A key sign of ICA dissection is ipsilateral "local signs," occurring in nearly half the patients. The most frequent local sign is Horner's syndrome. Painful Horner's syndrome occurs in up to 58% of cases, and it is the only clinical manifestation of ICA dissection in about 10% (Fisher, 1982; Mokri et al., 1986; Biousse et al., 1994; Silbert et al., 1995). Other signs and symptoms include pulsatile tinnitus, present in 5% to 10% of cases; lower cranial nerve palsies (XII with or without involvement of XI, X, and IX), present in 5.2% of cases; trigeminal involvement, present in 3.7% of cases; ocular motor palsies, present in 2.6% (III, IV, or VI); and dysgeusia, present in 2% (involvement of the chorda tympani nerve). Some of these local signs (Horner's syndrome, tinnitus, lower cranial nerve palsies) immediately suggest ICA dissection when associated with ipsilateral head pain; others, such as painful ophthalmoplegia, do not since ICA dissection is an extremely rare cause of this syndrome.

Investigations

Once dissection is suspected, appropriate investigations should be performed as rapidly as possible in order to start treatment and not miss the diagnosis if rapid recanalization occurs. Investigations include duplex scanning, MRI, MRA, helical CT, and, in doubtful cases, conventional angiography. Ultrasound investigations are often performed first, on an emergency basis. They are usually abnormal, showing direct and/or indirect signs of stenosis or occlusion; but they are rarely specific, requiring other investigations to confirm the diagnosis. The MRI is pathognomonic if it shows a narrowed lumen with an increase in external diameter and a semilunar-shaped eccentric hypersignal of the vessel wall (mural hematoma) (Ozdoba et al., 1996). The MRA is diagnostic of dissection if it shows sequential narrowing or a lack of arterial signal and an abnormal signal along the length of the dissection site (hematoma) with an increase in the external diameter of the vessel (Levy et al., 1991). Combined MRA and MRI has a remarkable diagnostic yield in extracranial ICA dissections. For VA, basilar artery, or intracranial ICA dissection, angiography is often required.

Treatment

Treatment is aimed at preventing ocular and cerebral infarction. Although no controlled study of cervical artery dissection treatment has been conducted, heparin (partial thromboplastin time 1.5–2.5 × control) is usually prescribed to prevent subsequent emboli. The risk of hemodynamic stroke in dissections associated with occlusion or severe stenosis is unpredictable; therefore, bedrest is recommended until the artery is reopened or effective collateral circulation develops. This is assessed by noninvasive procedures such as cervical duplex scanning and transcranial Doppler (Guillon et al., 1998b). Warfarin (international normalized ratio 2 to 3.5) is usually started after a few days of IV heparin. There is no consensus as to the duration of anticoagulant therapy; our preference is to stop warfarin when the luminal diameter has returned to normal (which occurs by 6 months in 70% to 90% of cases) or if the occlusion is stable after 6 months. In the rare case of persistent stenosis, warfarin should be continued; aspirin is substituted for warfarin when a patient has a persisting aneurysm that has a good prognosis (Guillon et al., 1999). Other treatment modalities include angioplasty with stenting (Marks et al., 1999), but their usefulness and risk/benefit ratio need rigorous evaluation.

HEADACHES ASSOCIATED WITH VASCULAR PROCEDURES

Post-Carotid Endarterectomy Headache

Post-carotid endarterectomy headache is recognized as an entity in the IHS classification; it is defined as an ipsilateral headache that begins within 2 days of carotid endarterectomy, in the absence of carotid occlusion or dissection. A critical review of the literature does not permit isolation of a group of patients who completely satisfy these criteria for two reasons. First, carotid angiography or ultrasonography has not been systematically performed. Second, bilateral headaches, as well as headaches occurring after 2 days, have been included in postendarterectomy headache series (Tehindrazanarivelo et al., 1992; Biousse et al., 1992).

The most frequent type of headache that occurs after carotid endarterectomy is a mild, diffuse, nonspecific headache that is not associated with focal deficits, seizures, or an increase in systemic blood pressure (Tehindrazanarivelo et al., 1991). It is present in up to 60% of cases, usually occurs in the 5 days following surgery, and is particularly frequent in the first 2 postoperative days. It is more commonly bilateral than unilateral and is preferentially located in the frontal region.

Described as a sensation of pressure or heaviness, it is usually mild or moderate and requires no treatment. Its temporal profile is highly variable and may be continuous or intermittent, with a mean duration of 3 days (Tehindrazanarivelo et al., 1991). Although acknowledged in the past (Messert and Black, 1978; Mitsias and Ramadan, 1992a,b), this variety of headache is rarely mentioned, probably because it is a benign, self-limiting condition devoid of any specific characteristic. The fact that it can occur in patients with no past history of headache suggests a direct relationship with the surgical procedure.

The second type of post-carotid endarterectomy headache is a "cluster-like" pain, considered rare by some (Leviton et al., 1975; Pearce, 1976; Tehindrazanarivelo et al., 1991) and common (up to 30% of cases) by others (de Marinis et al., 1991). It is an ipsilateral headache, occurring from 12 to 120 hours after carotid surgery (mean 49.5 hours). It consists of attacks that occur once or twice a day and last 2 to 3 hours. There are no prodromata. The pain is pulsating, moderate or severe, and located mainly in the retro-ocular and temporoparietal regions. It is sometimes associated with ipsilateral conjunctival injection, lacrimation, rhinorrhea, nasal stuffiness, and Horner's syndrome. In most cases, the pain resolves spontaneously in 2 to 25 days (mean 14 days). This headache has been related, on the basis of pharmacologic pupillary testing, to decreased sympathetic activity (de Marinis et al., 1991).

The third type of headache is part of the "cerebral hyperperfusion syndrome," which occurs mainly after correction of a very high-grade stenosis in patients with chronic cerebral ischemia (Leviton et al., 1975; Dolan and Mushlin, 1984; Bernstein et al., 1984; Reigel et al., 1987; Breen et al., 1996; Ille et al., 1995). It is a severe, unilateral, throbbing pain that begins after a mean latent interval of 3 days after surgery. It often precedes the onset of seizures, contralateral focal deficits, and an increase in systemic blood pressure on around the seventh postoperative day. This association of symptoms can herald cerebral hemorrhage (Bernstein et al., 1984; Reigel et al., 1987), but it has mainly been reported in the absence of stroke (Leviton et al., 1975;

Reigel et al., 1987). Often, CT scans are normal, but they can show diffuse, patchy edema consistent with hyperperfusion (Breen et al., 1996). This syndrome, which deserves careful management, is rare; it was not encountered in a prospective series of 50 carotid endarterectomies (Tehindrazanarivelo et al., 1991).

Another headache that can occur after carotid endarterectomy is the one that accompanies a postoperative stroke. It can happen in the absence of occlusion or dissection but is always associated with focal deficits; therefore, it should not be included in so-called postendarterectomy headache. Other types of post-carotid endarterectomy headache or pain include severe hemicranias, delayed cluster headache, chronic paroxysmal hemicrania, carotidynia, and the elongated styloid process syndrome (Eagle syndrome) (Messert and Black, 1978). These cases poorly documented prior headaches, time course of pain, and assessment of carotid patency.

In summary, a critical literature review shows that there is no such entity as postendarterectomy headache. There is a very rare "hyperperfusion injury syndrome" headache, and there is a frequent, mild, diffuse, self-limited headache that does not incapacitate the patient. Reports of other varieties of headache occurring after carotid surgery are anecdotal.

Headache Associated with Percutaneous Angioplasty and Stenting

Randomized trials comparing percutaneous angioplasty (PTA) and stenting to surgery are in progress (Brown et al., 1997). Headache is not mentioned as a complication of carotid angioplasty and stenting in current large series (Roubin et al., 1996; Eckert et al., 1996; Gil-Peralta et al., 1996; Yadav et al., 1997; Dietrich et al., 1996). An early series of 53 patients who underwent angioplasty (Munari et al., 1994) reported cervical pain in 51% of patients, with radiation to the face and scalp in 33%. The pain occurred with balloon inflation and was considered mild in 18% of cases, moderate in 59%, and severe in 22%. Different segments of the ICA next to the bifurcation were associated with different patterns of radiation. The pain typically disappeared within a few seconds of balloon deflation; the pain lasted several minutes in seven patients and up to 3 hours in two subjects, in the absence of dissection. The pain was interpreted as true carotid pain, clearly distinguishable from the pain induced by infusing hyperosmolar contrast medium through the carotid artery during a standard angiogram (Edvinsson et al., 1987).

A "hyperperfusion injury syndrome" similar to that observed after carotid endarterectomy has been reported following PTA/stenting of the ICA and various other cervical arteries. Headache was a prominent symptom in three patients, at times associated with seizures, hypertension, and intracerebral hemorrhage (Bergeron et al., 1996; Benichou and Bergeron, 1996; Schoser et al., 1997; McCabe et al., 1999).

Headache During Intracranial Endovascular Procedures

A specific variety of headache has been reported after balloon inflation or embolization of arteriovenous malformations or aneurysms (Nichols et al., 1990; Martins et al., 1993). It is a severe, unilateral pain of abrupt onset that occurs shortly after the procedure and is ipsilateral to the occluded artery. It is localized to specific areas according to the artery involved: the temple for the proximal middle cerebral artery, the retro-orbital area for the middle of the middle cerebral artery stem, the lateral part of the neck for the upper vertebral artery, and the vertex and occiput for the inferior portion of the basilar artery. This pain is nonthrobbing and is not associated with other symptoms. It is most likely due to distention of the arterial wall and provides a good model of pure vascular headache. By contrast, pain is not mentioned in the largest series (23 patients) so far published of angioplasty for atherosclerotic intracranial stenosis (Marks et al., 1999).

ANGIITIS OF THE CENTRAL NERVOUS SYSTEM

Angiitis (vasculitis) is a pathologic process characterized by inflammation of blood ves-

sels. Although much of the evidence is indirect and may reflect epiphenomena rather than true causality, inflammation is thought to be mediated by immunopathogenetic mechanisms. Blood vessels of any type (e.g., arteries and veins) or size (e.g., large, medium, and small) may be involved, at any site or combination of sites (e.g., skin, kidney, and brain). Inflammation may be a primary process (primary angiitis) or a complication of another process, such as infection or carcinoma (secondary angiitis). Primary and widespread angiitis is called primary systemic angiitis (or vasculitides) (Savage et al., 2000; Hankey, 1998; Jenette and Falk, 1997). Definitive classification of systemic vasculitis is unsatisfactory since etiology and pathogenesis are rarely known and clinical and histologic features overlap (Table 15–4) (Savage et al., 2000).

Angiitis in the central nervous system (CNS) may therefore be restricted to the CNS (isolated angiitis) or associated with more widespread angiitis (systemic angiitis). It may also be primary or secondary (Table 15–5). Headache is a prominent symptom when inflammation affects head vessels either extracranially, as in temporal arteritis, or intracranially, as in CNS angiitis. Headache associated with temporal arteritis is due to inflammation of the involved arteries; it improves dramatically with steroid treatment. In CNS angiitis, the pathogenesis of the headache is multifactorial: inflammation, stroke

Table 15–4 Classification of systemic angiitis

- Large vessel angiitis
   Giant cell arteritis (temporal arteritis)
   Takayasu's arteritis
- Medium vessel angiitis
   Polyarteritis nodosa
   Kawasaki syndrome
- Small vessel angiitis
   With antineutrophil cytoplasmic antibodies
      Wegener's granulomatosis
      Microscopic polyangiitis (microscopic
         polyarteritis)
      Churg-Strauss syndrome
   Without antineutrophil cytoplasmic antibodies
      Henoch-Schönlein purpura
      Cryoglobulinemic vasculitis
      Isolated cutaneous leukocytoclastic vasculitis
      Goodpasture's disease

Table 15–5 Angiitis of the central nervous system

1. Primary angiitis of the CNS
2. Systemic angiitis with CNS involvement
3. Secondary angiitis due to
   - Infections (viral, bacterial, fungal, rickettsial, mycoplasmal, protozoal, etc.)
   - Connective tissue diseases and other systemic diseases (outside angiitis)
   - Drugs and toxics (sympathomimetics, cocaine, radiations, etc.)
   - Malignancies

(ischemic or hemorrhagic), elevated intracranial pressure, meningitis, or SAH. The beneficial effect of treatment is far less dramatic.

Of the many forms of angiitis listed in Tables 15–4 and 15–5, the most frequent cause of headache is giant cell arteritis (see Chapter 24). Headache is also a prominent symptom of CNS angiitis, whatever the cause. In this chapter, we concentrate on primary isolated angiitis of the CNS, a very rare, often misdiagnosed, but potentially treatable condition.

Primary Angiitis of the Central Nervous System

Primary angiitis of the CNS (PACNS) is also called noninfectious granulomatous angiitis, isolated angiitis, primary angiitis, and primary vasculitis of the CNS; it is a noninfectious granulomatous angiitis with a predilection for small (200 to 500 μ) leptomeningeal and intraparenchymal arteries of the CNS with no systemic involvement (Cravioto and Feigin, 1959). It is characterized by fibroid necrosis and infiltration of the vessel walls by lymphocytes, histiocytes, and/or multinucleated giant cells (Chu et al., 1998; Lie, 1992; Parisi and Moore, 1994).

The pathogenesis of PACNS is unknown. It may be due to an immunopathologic inflammatory reaction to an unknown antigen or disease. Numerous viral, bacterial, or mycotic agents have been suspected to cause the disorder (Calabrese and Mallek, 1987; Calabrese et al., 1997; Moore, 1989, 1994). A few cases have been reported in association with cerebral amyloid angiopathy (Gray et al., 1990; Fountain and Eberhard, 1996; Case

Records of the MGH, 2000), raising the possibility that the angiitis might, in part, represent a foreign body reaction to A4 amyloid deposition.

Primary angiitis of the CNS can occur at any age, with a slight preponderance in young adults. There is no sex preponderance.

Headache in Primary Angiitis of the Central Nervous System

Headache is the most frequent symptom of PACNS. It was present in 63% of the eight cases reported by Calabrese and Mallek (1987), in 50% of the ten cases reported by Chu et al. (1998), in 56% of the 40 cases reviewed by Calabrese, and in six of nine case reports published since 1998 (Case Records of the MGH, 2000; Börnke et al., 1999; Sudo and Tashiro, 1998; Berger et al., 1998; Kruisdijk and Vanneste, 1998; Masson et al., 1998; Reimer et al., 1999a,b). Headache frequency varies according to the diagnostic criteria used. Headache occurs in 56% of pathologically documented cases and in 78% of angiographically diagnosed cases (Calabrese et al., 1997). This reflects the more benign presentation of cases that are not pathologically documented and the inclusion of other disorders, such as benign angiopathy of the CNS (Calabrese et al., 1993).

Headache in PACNS has no specific pattern: it is variable in location (although most often diffuse), severity (from mild to excruciating), and temporal profile (from chronic to hyperacute, with occasional spontaneous remissions) (Calabrese et al., 1997). It can precede the onset of other neurologic symptoms by days or weeks, but it never remains isolated. Except for headache associated with stroke or SAH (Kumar et al., 1997), the exact mechanism remains undetermined.

Given its nonspecific characteristics, headache has very little positive diagnostic value. By contrast, CSF pleocytosis with no headache makes a diagnosis of PACNS less likely. In a study of 61 patients who underwent a brain biopsy for suspected PACNS, CSF pleocytosis and headache were the only features that differentiated patients with (36%) and without PACNS: of the nine patients who lacked CSF pleocytosis and headache, none had PACNS; of the 43 who had CSF pleocytosis and/or headache, 21 (49%) had PACNS. However, the presence of both pleocytosis and headache was not significantly associated with a PACNS-positive biopsy (Alrawi et al., 1999).

Other Signs

The fact that virtually any neurologic sign can be encountered reflects the wide distribution of CNS involvement: there can be focal neurologic deficits (motor, sensory, visual, aphasia), cerebellar signs, cranial nerve palsies, generalized or focal seizures, altered cognition, dementia, and disorders of consciousness. The mode of onset varies, from acute to slowly progressive. The mean duration of symptoms before diagnosis is 5 months, but many patients have much longer documented prodromal periods (Hankey, 1998; Cravioto and Feigin, 1959; Calabrese et al., 1997; Calabrese and Mallek, 1987; Moore, 1994).

Various multiple patterns of presentation occur in which headache may or may not be present: diffuse encephalopathy with decreased consciousness or subacute-onset dementia related to the involvement of multiple small arteries; focal cerebral syndromes with focal deficits and seizures, either of acute onset, related to an ischemic or hemorrhagic stroke, or of progressive onset, mimicking a mass lesion (Johnson et al., 1989; Valavanis et al., 1979); spinal cord syndromes (Caccamo et al., 1992), in which headache is usually absent.

Investigations

The diagnosis of PACNS is difficult because of its variable clinical manifestations and modes of onset and the absence of specific features, but a prompt diagnosis is important because the outcome may be fatal when treatment is delayed.

There is no consensus regarding the use of MRI, angiography, and leptomeningeal brain biopsy for the diagnosis of PACNS (Chu et al., 1998; Calabrese et al., 1992, 1997; Moore, 1989, 1994; Koo and Massey, 1988; Cupps et

al., 1983; Harris et al., 1994; Stone et al., 1994; Alhalabi and Moore, 1994; Vollmer et al., 1993).

Almost always, CT scan and MRI of the brain are abnormal in histologically documented cases, but the findings are nonspecific: multiple small T2 lesions in both gray and white matter are the most frequent findings; but hemorrhages, mass lesions, leptomeningeal enhancement, or even diffuse, extensive white matter lesions can be seen (Sudo and Tashiro, 1998; Berger et al., 1998; Cupps et al., 1983; Harris et al., 1994; Stone et al., 1994; Greenan et al., 1992; Ehsan et al., 1995; Finelli et al., 1997). Thus, CT and MRI are mainly useful to rule out other conditions and to guide eventual biopsy.

A CSF examination is crucial, but the findings are not specific: examination is abnormal in 80% to 90% of histologically diagnosed cases and in 50% to 53% of angiographically diagnosed cases (Calabrese et al., 1997; Moore, 1989, 1994). The findings usually reflect aseptic meningitis with a modest pleocytosis and elevated protein levels. The CSF analysis should include appropriate stains, cultures, and serologic tests for CNS infections that would point to a secondary CNS angiitis. Thus, CSF examination is essential to rule out other conditions and because of its negative predictive value when it is normal.

The role of angiography in the diagnosis of PACNS is debatable (Chu et al., 1998; Calabrese et al., 1993, 1997; Koo and Massey, 1988; Harris et al., 1994; Alhalabi and Moore, 1994; Vollmer et al., 1993; Greenan et al., 1992). Many cases have been diagnosed by angiography alone. However, the changes that are attributed to PACNS (alternating areas of stenosis and ectasia in multiple vascular distributions) occur in less than 40% to 50% of histologically proven cases (Chu et al., 1998; Calabrese et al., 1997), and more than 50% of patients with these classical changes have other conditions, such as distal atheroma or spasm (Chu et al., 1998; Calabrese et al., 1997). Thus, angiography, although useful, lacks sensitivity and specificity. Cases of PACNS diagnosed on angiography are different from those that have been confirmed histologically; they have a more benign presentation and a more benign outcome. Most likely, a number of cases of benign angiopathy of the CNS (BACNS) were included among angiitis cases that were diagnosed angiographically.

Histologic confirmation remains the gold standard for the diagnosis of PACNS. Brain biopsy is crucial to rule out other conditions that can mimic PACNS, such as lymphoproliferative diseases, certain infections, and sarcoidosis (Chu et al., 1998; Parisi and Moore, 1994; Calabrese et al., 1997); however, its sensitivity is poor since biopsies are negative in as many as 25% of autopsy-documented cases of PACNS (Calabrese et al., 1992). The yield of the biopsy is increased by sampling the leptomeninges as well as the underlying cortex in a lesion with gadolinium enhancement (Calabrese et al., 1997). Despite its morbidity (0.2% to 2% complication rate), biopsy is crucial before starting aggressive treatment.

Outcome and Treatment

Once thought to be uniformly fatal, PACNS has a variable prognosis; some acute cases lead to death in a few months, and others slowly progress with spontaneous remissions. In the absence of treatment, 80% of patients die in the first year and nearly 100% in 4 years (Hankey, 1998). There are no controlled trials of PACNS treatment. A small series (Cupps et al., 1983) suggested that aggressive combination of cyclophosphamide (3 to 5 mg/kg daily) and prednisone (1 mg/kg daily) was beneficial. This is the recommended treatment, although in some benign presentations with angiographic changes but no histologic confirmations, some would start with steroids alone (Calabrese et al., 1997).

Conclusion

Primary angiitis of the CNS is a rare, challenging neurologic disorder that is difficult to diagnose and treat and requires a rigorous diagnostic approach. The first step is to rule out conditions that can mimic PACNS clinically or at neuroimaging. The most difficult differential diagnosis is BACNS (see below). The second step is to rule out the many systemic diseases that can cause secondary angiitis of the CNS. If there is a high degree of suspicion of PACNS, a brain and meningeal biopsy is required before embarking on an aggressive immunosuppressive/steroid treatment.

BENIGN ANGIOPATHY OF THE CENTRAL NERVOUS SYSTEM AND POSTPARTUM CEREBRAL ANGIOPATHY

Benign angiopathy of the CNS is not a disease but a clinical angiographic syndrome characterized by the acute onset of headache and other neurologic signs and angiographically by reversible multiple segmental stenosis (Calabrese, 1999).

Similar symptoms have been reported under different names, such as isolated benign cerebral vasculitis (Snyder and McClelland, 1978), benign acute cerebral angiopathy (Michel et al., 1985), reversible cerebral segmental vasoconstriction (Call et al., 1988), CNS pseudovasculitis (Razavi et al., 1999), and nonaneurysmal thunderclap headache with diffuse, multifocal, segmental, reversible vasospasm (Dodick et al., 1999). Of these eponyms, the most widely used are BACNS and isolated benign cerebral vasculitis. However, neither of these is satisfactory since some cases are not benign and there was no evidence of vasculitis in the few cases that underwent biopsy (Call et al., 1988; Serdaru et al., 1984). The terms "reversible cerebral segmental vasoconstriction" and "reversible cerebral angiopathy" have the advantage of being purely descriptive, but they lack specificity since they include cases of angiitis, which may be reversible after treatment and the vasospasm that occurs after SAH.

The syndrome of headache with or without other neurologic signs and diffuse, reversible, segmental arterial narrowings also occurs after delivery and is called postpartum cerebral angiopathy (Rascol et al., 1980; Dupuy et al., 1979; Rousseaux et al., 1983; Bogousslavsky et al., 1989; Chartier et al., 1997; Comabella et al., 1996; Garner et al., 1990; Janssens et al., 1985; Gelford et al., 1967; Lucas et al., 1996; Raps et al., 1993a; Raroque et al., 1993;

Trommer et al., 1988; Ursell et al., 1998; Granier et al., 1999).

Headache is a constant feature of this syndrome. It is usually severe, diffuse, and pulsatile. It has an acute onset, reaching its maximum in minutes or hours; but it can also be extremely sudden, mimicking SAH or thunderclap headache (Dodick et al., 1999), or progressive over days or weeks (Call et al., 1988). The headache is usually nonremitting, but a few cases of a relapsing course over a few hours or days, with relapses occasionally triggered by emotional stress, physical exercise, or change in position, have been reported (Iglesias and Baron, 1994; Silbert et al., 1989).

Headache may be the only symptom of this syndrome, but it is usually associated with nausea and vomiting and frequently with other neurologic signs, such as phonophobia, photophobia, seizures, or focal deficits. These signs usually occur acutely within a few hours or days of headache onset, but they can be delayed or have a fluctuating course. Other signs include redness and sweating of the face and increased blood pressure (Michel et al., 1985).

The outcome is generally favorable, with full resolution of the headache and other neurologic signs in 2 weeks to 4 months (usually 1 month). Some of the cases that had the longest duration and residual neurologic signs were treated with steroids and may well have been true cases of CNS angiitis (Snyder and McClelland, 1978; Michel et al., 1985; Call et al., 1988).

In most reported cases, CSF in BACNS is usually normal (Calabrese, 1999); but reports of slight pleocytosis (Michel et al., 1985), mild increase in protein (Call et al., 1988), or even blood in the CSF (Iglesias and Baron, 1994; Roh and Park, 2000) exist. These abnormal findings suggest the diagnosis of angiitis and/or SAH.

Angiography is crucial to the diagnosis, although it may aggravate neurologic signs (Comabella et al., 1996). It typically shows diffuse, multifocal, segmental narrowings involving large and medium-sized arteries in the anterior and posterior circulations, with occasional dilated segments (like "sausage strings"). Cases with more localized abnormalities have been reported, particularly in the basilar territory (Lee et al., 2000). These segmental narrowings are not specific, and a similar angiographic appearance is seen in CNS angiitis (see above). Transcranial Doppler is extremely useful for the assessment and follow-up of this vasoconstriction (Bogousslavsky et al., 1989; Lee et al., 2000). By definition, arteries spontaneously normalize within a few days to several months.

The angiographic pattern of reversible, multifocal, segmental narrowings, which is the hallmark of this condition, is thought to be due to a widespread arterial vasoconstriction (spasm) that may be due to, or triggered by, a variety of substances or conditions, often but not always inducing acute hypertension. These include pheochromocytoma (Razavi et al., 1999; Armstrong and Hayes, 1961; McColl and Fraser, 1995), eclampsia (Raps et al., 1993a; Trommer et al., 1988; Will et al., 1987), sympathomimetic drugs (amphetamine) (Margolis and Newton, 1971), ephedrine (Mourand et al., 1999), phenylpropanolamine (Mueller, 1983; le Coz et al., 1988), isometheptene (Raroque et al., 1993), nicotine (Jackson, 1993), ergot alkaloid derivatives (particularly lisuride) (Roh and Park, 2000), bromocriptine when used to suppress lactation (Comabella et al., 1996; Janssens et al., 1985; Lucas et al., 1996), ergonovine (Barinagarrementeria et al., 1992b), other ergot derivatives (Henry et al., 1984; Senter et al., 1976), and sumatriptan [in association with cocaine in one case (Rousseaux et al., 1983) and with dihydroergotamine in another (Granier et al., 1999)]. Migrainous vasospasm has been suspected in a few cases (Serdaru et al., 1984; Lieberman et al., 1984; Schon and Harrison, 1987; Solomon et al., 1990), and in others, arterial changes have been attributed to thunderclap headache (Dodick et al., 1999); however, it may be that both migrainous headache and thunderclap headache were due to a reversible angiopathy of unknown origin. Some cases have been reported in which the onset of headache was triggered by physical exercise or sexual intercourse, suggesting a possible link between BACNS and exertional headache (Iglesias and Baron,

1994; Silbert et al., 1989; Kappor et al., 1990). Finally, in a number of cases, no cause or trigger factor is found; idiopathic cases are more frequent in young women, whether occurring postpartum or not (Calabrese, 1999; Snyder and McClelland, 1978; Michel et al., 1985; Call et al., 1988; Geraghty et al., 1991).

There is no accepted treatment for this condition: symptomatic treatment includes analgesics and nimodipine, with antiepileptic and antihypertensive drugs added on a case-by-case basis. The role of steroids is uncertain since these drugs may mask CNS angiitis and not be sufficient to treat it. Some prescribe steroids as soon as a diffuse vasoconstriction is found, while others prefer to delay steroid treatment as much as possible according to the clinical status and to raise the question of a brain biopsy if the patient worsens. This wait-and-see attitude particularly applies to cases in which a treatable cause or a precipitating factor (such as a drug) for BACNS is present. It also usually applies to postpartum angiopathy.

MIGRAINE AND STROKE

A close relationship between migraine and stroke has long been suspected. Over a century ago, Charcot insisted that "any of the symptoms occurring during—or associated with—'migraine ophthalmique' (migraine with visual aura) can persist for a variable length of time or even become permanent" (Féré, 1881). Fere himself reported ten cases of *migraine ophthalmique*; four of these patients had permanent neurologic deficits (hemianopia in three and aphasia in one). Two years later, Féré (1883) reported a case of *migraine ophthalmique à accès répétés et suivis de mort* (ophthalmic migraine with repeated attacks followed by death). Since childhood this "very distinguished 53-year-old barrister" had suffered typical attacks of migraine with ophthalmic and dysphasic aura. Beginning in early October 1882, he had recurrent attacks of left-sided headache, visual disturbances, right or left hemiplegia, seizures, and dysphasia; and he died 2 months later. There was no autopsy, but Féré (1883) thought that this patient died of "bilateral brain lesions due to the permanent constriction of supplying vessels."

Although this case might well have been a case of "symptomatic migraine" due, e.g., to an arteriovenous malformation, it is usually referred to as the first reported case of lethal migrainous stroke. Since then, numerous cases of "migrainous infarcts" have been reported, and this arterial complication of migraine has long been thought to summarize the relationship between migraine and stroke. Migraine was viewed as a purely vasospastic disorder, with arterial constriction and decreased cerebral blood flow during the aura and dilation during the headache. Sometimes the vasoconstriction was so severe that blood flow decreased below the threshold of ischemia, thus inducing a stroke designated as "migrainous infarct."

The diversity of migraine, the heterogeneity of stroke, and their complex relationships have been demonstrated. Neuronal factors have been identified in migraine (cortical spreading depression, the trigeminovascular system, the calcium channel gene), but it is still not established whether the neuronal or the vascular factors are primary. It is uncertain if migraine is a single entity, a syndrome, or a group of related disorders. Stroke includes intracerebral hemorrhage (20%) and infarction (80%). In infarction (ischemic stroke), there is a tremendous etiologic heterogeneity, the three main varieties being atherosclerosis (30%), small arterial diseases (20%), and cardiac emboli (20%). Some 100 other causes have been identified, but despite extensive investigations, the cause of stroke, particularly in the young, cannot be determined in up to 40% of cases.

Given the diversity and heterogeneity that characterize these two conditions, it is not surprising that their relationships are far more complex than the mere ischemic consequence of an unusually pronounced vasoconstriction (Bousser, 1999b; Bousser et al., 1985; Iglesias and Bousser, 1990; Welch et al., 1998a; Welch, 1994; Welch and Levine, 1990). Migraine is a risk factor and not just a cause for cerebral infarction. Cerebral ischemia can induce a migrainous aura, and it has even been suggested that "ischemia-induced migraine" might be more frequent than "migraine-induced ischemia." A number of conditions have both migraine attacks and ischemic strokes as part of their symptom complex. Therefore, when these two diseases coexist, particularly in young subjects, the possibility of a common underlying disorder should be considered.

Migrainous Infarction, Classical Description

Although a few cases of intracerebral hemorrhage have been reported in migraineurs (Cole and Aube, 1990; Dunning, 1942; Shuaib et al., 1989), there is no good evidence linking migraine and hemorrhagic stroke. By contrast, there is an abundant literature devoted to migrainous infarcts describing their incidence, anatomic features, clinical presentation, neuroimaging characteristics, and pathophysiology (Featherstone, 1986; Tatemichi and Mohr, 1992; Welch et al., 1998a; Welch and Levine, 1990; Bousser, 1999b; Bousser et al., 1985; Iglesias and Bousser, 1990).

In hospital-based studies of stroke in the young, migraine is said to be the cause of stroke in up to 27% of cases, and several hundred reports of "migrainous stroke" or "migrainous infarcts" have been published (Iglesias and Bousser, 1990; Welch et al., 1998a; Bogousslavsky et al., 1988). In the Oxfordshire Community Stroke Project, 7 (3%) of 244 first cerebral infarctions were reported to be due to migraine, corresponding to a yearly incidence of 3.36/100,000 and to an absolute number of 1,700 new cases of migrainous infarcts each year in the United Kingdom (Henrich et al., 1986). However, of the seven strokes attributed to migraine, only two had CT scan evidence of infarct, only one underwent cerebral angiography, only one had echocardiography, three were hypertensive, and one had severe widespread atheroma. It is wrong to consider these seven cases "migrainous infarcts" and to use them to calculate incidence rates.

A dozen cases of "fatal migraine" have been reported since Fere's (1883) report (Sinclair, 1959; Buckle et al., 1964; Guist and Woolf, 1964; Neligan et al., 1977; Selby and Gryer, 1984; Lindboe et al., 1989). It is remarkable that there was no single consistent pattern of infarction. Infarcts were large or small, single or multiple, and cortical or subcortical, and they involved the carotid and/or the basilar territories. There was no consistent pattern either of arterial changes: thrombosis, embolism, spasm, dissection, and normal arteries have been reported in these lethal cases of migraine.

Such inconsistency equally applies to the clinical descriptions of these infarcts. The most frequent clinical sign is a homonymous field defect such as hemianopia or hemianopic scotoma due to a posterior cerebral artery infarct. However, the clinical presentation is highly variable since migrainous infarcts have also been reported in the territories of all large arteries (middle cerebral, anterior cerebral, basilar) and of their branches. Single or multiple small infarcts affecting any cortical or subcortical structure have also been reported. All varieties of retinal infarcts as well as anterior or posterior ischemic neuropathies with unilateral loss of vision have also been described as a complication of retinal migraine.

This extreme diversity holds true for the neuroimaging findings in migrainous infarcts. Vasospasm during a migraine attack was documented on angiography by Dukes and Vieth in 1964. The patient was a 44-year-old man who had poor filling of the intracranial carotid system while experiencing a left hemianopia and numbness. During the headache phase that followed, there was again good filling of the internal carotid system. Other cases showed large- or small-artery occlusion. Besides spasm and occlusion, other abnormalities, such as dissections and aneurysms, have been reported; but they obviously raise the question of symptomatic migraine rather than migrainous infarcts (Rascol et al., 1979; Solomon et al., 1990). In most reported cases, angiography was normal (Garnic and Schellinger, 1983; Rascol et al., 1979; Masuzawa et al., 1983). Also, CT scan and MRI findings are remarkably diverse. While most cases have occipital infarcts, infarcts of any size and location, single or multiple, have been reported (Cala and Mastaglia, 1976; Hungerford et al., 1976; Rascol et al., 1979; Soges et al., 1988; Fazekas et al., 1992).

Given this wide variety of infarct types and arterial changes, no single mechanism can account for every case (Welch et al., 1998a). The prevailing idea was that of a primarily vascular mechanism, such as spasm (Dukes and Vieth, 1964; Solomon et al., 1990); vessel wall hyperplasia, as in the lethal case reported by Neligan et al. (1977); embolism, as suggested in a number of cases of sudden onset in the absence of arterial wall disease (Rascol et al., 1979); or local arterial dissection (Sinclair, 1959). As a result of the arterial change, focal ischemia ensued, leading to an infarct. This is not consistent with cerebral blood flow (CBF) (Olesen et al., 1981; Lauritzen et al., 1983), PET (Woods et al., 1994), and functional MRI (Welch et al., 1998b; Cutrer et al., 1998) techniques, which have shown that the maximum decrease in CBF is 37%. This is well above the threshold associated with ischemic injury (>50%) and is not accompanied by a decrease in diffusion (Cutrer et al., 1998; Sanchez-del Rio et al., 1999). Neuronal spreading depression is associated with oligemia and may play a role in migraine aura, but its relationship to migrainous infarcts is unclear.

Acute or prophylactic medication was suspected to play a role in some cases by acting as an aggravating factor for the mechanisms that lead to stroke. Ergotamine was a suspect, even though, in therapeutic doses, it usually has no effect on CBF (Lindboe et al., 1989). Strokes have been reported in patients taking sumatriptan, but the drug was usually given for a wrong indication, such as CVT with migraine-like symptoms (Cavazos et al., 1994). β-Blockers have been associated with some migrainous infarcts (Bardwell and Trott, 1987). Although there are no firm data supporting a link between β-blockers and migrainous infarcts, some experts believe that this pharmacologic class of drugs should be avoided in migraine with prolonged aura because it may increase the frequency and duration of attacks.

Cerebral angiography, a well-known inducer of migraine attacks, might trigger cerebral ischemia. In large series of carotid angiographies, there was a 1% risk of stroke. This risk is not higher in migraineurs (Shuaib and Hachinski, 1988), but the risk of angiography is higher in patients with familial hemiplegic migraine; it can precipitate dramatic attacks leading to stroke (Harrison, 1981).

Migrainous Infarction is Overdiagnosed

What has been reported as "migrainous infarct" is nothing more than a potpourri of a variety of conditions, such as strokes occurring in migraineurs, strokes with migrainous features in non-migraineurs, sometimes any stroke with headache, or even no stroke but a long-lasting deficit in migraine with aura. This is clearly due to a total lack of consistency, not only in the definition of migrainous infarct but also in the definition of migraine itself and sometimes that of stroke.

The classification proposed in 1988 by the IHS has clarified this issue by suggesting a restricted definition that includes four major criteria: (1) the patient previously had a migraine with aura; (2) the present attack is typical of previous attacks, which means that the symptoms of the infarct are, at least partly, those of the aura; (3) neurologic deficits are not completely reversible within 7 days and/or neuroimaging demonstrates ischemic infarction in relevant area; (4) other causes of infarction are ruled out by appropriate investigations.

This definition is a major improvement, although the 7-day rule is objectionable since it leads to the inclusion of cases with long-lasting deficits without cerebral infarction (see below). The crucial issue is the need for appropriate investigations to rule out other causes of cerebral infarction: which investigations and when should they be performed? We performed an extensive review of over 200 cases of migrainous infarcts reported before 1988. When we applied IHS criteria, requiring minimum "appropriate investigations" [transthorasic echocardiography (TTE) and cerebral angiogaphy (any variety)], the number of migrainous infarcts dramatically shrank to 40 (Iglesias and Bousser, 1990). This would further decrease if blood tests such as anti-phospholipid antibodies (APLs) were required as "appropriate investigations." The absence of another cause does not imply, by default, that migraine is the cause. Half of all cases of ischemic stroke in the young have no detectable, undisputable cause, and sometimes years later another potential cause is detected (Mas et al., 1986; Bousser et al., 1980; Tourbah et al., 1988). Always be reluctant to diagnose a migrainous infarction, even after an extensive negative etiologic workup. There are, however, documented cases that satisfy IHS criteria and occur in the absence of other causes, even after a long follow-up. One illustrative case (Polyak, 1957) is that of the pathologist Frank Mallory who, at age 47, suffered one of his typical attacks of migraine with a scintillating scotoma in the left visual field. Instead of totally recovering as usual, he was left with an upper left quadrant defect. He died 30 years later and, at autopsy, his co-worker, Polyak, found an old, small infarct confined to the right lower calcarine lip, without arterial disease or any other cause.

Migrainous infarcts exist, but they are rare and vastly overdiagnosed (Bousser, 1999b; Bousser et al., 1985; Fisher, 1986; Iglesias and Bousser, 1990; Welch, 1994; Welch and Levine, 1990; Varelas et al., 1999). Until we have specific diagnostic tools for migraine, it is good clinical practice to use restrictive criteria so as not to overlook other potentially treatable causes. The following criteria are suggested:

1. A documented infarct, not just a long-lasting deficit
2. Occurs during an attack of migraine with aura
3. Subject has a history of migraine with aura
4. Characterized clinically by the persistence of all or some of the symptoms of the aura
5. Another cause ruled out after extensive and repeated etiologic investigations, including at least ultrasound studies, angiography (MRA or conventional), TTE (and preferably transesophageal) and antiphospholipid antibodies (APL)

Migrainous infarcts so defined frequently involve the posterior cerebral artery (PCA) territory and are likely to be due to an unusually severe hypoperfusion during the aura, the precise mechanism of which remains unknown.

Migraine as a Risk Factor for Stroke

The issue of migraine as a risk factor for stroke has been addressed in two cohort (Buring et al., 1995; Merikangas et al., 1997) and seven case-control (Collaborative Group for the Study of Stroke in Young Women, 1975; Henrich and Horowitz, 1989; Tzourio et al., 1993, 1995; Tzourio et al., 1995; Lidegaard, 1995; Carolei et al., 1996; Chang et al., 1999) studies. In the Physicians Health Study (Buring et al., 1995) and the National Health and Nutrition Examination Survey (NHANES) study (Merikangas et al., 1997), the risk of ischemic stroke was slightly more than doubled in subjects with migraine. These studies suffer major shortcomings in the diagnosis of both migraine and stroke, but they have less potential bias due to selection of a control group and the assessment of migraine before stroke. The five most recent case-control studies, summarized in Table 15–6, suggest that migraine is a risk factor for ischemic stroke in young women, with a relative risk (RR) of around 3 (Tzourio et al., 1993, 1995; Lidegaard, 1995; Carolei et al., 1996; Chang et al., 1999). The risk is higher in migraine with aura, with RRs ranging from 4 (Chang et al., 1999) to 6 (Tzourio et al., 1995) to 9 (Carolei et al., 1996). It is markedly increased by smoking (RR = 10) and by oral contraceptive (OC) use (RR = 16) (Tzourio et al., 1995; Chang et al., 1999). These risk factors seem to have more than an additive effect since the odds ratio for ischemic stroke in young female migraineurs who take OCs and smoke reaches 34.4 (95% confidence interval 3.27–361) (Chang et al., 1999).

The absolute risk of stroke, which is normally low in young women, increases with increased RR. Therefore, young migrainous women should be considered a target group for stroke prevention. Other vascular risk factors and potential protective factors need to be considered. Blood pressure should be con-

Table 15–6 Association between migraine and stroke in young women: recent case-control studies

Study	Patients	Diagnosis of migraine	Risk of stroke in migraine patients
Tzourio et al. (1993)	212 patients aged 15 to 80 years with ischemic stroke 212 hospitalized controls matched for sex, age, and history of hypertension	Direct interview by neurologists, IHS criteria	OR = 4.3 (1.2–16.3) in women <45 years
Tzourio et al. (1995)	72 women aged 15 to 44 years and hospitalized for an ischemic stroke 173 hospitalized controls matched for age	Direct interview by neurologists, IHS criteria	MWA: OR = 3.0 (1.5–5.8) MA: OR = 6.2 (2.11–18.0)
Lidegaard (1995)	692 women aged 15 to 44 years in a national registry of ischemic stroke 1,584 population-based controls matched for age	Questionnaire	OR = 2.8 (p < 0.001)
Carolei et al. (1996)	308 patients aged 15 to 44 years and hospitalized for transient ischemic attack or stroke 591 hospitalized controls	Direct interview by neurologists, IHS criteria	OR = 3.7 (1.5–9) in women <35 years MA: OR 8.6 (1–75)
Chang et al. (1999)	291 women aged 20–44 with stroke 736 age- and hospital-matched controls	Questionnaire, modified IHS criteria	OR = 3.5 (1.3–9.6) MWA: OR = 2.9 (0.6–13.5) MA: OR = 3.8 (1.2–11.5)

Key to abbreviations: IHS, International Headache Society; OR, odds ratio (95% confidence interval); MWA, migraine without aura; MA, migraine with aura.

trolled, and other diseases (hyperlipemia, diabetes, familial thrombophilia) that might increase the risk of stroke should be searched for and appropriately treated when present.

Some specialists consider migraine with aura to be an absolute contraindication to OC use (Steiner et al., 1998). We believe that a less rigid position can be taken for two reasons. First, OC use has obvious benefits for many young women. Second, there is a low absolute risk of stroke, provided that migrainous women (even those with auras) who take the pill do not smoke. Smoking, not OC use, is the single most important modifiable stroke risk factor in the young. If OCs are used, low estrogen-content pills or even progestin-alone pills should be advised, particularly for women who have migraine with aura (Becker, 1999). We discourage OC use only for older women who have migraine with aura or for patients who develop new aura symptoms while taking OCs (Bousser, 1999a; Becker, 1999).

We do not favor the systematic use of daily aspirin for stroke prevention because of the increased risk of gastric ulcers and bleeding (particularly intracranially) and because of its lack of efficacy in primary stroke prevention (Antiplatelet Trialists' Collaboration, 1994; Olesen et al., 1993b). We only recommend aspirin for the rare patients who have very frequent attacks of migraine with aura, more for its preventive effect on migraine itself (Buring et al., 1990) than for stroke prevention. Regular physical activity, which has been shown to decrease the risk of stroke, and other protective measures should be encouraged (Shinton and Sagar, 1993; Abbott et al., 1994).

In contrast to young women, there is no strong evidence that migraine is a risk factor in older age groups. Data from the Framingham cohort based on 2,100 subjects examined during 1971–1989 confirm this. Visual migrainous auras were present in 1.23% and began at a mean age of 56.2 ± 18.7 years. In contrast to subjects with transient ischemic attacks (TIAs), those with migrainous visual accompaniments had no increased risk of stroke compared to subjects without either

TIAs or migrainous visual accompaniments (Wijman et al., 1998).

How migraine increases the risk of ischemic stroke in young women is unknown. Migraine is not associated with an increase in the major conventional risk factors for ischemic stroke (Launer et al., 1999), but conflicting reports suggest an association with equivocal or newly suggested risk factors, such as mitral valve prolapse (Welch et al., 1998a), patent foramen ovale (del Sette et al., 1998), hereditary thrombophilia (D'Amico et al., 1998), particularly factor V Leiden mutation (Kontula et al., 1995; Haan et al., 1997; Sorani et al., 1998), or increased platelet aggregation (Couch and Hassanein, 1977). Up to 40% of strokes in migrainous women are reported to be migrainous infarcts (Chang et al., 1999), but this was found only in the recent WHO study (Chang et al., 1999), which failed to use strict criteria to define migrainous infarcts. In other case-control studies, the increased risk of ischemic stroke was not explained by the occurrence of migrainous infarcts. A possible link between migraine and cerebral infarction is cervical artery dissection. In a number of cases of so-called migrainous infarcts, a carotid narrowing was seen at angiography; this was interpreted as spasm but was strikingly similar to the characteristic "string sign" of carotid dissection (Bousser et al., 1986; Shuaib, 1991). In one case-control study, migraine was a risk factor for dissection (d'Anglejan-Chatillon et al., 1989). The association between migraine and dissection needs further study.

Differential Diagnosis: Migraine Auras or Transient Ischemic Attacks?

Transient ischemic attacks and migraine auras are characterized by temporary focal neurologic deficits that usually last less than 1 hour. By definition, TIAs are related to ischemia, as indicated by the fact that up to 40% of TIAs that last less than 24 hours reveal a small infarct on CT or MRI. By contrast, migraine auras are not ischemic. Recent MRI studies have shown a decrease in regional perfusion and cerebral blood volume but no change in water diffusion during the aura, suggesting a primary neuronal dysfunction underlying the hypoperfusion (Cutrer et al., 1998). The distinction between migraine aura and a TIA is crucial because TIAs are well-established warning signs of stroke, particularly atherothrombotic stroke (Fisher, 1968, 1971, 1980).

The distinction between migraine aura and TIA, based exclusively on the patient's description of the symptoms, is easy when symptoms are typical. Symptoms of the migraine aura progress gradually over several minutes or occur in succession, last around 30 minutes, and are often followed by a severe, throbbing, unilateral headache associated with phonophobia, photophobia, nausea, or vomiting. A TIA is characterized by a focal deficit of sudden onset that lasts, by definition, less than 24 hours but typically lasts less than 15 minutes. Migraine with aura often starts in childhood, whereas TIAs are usually late-life events. However, migraine auras can occur for the first time after 40 years of age, headache can occasionally be absent, and TIAs, particularly basilar TIAs, can sometimes be associated with headache. The crucial distinctive feature is the mode of onset (Fisher, 1968, 1971). In 68 patients with migraine, there was a typical "migrainous march" with slow progression of symptoms in 52 cases; this progression was always absent in 57 cases of posterior cerebral artery occlusion and in 40 cases of pure sensory stroke. A distinctive feature of the migraine aura is the presence of "positive" phenomena, such as fortifications, scintillations, flashes, or flickering spots. A typical scintillating scotoma is not produced by a TIA. However, a migraine aura can be limited to a hemianopia, and if this hemianopia is of sudden onset and not followed by headache, it is indistinguishable from a TIA (Fisher, 1968, 1971, 1980; Martsen et al., 1990; Bousser et al., 1980; Caplan, 1991). Since migraine auras can thus be mistaken for TIAs, studies that have mixed TIAs in with stroke to evaluate the frequency of migraine in stroke subjects are likely to have introduced a bias in favor of migraine.

The same difficulty arises in the differentiation of "retinal migraine" from transient monocular blindness (TMB). Fisher (1971) has commented on the frequency of positive phenomena in migraine and their rarity in embolic TMB. Since retinal migraine is a rare, poorly defined entity, all patients with transient unilateral visual disturbances should have a full ophthalmologic, neurologic, and vascular workup (Troost and Tomsak, 1993). This also applies in all cases of migraine aura that cannot be differentiated from TIA. If no vascular cause is found, long-term aspirin use should be considered since it is effective for migraine prophylaxis and secondary stroke prevention.

Differential Diagnosis: Migrainous Infarction or Prolonged Migrainous Deficits Without Infarcts

Migrainous infarcts should be differentiated from very long-lasting deficits that can occur after a migrainous attack without CT scan or MRI evidence of infarcts and with complete recovery. This has been documented in migraine with aura (Marchioni et al., 1995), particularly in familial hemiplegic migraine (FHM), an autosomal dominant variety of migraine with aura in which hemiplegia, often associated with aphasia, hemianopia, drowsiness, and sometimes coma, can last up to several weeks and then resolve without sequelae (Whitty, 1953; Harrison, 1981; Baron et al., 1983; Fitzsimons and Wolfenden, 1985; Mtinte and Miiler-Vahl, 1990; Joutel et al., 1993). During severe attacks of FHM that mimic a massive middle cerebral artery infarction, there is major swelling of the hemisphere and severe electroencephalographic (EEG) disturbances (Harrison, 1981; Baron et al., 1983). In one case, PET showed a diffuse metabolic depression with a relative increase in CBF, a major decrease in oxygen extraction fraction, and a moderate decrease in the cerebral metabolic rate of oxygen ($CMRO_2$) (Baron et al., 1983). This pattern is not that of an infarct; it is a unique example of a severe neuronal dysfunction with a preserved $CMRO_2$. Another case recently studied by magnetic resonance diffusion-weighted imaging (MR-DWI) showed extensive restricted diffusion in the white matter of the left hemisphere during a prolonged attack characterized by right hemiplegia, aphasia,

and hemianopia (Soman et al., 1999). Abnormalities on DWI completely resolved on day 9, and the patient recovered in 3 weeks. This transient DWI decrease is very different from what is observed in ischemic stroke, and it may represent abnormal energy metabolism in the affected hemisphere during the attack. These cases demonstrate that very long-lasting deficits can occur in migraine without cerebral infarction and that the time limit of 7 days suggested by the IHS classification (Headache Classification Committee of the International Headache Society, 1988) is far too short. Whether these long-lasting deficits are specifically related to the involvement of the calcium channel gene CACNA1A, implicated in 50% of FHM families, or to other genes remains to be determined (Joutel et al., 1993; Ophoff et al., 1994; Ducros et al., 1997).

Ischemia-Induced Migraine

The idea that stroke can induce migraine was proposed by Olesen et al. (1993a), who suggested that "ischemia-induced symptomatic migraine attacks may be more frequent than migraine-induced ischemic insults." They described a few cases of ischemic stroke causing single or recurrent attacks of migraine with aura and a few other cases of severe carotid stenosis or occlusion with decreased CBF causing a flurry of attacks of migraine with aura. Two of these cases had carotid dissection, which is a great mimic of so-called migrainous infarction (Bousser et al., 1986; Shuaib, 1991; Biousse et al., 1994). The possible triggering of an attack of migraine with aura by focal ischemia is further supported by animal studies showing that cerebral ischemia can induce cortical spreading depression. Attacks of symptomatic migraine with aura can be triggered by acute focal ischemia, but there is no evidence that migraine can be the consequence of cerebral ischemia.

Migraine and Stroke Sharing a Common Cause

There are a number of conditions, local and general, that can cause stroke and are associated with a high frequency of migraine. The most classical local cause is arteriovenous malformation (AVM), which has long been thought to be a cause of migraine (symptomatic migraine) (Waltimo et al., 1975; Bruyn, 1984). The situation is not clear because of the lack of large-scale, well-conducted case-control studies and because of the unpredictable effect AVM treatment has on migraine. There are well-documented cases of migraine attacks satisfying all IHS criteria that stopped after AVM removal (Troost et al., 1979), but there are equally well-documented cases of attacks that persisted unchanged after surgery (Haas, 1991). An argument in favor of a causal relationship is the overwhelming correlation between the side of the aura (contralateral to the AVM) and the headache (ipsilateral) and the side of the AVM. Haas (1991), in a review of the literature, found that only one patient out of 15 experienced aura ipsilateral to the malformation and one out of 11 had unilateral headache contralateral to the AVM. This suggests that AVM can trigger attacks of migraine, particularly migraine with aura. By contrast, the relation of migraine to saccular aneurysm remains poorly substantiated, provided that thunderclap headache (Day and Raskin, 1986) and sentinel headache (Ostergaard, 1991) are not mistaken for migraine. A number of other local conditions can manifest themselves as stroke and/or more or less typical migraine attacks: leptomeningeal angiomatosis of the Sturge-Weber type (Cambon et al., 1987; Chabriat et al., 1996; Klapper, 1994); lymphocytic meningitis, which always raise the question of migraine attacks with pleiocytosis (Fitzsimons and Wolfenden, 1985); and some rare cases of CVT (Newman et al., 1989).

Many general conditions are also characterized by both migraine attacks, most commonly with aura, and ischemic strokes: essential thrombocytemia (Bousser et al., 1980), thrombocytopenia (Damasio and Beck, 1978), leukemia (Geller and Wen, 1995), systemic lupus erythematosus (Isenberg et al., 1982), antiphospholipid antibodies syndrome (Tietjen et al., 1992; Levine et al., 1990), hereditary hemorrhagic telangiectasia (Steele et al., 1993), and mitochondrial cytopathies

(Pavlakis et al., 1984; Andermann et al., 1986; Klopstock et al., 1996; Koo et al., 1993; Ojaimi et al., 1998). Stroke and migraine are major features of the syndrome of mitochondrial encephalopathy, lactic acidosis, and stroke-like episodes (MELAS), which is associated with the 3243 point mitochondrial DNA mutation in the tRNA *Leu* (UUR) gene. The frequency of migraine attacks with this condition has led to the hypothesis that mitochondrial mutations could play a role in migraine with aura and in "migrainous stroke," but the 3243 mutation was not detected in two groups of subjects with migraine with aura (Klopstock et al., 1996; Ojaimi et al., 1998). However, other mutations that have not yet been detected on this huge gene could play a role in both migraine and ischemic stroke.

Cerebral Autosomal Dominant Arteriopathy with Subcortical Infarcts and Leukoencephalopathy

Cerebral autosomal dominant arteriopathy with subcortical infarcts and leukoencephalopathy (CADASIL) is a condition that can cause migraine and stroke. In 1993, we suggested this acronym to designate an autosomal dominant, small-artery disease of the brain that is characterized clinically by recurrent, small, deep infarcts; subcortical dementia; mood disturbances; and migraine with aura (Tournier-Lasserve et al., 1991, 1993; Baudrimont et al., 1993; Chabriat et al., 1995). When CADASIL is present, migraine is usually the first symptom of the disease, appearing at a mean age of 30, some 15 years before the first ischemic stroke. Symptoms of migraine correspond clinically to those defined as migraine with aura by the IHS, with an unusual frequency of attacks with prolonged aura and attacks of acute-onset aura without headache that are sometimes indistinguishable from TIAs (Tournier-Lasserve et al., 1991; Chabriat et al., 1995). However, MRI in CADASIL is always abnormal, showing striking white matter abnormalities on T2-weighted images and, later in the disease, small subcortical areas of hyposignal on T1-weighted images suggestive of small, deep infarcts. These abnormalities should not be interpreted just as white matter changes related to migraine, which have been reported to be particularly frequent in migraine with aura (Igarashi et al., 1991; Pavese et al., 1994). The finding of white matter abnormalities in subjects who suffer from migraine with aura and have a family history of stroke or dementia is suggestive of CADASIL. In some families, however, the migraine phenotype may be preponderant, leading to greater diagnostic difficulties (Chabriat et al., 1995; Verin et al., 1995). The CADASIL gene has now been identified as *Notch3*. The mutations are remarkably stereotyped (missense mutations leading to an unpaired number of cysteine residues) and clustered within the epidermal growth factor (EGF)-like repeats, mostly in the extracellular domain of exons 3 and 4. This allows a diagnostic test that detects the pathogenic mutation in about 75% of subjects with a clinical and MRI pattern suggestive of CADASIL (Joutel et al., 1996, 1997). This disease, the effects of which include changes in small cerebral and leptomeningeal arteries, is a fascinating model, enabling one to speculate about the relationships between migraine with aura and ischemic stroke. It is unlikely that migraine is the consequence of ischemia since the infarcts are subcortical, whereas the visual aura typically points to the occipital lobe. In addition, infarcts occur some 15 to 20 years after the onset of migraine. Both migraine and ischemic stroke might be due to the arteriopathy itself. At an early stage, activation of smooth-muscle cells may be responsible for migraine; at a later stage, destruction of smooth-muscle cells with thickening of the arterial wall may be responsible for stroke. A third hypothesis would be that the arteriopathy causes the ischemic strokes but migraine is directly due to *Notch3* alterations, which might modulate the calcium channel gene involved in migraine. This is totally speculative, but an understanding of the exact role of *Notch3* mutations might be crucial for the elucidation of the pathogenesis of migraine with aura and of the migraine–stroke connection.

Thus, there are many local or general conditions that can induce both migraine ("symptomatic migraine") and stroke. These conditions should always be carefully looked for when a migrainous subject suffers a stroke, particularly at a young age and in the absence of an obvious cause or of the classical vascular risk factors.

Therapeutic Implications

Young female migraineurs should be considered as a target group for stroke prevention, and smoking should be discouraged. There is no general contraindication for OC use in migraine without aura, but caution is required in migraine with aura (see above).

There are no data to suggest that migraine prophylaxis decreases the risk of migrainous infarcts. For the acute treatment of migraine attacks, there is a case, particularly in migraine with aura, for trying analgesics and nonsteroidal anti-inflammatory drugs before turning to ergot derivatives and triptans, which are ineffective when taken during the aura and should be used only during the headache phase of migraine.

There is no specific treatment for migrainous infarcts. The treatment and the investigations should be those of any cerebral infarct in the young, according to its severity and presumed mechanism. After the infarct, the usual measures of secondary stroke prevention should be taken: cessation of OCs, cessation of smoking, daily use of antiplatelet drugs such as aspirin (Antiplatelet Trialists' Collaboration, 1994) or clopidogrel (CAPRIE Steering Committee, 1996), and regular monitoring of blood pressure, glycemia, and cardiac status. Some would avoid persantine because headache is a major side effect; others might use it. Ergot derivatives and triptans should not be used for migraine treatment after a cerebral infarct. Preventive treatment may be unnecessary because of aspirin's prophylactic effect on migraine.

In conclusion, migrainous infarcts (i.e., infarcts due to a severe attack of migraine with aura in the absence of other causes) are extremely rare and should be diagnosed only by exclusion. The workup and treatment should be identical to that for stroke in nonmigraineurs. The debate over the risk of angiography, which was not increased in migraineurs (Shuaib and Hachinski, 1988) except in those with FHM (Chabriat et al., 1995), is now moot because of the widespread use of ultrasound and MRA. Many conditions, such as prolonged aura symptoms and ischemia-induced migraine attacks, can mimic migrainous infarcts; and other conditions, such as AVM, mitochondrial cytopathies, and CADASIL, can induce both ischemic stroke and migraine attacks. Migraine, particularly migraine with aura, is an established risk factor for ischemic stroke in young women, through an unknown mechanism. Young migrainous women thus constitute an important target group for stroke prevention and should strongly be advised not to smoke.

ARTERIAL HYPERTENSION

Hypertension is the sustained elevation of diastolic blood pressure at or above 90 mm Hg or a systolic blood pressure at or above 140 mm Hg. It is estimated that 10% to 20% of the population is hypertensive and the association with headache is usually coincidental.

Headache may be associated with hypertension in several ways. First, headache is associated with acute or severe hypertension. Second, there may be a reactive rise in blood pressure in response to severe pain, including headache. Third, headache may be a side effect of antihypertensive treatment, particularly rapid-acting calcium antagonists (Abernethy and Schwartz, 1999).

Headache was believed to be associated with hypertension across the entire range of blood pressure (Walker, 1959). However, reports such as this may be due to *Berkson's bias*, the observation that individuals who seek medical care are more likely to have a high rate of concordance of two medical conditions, which may be independent in the general population (Berkson, 1946). Even general population studies, based on self-report of physician-diagnosed hypertension and migraine (Merikangas et al., 1997), are susceptible to this bias. In the Physicians Health Study (Buring et al., 1995), where a uniformly high degree of medical care would

be expected, there was no association between migraine and hypertension. In support of this position, studies based on representative population samples and actual blood pressure measurements have not shown an association of blood pressure level with headache (Waters, 1971; Weiss, 1972). In a Danish population study, no difference was found in migraine or tension-type headache prevalence in hypertensives compared with controls (Rasmussen and Olesen, 1992). However, these studies have not included sufficient numbers of persons with severe hypertension (Janeway, 1913) to allow detection of threshold effects.

Pathophysiology

Several mechanisms may contribute to headache in severe hypertension as listed in the IHS classification (Strandgaard and Henry, 1993). Headache may be caused by hypertensive dilation of resistance vessels. For example, in one study published before the advent of modern antihypertensives, IV injection of aminophylline, a cerebral vasocontrictor, as well as caffeine into severely hypertensive patients caused immediate relief of headache (Moyer et al., 1952). Another mechanism for hypertensive headache, particularly in the context of malignant hypertension (Chester et al., 1978) or eclampsia, is the failure of autoregulation and the development of raised intracranial pressure.

Main Patterns of Presentation and Headache Characteristics

Based on a literature review and clinical experience, the IHS detailed diagnostic criteria for four subgroups of headache associated with severe hypertension (Headache Classification Committee of the International Headache Society, 1988):

1. Acute pressor response to exogenous agent
   A. Headache occurs with acute rise (>25%) of diastolic blood pressure
   B. Evidence of appropriate toxin or medication

C. Headache disappears within 24 hours after normalization of blood pressure

2. Pheochromocytoma

A. Headache occurs with acute rise (>25%) of diastolic blood pressure

B. At least one of the following:
   (1) Sweating
   (2) Palpitation
   (3) Anxiety

C. Pheochromocytoma proved by biologic upon imaging tests or surgery

D. Headache disappears within 24 hours after normalization of blood pressure

3. Malignant (accelerated) hypertension (including hypertensive encephalopathy)

A. Headache associated with grade 3 or 4 retinopathy

B. Diastolic blood pressure persistently above 120 mm Hg

C. Appropriate investigations rule out vasopressor toxins, medication, and pheochromocytoma as causative factors

D. Headache is temporally related to rise in blood pressure and disappears within 2 days after reduction of blood pressure; if hypertensive encephalopathy is present, headache may persist for up to 7 days after reduction of blood pressure.

4. Pre-eclampsia and eclampsia

A. Headache during pregnancy

B. Edema or proteinuria and blood pressure rise from prepregnant level (not necessarily markedly increased but at least a mean elevation of 15 mm Hg or diastolic of 90 mm Hg)

C. Appropriate investigations rule out vasopressor toxins, medication, and pheochromocytoma as causative factors

D. Headache occurs with rise in blood pressure and disappears within 7 days after blood pressure reduction or after termination of pregnancy.

The classic description of hypertensive headache (Janeway, 1913; Moser et al., 1962) is one which appears on wakening or wakes the patient during the early morning hours, has its greatest intensity before arising, and tends to subside over hours. The most frequent location was frontal or occipital. Other headache characteristics, such as frontal or occipital location or throbbing quality, were less consistent. Brief duration has been described as an important feature of pheochromocytoma-associated headaches (Raskin and Appenzeller, 1980).

Treatment

The treatment of headache due to markedly or acutely elevated blood pressure is blood pressure reduction. If the headache is not due to another coincident cause, it should be relieved within 24 hours of treatment, although headache may persist for several days in cases of hypertensive encephalopathy (Strandgaard and Henry, 1993).

REFERENCES

Abbott, R.D., B.L. Rodriguez, C.M. Burchfiel et al. (1994). Physical activity in older middle-aged men and reduced risk of stroke: The Honolulu Heart Program. *Am. J. Epidemiol. 139*:881–893.

Abernethy, D.R. and J.B. Schwartz (1999). Drug therapy: Calcium-antagonist drugs. *N. Engl. J. Med. 34*:1447–1457.

Adams, H.P., T.G. Brott, R.M. Crowell et al. (1994). Guidelines for the management of patients with acute ischemic stroke. A statement for healthcare professionals from a special writing group of the Stroke Council, American Heart Association. *Circulation 90*:1588–1601.

Adams, H.P., T.G. Brott, A.J. Furlan et al. (1996). Guidelines for thrombolytic therapy for acute stroke: A supplement to the guidelines for the management of patients with acute ischemic stroke. A statement for healthcare professionals from a special writing group of the Stroke Council, American Heart Association. *Circulation 94*:1167–1174.

Adams, H.P., D.D. Jergenson, N.F. Kassell et al. (1980). Pitfalls in the recognition of subarachnoid hemorrhage. *JAMA 244*:794–796.

Aidi, S., M.P. Chaunu, V. Biousse et al. (1999). Changing pattern of headache pointing to cerebral venous thrombosis after lumbar puncture and intravenous high dose corticosteroids. *Headache 39*:559–564.

Albers, G.W., M.G. Lansberg, A.M. Norbash et al. (2000). Yield of diffusion-weighted MRI for detection of potentially relevant findings in stroke patients. *Neurology 54*:1562–1567.

Alhalabi, M. and P.M. Moore (1994). Serial angiography in isolated angiitis of the central nervous system. *Neurology* 44:1221–1226.

Alrawi, A., J.D. Trobe, M. Blaivas et al. (1999). Brain biopsy in primary angiitis of the central nervous system. *Neurology* 53:858–860.

Ameri, A. and M.G. Bousser (1992). Cerebral venous thrombosis. *Neurol. Clin.* 10:87–111.

Andermann, F., E. Lugaresi, G.S. Dvorkin et al. (1986). Malignant migraine: The syndrome of prolonged classical migraine, epilepsia partialis continua, and repeated strokes: A clinically characteristic disorder probably due to mitochondrial encephalopathy. *Funct. Neurol.* 1: 481–486.

Andreoli, A., G. Dipasquale, G. Pinelli et al. (1987). Subarachnoid hemorrhage: Frequency and severity of cardiac arrhythmias. A survey of 70 cases studied in the acute phase. *Stroke* 18: 558–564.

Antiplatelet Trialists' Collaboration (1994). Prevention of death, myocardial infarction, and stroke by prolonged antiplatelet therapy in various categories of patients. Collaborative review of randomized trials of antiplatelet therapy. *BMJ* 308:81–106.

Arboix, A., J. Massons, M. Oliveres et al. (1994). Headache in acute cerebrovascular disease: A prospective clinical study in 240 patients. *Cephalalgia* 14:37–40.

Armstrong, F.S. and G.J. Hayes (1961). Segmental cerebral arterial constriction associated with pheochromocytoma. *J. Neurosurg.* 18:843–846.

Ausman, J.I., F.G. Diaz, G.M. Malik et al. (1989). Management of cerebral aneurysms: Further facts and additional myths. *Surg. Neurol.* 32:21–35.

Bardwell, A. and J. Trott (1987). Stroke in migraine as a consequence of propranolol. *Headache* 27:381–383.

Barinagarrementeria, F., C. Cantu, and H. Arredondo (1992a). Aseptic cerebral venous thrombosis: Proposed prognostic scale. *J. Stroke Cerebrovasc. Dis.* 2:34–39.

Barinagarrementeria, F., C. Cantu, and J. Balderrama (1992b). Postpartum cerebral angiopathy with cerebral infarction due to ergonovine use. *Stroke* 23:1366.

Baron, J.C., M. Serdaru, P. Lebrun-Gandrie et al. (1983). Debit sanguine cerebral et consommation d'oxygene locale au cours migraine hemiplegique prolongee. In *Migraine et Cephales*, Sandoz Editions, pp. 33–43. Colloque de Marseille, Marseille.

Bartleson, J.D., J.W. Swanson, and J.P. Whisnant (1981). A migrainous syndrome with cerebrospinal fluid pleocytosis. *Neurology* 31:1257–1262.

Bassi, P., R. Bandera, M. Loiero et al. (1991). Warning signs in subarachnoid hemorrhage: A

cooperative study. *Acta Neurol. Scand.* 84:277–281.

Baudrimont, M., F. Dubas, A. Joutel et al. (1993). Autosomal dominant leukoencephalopathy and subcortical ischemic stroke. A clinicopathological study. *Stroke* 24:122–125.

Becker, W.J. (1999). Use of oral contraceptives in patients with migraine. *Neurology* 53:519–525.

Benichou, H. and P. Bergeron (1996). Carotid angioplasty and stenting: Will periprocedural transcranial doppler monitoring be important? *J. Endovasc. Surg.* 3:217–223.

Berger, J.T., T. Wei, and D. Wilson (1998). Idiopathic granulomatous angiitis of the CNS manifesting as white matter disease. *Neurology* 51: 1774–1775.

Bergeron, P., P. Chambran, H. Benichou et al. (1996). Recurrent carotid disease: Will stents be an alternative to surgery? *J. Endovasc. Surg.* 3: 76–79.

Berkson, J. (1946). Limitations of the application of four-fold table analysis to hospital data. *Biometrics* 2:47–53.

Bernstein, M., J.F. Fleming, and J.H. Deck (1984). Cerebral hyperperfusion after carotid endarterectomy: A cause of cerebral hemorrhage. *Neurosurgery* 15:50–56.

Biousse, V., A. Ameri, and M.G. Bousser (1999). Isolated intracranial hypertension as the only sign of cerebral venous thrombosis. *Neurology* 53:1537–1542.

Biousse, V. and M.G. Bousser (1994). The myth of carotidynia. *Neurology* 44:993–995.

Biousse, V., J. d'Anglejan-Chatillon, H. Massiou et al. (1994). Head pain in nontraumatic carotid artery dissection: A series of 65 patients. *Cephalalgia* 14:33–36.

Biousse, V., J. d'Anglejan-Chatillon, P.J. Touboul et al. (1995). Time course of symptoms in extracranial carotid artery dissections. A series of 80 patients. *Stroke* 26:235–239.

Biousse, V., F. Woimant, P. Amarenco et al. (1992). Pain as the only manifestation of internal carotid artery dissection. *Cephalalgia* 12:314–317.

Bogousslavsky, J., P.A. Despland, F. Regli et al. (1989). Postpartum cerebral angiopathy: Reversible vasoconstriction assessed by transcranial Doppler ultrasound. *Eur. Neurol.* 29:102–105.

Bogousslavsky, J., F. Regli, G. VanMelle et al. (1988). Migraine stroke. *Neurology* 38:223–227.

Bonita, R. and S. Thomson (1985). Subarachnoid hemorrhage: Epidemiology, diagnosis, management, and outcome stroke. *Stroke* 16:591–594.

Börnke, C., N. Heye, and T. Büttner (1999). Rapidly progressive dementia. *Lancet* 353:1150.

Bousser, M.G. (1999a). Migraine, female hormones and stroke. *Cephalalgia* 19:75–79.

Bousser, M.G. (1999b). Migrainous stroke. Diagnosis and treatment. In *Prevention of Ischemic Stroke* (C. Fieschi and M. Fisher, eds.), pp. 253–264. M. Dunitz, London.

Bousser, M.G. (1999c). Cerebral venous thrombosis. Nothing, heparin, or local thrombolysis? *Stroke* 30:481–483.

Bousser, M.G., J.C. Baron, and J. Chiras (1985a). Ischemic strokes and migraine. *Neuroradiology* 27:583–587.

Bousser, M.G., J.C. Baron, M.T. Iba-Zizen et al. (1980). Migrainous cerebral infarction; a tomographic study of cerebral blood flow and oxygen extraction fraction with the oxygen-15 inhalation technique. *Stroke* 11:145–148.

Bousser, M.G., J.C. Baron, and J.L. Mas (1986). More on unusual angiographic appearance during an attack of hemiplegic migraine [letter]. *Headache* 26:487.

Bousser, M.G., J. Chiras, B. Sauron et al. (1985b). Cerebral venous thrombosis. A review of 38 cases. *Stroke* 16:199–213.

Bousser, M.G. and R.R. Russell (1997). Cerebral venous thrombosis. In *Major Problems in Neurology* (M.G. Bousser and R.R. Russell, eds.), p. 175. W.B. Saunders, London.

Breen, J.C., L.R. Caplan, L.D. deWitt et al. (1996). Brain edema after carotid surgery. *Neurology* 46:175–181.

Brillman, J. (1979). Acute hydrocephalus and death one month after nonsurgical treatment for acute cerebellar hemorrhage. *J. Neurosurg.* 50:374–376.

Brown, M.M., G. Venables, A. Clifton et al. (1997). Carotid endarterectomy versus carotid angioplasty. *Lancet* 349:880–881.

Bruyn, G.W. (1984). Intracranial arteriovenous malformation and migraine. *Cephalalgia* 4:191–207.

Buckle, R.M., G. duBoulay, and B. Smith (1964). Death due to cerebral vasospasm. *J. Neurol. Neurosurg. Psychiatry* 27:440–444.

Buonanno, F.S., D.M. Moody, and R.M. Ball (1982). CT scan findings in cerebral sinovenous occlusion. *Neurology* 12:288–292.

Buring, J.E., P. Hebert, J. Romero et al. (1995). Migraine and subsequent risk of stroke in the Physicians' Health Study. *Arch. Neurol.* 52:129–134.

Buring, J.E., R. Peto, and C.H. Hennekens (1990). Low-dose aspirin for migraine prophylaxis. *JAMA* 264:1711–1713.

Caccamo, D.V., J.H. Garcia, and K.L. Ho (1992). Isolated granulomatous angiitis of the spinal cord. *Ann. Neurol.* 32:580–582.

Cala, L.A. and F.L. Mastaglia (1976). Computerized axial tomography findings in patients with migrainous headaches. *BMJ* 2:149–150.

Calabrese, L.H. (1999). Angiographically defined primary angiitis of the CNS: Is it really benign? *Neurology* 52:1302.

Calabrese, L.H., G.F. Duna, and J.T. Lie (1997). Vasculitis in the central nervous system. *Arthritis Rheum.* 40:1189–1201.

Calabrese, L.H., A.H. Furlan, L.A. Gragg et al. (1992). Primary angiitis of the central nervous system: Diagnostic criteria and clinical approach. *Cleve. J. Med.* 59:293–306.

Calabrese, L.H., L.A. Gragg, and A.J. Furlan (1993). Benign angiopathy: A distinct subset of angiographically defined primary angiitis of the central nervous system. *J. Rheumatol.* 20:2046–2050.

Calabrese, L.H. and J.A. Mallek (1987). Primary angiitis of the central nervous system: Report of eight new cases, review of the literature, and proposal for diagnostic criteria. *Medicine* 67:20–39.

Call, G.K., M.C. Fleming, S. Sealfon et al. (1988). Reversible cerebral segmental vasoconstriction. *Stroke* 19:1159–1170.

Cambon, H., J.L. Truelle, J.C. Baron et al. (1987). Ischemic chronique focale et migraine accompagne: Forme atypique d'une angiomatose de Sturge-Weber. *Rev. Neurol.* 143:588–594.

Cantu, C. and F. Barinagarrementeria (1993). Cerebral venous thrombosis associated with pregnancy and puerperium: Review of 67 cases. *Stroke* 24:1880–1884.

Caplan, L. (1988). Intracerebral hemorrhage revisited. *Neurology* 38:624–627.

Caplan, L.R. (1991). Migraine and vertebrobasilar ischemia. *Neurology* 41:55–61.

Caplan, L.R. (1993). *Stroke: A Clinical Approach*. Butterworth-Heinemann, Boston.

CAPRIE Steering Committee (1996). A randomized, blinded trial of clopidogrel versus aspirin in patients at risk of ischemic events (CAPRIE). *Lancet* 348:1329–1339.

Carolei, A., C. Marini, C. DeMatteis et al. (1996). History of migraine and risk of cerebral ischemia in young adults [abstract]. *Lancet* 343:1503–1506.

Case Records of the MGH (2000). Case 10-2000. *N. Engl. J. Med.* 342:957–965.

Cavazos, J.E., J.B. Caress, V.R. Chilukuri et al. (1994). Sumatriptan-induced stroke in sagittal sinus thrombosis. *Lancet* 343:1105–1106.

Chabriat, H., S. Pappata, L. Traykov et al. (1996). Angiomatose de Sturge-Webber responsable d'une hemiplegie sans infarctus cerebral en fin de grossesse. *Rev. Neurol.* 152:536–541.

Chabriat, H., E. Tournier-Lasserve, K. Vahedi et al. (1995). Autosomal dominant migraine with MRI white-matter abnormalities mapping to the CADASIL locus. *Neurology* 45:1086–1091.

Chang, C.L., M. Donaghy, and N. Poulter (1999). Migraine and stroke in young women: Case-control study. The World Health Organization Collaborative Study of Cardiovascular Disease and Steroid Hormone Contraception. *BMJ* 318:13–18.

Chartier, J.P., J.Y. Bousique, A. Teisseyre et al. (1997). Angiopathie cerebrale du postpartum d'origine iatrogene. *Rev. Neurol.* 153:212–214.

Chen, Z.M., P. Sandercock, H.C. Pan et al. (2000). Indications for early aspirin use in acute ischemic stroke: A combined analysis of 40,000 randomized patients from the Chinese Acute Stroke Trial and the International Stroke Trial. On behalf of the CAST and IST Collaborative Groups. *Stroke* 31:1240–1249.

Chester, E.M., D.P. Agamanolis, B.Q. Banker et al. (1978). Hypertensive encephalopathy: A clinicopathologic study of 20 cases. *Neurology* 28: 928–939.

Chu, C.T., L. Gray, L.B. Goldstein et al. (1998). Diagnosis of intracranial vasculitis: A multidisciplinary approach. *J. Neuropathol. Exp. Neurol.* 57:30–38.

Cole, A.J. and M. Aube (1990). Migraine with vasospasm and delayed intracerebral hemorrhage. *Arch. Neurol.* 47:53–56.

Collaborative Group for the Study of Stroke in Young Women (1975). Oral contraceptives and stroke in young women. *JAMA* 231:718–722.

Comabella, M., J. Alvarez-Sabin, A. Rovira et al. (1996). Bromocriptine and postpartum cerebral angiopathy. A causal relationship? *Neurology* 46:1754–1756.

Couch, J.R. and R.S. Hassanein (1977). Platelet aggregability in migraine. *Neurology* 27:843–848.

Crassard, I., V. Biousse, M.G. Bousser et al. (1997). Hearing loss and headache revealing lateral sinus thrombosis in a patient with factor V Leiden mutation. *Stroke* 28:876–877.

Cravioto, J. and I. Feigin (1959). Noninfectious granulomatous angiitis with a predilection for the nervous system. *Neurology* 9:599–609.

Cupps, T.R., P.M. Moore, and A.S. Fauci (1983). Isolated angiitis of the central nervous system: Prospective diagnostic and therapeutic experience. *Am. J. Med.* 74:97–105.

Cutrer, F.M., A.G. Sorenson, R.M. Weisskoff et al. (1998). Perfusion-weighted imaging defects during spontaneous migrainous aura. *Ann. Neurol.* 43:25–31.

Daif, A., A. Awada, S. al Rajeh et al. (1995). Cerebral venous thrombosis in adult. A study of 40 cases from Saudi Arabia. *Stroke* 26:1193–1195.

Damasio, H. and D. Beck (1978). Migraine, thrombocytopenia and serotonin metabolism. *Lancet* 2:240–241.

D'Amico, D., F. Moschiano, M. Leone et al. (1998). Genetic abnormalities of the protein C system: Shared risk factors in young adults with migraine with aura and with ischemic stroke? *Cephalalgia* 18:618–621.

d'Anglejan-Chatillon, J., V. Ribeiro, J.L. Mas et al. (1989). Migraine: A risk factor for dissection of cervical arteries. *Headache* 29:560–561.

Day, J.W. and N.H. Raskin (1986). Thunderclap headache: Symptom of unruptured cerebral aneurysm. *Lancet* ii:1247–1248.

de Bray, J.M., I. Penisson-Besnier, F. Dubas et al. (1997). Extracranial and intracranial vertebrobasilar dissections: Diagnosis and prognosis. *J. Neurol. Neurosurg. Psychiatry* 63:46–51.

de Bruijn, S.F., J. Stam, and U. Kappelle (1996). Thunderclap headache as first symptom of cerebral venous sinus thrombosis. For the CVST Study Group. *Lancet* 348:1623–1625.

de Bruijn, S.F. and J. Stam (1999). Randomized, placebo-controlled trial of anticoagulant treatment with low molecular weight heparin for cerebral sinus thrombosis. For the Cerebral Venous Sinus Thrombosis Group. *Stroke* 30:484–488.

de la Sayette, V., F. Leproux, and P.H. Letellier (1999). Cervical cord and dorsal medullary infarction presenting with retroorbital pain. *Neurology* 53:632–634.

del Sette, M., S. Angeli, M. Leandri et al. (1998). Migraine with aura and right-to-left shunt on transcranial doppler: A case-control study. *Cerebrovasc. Dis.* 8:327–330.

de Marinis, M., A. Zaccaria, V. Faraglia et al. (1991). Postendarterectomy headache and the role of the oculosympathetic system. *J. Neurol. Neurosurg. Psychiatry* 54:314–317.

Dietrich, E.B., M. Ndiaye, and D.B. Reid (1996). Stenting in the carotid artery. Experience in 110 patients. *Endovasc. Surg.* 3:42–62.

Dodick, D.W., R.D. Brown, J.W. Britton et al. (1999). Nonaneurysmal thunderclap headache with diffuse, multifocal, segmental, and reversible vasospasm. *Cephalalgia* 19:118–121.

Dolan, J.G. and A.L. Mushlin (1984). Hypertension, vascular headaches, and seizures after carotid endarterectomy. *Arch. Intern. Med.* 144: 1489–1491.

Dormont, D., R. Anxionnat, S. Evrard et al. (1994). MRI in cerebral venous thrombosis. *J. Neuroradiol.* 21:81–99.

Ducros, A., A. Joutel, and K. Vahedi (1997). Mapping of a second locus for familial hemiplegic migraine to 1q21-q23 and evidence of further heterogeneity. *Ann. Neurol.* 42:885–890.

Duffy, G.P. (1983). The "warning leak" in spontaneous subarachnoid hemorrhage. *Med. J. Aust.* 1:514–516.

Dukes, H.T. and R.G. Vieth (1964). Cerebral arteriography during migraine prodrome and headache. *Neurology* 14:636–639.

Dunning, H.S. (1942). Intracranial and extracranial vascular accidents in migraine. *Arch. Neurol. Psychiatr.* 48:396–406.

Dupuy, B., B. Lechevalier, D. Lechevalier et al. (1979). Complications vasculaires a rechute liees a la prise de methergin en milieu obstetrical. *Rev. Otoneuroophthalmol.* 51:293–299.

Duyff, R.F., C.J. Snidjers, and J.A. Vanneste (1997). Spontaneous bilateral internal carotid artery dissection and migraine: A potential diagnostic delay. *Headache* 37:109–112.

Eckert, B., F.E. Zanella, A. Thie et al. (1996). Angioplasty of the internal carotid artery: Results, complications, and followup in 61 cases. *Cerebrovasc. Dis.* 6:97–105.

Edlow, J.A. and L.R. Caplan (2000). Avoiding pitfalls in the diagnosis of subarachnoid hemorrhage. *N. Engl. J. Med.* 342:29–36.

Edvinsson, L., K. Golman, and I. Jansen (1987). Site of action of contrast media on cerebral vessels. *Cephalalgia* 7:83–85.

Ehsan, T., S. Hasan, J.M. Powers et al. (1995). Serial magnetic resonance imaging in isolated angiitis of the central nervous system. *Neurology* 45:1462–1465.

Einhaupl, K.M., A. Villringer, W. Meister et al. (1991). Heparin treatment in sinus venous thrombosis. *Lancet* 338:597–600.

Evans, R.W. (1996). Diagnostic testing for the evaluation of headaches. *Neurol. Clin.* 14:1–26.

Fay, T. (1927). Atypical facial neuralgia. *Arch. Neurol. Psychiatry* 18:309–315.

Fazekas, F., M. Koch, R. Schmidt et al. (1992). The prevalence of cerebral damage varies with migraine type: A MRI study. *Headache* 32:287–291.

Featherstone, H.J. (1986). Clinical features of stroke in migraine. A review. *Headache* 26:128–133.

Féré, C. (1881). Contribution a l'etude de la migraine ophthalmique. *Rev. Med. Paris* 1:625–647.

Féré, C.H. (1883). Note sur un cas de migraine ophthalmique à accés répétés et suivis de mort. *Rev. Med. Paris* 3:194–201.

Ferro, J.M., T.P. Melo, and M. Guerreiro (1998). Headaches in intracerebral hemorrhage survivors. *Neurology* 50:203–207.

Ferro, J.M., T.P. Melo, V. Oliveira et al. (1995). A multivariate study of headache associated with ischemic stroke. *Headache* 35:315–319.

Findlay, J.M. (1997). Canadian Neurosurgical Society Practice Guidelines Review Group. Current management of aneurysmal subarachnoid hemorrhage guidelines from the Canadian Neurosurgical Society. *Can. J. Neurol. Sci.* 24:161–170.

Finelli, P.F., H.C. Onyiuke, and D.F. Uphoff (1997). Idiopathic granulomatous angiitis of the CNS manifesting as diffuse white matter disease. *Neurology* 49:1696–1699.

Fisher, C.M. (1968). Migraine accompaniments versus arteriosclerotic ischemia. *Trans. Am. Neurol. Assoc.* 93:211–213.

Fisher, C.M. (1971). Cerebral Ischemia: Less familiar types. *Clin. Neurosurg.* 18:267–336.

Fisher, C.M. (1980). Late life migraine accompaniments as a cause of unexplained transient ischemic attacks. *Can. J. Neurol. Sci.* 7:9–17.

Fisher, C.M. (1982). The headache and pain of spontaneous carotid dissection. *Headache* 22:60–65.

Fisher, C.M. (1986). An unusual case of migraine accompaniments with permanent sequelae. A case report. *Headache* 26:266–270.

Fisher, C.M., E.H. Picard, P. Polak et al. (1965). Acute hypertensive cerebellar hemorrhage: Diagnosis and surgical treatment. *J. Nerv. Ment. Dis.* 140:38–57.

Fitzsimons, R.B. and W.H. Wolfenden (1985). Migraine coma. Meningitic migraine with cerebral edema associated with a new form of autosomal dominant cerebellar ataxia. *Brain* 108:555–577.

Fontanarosa, P.B. (1989). Recognition of subarachnoid hemorrhage. *Ann. Emerg. Med.* 18:1119–1205.

Fountain, N.B. and D.A. Eberhard (1996). Primary angiitis of the central nervous system associated with cerebral amyloid angiopathy: Report of two cases and review of the literature. *Neurology* 46:190–197.

Frey, J.L., G.J. Muro, C.G. McDougall et al. (1999). Cerebral venous thrombosis, combined intrathrombus rtPA, and intravenous heparin. *Stroke* 30:489–494.

Ganesan, V. and F.J. Kirkham (1997). Carotid dissection causing stroke in a child with migraine. *BMJ* 314:291–292.

Garner, B.F., P. Burns, R.D. Bunning et al. (1990). Acute blood pressure elevation can mimic arteriographic appearance of cerebral vasculitis (a postpartum case with relative hypertension). *J. Rheumatol.* 17:93–97.

Garnic, J.D. and D. Schellinger (1983). Arterial spasm as a finding intimately associated with onset of vascular headache. *Neuroradiology* 24:273–276.

Gelford, G.H., A.J. Wilets, D. Nelson et al. (1967). Retroperitoneal fibrosis and methysergide. Report of three cases. *Radiology* 88:976–981.

Geller, E.B. and P.Y. Wen (1995). Migraine with aura as the presentation of leukemia. *Headache* 35:560–562.

Geraghty, J.J., D.B. Hoch, M.E. Robert et al. (1991). Fatal puerperal cerebral vasospasm and stroke in a young woman. *Neurology* 41:1145–1147.

Gil-Peralta, A., A. Mayol, G.J. Marcos et al. (1996). Percutaneous transluminal angioplasty of the symptomatic atherosclerotic carotid arteries: Results, complications, and follow-up. *Stroke* 27:2271–2273.

Gorelick, P.B. (1993). Ischemic stroke and intracranial hematoma. In *The Headaches* (J. Olesen, P. Tfelt-Hansen, and K.M.A. Welch, eds.), 639–645. Raven Press, New York.

Gorelick, P.B., D.B. Hier, L.R. Caplan et al. (1986). Headache in acute cerebrovascular disease. *Neurology* 36:1445–1450.

Granier, I., E. Garcia, A. Geissler et al. (1999). Postpartum cerebral angioplasty associated with the administration of sumatriptan and dihydroergotamine: A case report. *Intensive Care Med.* 25:532–534.

Gray, F., H.V. Vinters, H. le Noan et al. (1990). Cerebral amyloid angiopathy and granulomatous angiitis: Immunohistochemical study using antibodies to the Alzheimer A4 peptide. *Hum. Pathol.* 21:1290–1293.

Greenan, T.J., R.I. Grossman, and H.I. Goldberg (1992). Cerebral vasculitis: MR imaging and angiographic correlation. *Radiology* 182:65–72.

Greenberg, M.S. (1994). *Handbook of Neurosurgery.* Greenberg Graphics, Lakeland, Florida.

Greselle, J.F., M. Zenteno, P. Kien et al. (1987). Spontaneous dissection of vertebrobasilar system. *J. Neuroradiol.* 14:115–123.

Guillon, B., V. Biousse, H. Massiou et al. (1998a). Orbital pain as an isolated sign of internal carotid artery dissection. A diagnostic pitfall. *Cephalalgia* 18:222–224.

Guillon, B., L. Brunereau, V. Biousse et al. (1999). Long-term follow-up of aneurysms developed during extracranial internal carotid artery dissection. *Neurology* 53:117–122.

Guillon, B., C. Levy, and M.G. Bousser (1998b). Internal carotid artery dissection: An update. *J. Neurol. Sci.* 153:146–158.

Guist, I.A. and A.L. Woolf (1964). Fatal infarction of the brain in migraine. *BMJ* 18:267–336.

Haan, J., L.J. Kappelle, H. deRonde et al. (1997). The factor V Leiden mutation (R506Q) is not a major risk factor for migrainous cerebral infarction. *Cephalalgia* 17:605–607.

Haas, D.C. (1991). Arteriovenous malformations and migraine: Case reports and an analysis of the relationship. *Headache* 31:509–513.

Hankey, G.J. (1998). Necrotizing and granulomatous angiitis of the CNS. In *Cerebrovascular Disease: Pathophysiology, Diagnosis, and Management* (M.D. Ginsberg and J. Bogousslavsky, eds.), pp. 1647–1683. Blackwell Science, London.

Harling, D.W., R.C. Peatfield, P.T. Van Hille et al. (1989). Thunderclap headache: Is it migraine? *Cephalalgia* 9:87–90.

Harris, K.G., D.D. Tran, W.J. Sickels et al. (1994). Diagnosing intracranial vasculitis: The roles of MR and angiography. *Am. J. Neuroradiol.* 15:317–330.

Harrison, M.J. (1981). Hemiplegic migraine. *J. Neurol. Neurosurg. Psychiatry* 44:652–653.

Headache Classification Committee of the International Headache Society (1988). Classification and diagnostic criteria for headache disorders, cranial neuralgia, and facial pain. *Cephalalgia* 8:1–96.

Henrich, J.B. and R.I. Horowitz (1989). A controlled study of ischemic stroke risk in migraine patients. *J. Clin. Epidemiol.* 42:773–780.

Henrich, J.B., P.A.G. Sandercock, C.P. Warlow et al. (1986). Stroke and migraine in the Oxfordshire Community Stroke Project. *J. Neurol.* 233:257–262.

Henry, P.Y., P. Larre, M. Aupy et al. (1984). Reversible cerebral arteriopathy associated with the administration of ergot derivatives. *Cephalalgia* 4:171–178.

Heros, R.C. (1982). Cerebellar hemorrhage and infarction. *Stroke* 13:106–109.

Hess, D.C., A.M. Demchuk, L.M. Brass et al. (2000). HMG-CoA reductase inhibitors (statins): A promising approach to stroke prevention. *Neurology* 54:790–796.

Hillman, J. (1986). Should computed tomography scanning replace lumbar puncture in the diagnostic process in suspected subarachnoid hemorrhage? *Surg. Neurol.* 26:547–550.

Hop, J.W., G.J. Rinkel, A. Algra et al. (2000). Randomized pilot trial of postoperative aspirin in subarachnoid hemorrhage. *Neurology* 22:872–878.

Hosoya, T., M. Adachi, K. Yamaguchi et al. (1999). Clinical and neuroradiological features of intracranial vertebrobasilar artery dissection. *Stroke* 30:1083–1090.

Hubbert, C.H. (1987). Dural puncture headache suspected, cortical vein thrombosis diagnosed. *Anesth. Anal.* 66:285

Hughes, R.L. (1992). Identification and treatment of cerebral aneurysms after sentinel headache. *Neurology* 42:1118–1119.

Hungerford, G.D., G.H. du Boulay, and K.J. Zilkha (1976). Computerized axial tomography in patients with severe migraine: A preliminary report. *J. Neurol. Neurosurg. Psychiatry* 39:990–994.

Igarashi, H., F. Sakai, S. Kan et al. (1991). Magnetic resonance imaging of the brain in patients with migraine. *Cephalalgia* 11:69–74.

Iglesias, S. and J.C. Baron (1994). Circonstance declenchante inhabituelle de l'angiopathie cerebrale aigue benigne: Lien avec les cephalee d'effort. *Rev. Neurol.* 3:241–244.

Iglesias, S. and M.G. Bousser (1990). Migraine et infarctus cerebral. *Circ. Metab. Cerveau* 7:237–249.

Ille, O., F. Woimant, A. Pruna et al. (1995). Hypertensive encephalopathy after bilateral carotid endarterectomy. *Stroke* 26:488–491.

Isenberg, D.A., D.M. Thomas, M.L. Snaith et al. (1982). A study of migraine in systemic lupus erythematosis. *Ann. Rheum. Dis.* 41:30–32.

Jackson, M. (1993). Cerebral arterial narrowing with nicotine patch. *Lancet* 342:236–237.

Janeway, T.C. (1913). A clinical study of hypertensive cardiovascular disease. *Arch. Intern. Med.* 12:755–798.

Janssens, E., M. Hommel, F. Mounier-Vehier et al. (1985). Postpartum cerebral angiopathy possibly due to bromocriptine therapy. *Stroke 26*: 128–130.

Jenette, J.C. and R.J. Falk (1997). Small vessel vasculitis. *N. Engl. J. Med.* 337:1512–1523.

Johnson, M., R. Maciunas, P. Dutt et al. (1989). Granulomatous angiitis masquerading as a mass lesion. *Surg. Neurol.* 31:49–53.

Joutel, A., M.G. Bousser, and V. Biouse (1993). A gene for familial hemiplegic migraine maps to chromosome 19. *Nat. Genet.* 5:40–45.

Joutel, A., C. Corpechot, A. Ducros et al. (1996). Notch3 mutations in CADASIL, a hereditary adult-onset condition causing stroke and dementia. *Nature* 383:707–710.

Joutel, A., K. Vahedi, C. Corpechot et al. (1997). Strong clustering and stereotyped nature of Notch3 mutations in CADASIL patients. *Lancet* 350:1511–1515.

Juvela, S. (1995). Aspirin and delayed cerebral ischemia after aneurysmal subarachnoid hemorrhage. *J. Neurosurg.* 82:945–952.

Kappor, R., B.E. Kendal, and M.J. Harrison (1990). Persistent segmental cerebral artery constrictions in coital cephalalgia. *J. Neurol. Neurosurg. Psychiatry* 53:266.

Kase, C.S., J.P. Mohr, and L.R. Caplan (1998). Intracerebral hemorrhage. In *Stroke: Pathophysiology, Diagnosis, and Management* (H.J. Barnett, J.P. Mohr, B.M. Stein et al., eds.) pp. 649–700. Churchill Livingstone, New York.

Kassell, N.F., J.C. Torner, E.C. Haley et al. (1990). The international cooperative study on the timing of aneurysm surgery. Part I: Overall management results. *J. Neurosurg.* 73:18–36.

Kawamura, J. and J.S. Meyer (1991). Headache due to cerebrovascular disease. *Med. Clin. North Am.* 75:617–630.

Kidwell, C.S., J.R. Alger, F. diSalle et al. (1999). Diffusion MRI in patients with transient ischemic attacks. *Stroke* 30:1174–1180.

King, R.B. and M.I. Saba (1974). Forewarnings of major subarachnoid hemorrhage. *N.Y. State J. Med.* 74:638–639.

Klapper, J. (1994). Headache in Sturge-Weber syndrome. *Headache* 34:521–522.

Klopstock, T., A. May, P. Seibel et al. (1996). Mitochondrial DNA in migraine with aura. *Neurology* 46:1735–1738.

Kontula, Y., A. Ylikorkala, H. Miettinen et al. (1995). Arg 506 factor V mutation (factor V Leiden) in patients with ischemic cerebrovascular disease and survivors of myocardial infarction. *Thromb. Haemost.* 73:558–560.

Koo, B., L. Becker, S. Chuang et al. (1993). Mitochondrial encephalomyopathy, lactic acidosis, stroke-like episodes (MELAS) clinical, radiological, pathological, and genetic observations. *Ann. Neurol.* 34:25–32.

Koo, E.H. and E.W. Massey (1988). Granulomatous angiitis of the central nervous system: Protean manifestations and response to treatment. *J. Neurol. Neurosurg. Psychiatry* 51:1126–1133.

Kruisdijk, J.J. and J.A. Vanneste (1998). Acute primary cerebral angiitis mimicking basilar artery dissection. *Eur. J. Neurol.* 5:95–98.

Kumar, R., E.F. Wijdicks, R.D. Brown et al. (1997). Isolated angiitis of the CNS presenting as subarachnoid hemorrhage. *J. Neurol. Neurosurg. Psychiatry* 62:649–651.

Launer, L.J., G.M. Terwindt, N.J. Nagelkerke et al. (1999). Risk factors for stroke in female migraineurs and nonmigraineurs: The GEM study. *Neurology* 52:123

Lauritzen, M., T.S. Olsen, N.A. Lassen et al. (1983). Changes in regional cerebral blood flow during the course of classic migraine attacks. *Ann. Neurol.* 13:633–641.

Leblanc, R. (1987). The minor leak preceding subarachnoid hemorrhage. *J. Neurosurg.* 66:35–39.

le Coz, P., F. Woimant, D. Rougemont et al. (1988). Angiopathies cerebrales benignes et phenylpropanolamine. *Rev. Neurol.* 144:295–300.

Lee, K.Y., Y.J. Sohn, S.H. Kim et al. (2000). Basilar artery vasospasm in postpartum cerebral angiopathy. *Neurology* 54:2003–2005.

Leker, R.R. and I. Steiner (1999). Features of dural sinus thrombosis simulating pseudotumor cerebri. *Eur. J. Neurol.* 6:601–604.

Leow, K. and J.A. Murie (1988). New information on several painful conditions: Thunderclap headache mimicking subarachnoid hemorrhage. *Neurol. Alert* 7:5–6.

Levine, S.R., M.J. Deegan, N. Futrell et al. (1990). Cerebrovascular and neurologic disease associated with antiphospholipid antibodies: 48 cases. *Neurology* 40:1181–1189.

Levine, S.R., R.E. Twyman, and S. Gilman (1988). The role of anticoagulation in cavernous sinus thrombosis. *Neurology* 38:521

Leviton, A., L. Caplan, and E. Salzmen (1975). Severe headaches after carotid endarterectomy. *Headache* 15:207–210.

Lidegaard, O. (1995). Oral contraceptives, pregnancy, and the risk of cerebral thromboembolism: The influence of diabetes, hypertension, migraine, and previous thrombotic disease. *Br. J. Obstet. Gynaecol.* 102:153–159.

Lie, J.T. (1992). Primary (granulomatous) angiitis of the central nervous system: A clinicopathologic analysis of 15 new cases and a review of the literature. *Hum. Pathol.* 23:164–171.

Lieberman, A.N., S. Jonas, and W.K. Hass (1984). Bilateral cervical carotid and intracerebral vasospasm causing cerebral ischemia in a migrainous patient: A case of diplegic migraine. *Headache* 24:245–248.

Lindboe, C.F., T. Dahl, and B. Rostad (1989). Fatal stroke in migraine: A case report with autopsy findings. *Cephalalgia* 9:277–280.

Linn, F.H., G.J. Rinkel, A. Algra et al. (1998). Headache characteristics in subarachnoid hemorrhage and benign thunderclap headache. *J. Neurol. Neurosurg. Psychiatry* 65:791–793.

Linn, F.H., E.F. Wijdicks, Y. van der Graaf et al. (1994). Prospective study of sentinel headache in aneurysmal subarachnoid hemorrhage. *Lancet* 344:590–593.

Little, J.R., D.E. Tubman, and R. Ethier (1978). Cerebellar hemorrhage in adults. Diagnosis by computerized tomography. *J. Neurosurg.* 48: 575–579.

Lucas, C., D. Deplanque, A. Salhi et al. (1996). Angiopathie benigne du postpartum: Un cas clinicoradiologique associé à la prise de bromocriptine. *Rev. Med. Interne.* 17:839–841.

Marchioni, E., A. Galimberti, D. Soragna et al. (1995). Familial hemiplegic migraine versus migraine with prolonged aura: An uncertain diagnosis in a family report. *Neurology* 45:33–37.

Margolis, M.T. and T.H. Newton (1971). Methamphetamine ("speed") arteritis. *Neuroradiology* 2:179–182.

Marks, M.P., M. Marcellus, A.M. Norbash et al. (1999). Outcome of angioplasty for atherosclerotic intracranial stenosis. *Stroke* 30:1065–1069.

Markus, H.S. (1992). A prospective follow-up of thunderclap headache mimicking subarachnoid hemorrhage. *J. Neurol. Neurosurg. Psychiatry* 54:117–1125.

Martins, I.P., E. Baeta, T. Paiva et al. (1993). Headaches during intracranial endovascular procedures: A possible model of vascular headache. *Headache* 33:227–233.

Martsen, B.H., P.S. Sorensen, and J. Marquardsen (1990). Transient ischemic attacks in young patients: A thromboembolic or migrainous manifestation? A ten-year follow-up of 46 patients. *J. Neurol. Neurosurg. Psychiatry* 53:1029–1033.

Mas, J.L., J.C. Baron, M.G. Bousser et al. (1986). Stroke, migraine, and intracranial aneurysm: A case report. *Stroke* 17:1019–1021.

Mas, J.L., M.G. Bousser, D. Hasboun et al. (1987). Extracranial vertebral artery dissections: A review of 13 cases. *Stroke* 18:1037–1047.

Mas, J.L., D. Henin, M.G. Bousser et al. (1989). Dissecting aneurysm of the vertebral artery and cervical manipulation. *Neurology* 39:512–515.

Masson, C., D. Henin, J.M. Colombani et al. (1998). Un cas d'angéite cérébrale à cellules géantes associée à une angiopathie amyloide cérébrale. *Rev. Neurol.* 154:695–698.

Masuzawa, T., S. Shinoda, M. Furuse et al. (1983). Cerebral angiographic changes on serial examination of a patient with migraine. *Neuroradiology* 24:277–281.

Mattle, H., R.R. Edelkman, M.A. Reis et al. (1990). Flow quantification in the superior saggittal sinus using magnetic resonance. *Neurology* 40:813–815.

Mayberg, M.R., H.H. Batjer, R. Dacey et al. (1994). Guidelines for the management of aneurysmal subarachnoid hemorrhage: A statement for healthcare professionals from a special writing group of the Stroke Council, American Heart Association. *Stroke* 25:2315–2328.

McCabe, D.J., M.M. Brown, and A. Clifton (1999). Fatal cerebral reperfusion hemorrhage after carotid stenting. *Stroke* 30:2483–2486.

McColl, G.J. and K. Fraser (1995). Pheochromocytoma and pseudovasculitis. *J. Rheumatol.* 22: 1441–1442.

Melo, T.P., A.N. Pinto, and J.M. Ferro (1996). Headache in intracerebral hematomas. *Neurology* 47:494–500.

Merikangas, K.R., B. Fenton, S.H. Cheng et al. (1997). Association between migraine and stroke in a large-scale epidemiological study of the United States. *Arch. Neurol.* 54:362–368.

Messert, B. and J.A. Black (1978). Cluster headache, hemicrania, and other head pains: Morbidity of carotid endarterectomy. *Stroke* 9:559–562.

Michel, D., C. Vial, J.C. Antoine et al. (1985). Benign acute cerebral angiopathy: Four cases. *Rev. Neurol. (Paris)* 141:786–792.

Mitsias, P. and N.M. Ramadan (1992a). Headache in ischemic cerebrovascular disease. Part I: Clinical features. *Cephalalgia* 12:269–274.

Mitsias, P. and N.M. Ramadan (1992b). Headache in ischemic cerebrovascular disease. Part II: Mechanisms and predictive value. *Cephalalgia* 12:341–344.

Mokri, B., T.M. Sundt, O.W. Houser et al. (1986). Spontaneous dissection of the cervical internal carotid artery. *Ann. Neurol.* 19:126–138.

Moore, P.M. (1989). Diagnosis and management of isolated angiitis of the central nervous system. *Neurology* 39:167–173.

Moore, P.M. (1994). Vasculitis of the central nervous system. *Semin. Neurol.* 14:313–319.

Morgenstern, L.B., H. Luna-Gonzales, J.C. Huber et al. (1998). Worst headache and subarachnoid hemorrhage: Prospective modern computed tomography and spinal fluid analysis. *Ann. Emerg. Med.* 32:297–304.

Moser, M., H. Wish, and A.P. Friedman (1962). Headache and hypertension. *JAMA* 180:115–120.

Moskowitz, M.A. (1984). The neurobiology of vascular head pain. *Ann. Neurol.* 16:157–168.

Moskowitz, M.A., M.G. Buzzi, D.E. Sakas et al. (1989). Pain mechanisms underlying vascular headaches: Progress report. *Rev. Neurol.* 145: 181–193.

Mourand, I., X. Ducrocq, J.C. Lacour et al. (1999). Acute reversible cerebral arteritis associated with parenteral ephedrine use. *Cerebrovasc. Dis.* 9:355–357.

Moyer, J.H., A.B. Tashnek, S.I. Miller et al. (1952). The effect of theophylline with ethylenediamine (aminophylline) and caffeine on cerebral hemodynamics and cerebrospinal fluid pressure in patients with hypertensive headaches. *Am. J. Med. Sci.* 224:377–385.

Mtinte, T.F. and H. Miiler-Vahl (1990). Familial migraine coma: A case study. J. Neurol. 237:59–61.

Mueller, S.M. (1983). Neurologic complications of phenylpropanolamine use. *Neurology* 33:650–652.

Munari, L.M., G. Belloni, L. Moschini et al. (1994). Carotid pain during percutaneous angioplasty. Pathophysiology and clinical features. *Cephalalgia* 14:127–131.

Nakatomi, H., K. Nagata, S. Kawamoto et al. (1997). Ruptured dissecting aneurysm as a cause of subarachnoid hemorrhage of unverified etiology. *Stroke* 28:1278–1282.

National Cholesterol Education Program (1988). Report of the National Cholesterol Education Program Expert Panel on Detection, Evaluation, and Treatment of High Blood Cholesterol in Adults. *Arch. Intern. Med.* 148:36–69.

Neligan, P., D.G. Harriman, and J. Pierce (1977). Respiratory arrest in familial hemiplegic migraine. *BMJ* 11:732–734.

Newman, D.S., S.R. Levine, V.L. Curtis et al. (1989). Migraine-like visual phenomena associated with cerebral venous thrombosis. *Headache* 29:82–85.

Ng, P.K. and S.M. Pulst (1992). Not so benign "thunderclap headache." *Neurology* 260:42

Nichols, F.T., M. Mawad, J.P. Mohr et al. (1990). Focal headache during balloon inflation in the internal carotid and middle cerebral arteries. *Stroke* 21:555–559.

Ogawa, T., A. Inugami, E. Shimosegawa et al. (1993). Subarachnoid hemorrhage: Evaluation with MR imaging. *Radiology* 186:345–351.

Ojaimi, J., S. Katsabanis, S. Bower et al. (1998). Mitochondrial DNA in stroke and migraine with aura. *Cerebrovasc. Dis.* 8:102–106.

Olesen, J., L. Friberg, T.S. Olsen et al. (1993a). Ischemia-induced (symptomatic) migraine attacks may be more frequent than migraine-induced ischemic insults. *Brain* 116:187–202.

Olesen, J., B. Larsen, and M. Lauritzen (1981). Focal hyperemia followed by spreading oligemia and impaired activation of rCBF in classic migraine. *Ann. Neurol.* 9:344–352.

Olesen, J., K.M.A. Welch, A. Carolei et al. (1993b). Treatment to prevent migraine-related stroke. *Cerebrovasc. Dis.* 3:244–247.

Ophoff, R.A., R. Van Eijk, L.A. Sandkuijl et al. (1994). Genetic heterogeneity of familial hemiplegic migraine. *Genomics* 22:21–26.

Ostergaard, J.R. (1991). Headache as a warning symptom of unpending aneurysmal subarachnoid hemorrhage. *Cephalalgia* 11:53–55.

Ott, K.H., C.S. Kase, R.G. Ojemann et al. (1974). Cerebellar hemorrhage: Diagnosis and treatment. A review of 56 cases. *Arch. Neurol.* 31:160–167.

Ozdoba, C., M. Sturzenegger, and G. Schroth (1996). Internal carotid artery dissection: MR imaging features and clinical-radiologic correlation. *Radiology* 199:191–198.

Padayachee, T.S., J.B. Bingham, M.J. Grave et al. (1991). Dural sinus thrombosis. Diagnosis and follow-up by magnetic resonance angiography and imaging. *Neuroradiology* 33:165–167.

Parisi, J.E. and P.M. Moore (1994). The role of biopsy in vasculitis of the central nervous system. *Neurology* 14:341–348.

Pavese, N., R. Canapicchi, A. Nuti et al. (1994). White matter MRI hyperintensities in 129 consecutive migraine patients. *Cephalalgia* 14:342–345.

Pavlakis, S.G., P.C. Phillips, S. DiMauro et al. (1984). Mitochondrial myopathy, encephalopathy, lactic acidosis and stroke-like episodes: A distinct clinical syndrome. *Ann. Neurol.* 16:481–488.

Pearce, J. (1976). Headache after carotid endarterectomy. *BMJ* 2:85–86.

Pickard, J.D., G.D. Murray, R. Illingworth et al. (1989). Effect of oral nimodipine on cerebral infarction and outcome after subarachnoid hemorrhage. British Aneurysm Nimodipine Trial. *BMJ* 298:636–642.

Polyak, S. (1957). *The Vertebrate Visual System.* University of Chicago Press, Chicago.

Portenoy, R.K., C.J. Abissi, R.B. Lipton et al. (1984). Headache in cerebrovascular disease. *Stroke* 25:1009–1012.

Preter, M., C.H. Tzourio, A. Ameri et al. (1996). Long-term prognosis in cerebral venous thrombosis. A follow-up of 77 patients. *Stroke* 27:243–246.

Radanov, B.P., M. Sturzenegger, and G. DiStefano (1995). Long-term outcome after whiplash injury: A 2-year follow up considering features of injury mechanism and somatic, radiologic, and psychosocial findings. *Medicine* 74:281.

Ramadan, N.M., G.E. Tietjen, S.R. Levine et al. (1991). Scintillating scotomata associated with internal carotid dissection: A report of three cases. *Neurology* 41:1084–1087.

Ramirez-Lassepas, M., C.E. Espinosa, J.J. Cicero et al (1997). Predictors of intracranial pathologic findings in patients who seek emergency care because of headache. *Arch. Neurol.* 54:1506–1509.

Raps, E.C., S.L. Galetta, M. Broderick et al. (1993a). Delayed peripartum vasculopathy: Cerebral eclampsia revisited. *Ann. Neurol.* 33:222–225.

Raps, E.C., J.D. Rogers, S.L. Galetta et al. (1993b). The clinical spectrum of unruptured intracranial aneurysms. *Arch. Neurol.* 50:265–268.

Raroque, H.G., G. Tefsa, and P. Purdy (1993). Postpartum cerebral angiopathy: Is there a role for sympathomimetic drugs. *Stroke* 24:2108–2110.

Rascol, A., J. Cambier, B. Guiraud et al. (1979). Accidents ischemiques cerebraux aucours des crises migraineuses. A propos des migraines compliques. *Rev. Neurol.* 135:867–884.

Rascol, A., B. Guiraud, C. Manelfe et al. (1980). Accidents vasculaires cerebraux de la grossesse et du postpartum. In *2e Conference de la Salpetriere sur les Maladies Vasculaires Cerebrales*. J.B. Bailliere, Paris.

Raskin, N.H. and O. Appenzeller (1980). *Headache*. W.B. Saunders, Philadelphia.

Rasmussen, K.R. and J. Olesen (1992). Symptomatic and nonsymptomatic headaches in a general population. *Neurology* 42:1225–1231.

Rasmussen, P., H. Busch, J. Haase et al. (1981). Intracranial saccular aneurysms. Results of treatment in 851 patients. *Acta Neurochir.* 53:1–17.

Razavi, M., B. Bendixen, J.E. Maley et al. (1999). CNS pseudovasculitis in a patient with pheochromocytoma. *Neurology* 52:1088–1090.

Reigel, M.M., L.H. Hollier, T.M. Sundt et al. (1987). Cerebral hyperperfusion syndrome: A cause of neurologic dysfunction after carotid endarterectomy. *J. Vasc. Surg.* 5:628–634.

Reimer, G., K. Lamszus, R. Zschaber et al. (1999a). Control of primary angiitis of the CNS associated with cerebral amyloid angiopathy by cyclophosphamide alone. *Neurology* 52:660–662.

Reimer, G., K. Lamszus, R. Zschaber et al. (1999b). Isolated angiitis of the central nervous system: Lack of inflammation after long-term treatment. *Neurology* 52:196–199.

Rippe, D.J., O.B. Boyko, C.E. Spritzer et al. (1990). Demonstration of dural sinus occlusion by the use of MR angiography. *Am. J. Neuroradiol.* 11:199–201.

Roh, J.K. and K.S. Park (2000). Postpartum cerebral angiopathy with intracerebral hemorrhage in a patient receiving lisuride. *Neurology* 54:2003–2005.

Roubin, G.S., S. Yadav, S. Lyer et al. (1996). Carotid stent supported angioplasty: A neurovascular intervention to prevent stroke. *Am. J. Cardiol.* 78:8–12.

Rousseaux, P., B. Scherpereel, M.H. Bernard et al. (1983). Angiopathie cerebrale aigue benigne: Six observations. *Presse Med.* 12:2163–2168.

Sames, T.A., A.B. Storrow, J.A. Finkelstein et al. (1996). Sensitivity of new generation computed tomography in subarachnoid hemorrhage. *Acad. Emerg. Med.* 3:16–20.

Sanchez-del Rio, M., D. Bakker, O. Wu et al. (1999). Perfusion weighted imaging during migraine: Spontaneous visual aura and headache. *Cephalalgia* 19:701–707.

Savage, C.O., L. Harper, P. Cockwell et al. (2000). ABC of arterial and vascular disease: Vasculitis. *BMJ* 320:1325–1328.

Schievink, W.I. (1997). Intracranial aneurysms. *N. Engl. J. Med.* 336:28–40.

Schon, R. and M.J. Harrison (1987). Can migraine cause multiple segmental cerebral artery constrictions? *J. Neurol. Neurosurg. Psychiatry* 50:492–494.

Schoser, B.J., C. Heesen, B. Eckert et al. (1997). Cerebral hyperperfusion injury after percutaneous transluminal angioplasty of extracranial arteries. *J. Neurol.* 244:101–104.

Selby, G. and J.A. Gryer (1984). Fatal migraine. *Clin. Exp. Neurol.* 20:85–92.

Senter, H.J., A.N. Lieberman, and R. Pinto (1976). Cerebral manifestations of ergotism, report of a case and review of the literature. *Stroke* 7:88–92.

Serdaru, M., J. Chiras, M. Cujas et al. (1984). Isolated benign cerebral vasculitis or migrainous vasospasm? *J. Neurol. Neurosurg. Psychiatry* 47:73–76.

Seymour, J.J., R.M. Moscati, and D.V. Jehle (1995). Response of headaches to nonnarcotic analgesic resulting in missed intracranial hemorrhage. *Am. J. Emerg. Med.* 13:43–45.

Shinton, R. and G. Sagar (1993). Life-long exercise and stroke. *BMJ* 307:231–234.

Shuaib, A. (1991). A stroke from other etiologies masquerading as a migraine-stroke. *Stroke* 22:1068–1074.

Shuaib, A. and V. Hachinski (1988). Migraine and the risks from angiography. *Arch. Neurol.* 45:911–912.

Shuaib, A., L. Metz, and T. Hing (1989). Migraine and intracerebral hemorrhage. *Cephalalgia* 9:59–61.

Silberstein, S.D. (1992). Evaluation and emergency treatment of headache. *Headache* 32:396–407.

Silbert, P.L., B. Mokri, and W.I. Schievink (1995). Headache and neck pain in spontaneous internal carotid and vertebral artery dissections. *Neurology* 45:1517–1522.

Silbert, P.L., D.A. Prentice, G.J. Hankey et al. (1989). Angiographically demonstrated arterial spasm in a case of benign sexual headache and benign exceptional headache. *Aust. N. Z. J. Med.* 19:466–468.

Sinclair, W. (1959). Dissecting aneurysm of the middle cerebral artery associated with migraine syndrome. *Am. J. Pathol.* 29:1083–1091.

Smith, T.P., R. Higashida, S. Barnwell et al. (1994). Treatment of dural sinus thrombosis by urokinase infusion. *Am. J. Neuroradiol.* 15:801–807.

Snyder, B.D. and R.R. McClelland (1978). Isolated benign cerebral vasculitis. *Arch. Neurol.* 35:612–614.

Soges, L.J., E.D. Cacayorin, G.R. Petro et al. (1988). Migraine evaluation by MR. *Am. J. Neuroradiol.* 9:425–429.

Solomon, S., R.B. Lipton, and P.Y. Harris (1990). Arterial stenosis in migraine spasm or arteriopathy. *Headache* 30:51–61.

Soman, T.B., A.B. Singhal, B. Wang et al. (1999). Reversible white matter hyperintensity on diffusion weighted imaging (DWI) in a patient with hemiplegic migraine [abstract]. *Neurology* 52:87.

Sorani, S., C. Borgna-Pignatti, E. Trabetti et al. (1998). Frequency of factor V Leiden in juvenile migraine with aura. *Headache* 38:779–781.

Steele, J.G., P.U. Nath, J. Burn et al. (1993). An association between migrainous aura and hereditary hemorrhagic telangiectasia. *Headache* 33: 145–148.

Steiner, T.J., F. Ahmed, L.J. Findley et al. (1998). S-Fluoxetine in the prophylaxis of migraine: A phase II double-blind randomized placebo-controlled study. *Cephalalgia* 18:283–286.

Stone, J.H., M.G. Pomper, R. Roubenoff et al. (1994). Sensitivities of noninvasive tests for central nervous system vasculitis: A comparison of lumbar puncture, computed tomography, and magnetic resonance imaging. *J. Rheumatol.* 21: 1277–1282.

Strandgaard, S. and P. Henry (1993). Arterial hypertension. In *The Headaches* (J. Olesen, P. Tfelt-Hansen, and K.M.A. Welch, eds.), pp. 675–678. Raven Press, New York.

Sturzenegger, M. (1994). Headache and neck pain. The warning symptoms of vertebral artery dissection. *Headache* 34: 187–193.

Sturzenegger, M. (1995). Spontaneous internal carotid artery dissection: early diagnosis and management in 44 patients. *J. Neurol.* 242:231–238.

Sudo, K. and K. Tashiro (1998). Idiopathic granulomatous angiitis of the CNS manifesting as white matter disease. *Neurology* 51:1774.

Tatemichi, T.K. and J.P. Mohr (1992). Migraine and stroke. In *Stroke: Pathophysiology, Diagnosis and Management* (H.J.M. Barnett, J.P. Mohr, B.M. Stein et al., eds.), pp. 761–785. Churchill-Livingstone, New York.

Tehindrazanarivelo, A., G. Lutz, C. Petitjean et al. (1991). Headache following carotid endarterectomy: A prospective study. *Cephalalgia* 11:353.

Tehindrazanarivelo, A.D., S. Evrard, M. Schaison et al. (1992). Prospective study of cerebral sinus venous thrombosis in patients presenting with benign intracranial hypertension. *Cerebrovasc. Dis.* 2:22–27.

Tietjen, G.E., S.R. Levine, and K.M.A. Welch (1992). Migraine and antiphospholipid antibodies. In *Current Neurology* (S.H. Appel, ed.), pp. 201–213. Mosby Year Book, Chicago.

Tourbah, A., J.L. Mas, J.C. Baron et al. (1988). Complicated migraine, migrainous infarction or what? *Headache* 28:689.

Tournier-Lasserve, E., M.T. Iba-Zizen, N. Romero et al. (1991). Autosomal dominant syndrome with stroke-like episodes and leukoencephalopathy. *Stroke* 22:1297–1302.

Tournier-Lasserve, E., A. Joutel, and J. Melki (1993). Cerebral autosomal dominant arteriopathy with subcortical infarcts and leukoencephalopathy maps to chromosome 19q12. *Nat. Genet.* 3:256–259.

Trommer, B.C., D. Homer, and M.A. Mikhael (1988). Cerebral vasospasm and eclampsia. *Stroke* 19:326–329.

Troost, B.T., L.E. Mark, and J.C. Maroon (1979). Resolution of classic migraine after removal of an occipital lobe arteriovenous malformation. *Ann. Neurol.* 5:199–201.

Troost, B.T. and R.L. Tomsak (1993). Ophthalmoplegic migraine and retinal migraine. In *The Headaches* (J. Olesen, P. Tfelt-Hansen, and K.M.A. Welch, eds.), pp. 421–426. Raven Press, New York.

Tsai, F.Y., A.M. Wang, V.B. Matovich et al. (1995). MR staging of acute dural sinus thrombosis: Correlation with venous pressure measurements and implications for treatment and prognosis. *Am. J. Neuroradiol.* 16:1021–1029.

Tzourio, C., S. Inglesias, J.B. Hubert et al. (1993). Migraine and risk of ischemic stroke: a case control study. *BMJ* 307:289–292.

Tzourio, C., A. Tehindrazanarivelo, S. Iglesias et al. (1995). Case-control study of migraine and risk of ischemic stroke in young women. *BMJ* 310:830–833.

Ursell, M.R., C.L. Marras, R. Farb et al. (1998). Recurrent intracranial hemorrhage due to postpartum cerebral angiopathy. Implications for management. *Stroke* 29:1995–1998.

Valavanis, A., R. Friede, O. Schubiger et al. (1979). Cerebral granulomatous angiitis simulating brain tumor. *J. Comput. Assist. Tomogr.* 3:536–538.

van der Wee, N., G.J. Rinkel, D. Hasan et al. (1995). Detection of subarachnoid hemorrhage on early CT: Is lumbar puncture still needed after a negative scan? *J. Neurol. Neurosurg. Psychiatry* 58:357–359.

Varelas, P.N., C.A. Wojman, and P. Fayad (1999). Uncommon migraine subtypes and their relation to stroke. *Neurologist* 5:135–144.

Verin, M., Y. Rolland, F. Landgraf et al. (1995). New phenotype of the cerebral autosomal dominant arteriopathy mapped to chromosome 19; migraine as the prominent clinical feature. *J. Neurol. Neurosurg. Psychiatry* 59:579–585.

Vermeulen, M. (1996). Subarachnoid hemorrhage: Diagnosis and treatment. *J. Neurol.* 243:496–501.

Vermeulen, M., D. Hasan, B.G. Blijenberg et al. (1989). Xanthochromia after subarachnoid hemorrhage needs no revisitation. *J. Neurol. Neurosurg. Psychiatry* 52:826–828.

Vermeulen, M. and J. Van Gijn (1990). The diagnosis of subarachnoid hemorrhage. *J. Neurol. Neurosurg. Psychiatry* 53:365–372.

Verweij, R.D., E.F. Wijdicks, and J. Van Gijn (1988). Warning headache in aneurysmal subarachnoid hemorrhage: A case-control study. *Arch. Neurol.* 45:1019–1020.

Vestergaard, K., G. Andersen, M.I. Nielsen et al. (1993). Headache in stroke. *Stroke* 24:1621–1624.

Vijayan, N. and C. Watson (1986). Raeder's syndrome, pericarotid syndrome and carotidynia. In *Headache* (P.J. Vinken and G.W. Bruyn, eds.), pp. 329–341. North Holland Publishing, Amsterdam.

Villringer, A., S. Mehraein, and K.M. Einhdupl (1994). Treatment of sinus venous thrombosis beyond the recommendation of anticoagulation. *J. Neuroradiol.* 21:72–80.

Virapongse, C., C. Cazenave, R. Quisling et al. (1987). The empty delta sign: Frequency and significance in 76 cases of dural sinus thrombosis. *Radiology* 162:779–785.

Vollmer, T.L., J. Guarnaccia, W. Harrington et al. (1993). Idiopathic granulomatous angiitis of the central nervous system: Diagnostic challenges. *Arch. Neurol.* 50:925–930.

Waga, S., K. Ohtsubo, and H. Handa (1975). Warning signs in intracranial aneurysms. *Surg. Neurol.* 18:119–1205.

Walker, C.H. (1959). Migraine and its relationship to hypertension. *BMJ* 2:1430–1433.

Waltimo, O., E. Hokkanen, and R. Pirskanen (1975). Intracranial arteriovenous malformations and headache. *Headache* 15:133–135.

Waters, W.E. (1971). Headache and blood pressure in the community. *BMJ* 1:142–143.

Weir, B. (1998). Diagnostic aspects of subarachnoid hemorrhage. In *Subarachnoid Hemorrhage: Causes and Cures* (B. Weir, ed.), pp. 144–176. Oxford University Press, New York.

Weiss, N.S. (1972). Relation of high blood pressure to headache, epistaxis, and selected other symptoms. *N. Engl. J. Med.* 287:631–633.

Welch, K.M.A. (1994). Relationships of stroke and migraine. *Neurology* 44:33–36.

Welch, K.M., T.K. Tatemichi, and J.P. Mohr (1998a). Migraine and stroke. In *Stroke, Pathophysiology, Diagnosis, and Management* (H.J. Barnett, J.P. Mohr, B.M. Stein et al., eds.), pp. 845–867. Churchill Livingstone, Philadelphia.

Welch, K.M.A., Y. Cao, S. Aurora et al. (1998b). MRI of the occipital cortex, red nucleus, and substantia nigra during visual aura of migraine. *Neurology* 51:1465–1469.

Welch, K.M.A. and S.R. Levine (1990). Migraine-related stroke in the context of the International Headache Society classifications of migraine. *Arch. Neurol.* 47:458–462.

Whitty, C.W. (1953). Familial hemiplegic migraine. *J. Neurol. Neurosurg. Psychiatry* 16:172–177.

Wijdicks, E.F.M., H. Kerkhoff, and H. VanGijn (1988). Long-term follow-up of 71 patients with thunderclap headache mimicking subarachnoid hemorrhage. *Lancet* 2:68–70.

Wijman, C., P.A. Wolf, C.S. Kase et al. (1998). Migrainous visual accompaniments are not rare in late life: The Framingham Study. *Stroke* 29:1539–1543.

Will, A.D., K.L. Lewis, D.B. Hinshaw et al. (1987). Cerebral vasoconstriction in toxemia. *Neurology* 37:1555–1557.

Woods, R.P., M. Iacoboni, and J.C. Mazziotta (1994). Bilateral spreading cerebral hypoperfusion during spontaneous migraine headaches. *N. Engl. J. Med.* 331:1689–1692.

Yadav, J.S., G.S. Roubin, S. Iyer et al. (1997). Elective stenting of the extracranial carotid arteries. *Circulation* 95:376–381.

Yusuf, S., P. Sleight, J. Pogue et al. (2000). Effects of an angiotensin-converting enzyme inhibitor, ramipril, on cardiovascular events in high-risk patients. *N. Engl. J. Med.* 342:145–153.

16

Headache Associated with Abnormalities in Intracranial Structure or Function: High Cerebrospinal Fluid Pressure Headache and Brain Tumor

MICHAEL WALL
STEPHEN D. SILBERSTEIN
ROBERT D. AIKEN

Headache is one of the most common clinical manifestations of altered intracranial pressure (ICP). Any disruption of cerebrospinal fluid (CSF) production, flow, or absorption may lead to alterations in ICP and headache. Clinical syndromes include post-lumbar puncture (LP) headache, spontaneous intracranial hypotension (ICH), brain tumor, idiopathic intracranial hypertension (IIH), hydrocephalus, intracranial hemorrhage, and subdural hematoma. Mass lesions can produce traction on pain-sensitive intracranial structures, impede CSF flow, or directly increase pressure by mass effect, all of which can produce headache. Some disorders produce unique symptoms that aid in their diagnosis, e.g., the cough headache associated with hindbrain abnormalities. The International Headache Society (IHS) (Headache Classification Committee of the International Headache Society, 1988) classifies these disorders as "headache associated with nonvascular intracranial disorder" (Table 16–1). Patients may have a worsening of a pre-existing headache or may develop a new form of headache (including migraine, tension-type headache, or cluster headache) in close temporal relationship to a nonvascular intracranial disorder. Causality is not necessarily implied.

CEREBROSPINAL FLUID

Galen first described the ventricular cavities in the second century, but it was left to Contugno, in 1764, to describe the CSF. Magendie, in 1825, named the CSF and discovered, between the fourth ventricle and the subarachnoid space, the foramen that bears his name (Fishman, 1992). Dandy's work supported the view that the CSF originated from the choroid plexus and the perivascular

Table 16–1 Headache associated with nonvascular intracranial disorder

Diagnostic criteria
  Symptoms and/or signs of intracranial disorder
  Confirmation by appropriate investigation
  Headache as a new symptom or of a new type
    occurs temporally related to intracranial disorder

Table 16–2 Factors determining cerebrospinal fluid (CSF) pressure

CSF secretion pressure
CSF absorption rate
Intracranial arterial pressure
Intracranial venous pressure
Brain bulk
Hydrostatic pressure
Presence of intact/surrounding coverings

spaces of the brain. Key and Retzius demonstrated that the CSF passes from the subarachnoid space through the Pacchionian bodies into the cerebral venous sinuses (Fishman, 1992). Lumber puncture was introduced by Quinke in 1891. Using a percutaneous needle with a stylet, he measured the components of CSF and its pressure in normal and disease states. Bier first described post-LP headache in 1898, when he injected cocaine into his own subarachnoid space and developed a violent postspinal headache (Morewood, 1993). Schaltenbrand (1938) was the first to describe spontaneous ICH, using the term "spontaneous aliquorrhea."

The major source of CSF is the choroid plexus; however, some CSF is formed in extrachoroidal sites. The estimated rate of CSF formation in humans is 0.37 ml/min, which represents a formation rate of 500 ml/day. The total CSF volume is renewed every 6 to 8 hours.

In humans, in the lateral recumbent position, the average CSF pressure is 150 mm H_2O, with a range of 70 to 200 mm (Fishman, 1992; Milhorat, 1972). Corbett and Mehta (1988) recorded CSF pressures of up to 250 mm of H_2O in normal obese controls, suggesting that the upper limit of normal may be 250 mm H_2O in obese patients. When CSF pressure falls below 50 to 90 mm H_2O, symptoms of ICH occur. At times, the CSF pressure is not measurable and CSF can be obtained only by aspiration (Fishman, 1992; Milhorat, 1972; Gamache et al., 1987). If simultaneous pressures are taken from the cerebral ventricles, the cisterna magna, and the lumbar sac during a change from the recumbent to the erect posture, there is a significant change in pressure throughout the system. The pressure rises to 375 to 565 mm in the lumbar sac, becomes 0 at the level the cis-

terna magna, and can fall to −85 mm H_2O in the ventricles (Milhorat, 1972; Von Storch et al., 1937; Loman, 1934; Loman et al., 1935; Freemont-Smith and Kubie, 1929).

Transmitted venous pressure is the most important of the factors that determine CSF pressure (Table 16–2) (Milhorat, 1972). Intracranial pressure can be elevated by any of the mechanisms listed in Table 16–3. A mass lesion can produce elevated ICP when it (1) reaches a critical size; (2) obstructs the intracranial venous system, producing increased venous pressure; or (3) obstructs the CSF pathways. According to the Monro-Kellie doctrine, any increase in intracranial volume leads to increased ICP; since an adult's skull has rigid walls, it forms a closed chamber, with a small exit, the foramen magnum, providing the only outlet for CSF into the vertebral canal.

INTRACRANIAL HYPERTENSION

Intracranial hypertension may be either (1) *idiopathic*, with no clear identifiable cause, or (2) *symptomatic*, a result of other causes such as venous sinus occlusion, mass lesion, meningitis, trauma, radical neck dissection, hy-

Table 16–3 Mechanisms for elevated intracranial pressure

Increased CSF production or secretion pressure
Decreased CSF absorption
Increased venous pressure
Obstruction of normal CSF flow
Increase in brain bulk
Mass lesion/cerebral edema
Increased bulk or pressure in dura
Combination of above

Key to abbreviations: CSF, cerebrospinal fluid.

Table 16–4 Syndromes of increased intracranial pressure

Primary
  Idiopathic intracranial hypertension
Secondary
  A. Hydrocephalus
  B. Mass lesion
    1. Neoplasm
    2. Stroke, hematoma
  C. Meningitis/encephalitis
  D. Trauma
  E. Major intracranial and extracranial venous
     obstruction
  F. Drugs
    1. Vitamin A
    2. Nalidixic acid
    3. Anabolic steroids
    4. Steroid withdrawal
  G. Systemic disease
    1. Renal disease
    2. Hypoparathyroidism
    3. Systemic lupus erythematosus

poparathyroidism, vitamin A intoxication, systemic lupus, renal disease, or drug side effects (nalidixic acid, danocrine, steroid withdrawal) (Table 16–4) (Corbett and Thompson, 1989). Intracranial venous outflow obstruction can be caused by chronic otitis, head trauma, tumors, hypercoagulable states, and cerebral edema (Johnston et al., 1991). Extracranial venous outflow obstruction occurs with surgical ligation and further compression of venous outflow. Cranial venous outflow hypertension can also occur without obstruction in patients with arteriovenous malformations, cardiac failure, and pulmonary failure. Increased ICP is not always associated with either headache or papilledema, and there is no direct correlation between the degree of pressure elevation and the presence of headache. Postulated mechanisms for headache are listed in Table 16–5. A convexity meningioma may distort the

Table 16–5 Mechanisms for headache with increased intracranial pressure

Traction on pain-sensitive intracerebral vessels (venous sinuses and arteries at the base of the brain)
Transient herniation of hippocampal gyri
Traction on cranial or cervical nerves or elevation of intracranial pressure

adjacent middle meningeal artery and cause pain, which may be referred to the ipsilateral frontotemporal region. A posterior fossa tumor may impinge upon the seventh cranial nerve, producing a headache that is referred to the ipsilateral ear.

Although increased CSF pressure is not necessary for headache development, it clearly plays a role in some patients with CNS neoplasms, acute obstructive hydrocephalus, and idiopathic intracranial hypertension. The rate of the change in pressure may be critical. Sudden increases in ICP by tumors obstructing the foramen of Monro or the cerebral aqueduct may cause abrupt, severe headache associated with gait disturbance, syncope, incontinence, or visual obscurations.

INTRACRANIAL NEOPLASMS

Headaches are initially present in 20% of patients with brain tumor and rise to about 60% during the disease (Jaeckle, 1993). Headache is a rare initial symptom in patients with pituitary tumors, craniopharyngiomas, or cerebellopontine angle tumors (Jaeckle, 1991; Lavyne and Patterson, 1987). It is a very common initial symptom with infratentorial tumors (other than cerebellopontine angle tumors), occurring in 80% to 85% of patients (Kunkle et al., 1942b; Northfield, 1938). Elevation of ICP is not necessary for its production. In one older, pre-computed tomography (CT) series of 72 brain tumor patients, headache occurred in those patients without elevated ICP as often as it did in those with increased ICP (Lavyne and Patterson, 1987).

The headache is usually bilateral, but it can be on the side of the tumor (Jaeckle, 1991; Lavyne and Patterson, 1987). Supratentorial tumors that impinge on structures innervated by the ophthalmic division of the fifth cranial nerve may produce frontotemporal headache, while posterior fossa tumors may compress the ninth and tenth cranial nerves and produce occipitonuchal pain. Metastatic brain tumors may invade the meninges (meningeal carcinomatosis) and produce generalized headache and other signs of meningeal irritation. Occasionally, brain tumors produce a migraine-like headache, even with a visual aura. Nausea and/or vomiting accompany the headache in 50% of patients. The mild, early-morning, frontal headache that resolves within 30 to 60 minutes after waking is uncommon in brain tumor patients (Forsyth and Posner, 1993). The severe headaches they experience can be aggravated by Valsalva, change in position, or exertion and probably result from sudden increases in ICP or traction on pain-sensitive structures such as the dura, cranial nerves, or large venous sinuses (Ray and Wolff, 1940).

The headache most commonly described is similar to a tension-type headache and is typically described as a dull ache or pressure. These headaches are usually bifrontal and worse on the side ipsilateral to the tumor. They generally have little radiation, except in posterior fossa tumors, and often spare the posterior head region. They are worse in the morning in about one-third of patients and day-long in a similar number.

The features associated with brain tumor headache are increased ICP, tumor size and amount of midline shift, and a prior history of headache (Forsyth and Posner, 1993). Increased ICP (mostly from posterior fossa and leptomeningeal tumors) usually produces headaches. It is more commonly an isolated symptom in patients who have multiple metastases than in those with single lesions.

Tumor size and degree of midline shift are congruent with the observation in intracranial stimulation experiments (Kunkle et al., 1942a) that brain tumor headaches result from traction on intracranial pain-sensitive structures. Traction by the tumor mass may distort pain-sensitive structures or act distantly by causing brain displacement or hydrocephalus. Frontal and periorbital headache is common in supratentorial tumors because of irritation of trigeminal sensory afferents. Posterior fossa tumors irritate the tissues supplied by the sensory branches of cranial nerves IX and X and the upper cervical nerves. One pre-CT/magnetic resonance imaging (MRI) series looked at the characteristic headache features of 221 patients who had brain tumors, only 60% of whom had headache (Rushton and Rooke, 1962). Tumor

location had no significant bearing on the presence or absence of headache. Pain intensity was mild to moderate in 63% of patients and severe in 37%. Headaches were intermittent in 85%, throbbing in 15%, and aggravated by changing position in 20%, by coughing or exertion in 25%, and on the side of the tumor in 30%. Five patients had exertional headache. Half of the patients had nausea or vomiting. Twenty-five percent had headache during sleep, on arising, or both. Increased ICP was observed in 42% of patients with headache and in 6% of patients without headache.

In a survey of 778 patients with cerebral tumor, headache was the earliest or principal symptom in 54%. No difference in headache frequency was noted between rapidly growing and slowly growing tumors. The headache can occur intermittently and mimic migraine (Heyck, 1968).

Patients who have a history of headaches are more likely to have headaches with their brain tumor. In many cases, this headache is similar in character to the prior headache but more severe, more frequent, or associated with neurologic signs or symptoms. Vazquez-Barquero et al. (1994) found that only 8% of patients with brain tumor had headache as their first and isolated clinical manifestation at the time of diagnosis. Thirty-one percent had headache, but only one of the original patients continued to have headache as an isolated symptom (Vazquez-Barquero et al., 1994). The prevalence of headache as an initial symptom of brain tumor has decreased in many series due to earlier detection by neuroimaging.

UNCOMMON HEADACHES IN BRAIN TUMOR PATIENTS

Paroxysmal headaches are a unique feature of some patients who have a colloid cyst of the third ventricle or other pedunculated tumor that may obstruct CSF flow. These headaches are generally of sudden onset, reach peak intensity in seconds, and are brief. They may also resolve quickly and may be suddenly precipitated (and relieved) by changes in position. They may be a cause of brief losses of consciousness or "drop attacks." Patients may walk unsteadily between headaches.

Cough or exertional headache is a transient, severe headache precipitated by Valsalva maneuver or running. These headaches are brief and poorly localized. Brain tumors have been identified in 2% to 11% of patients who have these types of headache (Symonds, 1956; Rooke, 1968).

Headaches may be caused by base-of-skull metastasis. Five distinct syndromes have been defined according to location (Greenberg et al., 1981). These include (1) orbital syndrome, (2) parasellar syndrome, (3) gasserian ganglion syndrome, (4) jugular foramen syndrome, and (5) occipital condyle syndrome. The orbital syndrome results from orbital metastases and consists of a dull supraorbital ache. It may be followed by diplopia, proptosis, and, in its later stages, deteriorating visual acuity. The parasellar syndrome is caused by metastasis to the sella turcica. The tumor (metastases) erodes into the cavernous sinus and produces unilateral frontal headache, periorbital edema, ocular paresis, and ophthalmic trigeminal sensory loss. The gasserian ganglion syndrome is characterized by a dull ache in the cheek, jaw, or forehead and occasional trigeminal neuralgia-like pain. Loss of sensation is present in the V_2 and V_3 sensory distribution. Jugular foramen metastases produce a unilateral, dull, aching, retroauricular pain, hoarseness, and dysphagia. Occipital condyle metastases cause severe, unilateral, occipital headaches that are aggravated by neck flexion. Patients may also complain of dysarthria and dysphagia. Ipsilateral tongue atrophy is also commonly seen.

Headaches are a more common symptom of brain tumor in children (>90%) than in adults (ca. 60%), due in part, perhaps, to the greater prevalence of posterior fossa tumors (Zulch et al., 1974). The following characteristics occur frequently: headache awakening the child or present on awakening, severe or prolonged headache, increased severity or frequency of headache, and increased frequency of vomiting. Most children (94%) with headache had neurologic signs. In 96%, diagnostic clues appeared within 4 months of the onset of headache (Honig and Charney, 1982).

The Childhood Brain Tumor Consortium published their retrospective record review on the incidence of headache in children with central nervous system tumors. The overall incidence of headache was 62%, ranging from 70% with infratentorial lesions to 58% with supratentorial tumors to 35% in patients with spinal canal tumors, approximately the incidence of benign headache in elementary school children. Headache was typically associated with other signs or symptoms and was rarely an isolated symptom (<1%). Symptoms of intracranial tumor included abnormal academic performance, difficulty walking, back or abdomen pain, bladder symptoms, increasing head circumference, and failure to thrive. Headache frequency increased through age 7 and leveled off regardless of tumor location. The low percentage of headache in the very young may be due to the expansile nature of the infant skull or may be an artifact of the inability of young children to communicate the source of their discomfort (Childhood Brain Tumor Consortium, 1991).

Following successful combined whole-brain radiotherapy and chemotherapy of posterior fossa or pineal tumors (14 to 32 months after termination of therapy), four children developed episodic, severe hemicranial headaches associated with nausea and transient visual loss, hemisensory deficit, dysphasia, or hemiparesis (Shuper et al., 1995). These children had no prior history of similar headaches, no family history of migraine, and no evidence of tumor recurrence. It is unclear what produces these migrainous manifestations. The occurrence of headaches in treated brain tumor patients does not necessarily mean tumor recurrence.

There is a significant overlap between the headache of brain tumor and migraine or tension-type headache (TTH). A headache of recent onset, a headache that has changed in character, or a headache accompanied by a neurologic sign or symptom that cannot be easily explained by the aura of migraine requires a thorough evaluation, particularly if it is severe or occurs with nausea or vomiting.

Morning or nocturnal headache associated with vomiting and increased headache frequency can be seen with both migraine and brain tumor. Brain tumor headache is more common in patients with a history of prior headache, increased ICP, and large tumors with a midline shift.

In other space-occupying lesions, such as subdural hematomas and brain abscesses, headache is an earlier and more frequent symptom. Eighty-one percent of McKissock's (1960) 216 patients with chronic subdural hematoma had headache; only 11% of acute and 53% of subacute subdural hematoma patients had headache. The difference in headache prevalence between tumor and subdural hematoma is believed to be due to the more rapid evolution and greater extent of the hematomas. The lesser occurrence of headache in acute and subacute subdural hematomas compared with chronic subdural hematoma may be due to the underlying traumatic cerebral changes in the former, affecting consciousness early and making it difficult to elicit a history of headache.

In brain abscesses, a progressively severe, intractable headache is common. In published clinical series, headache was present in 70% to 90% of patients (Britt, 1985) (Fig. 16–1). The higher headache prevalence in patients with abscesses compared to tumors may be due to the faster evolution, the associated meningeal reaction, and the occasional fever that may accompany abscess.

IDIOPATHIC INTRACRANIAL HYPERTENSION

Idiopathic intracranial hypertension (IIH), also called pseudotumor cerebri or benign intracranial hypertension, is a disorder of elevated CSF pressure, usually of women in the childbearing years. Its primary presenting symptom is headache. The disorder is characterized by the symptoms and signs of increased ICP in an alert and oriented patient but without localizing neurologic findings. There is no evidence of deformity or obstruction of the ventricular system, and neurodiagnostic studies are otherwise normal except for increased CSF pressure (>200 mm of water in the nonobese and >250 mm of water in the obese patient) (Corbett and Mehta, 1983). In addition, no secondary cause of generalized ICP is present. These comprise the modified Dandy criteria for IIH (Smith, 1985) (Table 16–6). The common signs and symptoms of increased ICP are headache, transient episodes of visual loss (transient visual obscurations), and pulse-synchronous tinnitus; visual findings are diplopia due to

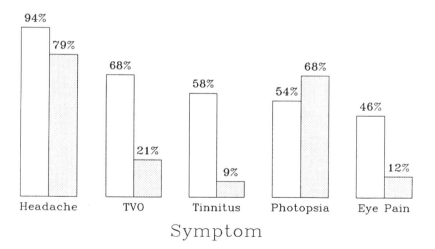

Figure 16–1 Frequency in percent of symptoms of patients with idiopathic intracranial hypertension (IIH) compared with a control group. *TVO*, transient visual obscurations. Reprinted with permission from Giuseffi, V., M. Wall, P.Z. Siegal et al. (1991). Symptoms and disease associations in idiopathic intracranial hypertension (pseudotumor cerebri): A case-control study. *Neurology* 41:239–244.

Table 16–6 Modified Dandy criteria for the diagnosis of increased intracranial pressure

Signs and symptoms of increased intracranial pressure
Absence of localizing findings on neurologic examination
Absence of deformity, displacement, or obstruction of the ventricular system and otherwise normal neurodiagnostic studies except for increased cerebrospinal fluid pressure (>250 mm H_2O in the obese patient)
Awake and alert patient
No other cause of increased intracranial pressure present

sixth cranial nerve paresis and papilledema with its associated loss of sensory visual function.

Epidemiology

The annual incidence of IIH is 0.9/100,000 persons and 3.5/100,000 in women 15 to 44 years of age (Durcan et al., 1988; Radhkrishnan et al., 1993). More than 90% of IIH patients are obese, and over 90% are women. The mean age at the time of diagnosis is 32 years.

Studies of conditions associated with IIH are mostly uncontrolled and retrospective. This has led to erroneous conclusions because investigators have reported chance and spurious associations with common medical conditions and medications as well as many case reports of associations with IIH where the cases do not meet the modified Dandy criteria of IIH. A critical review of these associations can be found elsewhere (Giuseffi et al., 1991; Wall, 1991) (Table 16–7).

Any disorder that causes decreased flow through the arachnoid granulations or obstructs the venous pathway from the granulations to the right heart is accepted as a cause of ICH. Arteriovenous malformations or dural fistulae with high flow may overload venous return and result in elevation of ICP.

Although steroid withdrawal and Addison's disease are clearly associated with IIH, as is hypoparathyroidism, links to other endocrine abnormalities remain unproven. For example, corticosteroid use has been associated with

many suspected cases of IIH; however, none fulfills the modified Dandy criteria of IIH.

Several other associations with IIH have been refuted by controlled studies (Digre and Corbett, 1988; Ireland et al., 1990; Giuseffi et al., 1991; Williams, 1976). Pregnancy, irregular menses, and oral contraceptive use have been shown to be chance associations. In case-control studies, no association has been found between IIH and multivitamin, oral contraceptive, corticosteroid, or antibiotic use. However, case reports associating some drugs appear convincing: nalidixic acid (Deonna and Guignard, 1974), nitrofurantoin (Mushet, 1977), indomethacin (Konomi et al., 1978) or ketoprofen (Larizza et al., 1979) in Bartter's syndrome, vitamin A (Feldman and Schlezinger, 1970), isotretinoin (Spector and Carlisle, 1984), thyroid replacement therapy in hypothyroid children (Van Dop et al., 1983), lithium (Saul et al., 1985), and anabolic steroids (Shah et al., 1987).

A case-control study has found strong associations between IIH and obesity and weight gain during the 12 months before diagnosis (Giuseffi et al., 1991). In this study, there was no evidence that IIH was associated with any other medical conditions, pregnancy, or consumption of any medications. In summary, other than obesity and recent weight gain, many conditions associated with IIH are common disorders of women in childbearing years and are likely chance associations.

Pathogenesis

The most popular hypothesis is that IIH is a syndrome of reduced CSF absorption. Reduced conductance to CSF outflow may be due to dysfunction of the absorptive mechanism of the arachnoid granulations. Intracranial pressure then must rise for CSF to be absorbed. There are conflicting results regarding the presence of any brain edema (Sahs and Joynt, 1956) but it is likely that significant brain edema does not occur (Wall et al., 1995). Malm et al. (1992) believe, but it is not yet certain, that increased CSF pressure in IIH is a result of either a rise in venous sagittal sinus pressure secondary to ex-

Table 16–7 Differential diagnosis of idiopathic intracranial hypertension

Highly likely
    Decreased flow through arachnoid granulations
        Scarring from previous inflammation (e.g., meningitis, sequel to subarachnoid
        hemorrhage)
    Obstruction to venous drainage
        Venous sinus thromboses
            Hypercoagulable states
            Contiguous infection (e.g., middle ear or mastoid, otitic hydrocephalus)
        Bilateral radical neck dissections
        Superior vena cava syndrome
        Increased right heart pressure
    Endocrine disorders
        Addison's disease
        Hypoparathyroidism
        Obesity
        Steroid withdrawal
    Nutritional disorders
        Hypervitaminosis A (vitamin, liver, or isotretinoin intake)
        Hyperalimentation in deprivation dwarfism
    Arteriovenous malformations and dural shunts
Probable causes
    Anabolic steroids (may cause venous sinus thrombosis)
    Chlordecone (kepone)
    Ketoprofen or indomethacin in Bartter's syndrome
    Systemic lupus erythematosus
    Thyroid replacement therapy in hypothyroid children
    Uremia
Possible causes
    Amiodarone
    Diphenylhydantoin
    Iron-deficiency anemia
    Lithium carbonate
    Nalidixic acid
    Sarcoidosis
    Sulfa antibiotics
    Tetracycline
Causes frequently cited that are unproven
    Corticosteroid intake
    Hyperthyroidism
    Hypovitaminosis A
    Menarche
    Menstrual irregularities
    Multivitamin intake
    Oral contraceptive use
    Pregnancy

The table lists the etiologies of intracranial hypertension that meet the modified Dandy criteria except that a cause is associated. The highly likely category is a list of cases with many reports of the association with multiple lines of evidence. Probable causes have reports with some convincing evidence. Possible causes have suggestive evidence or are common conditions or medications with intracranial hypertension as a rare association. Also listed are some frequently cited but poorly documented or unlikely causes; three case-control studies suggest that this group of associations is not valid.

tracellular edema causing venous obstruction or a low conductance for CSF reabsorption producing a compensatory increase in CSF pressure. King et al. (1995) evaluated nine IIH patients with cerebral venography and manometry. Elevated venous pressure was found in the superior sagittal and proximal transverse sinuses, which dropped at the level of the lateral third of the transverse sinus. The abnormality, not as well demonstrated on venography, resembled mural thrombosis. Two patients with ICH due to minocycline did not have venous hypertension.

Karahalios et al. (1996) studied ten patients with IIH using angiography and manometry. Five patients had dural venous outflow obstruction on venography, while five had normal anatomy. Pressure was elevated in the superior sagittal sinus in all patients. In those with obstruction, there was a high pressure gradient across the stenosis. In those without obstruction, the right atrial pressure was elevated. Angioplasty or infusion of thrombolytic agents improved outlet obstruction but not the clinical picture. The authors suggested that elevated venous ICP may be the universal mechanism of IIH and that all cases are symptomatic. Our major concerns with this observation is the absence of any sign of right-heart failure in patients with elevated right atrial pressure. And, papilledema is rare in patients with right-heart failure, a condition that elevates CSF venous pressure.

Symptoms

Fifty patients in a case-control study answered a questionnaire at the time of their initial office visit. Their symptoms were compared to 100 age-matched controls (Giuseffi et al., 1991). The symptoms most commonly reported by IIH patients were headache (94%), transient visual obscurations (68%), pulse-synchronous tinnitus (58%), photopsia (54%), and retrobulbar pain (44%). The frequency of these symptoms compared to controls is shown in Figure 16–1. Diplopia (38%), visual loss (30%), and retrobulbar pain on eye movement (22%) were less common accompaniments of IIH and were not reported by any of the controls. Of these common symptoms, all except headache and photopsia occurred much more frequently in cases than controls.

Headache

The presence of headache is nearly ubiquitous in patients with IIH and is the usual presenting symptom. Experimentally induced increased ICP in humans produced by CSF infusion can cause pulsatile pain that is usually frontal or temporal in location. It may be associated with vomiting. More commonly, however, the infusion provoked variable headache responses (Fay, 1940). Johnston and Paterson (1974) monitored ICP in 20 patients us-

ing an intraventricular catheter. Thirteen cases had plateau waves. Eight cases had plateau-like waves. Neither type of wave was related to headache or, for that matter, any change in clinical symptoms. Therefore, the trigger for headache due to raised ICP is unknown.

The headache profile of the IIH patient based on prospective data collection (Wall, 1990) is that of severe daily headaches described as pulsatile pain that gradually increased in intensity. Nausea was common and vomiting less frequent. Most of those with headache reported that it was the worst head pain ever and different from previous headaches. The headache commonly awakened the patient. Postural aggravating factors were uncommon. The cephalalgia usually lasted hours. Although uncommon, the presence of retrobulbar pain accentuated by eye movements or pain radiating in a nerve root distribution, possibly from dilation of spinal nerve root sleeves, may aid in separation of this headache syndrome. Neck stiffness is found in about half of patients. The frequency of these headache characteristics with respect to a control population is shown in Table 16–8.

Transient Visual Obscurations

Visual obscurations are episodes of transient visual loss usually lasting less than 30 seconds.

Table 16–8 Frequency of symptoms associated with headache in cases and controls (Wall, 1990)

Symptom	Cases	Controls
Most severe	91%	1%
Different from previous	85%	1%
Radicular pain	19%	0%
Vomiting	36%	3%
One-sided	62%	9%
Awaken patient	62%	13%
Nausea	60%	14%
Neck stiffness	51%	13%
Pulsatile	79%	38%
Retro-orbital pain	47%	15%
on eye movement	23%	0%
Last longer than 1 hour	85%	53%
Generalized	47%	25%
Intensity slowly increases	70%	54%
Focal	49%	75%

Reproduced with permission from Wall, M. (1990). The headache profile of idiopathic intracranial hypertension. *Cephalagia* 10:331–335.

Visual obscurations occur in about three-fourths of IIH patients (Wall and George, 1991). The attacks may be monocular or binocular. They are not correlated with the degree of ICH or with the extent of disc edema (Hayreh, 1977). The cause of these episodes is thought to be transient ischemia of the optic nerve head due to increased tissue pressure (Sadun et al., 1984). Visual obscurations do not appear to be associated with poor visual outcome (Corbett, 1983; Rush, 1980; Wall and George, 1991).

Pulse-Synchronous Tinnitus

Pulse-synchronous tinnitus, or pulsatile intracranial noise, occurs in about two-thirds of patients with IIH. The sound is often unilateral, with neither side predominating. In patients with ICH, jugular compression ipsilateral to the sound abolishes it. Sismanis (1987) found pulsatile tinnitus in each of 20 IIH patients. It was synchronous with the heartbeat and disappeared immediately, but temporarily, following LP. He attributed the noise to transmission of intensified vascular pulsations via CSF under high pressure to the walls of the venous sinuses. The periodic compres-

sions were thought to convert the laminar blood flow to turbulent.

Signs

Ophthalmoscopic Examination

Papilledema is the hallmark sign of IIH, but rare patients with increased ICP do not have papilledema (Wang et al., 1998; Spence et al., 1980; Mathew et al., 1996). Dilated examination of the ocular fundus using indirect ophthalmoscopy is necessary to be certain there is no optic disc edema. Although IIH can occur without papilledema, the reports above suffer from lack of indirect ophthalmoscopy.

Recognition of early papilledema can be difficult. The earliest sign of papilledema is optic disc elevation. Unfortunately, this sign may also occur as a normal variant. The earliest objective signs of papilledema are (1) edema in the peripapillary region obscuring the details of the adjacent nerve fiber layer (Figure 16–2), (2) irregularity and coarsening of this nerve fiber layer, (3) loss of spontaneous venous pulsations after previous documentation of their presence, and (4) associ-

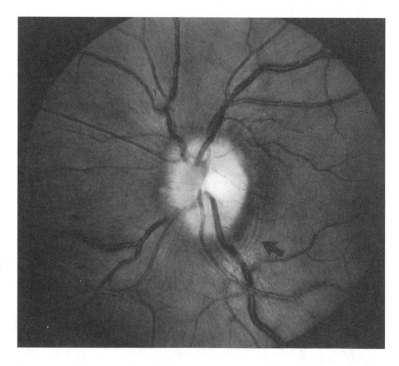

Figure 16–2 Optic disc with early papilledema showing a characteristic "C-shaped halo" with a temporal gap surrounding the disc. Also, note the choroidal folds (*arrow*).

ated choroidal folds (Figure 16–2). When the presence of papilledema is difficult to determine, repeated examinations or serial optic disc stereo photographs are useful.

Papilledema is the cause of most of the visual loss of IIH. Although there is a significant correlation between high-grade papilledema and atrophic papilledema and visual loss (Wall and White, 1998; Orcutt et al., 1984), in the individual patient the severity of visual loss cannot be predicted from the severity of the papilledema. A partial explanation for this is that, with axonal death from compression of the optic nerve, the amount of papilledema decreases.

Ocular Motility Disturbances

Horizontal diplopia occurs in about one of three IIH patients, and sixth nerve palsies are documented in 10% to 20% in large series. Motility disturbances other than sixth nerve palsies have been reported. Some of these reflect erroneous conclusions from the small vertical ocular motor imbalance known to accompany sixth nerve palsies. A diagnosis of IIH should be questioned in patients with ocular motility disturbances other than sixth nerve palsies.

Pupil Examination

A relative afferent pupillary defect is a sensitive sign of a unilateral optic neuropathy. It occurs in about 25% of IIH patients. It is usually absent in IIH since its existence depends on asymmetric visual loss and the optic neuropathy of IIH is most often fairly symmetric.

Central Visual Function

Visual acuity is usually unaffected in patients with papilledema except when the condition is long-standing or severe. Although commonly used, Snellen acuity testing is insensitive to the amount of visual loss compared to perimetry (Wall and George, 1991).

A better measure of central visual loss is contrast sensitivity testing. As opposed to Snellen acuity, it reveals deficits in 50% to 75% of eyes tested. In a study emphasizing visual function testing, it was the only visual parameter that significantly correlated with the symptom of sustained visual loss (Verplanck et al., 1988). Color vision testing has been disappointing as a method of detecting visual loss and following patients with IIH.

Perimetry

Most patients (up to 94%) with papilledema have visual loss (Wall and George, 1991). In 25% to 50%, this visual loss is asymptomatic. However, it is important to measure since it serves as a marker for therapeutic intervention. Perimetry is the main measure used to determine the course of therapy.

The visual field defects found in IIH are the same types as those that occur in papilledema from other causes. These "disc-related defects" are the same types as those found in glaucoma. The most common defects are enlargement of the physiologic blind spot, loss of inferonasal portions of the visual field (Fig. 16–3), and constriction of isopters. Other defects are central, paracentral, and cecocentral scotomas; arcuate scotomas; altitudinal patterns of loss; and other nerve fiber bundle defects. The loss of visual field may be progressive and severe, leading to blindness. The progression of visual loss is usually gradual.

The size of the blind spot has been used to monitor therapy. Since refraction using plus lenses often eliminates this defect, blind spot enlargement should not be considered significant visual loss unless it encroaches on fixation. Also, since blind spot size is so dependent on refraction and the patient's accommodation, it is a poor candidate to follow the course of therapy.

With treatment, there is significant improvement in the visual field in about half of patients (Wall and George, 1991). This reversibility of visual field loss in IIH is not widely appreciated. Those at risk for severe visual loss are patients with recent marked weight gain, African-American men, patients with glaucoma, those with severe systemic arterial hypertension, and patients rapidly tapered off corticosteroids.

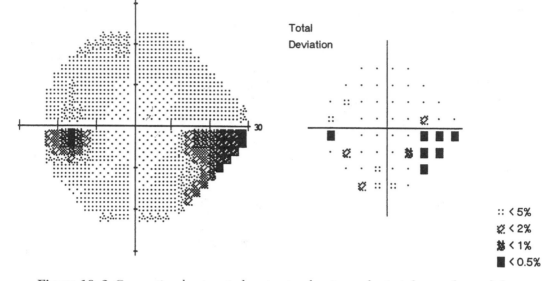

Figure 16–3 Conventional automated perimetry showing a classic inferonasal step defect.

Mechanisms of Visual Loss

Visual loss in IIH is due to optic nerve head damage. This is most likely due to the stasis of axoplasmic flow found in papilledema with resultant intraneuronal ischemia. Another mechanism to account for the rarely seen central scotomas is extension of edema from the disc into the macula. In addition, macular hemorrhages, macular pigment epithelial changes, and neovascular membrane formation have been reported in cases of papilledema.

Enlargement of the blind spot is due primarily to the peripapillary retina being hyperopic. Detachment of peripapillary retina and choroidal folds also produces defects contiguous with the blind spot. Defects from choroidal folds result from an angular misalignment of photoreceptors (Stiles-Crawford effect).

Idiopathic Intracranial Hypertension Without Papilledema

Intracranial hypertension can occur without papilledema (Wang et al., 1998; Marcelis and Silberstein, 1991; Spence et al., 1980; Scanari et al., 1979; Lipton and Michelson, 1972). The clinical, historical, radiographic, and demographic characteristics are identical to patients with papilledema, except for (1) possible association with prior head trauma or meningitis; (2) extended delay in diagnosis, which requires LP in the absence of papilledema; and, (3) no evidence of visual loss as seen in patients with IIH with papilledema. It is very rare and should not be accepted without careful indirect ophthalmoscopic examination. Patients, particularly obese women, with chronic daily headache and symptoms of increased ICP, i.e., pulsatile tinnitus, a history of head trauma or meningitis, an empty sella on neuroimaging studies, or a headache that is unrelieved by standard therapy, should have a diagnostic LP.

Why papilledema is absent in these cases of ICH is not known. Congenital or acquired optic nerve sheath defects possibly from arachnoid scanning is possible. Alternatively, ICP may not be present for a long enough period of the day to cause axoplasmic flow stasis. Unless the examination has been done with a 14-diopter lens, documented with fundus photos, and evaluated by a neuro-ophthalmologist, early papilledema is very easily missed.

In a case-control study conducted at a tertiary headache center, 25 consecutive patients with chronic daily headache (24 women, 1 man; 38 ± 6 years) who had IIH without papilledema were diagnosed between June 1989 and June 1996 (CSF pressure was $\geq$ 200 mm on two occasions, and there was no obvious papilledema). Control subjects consisted of patients with refractory chronic daily headache who had normal CSF pressure on LP (n = 60, 50 women, 10 men; 36 $\pm$ 11 years). Significant predictors of IIH without papilledema in chronic daily headache patients included pulsatile tinnitus (odds ratio = 13.0) and obesity (odds ratio = 4.4) (Wang et al., 1998). Thus, a small subset of patients with chronic daily headache, who fit the stereotype of the obese female of childbearing age, may have IIH without papilledema. These patients may respond to CDH treatment but often, although not always, respond better if the elevated CSF pressure is treated (Wang et al., 1998). These patients would not have been identified without an LP (Silberstein and Corbett, 1993a).

Therapy for Idiopathic Intracranial Hypertension

The management of patients with IIH is divided into symptomatic treatment and treatment of raised ICP. Symptomatic treatment, for the most part, is treatment of headache. Most of the migraine drugs can be used to treat the headache of IIH. However, problems that are encountered include weight gain associated with tricyclic antidepressants or valproic acid, hypotension associated with β blockers, and use of analgesics, often on a daily basis, with resultant "rebound headaches."

Medical Treatment

There are both medical and surgical treatments of raised ICP. Treatment is aimed at lowering ICP. Unfortunately, all reports to date are anecdotal as there have not been any controlled clinical treatment trials for IIH. The mainstays of medical treatment are diet and diuretics. Most IIH patients can be controlled with medical interventions.

WEIGHT LOSS

Weight loss is a cornerstone in the management of IIH. Newborg (1974) reported re-

mission of papilledema in all nine patients placed on a strict diet. She used a low-calorie rice diet with intake of 400 to 1,000 calories/day. Fluids and salt were restricted. All patients had reversal of their papilledema. Unfortunately, there was no mention of the patients' visual testing. It is unclear whether patients benefitted from weight loss, fluid restriction, sodium reduction, or a combination of these factors.

Kupersmith et al. (1998) retrospectively reviewed the charts of 56 medically treated IIH patients from two centers that had at least 6 months of follow-up. The mean time to improve one papilledema grade (of Frisén) was about 4 months in patients with weight loss compared with about 1 year in patients without weight loss. Papilledema resolved in 28/38 patients with weight loss compared with 8/20 without weight loss.

Johnson et al. (1998) retrospectively studied 15 IIH patients treated with acetazolamide and weight loss for 24 weeks. They reported an average of 3.3% weight loss in patients having one papilledema grade of improvement. Our experience has also been that improvement often occurs with only modest degrees of weight loss. Greer (1965), however, reported a group of six obese patients who became asymptomatic without weight loss.

Resolution of IIH in a patient following surgically induced weight loss (gastric exclusion procedure) was first reported by Amaral et al. (1987). Sugerman et al. (1999) performed gastric weight reduction surgery in 24 morbidly obese women with IIH. Five patients were lost to follow-up. Symptoms resolved in all but one patient within 4 months of the procedure. Two patients regained weight associated with return of their symptoms. There were many significant but treatable surgically related complications.

As Friedman and Streeten (1998) have shown, there is a subset of IIH patients with orthostatic edema. Low-salt diets and fluid restriction appear to be beneficial for many IIH patients. This may be especially true in patients who lose only a few percent of their total body mass yet have resolution of their optic disc edema. It is not yet clear whether improvement occurs because of weight loss per se or other changes in diet, such as fluid or sodium restriction.

LUMBAR PUNCTURE

Repeated LPs, although still occasionally performed, have unproven efficacy. Reduction of CSF pressure with LP has only short-lived effects. Johnston and Paterson (1974) found a return of pressure to pre-tap level after only 82 minutes. Also, repeated LPs measure CSF pressure at only one point in time. Since CSF pressure fluctuates considerably, this information has only limited clinical use for modifying treatment plans.

CORTICOSTEROIDS

Corticosteroids have been used for treating IIH since the 1960s (Paterson et al., 1961). Weisberg (1975) also has reported successfully treating patients with corticosteroids. Of those responding favorably to corticosteroid therapy, improvement of symptoms or signs occurred within 4 days.

Corticosteroids are still used to treat IIH, but their mechanism of action remains unclear. The side effects of weight gain, striae, and acne are troublesome for these obese patients. Although patients treated with steroids often respond well, there may be recurrence of papilledema with rapid tapering of the dose. This may be accompanied by severe worsening of visual function. A prolonged tapering may prevent return of symptoms and signs in some patients.

DIURETICS

Acetazolamide, a strong carbonic anhydrase inhibitor that reduces CSF production, appears effective in the treatment of IIH. Gucer and Viernstein (1978), using ICP monitoring, showed that acetazolamide lowered ICP in doses of 2 to 4 g a day. Tomsak et al. (1988) documented resolution of papilledema with photographs of the optic disc in patients treated with 1 g of acetazolamide a day. Acetazolamide is initiated with a dose of 250 mg PO BID, and the dosage is gradually increased to 1 to 2 g/day. Doses as high as 4 g/day can be used.

Furosemide has also been used to treat IIH (Corbett, 1983). It has been well documented that furosemide (Lasix) can lower ICP (Pollay et al., 1983; Roberts et al., 1987; Vogh and Langham, 1981). It appears to work by both diuresis and reducing sodium transport into the brain (Buhrley and Reed, 1972). It has also been shown to effectively lower CSF pressure when combined with acetazolamide (Schoeman, 1994). Furosemide is started at doses of 20 mg PO BID and gradually increased to a maximum dose of 40 mg PO TID. Potassium supplementation is often necessary.

Surgical Treatment

SHUNTING PROCEDURES

Current surgical therapies are various shunting and decompression procedures: lumbar subarachnoid–peritoneal shunt and optic nerve sheath fenestration. Lumbar subarachnoid–peritoneal shunting is a definitive CSF pressure–lowering procedure. It can be effective in selected patients (Eggenberger et al., 1996; Burgett et al., 1997). However, the shunting procedure may be complicated by occlusion of the tubing, sciatica, or infection. Because of high rates of shunt failure and high incidence rates of acquired Chiari I defects and syringomyelia, the procedure should not be used as a primary treatment (Rosenberg et al., 1993). Unfortunately, when shunts fail, severe visual loss can occur.

OPTIC NERVE SHEATH FENESTRATION

Optic nerve sheath fenestration is an effective method for reversing visual loss and protecting the optic nerve from further damage (Sergott et al., 1988, 1990; Corbett et al., 1988; Spoor et al., 1991; Brourman et al., 1988; Keltner, 1988; Acheson et al., 1994). Although uncommon, patients can lose vision in the perioperative period. This treatment is preferred for the patient with progressive visual loss with mild to moderate or easily controlled headaches. About half of patients with optic nerve sheath fenestration obtain adequate headache control. Since improvement in papilledema may occur in the unoperated eye and fistula formation has been demonstrated, Keltner (1988) proposed that the mechanism of action of fenestration is local decompression of the subarachnoid space. Occasional failure of the fellow eye to improve and the asymmetry of the papilledema may be explained by the resistance to CSF flow produced by the trabeculations of the subarachnoid space or tightness of the optic canal. In addition to orbital drainage (Hamed et al., 1992), the long-term mechanism of action of optic nerve sheath fenestration is unresolved but may involve closure by scarring of the subarachnoid space in the retrolaminar optic nerve or continuous function of the fistula (Smith and Orcutt, 1986).

Spoor et al. (1991) have raised the issue that patients undergoing optic nerve sheath fenestration have substantial failure rates. However, the high variability of conventional automated perimetry makes this study difficult to evaluate. Our experience has been considerably different, with few failures.

Treatment Recommendations

Patients first are educated about IIH, with an explanation of the risk of blindness as a potential outcome. This may provide the motivation to lose weight. A treatment decision algorithm that uses changes in visual function to determine the type of intervention is recommended (Fig. 16–4). Since in individual patients, symptoms and the degree of papilledema may not correlate well with loss of visual function, treatment decisions should be based primarily on the results of perimetry.

Details of treatment are beyond the scope of this monograph and can be found in other sources (Corbett and Thompson, 1989; Chou and Digre, 1999; Wall, 1991). In summary, weight loss is strongly encouraged. The patient is asked to follow a low-salt diet and to avoid excessive fluid intake. A goal of 1 pound a week of weight loss for 2 months is set. This modest amount (usually about 5% of total body weight) may be adequate to control the disease. If visual loss is present, acetazolamide or, secondarily, furosemide is used. If patients lose vision in spite of full medical therapy, optic nerve sheath fenestration is

recommended. If refractory headache is the main symptom, symptomatic therapy is given. Caffeine and frequent analgesic use is eliminated. If incapacitating headache remains, a lumbar shunt is recommended. Treatment of IIH is multifactorial and can be complex. Patients who do not respond to standard therapeutic regimens should be referred to physicians with experience in treating the disease.

EXERTIONAL AND COUGH HEADACHES

Although coughing and exertion rarely provoke headache, these maneuvers can aggravate any type of headache. However, transient, severe head pain upon coughing, sneezing, weight-lifting, bending, straining at stool, or stooping defines cough headache. Originally described by Tinel (1932b) as *la céphalée à l'effort* and later by Symonds (1956), cough headache affects mainly middle-aged men. It runs its course over a few years and is uncommon in the clinic: only 93 diagnoses were made at the Mayo Clinic over a 14-year period by Rooke (1968). He proposed the broader term "benign exertional headache" for any headache that is precipitated by exertion, has an acute onset, and is unassociated with structural central nervous system disease, thus combining cough and exertional headache. In a population-based study (Rasmussen et al., 1991), benign cough headache and benign exertional headache each had a prevalence of about 1%.

The most recent classification of these disorders was done by the IHS (Headache Classification Committee of the International Headache Society, 1988) (Tables 16–9, 16–10). The IHS separates benign cough headache and benign exertional headache since these entities have different clinical features, diagnostic evaluations, and treatment responses (Pascual et al., 1996; Sands et al., 1991).

Benign Cough Headache

Benign cough headache is infrequent. The mean age at onset is 55, with a range of 19

Perimetry

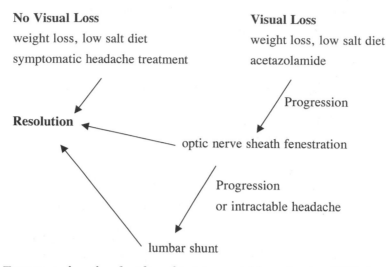

No Visual Loss

weight loss, low salt diet

symptomatic headache treatment

Visual Loss

weight loss, low salt diet

acetazolamide

Progression

Resolution

optic nerve sheath fenestration

Progression

or intractable headache

lumbar shunt

Figure 16–4 Treatment algorithm for idiopathic intracranial hypertension (IIH). Decisions are made for IIH therapy mainly on the results of perimetry. Visual loss does not include enlargement of the blind spot unless it is compromising vision. Optic nerve sheath fenestration is preferred over steroids. (Reprinted with permission from Wall, M. (1991). Idiopathic intracranial hypertension. *Neurol. Clin.* 9: 73–95.)

to 73 years. It is twice as common in patients over 40 years of age and is four times more common in men than in women (Rooke, 1968). The pain begins immediately (Symonds, 1956; Nick, 1980) or within seconds after coughing, sneezing, or a Valsalva maneuver (lifting, straining at stool, blowing, crying, or singing) (Tinel, 1932a,b; Nightingale and Williams, 1987). The pain is severe in intensity, with a bursting, explosive, or splitting quality that lasts a few seconds or minutes. The headache is usually bilateral, with maximal pain at the vertex or in the occipital, frontal, or temporal region. Bending the head or lying down may be impossible (Mathew, 1981). The headache is not generally associated with nausea or vomiting, and the neurologic examination is usually normal. Vom-

iting suggests an organic basis for the headache (Sands et al., 1991). As many as 25% of cases have an antecedent respiratory infection (Symonds, 1956; Rooke, 1968; Raskin, 1988). Most patients are pain-free between attacks of head pain, but in some cases the paroxysms are followed by dull, aching pain that may persist for hours; 5/21 patients reported by Symonds (1956) had such additional headaches. As these patients often express their complaint as a continuous headache, they should be asked directly about the role of exertion as a trigger factor.

Symptomatic Cough Headache

Age at onset is significantly lower for symptomatic cough headache than for benign cough headache (Table 16–9). Pascual et al. (1996) found that symptomatic cough headache could be precipitated by laughing, weight-lifting, or acute body or head postural changes in addition to coughing. Symptomatic cough headache can be caused by hindbrain abnormalities, posterior fossa meningioma, midbrain cysts, basilar impression,

Table 16–9 Benign cough headache

Bilateral headache of sudden onset, lasting less than 1 minute, precipitated by coughing

May be prevented by avoiding coughing

May be diagnosed only after structural lesions such as posterior fossa tumor have been excluded by neuroimaging

Table 16–10 Benign exertional headache

Specifically brought on by physical exercise
Bilateral, throbbing in nature at onset, and may
  develop migrainous features in patients susceptible to migraine
Lasts from 5 minutes to 24 hours
Prevented by avoiding excessive exertion, particularly
  in hot weather or at high altitude
Not associated with any systemic or intracranial
  disorder

acoustic neurinoma, and brain tumor such as Arnold-Chiari malformation (Williams, 1980; Rushton and Rooke, 1962; Raskin, 1978). In the series of Pascual et al. (1996), headache was the only symptom, at first, of Arnold-Chiari type I malformation in three patients; however, all patients had or eventually developed posterior fossa signs or syringomyelia. Besides beginning earlier in life than benign cough headache, symptomatic cough headache does not respond to indomethacin. If a patient does not respond to indomethacin, has posterior fossa signs, or is younger than 50, MRI must be done.

Cough headache can be confused with other disorders, such as exertional headache, effort migraine, and coital headache (Raskin, 1988; Ekbom, 1986). In fact, 40% of patients with coital headache of the vascular type had exertional headache, suggesting a relationship between these entities (Silbert et al., 1991).

Benign Exertional Headache

Benign exertional headache begins significantly earlier than benign cough headache (p < 0.005), by almost 40 years. It is typically throbbing, lasts from 5 minutes to 24 hours, and is provoked by physical exercise (Table 16–10). The pain usually begins during exertion, is nonexplosive, and can be either bilateral or unilateral.

Symptomatic Exertional Headache

Symptomatic exertional headache is usually acute in onset, severe, and bilateral. Twelve of Pascual et al.'s (1996) patients presented because of acute headache that coincided with physical exercise. Etiologies included subarachnoid hemorrhage (SAH), sinusitis, and brain mass.

Benign Sexual Headache

Benign sexual headache (type 2) begins later than benign exertional headache and earlier than benign cough headache. The headache is usually bilateral, but it can be unilateral. It is usually severe and explosive, with occasional throbbing and stabbing. Its duration varies, lasting from less than 1 minute to 3 hours (average 30 minutes). The frequency of the episodes was directly related to that of sexual intercourse or masturbation. Up to one-third of patients have similar episodes with physical exertion (Table 16–12).

Symptomatic Sexual Headache

Explosive headache that occurs during coitus is usually symptomatic of SAH. Rooke (1968) followed 103 patients who had exertional headache but no detectable intracranial disease on initial examination. After 3 or more years of follow-up, ten patients subsequently developed organic intracranial lesions. Thirty of the remaining 93 had complete headache relief within 5 years. The remainder improved or were headache-free after 10 years. This pre-CT era study emphasizes the importance of careful evaluation for organic disease.

Overview

Apart from that of Rooke (1968), the largest series of headaches of sudden onset provoked by cough, physical exercise, or sexual excitement was performed by Pascual et al. (1996). Benign and symptomatic cases differed in several clinical aspects (Table 16–11). Symptomatic cough headache began earlier in life, tended to last longer, and was more frequent than benign cough headache. Chiari type I malformation was the only cause found. Sinusitis, SAH, and brain metastases were the causes of symptomatic exertional headache.

Of the 219 cases of exertional and cough headache reviewed by Sands et al. (1991), 48 had an identifiable organic etiology (Table

Table 16-11 Exertional and cough headaches

	Cough headache		Exertional headache		Sexual headache	
	Benign	Symptomatic	Benign	Symptomatic	Benign	Symptomatic
Number	13	17	16	12	13	1
Age (years), range	67±11, 44–81	39±14, 15–63	24±11, 10–48	42±14, 18–61	41±9, 24–57	60
Sex (% men)	77%	59%	88%	43%	85%	100%
Duration	Seconds to 30 minutes	Seconds to days	Minutes to 2 days	1 day to 1 month	1 minute to 3 hours	10 days
Bilateral localization	92%	94%	56%	100%	77%	Yes
Quality	Sharp, stabbing	Bursting, stabbing	Pulsating	Explosive, pulsating	Explosive, pulsating	Explosive, pulsating
Other manifestations	No	Posterior fossa signs	Nausea, photophobia	Nausea, vomiting, double vision, neck rigidity	None	Vomiting, neck rigidity
Diagnosis	Idiopathic	Chiari type I malformation	Idiopathic	Subarachnoid hemorrhage, sinusitis, brain metastases	Idiopathic	Subarachnoid hemorrhage

Modified from Pascual, J., F. Igessias, A. Oterino et al. (1996). Cough, exertional and sexual headaches: An analysis of 72 benign and symptomatic cases. *Neurology 46*:1520–1524.

16–13). Sands et al. (1991) summarizes cases of cough and exertional headache, grouping together etiologically related cases from several selected series. The group with posterior fossa space–occupying lesions includes cases with Arnold-Chiari deformity and hindbrain herniation. Post-traumatic and postcraniotomy cases were also grouped together. From his review, one cannot accurately estimate how many patients with exertional headache have structural disease (Tinel, 1932b; Symonds, 1956; Rooke, 1968; Nick, 1980; Nightingale and Williams, 1987; Mathew, 1981; Williams, 1980; Ekbom, 1986; Silbert et al., 1991; Ibbotson, 1987; Paulson, 1983; Powell, 1982). Headache associated with sexual activity is usually bilateral and precipitated by masturbation or coitus. It usually occurs in the absence of any intracranial disorder. Benign sexual headache is now a well-defined entity, with three types recognized in the IHS classification (Table 16–12) (Headache Classification Committee of the International Headache Society, 1988). They are described according to the presumed clinical pathophysiologic mechanism. The most frequent, type 2, begins suddenly at the time of orgasm and is thought to be related to hemodynamic changes. It is often associated with exertional headache.

Symptomatic exertional and sexual headaches begin later in life and last longer than benign exertional and sexual headaches. Male predominance is not present in the symptomatic exertional headache group. Furthermore, all patients with symptomatic headaches had manifestations of meningeal irritation or ICH. Patients with subarachnoid hemorrhage had only had one headache episode. Although neuroradiologic studies could be avoided in cases with clinically typical benign sexual or exertional headaches (men around the third decade of life, with a normal examination and short-duration, multiple episodes of pulsating pain that responded to ergotamine or to preventive β blockers), the remaining patients must have a brain CT (and a CSF examination if the CT scan is normal).

Benign cough headache and benign exertional headache are separate conditions. Besides the different precipitants (sudden Val-

Table 16–12 Headache associated with sexual activity

Precipitated by sexual excitement
Bilateral at onset
Prevented or eased by ceasing sexual activity before orgasm
Not associated with any intracranial disorder such as aneurysm
Dull type
   A dull ache in the head and neck that intensifies as sexual excitement increases
Explosive type
   A sudden, severe ("explosive") headache occurring at orgasm
Postural type
   Postural headache resembling that of low cerebrospinal fluid pressure developing after coitus

salva maneuvers and sustained physical exercise, respectively), benign cough headache begins later than benign exertional headache. Cough headache starts 43 years later, on average, than exertional headache, and while the youngest patient with benign cough headache in this series was 44 years old, the oldest patient with benign exertional headache was 48. Benign cough headache tended to be shorter than benign exertional headache, and the pain quality and response to treatment were different. Benign cough headache was described as sharp or stabbing and responsive to indomethacin, whereas benign exertional headache was pulsating, tended to last longer, and improved with ergotamine or propranolol. It is not uncommon for patients to experience both benign sexual headache and benign exertional headache; this occurred in 31% of patients in the series of Pascual et al. (1996).

Other types of headache may be exacerbated by exertion. Severe migraine, post-LP

Table 16–13 Etiologies for cough and exertional headache in literature

Structural (organic)	48
Posterior fossa space–occupying lesions	18 (37.5%)
After trauma or after craniotomy	13 (27.0%)
Supratentorial space–occupying lesions	9 (18.7%)
Basilar impression/platybasia	6 (12.5%)
Syrinx	2 (4.2%)
Benign exertional headache	171
Total	219

headache, and, rarely, pseudotumor cerebri may be aggravated by coughing (Silberstein and Marcelis, 1993). Paroxysmal headache may also occur in patients with third ventricular colloid cysts, which may produce intermittent obstruction of CSF flow through the foramen of Monroe, resulting in abrupt increases of ICP. Similar headache has also been experienced by patients who have lateral ventricular tumors, craniopharyngiomas, pinealomas, and tumors of the cerebellum and cerebrum. Pheochromocytomas (Silberstein and Marcelis, 1993; Lance and Hinterberger, 1976; Paulson et al., 1979) may also cause paroxysmal headache, especially during exercise. In Rooke's (1968) series of 303 patients with intracranial lesions, however, none of the 27 patients with an unruptured cerebral aneurysm or vascular anomaly complained of exertional headache.

Van den Bergh (1987) reported two patients with Arnold-Chiari malformation who had headache paroxysms brought on by coughing, sneezing, and laughing. In Arnold-Chiari malformation, a ball-valve mechanism may be responsible for CSF passing more easily from the spine to the cranium than vice versa. Lumbar CSF pressure waves following a cough occur sooner and rise higher than cisternal pressure waves; the lumbar pressure waves also fall sooner and lower. Therefore, there is a phase during which the lumbar pressure exceeds the cisternal pressure, followed by a phase in which the cisternal pressure is greater than the lumbar pressure; this is aggravated by the ball-valve effect and is thought to produce cough headache (Van den Bergh et al., 1987; Williams, 1976).

Stevens et al. (1993) retrospectively studied 141 patients with adult Arnold-Chiari malformation (defined as descent of the hind-brain into the cervical canal, with meningomyelocele absent and hydrocephalus rare). Headache was present in 41 patients and considered a symptom only if exacerbated by head movement, exercise, or coughing.

The long-term course of preoperative cough and posture-related headache showed no relationship to tonsillar descent or any other imaging parameter, including the size of the cisterna magna, yet the latter. feature

was significantly improved in 62.6% of cases. Posture- and cough-related headaches, like drop attacks, are thought to result from intermittent tonsillar impaction in the foramen magnum. Therefore, the lack of association of such features with small or obliterated cisterna magna or low-lying tonsils both pre- and postoperatively suggests that the origin of these symptoms is more complex (Stevens et al., 1993).

The long-term outlook for these patients is favorable. If the headaches are frequent or severe, prophylactic therapy is required as the short duration of the headaches renders abortive therapy impractical. Some patients respond dramatically to indomethacin in doses of 25 to 150 mg daily (Mathew, 1981). If there is gastrointestinal intolerance to indomethacin, concomitant treatment with misoprostol, sucralfate, or antacids may be helpful. When indomethacin fails, Raskin (1988) reports that naproxen, ergonovine, and phenelzine are useful but propranolol is not.

Symonds (1956) performed four LPs or pneumoencephalograms on each of 21 patients with benign cough headache syndrome. One patient developed a typical post-LP headache, but her cough headache syndrome remitted for 3 weeks and then recurred. Some patients with benign cough headache respond to LP (Raskin, 1995).

Headache associated with abnormalities in intracranial structure or function comprises an interesting and important group of diseases and syndromes. While there is some overlap with migraine and tension type headaches, there are usually features of the clinical presentation that alert the clinician that a less common headache syndrome is present. These identifying features of the clinical presentation are often found in the history but may also occur with the examination. Alternatively, one should consider these headache syndromes when the IHS criteria for migraine or tension type headache are not met. Diagnosis of entities associated with abnormalities in intracranial structure or function is important because it may signal an important underlying condition having a specific treatment.

REFERENCES

Acheson, J.F., W.T. Green, and M.D. Sanders (1994). Optic nerve sheath decompression for the treatment of visual failure in chronic raised intracranial pressure. *J. Neurol. Neurosurg. Psychiatry* 57:1426–1429.

Amaral, J., W. Tsiaris, T. Morgan et al. (1987). Reversal of benign intracranial hypertension by surgically induced weight loss. *Arch. Surg. 122*: 946–949.

Britt, R.H. (1985). Brain abscess. In *Neurosurgery* (R.H. Wilkins and S.S. Rengachary, eds.), pp. 1928–1956. McGraw-Hill, New York.

Brourman, N.D., T.C. Spoor, and J.M. Ramocki (1988). Optic nerve sheath decompression for pseudotumor cerebri. *Arch. Ophthalmol. 106*: 1378–1383.

Buhrley, L.E. and D.J. Reed (1972). The effect of furosemide on sodium-22 uptake into cerebrospinal fluid and brain. *Exp. Brain Res. 14*:503–510.

Burgett, R.A., V.A. Purvin, and A. Kawasaki (1997). Lumboperitoneal shunting for pseudotumor cerebri. *Neurology 49*:734–739.

Childhood Brain Tumor Consortium (1991). The epidemiology of headache among children with brain tumor: Headache in children with brain tumors. *J. Neurooncol. 10*:31–46.

Chou, S.Y. and K.B. Digre (1999). Neuroophthalmic complications of raised intracranial pressure, hydrocephalus, and shunt malfunction. *Neurosurg. Clin. N. Am. 10*:587–608.

Corbett, J.J. (1983). Problems in the diagnosis and treatment of pseudotumor cerebri. The 1982 Silversides Lecture. *Can. J. Neurol. Sci. 10*:221–229.

Corbett, J.J. and M.P. Mehta (1983). Cerebrospinal fluid pressure in normal obese subjects and patients with pseudotumor cerebri. *Neurology* 33:1386–1388.

Corbett, J.J. and M.P. Mehta (1988). Cerebrospinal fluid pressure in normal obese subjects and patients with pseudotumor cerebri. *Neurology* 33:1386–1388.

Corbett, J.J., J.A. Nerad, D.T. Tse et al. (1988). Results of optic nerve sheath fenestration for pseudotumor cerebri. The lateral orbitotomy approach. *Arch. Ophthalmol. 106*:1391–1397.

Corbett, J.J. and H.S. Thompson (1989). The rational management of idiopathic intracranial hypertension. *Arch. Neurol. 46*:1049–1051.

Deonna, T. and J.P. Guignard (1974). Acute intracranial hypertension after nalidixic acid administration. *Arch. Dis. Child. 49*:743.

Digre, K.B. and J.J. Corbett (1988). Pseudotumor cerebri in men. *Arch. Neurol. 45*:866–872.

Durcan, F.J., J.J. Corbett, and M. Wall (1988). The incidence of pseudotumor cerebri: Population studies in Iowa and Louisiana. *Arch. Neurol. 45*: 875–877.

Eggenberger, E.R., N.R. Miller, and S. Vitale (1996). Lumboperitoneal shunt for the treatment of pseudotumor cerebri. *Neurology 46*: 1524–1530.

Ekbom, K. (1986). Cough headache. In *Headache (Handbook of Clinical Neurology)* (P.J. Vinkin, G.W. Bruyn, and H.L. Klawans, eds.), pp. 67–371. Elsevier, New York.

Fay, T. (1940). A new test for the diagnosis of certain headaches; the cephalogram. *Dis. Nerv. Syst. 1*:312–315.

Feldman, M.H. and N.S. Schlezinger (1970). Benign intracranial hypertension associated with hypervitaminosis A. *Arch. Neurol.* 22:1–7.

Fishman, R.A. (1992). *Cerebrospinal Fluid in Diseases of the Nervous System.* W.B. Saunders, Philadelphia.

Forsyth, P.A. and J.B. Posner (1993). Headaches in patients with brain tumors. A study of 111 patients. *Neurology 43*:1678–1683.

Freemont-Smith, F. and L. Kubie (1929). Relation of vascular hydrostatic pressure and osmotic pressure to cerebrospinal fluid pressure. *Assoc. Res. Nerv. Dis. Proc. 8*:154.

Friedman, D.I. and D.H. Streeten (1998). Idiopathic intracranial hypertension and orthostatic edema may share a common pathogenesis. *Neurology 50*:1099–1104.

Gamache, F.W., R.H. Patterson, and J.F. Alksne (1987). Headache associated with changes in intracranial pressure. In *Wolff's Headache and Other Head Pain* (D.J. Dalessio, ed.), pp. 352–355. Oxford University Press, New York.

Giuseffi, V., M. Wall, P.Z. Siegal et al. (1991). Symptoms and disease associations in idiopathic intracranial hypertension (pseudotumor cerebri): A case control study. *Neurology 41*:239–244.

Greenberg, H.S., M.D. Deck, B. Vikram et al. (1981). Metastasis to the base of the skull: Clinical findings in 43 patients. *Neurology 31*:530–537.

Greer, M. (1965). Benign intracranial hypertension. VI: Obesity. *Neurology 15*:382–388.

Gucer, G. and L. Vierenstein (1978). Long-term intracranial pressure recording in management of pseudotumor cerebri. *J. Neurosurg. 49*:256–263.

Hamed, L.M., D.T. Tse, J.S. Glaser et al. (1992). Neuroimaging of the optic nerve after fenestration for management of pseudotumor cerebri. *Arch. Ophthalmol. 110*:636–639.

Hayreh, S.S. (1977). Optic disc edema in raised intracranial pressure. V: Pathogenesis. *Arch. Ophthalmol.* 95:1553–1565.

Headache Classification Committee of the International Headache Society (1988). Classification and diagnostic criteria for headache disorders, cranial neuralgia, and facial pain. *Cephalalgia 8:* 1–96.

Heyck, H. (1968). Examinations and differential diagnosis of headache. In *Handbook of Clinical Neurology* (H. Heyck, ed.), pp. 25–36. Elsevier, New York.

Honig, P.J. and E.B. Charney (1982). Children with brain tumor headaches. *Am. J. Dis. Child.* 136:121–124.

Ibbotson, S. (1987). Weight-lifter's headache. *Br. J. Sports Med.* 3:138.

Ireland, B., J.J. Corbett, and R.B. Wallace (1990). The search for causes of idiopathic intracranial hypertension: A preliminary case-control study. *Arch. Neurol.* 47:315.

Jaeckle, K.A. (1991). Clinical presentations and therapy of nervous system tumors. In *Neurology in Clinical Practice* (W.G. Bradley, R.B. Daroff, G.M. Fenichel et al., eds.), pp. 1008–1030. Butterworth-Heinemann, Boston.

Jaeckle, K.A. (1993). Causes and management of headaches in cancer patients. *Oncology* 7:27–31.

Johnson, L.N., G.B. Krohel, R.W. Madsen et al. (1998). The role of weight loss and acetazolamide in the treatment of idiopathic intracranial hypertension (pseudotumor cerebri). *Ophthalmology* 105:2313–2317.

Johnston, I., S. Hawke, M. Kalmagyi et al. (1991). The pseudotumor syndrome. *Arch. Neurol.* 48:740–747.

Johnston, I. and A. Paterson (1974). Benign intracranial hypertension II. CSF pressure and circulation. *Brain* 97:301–312.

Karahalios, D.G., H.L. Rekate, M.H. Khayata et al. (1996). Elevated intracranial venous pressure as a universal mechanism in pseudotumor cerebri of varying etiologies. *Neurology* 46:198–202.

Keltner, J. (1988). Optic nerve sheath decompression: How does it work? Has its time come? *Arch. Ophthalmol.* 106:1378–1383.

King, J.O., P.J. Mitchell, K.R. Thomson et al. (1995). Cerebral venography and manometry in idiopathic intracranial hypertension. *Neurology* 45:2224–2228.

Konomi, H., M. Imai, K. Nihei et al. (1978). Indomethacin causing pseudotumor cerebri in Bartter's syndrome. *N. Engl. J. Med.* 298:855.

Kunkle, E.C., S.R. Bronson, and H.G. Wolff (1942a). Studies on headache: The mechanisms and significance of the headache associated with brain tumor. *Bull. N.Y. Acad. Med.* 18:400–422.

Kunkle, E.C., J.B. Pfeiffer, W.M. Wilholt et al. (1942b). Recurrent brief headache in "cluster" pattern. *Trans. Am. Neurol. Assoc.* 77:240–243.

Kupersmith, M.J., L. Gamell, R. Turbin et al. (1998). Effects of weight loss on the course of idiopathic intracranial hypertension in women. *Neurology* 50:1094–1098.

Lance, J.W. and H. Hinterberger (1976). Symptoms of pheochromocytoma with particular reference to headache correlated with catecholamine production. *Arch. Neurol.* 33:281–288.

Larizza, D., A. Colombo, R. Lorini et al. (1979). Ketoprofen causing pseudotumor cerebri in Bartter's syndrome. *N. Engl. J. Med.* 300:796.

Lavyne, M.H. and R.H. Patterson (1987). Headache and brain tumor. In *Wolff's Headache and Other Head Pain* (D.J. Dalessio, ed.), pp. 343–349. Oxford University Press, New York.

Lipton, H.L. and P.E. Michelson (1972). Pseudotumor cerebri syndrome without papilledema. *JAMA* 220:1591–1592.

Loman, J. (1934). Components of cerebrospinal fluid pressure as affected by changes in posture. *Arch. Neurol. Psychiatry* 31:679–681.

Loman, J., A. Myerson, and D. Goldman (1935). Effects of alteration of posture on cerebrospinal fluid pressure. *Arch. Neurol. Psychiatry* 33:1279–1284.

Malm, J., B. Kristensen, P. Markgren et al. (1992). CSF hydrodynamics in idiopathic intracranial hypertension: A long-term study. *Neurology* 42:851–858.

Marcelis, J. and S.D. Silberstein (1991). Idiopathic intracranial hypertension without papilledema. *Arch. Neurol.* 48:392–399.

Mathew, N.T. (1981). Indomethacin responsive headache syndromes. *Headache* 21:147–150.

Mathew, N.T., K. Ravinshankar, and L.C. Sanin (1996). Coexistence of migraine and idiopathic intracranial hypertension without papilledema. *Neurology* 46:1226–1230.

McKissock, W. (1960). Subdural hematoma. A review of 389 cases. *Lancet* 1:1365–1370.

Milhorat, T.H. (1972). *Hydrocephalus and the Cerebrospinal Fluid*. Williams and Wilkins, Baltimore.

Morewood, G.H. (1993). A rational approach to the cause, prevention and treatment of postdural puncture headache. *Can. Med. Assoc. J.* 148:1087–1093.

Mushet, G.R. (1977). Pseudotumor and nitrofurantoin therapy. *Arch. Neurol.* 34:257.

Newborg, B. (1974). Pseudotumor cerebri treated by rice reduction diet. *Arch. Intern. Med.* 133:802–807.

Nick, J. (1980). La céphalée d'effort. A propos d'une série de 43 cases. *Semin. Hop. Paris* 56:621–628.

Nightingale, S. and B. Williams (1987). Hindbrain hernia headache. *Lancet* 1:731–734.

Northfield, D.W.C. (1938). Some observations on headache. *Brain* 77:240–243.

Orcutt, J.C., N.G. Page, and M.D. Sanders (1984). Factors affecting visual loss in benign intracranial hypertension. *Ophthalmology* 91:1303–1312.

Pascual, J., F. Igessias, A. Oterino et al. (1996). Cough, exertional, and sexual headaches: An analysis of 72 benign and symptomatic cases. *Neurology* 46:1520–1524.

Paterson, R., N. DePasquale, and S. Mann (1961). Pseudotumor cerebri. *Medicine* 40:85–99.

Paulson, G.W. (1983). Weightlifters headache. *Headache* 23:193–194.

Paulson, G.W., R.E. Zipf, and J.F. Beekman (1979). Pheochromocytoma causing exercise-related headache and pulmonary edema. *Ann. Neurol.* 5:96–99.

Pollay, M., C. Fullenwider, P.A. Roberts et al. (1983). Effect of mannitol and furosemide on blood–brain osmotic gradient and intracranial pressure. *J. Neurosurg.* 59:945–950.

Powell, B. (1982). Weight lifter's cephalalgia. *Ann. Emerg. Med.* 11:449–451.

Radhkrishnan, K., J.E. Ahlskog, S.A. Cross et al. (1993). Idiopathic intracranial hypertension (pseudotumor cerebri). Descriptive epidemiology in Rochester, Minnesota, 1976 to 1990. *Arch. Neurol.* 50:78–80.

Raskin, N. (1978). Headaches associated with organic diseases of the nervous system. *Med. Clin. N. Am.* 62:459–466.

Raskin, N.H. (1988). The indomethacin-responsive syndromes. In *Headache* (N.H. Raskin, ed.), pp. 255–268. Churchill Livingstone, New York.

Raskin, N.H. (1995). The cough headache syndrome. *Neurology* 45:1784.

Rasmussen, B.K., R. Jensen, M. Schroll et al. (1991). Epidemiology of headache in a general population—a prevalence study. *J. Clin. Epidemiol.* 44:1147–1157.

Ray, B.S. and H.G. Wolff (1940). Experimental studies on headache. Pain sensitive structures of the head and their significance in headache. *Arch. Surg.* 41:813–856.

Roberts, P.A., M. Pollay, C. Engles et al. (1987). Effect on intracranial pressure of furosemide combined with varying doses and administration rates of mannitol. *J. Neurosurg.* 66:440–446.

Rooke, E.D. (1968). Benign exertional headache. *Med. Clin. N. Am.* 52:801–808.

Rosenberg, M.L., J.J. Corbett, C. Smith et al. (1993). Cerebrospinal fluid diversion procedures in pseudotumor cerebri. *Neurology* 43:1071–1072.

Rush, J.A. (1980). Pseudotumor cerebri: Clinical profile and visual outcome in 63 patients. *Mayo Clin. Proc.* 55:541–546.

Rushton, J.G. and E.D. Rooke (1962). Brain tumor headache. *Headache* 2:147–152.

Sadun, A.A., J.N. Currie, and S. Lessell (1984). Transient visual obscurations with elevated optic discs. *Ann. Neurol.* 16:489–494.

Sahs, A.L. and R.J. Joynt (1956). Brain swelling of unknown cause. *Neurology* 6:791–803.

Sands, G.H., L. Newman, and R. Lipton (1991). Cough, exertional, and other miscellaneous headaches. *Med. Clin. N. Am.* 75:733–746.

Saul, R.F., H.A. Hamburger, and J.B. Selhorst (1985). Pseudotumor cerebri secondary to lithium carbonate. *JAMA* 253:2869–2870.

Scanari, M., S. Mingrino, D. d'Avella et al. (1979). Benign Intracranial hypertension without papilledema: A case report. *Neurosurgery* 5:373–377.

Schaltenbrand, G. (1938). Neure Anschauen zor Pathophysiologie der Liquorzirkulation. *Zentralbl. Neurochir.* 3:290–300.

Schoeman, J.F. (1994). Childhood pseudotumor cerebri: Clinical and intracranial pressure response to acetazolamide and furosemide treatment in a case series. *J. Child Neurol.* 9:130–134.

Sergott, R.C., P.J. Savino, and T.M. Bosley (1988). Modified optic nerve sheath decompression provides long-term visual improvement for pseudotumor cerebri. *Arch. Ophthalmol.* 106:1391–1397.

Sergott, R.C., P.J. Savino, and T.M. Bosley (1990). Optic nerve sheath decompression: A clinical review and proposed pathophysiologic mechanism. *Aust. N.Z. J. Ophthalmol.* 18:365–373.

Shah, A., T. Roberts, I.N. McQueen et al. (1987). Danazol and benign intracranial hypertension. *BMJ* 294:1323.

Shuper, A., R.J. Packer, and L.G. Vezina (1995). Complicated migraine-like episodes in children following cranial irradiation and chemotherapy. *Neurology* 45:1837–1840.

Silberstein, S.D. and J.J. Corbett (1993). The forgotten lumbar puncture. *Cephalalgia* 13:212–213.

Silberstein, S.D. and J. Marcelis (1993). Headache associated with abnormalities in intracranial structure or pressure. In *Wolff's Headache and Other Head Pain* (D.J. Dalessio and S.D. Silberstein, eds.), pp. 438–461. Oxford University Press, New York.

Silbert, P.L., R.H. Edis, E.G. Stewart-Wynne et al. (1991). Benign vascular sexual headache and exertional headache: Interrelationships and long term prognosis. *J. Neurol. Neurosurg. Psychiatry* 54:417–421.

Sismanis, A. (1987). Otologic manifestations of benign intracranial hypertension syndrome: Diagnosis and management. *Laryngoscope* 97:1–17.

Smith, C.H. and J.C. Orcutt (1986). Surgical treatment of pseudotumor cerebri. *Int. Ophthalmol. Clin.* 26:265–275.

Smith, J.L. (1985). Whence pseudotumor cerebri? *J. Clin. Neuroophthalmol.* 5:55–56.

Spector, R.H. and J. Carlisle (1984). Pseudotumor cerebri caused by a synthetic vitamin A preparation. *Neurology* 34:1509–1511.

Spence, J.D., A.L. Amacher, and N.R. Willis (1980). Benign intracranial hypertension without papilledema: Role of 24 hour cerebrospinal fluid pressure monitoring in diagnosis and management. *Neurosurgery* 7:326–336.

Spoor, T.C., J.M. Ramocki, M.P. Madion et al. (1991). Treatment of pseudotumor cerebri by primary and secondary optic nerve sheath decompression. *Am. J. Ophthalmol. 112*:177–185.

Stevens, J.M., W.A.D. Serva, B.E. Kendall et al. (1993). Chiari malformation in adults: Relation of morphological aspects to clinical features and operative outcome. *J. Neurol. Neurosurg. Psychiatry 56*:1072–1077.

Sugerman, H.J., W.L. Felton, A. Sismanis et al. (1999). Gastric surgery for pseudotumor cerebri associated with severe obesity. *Ann. Surg. 229:* 634–640.

Symonds, C. (1956). Cough headache. *Brain 79:* 557–568.

Tinel, J. (1932a). La cephalee a l'effort. Syndrome de distension douloureuse des veines intracraniennes. *Medicine (Paris) 13*:113–118.

Tinel, J. (1932b). Un syndrome d'algie veineuse intracranienne. La cephalee a l'effort. *Prat. Med. Fr. 13*:113–119.

Tomsak, R.L., A.S. Niffenegger, and B.F. Remler (1988). Treatment of pseudotumor cerebri with Diamox (acetazolamide). *J. Clin. Neuroophthalmol. 8*:93–98.

Van den Bergh, V., W.K. Amery, and J. Waelkens (1987). Trigger factors in migraine: A study conducted by the Belgian migraine society. *Headache 27*:191–196.

Van Dop, C., F.A. Conte, T.K. Koch et al. (1983). Pseudotumor cerebri associated with initiation of levothyroxine therapy for juvenile hypothyroidism. *N. Engl. J. Med. 308*:1076–1080.

Vazquez-Barquero, A., F.J. Ibanez, and S. Herrera (1994). Isolated headache as the presenting clinical manifestation of intracranial tumor: A perspective study. *Cephalalgia 14*:270–272.

Verplanck, M., D.I. Kaufman, T. Parsons et al. (1988). Electrophysiology versus psychophysics in the detection of visual loss in pseudotumor cerebri. *Neurology 38*:1789–1792.

Vogh, B.P. and M.R. Langham (1981). The effect of furosemide and bumetanide on cerebrospinal fluid formation. *Brain Res. 221*:171–183.

Von Storch, T., A. Carmichael, and T. Banks (1937). Factors producing lumbar cerebrospinal fluid pressure in many in the erect position. *Arch. Neurol. Psychiatry 38*:1158.

Wall, M. (1990). The headache profile of idiopathic intracranial hypertension. *Cephalalgia 10*:331–335.

Wall, M. (1991). Idiopathic intracranial hypertension. *Neurol. Clin. 9*:73–95.

Wall, M., J.D. Dollar, A.A. Sadun et al. (1995). Idiopathic intracranial hypertension: Lack of histologic evidence for cerebral edema. *Arch. Neurol. 52*:141–145.

Wall, M. and D. George (1991). Idiopathic intracranial hypertension: A prospective study of 50 patients. *Brain 114*:155–180.

Wall, M. and W.N. White (1998). Asymmetric papilledema in idiopathic intracranial hypertension: Prospective interocular comparison of sensory visual function. *Invest. Ophthalmol. Vis. Sci. 39*:134–142.

Wang, S.J., S.D. Silberstein, S. Patterson et al. (1998). Idiopathic intracranial hypertension without papilledema: A case-control study in a headache center. *Neurology 51*:245–249.

Weisberg, L.A. (1975). Benign intracranial hypertension. *Medicine 54*:197–207.

Williams, B. (1976). Cerebrospinal fluid pressure changes in response to coughing. *Brain 99*:331–346.

Williams, B. (1980). Cough headache due to craniospinal pressure dissociation. *Arch. Neurol. 37*:226–230.

Zulch, K.J., H.D. Mennel, and V. Zimmerman (1974). Intracranial hypertension. In *Handbook of Clinical Neurology* (K.J. Zulch, H.D. Mennel, and V. Zimmerman, eds.), pp. 89–149, Elsevier, New York.

17

Headache Associated with Abnormalities in Intracranial Structure or Function: Low Cerebrospinal Fluid Pressure Headache

BAHRAM MOKRI

Cerebrospinal fluid (CSF) is a circulating body fluid, sometimes referred to as the "third circulation" (Cushing, 1926). Most of the CSF is formed by the choroid plexus, which has structural and functional similarities to the distal and collecting tubules of the kidneys and maintains the compositional integrity of the CSF (Rowland et al., 1991). Only a minor portion of the CSF is secreted by the brain capillaries, entering the ventricular system through the ependyma. For many years, on the basis of data from autopsies, the CSF volume was estimated to be 150 ml. More recent volumetric studies based on magnetic resonance imaging (MRI) techniques suggest an average volume of about 210 ml in adults (Hogan et al., 1996; Matsumae et al., 1996). This, however, shows significant variation. Cranial CSF volume is smaller for women and for younger persons than for older persons, who have larger ventricular volumes and more generous CSF cisterns and subarachnoid spaces (Matsumae et al., 1996). Spinal CSF volume is significantly less in obese than nonobese persons (Hogan et al., 1996).

The rate of CSF formation is about 0.35 ml per minute, or about 500 ml per day. Therefore, the entire CSF volume is turned over a few times each day.

CSF is absorbed via the arachnoid villi into the cerebral venous sinuses and veins through a valve-like direct-flow mechanism termed "bulk flow" (Tripathi, 1973; Tripathi and Tripathi, 1974). Only a very minor portion of the CSF is absorbed through simple diffusion into the cerebral vessels.

Although increases or decreases in the rate of CSF formation have been obtained under experimental conditions in laboratory animals, human data are limited. In general, however, the rate of formation of CSF in humans is relatively constant (Fishman, 1992). There is no solid evidence to indicate that increases in CSF formation sufficient to cause intracranial hypertension occur in any condition other than choroid plexus papilloma. The effect of increased CSF pressure (hydrocephalus, or increased intracranial pressure) on CSF formation is complex. The rate of CSF formation under these conditions can likely be reduced if the intraventricular pressure is increased to a sufficient degree for a sufficient duration (Welch, 1975), although the critical limits of pressure and duration in these situations are not clearly defined.

In the horizontal position, the lumbar, the cisternal, and presumably the intracranial or vertex CSF pressures are equal, approximately 60 to 180 mm H_2O. In the erect posture, these pressures diverge and the vertex pressure becomes negative.

The relationship between CSF pressure and volume is exponential (Miller, 1975). Kunkle et al. (1943), in a study of induction of headache by CSF drainage in subjects in the erect posture, noted that headache was regularly induced when 10% of the estimated total volume of the CSF was withdrawn. This caused a decrease of more than 40% in already negative vertex CSF pressure.

HISTORICAL ASPECTS

The ventricular system of the brain and its contents have been sources of curiosity for centuries (Lyons and Meyer, 1990). Galen, a second century Greek physician and teacher, described a gas-like "spirituous animalis," or vital spirit, filling the cerebral ventricles. This concept survived for many centuries. When Vesalius, an anatomist in Padua in the 16th century, described fluid within the ventricles, he was not believed. Even as late as the early 19th century, Romberg thought that brain cavities were filled with "humid gas." It was François Magendie, a French physiologist, who, in the 19th century, convinced others of the presence of CSF.

Lumbar puncture was introduced in the 19th century by Quincke (Silberstein and Marcelis, 1992). Bier experienced headaches after lumbar puncture and was the first to report them (Raskin, 1990).

Schaltenbrand, a German neurologist, in an article in German in 1938 and an article in English in 1953, emphasized two terms: "liquorrhea" and "aliquorrhea." *Liquorrhea*, a condition mimicking brain tumor, involves headaches and papilledema. This later came to be known as pseudotumor cerebri and has not been shown to be due to excess CSF production. *Aliquorrhea* is a condition associated with very low, unobtainable, or even negative CSF pressures and clinically manifested by orthostatic headaches and other features that are now recognized as the clinical picture of intracranial hypotension. Recent evidence fails to show decreased CSF production, or aliquorrhea, in this condition; instead, a CSF leak is present. Before Schaltenbrand's descriptions, this syndrome had been described in the French literature as "hypotension of spinal fluid" or "ventricular collapse" (Schaltenbrand, 1953). Schaltenbrand continued to think that the cause of the syndrome was decreased CSF production; even when he discussed the appearance of the same syndrome after lumbar puncture, he speculated that lumbar puncture caused a decrease in CSF pressure and, thus, exerted a strong stimulus to the choroid plexus, causing a sudden cessation of CSF production (Schaltenbrand, 1953). He did not consider CSF leak the cause. As addressed by Fishman (1992), the technology of the time would not have allowed him or his contemporaries to assess patients adequately for CSF leak.

In the United States, as early as 1940, Woltman, at the Mayo Clinic, wrote about "headaches associated with decreased intracranial pressure," stating that "occasionally an occipital or frontal headache comes on only when the patient is up and about and leaves when the patient lies down. Such a headache is often associated with low pressure of the spinal fluid. Thus, it resembles postpuncture headache."

From the 1960s to early 1990s, several publications described the clinical manifestations of the syndrome of intracranial hypotension, or CSF leak (Baker, 1983; Bell et al., 1960; Huber, 1970; Lasater, 1970; Marcelis and Silberstein, 1990; Rando and Fishman, 1992). Furthermore, with introduction of radioisotope cisternography (Front and Penning, 1974; Labadie et al., 1976; Molins et al., 1990; Murros and Fogelholm, 1983; Weber et al., 1991) and water-soluble myelography and computed tomography (CT)-myelography, clinicians were provided with more effective tools to discover CSF leaks.

In the early 1990s, the MRI features of intracranial hypotension and CSF leaks were recognized (Fishman and Dillon, 1993; Hochman et al., 1992; Mokri et al., 1991, 1993; Pannullo et al., 1993; Sable and Ramadan, 1991). Magnetic resonance imaging of the head and spine has revolutionized the knowledge regarding this disorder, broadened the clinical and imaging spectrum of the syndrome (Mokri, 1999), and led to detection of far more cases than before. Many experienced clinicians have evaluated more cases of intracranial hypotension, or CSF leak, in the past decade than they had throughout all the previous years. There is little doubt that the diagnosis was missed in many patients before the use of MRI. Some of the patients improved spontaneously, whereas others had to live with a substantially compromised quality of life and sought care from various specialists or chronic pain–management facilities.

ETIOLOGY

Systemic conditions that cause a true hypovolemic state, or reduced total body water, also can lead to decreased CSF volume. Shunt overdrainage (Table 17–1) is a complication that is not uncommon in the practice of neurosurgery and neurology and can lead to orthostatic headaches and diffuse pachymeningeal gadolinium enhancement.

Traumatic causes of CSF leak, including head or spine trauma related to various accidents, cranial or spinal surgery, or lumbar puncture, are well recognized. Post-traumatic or postsurgical leaks may lead to frank CSF otorrhea or rhinorrhea.

Spontaneous CSF leaks are the most intriguing and the most common cause of spontaneous CSF volume depletion leading to orthostatic headaches and diffuse pachymeningeal gadolinium enhancement. Although the spontaneous leak may occur at the level of the skull base, in the overwhelming majority of patients it occurs at the spinal level, particularly the thoracic spine or cervicothoracic junction.

The exact cause of so-called spontaneous CSF leaks will remain unknown in the majority of patients. However, in a significant minority, two important contributory etiologic factors are frequently suspected: (1) weakness of the meningeal sac in certain regions and (2) trivial trauma. Meningeal diverticulae, sometimes multiple, are not uncommon. Furthermore, in some patients who have had surgery to stop the leak, patches of attenuated dura of various size have been noted. Spontaneous CSF leaks have been observed in heritable disorders of the connective tissue, such as Marfan syndrome (Davenport et al., 1995). Furthermore, some patients with spontaneous CSF leaks have stigmata of connective tissue disorders, such as hyperflexible joints, marfanoid features, or retinal detachment at a young age. Abnormalities of elastin or fibrillin or both are suspected in these patients (Mokri et al., 1997). Occasional dural tears resulting from spondylotic spurs may lead to CSF leak (Vishteh et al., 1998). Many patients report a history of trivial trauma. In some, trivial trauma likely might have started a CSF leak in the presence of an abnormality of fibrillin or elastin and of weakened and attenuated dural zones or meningeal diverticulae.

Despite speculations in the older literature (Schaltenbrand, 1938, 1953), there is very little evidence to indicate that CSF volume de-

Table 17–1 Etiology of cerebrospinal fluid (CSF) volume depletion

A. True hypovolemic state (reduced total body water)
B. CSF shunt overdrainage
C. CSF leaks
  1. Traumatic
    a. After definite trauma (e.g., sports, motor vehicle accidents)
    b. After surgical procedure
    c. After lumbar puncture
  2. Spontaneous
    a. Unknown cause (often)
    b. Meningeal diverticulae
    c. Weak, attenuated dura
    d. Connective tissue disorders (may also relate to b and c)
      (1) Marfan syndrome
      (2) Marfanoid features
      (3) Hyperflexible joints
      (4) Retinal detachment at young age
      (5) Elastin or fibrillin abnormalities
    e. Spondylitic-dural tear
    f. "Trivial" trauma

pletion is ever caused by CSF hyperabsorption or by decreased CSF formation (Mokri, 1999).

CLINICAL MANIFESTATIONS

Headache is the main clinical feature. It is typically an orthostatic headache that is present when the patient is upright and is relieved by recumbency. It may be throbbing, but often it is nonthrobbing. The location of the headache may be occipital, bifrontal, bifrontal–occipital, or holocephalic. The variability, however, is considerable. In some patients in the early or active stages of the disease, the headache is typically orthostatic, but with chronicity the orthostatic features may blur and the headache may take the form of a lingering chronic daily headache that is often, although not invariably, worse when the patient is upright and less pronounced with recumbency.

Sometimes it may start as a chronic lingering headache, and after days or a few weeks, typical orthostatic headaches develop. Other patients may start with intrascapular or posterior neck pains, which may or may not be orthostatic, and after a few to several days, typical orthostatic headaches may develop.

In intermittent CSF leaks, the headaches, with whatever features they might have, may appear and disappear for variable periods.

A small group of patients with CSF volume depletion, whether due to CSF shunt overdrainage or to CSF leak, may have no headaches at all (Mokri, 1999).

Associated Clinical Manifestations

Although headache, and typically orthostatic headache, is the sole manifestation in many patients with CSF volume depletion, many have additional clinical manifestations (Table 17–2). Occasional patients may have an unusual clinical presentation, such as stupor and encephalopathy (Beck et al., 1998) or parkinsonism, ataxia, and bulbar weakness (Pakiam et al., 1999).

Table 17–2 Clinical manifestations, other than headache, in cerebrospinal fluid volume depletion

Pain or stiff feeling of neck, sometimes orthostatic
Nausea, sometimes emesis, often orthostatic
Diplopia, typically horizontal (6th nerve palsy)
Dizziness
Change in hearing (muffled, distant, distorted, echoes)
Visual blurring
Photophobia
Visual field cut (superior binasal) (Horton and Fishman, 1994)
Interscapular pain
Face numbness or weakness
Galactorrhea (Yamamoto et al., 1993)
Radicular upper limb symptoms
Stupor (?), diencephalic compression (single case report) (Pleasure et al., 1998)
Parkinsonism, ataxia, bulbar symptoms (single case report) (Beck et al., 1998)
Encephalopathy (single case report) (Pakiam et al., 1999)

Mechanism of Clinical Manifestations

The headache of CSF volume depletion is a consequence of descent of the brain. By its buoyant effect, the CSF reduces the weight of the floating brain within the cranial cavity to <50 g. Even at this reduced weight, the brain must be supported within the cranium. Some of the weight is shared by suspension from above, mostly by the cerebral veins ending in the sagittal sinus and, to a lesser extent, by cerebellar veins ending in the transverse and straight sinuses. Cerebellar tentorium, large vessels of the base, and skull base provide support from below. Various anchoring structures of the brain are pain-sensitive, and pain can be provoked when these structures are subjected to traction or distortion (Fay, 1937). Sinking of the brain leads to traction or distortion of these structures and, therefore, to the appearance of orthostatic or primarily orthostatic headaches.

The same mechanism may be responsible for the cranial nerve palsies, visual blurring or visual field defects, or even dizziness or altered hearing, which is fairly common in affected patients. Another possible mechanism for the dizziness or disturbed hearing, however, may be an altered pressure in the perilymphatic fluid. Stupor, encephalopathy, cerebellar size, and parkinsonism may result

Table 17–3 Mechanisms of clinical manifestations of cerebrospinal fluid volume depletion

Clinical manifestation	Mechanism
Headache	Sinking of the brain, stretch and distortion of pain-sensitive suspending structures
Cranial nerve palsies (5th, 6th, 7th, chorda tympani)	Stretching and distortion of these nerves
Visual blurring, visual field cuts	Compression or vascular congestion of intracranial portions of optic nerves
Dizziness, change in hearing	Stretching of 8th cranial nerve or pressure changes in perilymphatic fluid of the inner ear
Galactorrhea and increased prolactin	Distortion of pituitary stalk
Radicular upper limb symptoms	Stretching of cervical nerve roots or structural anomalies at nerve root sleeve level
Stupor or encephalopathy°	Diencephalic compression
Cerebellar ataxia, parkinsonism°	Compression of posterior fossa and deep midline structures

°Single case reports.

from compression of the diencephalon, posterior fossae, and midline structures. Various clinical manifestations and their proposed mechanisms are listed in Table 17–3.

Pain at different levels of the spine (cervical, thoracic, lumbar) is not uncommon. In some cases, it is tempting to use the level of the pain or the radicular symptoms as clinical indicators of the level of the leak. In my experience, these "localizing signs" have been accurate in only a small minority of patients and have been "false-localizing signs" in the majority.

DIAGNOSIS

Cerebrospinal Fluid Examination

The CSF opening pressure is typically very low (sometimes atmospheric or unmeasurable, very occasionally even negative). There is, however, considerable variability. In some patients, the pressure may be "low-normal," whereas some others, despite persistent symptomatic CSF leaks, may have opening CSF pressures that are consistently within the limits of normal (Mokri et al., 1998). Some patients with intermittent or variable leaks may have pressures that are sometimes very low, sometimes low-normal, and sometimes entirely normal.

Analysis of CSF typically reveals a clear and colorless fluid, but occasionally the fluid is xanthochromic. Some patients who have undergone multiple CSF examinations in a span of a few years have had xanthochromic fluid in some tests and clear fluid in most of them.

The CSF protein level may be normal or high. The variability is considerable. When increased, the protein concentration is often <100 mg/dl. However, not uncommonly, protein concentrations range from 100 to 200 mg/dl or more. My colleagues and I have seen CSF protein concentrations as high as 1,000 mg/dl (Mokri et al., 1997).

The CSF cell counts also show considerable variability. The CSF erythrocyte count may be normal or increased to as high as a few or several hundreds. The CSF leukocyte count (typically lymphocytes) may be normal or increased. It is not unusual to note a pleocytosis with cell counts from 10 to 50/mm^3. Higher values are not rare, however. We have seen CSF pleocytosis with a cell count as high as 220/mm^3 in documented CSF leak without any evidence of meningeal infection or inflammation (Mokri et al., 1995, 1997).

Cytologic and microbiologic test results are always negative, and CSF glucose concentration is never low in proportion to plasma glucose concentration.

Computed Tomography of the Head

Computed tomography is typically negative. Sometimes it shows subdural fluid collections, increased tentorial enhancement, or small ventricular size (Pavlin et al., 1979; Sipe et al., 1981).

Radioisotope Cisternography (Indium-111)

In CSF leaks, typically the radioactivity does not reach cerebral convexities, even at 24 or 48 hours. Focal extension of radioactivity beyond the dural sac may be noted, pointing to the level of the CSF leak (Fig. 17–1). Meningeal diverticula, if large enough, also may be detected by this test. Another important finding in CSF leaks is early appearance of radioactivity in the kidneys and urinary bladder (in <4 hours vs. the normal 6 to 24 hours). This finding should not be interpreted as a manifestation of increased reabsorption of the CSF causing intracranial hypotension (Molins et al., 1990; Weber et al., 1991).

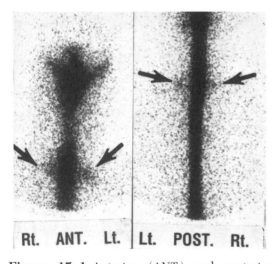

Figure 17–1 Anterior (*ANT.*) and posterior (*POST.*) views of upper cervical spine as noted in indium-111 cisternography, approximately 4 hours after spinal intrathecal injection of the radioisotope. The study shows extra-arachnoid accumulation of radioisotope in the upper thoracic spine, which extends laterally on both sides of the spinal canal (*arrows*). Note accumulation of radioisotope in the basal cisterns (upper part of the anterior view). The radioactivity never reached the cerebral convexities, even at 24 or 48 hours. (From Mokri, B., D.G. Piepgras, and G.M. Miller (1997). Syndrome of orthostatic headaches and diffuse pachymeningeal gadolinium enhancement. *Mayo Clin. Proc.* 72:400–413. By permission of Mayo Foundation for Medical Education and Research.)

Rather, it is an indication of CSF leak that has led to extravasation of radioisotope in the paraspinal tissues and its early entrance into the venous system, thus its early clearance by the kidneys and early appearance in the urinary bladder.

Magnetic Resonance Imaging

It is hardly a decade since the first report on meningeal gadolinium enhancement in CSF leaks appeared in the literature (Mokri et al., 1991). Magnetic resonance imaging of the head and spine has revolutionized identification, diagnosis, management, and follow-up of patients with spontaneous CSF leaks, and it has increased our overall understanding of CSF volume depletion.

Head Abnormalities

Diffuse pachymeningeal enhancement is the most common head MRI abnormality in CSF leaks and CSF volume depletion (Table 17–4). This is limited to pachymeninges without any evidence of leptomeningeal involvement. The enhancement is both supertentorial and infratentorial (Figs. 17–2, 17–3). It is nonnodular, linear, and typically uninterrupted (Mokri et al., 1995; Pannullo et al., 1993). It is of variable thickness, often being thick and obvious, but sometimes it is very thin.

Descent of the brain, or "sagging" or "sinking" of the brain, is also a common finding

Table 17–4 Abnormalities on magnetic resonance imaging in cerebrospinal fluid leaks

Head
    Diffuse pachymeningeal enhancement
    Sinking (sagging of the brain)
    Subdural fluid collections
    Decrease in size of ventricles ("ventricular collapse")
    Enlarged pituitary
    Engorged venous sinuses
    Elongation of brain stem in anteroposterior plane
Spine
    Extra-arachnoid fluid (often extending to several levels)
    Extradural fluid (extending to paraspinal soft tissues)
    Diverticula
    Level of the leak
    Pachymeningeal enhancement
    Engorgement of epidural venous plexus

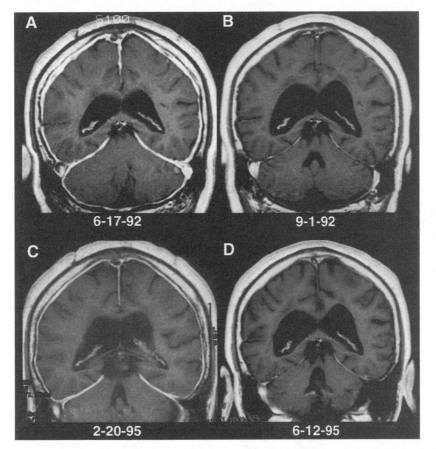

Figure 17–2 Post-contrast coronal T1-weighted magnetic resonance images through parietal lobes and fourth ventricle in a patient who had undergone shunting for normal-pressure hydrocephalus. *A*: Image obtained after insertion of shunt shows symmetric pachymeningeal gadolinium enhancement. At this stage, the patient had significant orthostatic headaches. *B*: After shunt revision, the ventricular system is larger, but pachymeningeal enhancement has resolved. The orthostatic headaches disappeared, but the gait disturbance related to normal-pressure hydrocephalus again increased. *C*: Shunt was revised again because of increasing ataxia and confusion. These improved, but headaches and abnormal meningeal enhancement returned. Ventricles are now slightly smaller. *D*: Ventricles are slightly larger again, but meningeal enhancement has resolved after another shunt revision. Also note engorged and enlarged sagittal sinus in *A* and *C* (compare with *B* and *D*) during periods of shunt overdrainage. (From Mokri, B., D.G. Piepgras, and G.M. Miller (1997). Syndrome of orthostatic headaches and diffuse pachymeningeal gadolinium enhancement. *Mayo Clin. Proc.* 72:400–413. By permission of Mayo Foundation for Medical Education and Research.)

and is manifested by descent of the cerebellar tonsils (Fig. 17–3) (which may sometimes mimic type I Chiari malformation) (Atkinson et al., 1998), decrease in the size of the prepontine cistern, inferior displacement of the optic chiasm (Fig. 17–4), effacement of perichiasmatic cisterns, and crowding of the posterior fossa.

Subdural fluid collections are usually but not always bilateral. These are thin, often measuring 2 to 7 mm in maximal thickness, without compression or effacement of the underlying sulci. Subdural fluid collections display variable signal intensity depending on the composition of the fluid (protein concentration, blood) (Fig. 17–5).

Decrease in the size of the ventricles, or "ventricular collapse," is sometimes obvious and sometimes subtle and is best noted when a head MRI obtained after recovery is compared with a previous MRI taken during the symptomatic phase (Figs. 17–3, 17–4).

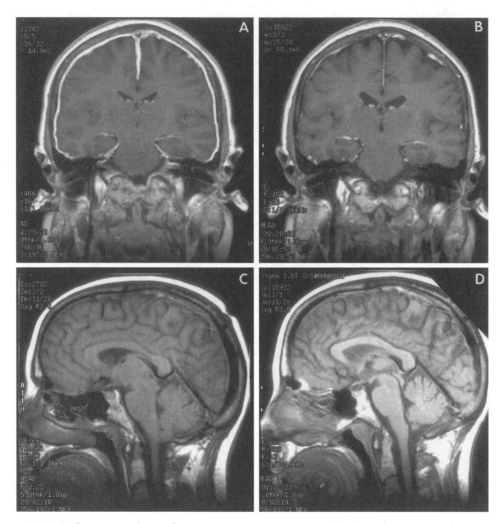

Figure 17–3 Gadolinium-enhanced magnetic resonance images (*A, B*) and unenhanced T1-weighted sagittal images (*C, D*) in a patient with cerebrospinal fluid (CSF) leak. During a symptomatic phase (*A, C*) and after treatment of the leak (*B, D*), which caused resolution of symptoms. During the symptomatic phase and active leak, there was diffuse pachymeningeal enhancement (*A*) and crowding of the posterior fossa with the tip of the cerebellar tonsils below the foramen magnum (*C*). All of these abnormalities resolved after surgical treatment of the CSF leak (*B, D*). (From Mokri, B. (1999). Spontaneous cerebrospinal fluid leaks: From intracranial hypotension to cerebrospinal fluid hypovolemia—evolution of a concept. *Mayo Clin. Proc.* 74:1113–1123. By permission of Mayo Foundation for Medical Education and Research.)

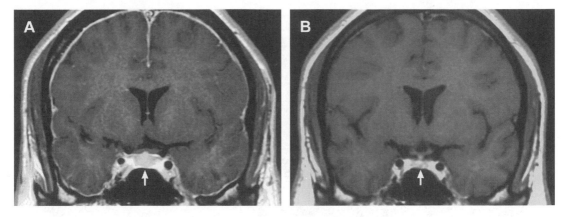

Figure 17–4 Contrast-enhanced T1-weighted coronal magnetic resonance images (MRI) of a patient with cerebrospinal fluid (CSF) leak during the symptomatic phase and active leak (*A*) and after recovery and resolution of clinical symptoms and MRI abnormalities (*B*). *A*: Several abnormalities are present, including diffuse pachymeningeal enhancement, flattening of the optic chiasm, partial obliteration of perichiasmatic cisterns, mild decrease in size of the lateral ventricles, and enlarged pituitary gland (*arrow*). *B*: Resolution of abnormalities after cessation of the CSF leak and disappearance of the clinical manifestations. (From Mokri, B. and J.L.D. Atkinson (2000). False pituitary tumor in CSF leaks. *Neurology* (in press). By permission of the American Academy of Neurology.)

Other abnormalities noted on the MRI of the head include pituitary enlargement (Mokri and Atkinson, 1999), sometimes mimicking pituitary adenoma or hyperplasia (Fig. 17–4); engorged venous sinuses (Bakshi et al., 1999) (Figs. 17–2, 17–3); and elongation of the brain stem in the anteroposterior plane (Pakiam et al., 1999).

Spine Abnormalities

Spine MRI may reveal extra-arachnoid or extradural fluid (Mokri et al., 1997; Rabin et al., 1998). This fluid may extend to the paraspinal soft tissues or present as elongated, localized collections in the epidural space within the spinal canal (Fig. 17–6C), which on axial sections appear to be located ventral or dorsal to the thecal sac (Dillon and Fishman, 1998). Spine MRI sometimes shows the diverticula (Fig. 17–6B) or, less frequently, may even identify the location of the leak. Other spine MRI abnormalities in CSF leak and CSF volume depletion include dural enhancement (Moayeri et al., 1998) and engorgement or prominence of the epidural venous plexus (Mokri, unpublished data).

Head MRI abnormalities appear to be the consequences of CSF volume depletion. Loss of CSF volume leads to sinking of the brain and to descent of cerebellar tonsils, collapse and decrease in the size of ventricles, decrease in the size of subarachnoid cisterns, flattening of the optic chiasm, and crowding of the posterior fossa. Furthermore, in the presence of an intact skull, according to the Monro-Kellie doctrine (Schaltenbrand, 1953), the loss of CSF volume has to be compensated for by an increase in intracranial blood volume. The latter is primarily reflected on the venous system and is manifested by meningeal venous hyperemia. Because leptomeninges have blood–brain barriers and pachymeninges do not, it is the pachymeninges that enhance with gadolinium (Fishman and Dillon, 1993; Haines et al., 1993; Mokri, 1999). Other manifestations of compensatory venous hypervolemia include engorgement of the venous sinuses and pituitary gland and prominence and engorgement of the spinal epidural venous plexus.

Myelography and Computed Tomography-Myelography

Myelography with water-soluble contrast material, especially when followed by CT scanning (CT-myelography), so far is the most ac-

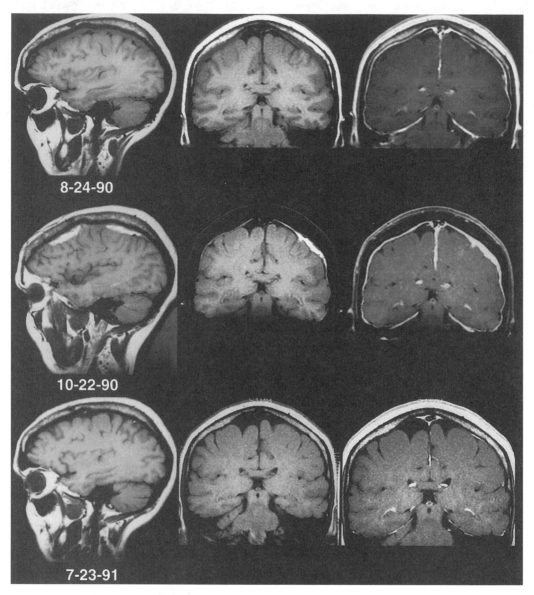

Figure 17–5 Non-contrast-enhanced T1-weighted parasagittal (*left vertical row*) and coronal (*middle vertical row*) magnetic resonance images and post-contrast T1-weighted coronal images (*right vertical row*) in same patient on three separate occasions. On August 24, 1990, non-contrast-enhanced images (*upper horizontal row*), subdural fluid collections are evident over both cerebral convexities. Diffuse pachymeningeal enhancement is noted in contrast-enhanced image. On October 22, 1990, images (*middle horizontal row*), while the patient was still symptomatic, extracerebral fluid collection on the right has resolved, whereas left-sided subdural collection now contains high-protein fluid or blood products and displays bright signals. The meningeal enhancement is unchanged. On July 23, 1991, images (*lower horizontal row*), with the headaches now resolved, the extracerebral fluid collections and abnormal meningeal enhancement have also completely resolved. (From Mokri, B., D.G. Piepgras, and G.M. Miller (1997). Syndrome of orthostatic headaches and diffuse pachymeningeal gadolinium enhancement. *Mayo Clin. Proc.* 72:400–413. By permission of Mayo Foundation for Medical Education and Research.)

curate test for demonstrating the site of CSF leaks (Mokri et al., 1997) (Fig. 17–6D, E, G). It can demonstrate extra-arachnoid or extra-dural contrast as well as penetration of contrast (and therefore the leaked CSF) in the paraspinal soft tissues. This sometimes may present as elongated collections in the epidural space within the spinal canal and on axial CT cuts may appear as "dog ear"–shaped collections located ventral or dorsal to the thecal sac (Fig. 17–7). Also, CT and CT-myelography show meningeal diverticula of various sizes. Depending on the nature of the leak (quick profuse vs. small and slow), both early and delayed CT cuts may be needed. If previous neurodiagnostic studies, such as MRI or cisternography or even myelography itself, have demonstrated an approximate level of the leak, the CT cuts may be concentrated to the suspected zone. Otherwise, thin CT cuts should be obtained at each spinal level from the foramen magnum to the sacrum.

Myelography also provides an opportunity to measure the CSF opening pressure and to obtain fluid for analysis.

Biopsy

With the current knowledge on clinical and imaging features of CSF volume depletion and CSF leaks, there is no justification for subjecting patients to meningeal biopsy. The information on biopsy dates back to the initial observations of meningeal enhancement on MRI, when the clinicians were not confident about the association of pachymeningeal enhancement and CSF leaks or intracranial hypotension. Then, understandably, patients were vigorously investigated for various types of meningeal disease, particularly meningeal inflammation, infection, and meningeal carcinomatosis.

Meningeal biopsy has shown normal appearance of the dura on gross examination. Leptomeninges also appear normal, except in some of the long-standing cases, in which the arachnoid may appear thickened or opaque. Microscopically, the dura appears entirely normal on its epidural aspect. However, a fairly thin zone of fibroblasts and thin-walled

blood vessels in an amorphous matrix is typically noted in the subdural aspect of the dura, resembling an organized hygroma. Hyperplasia of arachnoidal cells may be seen in some long-standing cases. No particular cellular infiltration or inflammatory change is noted. The pathologic findings support the notion that the dural meningeal abnormalities represent secondary reactive phenomena likely related to the changes in CSF volume or pressure (Mokri et al., 1995).

TREATMENT

Various treatments have been used for patients with spontaneous CSF leaks, but there is no definite or agreed-on standard approach. Some of these approaches are listed in Table 17–5.

Many patients, fortunately, improve spontaneously. Bed rest and increased fluid intake have been advocated. Because the majority of patients have significant orthostatic headaches, they nevertheless stay recumbent and in bed. Although hydration or overhydration was recommended in some older studies (Tourtellotte et al., 1964), its effectiveness has not been definitely established. The effectiveness of the cerebral vasoconstrictors caffeine and theophylline has been shown in some studies (Grant et al., 1989); however, the efficacies of caffeine and theophylline are often unimpressive, and durable beneficial effect is doubtful. The efficacy of steroids is unproved and mostly anecdotal. One might see an occasional patient who reports partial improvement with steroids, but substantial lasting effects are doubtful.

Epidural saline infusion has produced variable results (Gibson et al., 1988; Rice and Dabbs, 1950; Usubiaga et al., 1967). It can be tried with limited expectations in some patients in whom repeated blood patches have failed and when studies have not shown the site of the leak that can be approached surgically.

Epidural blood patch is an effective technique that can be considered the treatment of choice for patients in whom the initial trial of conservative management has failed

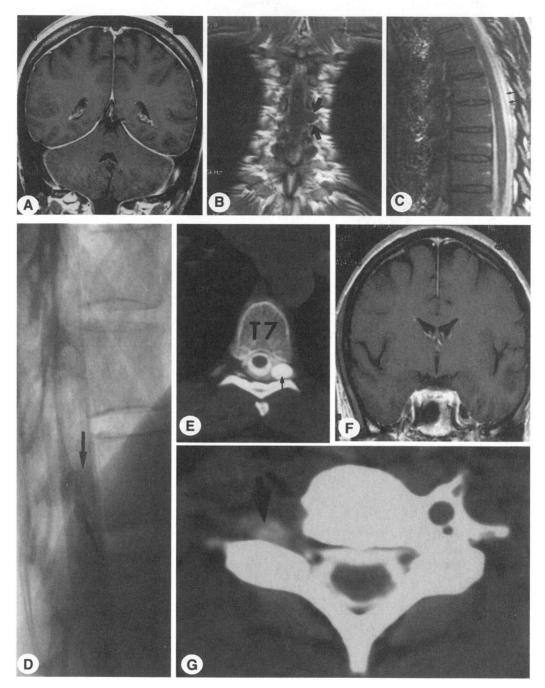

Figure 17–6 *A*: Gadolinium-enhanced coronal magnetic resonance imaging (MRI) shows diffuse pachymeningeal enhancement. *B*: Spine MRI shows a left T7 root sleeve diverticulum (*arrows*). *C*: T2-weighted spine MRI shows subdural cerebrospinal fluid (CSF) in the posterior aspect of the thoracic canal. *D* and *E*: Myelogram and computed tomography (CT)-myelogram confirm the left T7 root sleeve diverticulum (*arrows*) but do not show frank extravasation of CSF extradurally. *F*: Gadolinium-enhanced coronal head MRI obtained about 2 months later shows resolution of pachymeningeal gadolinium enhancement. *G*: Subsequent CT-myelogram demonstrates the site of CSF leak with contrast material exiting through the right C6 neural foramen into the soft tissues (*arrow*). This case not only demonstrates some of the imaging features of CSF leaks but also points to two important observations: (1) despite proven and persistent CSF leak (*G*), head MRI may fail to show pachymeningeal and gadolinium enhancement (*F*); (2) the presence of a meningeal diverticulum, even when obvious and large, may not

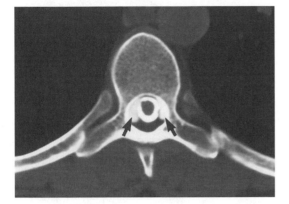

Table 17–5 Treatment of cerebrospinal fluid leaks

Bed rest
Caffeine
Steroids
Abdominal binder
Epidural blood patch
Continuous epidural saline infusion
Epidural infusion of dextran
CSF shunting
Surgical repair

Figure 17–7 Post-myelographic computed tomographic section through thoracic level in a patient with cerebrospinal fluid leak and extra-arachnoid accumulation of contrast material. Note the accumulation of fluid on both sides, exerting a bilateral mass effect on the dural sac. These longitudinal accumulations of fluid on cross-sections produce a characteristic "dog-ear" appearance (*arrows*). (From Mokri, B., D.G. Piepgras, and G.M. Miller (1997). Syndrome of orthostatic headaches and diffuse pachymeningeal gadolinium enhancement. *Mayo Clin. Proc.* 72:400–413. By permission of Mayo Foundation for Medical Education and Research.)

(Crawford, 1985; Di Giovanni et al., 1972; Geurts et al., 1990; Gormley, 1960; Rosenberg and Heavner, 1985; Seebacher et al., 1989; Szeinfeld et al., 1986; Vakharia et al., 1997). For relieving orthostatic headaches, this procedure essentially has two different aspects; the first is the immediate effect, simply related to volume replacement (by compressing the dura); the second is the latent effect, related to sealing of the dural defect. The interval between these two effects varies considerably, but sometimes (especially when the blood patch is used for headaches that occur after lumbar puncture) these two effects almost fuse temporarily. For headaches that occur after lumbar puncture, a single epidural blood patch gives relief in an over-

whelming majority of patients. In the small minority who do not respond to the first epidural blood patch, a second blood patch almost always gives relief. In spontaneous CSF leaks, success is less impressive. Many patients require more than one blood patch, and in our experience some have required as many as four to six blood patches. This difference in success rate in the two groups likely results from two factors: (1) as opposed to headaches after lumbar puncture, in spontaneous CSF leaks the level of the epidural blood patch may be distant from the level of the leak, and this factor may render the procedure less effective; (2) in many spontaneous CSF leaks, the nature and anatomy of the leak are much different from a simple hole or rent produced by the spinal tap needle. In spontaneous CSF leaks, many of the dural defects are in the anterior aspect of the dura or in the root sleeves. In addition, the defect may not be a simple hole or a single rent but a congenitally attenuated zone or patch of the dura with the underlying arachnoid that has finally given way and is oozing CSF from one or more points. In cases such as these, blood patches fail altogether.

In well-selected cases, operation is effective and can be tried when conservative and less invasive approaches, such as epidural blood patch, have failed (Mokri et al., 1997;

necessarily correspond to the site of CSF leak. It is important to demonstrate the site of extravasation of the fluid, which may prove to be at a level distant from a diverticulum, which would have been suspected to be the source of the leak (*E* and *G*). (From Mokri, B. (1999). Spontaneous cerebrospinal fluid leaks: From intracranial hypotension to cerebrospinal fluid hypovolemia—evolution of a concept. *Mayo Clin. Proc.* 74:1113–1123. By permission of Mayo Foundation for Medical Education and Research.)

Schievink et al., 1998). However, the surgical approach is not entirely straightforward. The ideal cases are those in which a structural abnormality or focal leak has been shown by imaging techniques. Sometimes the surgeon may find that the CSF has leaked but will be unable to locate the exact site of the leak and, therefore, may pack the area with, e.g., blood-soaked absorbable gelatin sponge (Gelfoam) or muscle and hope for the best. Although it is not uncommon that a CSF leak develops from the weakened wall of a meningeal diverticulum, sometimes more than one diverticulum is present. The diverticula may be of different sizes, and the largest diverticulum may not necessarily be the site of the leak. In addition, we have seen patients with meningeal diverticula, even large ones, who had leak from a site remote from the diverticula (Mokri, 1999). Preoperatively, it is essential to demonstrate the actual site of CSF leak. So far, CT-myelography is the most reliable test for this purpose.

Sometimes the surgeon is faced with a dural defect with borders that are markedly attenuated and may not yield to suturing. Occasionally, patients have leak from more than one site at different levels; this possibility emphasizes the importance of thorough preoperative studies and their accurate interpretation.

BROADENING THE CLINICAL-IMAGING SPECTRUM OF CEREBROSPINAL FLUID VOLUME DEPLETION

Since the recognition of MRI abnormalities in intracranial hypotension and CSF leaks, a much larger number of patients have been identified and a broader clinical and imaging spectrum of the disorder has been recognized (Mokri, 1999). Thus far, at least four clinical-imaging syndromes in CSF volume depletion are recognized (Table 17–6). In the classic form, headaches (typically orthostatic), low CSF pressure, and typical MRI abnormalities are noted. Some patients have the typical clinical manifestations and imaging abnormalities but despite documented CSF leak

Table 17–6 Clinical-imaging syndromes in cerebrospinal fluid volume depletion

Type I	Classic
Type II	Normal pressure
Type III	Normal meninges
Type IV	Acephalgic

have CSF opening pressures that are consistently within limits of normal (the normal-pressure group) (Mokri et al., 1998). In yet another group, despite typical clinical manifestations and documented CSF leak and low CSF pressures, meninges appear normal on MRI (Mokri et al., 1999). In the acephalgic group, typical MRI abnormalities are present and CSF pressure is low but headaches are curiously absent despite documented CSF volume depletion as the result of CSF leak or CSF shunt overdrainage (Hochman and Naidich, 1999). The term "CSF volume depletion" appears to reflect this entire clinical-imaging spectrum more accurately because the term "intracranial hypotension" no longer appears to be broad enough to embrace all of the clinical and imaging variations that have emerged.

HEADACHES AFTER LUMBAR PUNCTURE

Lumbar puncture is well known to cause orthostatic headaches related to CSF leak from the puncture site. These typically begin within 2 days but may be delayed for as long as nearly 2 weeks. The headaches may be dull or throbbing and are clearly positional, provoked in the upright position, and relieved with recumbency. They may be frontal, occipital, fronto-occipital, or holocephalic. Nausea and neck stiffness or tightness may accompany the headache, and occasionally blurred vision, photophobia, tinnitus, change in hearing, or dizziness is reported (Raskin, 1990). Typically, the headaches resolve spontaneously within a few days. Because the diagnosis is often obvious, patients are not ordinarily subjected to neurodiagnostic techniques. Head MRI may show pachymeningeal gadolinium enhancement. Even subdural fluid collections have been reported.

Headaches occur after lumbar puncture in about one-third of patients who undergo CSF examination. In one-third of these patients, the headache is severe (in about 10% of the total number of patients); in one-third, it is moderate; and in one-third, it is mild (Kuntz et al., 1992). These figures are larger for patients with preceding headache and smaller for those without preceding headache.

Many investigators agree that the incidence of headaches after lumbar puncture would decrease if smaller-bore needles (e.g., 26-gauge) were used. In the usual practice of diagnostic lumbar puncture, whether in the outpatient or the inpatient setting, the narrower (25- to 29-gauge) needles are impractical because difficulties may be encountered in inserting the needle, measuring the opening pressure, and collecting the fluid. Young female patients with a low body mass index may be at higher risk than others for development of headaches after lumbar puncture. There are no established correlations between the CSF opening pressure, CSF composition, or position and recumbency period after lumbar puncture with the development of post-puncture headaches. Treatment of post-puncture headaches is often much less involved than treatment of spontaneous CSF leaks. The headache resolves spontaneously in the majority of patients with or without hydration, overhydration, or caffeine. Epidural blood patch is more effective than epidural saline (Di Giovanni et al., 1972). Epidural blood patch leads to relief in about 90% of patients. A second epidural blood patch brings relief in almost all of the remaining cases (Vilming and Titus, 1993).

REFERENCES

Atkinson, J.L., B.G. Weinshenker, G.M. Miller et al. (1998). Acquired Chiari I malformation secondary to spontaneous spinal cerebrospinal fluid leakage and chronic intracranial hypotension syndrome in seven cases. *J. Neurosurg.* 88:237–242.

Baker, C.C. (1983). Headache due to spontaneous low spinal fluid pressure. *Minn. Med.* 66:325–328.

Bakshi, R., L.L. Mechtler, S. Kamran et al. (1999). MRI findings in lumbar puncture headache syndrome: Abnormal dural-meningeal and dural venous sinus enhancement. *Clin. Imaging* 23: 73–76.

Beck, C.E., N.W. Rizk, L.T. Kiger et al. (1998). Intracranial hypotension presenting with severe encephalopathy. Case report. *J. Neurosurg.* 89: 470–473.

Bell, W.E., R.J. Joynt and A.L. Sahs (1960). Low spinal fluid pressure syndromes. *Neurology 10*: 512–521.

Crawford, J.S. (1985). Epidural blood patch [letter]. *Anaesthesia 40*:381.

Cushing, H. (1926). *Studies in Intracranial Physiology & Surgery; the Third Circulation, the Hypophysics, the Gliomas* (H. Milford, ed.). Oxford University Press, London.

Davenport, R.J., S.J. Chataway and C.P. Warlow (1995). Spontaneous intracranial hypotension from a CSF leak in a patient with Marfan's syndrome. *J. Neurol. Neurosurg. Psychiatry* 59: 516–519.

Di Giovanni, A.J., M.W. Galbert and W.M. Wahle (1972). Epidural injection of autologous blood for postlumbar-puncture headache. II. Additional clinical experiences and laboratory investigation. *Anesth. Analg.* 51:226–232.

Dillon, W.P. and R.A. Fishman (1998). Some lessons learned about the diagnosis and treatment of spontaneous intracranial hypotension [editorial]. *AJNR Am J Neuroradiol* 19:1001–1002.

Fay, T. (1937). Mechanism of headache. *Trans. Am. Neurol. Assoc.* 62:74–77.

Fishman, R.A. (1992). *Cerebrospinal Fluid in Diseases of the Nervous System*, 2nd ed. W.B. Saunders, Philadelphia.

Fishman, R.A. and W.P. Dillon (1993). Dural enhancement and cerebral displacement secondary to intracranial hypotension. *Neurology 43*: 609–611.

Front, D. and L. Penning (1974). Subcutaneous extravasation of CSF demonstration by scinticisternography. *J. Nucl. Med.* 15:200–201.

Geurts, J.W., M.C. Haanschoten, R.M. van Wijk et al. (1990). Post-dural puncture headache in young patients. A comparative study between the use of 0.52 mm (25-gauge) and 0.33 mm (29-gauge) spinal needles. *Acta Anaesthesiol. Scand.* 34:350–353.

Gibson, B.E., D.J. Wedel, R.J. Faust et al. (1988). Continuous epidural saline infusion for the treatment of low CSF pressure headache. *Anesthesiology* 68:789–791.

Gormley, J.B. (1960). Current comment: Treatment of postspinal headache. *Anesthesiology 21*: 565–566.

Grant, R., B. Condon, J. Patterson et al. (1989). Changes in cranial CSF volume during hypercapnia and hypocapnia. *J. Neurol. Neurosurg. Psychiatry* 52:218–222.

Haines, D.E., H.L. Harkey and O. al-Mefty (1993). The "subdural" space: A new look at an outdated concept. *Neurosurgery* 32:111–120.

Hochman, M.S. and T.P. Naidich (1999). Diffuse meningeal enhancement in patients with overdraining, long-standing ventricular shunts. *Neurology* 52:406–409.

Hochman, M.S., T.P. Naidich, S.A. Kobetz et al. (1992). Spontaneous intracranial hypotension with pachymeningeal enhancement on MRI. *Neurology* 42:1628–1630.

Hogan, Q.H., R. Prost, A. Kulier et al. (1996). Magnetic resonance imaging of cerebrospinal fluid volume and the influence of body habitus and abdominal pressure. *Anesthesiology* 84: 1341–1349.

Horton, J.C. and R.A. Fishman (1994). Neurovisual findings in the syndrome of spontaneous intracranial hypotension from dural cerebrospinal fluid leak. *Ophthalmology* 101:244–251.

Huber, M. (1970). Spontaneous hypoliquorrhea. Report on 7 personal observations [in German]. *Schweiz. Arch. Neurol. Neurochir. Psychiatr.* 106:9–23.

Kunkle, E.C., B.S. Ray, and H.G. Wolff (1943). Experimental studies on headache; analysis of the headache associated with changes in intracranial pressure. *Arch. Neurol. Psychiatry* 49: 323–358.

Kuntz, K.M., E. Kokmen, J.C. Stevens et al. (1992). Post-lumbar puncture headaches: Experience in 501 consecutive procedures. *Neurology* 42:1884–1887.

Labadie, E.L., J. van Antwerp and C.R. Bamford (1976). Abnormal lumbar isotope cisternography in an unusual case of spontaneous hypoliquorrheic headache. *Neurology* 26:135–139.

Lasater, G.M. (1970). Primary intracranial hypotension. The low spinal fluid pressure syndrome. *Headache* 10:63–66.

Lyons, M.K. and F.B. Meyer (1990). Cerebrospinal fluid physiology and the management of increased intracranial pressure. *Mayo Clin. Proc.* 65:684–707.

Marcelis, J. and S.D. Silberstein (1990). Spontaneous low cerebrospinal fluid pressure headache. *Headache* 30:192–196.

Matsumae, M., R. Kikinis, I.A. Morocz et al. (1996). Age-related changes in intracranial compartment volumes in normal adults assessed by magnetic resonance imaging. *J. Neurosurg. 84:* 982–991.

Miller, J.D. (1975). Volume and pressure in the craniospinal axis. *Clin. Neurosurg.* 22:76–105.

Moayeri, N.N., J.W. Henson, P.W. Schaefer et al. (1998). Spinal dural enhancement on magnetic resonance imaging associated with spontaneous intracranial hypotension. Report of three cases and review of the literature. *J. Neurosurg.* 88: 912–918.

Mokri, B. (1999). Spontaneous cerebrospinal fluid leaks: From intracranial hypotension to cerebrospinal fluid hypovolemia—evolution of a concept. *Mayo Clin. Proc.* 74:1113–1123.

Mokri, B. and J.L.D. Atkinson (2000). False pituitary tumor in CSF leaks. *Neurology* 55:573–575.

Mokri, B., J.L.D. Atkinson, D.W. Dodick et al. (1999). Absent pachymeningeal gadolinium enhancement on cranial MRI despite symptomatic CSF leak. *Neurology* 53:402–404.

Mokri, B., S.F. Hunter, J.L. Atkinson et al. (1998). Orthostatic headaches caused by CSF leak but with normal CSF pressures. *Neurology* 51:786–790.

Mokri, B., B.R. Krueger, G.M. Miller et al. (1991). Meningeal gadolinium enhancement in low pressure headaches [abstract]. *Ann. Neurol. 30:* 294–295.

Mokri, B., B.R. Krueger, G.M. Miller et al. (1993). Meningeal gadolinium enhancement in low-pressure headaches. *J. Neuroimaging* 3:11–15.

Mokri, B., J.E. Parisi, B.W. Scheithauer et al. (1995). Meningeal biopsy in intracranial hypotension: Meningeal enhancement on MRI. *Neurology* 45:1801–1807.

Mokri, B., D.G. Piepgras and G.M. Miller (1997). Syndrome of orthostatic headaches and diffuse pachymeningeal gadolinium enhancement. *Mayo Clin. Proc.* 72:400–413.

Molins, A., J. Alvarez, J. Sumalla et al. (1990). Cisternographic pattern of spontaneous liquoral hypotension. *Cephalalgia* 10:59–65.

Murros, K. and R. Fogelholm (1983). Spontaneous intracranial hypotension with slit ventricles. *J. Neurol. Neurosurg. Psychiatry* 46:1149–1151.

Pakiam, A.S., C. Lee and A.E. Lang (1999). Intracranial hypotension with Parkinsonism, ataxia, and bulbar weakness. *Arch. Neurol.* 56:869–872.

Pannullo, S.C., J.B. Reich, G. Krol et al. (1993). MRI changes in intracranial hypotension. *Neurology* 43:919–926.

Pavlin, D.J., J.S. McDonald, B. Child et al. (1979). Acute subdural hematoma—an unusual sequela to lumbar puncture. *Anesthesiology* 51:338–340.

Pleasure, S.J., A. Abosch, J. Friedman et al. (1998). Spontaneous intracranial hypotension resulting in stupor caused by diencephalic compression. *Neurology* 50:1854–1857.

Rabin, B.M., S. Roychowdhury, J.R. Meyer et al. (1998). Spontaneous intracranial hypotension: Spinal MR findings. *AJNR Am. J. Neuroradiol.* 19:1034–1039.

Rando, T.A. and R.A. Fishman (1992). Spontaneous intracranial hypotension: Report of two cases and review of the literature. *Neurology 42*: 481–487.

Raskin, N.H. (1990). Lumbar puncture headache: A review. *Headache 30*:197–200.

Rice, G.G. and C.H. Dabbs (1950). The use of peridural and subarachnoid injections of saline solution in the treatment of severe postspinal headaches. *Anesthesiology 11*:17–23.

Rosenberg, P.H. and J.E. Heavner (1985). In vitro study of the effect of epidural blood patch on leakage through a dural puncture. *Anesth. Analg. 64*:501–504.

Rowland, L.P., M.E. Fink, and L. Rubin (1991). Cerebrospinal fluid: blood–brain barrier, brain edema, and hydrocephalus. In *Principles of Neural Science*, 3rd ed. (E.R. Kandel, J.H. Schwartz and T.M. Jessell, eds.), pp. 1050–1060. Elsevier, New York.

Sable, S.G. and N.M. Ramadan (1991). Meningeal enhancement and low CSF pressure headache. An MRI study. *Cephalalgia 11*:275–276.

Schaltenbrand, G. (1938). Neuere Anschauungen zur Pathophysiologie der Liquorzirkulation. *Zentralbl. Neurochir. 3*:290–300.

Schaltenbrand, G. (1953). Normal and pathological physiology of the cerebrospinal fluid circulation. *Lancet 1*:805–808.

Schievink, W.I., V.M. Morreale, J.L. Atkinson et al. (1998). Surgical treatment of spontaneous spinal cerebrospinal fluid leaks. *J. Neurosurg. 88*:243–246.

Seebacher, J., V. Ribeiro, J.L. LeGuillou et al. (1989). Epidural blood patch in the treatment of post dural puncture headache: A double blind study. *Headache 29*: 630–632.

Silberstein, S.D. and J. Marcelis (1992). Headache associated with changes in intracranial pressure. *Headache 32*:84–94.

Sipe, J.C., J. Zyroff and T.A. Waltz (1981). Primary intracranial hypotension and bilateral isodense subdural hematomas. *Neurology 31*:334–337.

Szeinfeld, M., I.H. Ihmeidan, M.M. Moser et al. (1986). Epidural blood patch: Evaluation of the volume and spread of blood injected into the epidural space. *Anesthesiology 64*:820–822.

Tourtellotte, W.W., A.F. Haerer, G.L. Heller et al. (1964). *Post-lumbar Puncture Headaches*. Charles C. Thomas, Springfield, IL.

Tripathi, B.J. and R.C. Tripathi (1974). Vacuolar transcellular channels as a drainage pathway for cerebrospinal fluid. *J. Physiol. (Lond.) 239*:195–206.

Tripathi, R.C. (1973). Ultrastructure of the arachnoid mater in relation to outflow of cerebrospinal fluid. A new concept. *Lancet 2*:8–11.

Usubiaga, J.E., L.E. Usubiaga, L.M. Brea et al. (1967). Effect of saline injections on epidural and subarachnoid space pressures and relation to postspinal anesthesia headache. *Anesth. Analg. 46*:293–296.

Vakharia, S.B., P.S. Thomas, A.E. Rosenbaum et al. (1997). Magnetic resonance imaging of cerebrospinal fluid leak and tamponade effect of blood patch in postdural puncture headache. *Anesth. Analg. 84*:585–590.

Vilming, S.T. and F. Titus (1993). Low cerebrospinal fluid pressure. In *The Headache* (J. Olesen, P. Tfelt-Hansen, and K.M.A. Welch, eds.), pp. 687–695. Raven Press, New York.

Vishteh, A.G., W.I. Schievink, J.J. Baskin et al. (1998). Cervical bone spur presenting with spontaneous intracranial hypotension. Case report. *J. Neurosurg. 89*:483–484.

Weber, W.E., G.A. Heidendal and M.C. de Krom (1991). Primary intracranial hypotension and abnormal radionuclide cisternography. Report of a case and review of the literature. *Clin. Neurol. Neurosurg. 93*:55–60.

Welch, K. (1975). The principles of physiology of the cerebrospinal fluid in relation to hydrocephalus including normal pressure hydrocephalus. *Adv. Neurol. 13*:247–332.

Woltman, H.W. (1940). Headache: A consideration of some of the more common types. *Med. Clin. North Am. 24*:1159–1170.

Yamamoto, M., T. Suehiro, H. Nakata et al. (1993). Primary low cerebrospinal fluid pressure syndrome associated with galactorrhea. *Intern. Med. 32*:228–231.

18

Infectious, Toxic, and Metabolic Headache

LAWRENCE C. NEWMAN
SEYMOUR SOLOMON

The International Headache Society (IHS) classification (Headache Classification Committee of the International Headache Society, 1988) divides headaches into primary and secondary categories. *Secondary headaches*, those in which the headache is due to a structural or metabolic disease, are further subdivided into eight separate divisions. This chapter highlights those headache disorders caused by intracranial infection, metabolic disorders, and acute substance use or exposure. As with all forms of secondary headache, identification of the underlying problem is essential in determining the proper diagnosis and treatment.

INFECTIONS

The IHS classification separates infectious causes of headaches into three distinct categories: those associated with an intracranial infection, those associated with noncephalic (extracranial) infections, and those arising from disorders of the cranium and related regions.

Bacterial Meningitis

The most common organisms responsible for producing meningitis in the United States are *Haemophilus influenzae*, *Streptococcus pneumoniae*, and *Neisseria meningitidis*, which account for approximately 75% of all cases (Franke, 1987; Schlech et al., 1985; Schlech, 1992; Oliver and Harwood-Nuss, 1993; Carpenter and Petersdorf, 1963). *Listeria monocytogenes* is the fourth most common pathogen in adults. *Staphylococcus aureus* and group A streptococci, less common causes, are usually found in association with cerebral or epidural abscesses, head trauma, cranial thrombophlebitis, or neurosurgical interventions. Meningitis in newborns is usually caused by *Escherichia coli*, group B streptococci, and *Listeria* (Franke, 1987; Schlech et al., 1985; Schlech, 1992; Oliver and Harwood-Nuss, 1993; Carpenter and Petersdorf, 1963). Pathogens introduced during such medical interventions as lumbar puncture and spinal anesthesia include *Klebsiella*, *Proteus*, and *Pseudomonas* (Franke, 1987; Schlech et al., 1985; Schlech, 1992; Oliver and Harwood-Nuss, 1993; Carpenter and Petersdorf, 1963). Meningitis may be the result of more uncommon organisms in patients who are immunocompromised and receiving chemotherapy or other immunosuppression therapies; have lymphoma, leukemia, or acquired immunodeficiency syndrome (AIDS); or are malnourished. In these settings, *Mycobacterium tuber-*

culosis, Candida, Cryptococcus, Histoplasma, or other rare organisms may be the culprit (Isenberg, 1992; Tija et al., 1985; Bross and Gordon, 1991; Benson et al., 1988).

In the United States, acute bacterial meningitis has an annual incidence of five to ten cases per 100,000 (Nicolosi et al., 1986). Pneumococcal, *H. influenzae*, and meningococcal meningitis typically cause outbreaks during the fall, winter, and spring peak times. The majority of cases affect children less than 5 years old, although recently *H. influenzae* meningitis is being seen more commonly in adults over age 50. Pneumococcal meningitis usually affects the young and adults over age 40, whereas meningococcal meningitis strikes children and adolescents more commonly. Meningococcal meningitis occurs throughout adulthood but is rare after age 50.

The organisms most often responsible for causing bacterial meningitis are found in the nasopharynx in a large proportion of the general population. Why these organisms become blood-borne is not known; however, some patients report a previous viral upper respiratory infection. Pneumococcal meningitis often begins as pneumonia. Once they enter the bloodstream, these pathogens have an affinity for the meninges. Other routes by which organisms reach the meninges include craniotomy sites, skull fractures, dural tears, and the middle ear and paranasal sinuses. A cerebral abscess rupture into the subarachnoid space or ventricular system may also seed the meninges. Meningitis may be a secondary complication of miliary tuberculosis or endocarditis.

The earliest clinical manifestations of acute bacterial meningitis are fever, headache, alterations in consciousness, nuchal rigidity, and (rarely) convulsions. The headache is often the first symptom and usually progresses rapidly, increasing in severity over several minutes. The headache is typically generalized or frontal and radiates occipitally, into the neck and spine. The pain is severe, constant, and often associated with photophobia, phonophobia, nausea, vomiting, and pain with eye movements (Carpenter and Petersdorf, 1963; Isenberg, 1992). Young children often do not complain of headache, and the elderly suffer from headaches less often than young adults (Franke, 1987; Carpenter and Petersdorf, 1963; Lipton and Schafermeyer, 1993). Patients usually assume a flexed body posture, reflexively protecting their head and neck through spasm of the muscles of the neck and spine and keeping their head retracted (Carpenter and Petersdorf, 1963). Kernig's sign (inability to completely extend the legs) and Brudzinski's sign (forward flexion of the neck resulting in flexion at the hips and knees) often can be elicited. Alterations in mentation vary with the stage of infection. Drowsiness, delirium, stupor, or coma may occur. A petechial rash accompanies 50% of meningococcal infections (Tonjum et al., 1983). Seizures result most often from *H. influenzae* meningitis (Ferry et al., 1982).

Chronic meningitis is usually associated with tuberculosis (TB) or cryptococcal meningitis. Often, TB meningitis is associated with a severe headache and fever that begins subacutely, but it may present as a chronic headache with fever (Franke, 1987). Cryptococcal meningitis may present as a chronic headache that worsens over time, without associated fever or neurological deficits (Tija et al., 1985). Cryptococcal and TB meningitis are seen in patients who have Hodgkin's disease or AIDS or are receiving chemotherapy or other immunosuppressive therapy (Franke, 1987; Yu et al., 1988).

A subacute or chronic form of meningitis is seen in patients who are immunosuppressed. Nocardia meningitis presents as a subacute or chronic meningitis with fever, headache, and nuchal rigidity. Over 40% of patients develop brain abscesses (Bross and Gordon, 1991). *Listeria* is the pathogen most likely to cause meningitis in patients with leukemia and non-T-cell lymphomas (Franke, 1987).

If meningitis is clinically suspected, lumbar puncture should be performed emergently. A lumbar puncture may be undertaken without neuroimaging if no contraindications are present. Contraindications to lumbar puncture include increased intracranial pressure, mass lesions, coagulopathy, or a localized infection at the puncture site.

The cerebrospinal fluid (CSF) should be sent for Gram's stain and bacterial cultures. Determination of CSF glucose, protein, and cell counts should be performed, as well as assays for specific bacterial antigens and endotoxins. The CSF findings in acute bacterial meningitis include glucose <40 mg/dl, a protein level >45 mg/dl, and a marked pleocytosis with cell counts greater than 1,000/mm^3. Neutrophilic lymphocytes predominate in the early stages of infection. Measurements of CSF lactic dehydrogenase may be of diagnostic value as increased levels are consistently seen in patients with bacterial meningitis.

Patients with bacterial meningitis should have radiological studies of the chest, skull, and sinuses early in the workup, to identify foci of infection. The headache and meningitis in the acute phases of the infection are best managed with antibiotics or antifungal agents, analgesics, antipyretics and IV fluids.

Nonbacterial Meningitis

Aseptic meningitis is usually caused by enteroviruses (poliovirus, echovirus, and coxsackieviruses A and B). Less common pathogens include cytomegalovirus, herpes simplex, adenovirus, rubella, mumps, Epstein-Barr, herpes zoster, human immunodeficiency virus (HIV), influenza, and parainfluenza (Franke, 1987; Nicolosi et al., 1986; Beghi et al., 1984).

The annual incidence of viral meningitis in the United States is 11 to 27 per 100,000 (Beghi et al., 1984; Ponka and Pettersson, 1982). Because the enteroviruses grow in the intestinal tract and are spread by the fecal-oral route, familial outbreaks are common, the majority of cases occurring in children and young adults. The timing of the outbreak may give clues to the responsible agent. Enteroviral infections peak in August and September; mumps meningitis occurs throughout the year, with the highest incidence in late winter and spring.

Aseptic meningitis is manifested by a rapidly developing, severe headache associated with fever, malaise, anorexia, nuchal rigidity, photophobia, and phonophobia (Franke, 1987; Lepow et al., 1962; Davis, 1987). Every patient with viral meningitis suffers from a severe bilateral headache (Lamonte et al., 1995). The course of the disease is usually benign.

In viral meningitis, CSF findings reveal a mild pleocytosis with a predominance of polymorphonuclear cells early in the infection. The CSF protein is normal or mildly elevated, and glucose levels are normal or slightly decreased. The CSF should be sent for viral cultures and antigens, although the responsible agent is identified in only 11% to 12% of cases (Nicolosi et al., 1986; Beghi et al., 1984).

Amebic meningoencephalitis is rare. It is caused by amebas of the genus *Naegleria* and is acquired by swimming in freshwater lakes or ponds (Cleland et al., 1982). In the United States, most cases occur in the southwest; the majority are fatal. The disorder is characterized by an abrupt onset of severe headache, high fever, nausea, vomiting, and nuchal rigidity, followed by seizures, focal neurological deficits, stupor, and coma. Death typically occurs within a week (Seidel et al., 1982). Another rare form of aseptic meningitis, Mollaret's meningitis, is characterized by episodes of fever and other signs and symptoms of aseptic meningitis that recur every few days or weeks for many months to years. Studies of CSF demonstrate pleocytosis with large epithelioid cells (Bharrucha et al., 1991).

Encephalitis

Unlike meningitis, which is an inflammation of the meninges, encephalitis is an inflammation of the brain parenchyma. Encephalitis may be due to viral, bacterial, fungal, or parasitic agents, although most are secondary to viral infections. Whatever the cause, the syndrome of encephalitis consists of an acute febrile illness with evidence of meningeal involvement as well as some combination of seizures, mental status changes, aphasia or mutism, hemiparesis, reflex asymmetry, ataxia, myoclonic jerks, nystagmus, and weakness of facial and ocular muscles (Adams and Victor, 1993).

Viral Encephalitis

In the United States, the yearly incidence of viral encephalitis is 7.4 per 100,000 (Nicolosi et al., 1986; Beghi et al., 1984). Although viruses are the usual presumptive cause of encephalitis, the specific agent is identifiable in only 15% of cases (Nicolosi et al., 1986; Beghi et al., 1984). Common causes of viral encephalitis include herpes simplex virus, arbovirus, mumps, Epstein-Barr, influenza, and measles. Many viral encephalitides have a characteristic geographical and seasonal incidence and are usually due to arboviral infections. These infections are transmitted through the bites of infected mosquitoes and are, therefore, most common during the summer and fall months. These disorders are characterized by alternating cycles of viral infections in the mosquito and the host (usually horses and birds). In the United States, there are several common arthropod-borne encephalitides. St. Louis encephalitis, which can be found throughout the country but more commonly along the Mississippi River, usually occurs in the late summer. Eastern equine encephalitis is found in the eastern United States; western equine encephalitis occurs west of the Mississippi River. Venezuelan equine encephalitis occurs in the northeast and northern midwest states (Johnson, 1982). In 1999, the northeast states had an outbreak of West Nile encephalitis, the first time this illness occurred in the United States. During the 1999 outbreak 62 human cases of West Nile viral disease were documented, resulting in 7 deaths (CDC, 1999).

Clinically, arbovirus encephalitides are indistinguishable. Common symptoms include headache, fever, and nuchal rigidity. In infants, these disorders may present as a rapidly developing febrile illness with convulsions. Older children and adults may complain of a prodrome that lasts several days and consists of listlessness, mild headache, drowsiness, nausea, vomiting, and fever. These symptoms are followed by mental status changes, seizures, tremors, myalgias, photophobia, and focal neurological deficits (Johnson, 1982). Rarely, an abrupt-onset (thunderclap) headache may be the only presenting sign of acute encephalitis (Johnson, 1982). Of the arboviral infections found in the United States, eastern equine encephalitis is the most serious as most who become infected develop encephalitis and two-thirds of those patients die or have residual neurological deficits (Johnson, 1982).

Herpes simplex virus (HSV) is the most common cause of nonepidemic viral encephalitis and the most serious. There are approximately 2,000 cases yearly in the United States; 30% to 70% of these are fatal, and most of the survivors have serious neurological sequelae (Whitley, 1988). Encephalitis is caused most often by type 1 HSV; type 2 virus may cause acute encephalitis in the neonate if the mother has a genital herpes infection. Clinically, there is usually no identifiable prodrome, although some patients initially experience olfactory or gustatory hallucinations, personality changes, aphasia, bizarre behaviors, or seizures. A rapidly developing, severe, global headache associated with fever is seen in more than half of all patients. Mass effect due to the predilection of the virus to affect the temporal lobe occasionally leads to a focal headache. Other frequent clinical findings include fever (50% to 80%), meningismus (40% to 60%), focal neurological signs (80% to 90%), convulsions (45% to 60%), and coma (30% to 40%) (Davis and McLaren, 1983; Young et al., 1992; Kennedy, 1988; Silberstein, 1992). A subacute course, consisting of headache, fatigue, and lethargy progressing over 4 to 5 months, has also been reported (Young et al., 1992).

West Nile virus is a member of the Flavivirdae family. The disorder is transmitted through the bite of the mosquito Culex spp.; wild birds are the primary reservoir host. The incubation period is approximately 6 days (range 5–15 days). The most common symptoms reported during the New York outbreak consisted of fever, muscle weakness, headache, altered mental status, photophobia, myalgias, arthralgias, and rash (CDC, 1999; Cunha, 1999). Clinically, West Nile presented in a number of ways including encephalitis with or without muscle weakness, aseptic meningitis, and a mild form characterized by fever and headache (CDC, 1999; Cunha,

1999). A rare clinical presentation unique to the New York epidemic consisted of a Guillain-Barré-like syndrome with flaccid paralysis requiring ventilatory support and electromyographic evidence of an axonal neuropathy (Ahmed et al., 2000).

Bacterial Encephalitis

Although less common than viral encephalitis, bacterial causes of encephalitis do occur. Legionnaires' disease, caused by *Legionella pneumophilia*, was first described in 1976 when attendees at the annual convention of the American Legion became ill; many subsequently died. Various clinical presentations have been described and are characterized by pneumonia and extrapulmonary symptoms of headache, confusion, obtundation, high fever, cranial nerve palsies, tremors, and ataxia. The central nervous system (CNS) symptoms usually resolve quickly and without residual deficits (Lees and Tyrrell, 1978; Shetty et al., 1980; Baker et al., 1981). Encephalitis secondary to *L. monocytogenes* typically affects people who are immunosuppressed. A prodrome consisting of global headache, fever, and nausea is followed by ataxia, cranial nerve palsies, respiratory distress, and coma (Callea et al., 1985; Kohler et al., 1991). Encephalitis has also been reported in association with mycoplasma pneumonia (Fisher et al., 1983).

Brain Abscess

Brain abscess occurs with an incidence of about 1 per 100,000 and affects children and those older than 60 years most often (Chun et al., 1986; Molavi and Dinubile, 1988; Nicolosi et al., 1991). A brain abscess is almost always the result of an infection elsewhere in the body. In approximately 10% of cases, the abscess results from an outside source, such as a skull fracture, neurosurgical procedure, or penetrating injury (Chun et al., 1986; Brewer et al., 1982; Gates et al., 1950; Harris et al., 1985). Forty percent of all brain abscesses arise from infections of the paranasal sinuses, middle ear, or mastoid (Chatstrey et al., 1991; Kulay et al., 1990). About 10% of abscesses arise from pulmonary sites (Chun

et al., 1986; Harris et al., 1985), and congenital heart disease with infective endocarditis is responsible for approximately 20% of all cases (Ghosh et al., 1990). In the remaining 20%, no identifiable source is uncovered (Murphy et al., 1979).

Organisms commonly isolated from brain abscesses arising from otic or sinus sources include *S. aureus*, anaerobic or aerobic streptococci, *Enterobacter* sp., and *Bacteroides* sp. (Chun et al., 1986; Molavi and Dinubile, 1988; Nicolosi et al., 1991; Kaplan, 1985). Staphylococci, streptococci, and *Actinomyces* arise from pulmonary foci, whereas anaerobic streptococci and *S. aureus* are seen in association with endocarditis. *Streptococcus milleri* is frequently identified from brain abscesses as well (Chun et al., 1986; Kaplan, 1985).

Headache is the most common initial symptom of brain abscess and may occur alone or with symptoms referable to the primary infection (Takahashi, 1992). Other presenting signs and symptoms include drowsiness, confusion, seizures, and focal neurological deficits. The accompanying signs and symptoms will be determined by the primary site of the abscess as well as any mass effect that it produces. When arising from an otic source, the headache is usually preceded by temporal pain and chronic otitis (Kulay et al., 1990). Frontal headache is often reported by patients in whom the abscess began in the sinuses. Abscesses within the temporal lobe usually manifest with an ipsilateral frontotemporal headache; cerebellar abscesses cause suboccipital and retroauricular head pain radiating into the neck (De Marinis et al., 1993).

Fever and leukocytosis may occur early in the course of infection, resolving as the abscess becomes encapsulated. Nausea and vomiting usually begin 1 week after the onset of headache and may be secondary to increased intracranial pressure (Chun et al., 1986; Molavi and Dinubile, 1988). Papilledema is present in less than half of all patients at presentation (Chun et al., 1986).

The diagnosis of a brain abscess is made by demonstrating a middle ear, sinus, mastoid, pulmonary, or cardiac source of infection or the presence of a right-to-left cardiac shunt, increased intracranial pressure, focal neurological signs, and characteristic laboratory findings (Adams and Victor, 1993). Neuroimaging with computed tomography (CT) or magnetic resonance imaging (MRI) will confirm the diagnosis. Medical management requires aggressive antibiotic therapy, although surgical intervention is occasionally necessary.

Subdural Empyema

Subdural empyema is an intracranial infection between the inner surface of the dura and the outer portion of the arachnoid that usually arises in the frontal or ethmoid sinuses. Less common sites of origin include the sphenoid and maxillary sinuses, the middle ear, and the mastoids. The infection usually enters the subdural space by direct extension through the bone and dura or by thrombophlebitis of the venous sinuses (Bahndari and Sarkari, 1970; Coonrod and Dans, 1972). Common causative organisms include streptococci, staphylococi, bacteroides, and pseudomonas (Coonrod and Dans, 1972).

Clinically, patients report a recent exacerbation of chronic sinusitis or mastoiditis with local pain and purulent discharge. Fever, meningismus, and increasingly severe head pain herald the intracranial infection. The headache is localized initially, then intensifies and generalizes; it is frequently associated with vomiting (McIntyre et al., 1991). Alterations in consciousness and focal neurological deficits follow in rapid succession. Unlike brain abscesses, fever and leukocytosis are always present (McIntyre et al., 1991; Hodges et al., 1986; Sellik, 1989).

The diagnosis is confirmed by CT or MRI. Treatment consists of surgical drainage and IV antibiotics. Subdural empyema is often misdiagnosed as cerebral abscess. This is a fatal error, for without appropriate therapy the majority of patients will die within 1 to 2 weeks (McIntyre et al., 1991; Hodges et al., 1986; Sellik, 1989).

Intracranial Thrombophlebitis

The dural sinuses drain the cerebral venous blood into the jugular veins. Thrombophlebitis of these large vessels may result from infections of the middle ear, mastoids, paranasal sinuses, or facial structures. Infections may occur through direct trauma to the large veins or dural sinuses, although this is less common (Heineman et al., 1970). Streptococci and staphylococci are the most commonly implicated organisms. Thrombosis of the lateral sinus usually follows chronic infections of the mastoid, middle ear, or petrous bone.

Clinically, earache or tenderness of the mastoid region is replaced by a severe, global headache, often associated with papilledema and high fever. With propagation of the infection, IX, X, and XII cranial neuropathies; seizures; and focal deficits become apparent. Cavernous sinus thrombophlebitis follows ethmoid, maxillary, or sphenoid sinusitis or may be precipitated by infections of the skin surrounding the eyes and nose. It is clinically characterized by severe headache and high fevers. Characteristic local effects, such as chemosis, proptosis, eyelid edema, and swelling of the forehead and nose, may be observed (Adams and Victor, 1993). Cranial neuropathies involving III, IV, VI, and V_1 may also occur. Headaches, papilledema, and other signs of increased intracranial pressure, along with unilateral seizures and hemiplegia that may alternate sides, are seen with thrombophlebitis of the superior longitudinal sinus (Heineman et al., 1970).

Acquired Immunodeficiency Syndrome

Headache may be part of the clinical picture in a number of AIDS-related conditions. Headache is a prominent complaint in acute HIV infection and may last from a few days to about 1 month. The headache is often associated with typical features of a viral illness, such as fever, sore throat, myalgias, and arthralgias. During this acute infection, headache and photophobia are reported by 60% to 100% of patients (Denning, 1988). Infection with HIV may also present as an acute aseptic meningitis, and headache is associated with CSF lymphocytic pleocytosis and increased protein. This aseptic meningitis can occur during seroconversion or throughout the course of the disease. It may present clinically either as recurrent bouts of headache with fever, nausea, and meningismus lasting less than 1 month or as a persistent, chronic headache with pleocytosis that may or may not have other associated features (Hollander and Stringari, 1987).

Encephalidites occur in AIDS as part of the acute infection or as a subacute or chronic encephalitis that is part of the AIDS dementia complex. Herpes simplex virus and cytomegalovirus encephalidites are also seen in the disorder.

Headaches are also common in the secondary infections that affect patients with AIDS. Cerebral toxoplasmosis occurs in approximately 13% of patients with AIDS (Navia et al., 1986). Headache is a common complaint; it usually develops at the same time as other neurological symptoms but may on occasion precede them by many weeks. The headache associated with toxoplasmosis is typically bilateral, severe, and constant and often awakens the patient from sleep. Headaches accompany the meningidites that complicate AIDS. Cryptococcal meningitis occurs in 5% to 10% of patients with AIDS (Weinke et al., 1989). Tuberculosis meningitis and syphilitic meningitis are also common in this population.

Lyme Disease

Lyme disease is caused by the spirochete *Borrelia burgdorferi* and is transmitted through the bite of a deer tick (Steere, 1989). During the acute phase of the illness, patients may develop the classic cutaneous manifestation, erythema migrans, during which time between 38% and 54% of patients report headache (Berger, 1989; Scelsa et al., 1995). Headache may also be seen in any of the four neurological forms of Lyme disease (Halperin et al., 1996). Early in the course of infection, lymphocytic meningitis is associated with a bilateral throbbing headache that may be accompanied by nausea and often resembles migraine. A similar type of headache is described in the encephalomyelitic form of Lyme, which affects about 0.1% of patients

(Halperin et al., 1996). Headache is not a common complaint with the peripheral neuropathy that may complicate the disorder, but it is often seen with the encephalopathic form (Halperin et al., 1996). Rarely, chronic headache may be the most prominent manifestation of Lyme disease and may mimic tension-type headaches (Halperin et al., 1996; Brinck et al., 1993).

In general, routine screening for Lyme disease is not recommended in patients presenting with headache (Silberstein et al., 1998). In patients with atypical headaches or in whom headaches are associated with other features of *Borrelia* infection, serological testing by enzyme-linked immunosorbent assay is appropriate. The suggested workup and treatment options have been published (Halperin et al., 1996).

Fungal Infections

Fungal infections are significantly less common than bacterial or viral agents but occur with an increased frequency in patients who are immunosuppressed. Fungal meningitis develops slowly, over several days or weeks, and is characterized by chronic headache and cranial nerve pareses. Fungal meningitis may be complicated by cerebral infarcts, microabscesses, and hydrocephalus. Patients are often afebrile. Common fungal infections include cryptococcus, candidiasis, aspergillosis, and coccidiomycosis. Mucormycosis occurs in patients with diabetic acidosis, those treated with corticosteroids or cytotoxic drugs, and drug addicts. The infection starts in the nasal turbinates and sinuses, spreads retro-orbitally, and then invades the brain, where it causes multiple hemorrhagic infarcts (Walsh et al., 1985).

Protozoan Infections

Cysticercosis is the larval stage of infection with the pork tapeworm, *Taenia solium*. This disorder is one of the most common causes of epilepsy in countries of South and Central America. It is now being encountered more frequently in the United States because of emigration from those regions. The illness most commonly presents with seizures and headache. Other neurological features depend on the location of cysts in the cortex, subarachnoid space, and ventricles. The diagnosis is made by visualizing the cysts radiographically by CT or MRI. Treatment with the antihelminthic agent praziquantel may initially worsen the neurological symptoms before benefits are noticed (Watt et al., 1986; Sotelo et al., 1984).

Although a number of infectious disorders are characterized by headache and other neurological signs and symptoms, in general, resolution of the headache is correlated with proper treatment of the underlying infection. Symptomatic treatment with analgesics with or without opioids may be required pending complete eradication of the infectious process. Persistent headache following successful treatment of the underlying disorder should prompt a search for potential residual complications, such as hydrocephalus, cerebral edema, or other causes of increased intracranial pressure.

METABOLIC DISORDERS

The IHS classification contains a number of subcategories pertaining to headaches associated with metabolic disorders. These criteria mandate signs, symptoms, or both of a metabolic disorder; confirmation by laboratory investigations; headache intensity, frequency, or both related to variations in metabolic disorder with a specified time lag; and headache disappearance within 7 days after normalization of the metabolic state. The IHS guidelines describe the criteria for headaches associated with hypoxia, hypercapnia, mixed hypoxia and hypercapnia, hypoglycemia, hemodialysis, and other metabolic disorders, such as hangover and fever-associated headaches.

Hypoxia

Headaches associated with hypoxia may be the result of diseases that induce a hypoxic state, such as pulmonary diseases, congestive heart failure, or anemia, or may result from a variety of environmental conditions, such as high altitude and decompression sickness. The IHS criteria for hypoxic headache state that the headache occurs within 24 hours after the acute onset of hypoxia with a partial pressure of arterial oxygen (PaO_2) of 70 mm Hg or less or in patients with chronic hypoxia with a PaO_2 persistently at or below 70 mm Hg. The mechanism by which hypoxia induces headache is not clear, but in experimental models, hypoxia is associated with extreme vasodilation with subsequent increases in cerebral blood flow (Wolff and Lennox, 1930; Kuschinsky, 1989).

The high-altitude headache syndrome is a well-described form of hypoxic headache. The syndrome usually appears at altitudes above 10,000 feet, especially in unacclimatized subjects; headaches are universally present above 12,000 feet (Meyer and Dalessio, 1993). High-altitude headache is usually manifested within 24 hours of a sudden ascent above 10,000 feet (Appenzeller, 1972). The headache is often bifrontal and throbbing and worsened by coughing, straining, exertion, head movements, and lying down (Appenzeller, 1972; Kassirer and Such, 1989). The headache may be unilateral in one-fourth of patients (Raskin, 1988). High-altitude headaches may be associated with nausea, vomiting, vertigo, visual impairment, facial flushing, cyanosis, and impaired judgement (Meyer and Dalessio, 1993; Appenzeller, 1972; Singh et al., 1969). The best treatment of the disorder is to have the patient descend to a lower altitude. Dexamethasone and acetazolamide have been used (Rock et al., 1987; Mountain, 1983).

Approximately 42% of patients with decompression sickness experience a high-altitude-like headache (Wirjosemito et al., 1989). Decompression sickness occurs following a sudden change in the pressure of ambient gases to which the patient has been acclimatized (Appenzeller, 1972). The disorder is caused by the formation of nitrogen bubbles, which subsequently lodge in the small blood vessels and fatty tissue (Appenzeller, 1972). Neurological manifestations of decompression sickness vary with the affected region of the brain and spinal cord and include visual disturbances, confusion, seizures, and focal motor and sensory deficits. Patients typically report a bilateral throbbing headache (Erde and Edmonds, 1975; Kidd and Elliott, 1975). Decompression sickness is seen in aviators during rapid climbs and divers who ascend too rapidly (Erde and Edmonds, 1975; Kidd and Elliott, 1975).

Intracranial vasodilation is believed to be the underlying cause of headaches that are associated with anemia associated with hypoxia. Headache is likely to follow anemia that results from rapid blood loss but may occur in chronic anemia if the hemoglobin level is below 7 g (Graham, 1959).

Hypercapnia

Plasma carbon dioxide levels above 50 mm Hg commonly induce headaches in affected individuals, presumably through cerebral vasodilation. The headaches associated with hypercapnia are typically throbbing and global and increase with increasing partial pressure of CO_2 (P_{CO_2}) levels. Treatment consists of correcting the underlying metabolic abnormality.

Hypoglycemia

Although it is well established that low serum glucose levels may trigger migraine in susceptible patients, hypoglycemia may also produce headaches in hypopituitarism, adrenocortical insufficiency, hypothyroidism, and liver disease (Appenzeller, 1972). Hypoglycemic headache occurs at blood glucose levels below 2.2 mmol/l (Headache Classification Committee of the International Headache Society, 1988). Hypoglycemic headaches often resemble migraine and may be associated with mild nausea; resolution following carbohydrate ingestion is typical.

Hemodialysis

Headache is a well-recognized complication of hemodialysis treatment (Bana et al., 1972). Diagnostic criteria require the headache to occur during the course of dialysis and resolve within 24 hours after dialysis has ended.

Additionally, the headache should occur during at least half of the treatments, at least three previous times. The headache can be prevented by changing the dialysis parameters.

Other Metabolic Conditions

Headaches may be experienced by patients suffering from other metabolic disorders. Headache often accompanies dehydration and metabolic abnormalities that are seen in association with prolonged diarrhea, vomiting, heat exhaustion, diuresis, and postoperative fistulas (Appenzeller, 1972). Headaches associated with fever, hangovers, and fasting may also fall into this category.

TOXIC HEADACHES

Toxins

A wide array of substances have long been known to be capable of inducing headaches. These substances include drugs, chemicals, gases, food products, and additives. One of the most widely studied of the toxic headaches is that produced by histamine injections. Wolff and Lennox (1930) as well as other investigators (Clark et al., 1936; Schumaker et al., 1940) found that histamine infusions would first cause precipitous dips in blood pressure accompanied by the acute onset of a severe, diffuse headache lasting 6 to 8 minutes. Later studies documented that histamine infusions produced intracranial vasodilation and that the painful sensations were carried by the trigeminal nerve (Meyer and Dalessio, 1993; Schumacher et al., 1940). The IHS classification includes toxic headaches under the section "headache associated with substances or their withdrawal." These criteria for substance-induced headaches maintain that the headache must occur within a specified period of time following ingestion of the substance, a certain minimum dose is required, the headache follows at least half of the exposures (and at least three times), and the headache resolves when the substance is eliminated or within a specified time period.

Drugs that are commonly implicated in producing headaches include atenolol, metoprolol, propranolol, nifedipine, verapamil, cimetidine, ranitidine, danazol, tamoxifen, beclomethasone, ethinylestradiol, isosorbide dinitrate, methylprednisolone, indomethacin, diclofenac, monocycline, tetracycline, and trimethoprim-sulfamethoxazole (Askmark et al., 1989; Atkins, 1986; Pereira Monteiro, 1993).

Nitrates and Nitrites

Munition workers often complained of a bilateral, throbbing, frontotemporal headache that began several minutes to hours after exposure to dynamite. These headaches were often preceded by diplopia or monocular loss of vision and were determined to be the result of exposure to nitroglycerine (Schwartz, 1946). Nitroglycerine preparations and amyl nitrate used in the pharmacological treatment for angina frequently induce headaches in patients without prior headache history (Shively and Riegel, 1991) and can induce migraine and cluster headaches in patients with a known predisposition.

The "hot-dog" headache syndrome consists of a bilateral, throbbing headache that is occasionally associated with facial flushing and occurs in susceptible individuals within minutes to hours after eating cured meats such as hot dogs, sausages, or bacon. The headache is caused by nitrates and nitrites added to the food to impart a red color (Henderson and Raskin, 1972).

Monosodium Glutamate

The artificial flavor enhancer monosodium glutamate (MSG) is regularly added to a variety of foods and has been identified as the culprit responsible for Chinese restaurant syndrome (Schaumburg et al., 1969). Approximately 30% of people experience this syndrome after eating Chinese food (Reif-Lehrer, 1977). The syndrome is characterized by a generalized throbbing headache that develops 20 to 25 minutes following the ingestion of food containing MSG and associated with face and chest tightness; a burning sensation of the chest, neck, or shoulders; dizziness; and abdominal discomfort (Reif-Lehrer, 1977). An oral dose of 3 g of MSG (the amount found in a bowl of wonton soup) can produce these symptoms.

Carbon Monoxide

Carbon monoxide is a colorless, odorless gas that causes a variety of clinical symptoms at different levels of exposure. At low-level exposure, people report a dull, generalized, and suboccipital headache. As the concentration of the gas increases, so does the intensity of the head pain. At higher concentrations, nausea, vomiting, confusion, and finally coma and death occur.

Faulty oil burners or gas cooking appliances in poorly ventilated spaces are common sources of poisoning. Slow leaks of carbon monoxide may produce low-level headaches in family members occupying the same dwelling.

Alcohol

Alcohol-containing beverages can induce headaches within 30 to 45 minutes after ingestion in susceptible individuals. The mechanisms by which alcohol induces headache are believed to be both disruption of cerebral autoregulation and decreased cerebral turnover of serotonin, rather than vasodilation (Atkins, 1986). Alcohol is also a well-known trigger of migraine and cluster headaches.

Aspartame

Aspartame is an artificial sweetener found in many diet soft drinks, prepared foods, and desserts. Headache is the most common consumer complaint related to the ingestion of aspartame-containing products. Approximately 8% of migraine sufferers report aspartame as a headache trigger (Lipton et al., 1989). Conflicting results were obtained in two placebo-controlled trials, however (Schiffman et al., 1987; Koehler and Glaros, 1988). Nonetheless, aspartame should be considered a potential headache trigger, especially in people predisposed to migraine.

REFERENCES

Adams, R.D. and M. Victor (eds.) (1993). *Principles of Neurology.* McGraw-Hill, New York.

Ahmed, S., R. Libman, K. Wesson, F. Ahmed, and K. Einberg. (2000). Guillain-Barré syndrome: An unusual presentation of West Nile virus infection. *Neurology* 55:144–146.

Appenzeller, O. (1972). Altitude headache. *Headache* 12:126–130.

Askmark, H., P.O. Lundberg, and S. Olsson (1989). Drug related headache. *Headache* 29:441.

Atkins, F.M. (1986). A critical evaluation of clinical trials in adverse reactions to food in adults. *J. Allergy Clin. Immunol.* 78:174–182.

Bahndari, Y.S. and N.B.S. Sarkari (1970). Subdural empyema: A review of 37 cases. *J. Neurosurg.* 32:35–38.

Baker, P., T. Price, and C.D. Allen (1981). Brainstem and cerebellar dysfunction with Legionnaires' disease. *J. Neurol. Neurosurg. Psychiatry* 44:1054–1055.

Bana, D.S., A.U. Yap, and J.R. Graham (1972). Headache during hemodialysis. *Headache* 112:1–14.

Beghi, E., A. Nicolosi, L.T. Kurland et al. (1984). Encephalitis and aseptic meningitis, Olmstead County, Minnesota, 1950–1981: 1. Epidemiology. *Ann. Neurol.* 16:283–294.

Benson, C.A., A.A. Harris, and S. Levin (1988). Acute bacterial meningitis: General aspects. In: *Handbook of Clinical Neurology: Microbial Disease* (P.J. Vinken, G.W. Bruyn, H.L. Klawans et al., eds.), p. 119. Elsevier, Amsterdam.

Berger, B.W. (1989). Cutaneous manifestations of Lyme borreliosis. *Rheum. Dis. Clin. North Am.* 15:635–647.

Bharrucha, N.E., S.K. Bhaba, and E.P. Bharucha (1991). Infections of the nervous system. B. Viral infections. In *Neurology in Clinical Practice* (W.G. Bradley, R.B. Daroff, G.M. Fenichel et al., eds.), pp. 1085–1097. Butterworth-Heinemann, Stoneham.

Brewer, N.S., C.S. MacCarty, and W.E. Wellman (1982). Brain abscess: A review of recent experience. *Ann. Intern. Med.* 39:56–64.

Brinck, T., K. Hansen, and J. Olesen (1993). Headache resembling tension-type headache as the single manifestation of Lyme neuroborreliosis. *Cephalalgia* 13:207–209.

Bross, J.P. and G. Gordon (1991). Nocardial meningitis: Case reports and review. *Rev. Infect. Dis.* 13:160–165.

Callea, L., H. Donati, L. Faggi et al. (1985). Pontomedullary encephalitis and basal meningitis due to Listeria monocytogenes: Report of a case. *Eur. Neurol.* 254:217–220.

Carpenter, R.R. and R.G. Petersdorf (1963). The clinical spectrum of bacterial meningitis. *Am. J. Med.* 33:262–175.

CDC. (1999). Outbreak of West Nile-like viral encephalitis—New York. *MMWR* 48:845–849.

Chatstrey, S., A.G. Pfleiderer, and D.A. Moffat (1991). Persisting incidence and mortality of sinogenic cerebral abscess: A continuing reflection of late clinical diagnosis. *J. R. Soc. Med.* 84:193–195.

Chun, C.H., J.D. Johnson, M. Hofstettler et al. (1986). Brain abscess: A study of 45 consecutive cases. *Medicine* 65:415–431.

Clark, D., H. Hough, and H.G. Wolff (1936). Experimental studies on headache: observations on headache produced by histamine. *Arch. Neurol. Psychiatry* 35:1054–1069.

Cleland, P.G., R.G. Lawande, G. Onyemelukwe et al. (1982). Chronic amebic meningoencephalitis. *Arch. Neurol.* 39:56–58.

Coonrod, J.D. and P.E. Dans (1972). Subdural empyema. *Am. J. Med.* 53:85–88.

Cunha, B.A. (1999). West Nile encephalitis. *Infect. Dis. Practice* 23:85–90.

Davis, L.E. (1987). Acute viral meningitis and encephalitis. In: *Infections of the Nervous System* (P.G.E. Kennedy and R.T. Johnson, eds.), pp. 155–176. Butterworths, London.

Davis, L.E. and L.C. McLaren (1983). Relapsing herpes simplex encephalitis following antiviral therapy. *Ann. Neurol.* 26:192–195.

De Marinis, M., A.A. Kurdi, and K.M.A. Welch (1993). Headache associated with intracranial infection. In: *The Headaches* (J. Olesen, P. Tfelt-Hansen, and K.M.A. Welch, eds.), pp. 697–704. Raven Press, New York.

Denning, D.W. (1988). The neurological features of acute HIV infection. *Biomed. Pharmacother.* 42:11–14.

Erde, A.E. and C. Edmonds (1975). Decompression sickness: A clinical series. *J. Occup. Med.* 17:324–328.

Ferry, P.C., J.L. Culbertson, J.A. Cooper et al. (1982). Sequelae of *Haemophilus influenzae* meningitis: Preliminary report of a long-term follow-up study. In: Haemophilus influenzae—*Epidemiology, Immunology and Prevention of Disease* (S.H. Sell and P.F. Wright, eds.), pp. 111–116. Elsevier, New York.

Fisher, R.S., A.W. Clark, J.S. Wolinsky et al. (1983). Post infectious leukoencephalitis complicating *Mycoplasma pneumoniae* infection. *Arch. Neurol.* 40:109–110.

Franke, E. (1987). The many causes of meningitis. *Postgrad. Med.* 82:175–188.

Gates, E.M., J.W. Kernohan, and W. Craig (1950). Metastatic brain abscess. *Medicine* 29:71–73.

Ghosh, S., M.J. Chandy, and J. Abraham (1990). Brain abscess and congenital heart disease. *J. Indian Med. Assoc.* 88:312–314.

Graham, J.R. (1959). Headache in systemic disease. In: *Headache: Diagnosis and Treatment* (A.P. Friedman and H.H. Merritt, eds.), pp. 133–136. F.A. Davis, Philadelphia. Chapter 7.

Halperin, J.J., E.L. Logigian, M.F. Finel et al. (1996). Practice parameters for the diagnosis of patients with nervous system Lyme borreliosis (Lyme disease). *Neurology 46*:619–627.

Harris, L.F., D.A. Maccubbin, J.N. Triplett et al. (1985). Brain abscess: Recent experience at a community hospital. *South. Med. J. 78*:704–707.

Headache Classification Committee of the International Headache Society (1988). Classification and diagnostic criteria for headache disorders, cranial neuralgias and facial pain. *Cephalalgia 8*:S1–S96.

Heineman, H.S., A.I. Braude, and J.L. Osterholm (1970). Intracranial suppurative disease. *JAMA 218*:1542–1546.

Henderson, W.R. and N.H. Raskin (1972). "Hotdog" headache: Individual susceptibility to nitrite. *Lancet 2*:1162–1163.

Hodges, J., P. Anslow, and G. Gillet (1986). Subdural empyema: Continuing diagnostic problems in the CT scan era. *Q. J. Med. 59*:387–393.

Hollander, H. and S. Stringari (1987). Human immunodeficiency virus–associated meningitis. Clinical course and correlations. *Am. J. Med. 83*:813–816.

Isenberg H. (1992). Bacterial meningitis: Signs and symptoms. *Antibiot. Chemother. 45*:79–95.

Johnson, R.T. (1982). *Viral Infections of the Nervous System*. Raven Press, New York.

Kaplan, K. (1985). Brain abscess. *Med. Clin. North Am. 69*:345–360.

Kassirer, M.R. and R.V. Such (1989). Persistent high-altitude headache and aguesia without anosomia. *Arch. Neurol. 46*:340–341.

Kennedy, P.G.E. (1988). A retrospective analysis of forty-six cases of herpes simplex encephalitis seen in Glasgow between 1962 and 1985. *Q. J. Med. 68*:533–540.

Kidd, D.J. and D.H. Elliott (1975). Decompression disorders in divers. In: *The Physiology of Medicine of Diving and Compressed Air Work* (P.B. Bennett and D.H. Elliott, eds.), pp. 471–495. Williams and Wilkins, Baltimore.

Koehler, S.M. and A. Glaros (1988). The effect of aspartame on migraine headache. *Headache 28*:10–13.

Kohler, J., T. Winkler, and A.K. Wakhloo (1991). Listeria brainstem encephalitis: Two own cases and a literature review. *Infection 19*:36–40.

Kulay, A., N. Ozatik, and I. Topea (1990). Otogenic intracranial abscesses. *Acta Neurochir. 107*:140–146.

Kuschinsky, W. (1989). Coupling of blood flow and metabolism in the brain—the classical view. In: *Neurotransmission and cerebrovascular function*, Vol. 2 (J. Seylaz and R. Sercombe, eds.), pp. 331–342. Elsevier, Amsterdam.

Lamonte, M., S.D. Silberstein, and J.F. Marcelis (1995). Headache associated with aseptic meningitis. *Headache 35*:520–526.

Lees, A.W. and W.F. Tyrrell (1978). Severe cerebral disturbance in Legionnaires' disease. *Lancet 2*:1131–1132.

Lepow, M.L., N. Coyne, L.B. Yhompson et al. (1962). The clinical, epidemiological, and laboratory investigation of aseptic meningitis during the four-year period, 1955–1958. II. The clinical disease and its sequelae. *N. Engl. J. Med. 266*:1188–1193.

Lipton, J.D. and R.W. Schafermeyer (1993). Evolving concepts in pediatric bacterial meningitis. Part I: Pathophysiology and diagnosis. *Ann. Emerg. Med. 22*:1602–1615.

Lipton, R.B., L.C. Newman, J.S. Cohen et al. (1989). Aspartame as a dietary trigger of headache. *Headache 29*:90–92.

McIntyre, P.B., P.S. Lavercombe, R.J. Kemp et al. (1991). Subdural and epidural empyema: Diagnostic and therapeutic problems. *Med. J. Aust. 154*:653–657.

Meyer, J.S. and D.J. Dalessio (1993). Headache associated with chemicals, toxins, systemic infections, and metabolic disorders (toxic vascular headache). In: *Wolff's Headache and Other Head Pain*, 6th ed. (D.J. Dalessio and S.D. Silberstein, eds.), pp. 209–234. Oxford University Press, New York.

Molavi, A. and M.J. Dinubile (1988). Brain abscess. In: *Handbook of Clinical Neurology: Microbial Disease* (P.J. Vinken, G.W. Bruyn, H.L. Klawans et al., eds.), pp. 143–166. Elsevier, Amsterdam.

Mountain, R.D. (1983). Treatment of acute mountain sickness [letter]. *JAMA 250*:1392.

Murphy, F.K., P. Mackowiak, and J. Luby (1979). Management of infections affecting the nervous system. In: *The Treatment of Neurological Diseases* (R.N. Rosenberg, ed.), pp. 249–376. Spectrum, New York.

Navia, B.A., C.K. Petito, J.W.M. Gold et al. (1986). Cerebral toxoplasmosis complicating the acquired immune deficiency syndrome: Clinical and neuropathological findings in 27 patients. *Ann. Neurol. 19*:224–228.

Nicolosi, A., W.A. Hauser, E. Beghi et al. (1986). Epidemiology of central nervous system infections in Olmstead County, Minnesota, 1950–1981. *J. Infect. Dis. 154*:399–408.

Nicolosi, A., M.A. Hauser, Musicco et al. (1991). Incidence and prognosis of brain abscess in a defined population: Olmsted County, Minnesota, 1935–1981. *Neuroepidemiology 10*:122–131.

Oliver, L.G. and A.L. Harwood-Nuss (1993). Bacterial meningitis in infants and children: A review. *J. Emerg. Med. 11*:555–564.

Pereira Monteiro, J.M. (1993). Headache associated with single use of substances. In: *The Headaches* (J. Olesen, P. Tfelt-Hansen, and K.M.A. Welch, eds.), pp. 715–720. Raven Press, New York.

Ponka, A. and T. Pettersson (1982). The incidence and aetiology of central nervous system infections in Helsinki in 1980. *Acta. Neurol. Scand.* 66:529–535.

Raskin, N.H. (1988). *Headache.* Churchill-Livingstone, New York.

Reif-Lehrer, L. (1977). A questionnaire study of the prevalence of Chinese restaurant syndrome. *Fed. Proc.* 36:1617–1623.

Rock, P.B., T.S. Johnson, A. Cymerman et al. (1987). Effect of dexamethasone on symptoms of acute mountain sickness at Pikes Peak, Colorado (4,300 m). *Aviat. Space Environ. Med.* 58: 668–672.

Scelsa, S.N., R.B. Lipton, H. Sander et al. (1995). Headache characteristics in hospitalized patients with Lyme disease. *Headache* 35:125–130.

Schaumburg, H.H., R. Byck, and R. Gerstl (1969). Monosodium L-glutamate: Its pharmacology and role in the Chinese restaurant syndrome. *Science 163*:826–828.

Schiffman, S.S., C.E. Buckley, H.A. Sampson et al. (1987). Aspartame and susceptibility to headache. *N. Engl. J. Med. 317*:1181–1185.

Schlech, W.F. (1992). The epidemiology of bacterial meningitis. *Antibiot. Chemother.* 45:517.

Schlech, W.F., J.I. Ward, J.D. Band et al. (1985). Bacterial meningitis in the United States, 1978 through 1981. *JAMA 253*:1749–1754.

Schumacher, G.A., B.S. Roy, and H.E. Woff (1940). Experimental studies on headache and its pain pathways. *Arch. Neurol. Psychiatry 44*: 701–717.

Schwartz, A.M. (1946). The cause, relief and prevention of headaches arising from contact with dynamite. *N. Engl. J. Med. 135*:541–544.

Seidel, J.S., P. Harmatz, G.S. Visvesvara et al. (1982). Successful treatment of primary amebic meningoencephalitis. *N. Engl. J. Med. 306*:346–348.

Sellik, J.A. (1989). Epidural abscess and subdural empyema. *J. Am. Osteopath. Assoc.* 89:806–810.

Shetty, K.R., C.L. Cilvo, B.D. Starr et al. (1980). Legionnaires' disease with profound cerebellar involvement. *Arch. Neurol.* 37:379–380.

Shively, M. and B. Riegel (1991). Effect of nitroglycerine ointment placement on headache and facial flushing in healthy subjects. *Int. J. Nurs. Stud.* 28:153–161.

Silberstein, S.D. (1992). Evaluation and emergency treatment of headache. *Headache 32*: 396–407.

Silberstein, S.D., R.B. Lipton, and P.J. Goadsby (1998). *Headache in Clinical Practice.* Isis Medical Media, Oxford.

Singh, I., P.K. Khanna, and M.C. Srivastava (1969). Acute mountain sickness. *N. Engl. J. Med. 280*:175–184.

Sotelo, J., F. Escobedo, J. Rodriquez-Carbajal et al. (1984). Therapy of parenchymal brain cysticercosis with praziquantel. *N. Engl. J. Med. 310*: 1001–1003.

Steere, A.C. (1989). Lyme disease. *N. Engl. J. Med. 321*:586–596.

Takahashi, M. (1992). Infections of the central nervous system. *Curr. Opin. Neurol. Neurosurg.* 5:849–853.

Tija, T.L., Y.K. Yeow, and C.B. Tan (1985). Cryptococcal meningitis. *J. Neurol. Neurosurg. Psychiatry 48*:853–858.

Tonjum, T., P. Nilsson, J.N. Bruun et al. (1983). The early phase of meningococcal disease. *NIPH Annu.* 6:175–181.

Walsh, T.J., D.B. Hier, and L.R. Caplan (1985). Fungal infections of the central nervous system: Comparative analysis of risk factors and clinical signs in 57 patients. *Neurology 35*:1654–1657.

Watt, G., G.W. Long, and C.P. Renoa (1986). Praziquantel in the treatment of cerebral schistosomiasis. *Lancet ii*:529–531.

Weinke, T., G. Rogler, C. Sixt et al. (1989). Cryptococcosis in AIDS patients: Observations concerning CNS involvement. *J. Neurol. 236*:38–42.

Whitley, R.J. (1988). The frustrations of treating herpes simplex virus infections of the central nervous system. *JAMA 259*:1067–1072.

Wirjosemito, S.A., J.E. Touhey, and W.T. Workman (1989). Type II altitude decompression sickness (DCS): Air force experience with 133 cases. *Aviat. Space Environ. Med. 60*:252–262.

Wolff, H.G. and W.G. Lennox (1930). Cerebral circulation: 12. The effect on pial vessels of variation in the oxygen and carbon dioxide content of the blood. *Arch. Neurol. Psychiatry 23*:1097.

Young, C.A., D.M. Humphrey, E.J. Ghadiali et al. (1992). Short-term memory impairment as a presentation of herpes simplex encephalitis. *Neurology 42*:260–261.

Yu, Y.L., Y.N. Lau, B. Woo et al. (1988). Cryptococcal infection of the nervous system. *Q. J. Med.* 66:87–96.

19

Disorders of the Neck: Cervicogenic Headache

JOHN G. EDMEADS

Cervicogenic headache is a headache caused by disease or dysfunction of structures in the neck. Congenital anomalies of the craniovertebral junction, such as basilar invagination, atlanto-axial dislocation, separate odontoid, and occipitalization of the atlas may cause cervicogenic headache. In McRae's (1969) series, occipital headache was the presenting symptom in 26% of cases, and it occurred whether or not there were associated neural abnormalities, such as hydrocephalus, Arnold-Chiari malformation, or syringomyelia. These headaches were characterized by bursting suboccipital or occipital pains. They were triggered by flexing the neck or bending forward and eased by recumbency; sometimes they were accompanied by vomiting. Treatment of the anomaly relieved the headaches. Acquired lesions of the craniovertebral junction, such as foramen magnum meningiomas, or infections may also be causes. Paget's disease of the skull and upper cervical spine may present with similar symptoms (McRae, 1969). Rheumatoid arthritis and ankylosing spondylitis of the upper cervical spine may cause it (Conlon et al., 1966). Dissection of the vertebral and internal carotid arteries (which occurs mainly in the upper cervical region) may be a cause (Fisher et al., 1987). The pain is typically anterior if carotid and posterior if vertebral.

These examples of cervicogenic headache are indisputable because (1) a pain-sensitive structure within the neck is involved by an identifiable lesion or dysfunction (Table 19–1) and (2) this identifiable lesion or dysfunction is so located in the neck that the pain it generates can be referred to the head.

How can pain originating in the neck be referred to the head so that it is perceived as headache? There are many pathways:

- The second cervical nerve root (C2) gives rise to the occipital nerves; a lesion or dysfunction involving a neck structure innervated by C2 or the occipital nerves may produce occipital head pain. This is a well-known and universally accepted pathway of cervicocranial pain referral.
- The first cervical sensory nerve root (C1) is believed to contribute little or nothing to the sensory innervation of the head (Warwick and Williams, 1973), but Kerr (1961) stimulated this root during posterior fossa surgery and produced pain in the region of the vertex.
- The spinal nucleus of the trigeminal nerve (nucleus trigeminalis caudalis) descends to the level of C3–C4 and is in anatomic and functional continuity with the dorsal gray columns of these spinal segments. Stimuli applied to the upper cervical nerve roots excite potentials in the trigeminal apparatus (Kerr and Olafson, 1961). It is widely accepted that this "convergence" is the

Table 19–1 Cervicogenic headache

Pain-sensitive structure	Disease or dysfunction
Vertebral column	
Apophyseal and other synovial joints	Rheumatoid arthritis, ankylosing spondylitis, osteoarthritis, trauma, subluxation
Annulus fibrosus of intervertebral discs	Disc herniation, inflammation, trauma
Spinal ligaments	Postural strain, trauma, inflammation
Periosteum of vertebral body	Infection, Paget's disease, tumor
Cervical muscles	Postural strain, trauma, inflammation
Cervical roots and nerves	Compression by lesion (disc, tumor), stretching with subluxation of joints, direct injury from trauma, inflammation (e.g., herpes zoster)
Vertebral and carotid arteries	Dissection, thrombosis

mechanism through which lesions or dysfunctions in neck structures innervated by one or more of the first three or four cervical nerve roots may produce frontal or temporal head pain.

Thus, if a patient with headache has an identifiable lesion or dysfunction in a structure of the neck innervated by one or more of the C1–C4 nerve roots and if there is no other demonstrable cause for the headache, the headache may be cervicogenic. The causal relationship is more definite if the headache has characteristic features, such as occipital location and precipitation by neck movements, that are known to be associated with a headache with a cervical origin.

The Headache Classification Committee of the International Headache Society (1988) promulgated the following diagnostic criteria for cervicogenic headache:

A. Pain localized to neck and occipital region, may project to forehead, orbital region, temples, vertex, or ears
B. Pain is precipitated or aggravated by special neck movements or sustained neck posture
C. At least one of the following:
  1. Resistance to or limitation of passive neck movements
  2. Changes in neck muscle contour, texture, tone, or response to active and passive stretching and contraction
  3. Abnormal tenderness of neck muscles
D. Radiological examination reveals at least one of the following:

1. Movement abnormalities in flexion/extension
2. Abnormal posture
3. Fractures, congenital abnormalities, bone tumors, rheumatoid arthritis, or other distinct pathology (not spondylosis or osteochondrosis)

The criteria do not insist that the lesion be located within the neural territory of C1–C4 that has been identified as capable physiologically of referring pain to the head; it only must be in the neck. They do demand a neuroimaging abnormality and do not accept either cervical spondylosis or osteochondrosis as that abnormality, presumably because these conditions are common incidental findings in asymptomatic people (McRae, 1960).

CERVICOGENIC HEADACHE: EXPANDING THE CONCEPT

Several authors have proposed that headaches can be caused by problems in the neck that are not readily demonstrable by conventional diagnostic measures or are not located in the upper four cervical segments or both. Among the earliest such proposals were the *posterior cervical sympathetic syndrome of Barré* (1926) and the closely related *migraine cervicale of Bärtschi-Rochaix* (1949). Barré (1926) postulated that cervical osteophytes irritated the sympathetic nerves around the vertebral artery (which are sometimes called the vertebral nerve but are actually a series of neural arcades formed by communications between the gray rami of the sympathetic trunk and the ventral rami of C3–C7), producing vasoconstriction and ischemia. This produced a syndrome of headache, neck discomfort, dizziness, visual blurring, and psychological disturbances. Bartschi-Rochaix (1949) postulated that cervical osteophytes compress the vertebral artery, producing very similar symptoms. In terms of Barré's hypothesis, Bogduk et al. (1981) showed that electrically stimulating the vertebral artery sympathetic plexus and associated neural elements in the monkey reduced vertebral blood flow by only a trifling amount; and in terms of Bartschi-Rochaix's theory, Lance (1993) points out that only a minority of vertebrobasilar transient ischemic attacks produced by neck twisting are associated with headache. These two syndromes are now regarded by most as obsolete concepts.

Still current is the controversy over whether *cervical disc disease (cervical spondylosis)* is a common cause of headache. The controversy can be encapsulated in two statements, both made by the same author:

- "Cervical spondylosis is a common and important cause of headache beginning in middle-life or later" (Brain, 1963).
- "Since cervical spondylosis is not uncommon after middle-life and may be symptomless, there is danger that the discovery on radiography of cervical spondylosis in a patient suffering from some other disorder may lead to mistaken attribution of the symptoms to cervical spondylosis" (Brain et al., 1952).

Cervical spondylosis mainly involves the C5–C6 and C6–C7 intervertebral discs, well below the neural level that theory dictates can refer pain to the head, and this is an argument against cervical disc disease causing headache. Countering this is the argument that restricted movement of the lower neck caused by disc disease may result in increased movement at the upper cervical joints, particularly the facet joints, thus establishing a potentially painful dysfunction well within the C1–C4 territory. Such facet dysfunction may be extremely difficult to demonstrate by either physical examination or radiography.

Some clinicians have found headache to be a major symptom of cervical spondylosis. Peterson et al. (1975) found that headache was the chief complaint in 40% of their patients with symptomatic cervical disc disease (brachialgia or myelopathy) and a major symptom in 25%. The headaches associated with cervical spondylosis are typically occipital [Brain (1963) stated that "headaches sparing the occiput are not likely to be due to cervical spondylosis"] and unilateral [Peterson et al. (1975) commented that "if the headache is unilateral the likelihood of an organic cause is quite high"]. The headaches may spread anteriorly. Initially intermittent, they may become constant. They are aggravated by neck movements and occasionally by coughing and straining. Ideally, resolution of the headache by effective treatment of the cervical spondylosis would be evidence favoring a causal relationship, but cervical spondylosis can be quite difficult to treat and often involves modalities such as non-steroidal anti-inflammatory drugs (NSAIDs), which, because they are useful for other types of headaches, confound the picture. There are two isolated case reports (Michler et al., 1991; Fredriksen et al., 1999) in which surgical release of a lower cervical nerve root (C7 and C6, respectively) compressed by a herniated disc relieved long-standing ipsilateral headache, but the paucity of such positive reports in the context of the large number of surgical procedures done for disc protrusion suggests caution in drawing generalizable conclusions from them.

Until more evidence accumulates, it seems prudent when dealing with a patient who has headache and cervical spondylosis to treat the disc disease on its own merits, resorting to surgery if the patient has intractable brachialgia and/or myelopathy and a disc protrusion has been conclusively demonstrated by neuroimaging to be compressing the appropriate nerve root or the spinal cord. If the headache disappears, that will be a bonus.

Third occipital headache, described by Bogduk and Marsland (1986), is an important concept because it emphasizes the role of local anesthetic nerve blockade in the diagnosis of this (and other) cervicogenic headache entities. Prompted by clinical reports of headache resulting from disease or dysfunction of the C2–C3 zygapophysial joints and relieved by surgically removing an osteophyte compressing the third occipital nerve or by anesthetic blockade of the joint, the authors undertook a systematic study of the utility of anesthetic blockade of the third occipital nerve in diagnosing headache arising from the C2–C3 apophyseal joint. This joint is suspected of producing cervicogenic headache for two reasons. First, it is biomechanically vulnerable because, as a transitional joint between the C1 and C2 vertebrae, which rotate the head, and the C3 to C7 vertebrae, which flex and extend the neck, it bears both vectors of stress. Second, the lower joints cannot (at least in theory) refer pain to the head.

The third occipital nerve is the superficial medial branch of the C3 dorsal ramus. In its course, it crosses the C2–C3 zygoapophysial joint, to which it supplies sensory innervation. Disease of this joint may also compress the nerve. The nerve then supplies a part of the semispinalis capitus muscle and the skin of the suboccipital region. The anatomy of the third occipital nerve is stereotyped, and fluoroscopic control allows precise blockade with local anesthetic, which can be verified by the production of sensory loss in the C3 dermatome.

Bogduk and Marsland (1986) studied the effects of blockade of this nerve in ten consecutive patients whose headaches had characteristics suggesting a cervical origin. All had unilateral or bilateral suboccipital or occipital headache with anterior radiation; nearly all had precipitation by neck movements. Half of the patients had tenderness over the C2–C3 zygapophysial joints, and some had restricted neck movements. Blockade of the third occipital nerve relieved headache in seven of ten patients, with relief that persisted for the anesthetic's expected duration of action and was reproduced by subsequent blocks. Blockade of other cervical nerves and roots in five of these seven patients failed to affect the headaches. Of the three who did not respond, all had bilateral headaches (these received bilateral blocks), two had throbbing headaches (the other eight did not), and one had nausea, vomiting, and photophobia (none of the oth-

ers did). The authors commented that two of the three "failures" might well have had migraine (which will be a recurring theme as the discussion of cervicogenic headache continues). None of these patients demonstrated pathological changes in the C2–C3 zygapophysial joints radiographically, but these joints are notoriously difficult to visualize adequately using conventional techniques.

Bogduk and Marsland's (1986) contribution exemplifies how careful clinical selection of patients can narrow the candidacy for diagnostic nerve blocks and how diagnostic nerve blocks may assist in establishing that some headaches originate in the neck. There is a theoretical objection to what seems the eminently sensible assumption that relief of pain by blocking a nerve means that the pain must be emanating from a structure innervated by that nerve. The theory of modulatory effect holds that because the neurons of a sensory nucleus (such as the nucleus caudalis trigeminalis) are excited to a critical firing frequency, not by nociceptive impulses alone but by the combination of nociceptive and other sensory impulses impinging on them from all sources, then anything (such as a local anesthetic block) that reduces these ancillary impulses from other sources may reduce the firing frequency of the neurons to a level below threshold and reduce or eliminate the pain output of the nucleus. A modulatory effect may account for the observations of Anthony (1985), who found that injecting lidocaine and methylprednisolone (Depomedrol) into the ipsilateral occipital nerve in patients with cluster headache (a condition not generally believed in any way to emanate from the C2 segment) relieved the headaches for a mean of 20 days in 18 of 20 patients. Some might argue, however, that it was the systemic absorption of the steroid that terminated the cluster headaches. Less confounded examples of possible modulatory effect are the series of Bovim and Sand (1992) and of Caputi and Firetto (1997). Bovim and Sand (1992) performed occipital nerve blocks on migraine patients, tension-type headache patients, and clinically diagnosed cervicogenic headache patients. While the occipital blocks relieved the headaches in most of the clinically diagnosed cervicogenic headache patients, they relieved frontal headaches in only one each of the migraine and tension-type headache patients; clearly, there was no discernible modulatory effect in most of these patients. However, in that same series, supraorbital nerve blockade relieved occipital headache in about half the cervicogenic headache patients, which suggests that some modulatory effect was occurring. Caputi and Firetto (1997) found that 23 of their 27 patients with intractable migraine responded to a course of multiple injections of the supraorbital and occipital nerves; the authors attributed the improvement to "extinguishing foci of nociceptor discharges thus re-establishing normal central neurone sensitivity," i.e., a modulatory effect.

A modulatory effect, so far, has been neither proven nor disproven. It remains a theoretical but discomfiting deterrent to full acceptance of the thesis that relieving a headache by blocking a cervical nerve or nerve root proves that its origin is in the neck.

SJAASTAD'S CERVICOGENIC HEADACHE

The emergence of cervicogenic headache from relative obscurity into the spotlight of controversy has been effected largely by Sjaastad and colleagues (1983; 1998), who attempted to, first, define the clinical characteristics and diagnostic criteria for this entity and, second, establish that it is an extremely common headache syndrome.

It is important to understand that Sjaastad and colleagues do not propose cervicogenic headache as a *morbus sui generis*, a specific disease entity with a single etiology. Instead, they view cervicogenic headache generically as a syndrome or as a "reaction pattern," in which headache is the main, or sometimes only, symptom of a variety of dysfunctions or diseases in the neck. They identify certain features of the headache and certain findings on examination of the neck that they believe indicate the cervical origin of the headache (diagnostic criteria), and they state, on the basis of having applied these criteria to large populations of headache patients, that cervi-

cogenic headache is a very common and frequently undiagnosed entity. Controversy centers about the validity of the diagnostic criteria, the reliability and specificity of the physical examination findings, and the conclusion that cervicogenic headaches are common.

In their original version (Sjaastad et al., 1983), the criteria for diagnosing cervicogenic headache were recurrent, long-lasting attacks of moderately severe unilateral headache, beginning occipitally and radiating forward, which did not shift sides between attacks. This was sometimes associated with phonophotophobia, nausea, vomiting, irritability, dizziness, visual blurring on the side of the head pain, lacrimation, and conjunctival injection. It occurred in patients with signs of neck involvement, such as provocation of headache attacks by neck movements or ipsilateral neck, shoulder, or arm pain. Sjaastad et al. (1983) stipulated that these headaches should not cluster in time so that confusion with cluster headaches could be avoided, and Pfaffenrath et al. (1987) suggested that in some cases indomethacin needed to be given to avoid confusion with hemicrania continua or chronic paroxysmal hemicrania. A more pressing consideration, which aroused some controversy (Sjaastad and Bovim, 1991) was the observation (Edmeads, 1988) that some people who met these criteria for cervicogenic headache also fit the diagnostic criteria for common migraine of Vahlquist (1955) and Bousser et al. (1986) and for migraine without aura of the IHS (Headache Classification Committee of the International Headache Society, 1988). [Migraine headache may begin posteriorly; about 16% of people with migraine exhibit no side-shift of their headaches between attacks (Ekbom, 1970; Leone et al., 1993); migraine has been described as being triggered by movements or sustained postures of the neck (Liveing, 1873; Blau, 1987); and nausea, vomiting, phonophotophobia, etc. are seen very commonly in migraine.] Subsequently, Sjaastad and colleagues have taken the criteria for the diagnosis of cervicogenic headache through a number of iterations, the most recent (Sjaastad et al., 1998) is as follows:

Major Criteria

I. Symptoms and signs of neck involvement
   a. Precipitation of the usual headache by neck movement, by sustained awkward head positioning, and/or by external pressure over the upper cervical or occipital region on the symptomatic side
   b. Restriction of the range of motion in the neck
   c. Ipsilateral neck, shoulder, or arm pain
II. Confirmatory evidence by diagnostic anesthetic blockades
III. Unilaterality of pain, without side shift

Other Criteria

IV. Head pain characteristics
   a. Moderate to severe, nonthrobbing, and nonlancinating pain, usually starting in the neck (eventually spreading forward on symptomatic side)
   b. Episodes of varying duration (usually a few days to a couple of weeks, sometimes only an hour or two, but most frequently longer than in migraine without aura; marked intraindividual variation is characteristic)
   c. Fluctuating, continuous pain (while pain episodes seem to be typical of the early phase, generally continuous pain will prevail)
V. Other characteristics of some importance
   a. Only marginal or no effect from indomethacin (a negative diagnostic trial is not a prerequisite for the diagnosis of cervicogenic headache, but "an absolute indomethacin effect would undo the diagnosis")
   b. Only marginal or no effect from ergotamine and sumatriptan (at the time of publication of this reference, sumatriptan was the only triptan in general use)
   c. Female
   d. Not infrequent history of head or indirect neck trauma, usually of more than only medium severity
VI. Other characteristics of lesser importance: various attack-related phenomena, only occasionally present, and/or only moderately expressed when present

   a. Nausea
   b. Phonophobia and photophobia
   c. Dizziness
   d. Ipsilateral blurred vision
   e. Difficulty swallowing
   f. Ipsilateral edema, mostly periocular

Sjaastad et al. (1998) indicate that in their system only the major criteria are necessary for the diagnosis of cervicogenic headache: i.e., symptoms and signs of neck involvement (Ia,b,c), confirmatory evidence by diagnostic anesthetic blockades (II), and unilateral head pain without side shift (III). Even within these major criteria, the authors establish a hierarchy of importance. In terms of "symptoms and signs of neck involvement," they accept precipitation of the usual head pain by neck movements, posturing, or pressure as the prime criterion, sufficing alone to establish the presence of neck involvement, whereas restricted neck movement or ipsilateral neck or arm pain is insufficient alone to establish this (though both of them together are "provisionally" sufficient, even in the absence of precipitation of headache by neck movements, posturing, or pressure). The authors also draw a distinction between what combination of criteria suffice for "scientific work" and which lesser combination will do for "practical clinical work." For example, "for routine work, patients with bilateral headache ('unilaterality on two sides') may be acceptable. If so, patients with bilateral and unilateral pain should be compared. Great caution should be exercised in order not to include tension headache patients in cervicogenic headache series."

In terms of blockades, the authors urge positive blockade effect as a mandatory component of scientific and, preferably, of routine diagnostic workup. They require that with blockade the pain be drastically reduced in areas not anesthetized; e.g., frontotemporal pain must be reduced by cervical nerve blocks.

These criteria are multiple, complex, and sometimes relativistic. They are important, however, in that they represent a conscientious attempt to bring order to a confused area.

How well have the various schemata of diagnostic criteria worked in identifying cervicogenic headaches? In a Scandinavian study of headache patients, Nilsson (1995a) found 17.8% with cervicogenic headaches, and in a similar German study, Pfaffenrath and Kaube (1990) found 13.8%. However, in the Italian series of D'Amico et al. (1994), cervicogenic headache accounted for only 0.7% of 440 consecutive headache clinic patients and for only 4% of 74 consecutive patients with long-lasting, side-locked, unilateral pain (85% of these 74 patients had migraine and 11% had tension-type headaches as diagnosed by the IHS criteria). All of these groups used iterations of the criteria of Sjaastad et al. for the diagnosis of cervicogenic headache.

PROBLEMS IN DIAGNOSING CERVICOGENIC HEADACHE

Why is there such variation in the diagnosis of cervicogenic headache? There are a number of problems.

First, no specific qualities conclusively identify a headache as cervicogenic to the exclusion of other entities, such as migraine without aura or tension-type headache. For example, unilateral, occipitally originating, side-locked headaches are characteristic of cervicogenic headache; but all of these features may occasionally be present in migraine or tension-type headaches. Precipitation of the headache by neck movements or sustained postures of the neck are again characteristic of cervicogenic headache but do occur (admittedly much less commonly) in migraine and tension-type headache. As these characteristics of the headache accumulate in an individual patient, the diagnosis of cervicogenic headache will become more likely and the diagnoses of migraine and tension-type headache less likely, particularly if that patient's headaches fail to meet the IHS diagnostic criteria for the latter entities. The process, however, is as yet strongly empirical; firm, validated criteria are still "a work in progress."

Second, the evidence of neck involvement may be equivocal. There is no consensus on what constitutes an adequate physical examination of the neck, on the techniques for performing these examinations, or on what

findings are significant. Pöllmann et al. (1997) point to the diversity of "manual diagnostic findings" in various series of patients with cervicogenic and other types of headache. Jaeger (1989) gave a detailed protocol for assessing head posture, position and tenderness of the transverse processes of the atlas, functional movement of the first two cervical joints, and range of movement of the neck in forward flexion, extension, lateral flexion, and rotation; she also outlined the examination for myofascial trigger points. Maigne (1996) noted that "the only spinal sign showing the cervical origin of a headache is tenderness to palpation of the C2–3 facet joint on the affected side . . . a possible decrease in active or passive mobility has no particular value; it certainly demonstrates the existence of a cervical problem, but it does not establish the cervical origin of the headache." Maigne (1996) described certain craniofacial signs that also indicate the cervical origin of a headache, including the "friction sign of the scalp" in occipital headache, the painful pinch-roll "angle-of-the-jaw sign" in occipitotemporomaxillary headache, and the painful pinch-roll "eyebrow sign" in supraorbital headache. Other authors describe other combinations (Pöllmann et al., 1997), but in all of these, the problems of interobserver reliability (does Dr. Jones note the same degree of movement restriction and the same number of tender myofascial nodules as Dr. Smith when they examine the same patient?) and of the significance of findings once elicited (is Mrs. Smith's limitation of neck movements the key to her headaches, or does it just reflect that she's tense or has a bit of cervical spondylosis?) remain to be sorted out. Nor do imaging procedures aid in diagnosing cervicogenic headaches, except in that small minority of cases where there are clear-cut, appropriately located abnormalities. Most radiological examinations are not very sensitive. In the series of clinically diagnosed cervicogenic headache patients studied by Pfaffenrath et al. (1987), conventional radiographs of the skull and cervical spine did not distinguish between headache patients and controls; only a complex computer-based technique was able to show differences in mobility. There are insufficient data at this time to evaluate the contribution of magnetic resonance imaging (MRI) to the diagnosis of cervicogenic headache. The role of local anesthetic nerve blocks in imputing a cervical origin to headaches has already been discussed. Bogduk et al. (1985) note of nerve blocks that "this . . . procedure is not generally available and it would be impractical to apply it to every patient with suspected cervical headache," but Bogduk (1984) points out that in individual cases, particularly when combined with selective percutaneous stimulation of the cervical nerves to reproduce symptoms, it can be decisive in diagnosing cervicogenic headaches and in establishing the neural topography of the lesion or dysfunction.

Third, the apparent lack of any etiology in the neck may impede the diagnosis of cervicogenic headache. Not infrequently a patient may have a headache with characteristics strongly suggestive of cervicogenic headache: there may be a little limitation of neck movement and perhaps some tenderness over the C2–C3 apophysial joint, and the headache may be temporarily relieved by a C3 block. However, the patient may have no history of head or neck injury, her x-rays may be normal, and there may be no clinical or laboratory evidence of any inflammatory or degenerative process. What is causing the cervical dysfunction? Should the failure to establish its etiology invalidate the diagnosis? In general, it probably should not, but many physicians find the apparent lack of etiology (and even more so the frequent facile attempts to provide an etiology, such as "she was in a minor rear-end collision 3 weeks before her headache came on") a deterrent to embracing the diagnosis.

PRACTICAL CRITERIA FOR DIAGNOSING CERVICOGENIC HEADACHE

Cervicogenic headaches exist; nobody doubts this when the headache is otherwise unexplainable and a lesion, such as a separate odontoid or ankylosing spondylitis, is there for all to see on x-ray. Disbelief sets in when one attempts to attribute a cervical origin to a headache where the physical findings of neck involvement are equivocal and imaging evidence of cervical disease is absent. Doubtless, many cases of true cervicogenic headache are lost to diagnosis because of this disbelief, and doubtless many cases of migraine and tension-type headache are misdiagnosed as cervicogenic headaches when disbelief is suspended.

Perhaps the clinical diagnosis of a cervicogenic headache should begin when a patient has a headache similar to those seen in cases with indisputable lesions in the upper neck; these features of the headache should include *all* of the following:

- It originates in the occipital region, and while it may spread forward, there always remains an occipital component.
- It begins as a unilateral occipital pain, and while with the passage of time it may uncommonly become bilateral, it never switches sides.
- It may present initially as short episodes but evolve into long-continued and sometimes constant headache.
- It is triggered or conspicuously aggravated by specific neck movements and/or postures and by nothing else (except sometimes coughing, sneezing, and/or straining).
- It does not fulfil the IHS criteria for migraine or for any other type of headache.

With consideration of cervicogenic headache initiated by the characteristics of the headache, physical examination seeks to shore up the evolving diagnosis by eliciting some of the following signs of disease or dysfunction in the upper neck:

- Reproduction of the headache, consistently, by a specific passive movement of the neck or by pressure on a specific structure in the upper neck is a physical sign powerfully persuasive of cervicogenic headache.
- Persistent head tilt, limitation of rotation of head on neck (especially if painful), and abnormal mobility of the upper cervical spine in flexion or extension suggest the presence of a craniocervical lesion that could gen-

erate headaches (as do the findings of lower cranial nerve and/or cervical spinal cord deficits).

- Tenderness to deep pressure over the C2–C3 facet joint on the side of the headache, and nowhere else, suggests the presence of an arthropathy that could be generating headache.

There are some physical signs, adduced as evidence favoring a diagnosis of cervicogenic headache, which probably are not very dependable:

- Tenderness anywhere else in the neck, including the suboccipital triangle, is seen so frequently in other types of headache, including migraine and tension-type headache, that it is not a useful sign of cervicogenic headache.
- Similarly, limitation of movement of the lower cervical spine, whether painful or not, is so ubiquitous in and beyond middle age that it is valueless in diagnosing cervicogenic headache.
- Trigger points, nodules, and "pinch-and-roll" signs (Maigne, 1996) are highly subjective. Some clinicians find them in every patient; others have never elicited them. Until the former become more critical or the latter more adept, these signs are best not depended upon to make a diagnosis of cervicogenic headache.

At this point, with a headache description in hand that is strongly suggestive of cervicogenic headache and possibly some corroborative physical signs (but sometimes not), the clinician usually arranges for x-rays of the cervical spine, including the craniovertebral junction. Even with excellent radiographic technique and skilled radiological interpretation, these tests are seldom helpful in either establishing or excluding a cervicogenic basis for the headaches; nevertheless, they should be done because occasionally they show a lesion, or hypermobility or hypomobility, in spinal segments that could refer pain to the head. When suspicion is quite strong, recourse should be had to MRI or computerized tomographic (CT) imaging. When neuroimaging fails to show any relevant dysfunc-

tion or disease, local anesthetic blockade may be able to establish or exclude the cervicogenic basis of the headache and give a clue as to the segmental location of the problem. Certain caveats are crucial:

- The blockade should be of one particular nerve or nerve root, and it should relieve all aspects of the headache (i.e., if there is a frontal or temporal component of the headache, it must be relieved by the cervical block). While simultaneous blockade of multiple nerves and/or roots may relieve the headache, it is valueless in establishing the origin of the headache.
- There should be an "internal control" of the successful injection; i.e., another nerve or root should be blocked on a subsequent occasion, and this should not relieve the headache.
- The duration of relief from headache should approximate the duration of action of the local anesthetic used.

TREATMENT

The usual failure to demonstrate conclusively a specific disease or dysfunction of the neck is a powerful impediment to specific treatment for the patient believed, clinically, to have cervicogenic headache. What is the appropriate treatment when one knows only approximately where the trouble is and not what the trouble is?

Nevertheless, a number of treatments have been advocated:

- In *mobilization*, a joint or group of joints is taken passively to the limit of the usual physiological range of movement and then returned to the starting point, with this maneuver typically repeated; there is no "thrust." In *manipulation*, after the limit of the usual physiological range of movement has been attained, a thrust is administered to take the range slightly beyond the usual, typically with the accompaniment of a "cracking" noise. Where there is a suspicion that a particular facet joint in the neck is causing the headache, there are specific techniques for mobilizing or manipulating only that joint. Pöllmann et al. (1997) have summarized the published experience with manual therapy in various headache groups. Of the four studies cited that appeared to deal with patients with cervicogenic headache, two were uncontrolled; in one of the controlled studies, cervical manipulation gave relief, but so did deep massage and laser therapy; in the other controlled study, manual therapy was better than no therapy. In a general review, Vernon (1995) pointed to the methodological faults that almost always invest such studies. Cervical manipulation may cause stroke from dissection of vertebral or carotid arteries (Gotlib and Thiel, 1985). Though this is a rare complication, it gives pause when considering the employment of these essentially unproven techniques in conditions with essentially unproven etiology.

- *Massage, deep heat, and other physical methods* have the dual advantages of being harmless and giving comfort. In one study (Nilsson, 1995b), massage was as efficacious as manipulation.

- The idea that most cases of cervicogenic headache are due to mobility disturbances (too much or not enough) in the cervical spine and/or to fibromuscular dysfunction has tended to discourage *pharmacotherapy*, and no controlled studies have been published on the systematic use of medications. Frequently, NSAIDs are used, and the impression is that sometimes they bring partial and short-term relief of headaches.

- Though expertly administered *local anesthetic blocks* applied in a rational fashion can be of considerable diagnostic utility, their value as treatment for cervicogenic headache is much less clear. Controlled studies are difficult; placebo injections and control injections of inappropriate nerves or roots are ethically problematic. Depending on one's concept as to what the process is, the targets for injection in various studies range from nerves and roots through facet joints to "fibrositic nodules." In most studies, there are a few individuals with relief of symptoms that dramatically outlasts the expected duration of activity of the an-

esthetic used, but long-term relief is uncommon (Pöllmann et al., 1997). The addition of corticosteroid to the injection mix, usually outside of the context of a controlled study, further complicates the interpretation of results.

- Multiple surgical procedures have been employed for the treatment of cervicogenic headache. Sometimes the surgery is directed to the perceived lesion, e.g., fusion of cervical joints where hypermobility is believed to be etiological. More often, the surgery is aimed at interrupting pain pathways by section of nerves or roots. Most of the series are small, the diagnoses are often uncertain, and controls and long-term follow-up data are sparse. The conclusions of Pöllmann et al. (1997) seem reasonable: "until controlled studies on large and homogeneous groups of patients are performed, operative intervention cannot be recommended for cervicogenic headache."

CONCLUSIONS

Cervicogenic headache exists. Lesions in the neck can produce headache as their sole or major manifestation. What is unclear and controversial is this: in those with chronic posterior headaches triggered or exacerbated by neck movements and associated with only nonspecific and unconvincing evidence of disease or dysfunction of the neck, is the neck the cause of the headaches or just a bystander? Are cervicogenic headaches rare, and are most of the patients now diagnosed as having this condition simply people with stiff necks who have migraine or tension-type headache? Or are cervicogenic headaches common but underdiagnosed? Investigators are struggling to clarify this issue. Until they do, clinicians walk the line between intellectual rigidity and credulity, trying not to confuse an open mind with an empty head.

REFERENCES

Anthony, M. (1985). Arrest of attacks of cluster headache by local steroid injection of the occipital nerve. In: *Migraine: Clinical and Research Advances* (F. Rose, ed.), pp. 169–173. Karger, Basel.

Barré, J. (1926). Sur une syndrome sympathique cervical postérieur et sa cause fréquente, l'arthrite cervicale. *Rev. Neurol.* 33:1246–1248.

Bärtschi-Rochaix, W. (1949). *Migraine Cervicale: Das encephale Syndrom nach Halswirbeltrauma.* Medizinischer Verlag Hans Huber, Bern.

Blau, J. (1987). A clinicotherapeutic approach to migraine. In: *Migraine: Clinical, Therapeutic, Conceptual and Research Aspects* (J. Blau, ed.), p. 194. Chapman and Hall, London.

Bogduk, N. (1984). Headaches and the cervical spine. An editorial. *Cephalalgia* 4:7–8.

Bogduk, N., B. Corrigan, P. Kelly et al. (1985). Cervical headache. *Med. J. Aust.* 143:202–207.

Bogduk, N., G. Lambert, and J.W. Duckworth (1981). The anatomy and physiology of the vertebral nerve in relation to cervical migraine. *Cephalalgia* 1:11–24.

Bogduk, N. and O. Marsland (1986). On the concept of third occipital headache. *J. Neurol. Neurosurg. Psychiatry* 49:775–780.

Bousser, M., J. Elghozi, D. Lande et al. (1986). Urinary 5-HIAA is lowered in young adult female patients outside attacks. *Cephalalgia* 6:205–209.

Bovim, G. and T. Sand (1992). Cervicogenic headache, migraine without aura and tension-type headache. Diagnostic blockade of greater occipital and supraorbital nerves. *Spine* 51:43–48.

Brain, W. (1963). Some unsolved problems of cervical spondylosis. *BMJ* 1:771–777.

Brain, W., D. Northfield, and M. Wilkinson (1952). The neurological manifestations of cervical spondylosis. *Brain* 75:187–225.

Caputi, C. and V. Firetto (1997). Therapeutic blockade of greater occipital and supraorbital nerves in migraine patients. *Headache* 37:174–179.

Conlon, P., I. Isdale, and B. Rose (1966). Rheumatoid arthritis of the cervical spine: An analysis of 333 cases. *Ann. Rheum. Dis.* 25:120–126.

D'Amico, D., M. Leone, and G. Bussoni (1994). Side-locked unilaterality and pain localization in long-lasting headaches: Migraine, tension-type headache, and cervicogenic headache. *Headache* 34:526–530.

Edmeads, J.G. (1988). The cervical spine and headache. *Neurology* 38:1874–1878.

Ekbom, K. (1970). A clinical comparison of cluster headache and migraine. *Acta Neurol. Scand.* 46:1–48.

Fisher, C.M., R.G. Ojemann, and G. Robertson (1987). Spontaneous dissection of cervicocerebral arteries. *Can. J. Neurol. Sci.* 5:9–19.

Fredriksen, T., R. Salvesen, A. Stolt-Nielsen et al. (1999). Cervicogenic headache: Long term postoperative follow-up. *Cephalalgia* 19:897–900.

Gotlib, A. and H. Thiel (1985). A selected annotated bibliography of the core biomedical literature pertaining to stroke, cervical spine manipulation, and head-neck movement. *J. Can. Chiropract. Assoc.* 29:80–89.

Headache Classification Committee of the International Headache Society (1988). Classification and diagnostic criteria for headache disorders, cranial neuralgias and facial pain. *Cephalalgia* 8:1–96.

Jaeger, B. (1989). Are "cervicogenic" headaches due to myofascial pain and cervical spine dysfunction? *Cephalalgia* 9:157–164.

Kerr, F. (1961). A mechanism to account for frontal headache in cases of posterior fossa tumors. *J. Neurosurg.* 18:605–609.

Kerr, F. and R. Olafson (1961). Trigeminal and cervical volleys. *Arch. Neurol.* 5:171–178.

Lance, J. (1993). *Mechanism and Management of Headache.* Butterworth-Heineman, Oxford.

Leone, M., D. D'Amico, F. Frediani et al. (1993). Clinical considerations on side-locked unilaterality in long-lasting primary headaches. *Headache* 33:381–384.

Liveing, E. (1873). *On Megrim, Sick-Headache, and Some Allied Disorders: A Contribution to the Pathology of Nerve-Storms.* J & A Churchill, London.

Maigne, R. (1996). *Diagnosis and Treatment of Pain of Vertebral Origin.* Williams and Wilkins, Baltimore.

McRae, D. (1960). The significance of abnormalities of the cervical spine. Caldwell Lecture 1959. AJR Am. J. Roentgenol. 84:1–25.

McRae, D.L. (1969). Bony abnormalities at the craniospinal junction. *Clin. Neurosurg.* 16:356–375.

Michler, R.-P., G. Bovim, and O. Sjaastad (1991). Disorders in the lower cervical spine. A cause of unilateral headache? A case report. *Headache* 31:550–551.

Nilsson, N. (1995a). The prevalence of cervicogenic headache in a random population sample of 20–59 year olds. *Spine* 20:1884–1888.

Nilsson, N. (1995b). A randomized controlled trial of the effect of spinal manipulation in the treatment of cervicogenic headache. *J. Manipulative Physiol. Ther.* 18:435–440.

Peterson, D., G. Austin, and L. Dayes (1975). Headache associated with discogenic disease of the cervical spine. *Bull. L. A. Neurol. Soc. 40:* 96–100.

Pfaffenrath, V., R. Dandekar, and W. Pöllmann (1987). Cervicogenic headache—the clinical picture, radiological findings and hypotheses on its pathophysiology. *Headache* 27:495–499.

Pfaffenrath, V. and H. Kaube (1990). Diagnostics of cervicogenic headache. *Funct. Neurol.* 5:159–164.

Pöllmann, W., M. Keidel, and V. Pfaffenrath (1997). Headache and the cervical spine—a critical review. *Cephalalgia* 17:801–816.

Sjaastad, O. and G. Bovim (1991). Cervicogenic headache: The differentiation from common migraine. An overview. *Funct. Neurol.* 6:93–100.

Sjaastad, O., T. Fredricksen, and V. Pfaffenrath (1998). Cervicogenic headache; diagnostic criteria. *Headache* 38:442–445.

Sjaastad, O., C. Saunte, H. Hovdal et al. (1983). Cervicogenic headache: An hypothesis. *Cephalalgia* 3:249–256.

Vahlquist, B. (1955). Migraine. *Int. Arch. Allergy Appl. Immunol.* 7:348–355.

Vernon, H. (1995). The effectiveness of chiropractic manipulation in the treatment of headache: An exploration in the literature. *J. Manipulative Physiol. Ther.* 18:611–617.

Warwick, R. and P. Williams (1973). *Gray's Anatomy.* Longman, Edinburgh.

20

Disorders of the Eye

TIMOTHY J. MARTIN
JAMES J. CORBETT

Many patients with headache blame their eyes, given the ubiquitous belief that headaches are often the result of eye disease or the wrong glasses. In reality, the eyes are rarely the cause of common headaches (Martin and Soyka, 1993; Tomsak, 1991; Carlow, 1987; Romano, 1975; Waters, 1970; Newman and Burde, 1979).

In patients in whom eye disease is the cause of pain, the location and character of the pain, associated symptoms, and ocular signs are usually evident to the careful observer. Conjunctival injection, corneal edema, abnormal pupils, and decreased vision are hallmarks of such disorders (Behrens, 1978), and even the non-ophthalmologist should be able to readily identify and interpret these signs.

A thorough examination of the eyes and visual system may uncover important clinical clues about headaches that are primarily nonocular in origin but have prominent ocular signs, such as papilledema in idiopathic intracranial hypertension or homonymous visual field loss in stroke. In other circumstances, pain may be referred to the eyes from intracranial, dental, ear, throat, vascular, or sinus disease (Troost, 1998). Thus, the non-ophthalmologist investigating headache must become familiar with at least a basic examination of the eye and visual system (Table 20–1). On the other hand, ophthalmologists should have a systematic approach to evaluating patients with headache and a working knowledge of common (nonocular) headache syndromes so that appropriate referrals can be made (Gordon, 1966).

ASTHENOPIA

Asthenopia literally means "weak vision" but is frequently used to describe so-called eye-strain headaches that are thought to be the result of uncorrected (or improperly corrected) refractive errors or ocular misalignment. Afflicted patients describe a mild, bilateral, persistent brow ache that occurs when they must "strain" to clear a blurred (or possibly diplopic) image, especially with near tasks (Cameron, 1976; Romano, 1975). Such headaches are associated with extended and persistent close visual tasks and do not occur instantaneously with a visual challenge (Vincent et al., 1989).

Eye-strain headaches have been blamed on refractive errors (hyperopia, myopia, presbyopia) (Daum et al., 1988) and motility disorders (convergence insufficiency and other ocular misalignments). Of these, only uncorrected hyperopia (far-sightedness) and convergence insufficiency are likely to cause any significant degree of ocular or cranial discomfort.

Table 20–1 Eye examination (for the nonophthalmologist)

Evaluate *afferent* visual function
   Measure Snellen visual acuity in best correction (or
     with pinhole)
   Look for a relative afferent pupillary defect
   Perform confrontation visual fields
Evaluate *efferent* visual function
   Eyelids: look for ptosis, lid retraction
   Pupils: observe light reaction, anisocoria
   Ocular motility: observe ocular versions
Observe the structure of the eye and face
   Examine the conjunctiva, corneal reflex, and anterior
     segment with penlight
   Evaluate the red reflex and fundus with
     ophthalmoscope

Refractive Errors

To understand how refractive errors can cause eye strain, we present a brief (and simplified) review of the physiology of accommodation (or near-focusing). The ciliary muscle changes the shape of the lens to allow the eye to change its plane of focus. This muscle encircles and suspends the lens by numerous fibrous zonules that travel in a radial fashion from the ciliary body to the lens capsule (Fig. 20–1). When the ciliary muscle is relaxed, the zonules are tight and the lens is in its thinnest configuration, focusing distant light rays on

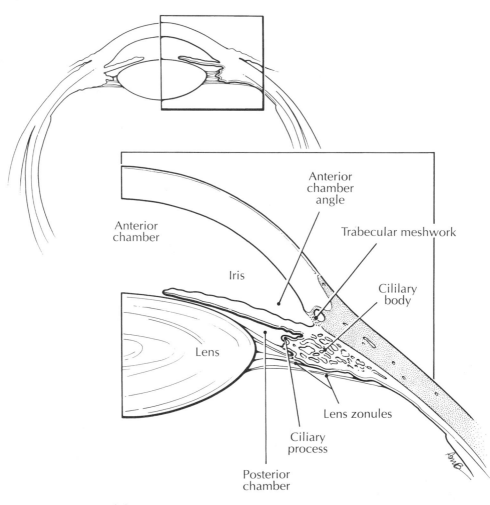

Figure 20–1 Anatomy of the anterior segment. This diagram illustrates cross section of the anterior segment. Observe how the lens zonules suspend the lens. Also note the normal path of aqueous humor: from the ciliary body, through the pupil, into the anterior chamber, into the anterior chamber angle, exiting through the trabecular meshwork. Courtesy of Martin, T.J. and D. Soyka (1993). Ocular causes of headache. In: *The Headaches* (J. Olesen, P. Tfelt-Hansen, and K.M.A. Welch, eds.), p. 748. Raven Press, New York.

the retina. To focus at near, the ciliary muscle contracts, reducing the diameter of its ring-like shape, which loosens the zonules and allows the lens to become more biconvex (fatter). This shape bends the light rays more strongly, allowing one to focus on a close-up object. Thus, individuals who are perfect *emmetropes* (i.e., have no refractive error) are able to relax their ciliary muscle most of the time (distant focus) and activate it only for near tasks.

Individuals who are *hyperopic* (far-sighted) do not have sufficient refractive power in a relaxed state to focus light rays from any plane, due to an eyeball that is too short relative to its optical power. When uncorrected, these subjects must keep their ciliary muscle "turned on" at all times to see clearly, even with distant focus. Attempts to focus at near require enormous effort. This requirement for constant contraction of the ciliary muscle can cause the "asthenopic" brow and eye ache, which intensifies with efforts to focus on near objects. It is not entirely clear whether the resulting asthenopic discomfort is due to fatigue of the ciliary muscles, traction on the scleral spur, or the action of accessory facial muscles (Cameron, 1976). Interestingly, hyperopic children do not usually experience this fatigue because their accommodative reserve is so great. Patients may not become symptomatic until they are in their thirties, when waning accommodative reserve creates eye fatigue and blur and their latent hyperopia is discovered by the eye doctor. Brow ache and frontal headache disappear when the hyperopia is corrected with glasses. Occasionally, overcorrected myopic individuals (see below) experience similar symptoms because their (too strong) glasses make them hyperopic.

Subjects with *myopia* (near-sightedness) have an eyeball that is too long for the amount of focusing power in the cornea and lens. These individuals can focus clearly at near with little or no contraction of the ciliary muscle but have blurry distant vision. Uncorrected myopes do not have problems with ciliary muscle overuse, but they may develop orbicularis muscle fatigue and discomfort from constant squinting.

Astigmatism refers to refractive errors that are not spherically uniform, but differ along a given meridian. Astigmatism can be the result of nonuniformity of the cornea or the lens. The word must sound intimidating as many patients ascribe all sorts of ills (including headache) to the discovery of their astigmatism. In truth, some degree of astigmatism is present in virtually everyone, and even a great amount of astigmatism (corrected, uncorrected, or improperly corrected) is not likely to cause significant headache. In a similar manner, *anisometropia* (a marked difference in the power of the lenses between the two eyes) is not likely to induce headaches.

The relative frequency of eye strain–induced headache was explored by Cameron (1976), who reviewed 50 patients referred to his ophthalmology practice with a chief complaint of headache. Only five patients had symptoms that could be attributed to visual effort and eye strain, and two of these five patients had relief of their discomfort after their refractive error was corrected.

Patients with headaches should have the benefit of a proper refraction, but corrective measures are unlikely to have a significant effect on most common headaches.

Presbyopia

As mentioned, accommodative amplitude declines steadily with age. This means that even emmetropic individuals will eventually need reading glasses to help them focus at near. However, this process of presbyopia is not a significant cause of ocular discomfort or headache. Cameron (1976) noted that only 6 of 50 patients with the onset of presbyopia described headache with near tasks and, of these, three improved with bifocals or reading glasses. Occasionally, medications with anticholinergic effects induce a pharmacologic pseudopresbyopia, but this tends to cause only symptoms of blurred vision, not pain.

Convergence Abnormalities

Three physiologic events occur when attention is directed from a distant to a near object, constituting the near synkinetic triad: (1) accommodation, (2) convergence, and (3) miosis. *Accommodation* results in an increase in the optical power of the eye, providing a clear image of a near object on the retina. *Convergence* is the inward movement of each eye, realigning the optical axis of the eyes from a parallel state (when focused at distance) to where the optical axis of each eye now intersects at the near object of regard. The pupil becomes more *miotic* (constricts), which also optically optimizes near focus. Abnormalities in this link between convergence and accommodative mechanisms are frequently implicated as a cause of eye pain and headache.

When *convergence insufficiency* is present, there is too little convergence for the required amount of accommodation; therefore, patients are exophoric or intermittently exotropic at near. Extra effort is required to maintain single binocular vision at near, which can cause fatigue and asthenopic symptoms or diplopia with extended near tasks (Mahto, 1972). Medications, head injuries, and some neurologic syndromes (such as Parkinson's disease) are associated with convergence insufficiency; but this condition is very common in the normal population as well. It is one of the few disorders of ocular alignment that may actually improve with ocular exercises to increase convergence strength. Although brow ache and ocular discomfort can occur as a result of convergence insufficiency, these symptoms occur only after a reasonable amount of near effort. Headache or ocular discomfort that occurs instantly upon glancing at a word on a page is nonphysiologic.

Convergence spasm is actually a spasm of the near synkinetic triad, with blurred vision from excessive accommodation, miotic pupils, and esotropia from excessive convergence. This uncomfortable condition occurs most often in young, anxious, but otherwise healthy students. It is usually transient and is more likely to occur in undercorrected hyperopes or overcorrected myopes. In isolation, convergence spasm is not usually associated with systemic diseases (and may be "functional" or deliberate), but it may also be one component of dorsal midbrain syndrome (in which case

the pupils are usually large) or other neurologic disorders. Convergence spasm can be distinguished from bilateral sixth nerve palsies by the presence of miotic pupils (as part of the synkinetic near reflex).

Strabismus

The diplopia that results from acquired cranial nerve palsies or orbital disorders does not generally cause headache, but the underlying condition may cause pain (such as orbital inflammatory pseudotumor). Small ocular deviations, especially those in which a patient can fuse with effort or with an abnormal head posture, may be associated with asthenopic symptoms. In one study, normal subjects who wore prisms to simulate an ocular muscle imbalance complained of brow ache and irritability (Eckhardt et al., 1943). In addition, chronic head positioning (like the head tilt in superior oblique palsies) can cause neck pain. Large deviations, in which fusion is not possible, are far less likely to cause headache or ocular pain. However, if patients have to keep one eye habitually closed to avoid diplopia, overworking the orbicularis can cause a tension-type headache. The use of an occluder (opaque plastic that clips onto one lens in the patient's glasses) can be a great relief when this situation occurs.

EYE DISEASES THAT CAUSE PAIN

Pain from eye diseases is usually localized to the offending eye. However, pain from an ocular source can be referred to any of the areas served by the ophthalmic division of the trigeminal nerve, such as the face (frontal sinuses, nasal cavity) or head (anterior meninges). In addition, tension-type headache may accompany eye pain.

Glaucoma

Glaucoma is not a single disease but a classification that includes many different disorders that usually (but not always) have three things in common: (1) elevated intraocular pressure, (2) optic nerve damage manifest as an enlarged central cup (optic disc cupping), and (3) optic disc–related visual field defects (usually peripheral). Eye pain is actually an uncommon symptom in most forms of glaucoma (Sherwood et al., 1988). However, many physicians are quick to associate glaucoma with pain because of the severe pain that occurs in a relatively uncommon (but memorable) form of glaucoma: acute angle-closure glaucoma.

The mechanism of intraocular pressure elevation is almost always decreased absorption of aqueous humor, rather than overproduction. The aqueous humor is produced by the ciliary body. This highly vascular structure is part of the *uvea* (the pigmented parts of the eye), contiguous with the choroid posteriorly and the iris anteriorly. The aqueous flows from the ciliary body (behind the iris) through the pupil into the anterior chamber and is absorbed at the trabecular meshwork located in the anterior chamber angle (Fig. 20–1). The glaucomas can be divided into those that mechanically block the flow of aqueous into the angle and trabecular meshwork (*angle-closure glaucoma*) and those that occur despite free access of aqueous to the angle (*open angle-glaucoma*) (Table 20–2).

Open-angle glaucomas are by far the most common, and the vast majority of patients in this group have *primary open angle glaucoma*

(POAG). Patients with POAG have a normal-appearing trabecular meshwork (as viewed by an ophthalmologist using the slit lamp and a gonioprism), moderately elevated intraocular pressure (characteristically 22–35), and evidence of optic nerve "cupping" (but not pallor, Fig. 20–2), with a tendency to develop visual field loss. Though usually bilateral, primary open-angle glaucoma can be very asymmetric. There is a strong hereditary predisposition for the disorder. The eye does not appear to be inflamed in POAG ("quiet" eye), and there are no obvious external signs. Patients with POAG are almost always entirely asymptomatic, with elevated intraocular pressure or optic disc cupping discovered on a routine or screening examination. The intraocular pressure in this chronic disorder elevates slowly over time and is usually moderate; very high intraocular pressures are unusual. Since pain is thought to correlate best with the rate and amount of rise in intraocular pressure, POAG alone does not cause eye pain or headache (Sherwood et al., 1988; Klein et al., 1993).

Primary open angle glaucoma is "primary" because the abnormal aqueous absorption occurs as an isolated defect and the pathophysiology is not well understood. There are a variety of *secondary open-angle glaucomas*, including disorders in which iris pigment

Table 20–2 Classifying the glaucomas

	Findings	Pain
Open-angle glaucomas		
Primary open-angle glaucoma	Normal-appearing eye except for increased cupping and possible visual field defects, intraocular pressure moderately elevated	No pain from the glaucoma but occasionally from topical drops (especially miotics)
Secondary open-angle glaucomas (pigment dispersion syndrome, traumatic hyphema, pseudoexfoliation of lens, lens-induced glaucoma)	Other signs are present but may be evident only on ophthalmologic examination	Can have episodes of pain with acute spikes in intraocular pressure
Angle-closure glaucomas		
Acute primary angle closure and secondary forms	Red painful eye, marked elevation in pressure (see Table 20–3)	Severe pain, may be confused with cluster headache
Intermittent angle closure glaucoma	Examination may be relatively unremarkable between episodes	Intermittent
Chronic angle-closure glaucoma	Eye may appear normal except for optic disc cupping	Asymptomatic or low-intensity brow or frontal headache
Normal-tension glaucoma	Cupping and visual field loss despite normal pressure	Questionable relationship to head pain

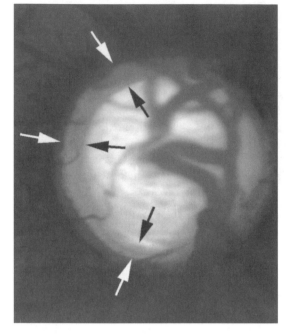

Figure 20–2 The optic disc in glaucoma. Glaucomatous optic atrophy occurs as an enlargement of the optic cup, presumably as axons in the neuroretinal rim die and drop out. An enlarged optic cup (*black arrows*) from primary open-angle glaucoma is pictured. Note that unlike most other forms of optic atrophy that cause optic disc pallor, the neuroretinal rim (*between arrowheads*) in glaucoma remains a normal pink color.

(pigment dispersion syndrome), inflammatory debris (uveitis), blood or degenerated red blood cells (traumatic hyphema), lens proteins (phacolytic glaucoma), or other material (pseudoexfoliation of the lens capsule) occlude an otherwise open, accessible angle. Pain from elevated intraocular pressure can occur in these forms of glaucoma if the pressure rises rapidly. Other ocular signs (by slit lamp) are invariably present in these cases.

Open-angle glaucomas are usually treated with topical medications, although oral agents (such as acetazolamide) or surgery (filters and tube shunts) may be required to treat recalcitrant disease. Interestingly, eyedrops are more likely to cause eye pain than most forms of open-angle glaucoma. Many topical medications can cause burning or a foreign-body sensation when applied. Pilocarpine can produce a more chronic type of eye and brow ache, thought to be caused by traction on the

scleral spur from this miotic agent. Pilocarpine and other miotics are now used less frequently, as many new (nonmiotic) agents are gaining in popularity (Shields, 1998).

Unlike POAG, *acute angle-closure glaucoma* presents with intense pain and photophobia, a red eye, and blurred vision, usually with accompanying nausea and vomiting. Though far less common than POAG, its often dramatic presentation is memorable. In the most common form of acute angle-closure glaucoma, the anterior chamber is anatomically shallow and the approach to the angle is narrow. Close apposition of the iris pupillary margin to the lens can cause a relative block to the flow of aqueous, ballooning the iris forward (iris bombe). This forward movement of the iris is sufficient to block access to the angle in predisposed eyes, driving the intraocular pressure up rapidly and severely (pressures of 50 to 70 mm Hg are not unusual). The result is a red eye (with ciliary flush), a "steamy" edematous cornea, blurred vision, a pupil that is often mid-dilated or irregular in shape (and poorly reactive to light), and severe pain (Fig. 20–3). The intense pain may radiate widely, and the nausea and vomiting may be equally severe. The globe feels very hard, especially when compared to palpation of the uninvolved eye, but be aware that the eye is exquisitely tender to touch. Misdiagnosis has led to tooth extractions (Joseph, 1999) and even laparotomies for the accompanying gastrointestinal complaints (Watson and Kirkby, 1989; Dayan et al., 1996).

Acute angle-closure glaucoma often occurs in patients over 60 years of age as the lens increases in the anterior–posterior dimension from cataract, further narrowing the anatomically predisposed anterior chamber angle. The mid-dilated pupil seems most prone to cause this cascade of events, so this condition may occur in the darkness of the movie theater or as the dilating drops are wearing off after a visit to the eye doctor. Some patients may have a history of previous, intermittent, self-aborting episodes.

Prompt diagnosis and referral is crucial since the condition can usually be quickly reversed by the ophthalmologist, with instantaneous relief of pain and nausea. Failure to

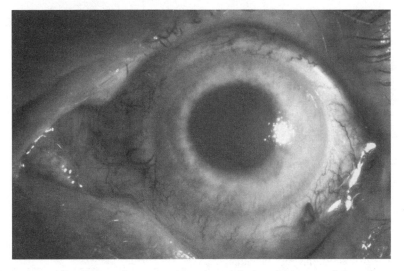

Figure 20–3 Acute angle-closure glaucoma. Many typical characteristics of the appearance of an eye with acute angle-closure glaucoma are seen in this clinical photograph. The cornea is edematous, as evidenced by a "steamy," dull light reflex. The pupil is mid-dilated and somewhat irregular in shape. The conjunctiva is injected, although this finding is less impressive in this photograph than in most cases.

treat can result in irreversible blindness. Since the fellow eye is usually likewise predisposed for an angle-closure attack, the ophthalmologist can also take steps to prevent this occurrence. Acute treatment includes the use of miotic eye drops and other pressure-lowering agents. Using a laser to create a hole in the iris (laser iridotomy) is curative as it allows an unobstructed alternate passage for the aqueous from the posterior to the anterior chamber. This procedure can be performed acutely if the corneal edema is not too severe and is routinely performed prophylactically in the fellow eye.

Acute angle-closure glaucoma can be confused with cluster headache (Prasad et al., 1991), and distinguishing these two disorders is crucial (Table 20–3). Therefore, all patients

Table 20–3 Cluster headache "look-alikes"

Acute angle-closure glaucoma	Cluster headache	Corneal erosion
Severe unilateral headache, nausea	Severe unilateral headache, nausea	Severe, sharp pain; nausea and vomiting unusual
Conjunctival injection is often intense, "ciliary flush" may be evident	Conjunctiva is only moderately injected	Conjunctiva is only moderately injected
Pupil usually mid-dilated and poorly reactive	Pupil may be smaller on affected side from Horner's syndrome but reactive to light	Pupil is normal
"Protective" ptosis (orbicularis activation) only, in response to pain	True 1–2 mm ptosis from Horner's syndrome may be present	"Protective" ptosis may narrow the fissure
Cloudy cornea with "grainy" light reflex and poor vision	Clear cornea with unaffected vision	Dull cornea with decreased vision
Intraocular pressure is very elevated during the attack (but may normalize quickly if attack has spontaneously reversed)	Intraocular pressure is normal (or slightly lower)	Intraocular pressure is normal
True emergency referral to ophthalmologist	Needs the care of a neurologist or other informed physician	Prompt referral to an ophthalmologist

with "red eyes" or vision loss must be examined by an ophthalmologist, even when the diagnosis of cluster headache seems convincing.

Intermittent angle-closure glaucoma consists of multiple, self-aborting episodes of angle closure with resultant intermittent eye pain. The typical signs and symptoms of angle-closure glaucoma may not be obvious between episodes, making the diagnosis difficult. In chronic angle-closure glaucoma, the intraocular pressure does not change rapidly and is, therefore, an unlikely cause of eye and head pain on the basis of intraocular pressure alone.

A common form of secondary angle-closure glaucoma is neovascular glaucoma, in which new blood vessels grow on the trabecular meshwork as a response to ischemia. This condition occurs in end-stage diabetic retinopathy or in ocular ischemic syndrome from carotid insufficiency. The pain that invariably accompanies this problem is deep, boring, unrelenting, and associated with a red eye and poor vision (Brown and Magargal, 1988).

In *normal-tension (or low-tension) glaucoma*, glaucomatous optic atrophy and progressive visual field loss occur despite intraocular pressure measurements being normal. Its cause is unknown, and it is unclear what relationship it bears to those glaucomas with elevated intraocular pressure. An association between low-tension glaucoma and headache has been proposed, but its significance is unclear (De Marinis et al., 1999; Pradalier et al., 1998; Wang et al., 1997; Ederer, 1986; Phelps and Corbett, 1985).

Ocular Inflammation

The fact that there are a myriad of clinical descriptors and classifications for ocular inflammation (Table 20–4) is evidence that inflammation of the eye can present in many ways and that there are a multitude of causes (many of which are not known or understood). As with glaucoma, pain is roughly proportional to the rate at which inflammation proceeds unchecked, as well as the severity of the inflammation. In addition, pain can be caused by the end result of inflammation,

Table 20–4 Various ways of classifying ocular inflammation

Duration and intensity: acute, subacute, chronic
Bilateral/unilateral
Type of inflammation: granulomatous/ non-granulomatous
Location: Scleritis
Keratitis
Uveitis
Anterior (iritis, cyclitis)
Posterior (vitritis, pars planitis, choroiditis)
Retinitis
Enophthalmitis
Etiology: Infectious
Specific agent if known or presumed
Source (endogenous exogenous)
Noninfectious (sterile)
Lens-induced
Traumatic
Sympathetic

such as high (inflammatory glaucoma) or low (hypotony) intraocular pressure. This section addresses a limited number of ocular inflammatory conditions that are important in the discussion of headache.

Acute nongranulomatous iritis is a relatively common form of intraocular inflammation that usually presents with a red, painful eye and decreased vision. The conjunctival injection is usually in the form of a "ciliary flush," in which dilated radial conjunctival vessels encircle the cornea at the limbus. Eye pain/headache is typical but ranges from a minimal persistent ache to overwhelming agony. Pain may be referred to the ear, teeth, or sinuses. Photophobia is a prominent symptom, and tearing and blepharospasm may also be present. Photophobia in this condition is thought by some to be caused by traction on the inflamed ciliary body as the pupil attempts to constrict to a light stimulus. Although photophobia is a common complaint among headache sufferers, the photophobia in unilateral iritis is unique in that a light stimulus to either eye will cause pain only in the involved eye (Au and Henkind, 1981). A definitive diagnosis can only be made with the ophthalmologist's slit lamp, which will reveal floating cells in the normally clear anterior chamber and flare (in which the slit beam is made visible in the anterior chamber by the products of inflammation and vascular permeability). The intraocular pressure may be low (from cyclitis) or high (from secondary inflammatory glaucoma). Acute nongranulomatous iritis can occur in isolation but may be associated with systemic diseases (such as collagen vascular diseases). The ophthalmologist's mainstay of treatment is steroids (topical, oral, or peri-ocular injection).

Granulomatous uveitis is characterized by a chronic, indolent, smoldering course, and the eye may not appear to be abnormal externally. The designation "granulomatous" is based on the slit lamp examination, in which characteristic large "mutton-fat" precipitates can be seen on the corneal endothelium (Fig. 20–4). The vision may be moderately affected, and pain is usually minimal but chronic. Common causes of granulomatous uveitis include sarcoidosis and tuberculosis, but many cases are idiopathic.

Posterior inflammation (retinitis, choroiditis, pars planitis, vitritis) is more likely to present as a decline in vision, rather than pain. In some cases, inflammatory cells and debris in the vitreous (vitritis) will manifest as a decrease in the red reflex of the involved eye (Nussenblatt and Palestine, 1989).

Scleritis presents as a painful red eye, with nodular or diffuse areas of intense injection of the scleral and conjunctival vessels. When scleritis is posterior, it can cause intense eye pain, decreased vision, and even a swollen optic disc, but the visible (anterior) sclera may appear normal (Benson, 1988).

Other ocular inflammatory conditions, such as herpes zoster opthalmicus and giant cell arteritis, are discussed in a later section.

Other Eye Diseases

Ocular surface disorders, such as dry eye syndrome, are a frequently overlooked cause of ocular discomfort. Patients may complain of a chronic, sandy, gritty, foreign-body sensation or occasional brief sharp eye pain that lasts only seconds. The vision may be intermittently blurred, and all symptoms typically worsen throughout the day. Not uncommonly, patients may paradoxically complain of frequent tearing, but this watery "reflex tearing" from ocular irritation lacks the tear film components that successfully adhere to and protect the ocular surface.

A corneal abrasion can cause excruciatingly severe eye pain and photophobia, often with radiation to other parts of the head or face. The eye is red, the corneal reflex is dull, and the vision is usually affected in this condition.

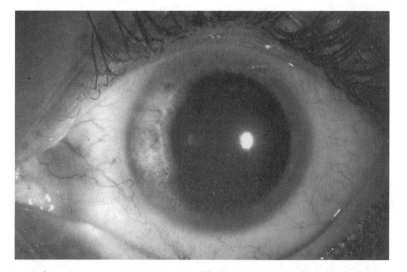

Figure 20–4 Granulomatous uveitis. A 46-year-old woman reported blurred vision and mild ocular discomfort. This clinical photograph demonstrates several characteristics of granulomatous uveitis, including (1) a relatively "quiet" eye (little conjunctival injection); (2) pigmented, "mutton-fat" keratic precipitates adhere to the endothelium of the inferior cornea; (3) the pupil is irregular as the iris is stuck to the lens capsule (posterior synechiae) from chronic inflammation.

Corneal abrasions are caused by trauma to the eye, with a resulting corneal epithelial defect; they may spontaneously heal within hours or days. However, treatment by the ophthalmologist with topical antibiotic ointment and patching speeds healing, reduces pain, reduces the risk of infection, and allows the physician to address other ocular trauma. Recurrent corneal erosions can occur from previous corneal trauma or corneal epithelial disorders. Corneal epithelial defects occur spontaneously, often during the night or on awakening, causing severe eye pain and photophobia. These recurrent episodes of pain and red eye should not be confused with cluster headache (Table 20–3). Corneal ulcers are deeper defects in the cornea that are often the result of infection and can lead to blindness if untreated.

Since the conjunctiva has fewer pain fibers than the cornea, conjunctivitis is generally less painful than corneal epithelial defects. Allergic conjunctivitis is characterized by itchy, red eyes with tearing. Viral conjunctivitis ("pink eye") is common and remarkably contagious. Since conjunctivitis presents with a red eye by definition, patients are usually appropriately referred to ophthalmologists.

Orbital Disorders

Orbital diseases may cause eye or facial pain even in the presence of a "quiet" (normal-appearing) eye. In many cases, other signs or symptoms are present to suggest an orbital etiology: motility disturbances and diplopia, proptosis, periocular edema, or decreased vision.

With regard to pain, idiopathic orbital inflammatory disorders are the most notable. *Myositis* is inflammation of one or more extraocular muscles, usually presenting with diplopia and pain that worsens with eye movement, somewhat like optic neuritis. However, myositis does not affect optic nerve function, and the visual acuity and visual field should be unaffected. *Trochleitis* is characterized by point tenderness over the trochlea (palpable along the superonasal internal orbital rim) and the absence of other orbital disease. Nonsteroidal anti-inflammatory agents are usually

successful in treating these low-grade inflammatory conditions.

In *orbital inflammatory pseudotumor*, the magnitude of pain and dysfunction is much greater than in myositis as inflammation may involve the extraocular muscles, the orbital fat, or even the optic nerve. This condition is usually accompanied by a motility disturbance, proptosis, or ocular injection. *Tolosa-Hunt syndrome* is an idiopathic inflammatory disorder of the orbital apex or cavernous sinus that causes cranial nerve dysfunction and a painful ophthalmoplegia. Tolosa-Hunt syndrome is most likely the same process as orbital inflammatory pseudotumor, just more posterior in location. Both of these conditions require thorough evaluations to rule out neoplastic diseases or other known inflammatory conditions, especially sarcoidosis and orbital metastases (Table 20–5). Steroids are the mainstay of treatment for orbital inflamma-

Table 20–5 Painful ophthalmoplegias

Orbit
   Inflammatory pseudotumor
   Contiguous sinusitis
   Mucormycosis or other fungal infections
   Tumors, local and metastatic
   Lymphoma
Superior orbital fissure–anterior cavernous sinus
   Nonspecific granulomatous inflammation (Tolosa-Hunt syndrome)
   Metastatic tumor
   Nasopharyngeal carcinoma
   Lymphoma
   Carotid-cavernous fistula
   Cavernous sinus thrombosis
Parasellar area
   Pituitary adenoma
   Intracavernous aneurysm
   Metastatic tumor
   Nasopharyngeal carcinoma
   Sphenoid sinus mucocele
   Meningioma, chordoma
   Petrositis (Gradenigo's syndrome)
Posterior fossa
   Posterior communicating artery aneurysm
   Basilar artery aneurysm (rare)
Miscellaneous
   Ischemic (diabetic) cranial mononeuropathy
   Ophthalmoplegic migraine
   Giant cell arteritis
   Herpes zoster

Adapted from Glaser J.S. (1990). *Neuro-ophthalmology*, 2nd ed., ch. xii, p. 577. Lippincott, Philadelphia.

tory pseudotumor and Tolosa-Hunt syndrome.

With *orbital Graves' disease*, eye pain and discomfort are usually minimal, especially compared to the obvious degree of dysfunction (proptosis, diplopia, eyelid retraction). However, ocular irritation from secondary-exposure keratopathy can cause a red eye, foreign body sensation, tearing, and eye pain.

NEURO-OPHTHALMIC DISORDERS ASSOCIATED WITH PAIN

The topics described below are discussed in great detail in other sections of this book. However, important points with regard to ocular signs and symptoms in the setting of headache are worth repeating.

Migraine

Aura

Not uncommonly, an aura of transient neurologic dysfunction precedes the headache in "classic" migraine. By far, visual disturbances are the most common type of aura experienced by migraine sufferers. Since this phenomenon usually originates in the occipital cortex, the visual aura is a homonymous phenomenon, appearing on the side opposite the affected visual cortex (and subsequent headache in most cases). Visual auras can be positive (visual scintillations or heat-wave sensations), negative (gray-, black-, or white-outs; hemianopia), or both. The classic *scintillating fortification scotoma* consists of colored, pulsating, jagged lines that begin as a small paracentral arc. Over 15 to 30 minutes, the angulated boundary enlarges and progresses toward the temporal visual field, leaving a scotoma in its wake. The time course and evolution of this visual phenomenon is thought to correspond to a slow, spreading wave of depression over the surface of the occipital cortex. Patients often do not understand the homonymous nature of the aura and are often insistent that the aura occurred only in the eye on the side of the homonymous visual phenomenon. Other common descriptions of

migraine aura include a "heat-wave" sensation or a visual distortion like water running down a windowpane. A severe, unilateral, throbbing headache (on the side opposite the visual aura) usually follows, although rarely the headache may occur before or during the aura.

Some patients, typically men over 50 years of age, may describe only a visual aura, without headache, that is termed *acephalgic migraine*. In many cases, these patients have a previous history of migraine headaches with or without aura (Hupp et al., 1989). The visual aura may be positive or negative and must be distinguished from amaurosis fugax or other causes of transient visual loss.

Rarely, arteriovenous malformations involving the occipital lobe can incite a migraine-like visual aura and cause headache. Magnetic resonance imaging (MRI) of the brain with gadolinium is indicated in patients whose visual phenomena are atypical in length or progression, who have other neurologic signs and symptoms, or who have persistent visual field defects. A visual aura that alternates sides is very likely to be caused by migraine rather than an occipital lobe lesion.

"Ocular" Migraine

Retinal (or ocular) migraine involves the retinal or posterior ciliary vasculature and, therefore, produces true monocular, rather than homonymous, visual disturbances. Episodes of transient monocular vision loss may last minutes to hours and may not be temporally related to the patient's headache. Patients are usually less than 44 years old and often have a history of other manifestations of migraine. Ocular migraine is a diagnosis of exclusion as other causes of transient vision loss must be considered in the differential diagnosis (such as embolic phenomenon and coagulopathies) (Corbett, 1983). Severe or repeated events can cause permanent visual field defects from retinal artery occlusion (Inan et al., 1994) or, more rarely, from anterior ischemic optic neuropathy (Lee et al., 1996).

Cluster Headache

Cluster headache is characterized by a sequence of abrupt-onset, short-lived episodes (60 to 90 minutes) of excruciating, unilateral, periorbital pain that are grouped temporally in "clusters." The severe retro-orbital pain typically occurs at night and is characterized by accompanying ipsilateral autonomic signs: tearing, rhinorrhea, and conjunctival injection (Corbett, 1983). This combination of lancinating pain and red eye can be confused with ocular disorders, such as acute glaucoma and recurrent corneal erosions (Table 20–3). A transient Horner's syndrome on the affected side may also occur in up to half of the cases; this may become permanent with repeated bouts (Curran, 1975).

Optic Neuritis

Demyelinating optic neuritis commonly presents with periocular pain on eye movement, in addition to vision loss (Optic Neuritis Study Group, 1991). The mechanism is believed to arise from the close attachments of the rectus muscles to the optic nerve sheath at the orbital apex. Contraction of the eye muscles with eye movement pulls on the inflamed optic nerve and causes pain (Lepore, 1991). The pain may precede symptomatic vision loss and usually resolves within days of onset.

Giant Cell Arteritis

Giant cell arteritis should always be considered in patients who are over the age of 50 and have new or different headaches. This systemic disease is commonly associated with weakness, malaise, and aches and pains of the proximal limbs. Ischemia results from vasculitic closure of extracranial small arteries causing scalp tenderness and jaw claudication. Blindness is a common and devastating complication of giant cell arteritis, which can present as anterior (or rarely posterior) ischemic optic neuropathy, central retinal artery occlusion, or ocular ischemic syndrome. Frequently, the disease is first suspected after unilateral vision loss. Prompt diagnosis and immediate treatment with steroids are required to prevent blindness in the second eye. Giant cell arteritis may also first manifest as diplopia, from an ischemic cranial neuropathy or extraocular muscle ischemia (Keltner, 1982).

There is evidence to suggest that high-dose IV steroids are of benefit when this diagnosis is suspected in the setting of acute vision loss. A suspicion of giant cell arteritis demands immediate laboratory studies (erythrocyte sedimentation rate, c-reactive protein, complete blood count), followed by immediate institution of steroids (oral or IV). A temporal artery biopsy should be performed within 2 weeks of beginning steriods (the earlier the better) (Ghanchi and Dutton, 1997). Treatment should not be delayed in anticipation of a temporal artery biopsy.

Carotid Dissection

A carotid dissection occurs when a tear in the intima of the carotid artery allows blood to dissect into the arterial wall, narrowing the lumen. Pain may involve the face, neck, and retroauricular areas on the side of the dissection and usually subsides within 3 to 4 days of onset (but can last weeks or even years). Pain may be the only symptom, but a postganlionic Horner's syndrome is present over half of the time. Additional neurologic symptoms can occur from thrombosis and occlusion of the internal carotid and its branches or from thromboembolism, causing cranial nerve dysfunction, stroke, and transient ischemic attacks. Cerebral angiography or magnetic resonance angiography (MRA) of the carotid system may be needed for diagnosis, but MRI alone is often diagnostic.

Idiopathic Intracranial Hypertension

Idiopathic intracranial hypertension (IIH) typically occurs in young, obese women, and headache is often the presenting complaint. Other causes of elevated intracranial hypertension, such as intracranial tumor or venous sinus thrombosis, are usually evident on MRI of the brain. The headache from elevated intracranial pressure is usually worse in the morning and is often made worse with coughing or Valsalva maneuver. Important findings with elevated intracranial pressure include papilledema and occasionally unilateral or bilateral sixth nerve palsies. Visual acuity is usually normal.

The visual fields are typically normal at first (except for enlargement of the blind spot), but insidious peripheral visual field loss can occur in the chronic stages of papilledema. Frequently, the headache severity does not correlate with the risk of vision loss. The management of IIH (and other causes of papilledema) requires the teamwork of a neurologist (to aid in diagnosis with a lumbar puncture and to help manage the headache) and an ophthalmologist (to monitor the visual fields and optic disc appearance).

Painful Ocular Motor Cranial Neuropathies

The Tolosa-Hunt syndrome and other inflammatory, infiltrative, or neoplastic processes involving the cavernous sinus or orbital apex can cause head and periorbital pain and multiple cranial neuropathies (Table 20–5). An ischemic mononeuropathy of the third, fourth, or sixth cranial nerve often presents with periorbital pain, typically in patients with diabetes, hypertension, or other vascular disease. In this setting, the pain is mild to moderate and dissipates within 1 or 2 weeks after onset.

A painful, isolated third nerve palsy can occur from an aneurysm. Intracranial aneurysms can expand and rupture with little or no warning, with catastrophic consequences. However, the close anatomic relationship of the oculomotor nerve (cranial nerve III) and the posterior communicating artery provides an early warning in some cases. Aneurysms that arise at the junction of the posterior communicating and internal carotid arteries may compress the oculomotor nerve, causing a third nerve palsy and pain before rupture. Bleeding or rupture of the aneurysm dramatically worsens the patient's prognosis. Therefore, the alert physician investigating a painful third nerve palsy has an opportunity to diagnose this condition early, before catastrophic consequences occur.

In many cases, the diagnosis is made by MRI, MRA, or cerebral angiography; but such tests may not be considered if the physician is not aware of the clinical signs that lead to suspicion. One important sign is the presence of relative pupillary involvement. Pupillomotor fibers travel superiolaterally on the subpial surface of the nerve, making them more vulnerable to external compressive forces (as opposed to ischemic events, which tend to affect the central "watershed" zone of the nutrient arteries and spare the superficial pupillary axons). Thus, an oculomotor palsy without pupillary involvement is likely to be ischemic and one with pupillary involvement (relative to the degree of extraocular weakness) is likely to be compressive, such as from an aneurysm. Although pain with symptomatic intracranial aneurysms is the rule, pain itself cannot reliably distinguish between ischemia and a third nerve palsy from aneurysmal compression (Table 20–5).

Pain Referred to the Eye from Intracranial Diseases

The trigeminal nerve carries pain and sensation from the eye, face, and many intracranial structures. The ophthalmic division of this nerve serves the eye and orbit. Interestingly, a tentorial–dural branch joins the ophthalmic division in the cavernous sinus, receiving sensory innervation from much of the intracranial dura, the arteries at the skull base, and the major venous structures (Burton, 1987). For this reason, pain from intracranial diseases, especially those involving the dura and cavernous sinus, may be referred to the eye and orbit. Inflammation, neoplasm, or ischemia involving intracranial structures may cause pain, which is often referred to the ipsilateral eye. Therefore, eye pain that remains unexplained after a thorough ophthalmic evaluation may require neuroimaging to rule out an intracranial disorder.

Herpes Zoster Ophthalmicus

Herpes zoster ophthalmicus (HZO) is caused by reactivation of latent herpes zoster virus in the gasserian ganglion, which typically involves the first division of the trigeminal nerve (ophthalmic division). The nasociliary branch of this nerve innervates intraocular structures, and intraocular inflammation (keratouveitis) can occur when this branch is involved. The risk of keratouveitis is greatest when vesicles are found in the cutaneous distribution of the nasociliary branch on the lateral aspect and the tip of the nose or the medial canthal area of the eye. Cranial neuropathies can also occur with HZO, usually weeks after the skin eruption (Fig. 20–5). Treating HZO with antiviral agents (acyclovir or famcyclovir) early in its course has greatly reduced the ocular morbidity of this potentially blinding disorder (Lavin, 1998).

OTHER TOPICS

"Atypical" Face Pain

The search for a diagnosis in the case of atypical facial pain is likely to involve a multidisciplinary team, including ophthalmologists, neurologists, dentists, otolaryngologists, and others. Lack of a definite diagnosis after an appropriate evaluation does not preclude treatment. Such patients require the services of a neurologist or anesthesiologist with expertise in pain control (Martin and Corbett, 2000).

Photophobia

Photophobia is the clinical term used to describe an abnormal intolerance to light, usually associated with eye pain. In some cases, the reason for discomfort seems apparent, such as the pain induced with pupillary constriction in iritis. In other cases, light exposure may cause the patient's vision to decrease (*hemeralopia*), as with cataract or cone–rod retinal dystrophies; but it is unclear why these patients frequently also describe ocular discomfort. Central mechanisms of photophobia are even less well understood. Thus, photophobia can occur in a number of very diverse clinical settings:

1. Anterior segment disorders of the eye, such as ocular surface disorders (dry eye syndrome), corneal disorders, uveitis, acute angle-closure glaucoma, and cataract (especially posterior subcapsular cataract)
2. Vitreoretinal disorders, such as albinism, achromatopsia, retinitis pigmentosa (cone–rod dystrophy), or cancer-associated retinopathy
3. Acquired optic neuropathies, such as optic neuritis
4. Intracranial diseases, such as migraine, meningeal inflammation, irritation, or infection; following intracranial trauma or surgery (Miller, 1985); and central photophobia, perhaps associated with thalamic

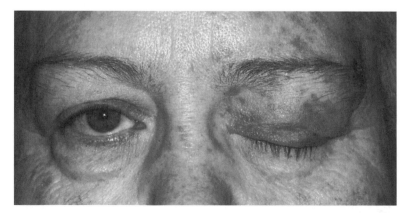

Figure 20–5 Herpes zoster ophthalmicus with a third cranial nerve palsy. A 71-year-old woman developed a left third nerve palsy several weeks after developing pain and vesicles in the distribution of the first division of the left trigeminal nerve. A complete ptosis is evident in this clinical photograph, along with the healing vesicles. (Courtesy of Martin, T.J. and J.J. Corbett (2000). *Requisites in Neuro-ophthalmology*, p. 230. Mosby, St. Louis.)

injury (Cummings and Gittinger, 1987) or trigeminal dysfunction (Gutrecht, et al., 1990)

5. Light deprivation, causing a "physiologic photophobia"

This last category may explain why photophobia can persist even after the exciting event is gone. The retina's sensitivity to light can increase dramatically when illumination is low. This dynamic, self-regulating feature of retinal sensitivity allows effective vision over a wide range of illumination conditions. However, patients who persist in living in low illumination (such as continuous wearing of dark sunglasses) may perpetuate photophobia even in the absence of disease.

Role of the Ophthalmologist in Evaluating Patients with Headache

When headache patients have visible eye or orbit abnormalities or concomitant complaints of diplopia, blurred vision, or pain in and around the eye, the importance of the ophthalmologist is obvious. Sometimes important clues suggesting nonocular causes of headache may be identified, such as Horner's syndrome in cluster headache or papilledema from elevated intracranial pressure. Patients without specific eye signs or symptoms can also be helped, even if all that is given is warranted reassurance after a thorough examination. Although patients with headache attributable to refractive error or muscle imbalance comprise only a small percentage of all headache patients, looking for refractive errors (especially latent hyperopia) and performing a quantitative examination of ocular motility and alignment (with particular attention to convergence abnormalities) is a necessity (Table 20–6). Refractive errors should be corrected, but this will help only a very few patients who present with headache (Daum et al., 1988). Beware of patients who bring their many pairs of "incorrect" glasses. Finding the cause of any ocular muscle imbalance must be given priority over rushing to attempt to correct the deviation with prisms or surgery (Hedges, 1979).

Table 20–6 Role of the ophthalmologist in evaluating headache

Look for eye and orbit diseases that can cause pain (corneal disease, acute glaucoma, uveitis, orbital inflammatory pseudotumor)
Perform a careful refraction and motility examination, looking especially for uncorrected hyperopia and convergence insufficiency
Be thorough as some nonocular causes of headache can be implicated by the eye exam
Communicate with the patient's other doctors, even when the exam is normal, so that the ongoing diagnosis or treatment of the patient's headache can continue

REFERENCES

Au, Y.-K. and P. Henkind (1981). Pain elicited by consensual pupillary reflex: A diagnostic test for acute iritis. *Lancet* 2:1254–1255.

Behrens, M.M. (1978). Headaches associated with disorders of the eye. *Med. Clin. North Am.* 62(3):507–521.

Benson W.E. (1988). Posterior scleritis. *Surv. Ophthalmol.* 32:297–316.

Brown, G.C. and L.E. Magargal (1988). The ocular ischemic syndrome. Clinical, fluorescein angiographic and carotid angiographic features. *Int. Ophthalmol.* 11:239–251.

Burton, H. (1987). Somatosensory features of the eye. In: *Adler's Physiology of the Eye, Clinical Applications*, 8th ed. (R.A. Moses and W.M. Hart, Jr., eds.), pp. 60–88. C.V. Mosby, St. Louis.

Cameron, M.E. (1976). Headaches in relation to the eyes. *Med. J. Aust.* 1:292–294.

Carlow, T.J. (1987). Headaches and the eye. In: *Wolff's Headache and Other Head Pain* (D.J. Dalessio, ed.), pp. 384–400. Oxford University Press, New York.

Corbett, J.J. (1983). Neuro-ophthalmic complications of migraine and cluster headaches. *Neurol. Clin.* 1:973–975.

Cummings, J.L. and J.W. Gittinger (1987). Central dazzle: A thalamic syndrome? *Arch. Neurol.* 38: 372–374.

Curran, R.E. (1975). Ophthalmic presentations of cluster headache. *Ann. Ophthalmol.* 7:1191–1194.

Daum, K.M., G. Good, and L. Tijerina (1988). Symptoms in video display terminal operators and the presence of small refractive errors. *J. Am. Optom. Assoc.* 59:691–697.

Dayan, M., B. Turner, and C. McGhee (1996). Acute angle closure glaucoma masquerading as systemic illness. *BMJ* 313:413–415.

De Marinis, M., J.P. Giraldi, A. de Feo et al. (1999). Migraine and ocular pain in "glaucoma suspect." *Cephalalgia* 19:243–247.

Eckhardt, L.B., J.M. McLean, and H. Goodell (1943). Experimental studies on headache. The genesis of pain from the eye. *Proc. Assoc. Res. Nerv. Ment. Dis.* 23:209–227.

Ederer, F. (1986). Migraine and low-tension glaucoma. A case control study. *Invest. Ophthalmol. Vis. Sci.* 27:632–633.

Ghanchi, F.D. and G.N. Dutton (1997). Current concepts in giant cell (temporal) arteritis. *Surv. Ophthalmol.* 42:99–123.

Glaser, J.S. (1990). *Neuro-ophthalmology*, 2nd ed., ch. xii, p. 577. Lippincott, Philadelphia.

Gordon, D.M. (1966). Some headaches in an ophthalmologist's office. *Headache* 6:141–146.

Gutrecht, J.A., I.M. Lessell, and A.A. Zamani (1990). Central dazzle in trigeminal sensory neuropathy. *Neurology* 40:722–723.

Hedges, T.R. (1979). An ophthalmologist's view of headache. *Headache* 19:151–155.

Hupp, S.L., L.B. Kline, and J.J. Corbett (1989). Visual disturbances of migraine. *Surv. Ophthalmol.* 33:221–236.

Inan, L.E., H. Uysal, U. Ergun et al. (1994). Complicated retinal migraine. *Headache* 34:50–52.

Joseph, A. (1999). A tooth for an eye: Dental procedures in unrecognized glaucoma. *J. R. Soc. Med.* 92:249.

Keltner, J.L. (1982). Giant-cell arteritis: Signs and symptoms. *Ophthalmology* 89:1101–1110.

Klein, B.E., R. Klein, S.M. Meuer et al. (1993). Migraine headache and its association with open-angle glaucoma: The Beaver Dam Eye Study. *Invest. Ophthalmol. Vis. Sci.* 34:3024–3027.

Lavin, P.J.M. (1998). Ocular and facial pain syndromes. In: *Neuro-ophthalmology* (E.S. Rosen, P. Eustace, H.S. Thompson et al., eds.), pp. 23.1–23.18. Mosby, St. Louis.

Lee, A.G., P.W. Brazis, and N.R. Miller (1996). Posterior ischemic optic neuropathy associated with migraine. *Headache* 36:506–509.

Lepore, F.E. (1991). The origin of pain in optic neuritis: Determinants of pain in 101 eyes with optic neuritis. *Arch. Neurol.* 48:748–749.

Mahto, R.S. (1972). Eye strain from convergence insufficiency. *BMJ* 2:564–565.

Martin, T.J. and J.J. Corbett (2000). *Requisites in Neuro-ophthalmology*, pp. 223–331. Mosby, St. Louis.

Martin, T.J. and D. Soyka (1993). Ocular causes of headache. In: *The Headaches* (J. Olesen, P. Tfelt-Hansen, and K.M.A. Welch, eds.), p. 748. Raven Press, New York.

Miller, N.R. (1985). Facial pain and neuralgia. In: *Walsh and Hoyt's Clinical Neuro-ophthalmology*, 4th ed., Vol. 2, p. 1071. Baltimore, Williams and Wilkins.

Newman, S. and R.M. Burde (1979). Headache and the ophthalmologist. *Sight Sav. Ref.* 49:99.

Nussenblatt, R.B and A.G. Palestine (1989). *Uveitis. Fundamentals and Clinical Practice*, pp. 54–75. Year Book Medical Publishers, Chicago.

Optic Neuritis Study Group (1991). The clinical profile of optic neuritis: Experience of the optic neuritis treatment trial. *Arch. Ophthalmol.* 109:1673–1678.

Phelps, C.D. and J.J. Corbett (1985). Migraine and low-tension glaucoma. A case-control study. *Invest. Ophthalmol. Vis. Sci.* 26:1105–1108.

Pradalier, A., P. Hamard, E. Sellem et al. (1998). Migraine and glaucoma: An epidemiologic survey of French ophthalmologists. *Cephalalgia* 18:74–76.

Prasad, P., R. Subramanya, and N.S. Upadhyaya (1991). Cluster headache or narrow angle glaucoma? *Indian J. Ophthalmol.* 39:181–182.

Romano, P.E. (1975). Pediatric ophthalmic mythology. *Postgrad. Med.* 58:146–150.

Sherwood, M.B., A. Garcia-Siekavizza, M.I. Meltzer et al. (1988). Glaucoma's impact on quality of life and its relation to clinical indicators. A pilot study. *Ophthalmology* 105:561–566.

Shields, M.D. (1988). Textbook of Glaucoma, 4th ed. Williams and Wilkins, Baltimore.

Tomsak, R.L. (1991). Ophthalmologic aspects of headache. *Med. Clin. North Am.* 75:693–706.

Troost, B.T. (1998). Headache and facial pain (excluding migraine). In *Walsh and Hoyt's Clinical Neuro-Ophthalmology*, 5th ed., Vol. 1 (N.R. Miller and N.J. Newman, eds.), pp. 1693–1758. Williams and Wilkins, Baltimore.

Vincent, A.J.P., E.L.H. Spierings, and H.B. Messinger (1989). A controlled study of visual symptoms and eye strain factors in chronic headache. *Headache* 29:523–527.

Wang, J.J., P. Mitchell, and W. Smith (1997). Is there an association between migraine headache and open-angle glaucoma? Findings from the Blue Mountain Eye Study. *Ophthalmology* 104:1714–1719.

Waters, W.E. (1970). Headache and the eye. A community study. *Lancet* 2:1–4.

Watson, N.J. and G.R. Kirkby (1989). Acute glaucoma presenting with abdominal symptoms. *BMJ* 299:254.

21

Disorders of the Mouth and Teeth

STEVEN B. GRAFF-RADFORD

Orofacial pain is a complex and often puzzling problem that clinicians are faced with on a daily basis. The International Association for the Study of Pain defines *pain* as "an unpleasant sensory and emotional experience associated with actual or potential tissue damage, or described in terms of such damage" (Mersky, 1986). This definition allows pain to be present without *nociception* (the recordable neural activity in A delta and C fibers) and encourages the clinician to assess the associated suffering and pain behavior when understanding and treating pain. Before one can treat facial pain, it is essential to have an accurate diagnosis. This requires a working knowledge of a classification system. This chapter describes a comprehensive classification system and addresses pains that present in the trigeminal nerve distribution.

CLASSIFICATION

The International Headache Society's (IHS) classification system can be used to describe many orofacial pains (Headache Classification Committee of the International Headache Society, 1988). This classification separates many conditions that may produce facial pain and classifies them independently. Table 21–1 provides an organ-based classification system that simplifies differential diagnosis.

The orofacial pains are divided into six categories and will be reviewed separately.

Extracranial

The eyes, ears, nose, throat, sinuses, teeth, lymph glands, and salivary glands may produce pain when noxious stimulation is triggered by infectious, degenerative, edematous, neoplastic, or destructive processes. Although the musculoskeletal system is included with the extracranial structures, it is separated in the classification as it commonly produces significant chronic pain.

Eye

Pain in and around the eye is usually caused by local disease, but it may also be referred from the teeth, jaw, or sinuses. Migraine and other neurovascular pains are often perceived in the eye. An inflammatory pseudotumor in the orbit associated with Tolosa-Hunt syndrome may produce eye pain. Eye pain may be differentiated into superficial or corneal pain, deep or inflammatory pain, and pain from excess retinal illumination. Pain quality is variable and depends on the cause of the pain or the location of the pathology. Localized eye pain should be evaluated by an ophthalmologist.

Table 21–1 Organ system classification for orofacial pain

Organ	Presence	Quality
Extracranial	Continuous	Dull
Intracranial	Continuous	Variable
Psychogenic	Variable	Variable
Neurovascular	Intermittent	Throbbing
Neuropathic	Intermittent	Sharp, shooting, electric
	Continuous	Burning
Musculoskeletal	Continuous	Dull, aching

Ear

Pain in the ear is often referred from musculoskeletal structures, such as the temporomandibular joint or muscles of mastication. The teeth may also refer pain to the ear. Pain referred from these structures is described as a dull, achey, or stopped-up sensation. Because the ear is innervated by cranial nerves V, VII, IX, and X and cervical roots C2 and C3, the source of the referred pain may be difficult to ascertain.

Nose

Pain in the nose may be referred from the teeth, sinuses, or other structures; but it is more likely to be caused by inflammation or local tumor. Referral to an ear, nose, and throat specialist is recommended if dental etiology is ruled out.

Throat

Throat pain is usually a local inflammatory reaction secondary to infection; however, other local problems, such as tumor, need to be considered. Other neurologic problems [glossopharyngeal neuralgia, stomatodynia (burning mouth syndrome), and Eagle's syndrome] will be included in the discussion of neurogenous pains later in this chapter.

Sinus and Paranasal Pain

Referred toothache is commonly due to inflammatory sinus disease. The problem is usually associated with the maxillary sinus, and pain is felt in the maxillary teeth on the involved side. The pain presents as a continuous, dull toothache, and the patient may state that the tooth feels extruded. Malaise, fever, and a purulent nasal discharge may accompany the pain. On examination, the sinus may be tender to palpation and the teeth sensitive to percussion. Four percent lidocaine, nasal spray or drops, often reduces the pain for the duration of the anesthesia. Radiographic sinus examination will demonstrate inflammatory change and is essential in finalizing the diagnosis. Seasonal changes, allergies, and barometric pressure changes may aggravate sinus problems. Sinus disease is classified as either acute or chronic. Acute sinusitis often follows an upper respiratory tract infection or dental disease and can produce nasal mucosal edema, preventing aeration and drainage through the ostia. Nociception will result from the inflammation. Chronic sinus disease usually is not painful. The acute sinusitis should be treated with antibiotics and systemic or topical decongestants. Surgical drainage may be required.

Teeth

The most common orofacial pain involves the teeth and their supporting structures. This pain is usually related to dental caries, presenting as a reversible pulpitis. The reversible pulpitis is characterized by poorly localized pain that may be sensitive to hot or cold stimuli. The reaction to the noxious stimulus (heat or cold) disappears soon after the stimulus is removed. When the carious lesion invades the pulp, an irreversible pulpitis begins. This is characterized by a lingering reaction to noxious stimuli. Periodontitis, which occurs if the micro-organisms and inflammatory products invade the periapical area (the area around the root apex), may present with toothache associated with chewing and sensitivity to touch and percussion. Periapical pathology may be observed as an area of increased radiolucency on radiograms. The tooth may have an abnormal response to pulp testing wherein heat, cold, or an electrical stimulus is not perceived. In clinical practice, it is difficult to differentiate reversible and irreversible pulpitis. When the diagnosis is not obvious, careful observation over days or weeks is recommended. Too often, endodontic therapy is performed when it is not indicated.

An intermittent pain that is triggered by biting on an offending tooth characterizes cracked-tooth syndrome. Unfortunately, the cracks are often difficult to find and do not appear on all x-ray images. The pain is often confused with that of pulpitis or trigeminal neuralgia, resulting in frustration and unnecessary treatment. Tomographic images 1 mm apart through the tooth's long axis may help define the crack. Further careful clinical examination, including staining or meticulous bite tests on each tooth cusp, may be useful. Graff-Radford et al. (1995) used thermography to study cracked teeth and found a difference in cracked-tooth pain and neuropathic facial pain. Patients who have cracked teeth have normal thermograms and patients who have neuropathic pain have asymmetrical thermograms. Chronic toothache may be a referred phenomenon. When no obvious local etiology is evident, neuropathic, muscular, or vascular etiologies should be considered (Graff-Radford et al., 1995).

Burning Mouth Syndrome

Burning mouth syndrome (BMS) is characterized by a burning sensation in one or several oral structures (Tourne and Fricton, 1992). Although no obvious cause has been established, numerous possibilities exist. The pathogenesis may be divided into local, systemic, and psychological etiologies. Local factors include contact allergy, denture irritation, oral habits, infection, and possibly reflux esophagitis. Systemic factors include menopause, vitamin and mineral deficiency, diabetes, oral infection, and chemotherapy. Psychogenic factors have often been cited but in an anecdotal fashion. It is essential to rule out a candidal infection. Although this may not be obvious to the eye, a swab and culture of the oral mucosa often reveals an incipient fungal infection. Patients with fungal infection respond quickly to antifungal preparations, such as clotrimazole or fluconazole. In

the author's experience, approximately half of patients with BMS have a candidal infection. This often follows steroid, antibiotic, or chemotherapy administration. When no systemic or local pathology is identified, the cause is probably neuropathic. Topical clonazepam (0.5 to 1.0 mg three times a day) effectively reduces burning oral pain (Woda et al., 1998). Patients are instructed to suck a tablet for 3 minutes (and then spit it out) three times a day for at least 10 days. Serum concentrations are minimal (3.3 ng/ml) 1 and 3 hours after application. Woda et al. (1998) hypothesized that clonazepam produces a peripheral, not a central, action that disrupts the neuropathologic mechanism. Additional treatments for BMS include tricyclic antidepressants, antiepileptic drugs, benzodiazepines, folic acid, and oral rinses. Treatment outcome is varied.

Intracranial

Intracranial pathology presenting as orofacial pain is exceedingly rare. The pain is usually associated with additional neurologic signs and symptoms. The meninges, cranial nerves, and blood vessels are the intracranial structures that are pain-sensitive. Traction, inflammation, distention, or pressure on these structures produces pain referral to distant sites.

Thalamic pain is described as "unilateral facial pain and dysesthesia attributed to a lesion of the quintothalamic pathway or thalamus. Symptoms may also involve the trunk and limbs of the affected side" (Mersky 1986). Infarcts in the thalamus involving the primary sensory nuclei or damage in other sensory pathways may lead to thalamic pain syndrome. The pain quality is moderate to severe burning or aching and localized to the contralateral face. Clinical presentation may include hemiplegia and associated allodynia, hyperesthesia, and hyperpathia. Magnetic resonance imaging (MRI) or computed tomography (CT) is used to confirm the diagnosis. Treatment is difficult, but patients respond best to the tricyclic antidepressants or membrane-stabilizing medications. Stimulation-produced analgesia, such as acupuncture, transcutaneous electrical nerve stimulation, or even deep brain stimulation, is a treatment option.

Intracranial neoplasms produce pain in approximately 60% of cases. This pain is typically dull, nonpulsatile, persistent, and aggravated by exertion or postural changes (Bulitt et al., 1986). Intracranial pathology must be considered when a patient presents with non-odontogenic face pain and other cranial nerve abnormalities. While certain intracranial tumors are more likely than others to produce neurologic problems, all do not have the same neurologic presentation (Rushton and Rooke, 1962). Tumors that produce facial pain include meningiomas, schwannomas, neurofibromas, acoustic neuromas, and cholesteatomas. Pituitary tumors may result in pain when they erode the sella or place pressure on the gasserian ganglion due to invasion of the cavernous sinus (Cueneo and Rand, 1952). Tumors arising from the trigeminal ganglion produce pain, and those arising from the root do not (Schisano and Olivercrona, 1960).

Psychogenic

Labeling a disease process psychogenic without clear documented objective criteria is grossly unfair to the patient. Fordyce and Steger (1990) pointed out that a patient's pain experiences are often labeled "psychogenic pain" when repeated failures using the biomedical model result in a lengthy medical history. They suggested that the system has not provided adequate diagnosis. Psychogenic pain may be interpreted in many ways. Some consider pain to be psychogenic when the pain behavior is excessive or varies from the physiological sensation or apparent nociceptive cause. A more useful method would use the psychogenic pain label when the emotional and psychological factors are the pain's primary manifestations. The latter alternative requires positive inclusion criteria, and Fordyce and Steger (1990) divide these into four groups: somatic delusions, somatization disorder, conversion, and depression. They point out that a psychogenic diagnosis is a philosophical one. The fact that the International Association for the Study of Pain (Mersky, 1986) defines pain as having an emotional

component should not allow one to confuse the emotional overlay with a psychogenic etiology.

A better term for pain problems in which no obvious pathology can be determined would be "idiopathic," rather than "psychogenic" or "atypical," pain. Further in-depth, systematic, objective study of these disorders needs to be carried out to understand their etiology. An ascribable diagnosis can usually be made if patients whose pain has been described as atypical or idiopathic are evaluated by someone with more experience (Fricton, 1999).

Neurovascular

All pain problems within the neurovascular organ system may not originate in this system, but all have the trigeminovascular pathway as the nociceptive mediator (Moskowitz et al., 1988). Neurovascular pains are largely intermittent and involve a complex mechanism that is still not fully understood. Table 21–2 lists the neurovascular pains that may present in the orofacial region.

Migraine, Exertional Headache, and Cough Headache

Although migraine is traditionally considered to present above the oculotragus line, facial migraine is well documented (Lovshin, 1960; Raskin and Prusiner, 1977). Migraine itself is discussed elsewhere in this volume. *Exertional migraine* is described as having "migraine symptoms lasting minutes and presenting with the other associated symptoms

Table 21–2 Orofacial pains of neurovascular origin

Migraine
   Migraine with aura
   Migraine without aura
   Exertional migraine
Cluster headache
Chronic paroxysmal hemicrania
Hemicrania continua
Severe unilateral neuralgiform headache with
   conjunctival injection and tearing, rhinorrhea and
   subclinical sweating (SUNCT)

attributed to migraine" (Rooke, 1968). Exertional migraine must be differentiated from benign cough headache and benign exertional headache. *Benign cough headache* is defined as intermittent pain, usually bilateral, with severe, bursting, explosive pain brought on by coughing. The pain location is usually in the vertex or the occipital, frontal, or temporal region, but it can also present in a tooth (Symonds, 1956; Moncada and Graff-Radford, 1993). This pain is responsive to indomethacin, 25 to 225 mg/day. This treatment should be maintained indefinitely since the symptoms will recur if the medication is decreased. Symonds (1956) emphasized the need to rule out intracranial pathology when evaluating benign cough headache.

Lovshin (1960) was the first to describe *facial migraine*, which is facial pain that occurs without a headache, a finding that was later confirmed by Raskin (1988). Facial migraine pain is described as dull pain with superimposed throbbing that occurs once to several times a week. Each attack lasts minutes to hours. Raskin (1988) describes ipsilatertal carotid tenderness, a finding also present when migraine presents in the head. This condition has also been referred to as carotidynia (Raskin and Prusiner, 1977). Raskin (1988) believes that dental trauma may be a precipitant.

Cluster Headache

Cluster headache is described (Headache Classification Committee of the International Headache Society, 1988) as:

Attacks of severe strictly unilateral pain orbitally, supraorbitally and/or temporally, lasting 15–180 minutes and occurring from once every other day to 8 times per day. The pains are associated with one or more of the following autonomic signs: conjunctival injection, lacrimation, nasal congestion, rhinorrhea, forehead and facial sweating, meiosis, ptosis, eyelid edema. Attacks occur in series lasting for weeks or months (so-called cluster periods) separated by remission periods usually lasting months or years. About 10 per cent of the patients have chronic symptoms.

Cluster headache has been called "periodic migrainous neuralgia" when it presents as or-ofacial pain (Brooke, 1978). Fifty-three percent of Brooke's (1978) facial cluster patients had toothache, and 47% had jaw pain. Bittar and Graff-Radford (1992) described 42 cluster headache patients, 42% of whom received unnecessary dental procedures. Cluster headache often presents in the orofacial region, especially in the maxilla. A sphenopalatine ganglion block with local anesthetic is useful as temporary abortive therapy.

Chronic paroxysmal hemicrania is described (Headache Classification Committee of the International Headache Society, 1988) as:

attacks with largely the same characteristics of pain and associated symptoms and signs as cluster headache, but they are shorter lasting, more frequent, occur mostly in females, and there is absolute effectiveness with indomethacin.

Chronic paroxysmal hemicrania may also involve the teeth or present as face pain. The clinical presentation is unchanged, as is the response to indomethacin (Delcanho and Graff-Radford, 1993).

Short-lasting unilateral neuralgiform headache attacks with conjunctival injection, tearing, rhinorrhea and subclinical sweating (SUNCT syndrome) was first described by Sjaastad et al. (1978). Most attacks are moderate to severe, with paroxysms of pain that last 30 to 120 seconds. Pain is usually localized to the eye and may occur in a cluster fashion with some quiet periods. Attack frequency may be up to 30 per day or many per hour (Sjaastad et al., 1989, 1991). Although SUNCT is clinically well identified, it is poorly treated. Carbamazepine may be effective at controlling some symptomatology, but this is not consistent (Sjaastad et al., 1991). Gabapentin may also offer relief to some patients (Graff-Radford, 2000b).

Neuropathic

Neuropathic pain suggests that tissue or nerve injury has occurred, with a permanent peripheral and/or central nervous system (CNS) change.

There are two types of neuropathic pain: transient and chronic. Short-lived pain that follows a stimulus that is potentially tissue-damaging, also referred to as acute pain, is a protective mechanism. Acute pain resolves in an appropriate time period, and then normal function is restored. What happens when the stimulus results in chronic pain? Although the injury appears to have healed, nonprotective pain remains. This may be due to central and peripheral nervous system changes (Ren and Dubner, 1999), which may include ongoing peripheral nociception, CNS sensitization, or downregulation of CNS inhibition.

Clinically, neuropathic pain can be classified as continuous or intermittent; these subtypes may present simultaneously or independently. Table 21–3 is a clinical classification of neuropathic facial pain.

Neuropathic pain presents clinically as an intermittent, bright, stimulating, electric, sharp, or burning pain. It is typically seen in trigeminal neuralgia, glossopharyngeal neuralgia, nervus intermedius neuralgia, and occipital neuralgia. These intermittent neuralgias are triggerable, usually by non-noxious stimuli. Vascular nerve compression is the proposed etiology (Fromm and Sessel, 1991). Compression may also be secondary to other structures, including tumors and bony growths, e.g., Eagle's syndrome (Janetta, 1977; Massey and Massey, 1979).

Trigeminal Neuralgia

Trigeminal neuralgia is described (Headache Classification Committee of the International Headache Society, 1988) as:

a painful unilateral affliction of the face, characterized by brief electric shock-like (lancinating) pain limited to the distribution of one or more divisions of the trigeminal nerve. Pain is commonly evoked by trivial stimuli including washing, shaving, smoking, talking and brushing the teeth, but may also occur spontaneously. The pain is abrupt in onset and termination may remit for varying periods.

Symptomatic trigeminal neuralgia is described as "pain indistinguishable from trigeminal neuralgia, caused by a demonstrable structural lesion." This lesion is usually a tumor, such as an acoustic neuroma, or demyelination, as seen in multiple sclerosis. If tissue or nerve injury is present, continuous trigeminal neuralgia may ensue; this is referred to as traumatic trigeminal neuralgia or trigeminal dysesthesia (Graff-Radford, 2000a).

Trigeminal neuralgia is usually unilateral; it occurs bilaterally in only 4% of subjects. There is no genetic link to the disorder. The average age at onset is between the sixth and seventh decades, with women slightly more affected than men, in a 3:2 ratio. The bright, stimulating pain is short-lived, lasting seconds to minutes. If the patient is not questioned carefully, he or she may report that the pain lasts all day as there is often a dull pain associated with trigeminal neuralgia or that sharp volleys come and go continuously. The author believes that the persistent aching pain may be secondary to reflex muscle splinting and can be controlled with stretching exercises and a vapocoolant spray. Mechanical maneuvering of the trigeminal sensory system usually triggers trigeminal neuralgia pain. The area from which the pain is activated has been described as a trigger zone. Characteristically, trigger zones occur around the supraorbital and infraorbital foramina, the inner canthus of the eye, lateral to the ala, and over the mental foramen. Trigger zones also occur intraorally. Pain is not elicited from the trigger zone if deep pressure is used or during a latency period between paroxysms. The second and third trigeminal nerve divisions are most commonly affected; the first division of the trigeminal nerve is affected in <5% of cases (Fromm and Sessel, 1991). Often, there is ipsilateral reflex facial spasm, hence the term, "tic douloureux," which has been used synonymously with trigeminal neuralgia (André, 1756).

Table 21–3 Neuropathic orofacial pain

Intermittent
  Trigeminal neuralgia
  Glossopharyngeal neuralgia
  Nervus intermedius neuralgia
  Occipital neuralgia
Continuous
  Trigeminal dysesthesia
  Trigeminal dysesthesia, sympathetically maintained

Trigeminal neuralgia may be due to trigeminal nerve focal demyelination at any point along its course. Posterior cranial fossa exploration reveals that in 60% to 88% of cases, trigeminal nerve root vascular compression is present in the posterior cranial fossa as it exits the pons (Gardner, 1962). This may set up a centrally mediated disinhibition of pain modulation and/or peripheral repetitive ectopic action potentials. Once there is sensitization, there may be increased afferent fiber activity and enhanced tactile stimulation, resulting in trigeminal nucleus interneuron discharge and trigeminothalamic neuron-producing pain. Taarnhoj (1982) described tumors as a possible cause in up to 6% of cases. These include acoustic neurinomas, cholesteatomas, meningiomas, osteomas, and angiomas. Aneurysms and adhesions have also been implicated. Although the pain may be typical of trigeminal neuralgia, there are usually additional symptoms or cranial deficits present. When patients between 20 and 40 years of age present with trigeminal neuralgia, multiple sclerosis should be ruled out. Fromm and Sessel (1991) suggest that all patients with trigeminal neuralgia should obtain a brain MRI or CT scan, with particular attention to the posterior cranial fossa.

Ratner et al. (1976, 1979) and Roberts et al. (1984) have proposed that bony cavities found in the alveolar bone are the cause of trigeminal neuralgia and that repetitive curettage of these cavities is curative. Using 15 half-maxillae and 12 half-mandibles from cadavers, Graff-Radford et al. (1988b) demonstrated that cavities larger than 2 mm in diameter occur throughout normal bone. The cavities do not appear to be unique to patients who have trigeminal neuralgia. This sheds doubt on the bony cavity theory and suggests that curettage may be effective through central mechanisms or peripheral denervation.

Trigeminal neuralgia treatment may be divided into pharmacologic and surgical types. Table 21–4 outlines the drugs that may be used in trigeminal neuralgia therapy.

The action of anticonvulsants in pain management is not well understood. Some, like carbamazepine, block sodium channels, inhibiting sustained repetitive firing. This reduces post-tetanic synaptic transmission potentiation and decreases synaptic transmission in the trigeminal nucleus, which may explain their effectiveness in facial pain. Valproic acid increases brain concentrations of gamma-aminobutyric acid (GABA), which affects sodium channels and is an inhibitory neurotransmitter in the CNS. Since phenobarbital's action is in the brain and not at the trigeminal nucleus, it is not effective for trigeminal neuralgia. Gabapentin may increase GABA by preventing its breakdown or may affect the N-methyl-D-aspartate (NMDA) receptor.

All drugs used in trigeminal neuralgia have side effects and must be used cautiously. Baclofen probably has the fewest side effects but is less effective than carbamazepine. Fromm et al. (1984) described the baclofen L isomer as the effective component. Therefore, non-response may be secondary to metabolizing the D isomer only. Baclofen should

Table 21–4 Common membrane-stabilizing drugs used in neuralgia therapy

Generic	Trade name	Dosage (mg/day)	Blood level (μg/ml)	Serum half-life (h)
Baclofen	Lioresal	10–80	—	
Carbamazepine	Tegretol (XR), Carbitrol	100–2000	4–12	12–17
Phenytoin	Dilantin	200–600	10–20	18–24
Valproic acid	Depakote	125–2,500	50–100	6–16
Gabapentin	Neurontin	100–5,000	—	
Lamotrigine	Lamictal	50–500	2–5	14–59
Clonazepam	Klonopin	0.5–8	—	22–33
Pimozide	Orap	2–12	—	55–154
Valproic acid	Depakote	125–2,000	50–100	6–16
Topiramate	Topamax	50–1,000	—	21

be started at a dose of 10 mg/day and increased every 2 days to a maximum of 80 mg/day, usually in four doses. Drowsiness and confusion are the major side effects, and many patients discontinue the drug for this reason. Carbamazepine is the most effective drug. Begin at a dose of 100 mg/day and increase by 100 mg every 2 days to a maximum of 1,200 mg/day. If no relief is obtained, a carbamazepine blood level should be obtained, to be sure the blood concentration is therapeutic. Trough level is usually in the range of 5 to 10 μg/ml. Aplastic anemia is a rare side effect of carbamazepine, and patients taking this drug need to have their blood levels watched carefully for this complication. Sustained preparations (Tegretol XR, Carbitrol) have improved compliance and reduce the medication's sedating side effects. Gabapentin, although not formally studied, has been useful in doses ranging from 300 to 3,000 mg/day. Phenytoin is a good alternative; doses range from 100 to 400 mg/day. Fromm and Sessel (1991) suggested using some of these drugs in combination, to either maximize their effects or minimize side effects. A double-blind crossover study using 48 subjects whose trigeminal neuralgia was refractory to medical treatment showed pimozide to be more effective than carbamazepine. Eighty-three percent of the subjects who received pimozide reported side effects that included physical and mental retardation, hand tremors, memory impairment, involuntary movements during sleep, and Parkinson-like symptoms. None of the patients stopped treatment because of side effects. The authors concluded that pimozide is effective but should be reserved for severe and intractable trigeminal neuralgia because of its possible adverse effects (Lechin et al., 1989).

The surgical treatments for trigeminal neuralgia are summarized in Table 21–5 (Burchiel, 1987). Less traditional treatments include curettage of the bony cavities as described above. Long-term success rates of 80% have been reported (Ratner et al., 1976, 1979; Roberts et al., 1984). A study of peripheral streptomycin and lidocaine injections was performed by Sokolovic et al. (1986). Twenty patients were given five injections of 2% lidocaine and 1g of streptomycin sulfate adjacent to peripheral nerves at 1-month intervals. Sixteen patients remained pain-free after 30 months. No side effects were reported, and the authors reported no loss of sensation after the local anesthetic wore off. Bittar and Graff-Radford (1993) completed a double-blind, placebo-controlled, crossover study using streptomycin, the results of which were not favorable. They also reported significant swelling associated with the injections.

Although not suggested as a therapeutic modality for trigeminal dysesthesia, surgery is an excellent alternative for trigeminal neuralgia. The most effective surgical approach remains microvascular decompression (Janetta, 1996). Microvascular decompression can now be performed using an endoscopic approach, which allows clearer observation and is less traumatic (Jarrahy et al., 2000). Gamma knife radiosurgery is a recent treatment for trigeminal neuralgia (Young et al., 1997). This technique offers a relatively noninvasive means to lesion the trigeminal nerve adjacent to the pons using a 4 mm collimator helmet. Complications are rare. To date, the author has seen one case of trigeminal dysesthesia attributed to the procedure.

Pretrigeminal Neuralgia

Sir Charles Symonds first described pretrigeminal neuralgia (Symonds, 1949). Mitchell (1980) later reviewed it. Fromm et al. (1990) described 16 patients who initially presented with a dull, continuous toothache in the upper or lower jaw and whose pain changed to classic trigeminal neuralgia. In seven cases, the continuous pain was successfully treated with traditional trigeminal neuralgia therapies. The diagnosis of pretrigeminal neuralgia is based on the following criteria: (1) pain is described as a dull toothache, (2) neurologic and dental examinations are normal, (3) CT or MRI scan of the head is normal. The pain of pretrigeminal neuralgia can be interrupted with somatic anesthetic blockade. Merrill and Graff-Radford (1992) described 61 patients who were treated for pretrigeminal or trigeminal neuralgia. Of these, 61% had been in-

Table 21–5 Surgical management of trigeminal neuralgia

Procedure	Effectiveness	Comment
Alcohol block	Excellent	Relief typically 8–16 months
		Paresthesia or dysesthesia occurs in 48%
Alcohol gangliolysis	88% at 4 years	Corneal anesthesia occurs in 15%
		Neuroparaletic keratitis occurs in 4–7%
		Postoperative paresthesia occurs in 55%
		Paresthesia occurs in 38%
		Herpetic outbreak occurs in 26%
		Transient masticatory muscle weakness occurs in 45%
Neurectomy	Excellent	Relief typically 26–38 months
		Anesthesia dolorosa and corneal anesthesia are rare
Glycerol gangliolysis	89%–96%	7%–10% have early recurrence
		7%–21% develop recurrence over extended follow-up
		Facial hyperesthesia occurs in 24%–80%
		Corneal anesthesia occurs in 9%
		Facial dysesthesia occurs in 8%–29%
Radiofrequency gangliolysis	78%–100%	1%–17% have early recurrence
		4%–32% develop recurrence over extended follow-up
		Masseter weakness occurs in 7%–23%
		Trigeminal dysesthesia occurs in 11%–42%
		Corneal hyperesthesia occurs in 3%–27%
		Neuroparalytic keratitis occurs in 1%–5%
		Anesthesia dolorosa occurs in 1%–4%
Microvascular decompression	96%–97%	16%–29% develop recurrence over extended follow-up
		Mortality occurs in 1%
		Morbidity occurs in 10%–23%
Rhizotomy	85%	15% develop recurrence over extended follow-up
		Mortality occurs in 0.5%–1.6%
		Facial weakness occurs in 7%–8%
		Paresthesia occurs as a minor complaint in 56%
		Paresthesia occurs as a major complaint in 5%
		Neuroparalytic keratitis occurs in 15%
Trigeminal tractotomy		Ipsilateral limb ataxia occurs in 10%
		Contralateral limb sensory loss occurs in 14%
Gamma knife	80%–95%	Onset may be 6 weeks or longer
		Facial numbness
		Trigeminal dysesthesia

correctly diagnosed and treated with traditional dental therapies. The clinician should be aware of pretrigeminal neuralgia before recommending surgery for a patient who has orofacial pain of unclear etiology.

Glossopharyngeal Neuralgia

The pain of glossopharyngeal neuralgia is similar in quality and characteristics to that of trigeminal neuralgia, but it occurs in the distribution of the glossopharyngeal nerve. It may be confused with Eagle's syndrome (Massey and Massey, 1979), which has a presentation similar to glossopharyngeal neuralgia but is associated with an elongated stylohyoid process that irritates or compresses the glossopharyngeal nerve. Rotation of the head, swallowing, and chewing are triggering factors. Patients may complain of a persistent sore throat. This pain can be decreased with neural blockade. Confirmation of the diagnosis requires that a calcified stylohyoid ligament be demonstrated on radiogram. Treatment is surgical resection of the ligament.

Nervus Intermedius Neuralgia

The pain of nervus intermedius neuralgia is described as similar to that of trigeminal neuralgia but localized to the middle ear. Patients often complain of feeling like a hot poker is in the ear (Walker, 1966). Treatment is similar to that for trigeminal neuralgia.

Occipital Neuralgia

Occipital neuralgia pain is located in the distribution of the greater and lesser occipital nerves. The pain is described as paroxysmal, sharp, and electric-like, and is usually associated with trauma at the onset. Graff-Radford et al. (1986) have described myofascial trigger points in the splenius cervicis and capitis muscles that may mimic occipital neuralgia. Trigger point injections can be used to help rule out this possibility. Surgical neurectomy has been employed for occipital neuralgia, but the results are often short-lived.

The neuropathic pain that sometimes follows tissue or nerve injury in the trigeminal nerve distribution is called *trigeminal dysesthesia*. Trigeminal dysesthesia is defined as a continuous pain following complete or partial damage to a peripheral nerve. The pain is described as a continuous, burning numbness and often pulling pain (Table 21–6).

The trauma that initiates trigeminal dysesthesia is usually quite obvious, e.g., wisdom tooth removal or dental implant placement. Trigeminal dysesthesia may occur with minor trauma, such as crown preparation, or following viral infection, such as herpes zoster. The discomfort can be self-limiting, depending on nerve regeneration. Campbell et al. (1990) stated that approximately 5% of patients who undergo root canal therapy have persistent pain that may be attributed to nerve damage. Ellies (1992) and Ellies and Hawker (1993) described 17% of patients with mandibular implants who developed persistent sensory change or pain. Thermographic studies reveal that all trigeminal dysesthesia patients have abnormal thermograms. Some are hot in the pain distribution and some are cold, none are normal. Graff-Radford et al. (1995a,b) described a hypothesis for these temperature changes that may be helpful in selecting a treatment.

Three peripheral mechanisms may be involved in chronic trigeminal neuropathic pain development: (1) nerve compression, (2) nerve regeneration, (3) sympathetically maintained pain.

1. *Nerve compression*: When a peripheral nerve is compressed or injured, there is a sus-

Table 21–6 Criteria for trigeminal dysesthesia

History of trauma
Continuous pain
Associated hyperalgesia and allodynia
Temperature change
Block effect (sympathetic vs. somatic)

tained firing that may be persistent. The closer the damage is to the CNS, the longer the spontaneous neural discharge. The pain that follows nerve compression can be temporarily relieved with local anesthetic blockade. Following neural trauma, receptor sprouting occurs on the damaged nociceptor, dorsal horn cells, and peripheral blood vessels. These may include α receptors, neuropeptide Y receptors, and possibly others. There is also increased release of trigeminal nucleus substance P, calcitonin gene–related peptide, and other neurotransmitters, resulting in further neurogenic inflammation and chronic pain (Bennett and Xie, 1988). When neural inflammation occurs, a neuritis ensues. The pain presents as a continuous, dull, burning pain with associated allodynia and hyperalgesia. A neuritis involving the facial nerve (cranial nerve VII) may be present (Bell's palsy). A painful Bell's palsy is usually due to herpes zoster involving the geniculate ganglion (Ramsay Hunt syndrome) with facial palsy and a herpes zoster eruption around the ear (Karnes, 1984).

2. *Nerve regeneration*: Neuroma formation is created by nerve regeneration where the path for regrowth is obstructed. The nerve resprouting and the continuous nerve irritation may result in pain. As in nerve compression, receptor sprouting and the presence of neurotransmitters increase the pain. Injecting the neuroma with local anesthetic will temporarily block the pain. Sprouting axons fire spontaneously and develop abnormal sensitization to cold, norepinephrine, and mechanical stimulation. This occurs in dorsal root ganglion cells as well as in peripheral terminals. Clinically, the neuroma may produce pain only after mechanical stimulation. The pain is aching and burning, with sharp volleys.

3. *Sympathetically maintained pain*: Campbell et al. (1992) states that the initial trauma to the peripheral nervous system activates nociceptors and produces sprouting of α-adrenergic receptors on the nociceptors. The initial sensory barrage sensitizes the CNS, causing sympathetic afferent activation and increased response to non-noxious stimuli. This causes peripheral norepinephrine release, which activates the peripheral nociceptors and keeps the cycle active. Sympathetic innervation in the dorsal root ganglia increases with age following neural injury (Roberts and Foglesong, 1988). It is not surprising that there is a higher incidence of neuropathic pain as we age. Sympathetically maintained pain is aggravated by non-noxious stimuli and can be interrupted temporarily by sympathetic block or α-adrenergic block with phentolamine.

Most orofacial trigeminal dysesthesia occurs in women who are in their fourth decade (Vickers et al., 1998; Solberg and Graff-Radford, 1988). Continuous dysesthesia is caused by a lesion in the trigeminal nervous system, either peripherally or centrally (Vickers et al., 1998). Sex-based differences are seen in many pain disorders. Although the role of sex hormones in the generation and perpetuation of central sensitization is not fully understood, it is important (Ren and Dubner, 1999). In a neuropathic pain model using partial sciatic nerve ligation, female rats were more likely than male rats to develop allodynia (Coyle et al., 1995). In studies of ovariectomized female rats, those with estrogen were more likely to develop allodynia after injury than those without estrogen (Coyle et al., 1996).

The therapy for trigeminal dysesthesia is aimed at reducing peripheral nociceptive inputs and simultaneously enhancing CNS pain-inhibitory systems (Graff-Radford, 1995a,b).

TOPICAL APPLICATIONS

Topical therapies have not been well studied. There is some evidence that capsaicin (Zostrix) applied regularly will result in desensitization and pain relief (Scrivani et al., 1999). The recommended dose is five times a day for 5 days, then three times a day for 3 weeks. If the patient cannot withstand the burning produced by the application, the addition of topical local anesthetic, either 4% lidocaine or EMLA, is useful. Clonidine can be applied to the hyperalgesic region by placing the proprietary subcutaneous delivery patch on the tender area. Alternatively, a 4% gel can be used over a larger area. A neurosensory stent can be used for local intraoral application. An oral impression is taken and an acrylic stent manufactured to cover the painful site (Graff-Radford, 1995a,b). The topical agent is applied to the gingival surface 24 hours a day.

Topical clonazepam (0.5 to 1.0 mg three times a day) effectively reduces burning oral pain (Woda et al., 1998). Patients were instructed to suck a tablet for 3 minutes (and then spit it out) three times a day for at least 10 days. Serum concentrations were minimal (3.3 ng/ml) 1 and 3 hours after application. Woda et al. (1998) hypothesized that there was peripheral, not central, action disrupting the neuropathologic mechanism.

PROCEDURES

Neural blockade is very effective at differentiating sympathetically maintained pain from sympathetically independent pain. It may also be effective at controlling sympathetically maintained pain if used repetitively. Stellate ganglion blocks, phentolamine infusion, and sphenopalatine blocks are useful in obtaining a chemical sympathetic block. The author has not had significant benefit using phentolamine infusion for facial pain. Scrivani et al. (1999), who used 30 mg infusions without benefit, supports this.

Lidocaine infusion (200 mg over 1 hour) may be used therapeutically for various forms of neuropathic pain (Boas et al., 1982; Rowbotham et al., 1991). Response to intravenous lidocaine may predict which patients will respond to the lidocaine analogue mexiletine. Sinnott et al. (1999) used an animal model to demonstrate the minimal lidocaine concentration (2.1 μg/ml) that will abolish allodynia. They also described a ceiling effect. Many animals with experimentally induced allodynia did not obtain persistent relief. They suggested that separate physiologic mechanisms,

Table 21–7 Common antidepressants used in trigeminal dysesthesia

Generic name	Route	Dosage (mg/day)
Amitriptyline	PO	10–150
Desipramine	PO	10–150
Doxepin	PO	10–150
Imipramine	PO	10–150
Nortriptyline	PO	10–150
Trazodone	PO	50–300

with differing pharmacologies, may account for the variability and postulate that there are different aspects of neuropathic pain.

PHARMACOLOGY

Tricyclic antidepressants are effective in many pain problems. Solberg and Graff-Radford (1988) have studied the response to amitriptyline in traumatic neuralgia. The effective range is 10 to 150 mg/day, usually taken in a single dose at bedtime. Many antidepressants may be used (Table 21–7).

Membrane stabilizers include anticonvulsants, lidocaine derivatives, and some muscle relaxants. They have been used for intermittent, sharp electric pains. Table 21–8 summarizes the common medications in this group and their doses.

BEHAVIORAL STRATEGIES

Before beginning therapy, a behavioral assessment and appropriate testing should be performed. Following the behavioral evaluation, attention is directed to the factors that may impact treatment and to determining the

Table 21–8 Common membrane stabilizers used in trigeminal dysesthesia

Generic name	Dosage (mg/day)
Baclofen	10–80
Carbamazepine	100–1,200
Gabapentin	300–3,000
Clonazepam	0.5–8
Lamotrigine	12.5–100
Pimozide	2–12
Phenytoin	100–400
Topiramate	25–200
Valproic acid	125–2,000

most appropriate interventions. Consideration should be given to the following: (1) behavioral or operant factors, (2) emotional factors, (3) characterologic factors, (4) cognitive factors, (5) side effects, (6) medication use, and (7) compliance. Cognitive and behavioral management techniques, relaxation, biofeedback, and psychotherapeutic and psychopharmacologic interventions may be useful.

SURGERY

Although not suggested as a therapeutic modality for trigeminal dysesthesia, surgery is an option for trigeminal neuralgia.

Postherpetic neuralgia (PHN) is a complex problem whose treatment has frustrated clinicians and patients (Loeser, 1986; Watson and Evans, 1986). Herpes zoster (HZ) is primarily a disease affecting older people, with some predilection for males (67% males 33% females to 53% males 47% females) (Molin, 1969). The localization of HZ in the face, including involvement of the facial nerve, is between 15% and 30% of reported cases (Molin, 1969). The duration of pain after vesicle outbreak varies, but the pain appears to last longer in older subjects. The number of subjects that go on to PHN (pain after the vesicles have healed) ranges from 14% of males to 25% of females, but almost all are older than 60 years (Molin, 1969). No studies to date have suggested that the subset of HZ patients who go on to PHN is predictable. The mechanism whereby the herpetic virus produces the neuralgic condition has not been determined. Reports by Head and Campbell (1900) and Denny-Brown and Adams (1944) reveal that changes occur in the skin and peripheral nerve endings that produce anesthesia or dysesthesia in the dorsal root ganglia characteristic of hemorrhage and lymphocytic infiltration. The adjacent proximal nerves and sensory nerve roots show demyelination, and rarely is cell death evident in the spinal cord. There are few controlled studies that assess treatment outcomes in this relentless disease. Watson and Evans (1986) have described the use of amitriptyline, which has by and large been the treatment of choice. This was confirmed by Max et al. (1988), who showed that amitriptyline, but not lorazepam, was effective in the treatment of PHN. Phenothiazines have been reported to be helpful in the treatment of chronic pain, and Taub (1973) reported five case studies in which the combination of amitriptyline and fluphenazine was effective. This report included a mix of acute cases (active lesions) and chronic cases (with pain lasting longer than 6 months). Graff-Radford et al. (2000c) studied the effects of amitriptyline and fluphenazine using a double-blind protocol and found no significant benefit in combining amitriptyline with fluphenazine. Sympathetic nerve block is considered by many to be effective at preventing PHN when used in the first 3 to 6 months following the outbreak of zoster. Depending on the effects, between one and six blocks should be performed. There is little purpose in doing more than three blocks if pain relief does not outlast the anesthetic effects. It may be more appropriate to place this in the autonomic nervous system category, but in some situations sympathetic block does not reduce the pain, which suggests a sympathetically independent pain.

MUSCULOSKELETAL SYSTEM

The musculoskeletal system is the most common origin of chronic orofacial pain. These may be divided into arthrogenous and muscular (temporomandibular) disorders. The temporomandibular joint (TMJ) is different from other body joints. The most recognizable difference between the TMJ and other synovial joints is its non-innervated, avascular, fibroconnective tissue articular covering. This is not hyaline in nature, possibly to aid in withstanding twisting, turning, and compressive forces. The fibroconnective tissue covering may also allow for significant remodeling to occur in the TMJ. Another significant difference is its diarthroidal structure. An intracapsular disk divides the joint into upper and lower compartments and provides for the complex hinge and gliding action. The mandible produces a reciprocal effect of one articulation on the other by joining the TMJs. Also interacting in this system is the dental

occlusion, which will result in altered forces on the system if it is not in equilibrium. The teeth provide a solid end point to joint movement, unlike any other joint, in which end range of motion is somewhat elastic. Due to the structure's nature, the intracapsular anatomy can remodel when subjected to extraneous forces. Such remodeling can be brought about through tooth loss, poor dental restoration, macro trauma, and parafunctional habits, such as tooth clenching and grinding. Remodeling may lead to dysfunction if the tissues are unable to compensate for the abnormal load. In addition, muscular hyperactivity may be initiated to compensate for the lack of equilibrium.

The joint's hinge action allows for about a 25 mm interincisal opening, which occurs primarily in the lower joint space (condylar rotation). The next 20 to 25 mm requires the disk condyle complex to slide down the temporal eminence, with the disk moving posterior relative to the condyle (translation). Remodeling resulting in a deviation in articular form may interrupt this rhythmic function. The articular tissues are usually characterized by smooth, rounded surfaces until subjected to extraneous forces, which produce remodeling (Solberg et al., 1985). The mechanical interferences produced by the remodeling may cause noise as they move over each other. Remodeling is an ongoing process and results in a disease continuum that begins with soft tissue change and progresses to involve the bony structures. One might view this as a failure of the adaptive process to compensate for the extraneous forces exerted on the joint. If there is sufficient change, the articular disk may become displaced. The usual direction for displacement is anteromedially (Ireland, 1953; Farrar, 1972), although posterior displacement has been reported (Blankestijn and Boering, 1985). The disk displacement may reduce if the individual can manipulate the condyle onto the disk, producing joint noise. This noise is usually heard after the initial 25 mm rotation in the opening movement and again just before the teeth occlude in the closing path. The closing noise is usually much quieter and may be produced by relocation of the disk in the anterior position. Joint noise occurs in 20% to 30% of individuals over 15 years of age (Egermark et al., 1981; Solberg et al., 1979). Pain associated with joint pathology is usually intermittent and associated with function. To confirm the diagnosis of an articular temporomandibular disorder, patients should display at least three of the following four criteria: (1) limited range of motion (less than 40 mm), (2) joint noise (clicking, popping, or crepitus), (3) tenderness to palpation, (4) functional pain. Continuous pain associated with an articular temporomandibular disorder is unusual and generally is produced by associated inflammation or secondary muscle pain. Pain emanating from the ligamentous attachments, the synovium, or the fibrous capsules is usually secondary to infection or trauma to these structures. The differences between synovitis and capsulitis are almost impossible to determine clinically (Bell, 1985).

Articular remodeling is a direct result of adaptive changes that help establish a status quo between joint form and function (Moffett et al., 1964). Osteoarthrosis results from destruction of articular tissues secondary to excessive strain on the remodeling mechanism. The problem is non-painful and usually produces only mechanical interferences. De Bont et al. (1985) suggested that the degenerative process is due to fatty degeneration and disruption of the collagen fiber network. Inflammation of the articular tissue does not occur due to the unvascularized surface. For inflammation to occur, a fundamental arthropathic change must occur, such as the proliferation of inflamed synovial membrane into the articular tissue or the exposure of innervated and vascularized osseous tissue (De Bont et al., 1985).

Osteoarthrosis is a common condition that progresses with age and affects more women than men (Davis, 1981). Osteoarthrosis is insidious in onset, usually not associated with systemic disease, but perhaps initiated through repetitive loading or a variety of factors that occur over a lifetime. The inflammation that occurs in osteoarthritis requires an innervated and vascular surface. This suggests that the adaptive remodeling that continues has been overwhelmed and the tissues

below the fibroconnective tissue surface are exposed, allowing the inflammatory process to begin.

Muscle Disorders

The disorders that involve muscles may be independent of articular problems but are usually involved when joint dysfunction exists. Their involvement may be mild and produce minimal dysfunction or it may be severe and markedly disabling. When muscle pain problems occur, the treatment may differ depending on the subgroup defined below.

Myofascial pain syndromes, as classified by the International Association for the Study of Pain Subcommittee on Taxonomy (Mersky, 1986), may be found in any voluntary muscle and are characterized by trigger points (TPs), which may cause referred pain and local and referred tenderness (Clark et al., 1981; Moller, 1981). When "active," TPs are painful to palpation and spontaneously refer pain and autonomic symptoms to remote structures in reproducible patterns characteristic for each muscle (Travell and Simons, 1984). This referred pain is usually the presenting complaint. When "latent," TPs are still locally tender but do not produce referred phenomena. The pain quality is pressing, tightening, deep, aching, and often poorly circumscribed (Travell and Simons, 1984). It may be associated with swelling, numbness, and stiffness. Pain, although usually constant, may fluctuate in intensity and shift anatomical sites (Travell and Simons, 1984). Associated symptoms may include autonomic phenomena, most commonly reactive hyperemia or erythema, although photophobia and phonophobia have been described (Butler et al., 1975).

The primary complaint for myofascial pain is referred pain. The referral patterns often do not make neurologic sense. As an example, pain from a TP in the trapezius muscle, which is innervated by cranial nerve XI, may refer to the forehead, which is innervated by cranial nerve V.

Mens (1994) described a hypothesis for muscle pain referral to other deep somatic tissues remote from the site of the original muscle stimulation or lesion. He criticized the convergence–projection pain referral theory by pointing out that there is little convergence in the dorsal horns associated with deep tissues. This hypothesis adds two new components to the convergence–projection theory. First, the convergent connections from deep tissues to dorsal horn neurons are opened only after nociceptive inputs from muscle are activated. The connections that are opened after muscle stimulus are called silent connections. Second, the referral to muscle outside the initially activated site is due to spread of central sensitization to adjacent spinal segments. The initiating stimulus requires a peripheral inflammatory stimulus. In the animal model described by Mens (1994), the noxious stimulus was bradykinin injected into the muscle. It is unclear what triggers the muscle referral in the clinical setting, where there is usually no obvious inflammation-producing incident.

The theory of Mens (1994) was used by Simons (1994) to discuss a neurophysiologic basis for TP pain. Simons (1994) hypothesized that neurotransmitters are released in the dorsal horn (trigeminal nucleus) when the tender area in the muscle is palpated, resulting in opening of nociceptive inputs that were previously silent. This causes distant neurons to produce a retrograde referred pain. This model accounts for most of the clinical presentation and therapeutic options seen in myofascial pain, but it does not account for initiation of the peripheral tenderness, which must be present to activate the silent connections.

Fields and Heinricher (1989) described a means whereby the CNS may switch on nociception. They described the presence of "on" cells which, when stimulated, may activate trigeminal nucleus nociceptors. Olesen (1991) used the Fields and Heinricher (1989) model to describe a hypothesis for tension-type headache. This model described the interaction of three systems: the vascular system, the supraspinal system, and the myogenic system. The proposed hypothesis suggests that perceived headache pain is facilitated by the CNS, depending on inputs from either muscle or blood vessel. In migraine, the inputs are primarily vascular,

whereas in tension-type headache, the inputs are primarily muscular. This model helps explain why the clinical presentation and therapeutic options in migraine and tension-type headache are often similar, as well as why there is temporary relief with peripheral treatments, such as TP injections.

The resultant hyperalgesia or TP sensitivity may represent peripheral sensitization related to serum levels of serotonin, or 5-hydroxytryptamine (5-HT). Ernberg et al. (1999) and Alstergen et al. (1999) showed a significant correlation with serum 5-HT and allodynia associated with muscular face pain. In rheumatoid temporomandibular pain, serum 5-HT concentrations correlated with pain. There was no correlation with circulating serum levels of neuropeptide Y or interleukin-1B.

Patients who present with facial pain of no obvious etiology should be presumed to have myofascial pain. Myofascial pain can be reproduced by digitally palpating the muscles and confirmed with TP injections using 1 to 2 cc of 1% procaine.

Myofascial pain is treated by enhancing central inhibition with pharmacologic or behavioral techniques and simultaneously reducing peripheral inputs with physical therapies, including exercises and TP-specific therapy (Travell and Simons, 1986; Graff-Radford et al., 1987; Davidoff, 1998). Patients must be aware that the goal of therapy is to manage the pain and not to cure it. Patients must also be aware of the role they themselves play in managing the perpetuating factors (Graff-Radford et al., 1987; Davidoff, 1998).

DISCUSSION

Evaluation of orofacial pain must begin with an in-depth medical history, which should include the chief complaint and a narrative history of the complaint, as well as its progression and prior treatment. Not all chronic pain conditions require a psychologic evaluation. However, all pain, no matter what its etiology, is subject to behavioral and emotional factors. These behavioral issues should be considered, and a psychologic evaluation is suggested when there is any doubt of what part they play. The psychologic evaluation is not done to determine whether the pain is psychogenic but, rather, to select specific cognitive and behavioral strategies that may be useful in pain management. Once these data are gathered, a neurologic screening examination, TMJ examination, and myofascial palpation should be carried out. At this time, a differential diagnosis can be established and the specific tests outlined above can be used to narrow the diagnosis. This process permits appropriate diagnosis and effective treatment.

REFERENCES

Alstergen, P., M. Ernberg, S. Kopp et al. (1999). TMJ pain in relation to circulating neuropeptide Y, serotonin, and interleukin-1B in rheumatoid arthritis. *Orofac. Pain* 13:49–55.

André, N. (1756). *Traité sur les Maladies de l'Urethre*, pp. 323–343. Delaguette, Paris.

Bell, W.E. (1985). *Orofacial Pains: Classification, Diagnosis, Management*, 3rd ed. Year Book Medical Publishers, Chicago.

Bennett, G.J. and Y.K. Xie. (1988). A peripheral mononeuropathy in rat that produces disorders of pain sensation like those seen in man. *Pain* 33:87–107.

Bittar, G. and S.B. Graff-Radford (1992). A retrospective study of patients with cluster headache. *Oral Surg. Oral Med. Oral Pathol.* 73: 519–525.

Bittar, G. and S.B. Graff-Radford (1993). The effect of streptomycin/lidocaine block on trigeminal and traumatic neuralgia. *Headache* 33:155–160.

Blankestijn, J. and G. Boering (1985). Posterior dislocation of the temporomandibular disk. *Int. J. Oral Surg.* 14:437–443.

Boas, R.A., B.G. Covino, and A. Shahnarian (1982). Analgesic responses to i.v. lignocaine. *Br. J. Anaesth.* 54:501–504.

Brooke, R.I. (1978). Periodic migrainous neuralgia: A cause of dental pain. *Oral Med.* 46:511–516.

Bulitt, E., J.M. Tew, and J. Boyd (1986). Intracranial tumors with facial pain. *J. Neurosurg.* 64: 865–871.

Burchiel, K.J. (1987). Surgical treatment of trigeminal neuralgia: Minor and major operative procedures. In *The Medical and Surgical Management of Trigeminal Neuralgia* (G.H. Fromm, ed.), pp. 71–101. Futura, New York.

Butler, J.H., L.E.A. Golke, and C.L. Bandt (1975). A descriptive survey of signs and symptoms associated with the myofascial pain dysfunction syndrome. *J. Am. Dent. Assoc.* 90:635–639.

Campbell, J.N., R. A. Meyer, K.D. Davis et al. (1992). Sympathetically mediated pain, a unifying hypothesis. In *Hyperalgesia and Allodynia* (W.D. Willis, ed.), pp. 141–149. Raven Press, New York.

Campbell, R.L., K.W. Parks, and R.N. Dodds (1990). Chronic facial pain associated with endodontic neuropathy. *Oral Surg. Oral Med. Oral Pathol.* 69:287–290.

Clark, G.T., P.L. Beemsterboer, and J.D. Rugh (1981). Nocternal masseter muscle activity and the symptoms of masticatory dysfunction. *J. Oral. Rehabil.* 8:279.

Coyle, D.E., C.S. Selhorst, and M.M. Behbehani (1996). Intact female rats are more susceptible to the development of tactile allodynia than ovariectomized female rats following partial sciatic nerve ligation (PSNL). *Neurosci. Lett.* 203: 37–40.

Coyle, D.E., C.S. Sehlorst, and C. Mascari (1995). Female rats are more susceptible to the development of neuropathic pain using the partial sciatic nerve ligation (PSNL) model. *Neurosci. Lett.* 186:135–138.

Cueneo, H.M. and C.W. Rand (1952). Tumors of the gasserian ganglion. Tumor of the left gasserian ganglion associated with enlargement of the mandibular nerve. A review of the literature and case report. *J. Neurosurg.* 9:423–432.

Davidoff, R.A. (1998). Trigger points and myofascial pain: Toward understanding how they affect headaches. *Cephalalgia* 18:436–438.

Davis, M.A. (1981). Sex differences in reporting osteoarthritic symptoms: A sociomedical approach. *J. Health Soc. Behav.* 22:293.

De Bont, L.G.M., G. Boering, R.S.B. Liem et al. (1985). Osteoarthritis of the temporomandibular joint: A light microscopic and scanning electron microscopic study of the articular cartilage of the mandibular condyle. *J. Oral Maxillofac. Surg.* 43:481–488.

Delcanho, R.E. and S.B. Graff-Radford (1993). Chronic paroxysmal hemicrania presenting as toothache. *J. Orofac. Pain* 7:300–306.

Denny-Brown, D., R.D. Adams, and P.J. Fitzgerald. (1944). Pathologic features of herpes zoster: a note on "geniculate herpes." *Arch. Neurol. Psychiatry* 51:216–231.

Egermark-Eriksson, I., G.E. Carlsson, and B. Ingervall (1981). Prevalence of mandibular dysfunction and orofacial parafunction in 7-, 11-, and 15-year-old Swedish children. *Eur. J. Orthod.* 3:163–172.

Ellies, L.G. (1992). Altered sensation following mandibular implant surgery: A retrospective study. *J. Prosthet. Dent.* 68:664–667.

Ellies, L.G. and P.B. Hawker (1993). The prevalence of altered sensation associated with implant surgery. *Int. J. Oral Maxillofac. Implants* 8:674–679.

Ernberg, M., B. Hadenberg-Magnusson, P. Alstergren et al. (1999). Pain, allodynia, and serum serotonin level in orofacial pain of muscular origin. *J. Orofac. Pain* 13:56–62.

Farrar, W.B. (1972). Differentiation of temporomandibular joint dysfunction to simplify treatment. *J. Prosthet. Dent.* 28:629–636.

Fields, H.L. and M. Heinricher (1989). Brainstem modulation of nociceptor-driven withdrawal reflexes. *Ann. N. Y. Acad. Sci.* 563:34–44.

Fordyce, W.E. and J.C. Steger (1978). Chronic pain. In *Behavior Medicine Theory and Practice* (D.F. Pomerteau and J.P. Brady eds.), p. 125. Williams and Wilkins, Baltimore.

Fricton, J.R. (1999). Critical commentary. A unified concept of idiopathic orofacial pain: Clinical features. *J. Orofac. Pain* 13:185–189.

Fromm, G.H., S.B. Graff-Radford, C.F. Terrence et al. (1990). Can trigeminal neuralgia have a prodrome. *Neurology* 40:1493–1495.

Fromm, G.H. and B.J. Sessel (1991). *Trigeminal Neuralgia. Current Concepts Regarding Pathogenesis and Treatment*. Butterworth-Heinemann Boston.

Fromm, G.H., C.F. Terrence, and A.S. Chattha (1984). Baclofen in the treatment of trigeminal neuralgia: Double blind study and long term follow up. *Ann. Neurol.* 15:240–244.

Gardner, W.J. (1962). Concerning mechanisms of trigeminal neuralgia and hemifacial spasm. *J. Neurosurg.* 19:947–957.

Graff-Radford, S.B. (1995a). Orofacial pain. In *Orofacial Pain and Temporomandibular Disorders* (J. Friction and R. Dubner, eds.), pp. 215–241. Raven Press, New York.

Graff-Radford, S.B. (1995b). Orofacial pain of neurogenous origin. In *Temporomandibular Disorders and Orofacial Pain* (R.A. Pertes and S.G. Gross, eds.), pp. 329–341. Quintessence, Chicago.

Graff-Radford, S.B.. (2000a). Facial Pain. *Curr. Opin. Neurol.* 13:291–296.

Graff-Radford, S.B. (2000b). SUNCT syndrome responsive to Gapbapentin (Neurontin). *Cephalalgia* 20:515–517.

Graff-Radford, S.B. L. Shaw, and B.N. Naliboff (2000c). Effects of fluphenazine and amitriptyline on postherpetic neuralgia. *Clinical J. Pain* 16:188–192.

Graff-Radford, S.B., B. Jaeger, and J.L. Reeves (1986). Myofascial pain may present clinically as occipital neuralgia. *Neurosurgery* 19:610–613.

Graff-Radford, S.B., M.-C., Ketelaer, B.M. Gratt et al. (1995). Thermographic assessment of neuropathic facial pain. *J. Orofac. Pain* 9:138–146.

Graff-Radford, S.B., J.L. Reeves, and B. Jaeger (1987). Management of headache: The effectiveness of altering factors perpetuating myofascial pain. *Headache* 27:186–190.

Graff-Radford, S.B., M. Simmons, L. Fox et al. (1988b). Are bony cavities exclusively associated with atypical facial pain or trigeminal neuralgia [abstract]? *Proc. West. USA Pain Soc.*

Head, H. and A.W. Campbell (1900). The pathology of herpes zoster. *Brain* 23:353–523.

Headache Classification Committee of the International Headache Society (1988). Classification and diagnostic criteria for headache disorders, cranial neuralgias, and facial pain. *Cephalalgia* 8:1–96.

Ireland, V.E. (1953). The problem of the clicking jaw. *J. Prosthet. Dent.* 3:200–212.

Janetta, P.J. (1996). Trigeminal neuralgia: Treatment by microvascular decompression. In *Neurosurgery* (R.H. Wilkins and S.S. Ragachary, eds.), pp. 3961–3968. McGraw-Hill, New York.

Janetta, P.J. (1977). Observation on the etiology of trigeminal neuralgia, hemifacial spasm, acoustic nerve dysfunction and glossopharyngeal neuralgia. Definitive microsurgical treatment and results in 117 patients. *Neurochirurgia* 20:145–154.

Jarrahy, R., G. Berci, and H.K. Shahinian (2000). Endoscopic-assisted microvascular decompression of the trigeminal nerve. *Otolaryngol. Head Neck Surg.* 123:218–223.

Karnes, W.E. (1984). Diseases of the seventh cranial nerve. In *Peripheral Neuropathy*, 2nd ed. (P.J. Dyke, P.K. Thomas, J.W. Griffin et al., eds.), pp. 1266–1299. W.B. Saunders, Philadelphia.

Lechin, F., B. Van der Dijs, M.E. Lechin et al. (1989). Pimozide therapy for trigeminal neuralgia. *Arch. Neurol.* 46:960–963.

Loeser, J.D. (1986). Herpes zoster and postherpetic neuralgia. *Pain* 25:149–164.

Lovshin, L.L. (1960). Vascular neck pain—a common syndrome seldom recognized: Analysis of 100 consecutive cases. *Cleve. Clin. Q.* 27:5–13.

Massey, E.W. and J. Massey (1979). Elongated styloid process (Eagle's syndrome) causing hemicrania. *Headache* 19:339–341.

Max, M.B., S.C. Schafer, M. Culnane et al. (1988). Amitriptyline, but not lorazepam, relieves post herpetic neuralgia. *Neurology* 38:1427–1432.

Mens, S. (1994). Referral of muscle pain new aspects. *Pain Forum* 3:1–9.

Merrill, R.L. and S.B. Graff-Radford (1992) Trigeminal neuralgia: How to rule out the wrong treatment. *J. Am. Dent. Assoc.* 123:63–68.

Mersky, H. (ed.) (1986). Classification of chronic pain: Description of chronic pain syndromes and definition of terms. *Pain* (Suppl. 3):S1.

Mitchell, R.G. (1980). Pretrigeminal neuralgia. *Br. Dent. J.* 149:167–170.

Moffett, B.C., L.C. Johnson, and J.B. McCabe (1964). Articular remodeling in the adult human temporomandibular joint. *Am. J. Anat. 115*: 119–130.

Molin, L. (1969). Aspects of the natural history of herpes zoster. *Acta Derm. Venereol.* 49:569–583.

Moller, E. (1981). The myogenic factor in headache and facial pain. In *Oral-facial Sensory and Motor Function* (Y. Kawamura and R. Dubner, eds.), p. 225. Quintessence, Tokyo.

Moncada, E. and S.B. Graff-Radford (1993). Cough headache presenting as toothache. *Headache* 33:240–243.

Moskowitz, M.A., B.M. Henrikson, S. Markowitz et al. (1988). Intra- and extravascular nociceptive mechanisms and the pathogenesis of head pain. In *Basic Mechanisms of Headache* (J. Olsen and L. Edvinsson, eds.), p. 429. Elsevier, Amsterdam.

Olesen, J. (1991). Clinical and pathophysiological observations in migraine and tension type headache explained by integration of vascular, supraspinal and myofascial inputs. *Pain* 46:125–132.

Raskin, N.H. (1988). *Headache*, 2nd ed. Churchill Livingstone, New York.

Raskin, N.H. and S. Prusiner (1977). Carotidynia. *Neurology* 27:43–46.

Ratner, E.J., P. Person, and D.J. Kleinman (1976). Oral pathology and trigeminal neuralgia. I Clinical experiences [abstract]. *J. Dent. Res. 55*: B299.

Ratner, E.J., P. Person, D.J. Kleinmann et al. (1979). Jawbone cavities and trigeminal and atypical facial neuralgias. *Oral Surg.* 48:3–20.

Ren, K. and R. Dubner (1999). Central nervous system plasticity and persistent pain. *J. Orofac. Pain* 13:155–163.

Roberts, A.M., P. Person, N.B. Chandran et al. (1984). Further observations on dental parameters of trigeminal and atypical facial neuralgias. *Oral Surg.* 58:121–129.

Roberts, W.J. and M.E. Foglesong (1988). Identification of afferents contributing to sympathetically evoked activity in wide-dynamic-range neurons. *Pain* 34:305–314.

Rooke, E.D. (1968). Benign exertional headache. *Med. Clin. North Am.* 52:801–808.

Rowbotham, M.C., L.A. Reisner-Keller, and H.L. Fields (1991). Both intravenous lidocaine and morphine reduce the pain of postherpetic neuralgia. *Neurology* 41:1024–1028.

Rushton, J.G. and E.D. Rooke (1962). Brain tumor headache. *Headache* 2:147–152.

Schisano, G. and H. Olivercrona (1960). Neuromas of the gasserian ganglion and trigeminal root. *J. Neurosurg.* 17:306.

Scrivani, S.J., A. Chaudry, R.J. Maciewicz et al. (1999). Chronic Neurogenic facial pain: Lack of response to intravenous phentolamine. *J Orofac. Pain* 13:89–96.

Simons, D.G. (1994). Neurophysiological basis of

pain caused by trigger points. *American Pain Society J.* 3:17–19.

Sinnott, C.J., J.M. Garfield, and G.R. Strichartz (1999) Differential efficacy of intravenous lidocaine in alleviating ipsilateral versus contralateral neuropathic pain in the rat. *Pain* 80:521–531.

Sjaastad, O., C. Saunte, R. Salvesen et al. (1989). Short lasting, unilateral neuralgia-form headache attacks with conjunctival injection, tearing, sweating and rhinorrhea. *Cephalalgia* 9:147–156.

Sjaastad, O., M. Vhaoj, P. Krusvewski et al. (1991). Short lasting unilateral neuralgia-form headache attacks with conjunctival injection, tearing, etc. (SUNCT): 3. Another Norwegian case. *Headache* 31:175–177.

Sjaastad, O., D. Russell, J. Horven, and U. Bunaes (1978). Multiple neuralgia-form unilateral headache attacks associated with conjunctival injection and tearing and clusters. Nosological problem. Proceedings of the Scandinavian Migraine Society, 31.

Sokolovic, M., L. Todorovic, Z. Stajcic et al. (1986). Peripheral streptomycin/lidocaine injections in the treatment of idiopathic trigeminal neuralgia. *J. Maxillofac. Surg.* 14:8–9.

Solberg, W.K. (1986). Masticatory myalgia and its management. *Br. Dent. J.* 160:351.

Solberg, W.K., and S.B. Graff-Radford (1988). Orodental considerations of facial pain. *Semin. Neurol.* 8:318–323.

Solberg, W.K., T.L. Hansson, and B.N. Nordstrom (1985). The temporomandibular joint in young adults at autopsy: A morphologic classification and evaluation. *J. Oral Rehabil.* 12:303–321.

Solberg, W.K., M.S. Woo, and J.B. Huston (1979). Prevalence of mandibular dysfunction in young adults. *J. Am. Dent. Assoc.* 98:25–34.

Symonds, C. (1956). Cough headache. *Brain 79*: 557–568.

Symonds, C. (1949). Facial pain. *Ann. R. Coll. Surg. Engl.* 4:206–212.

Taarnhoj, P. (1982). Decompression of the posterior trigeminal root in trigeminal neuralgia: A 30 year follow-up review. *J. Neurosurg.* 57:14–17.

Taub, A. (1973). Relief of postherpetic neuralgia with psychotropic drugs. *J. Neurosurg.* 39:235–239.

Tourne, L.P.M. and J.R. Fricton (1992). Burning mouth syndrome: Critical review and proposed clinical management. *Oral Surg. Oral Med. Oral Pathol.* 74:158–167.

Travell, J. and D.G. Simons (1984). *Myofascial Pain and Dysfunction. The Trigger Point Manual*. Williams and Wilkins, Baltimore.

Vickers, R.E., M.J. Cousins, S. Walker et al. (1998). Analysis of 50 patients with atypical odontalgia. A preliminary report on pharmacologic procedures for diagnosis and treatment.

Oral Surg. Oral Med. Oral Pathol. Oral Radiol. Endod. 85:24–32.

Walker, A.E. (1966). Neuralgias of the glossopharyngeal, vagus and nervous intermedius nerves. In *Pain* (P.R. Knighton and P.R. Dumke, eds.), pp. 421–429. Little Brown, Boston.

Watson, P.N. and R.J. Evans (1986). Postherpetic neuralgia: A review. *Arch. Neurol.* 43:836–840.

Woda, A., M.-L. Navez, P. Picard et al. (1998). A possible therapeutic solution for stomatodynia (burning mouth syndrome). *J. Orofac. Pain* 12: 272–278.

Young, R.F., S. Vermeulen, P. Grimm et al. (1997). Gamma knife radiosurgery for treatment of trigeminal neuralgia. Idiopathic and tumor related. *Neurology* 48:608–614.

22

Nasal Disease and Sinus Headache

STEPHEN D. SILBERSTEIN
THOMAS O. WILLCOX

Although sinus infections are much less common today than they were in the preantibiotic era, they are frequently overdiagnosed. Caldwell (1893) noted a functional relationship between the ostia of the sinuses and the development of sinusitis. Hajek (1926) emphasized that ostial stenosis was responsible for sinusitis. Hilding (1950) and Messerklinger (1978) demonstrated that ethmoid sinusitis is frequently a cause of frontal and maxillary sinusitis. Obstruction of the ostiomeatal complex, the common drainage pathway for the ethmoid, frontal, and maxillary sinuses, was later demonstrated to be involved in the development of sinus disease (McCaffrey, 1993).

EPIDEMIOLOGY

Sinusitis, which affects more than 31 million people in the United States, resulted in 16 million physician visits in 1989 (Moss and Parsons, 1986); by 1994, the National Health Interview Survey estimated that 35 million people were affected (Agency for Healthcare Policy and Research, 1999). A national health interview survey conducted in the United States between 1990 and 1992 found that chronic sinusitis was the second most frequent disease after orthopedic deformities, with an annual average of 33.1 million cases (Collins, 1997). The prevalence of acute sinusitis is increasing, according to data from the National Ambulatory Medical Care Survey, from 0.2% of diagnoses at office visits in 1990 to 0.4% of diagnoses at office visits in 1995 (Agency for Healthcare Policy and Research, 1999). About 0.5% of upper respiratory tract infections in adults are complicated by sinusitis (Diaz and Bamberger, 1995). Up to 38% of patients with symptoms of sinusitis in adult general medicine clinics may have acute bacterial rhinosinusitis. In otolaryngology practices, the prevalence was higher (50% to 80%). While sinusitis is generally more common in children than adults, frontal and sphenoid sinusitis are rare in children. Between 6% and 18% of children in the primary-care setting presenting with upper respiratory tract infections may have acute bacterial sinusitis (Agency for Healthcare Policy and Research, 1999). In the preantibiotic era, the sphenoid sinus was involved in up to 33% of cases of sinusitis. Today, its incidence is about 3% (Lew et al., 1983).

Overall health-care expenditures attributable to sinusitis in 1996 were estimated at $5.8 billion, of which $1.8 billion (30.6%) was for children 12 years or younger. A primary diagnosis of acute or chronic sinusitis accounted for 58.7% of all expenditures ($3.5 billion). About 12% each of the costs for asthma, chronic otitis media, and eustachian tube disorders were attributed to diagnosing and treating comorbid sinusitis. Nearly 90% of all expenditures ($5.1 billion) were associated with ambulatory or emergency department services (Ray et al., 1999). It is estimated that over $200 million is spent annually on cold and sinus prescription products; this does not include over-the-counter medications (Josephson and Gross, 1997).

ANATOMY AND DEVELOPMENT

The lateral nasal wall is composed of the ethmoid bone, a T-shaped structure that supports the ethmoid labyrinth. The horizontal limb of the T is formed by the cribriform plate, from which is suspended the ethmoid labyrinth, a complex structure with multiple bony septa and the medial projections of the superior and middle turbinates. Lateral to the uncinate process, a secondary projection of the ethmoid bone, is the infundibulum, a recess into which the maxillary sinus drains via the natural ostium. The frontal sinus drains into the frontal recess, which may drain into the middle meatus or the ethmoidal infundibulum. This region is known as the ostiomeatal complex (maxillary sinus ostium, infundibulum, hiatus semilunaris, middle turbinate, ethmoidal bulla, and frontal ostium) (McCaffrey, 1993). The sphenoidal sinus and posterior ethmoidal cells drain into the sphenoethmoidal recess (Fig. 22–1).

The sphenoid sinus is contained within the body of the sphenoid bone deep in the nasal cavity and is divided into two chambers by the intersphenoidal septum. Each sinus communicates with the sphenoethmoidal recess, located medial to the posterior superior aspect of the superior concha. The roof of the sphenoid sinus is related to the middle cranial fossa and the pituitary gland in the sella turcica; laterally is the cavernous sinus; posteriorly is the clivus and pons; anteriorly the posterior nasal cavity, posterior ethmoid cells, and cribriform plate; and inferiorly the na-

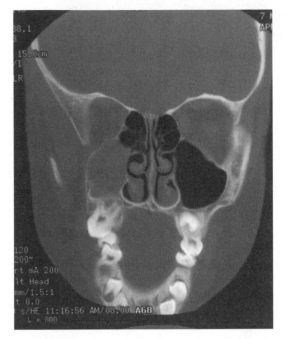

Figure 22–1 Coronal computed tomographic scan of the sinuses, demonstrating normal left-sided anatomy and right maxillary sinus opacification.

sopharynx. The cavernous sinus, which is lateral to the sphenoid sinus, contains the internal carotid arteries and the third, fourth, fifth, and sixth cranial nerves. The maxillary division of the fifth nerve may indent the wall of the sphenoid sinus. The sphenoid walls can be extremely thin, and sometimes the sinus cavity is separated from the adjacent structure by just a thin mucosal barrier. Because of the close proximity to the cortical venous system, cranial nerves, and meninges, infection may spread to these structures and present as a central nervous system infection or neurologic catastrophe (Lew et al., 1983; Sofferman, 1983).

The maxillary and ethmoid sinuses, both present at birth, are the most common sites of clinical infection in children. The sphenoidal sinuses are present as minute cavities at birth, and it is not until puberty that their main development occurs (Goss, 1959). The frontal sinus begins to develop from the anterior ethmoid sinus at about 6 years of age and continues to pneumatize into the late teens. Hypoplasia or aplasia of one or both

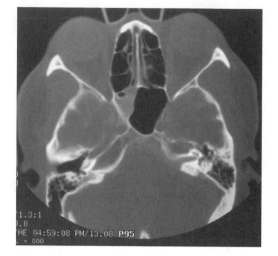

Figure 22–2 Axial computed tomographic scan of the sinuses, demonstrating isolated right sinusitis.

frontal sinuses has been reported to be between 2% and 20% (Lang, 1989), but true agenesis is rare (Schaefer, 1990). The frontal and sphenoid sinuses become clinically important in the teens and frequently become infected in pansinusitis. Isolated sphenoid sinusitis is rare (Reilly, 1990; Kennedy, 1990b) (Fig. 22–2).

PHYSIOLOGY

The primary functions of the nasal passages are humidification, warming, and removal of particulate material from the inspired air. The paranasal sinuses are air-filled cavities that communicate with the nasal airway. They are lined with pseudostratified, ciliated epithelium, which is covered by a thin layer of mucus that receives the largest deposits of inhaled large-particulate matter. The cilia and this mucous layer are in constant motion in a predetermined direction. Mucus and debris are transported toward the ostia by the beating of the cilia and are expelled into the nasal airway (Reilly, 1990; Zinreich, 1990; McCaffrey, 1993). This process is termed mucociliary clearance.

Bacterial contamination of the sinuses is effectively cleared by mucociliary clearance. If the sinus ostia are obstructed, mucociliary

flow is interrupted. Obstruction causes the oxygen tension within the sinus to decrease and the carbon dioxide tension to increase. This anaerobic, high-carbon dioxide, stagnant environment can facilitate bacterial growth (McCaffrey, 1993). Unobstructed flow through the sinus ostia and its narrow communicating passage within the ostiomeatal complex is integral to mucociliary clearance and sinus ventilation. Persistent low-grade inflammation in the ethmoid sinus may cause few localizing symptoms but can predispose to recurrent maxillary and frontal sinus infections (Reilly, 1990; McCaffrey, 1993).

Surgical drainage of the sinuses, avoiding the region of the natural ostia, was the treatment of choice for sinus infections for many years. This procedure alleviated the acute sinus infection but did not prevent reaccumulation of mucus within the sinus. Because the normal mucociliary clearance transports mucus toward the natural ostia, creating a new ostium at a site distant from the natural ostium fails to direct the flow of mucus to the new opening (McCaffrey, 1993).

Wolff (1948) showed that the sinuses themselves are relatively insensitive to pain. McAuliffe and associates (1943), using touch, pressure, and faradic stimulation, found that the nasal turbinates and sinus ostia were much more sensitive than the mucosal lining of the septum and the paranasal sinuses. Most of the pain elicited was referred. It was of increased intensity, longer duration, and referred to larger areas in subjects with swelling and engorgement of the nasal turbinates and the sinus ostia. Thus, the pain associated with sinusitis comes from engorged and inflamed nasal structures: nasofrontal ducts, turbinates, ostia, and superior nasal spaces.

All sinuses normally contain anaerobic bacteria, and more than one-third harbor both anaerobic and aerobic organisms. Ciliary dysfunction and retention of secretions, commonly a result of ostia obstruction, are necessary for bacterial proliferation and the development of sinus infection. Aerobes present in both normal and disease states include the gram-positive streptococci (alpha, 13, and *Streptococcus pneumoniae*) and *Staphylococcus aureus*, and the gram-negative *Moraxella catarrhalis*, *Haemophilus influenzae*, and *Escherichia coli*. Anaerobic organisms include the gram-positive *Peptococcus* and *Propionibacterium* species. The *Bacteroides* and *Fusobacterium* species also play a role in chronic sinusitis (Reilly, 1990; Kennedy, 1990a). *Streptococcus pneumoniae*, *H. influenzae*, and *M. catarrhalis* (Van Cauwenberge et al., 1997) cause most adult cases of acute maxillary sinusitis. While *S. aureus* is an infrequent cause of maxillary and ethmoid sinusitis, it is the major cause of acute sphenoid and frontal sinusitis. Sinusitis of dental origin is commonly due to mixed anaerobic infection with *Bacteroides* and anaerobic streptococcus (Diaz and Bamberger, 1995). Systemic diseases that predispose to sinusitis include cystic fibrosis (with impaired mucus production), immune deficiency, bronchiectasis, and immobile cilia syndrome (with impaired mucus transport). In one study, patients with recurrent sinusitis were unable to produce secretions with high concentrations of antimicrobial factors in response to cholinergic stimulation (Jeney et al., 1990). In purulent secretions of patients with sinusitis, the concentrations of immunoglobulin A (IgA), IgG, and IgM are decreased (Engquist et al., 1983). Local factors include upper respiratory tract infection (usually viral), allergic rhinitis, overuse of topical decongestants, hypertrophied adenoids, deviated nasal septum, nasal polyps, tumors, and cigarette smoke (Reilly, 1990). The most common predisposing factor is mucosal inflammation from viral upper respiratory tract infection or allergic rhinitis (Diaz and Bamberger, 1995). The sinuses are involved in nearly 90% of viral upper respiratory tract infections. In patients with a common cold and no previous history of rhinosinusitis, 87% had maxillary sinus abnormalities, 65% had ethmoid sinus abnormalities, and 30% to 40% had frontal or sphenoid sinus abnormalities on computed tomography (CT). The abnormalities are most likely due to highly viscid secretions in the sinuses. In 77% of patients, the infundibulum was occluded. In most patients, these abnormalities resolved spontaneously, but some developed secondary bacterial infections (Gwaltney et al., 1994). Foreign bodies are a common cause of ob-

struction in children, and 10% of sinus infections are of dental origin (Diaz and Bamberger, 1995). Loss of immunocompetence due to human immunodeficiency virus (HIV) infection, chemotherapy, post-transplant immunosuppression, insulin-dependent diabetes mellitus, and some connective tissue disorders predisposes patients to rhinosinusitis and increases the likelihood of its persistence. Rhinosinusitis is common in the intensive care unit (ICU) since prolonged supine positioning compromises mucociliary clearance and adds to the problems created by mucosal drying from transnasal supplemental oxygenation and sinus ostial obstruction from nasotracheal or nasogastric tubes. Rhinosinusitis occurred in 95.5% of bedridden ICU patients who had a nasogastric or nasotracheal tube in place for at least a week (Rouby et al., 1994).

Patients who are HIV-positive and deficient in both cell-mediated and humoral immunity are more susceptible to bacterial infection. Sinusitis occurs in 75% of those with acquired immunodeficiency syndrome (AIDS) and is often extensive and difficult to treat, especially if the CD4 count is less than 200/mm^3. As in HIV-negative patients, the ethmoid and maxillary sinuses are predominantly involved (Evans, 1998).

DIAGNOSTIC TESTING

The physical examination may not be helpful, particularly in sphenoid sinusitis. Not all patients are febrile, and sinus tenderness is not always present. Pus is not always seen in sphenoid sinusitis. Kibblewhite and associates (1988) found purulent exudate in only 3 of 14 patients. Transillumination of the sinuses has low sensitivity and specificity (Stafford, 1990), and routine anterior rhinoscopy performed with a headlight and nasal speculum allows only limited inspection of the anterior nasal cavity.

Standard Radiography

Standard radiography is inadequate for the evaluation of sinusitis as it does not evaluate the anterior ethmoid air cells, the upper two-thirds of the nasal cavity, or the infundibular, middle meatus, and frontal recess air passages (Zinreich, 1990). However, in a high-risk group of 300 patients with a clinical diagnosis of sinusitis, 68% had abnormal plain radiographs but none had sphenoid sinus abnormalities (Axelsson and Jensen, 1974).

Neuroimaging

The optimal radiographic study to accurately assess all of the paranasal sinuses for evidence of disease is CT. The mucosa of the normal noninfected sinus approximates the bone so closely that it cannot be visualized on CT. Therefore, any soft tissue seen within a sinus is abnormal (Schatz and Becker, 1984). Mucosal thickening, sclerosis, clouding, or air-fluid levels may be demonstrated. Imaging must be performed in the coronal plane to adequately demonstrate the ethmoid complex. It can reveal the extent of mucosal disease in the ostiomeatal complex. The test–retest reliability of CT in the assessment of chronic rhinosinusitis was high and stable in a prospective series of patients scheduled for endoscopic sinus surgery (Bhattacharyya, 1999). The prevalence of reversible sinus abnormalities on CT in patients with the common cold is high (Gwaltney et al., 1994). This suggests that CT may not be specific for bacterial infections (Diaz and Bamberger, 1995) (Fig. 22–3).

The appearance of normal nasal mucosa during the edematous phase of the nasal cycle in MRI scans (T2-weighted images) can resemble pathologic changes. Despite these problems with specificity, MRI is more sensitive than CT at detecting fungal infection (Zinreich, 1990). Maxillary mucosal thickening >6 mm, complete sinus opacification, and air-fluid levels on neuroimaging correlate to positive sinus cultures (Druce and Siavin, 1991). However, 30% to 40% of the normal population will exhibit mucosal thickening on CT evaluation (Havas et al., 1988). The Agency for Healthcare Policy and Research (1999) meta-analysis of six studies showed that sinus radiography has moderate sensitivity (76%) and specificity (79%) compared

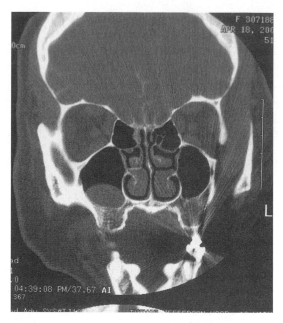

Figure 22–3 Coronal computed tomographic scan of the sinuses, demonstrating normal left-sided anatomy and right maxillary sinus soft tissue. The soft tissue may be mistaken for infection, but it represents a mucous retention cyst.

with sinus puncture in the diagnosis of acute bacterial rhinosinusitis.

Either CT or MRI is necessary to definitively diagnose sphenoid sinusitis because plain x-rays are nondiagnostic in about 26% of cases (Goldman et al., 1993). The gold standard for the diagnosis of sphenoid sinus disease is CT scanning; MRI is an adjunct. Lawson and Reino (1997) devised a system to categorize CT findings, which might better define the role of MRI. Type I findings are consistent with inflammatory lesions, such as acute and chronic sinusitis, as well as mucous retention cysts, polyps, and mucoceles, which do not routinely necessitate MRI. In acute sinusitis, an air-fluid level is present within the sinus cavity. With chronic disease, the cavity is partially or totally opacified by hypertrophic mucosa and secretions. A globular opacity partially filling the cavity generally represents a mucous retention cyst or polyp, similar to those present in the other paranasal sinuses. A superior or laterally based "polypoid" mass in the sphenoid sinus may represent such rare entities as an encephalocele or an internal carotid artery aneurysm (Lawson and Reino, 1997) (Fig. 22–4).

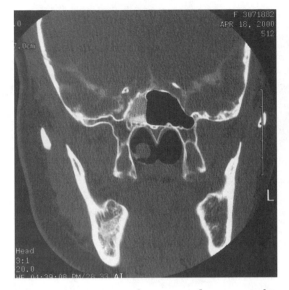

Figure 22–4 Coronal computed tomographic cysternogram of the sinuses, demonstrating contrast enhancement wihin the right sphenoid sinus secondary to a spontaneous atraumatic encephalocele.

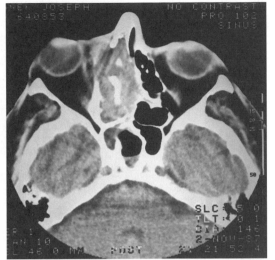

Figure 22–5 Soft-tissue window axial computed tomographic scan of the sinuses, demonstrating a right-sided inverting papilloma that is expanding the ethmoid labyrinth.

Type II findings include lesions that cause anatomic distortion of a sinus wall (i.e., thinning, expansion, or remodeling). Magnetic resonance imaging helps to differentiate between mucoceles and benign tumors. On MRI, a mucocele demonstrates a homogeneous, low signal intensity in the T1-weighted phase. A long-standing mucocele produces higher signal intensity in the T1-weighted and proton density images because of the concentration of proteinaceous secretions with loss of water. The T2-weighted signal remains high in most lesions until the protein concentration reaches 25% to 35%, which causes a decrease, first, in the T2-weighted signals, then in the T1-weighted signals. Tumors that are highly cellular show intermediate signal intensity in the T1-weighted phase, proton density images, and T2-weighted phase. With increased stromal components, the signal intensity becomes brighter and nonhomogeneous in the T2-weighted phase (Lawson and Reino, 1997) (Fig. 22–5).

Type III findings consist of total sinus opacification with sclerosis of the surrounding bone. If a mycetoma is suspected, fungal sinusitis may be diagnosed on MRI by demonstration of a signal void in the sinus cavity,

as opposed to the mixed signal pattern found in the cavity with fibro-osseous disorders (Lawson and Reino, 1997) (Fig. 22–6).

In type IV lesions, there is evidence of bone erosion. It is necessary to obtain information via MRI about the nature of the lesion and whether extrasinus extension is present. While most of these lesions are neoplastic, a mucocele may occasionally produce localized areas of bone destruction (7.89% of cases) (Lawson and Reino, 1997) (Fig. 22–7).

With type V findings there is perisinuous extension. The MRI delineates the extent of intracranial and skull base involvement. Bone erosion and extrasinal extension are hallmarks of malignant tumors (Fig. 22–8).

A-Mode Ultrasound

Although an A-mode ultrasound scan can demonstrate the presence of fluid or thickened mucosa in a sinus, operator experience plays a significant part and false-positive examinations are common. Ultrasound scans, similar to transillumination, are usually limited to frontal and antral disease and are most commonly used to follow the response to pharmacotherapy of a rhinosinusitis documented by nasal endoscopy or CT (Evans, 1994; Fergusen and Mabry, 1997; Wagner,

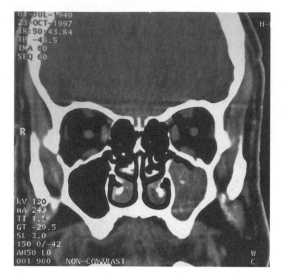

Figure 22–6 Soft-tissue window coronal computed tomographic scan of the sinus, demonstrating an aspergilloma (fungus ball) of the left maxillary antrum. There is heterogeneity of the soft tissue and thickening of the surrounding bone.

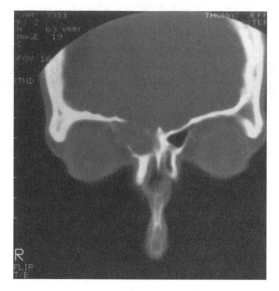

Figure 22–7 Coronal computed tomographic scan of the sinuses, demonstrating a right frontal mucocele with thinning of the floor of the anterior cranial fossa.

1996; Williams et al., 1992). Studies comparing sinus ultrasonography with puncture or sinus radiography were inconclusive in determining how well ultrasonography identifies patients with acute bacterial rhinosinusitis. The results of ultrasonography varied substantially, possibly because of differences in patient populations, ultrasonography techniques, or the medical personnel involved in diagnostic testing (Agency for Healthcare Policy and Research, 1999). Ultrasonography has lower sensitivity and specificity than sinus x-rays (Stafford, 1990).

Diagnostic Fiberoptic Nasal Endoscopy

Diagnostic endoscopy with rigid or flexible fiberoptic rhinoscopy allows direct visualization of the nasal passages and sinus drainage areas (ostiomeatal complex) and is complementary to CT or MRI. Infection is easily diagnosed if purulent material is seen emanating from the sinus drainage region. Mucosal sinus thickening is frequently present in normal, asymptomatic patients. In these cases, endoscopy should be positive before a diagnosis of sinusitis can be made (Kennedy, 1990b;

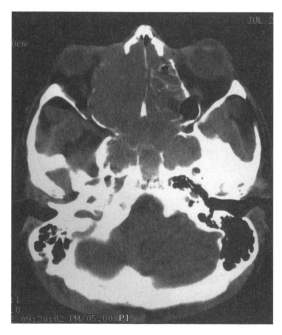

Figure 22–8 Soft-tissue axial window computed tomographic scan of the sinuses, demonstrating a poorly differentiated sinonasal carcinoma that has eroded much of the ethmoid labyrinth. There is also intracranial erosion of the coronal views.

McCaffrey, 1993). Sphenoid sinusitis is an exception to this generalization.

Nasal endoscopy should be considered when a sinus-related problem is suspected in a patient who fails to respond to conservative medical treatment and whose CT or MRI is inconclusive. Some use nasal endoscopy prior to neuroimaging. The combination of negative neuroimaging and nasal endoscopy usually, but not always, rules out sinus disease (Zinreich, 1990).

CLINICAL MANIFESTATIONS

In 1996, the American Academy of Otolaryngology–Head and Neck Surgery standardized the terminology for paranasal infections (Benninger et al., 1997). The term "rhinosinusitis" was felt to be more appropriate than "sinusitis" since rhinitis typically precedes sinusitis, purulent sinusitis without rhinitis is rare, the mucosa of the nose and sinuses are contiguous, and symptoms of nasal obstruction and discharge are prominent in sinusitis (Slavin, 1997). The diagnosis of rhinosinusitis is usually based on symptoms indicating maxillary or frontal sinus involvement. This may occur secondary to, and is frequently a result of, ethmoid disease. Obstruction of the sinus ostia is the usual precursor of sinusitis (Zinreich, 1990; Zinreich et al., 1987).

Rhinosinusitis is divided into four categories based on the temporal course and the signs and symptoms of the disease (Table 22–1) (Lanza and Kennedy, 1997). *Acute rhinosinusitis* is sudden in onset and lasts from 1 day to 4 weeks, with complete resolution of the symptoms. *Subacute rhinosinusitis* is continuous with acute rhinosinusitis and lasts from 4 to 12 weeks (Lanza and Kennedy, 1997). *Recurrent acute rhinosinusitis* requires four or more episodes of acute rhinosinusitis, lasting at least 7 days each, in any 1-year period. *Chronic rhinosinusitis* requires that signs or symptoms persist for 12 weeks or longer and may be punctuated by acute infectious episodes.

Facial tenderness and pain, nasal congestion, and purulent nasal discharge are common manifestations of acute sinus infection.

Other "classic" signs and symptoms include anosmia, pain upon mastication, and halitosis. An upper respiratory tract infection or a history of an upper respiratory tract infection is often present (Stafford, 1990). While fever is present in about 50% of adults and 60% of children and headache is common, the symptoms of headache, facial pain, and fever are often of minimal value in the diagnosis of sinusitis. Williams and associates (1992) looked at the sensitivity and specificity of individual symptoms in making the diagnosis of sinusitis. No single item was both sensitive and specific. Maxillary toothache was highly specific (93%), but only 11% of the patients had this symptom. Logistic regression analysis showed five independent predictions of sinusitis: maxillary toothache (odds ratio = 2.9), abnormal transillumination (odds ratio = 2.7, sensitivity 73%, specificity 54%), poor response to decongestants (odds ratio = 2.4), purulent discharge (odds ratio = 2.9), and colored nasal discharge (odds ratio = 2.2). Headache had an odds ratio of 1.0, with a 68% sensitivity and 30% specificity. The low specificity is due to lack of descriptive features of the headache. One proposed classification system is based on major and minor clinical criteria. The major symptoms are purulent anterior or posterior nasal discharge, nasal congestion, facial pain or pressure, and fever. Minor symptoms are cough, headache (not otherwise specified), halitosis, and earache (Shapiro and Rachelefsky, 1992). A diagnosis using these criteria requires two major criteria or one major and two minor criteria. However, none of these criteria alone is both sensitive and specific enough for diagnosis. It has been suggested that highly specific symptoms, such as facial erythema or maxillary toothache or symptoms that persist for more than 10 days warrant a diagnosis and treatment (International Rhinosinusitis Advisory Board, 1997). The Agency for Healthcare Policy and Research (1999) evidence report, based on limited evidence, suggested that clinical criteria (i.e., the presence of three or four of the following symptoms: purulent rhinorrhea with unilateral predominance, local pain with unilateral predominance, bilateral purulent rhinorrhea, and the presence of pus

Table 22–1 Classification of adult rhinosinusitis

Classification	Duration	Strong history	Include in differential	Special Notes
Acute	≤4 weeks	≥2 major factors, 1 major factor and 2 minor factors, or nasal purulence on examination	1 major factor or ≥2 minor factors	Fever or facial pain does not constitute a suggestive history in the absence of other nasal signs or symptoms; consider acute bacterial rhinosinusitis if symptoms worsen after 5 days, persist for >10 days, or are out of proportion to those typically associated with viral infection
Subacute	4–12 weeks	Same as chronic	Same as chronic	Complete resolution after effective medical therapy
Recurrent acute	≥4 episodes/year, with each episode lasting ≥7–10 days and no intervening signs or symptoms of chronic rhinosinusitis	Same as acute		
Chronic	≥12 weeks	≥2 major factors, 1 major factor and 2 minor factors, or nasal purulence on examination	1 major factor or ≥2 minor factors	Facial pain does not constitute a suggestive history in the absence of other nasal signs or symptoms
Acute exacerbations of chronic	Sudden worsening of chronic rhinosinusitis, with return to baseline after treatment			

in the nasal cavity) may have a diagnostic accuracy similar to that of sinus radiography.

Children with acute and chronic sinusitis almost always present with purulent nasal discharge, which is not characteristic in adults. Fever is infrequent even with acute sinusitis and is usually associated with complicated acute sinusitis (Muntz and Lusk, 1992).

The International Headache Society has established criteria for acute sinus headache (Headache Classification Committee of the International Headache Society, 1988) (Table 22–2). To qualify as acute sinus headache, there must be purulent discharge, abnormal neuroimaging, and simultaneous onset of headache and sinusitis. These criteria may not be valid for sphenoid sinusitis, however, as purulent discharge is often lacking and head-

ache may precede sinus drainage. Once drainage begins, obstruction is relieved and the headache may begin to abate.

Maxillary sinusitis pain is most typically located in the cheek, the gums, and the teeth of the upper jaw. Ethmoid sinusitis pain is generally felt between the eyes. The globe may be tender, and eye movement may aggravate pain. Frontal sinusitis pain is felt mainly in the forehead. Ethmoid and maxillary sinusitis are usually associated with rhinitis and are often referred to as rhinosinusitis.

Sphenoid sinusitis is an uncommon infection that accounts for approximately 3% of all cases of acute sinusitis. It is usually accompanied by pansinusitis; less commonly it occurs alone. In contrast to other paranasal sinus infections, sphenoid sinusitis is frequently

Table 22–2 Acute sinus headache

A. Purulent discharge in the nasal passage either spontaneous or by suction
B. Pathological findings on one or more of the following tests:
   1. X-ray examination
   2. Computed tomography or magnetic resonance imaging
   3. Transillumination
C. Simultaneous onset of headache and sinusitis
D. Headache location:
   1. Acute frontal sinusitis headache is located directly over the sinus and may radiate to the vertex or behind the eyes
   2. Acute maxillary sinusitis headache is located over the antral area and may radiate to the upper teeth or the forehead
   3. Acute ethmoiditis headache is located between the eyes and may radiate to the temporal area
   4. Acute sphenoiditis headache is located in the occipital area, the vertex, the frontal region, or behind the eyes
E. Headache disappears after treatment of acute sinusitis

misdiagnosed since the sphenoid sinus is not accessible to direct clinical examination even with the flexible endoscope and is not adequately visualized with routine sinus x-rays (Goldman et al., 1993). While sphenoid sinusitis is an uncommon cause of headache, it is potentially associated with significant morbidity and mortality and requires early identification and aggressive management (Lew et al., 1983; Kibblewhite et al., 1988; Goldman et al., 1993).

Headache is the most common symptom of acute sphenoid sinusitis: it is present in all patients who are able to complain about it. Standing, walking, bending, or coughing aggravates it; it often interferes with sleep and is poorly relieved by narcotics. Its location is variable: vertex headache is rare; frontal, occipital, or temporal headache or a combination of these locations is most common. Periorbital pain is common. This is in contrast to the common teaching that retro-orbital or vertex headache is the most common presenting symptom of sphenoid sinusitis (Lew et al., 1983; Kibblewhite et al., 1988; Urquhart et al., 1989; Nordeman and Lucid, 1990; Deans and Welch, 1991; Goldman et al., 1993).

Nausea and vomiting frequently occur dur-

ing an attack of acute sphenoid sinusitis, but nasal discharge, stuffiness, and postnasal drip are unusual. Fever occurs in over one-half of patients with acute sphenoid sinusitis. Isolated sphenoid sinusitis has been subclassified into four groups (inflammatory, neoplastic, fibro-osseous disorders, and miscellaneous) in a series of 132 cases (Lawson and Reino, 1997). Headache, visual loss, and cranial nerve palsy prevalence were determined in each group. Headache occurred in 98% of the inflammatory lesions, 90% of the benign tumors, and 71% of the malignant tumors. Visual disturbances (blurred vision and loss of visual acuity) were found in 12% of inflammatory lesions, 60% of benign tumors, and 50% of malignant neoplasms. Sixth cranial nerve palsy occurred in 6% of the inflammatory and 50% of the neoplastic cases. Eyelid ptosis (due to third-nerve involvement) occurred in 7.5% of cases. Other symptoms included cerebrospinal fluid leaks, epistaxis, meningitis, and proptosis. Four patients with fibro-osseous disorder presented with headache.

The diagnosis of acute or chronic sinusitis must be considered in an immunosuppressed patient who has fever, facial pain, swelling, and nasal crusting or ulceration. Plain x-rays may exhibit only slight mucosal thickening. Patients who fail to respond to medical treatment should have antral aspiration performed so that the causative organism can be identified and appropriate antibiotic treatment prescribed (Evans, 1998).

Hypertrophic turbinates, atrophic sinus membranes, and nasal passage abnormalities caused by septal deflection may cause headache; but these causes have not been validated by the International Headache Society. Whether nasal obstruction can lead to chronic headache is controversial (Schønsted-Madsen et al., 1986). Migraine and tension-type headaches are often confused with true sinus headache because of their similar locations. Recurrent episodic pain in the sinus areas is most likely migrainous in nature, with secondary (neurovascular) changes in the sinuses producing local symptoms.

The relationship between headache and subacute and chronic sinus disease is highly controversial (Faleck et al., 1988). Radio-graphic evidence of sinus disease is very common and does not establish the headache's etiology (Havas et al., 1988). A considerable proportion of adults not presenting with symptoms of sinusitis (39%, Lloyd et al., 1991; 42.5%, Havas et al., 1988; 15%, Calhoun et al., 1991) who had CTs for other reasons had coincidental CT findings suggestive of rhinosinusitis (International Rhinosinusitis Advisory Board, 1997). Headache associated with sinus disease is usually continuous, not intermittent. Chronic sinusitis is frequently associated with engorged and swollen nasal mucosa and a purulent or sanguinopurulent nasal discharge. The International Headache Society has not validated chronic sinusitis as a cause of headache or facial pain unless it relapses into an acute stage (Saunte and Soyka, 1993). Patients with rhinosinusitis and headache may not improve following treatment. One patient treated with functional endoscopic surgery for chronic sphenoidal sinusitis continued to have headaches postoperatively despite CT-documented absence of sinus disease (Gilain et al., 1994). This suggests that the headache and sinusitis were coincident, unrelated conditions.

Sphenoid sinusitis should be included in the differential diagnosis of acute or subacute headache. It may be mistaken for frontal or ethmoid sinusitis, aseptic meningitis, brain abscess, or septic thrombophlebitis. It can mimic trigeminal neuralgia, migraine, carotid artery aneurysm, or brain tumor (Lew et al., 1983; Kibblewhite et al., 1988; Goldman et al., 1993). Other causes of sphenoid sinus disease include mucoceles and benign and malignant tumors (Lawson and Reino, 1997).

The clinical features of a severe, intractable, new-onset headache that interferes with sleep, increases in severity, has no specific location, and is not relieved by simple analgesics should alert one to the diagnosis of sphenoid sinusitis. Pain or paresthesias in the facial distribution of the fifth nerve and photophobia or eye tearing are suggestive of sphenoid sinusitis (Lew et al., 1983; Turkewitz and Keller, 1987; Kibblewhite et al., 1988; Nordeman and Lucid, 1990; Deans and Welch, 1991; Goldman et al., 1993).

COMPLICATIONS

Sinus infection can result in acute suppurative meningitis, subdural or epidural abscess, and brain abscess. In addition, osteomyelitis and subperiosteal abscess can occur. Infection of the ethmoid and, to a lesser extent, the sphenoid sinuses is responsible for orbital complications, which include edema, orbital cellulitis, and subperiosteal and orbital abscess. Sinusitis thus can be a life-threatening condition and, if neglected or mismanaged, can lead to intracranial complications (Singh et al., 1995). In a review of patients admitted to the University of Virginia Health Sciences Center with a diagnosis of intracranial suppuration between 1992 and 1997, 15 patients were found who had 22 suppurative intracranial complications of sinusitis. These included epidural abscess (23%), subdural empyema (18%), meningitis (18%), cerebral abscess (14%), superior sagittal sinus thrombosis (9%), cavernous sinus thrombosis (9%), and osteomyelitis (9%). The diagnosis of suppurative intracranial complications of sinusitis requires a high index of suspicion and confirmation by imaging. Patients often present while on a regimen of antibiotics, which may mask or abolish neurologic as well as other symptoms and signs (Gallagher et al., 1998). A mucocele is a mucus-containing cyst located in the sinuses. These are most common (and benign) in the maxillary sinus (mucus retention cyst). Those located in the frontal, sphenoid, or ethmoid sinus can enlarge and erode into the surrounding structures. A pyocele is an infected mucocele (Hilger, 1989).

Sphenoid sinusitis is associated with most major complications, which include bacterial meningitis, cavernous sinus thrombosis, subdural abscess, cortical vein thrombosis, ophthalmoplegia, and pituitary insufficiency (Lew et al., 1983; Sofferman, 1983; Kibblewhite et al., 1988; Goldman et al., 1993). In addition, sphenoid sinusitis can present as an aseptic meningitis due to the presence of a parameningeal focus (Brook et al., 1982). Patients can present with the complications of sphenoid sinusitis, including visual loss mimicking optic neuritis, multiple cranial nerve palsies, or papilledema. Sudden onset, as a result of cavernous sinus thrombosis, can mimic a subarachnoid hemorrhage (Dale and Mackenzie, 1983).

Oktedalen and Lilleas (1992) reported on four patients with ethmoid sinusitis who were admitted to an infectious disease department with meningitis, sepsis, and orbital cellulitis. In the series of Lew et al. (1983), six of 16 acute cases had meningitis, five had cavernous sinus thrombosis, one had cortical vein thrombosis, one had unilateral ophthalmoplegia, and one had orbital cellulitis. Eight of the 14 patients studied by Kibblewhite et al. (1988) had complications on admission. None of the patients studied by Goldman et al. (1993) had complications. The difference in the complication rate is a result of selection bias: data for the latter study were retrieved from emergency room records; those for the other studies (Lew et al., 1983; Kibblewhite et al., 1988; Oktedalen and Lilleas, 1992) from inpatient records.

TREATMENT

Management goals for the treatment of sinusitis include (1) treatment of bacterial infection, (2) reduction of ostial swelling, (3) sinus drainage, and (4) maintenance of sinus ostia patency.

Uncomplicated sinusitis, other than sphenoid sinusitis, should be treated with a broad-spectrum oral antibiotic for 10 to 14 days. Nasal culture does not necessarily correlate with sinus pathogens; thus, initial treatment is empiric (Stafford, 1990). Steam and saline prevent crusting of secretions in the nasal cavity and facilitate mucociliary clearance. Locally active vasoconstrictor agents provide symptomatic relief by shrinking inflamed and swollen nasal mucosa. Their use should be limited to 3 to 4 days, to prevent rebound vasodilation. Oral decongestants should be used if prolonged treatment (longer than 3 days) is necessary. These agents are α-adrenergic agonists that reduce nasal blood flow without the risk of rebound vasodilation (Stafford, 1990). While phenylpropanolamine increased the nasal patency in controls, it was not more effective than placebo in patients with acute sinusitis (Aust et al., 1979). Nasal saline ir-

rigation, anticholinergics, antihistamines, expectorants, and mucolytics have not been prospectively studied, but most believe that antihistamines are not effective in the management of acute sinusitis (Diaz and Bamberger, 1995). Anti-inflammatory topical corticosteroids may help to maintain patency of the ostia. Intranasal flunisolide spray improved the symptoms of nasal obstruction in one controlled study (Metzger et al., 1993). Methods of prevention include using a humidifier, treating the underlying causes of sinus obstruction (polyps, adenoid hypertrophy, tumors of the nasopharynx, and nasal obstruction from allergic rhinitis), and smoking cessation (Hilger, 1989).

Treatment failure and recurrent infections are indications to use neuroimaging and endoscopy to search for a source of obstruction. Sinus sampling for culture should be considered. Endoscopic sinus surgery may be necessary to reopen and maintain the patency of the sinus ostia and ostiomeatal complex (Stafford, 1990).

Complications should be treated with high doses of intravenous antibiotics and surgical drainage, if appropriate, of any enclosed space.

Sphenoid sinusitis without complication may be managed with high-dose intravenous antibiotics and topical and systemic decongestants for 24 hours (Kibblewhite et al., 1988; Goldman et al., 1993). If the fever (if present) and the headache do not improve or if any complications are present or develop, sphenoid sinus drainage is indicated (Druce, 1990). Gilain and colleagues (1994) reviewed 12 cases of isolated sphenoid sinus disease secondary to chronic inflammatory sinusitis in seven patients, mucoceles in two, aspergillus lesions in two, and an isolated polyp in one. All patients in this series were treated with functional endoscopic sphenoidotomy and improved. All were treated with appropriate postoperative antibiotics, nasal irrigation, oral corticosteroids, and washing and cleaning of the nasal cavity weekly for 4 weeks.

NASAL HEADACHE

Many rhinologists believe that septal deformation, especially when it is traumatic in origin, may exert pressure on the sensitive structure of the lateral nasal wall, causing referred pain and "chronic headache."

Schønsted-Madsen and associates (1986) followed 444 patients with nasal obstruction, of whom 167 had headache that was usually localized to the forehead, the glabella, or above and around the eyes. If surgery relieved the nasal obstruction, 80% had headache relief. However, if the surgery failed, only 30% had headache relief. Treatment consisted of septoplastic surgery, reconstruction of the nasal pyramids, or submucosal conchotomy.

Clerico (1995) reported ten patients who had intractable migraine, tension-type headache, or cluster headache without significant nasal or sinus symptoms. Various intranasal and sinus abnormalities, such as anatomic variation or subclinical inflammation, were found on CT or nasal endoscopy. Patients were treated medically and/or surgically, and all improved. Low and Willatt (1995) reported on 106 patients who had a submucous resection for a deviated nasal septum. Almost half (47.4%) had recurring headaches preoperatively. Postoperatively, 63.6% had complete or partial relief at 18 months' follow-up. While 79.3% had headache relief when evaluated before 1 year, only 46.2% had relief after 1 year.

These studies do not account for the historical relationship between the onset of headache and the development of nasal obstruction or for the overuse of analgesics or decongestants, which may produce daily headache. In addition, any surgical procedure has a powerful placebo effect. It does suggest that a minority of patients with nasal obstruction have headache that is relieved by successful medical or surgical treatment. Since migraine prevalence in the population is about 12%, episodic tension-type headache prevalence about 90%, and chronic tension-type headache prevalence about 3%, these data are difficult to interpret. In addition, these studies had no control group, and only responders were reported in the study by Clerico (1995). In controlled trials of medication, the placebo effect can be quite large.

In a retrospective review of operative notes on 170 patients who underwent functional endoscopic sinus surgery, 50 patients (29%) who had a history of chronic headaches were identified. Thirty-seven met the predetermined inclusion criteria for this study: (1) history of chronic headaches; (2) rhinologic cause for headaches suggested by the presence of contact points as documented by nasal endoscopy and/or CT scans; (3) no other obvious origin or cause of headaches discernible after a thorough evaluation; and (4) surgical intervention that included relief of contact points by inferior, middle, and/or superior turbinoplasty. Following surgery, 29 of the 34 patients (85%) in the study group reported a decrease in headache frequency. However, there were many patients who had severe contact points on CT scan and did not complain of headaches. In fact, most patients with headaches and contact points also had concurrent chronic sinusitis, which served as the primary indication for surgery in this patient population (Parsons and Batra, 1998).

Other open studies (Chow, 1994; Salman and Rebeiz, 1994) and a review (Close and Aviv, 1997) have suggested that headache can be the only clinical presentation of sinus or nasal pathology. These studies do not use International Headache Society criteria for headache or the new diagnostic criteria for sinusitis. With the common involvement of the sinuses on CT with no symptoms of sinusitis, it is very difficult to comment favorably on these open trials.

REFERENCES

Agency for Healthcare Policy and Research (1999). Diagnosis and treatment of acute bacterial rhinosinusitis. Summary. Evidence Report/Technology Assessment 9. Agency for Healthcare Policy and Research, Rockville, MD.

Aust, R., B. Drettner, and B. Galck (1979). Studies of the effect of peroral phenylpropanolamine on the functional size of the human maxillary ostium. *Acta Otolaryngol. (Stockh.)* 88:455–458.

Axelsson, A. and A. Jensen (1974). The roentgenologic demonstration of sinusitis. *Am. J. Roentgenol. Rad. Ther. Neurol. Med.* 122:621–627.

Benninger, M.S., J. Anon, and R.L. Mabry (1997). The medical management of rhinosinusitis. Report of the Rhinosinusitis Task Force Committee Meeting. *Otolaryngol. Head Neck Surg. 117:* S41–S49.

Bhattacharyya, N. (1999). Test–retest reliability of computed tomography in the assessment of chronic rhinosinusitis. *Laryngoscope* 109:1055–1058.

Brook, I., G.D. Overturf, E.A. Steinberg et al. (1982). Acute sphenoid sinusitis presenting as aseptic meningitis: A pachymeningitis syndrome. *Int. J. Pediatr. Otorhinolaryngol.* 4:77–81.

Caldwell, G.W. (1893). The accessory sinuses of the nose: An improved method of treatment for suppuration of the maxillary antrum. *N. Y. Med. J.* 58:526.

Calhoun, K.H., G.A. Waggnespack, C.B. Simpson et al. (1991). CT evaluation of the paranasal sinuses in symptomatic and asymptomatic populations. *Otolaryngol. Head Neck Surg.* 104:480–483.

Chow, J.M. (1994). Rhinologic headaches. *Otolaryngol. Head Neck Surg.* 111:211–218.

Clerico, D.M. (1995). Sinus headaches reconsidered: Referred cephalgia of rhinologic origin masquerading as refractory primary headaches. *Headache* 35:185–192.

Close, L.G. and J. Aviv (1997). Headaches and disease of the nose and paranasal sinuses. *Semin. Neurol.* 17:351–354.

Collins, J.G. (1997). *Prevalence of selected chronic conditions*, series 10, pp. 1–89. U.S. Department of Vital and Health Statistics, Washington, D.C.

Dale, B.A.B. and I.J. Mackenzie (1983). The complications of sphenoid sinusitis. *J. Laryngol. Otol.* 97:661–670.

Deans, J.A.J. and A.R. Welch (1991). Acute isolated sphenoid sinusitis: A disease with complications. *J. Laryngol. Otol.* 105:1072–1074.

Diaz, I. and D.M. Bamberger (1995). Acute sinusitis. *Semin. Respir. Infect.* 10:14–20.

Druce, H.M. (1990). Adjuncts to medical management of sinusitis. *Otolaryngol. Head Neck Surg.* 103:880–883.

Druce, H.M. and R.G. Siavin (1991). Sinusitis: A critical need for further study. *J. Allergy Clin. Immunol.* 88:675–677.

Engquist, S., C. Lundberg, and P. Venge (1983). Effects of drainage in the treatment of acute maxillary sinusitis. *Acta Otolaryngol. (Stockh.)* 95:153–159.

Evans, K. (1994). Diagnosis and management of sinusitis. *BMJ* 309:1415–1422.

Evans, K.L. (1998). Recognition and management of sinusitis. *Drugs* 56:59–71.

Faleck, H., A.D. Rothner, G. Erenberg et al. (1988). Headache and subacute sinusitis in children and adolescents. *Headache* 28:96–98.

Fergusen, B.J. and R. Mabry (1997). Laboratory diagnosis. *Otolaryngol. Head Neck Surg. 117:* S12–S26.

Gallagher, R.M., C.W. Cross, and C.D. Phillips (1998). Suppurative intracranial complications of sinusitis. *Laryngoscope* 108:1635–1642.

Gilain, L., D. Aidan, A. Coste et al. (1994). Functional endoscopic sinus surgery for isolated sphenoid sinus disease. *Head Neck* 16:433–437.

Goldman, G.E., P.B. Fontanarosa, and J.M. Anderson (1993). Isolated sphenoid sinusitis. *Am. J. Emerg. Med.* 11:235–238.

Goss, C.M. (1959). *Gray's Anatomy of the Human Body*. Lea & Febiger, Philadelphia.

Gwaltney, J.M., C.D. Phillips, R.D. Miller et al. (1994). Computed tomographic study of the common cold. *N. Engl. J. Med.* 330:25–30.

Hajek, M. (1926). *Pathology and Treatment of Inflammatory Diseases of the Nasal Accessory Sinuses*. C.V. Mosby, St. Louis.

Havas, T.E., J.A. Motbey, and P.J. Gullane (1988). Prevalence of incidental abnormalities on computed tomographic scans of the paranasal sinuses. *Arch. Otolaryngol.* 114:856–859.

Headache Classification Committee of the International Headache Society (1988). Classification and diagnostic criteria for headache disorders, cranial neuralgia, and facial pain. *Cephalalgia* 8: 1–96.

Hilding, A.C. (1950). Physiologic basis of nasal operations. *Calif. Med.* 72:103–107.

Hilger, P.A. (1989). Diseases of the nose. In *Boies Fundamentals of Otolaryngology: A Textbook of Ear, Nose, and Throat Disease* (P.A. Hilger, ed.), pp. 206–248. W.B. Saunders, Philadelphia.

International Rhinosinusitis Advisory Board (1997). Infectious rhinosinusitis in adults: Classification, etiology, and management. *Ear Nose Throat J.* 76:S5–S22.

Jeney, E.V., G.D. Raphael, S.D. Meredith et al. (1990). Abnormal cholinergic responsiveness in the nasal muscosa of patients with recurrent sinusitis. *J. Allergy Clin. Immunol.* 86:8–10.

Josephson, G.D. and C.W. Gross (1997). Diagnosis and management of acute and chronic sinusitis. *Compr. Ther.* 23:708–714.

Kennedy, D.W. (1990a). Overview. *Otolaryngol. Head Neck Surg.* 103:847–854.

Kennedy, D.W. (1990b). Surgical update. *Otolaryngol. Head Neck Surg.* 103:884–886.

Kibblewhite, D.J., J. Cleland, and D.R. Mintz (1988). Acute sphenoid sinusitis: Management strategies. *J. Otolaryngol.* 17:159–163.

Lang, J. (1989). Clinical anatomy of the nose, nasal cavity and paranasal sinuses. Georg Thieme Verlag, Stutgart/New York.

Lanza, D.C. and D.W. Kennedy (1997). Adult rhinosinusitis defined. *Otolaryngol. Head Neck Surg.* 117:S1–S7.

Lawson, W. and A.J. Reino (1997). Isolated sphenoid sinus disease: An analysis of 132 cases. *Laryngoscope* 107:1590–1595.

Lew, D., F.S. Southwick, W.W. Montgomery et al. (1983). Sphenoid sinusitis: A review of 30 cases. *N. Engl. J. Med.* 19:1149–1154.

Lloyd, G.A., V.J. Lund, and G.K. Scadding (1991). CT of the paranasal sinuses and functional endoscopic surgery: A critical analysis of 100 symptomatic patients. *J. Laryngol. Otol.* 105: 181–185.

Low, W.K. and D.J. Willatt (1995). Headaches associated with nasal obstruction due to deviated nasal septum. *Headache* 35:404–406.

McAuliffe, G.W., H. Goodell, and H.G. Wolff (1943). Experimental studies on headache: Pain from the nasal and paranasal structures. *Res. Publ. Assoc. Res. Nerv. Ment. Dis.* 23:185–206.

McCaffrey, T.V. (1993). Functional endoscopic sinus surgery: An overview. *Mayo Clin. Proc.* 68: 675–677.

Messerklinger, W. (1978). *Endoscopy of the Nose.* Urban and Schwartzenberg, Baltimore.

Metzger, E.O., H.A. Orgel, J.W. Backhaus et al. (1993). Intranasal flunisolide spray as an adjunct to oral antibiotic therapy for sinusitis. *J. Allergy Clin. Immunol.* 92:812–823.

Moss, A.J. and V.L. Parsons (1986). Current estimates from the National Health Interview Survey United States 1985, series 10, pp. 1–182. U.S. Department of Vital and Health Statistics, Washington, D.C.

Muntz, H.R. and R.P. Lusk (1992). Signs and symptoms of chronic sinusitis. In *Pediatric Sinusitis* (R.P. Lusk, ed.), pp. 1–6. Raven Press, New York.

Nordeman, L. and E. Lucid (1990). Sphenoid sinusitis, a cause of debilitating headache. *J. Emerg. Med.* 8:557–559.

Oktedalen, O. and F. Lilleas (1992). Septic complications to sphenoidal sinus infection. *Scand. J. Infect. Dis.* 24:353–356.

Parsons, D.S. and P.S. Batra (1998). Functional endoscopic sinus surgical outcomes for contact point headaches. *Laryngoscope* 108:696–702.

Ray, N.F., J.N. Baraniuk, M. Thamer et al. (1999). Healthcare expenditures for sinusitis in 1996: Contributions of asthma, rhinitis, and other airway disorders. *J. Allergy Clin. Immunol.* 103: 408–414.

Reilly, J.S. (1990). The sinusitis cycle. *Otolaryngol. Head Neck Surg.* 103:856–862.

Rouby, J., P. Laurent, M. Gosnach et al. (1994). Risk factors and clinical relevance of nosocomial maxillary sinusitis in the critically ill. *Am. J. Respir. Crit. Care Med.* 150:776–783.

Salman, S.D. and E.E. Rebeiz (1994). Sinusitis and headache. *J. Med. Liban.* 42:200–202.

Saunte, C. and D. Soyka (1993). Headache related to ear, nose, and sinus disorders. In *The headaches* (J. Olesen, P. Tfelt-Hansen, and K.M.A. Welch, eds.), pp. 753–757. Raven Press, New York.

Schaefer, S.D. and L.G. Close (1990). Endoscopic management of frontal sinus disease. *Laryngoscope* 100:155–160.

Schatz, C.J. and T.S. Becker (1984). Normal CT anatomy of the paranasal sinuses. *Radiol. Clin. North Am.* 22:107–118.

Schønsted-Madsen, U., P. Stoksted, P.H. Christensen et al. (1986). Chronic headache related to nasal obstruction. *J. Laryngol. Otol.* 100:165–170.

Shapiro, G.G. and G.S. Rachelefsky (1992). Introduction and definition of sinusitis. *J. Allergy Clin. Immunol.* 90:417–418.

Singh, B., J. Van Dellen, S. Ramjettan et al. (1995). Sinogenic intracranial complications. *J. Laryngol. Otol.* 109:945–950.

Slavin, R.G. (1997). Nasal polyps and sinusitis. *JAMA* 278:1849–1854.

Sofferman, R.A. (1983). Cavernous sinus thrombophlebitis secondary to sphenoid sinusitis. *Laryngoscope* 93:797–800.

Stafford, C.T. (1990). The clinician's view of sinusitis. *Otolaryngol. Head Neck Surg.* 103:870–875.

Turkewitz, D. and R. Keller (1987). Acute headache in childhood: A case of sphenoid sinusitis. *Pediatr. Emerg. Care* 3:155–157.

Urquhart, A.C., G. Fung, and W.A. McIntosh (1989). Isolated sphenoiditis: A diagnostic problem. *J. Laryngol. Otol.* 103:526–527.

Van Cauwenberge, P.B., K.J. Ingels, C.L. Bachert et al. (1997). Microbiology of chronic sinusitis. *Acta Otorhinolaryngol. Belg.* 51:239–246.

Wagner, W. (1996). Changing diagnostic and treatment strategies for chronic sinusitis. *Cleve. Clin. J. Med.* 63:396–405.

Williams, J.W., D.L. Simel, L. Roberts et al. (1992). Clinical evaluation of sinusitis. *Ann. Intern. Med.* 117:705–710.

Wolff, H.G. (1948). *Wolff's Headache and Other Head Pain.* Oxford University Press, New York.

Zinreich, S.J. (1990). Paranasal sinus imaging. *Otolaryngol. Head Neck Surg.* 103:863–869.

Zinreich, S.J., D.W. Kennedy, A.E. Rosenbaum et al. (1987). Paranasal sinuses: CT imaging requirements for endoscopic surgery. *Radiology* 163:769–775.

23

Cranial Neuralgias and Atypical Facial Pain

TODD D. ROZEN
DAVID J. CAPOBIANCO
DONALD J. DALESSIO

Trigeminal neuralgia is a distinct, painful disorder of the face that is easily evoked by trivial stimuli and undergoes a relapsing, remitting course. There are about 15,000 new cases of trigeminal neuralgia per year. It is a disorder of the elderly and can cause severe disability. It is characterized by brief electric shock-like pain and is limited to one or more divisions of the trigeminal nerve. Patients who have experienced this disorder are continually fearful, while in pain remission, that the attacks will recur. Trigeminal neuralgia can be treated both medically and surgically. We review the epidemiology, diagnostic criteria, and pathophysiology and suggest a stepwise approach to treatment.

HISTORY

Trigeminal neuralgia was first clearly described in the 17th century, but it was probably initially recognized by the Greeks and Romans. The classic descriptions of trigeminal neuralgia came from Locke (1677), André (1756), and Fothergill (1773), (Zakrzewska, 1995e). They defined the clinical features of trigeminal neuralgia but did not recognize the paroxysmal profile of the disease. Trigeminal neuralgia has been recognized under various names, including trisma dolorificans, epileptiform neuralgia, dolor faciei Fothergillii, and the most recognized, tic douleureux, which is the term many still use today.

EPIDEMIOLOGY

Penman (1968) estimated the annual prevalence of trigeminal neuralgia to be 4.7 per one million men and 7.2 per one million women. Brewis et al. (1966) found an annual incidence rate of 2.1 cases per 100,000 individuals from only ten cases reported between 1955 and 1961 in Carlisle, England. Three incidence studies have been reported from Rochester, Minnesota: Kurland (1958) examined the period 1945 through 1956 and found four new cases per 100,000 population per year, Yoshimasu et al. (1972) studied the period 1945 through 1969 and found four new cases per 100,000 population per year (5/100,000 women and 2.7/100,000 men per year), and Katusic et al. (1990) studied the period 1945 through 1984 and found 4.3 new cases per 100,000 population per year (5.9/ 100,000 women and 3.4/100,000 men per year). Extrapolating the Rochester, Minnesota data to the United States population suggests an annual incidence of 15,000 new cases.

The peak incidence of idiopathic trigeminal neuralgia occurs in the fifth to seventh decade, with 90% of cases beginning after the age of 40. The gender distribution is uneven, with a female predominance (1.5 female cases to every 1 male case). The gender ratio varies in different populations, from 1.8:1 in the Rochester, Minnesota, population to 1.17: 1 in a Massachusetts population of 526 hospitalized patients (Rothman and Monson, 1973).

Familial cases of trigeminal neuralgia are very rare but have been reported. Harris (1926) found nine members of the same family with trigeminal neuralgia. Yoshimasu et al. (1972) found one of 36 patients with a family history of trigeminal neuralgia. Pollack et al. (1988) identified 33 cases of hereditary trigeminal neuralgia in 699 patients. Katusic et al. (1990) found four of 75 patients with a family history of trigeminal neuralgia. In these familial cases, trigeminal neuralgia presented earlier in each successive generation. Duff et al. (1999) identified a family with trigeminal neuralgia and contralateral hemifacial spasm. The transmission of trigeminal neuralgia in this family suggested an autosomal dominant inheritance.

CLINICAL CHARACTERISTICS

The pain of trigeminal neuralgia is a sharp, shooting, lightning-rod or electric shock-like sensation. It is extremely severe, with usual maximum intensity without latency. The pain typically lasts seconds, although it can last up to 2 minutes. Multiple attacks may occur daily for weeks or months at a time. Most individuals have short periods of pain-free time in between spikes of pain, but they may have difficulty detecting this remission and often state that their pain is constant. Others have continuous interictal pain, which is dull, burning, or throbbing in quality. These individuals may have a worse prognosis for successful treatment than those without interictal pain. Szapiro and Sindou (1985) found

that microvascular decompression was less successful in individuals who had a dull ache between trigeminal neuralgia attacks than in individuals without interictal pain: 95% without paroxysmal pain did well compared to 58% with interictal pain. Jassim (1994) completed a 3-year prospective study of individuals with interictal pain before they underwent radiofrequency thermocoagulation. These patients continued to have background pain and more side effects after radiofrequency than patients who had pain-free intervals between their trigeminal neuralgia attacks.

Trigeminal neuralgia pain occurs in the distribution of the trigeminal nerve. White and Sweet (1969) completed a literature review search of 8,124 patients and found that 61% had right-sided attacks and 36% had left-sided attacks. Most individuals experience the pain in the maxillary and mandibular divisions. It occurs much less frequently in the ophthalmic division (Table 23–1). Only 4% of trigeminal neuralgia cases are bilateral, and most of those individuals have multiple sclerosis. Trigeminal neuralgia never spreads across the midline, and bilateral cases are never synchronous. Trigeminal neuralgia is a paroxysmal disorder with a relapsing or remitting course. Over 50% of individuals will have at least a 6-month remission during their lifetime, and 24% will have a 12-month remission (Rushton and MacDonald, 1957).

Trigeminal neuralgia attacks can be triggered by trivial stimuli. The slightest touch, even the movement of a single fine hair, can trigger a volley of pain, as can cold air, chewing, talking, facial movement, brushing of teeth, and emotional distress. Rare triggers include auditory stimuli, acute infection, and trauma. Touch and vibration appear to trigger

Table 23–1 Pain distribution in trigeminal neuralgia

V_1 alone	4%
V_2 alone	17%
V_3 alone	15%
$V_2 + V_3$	32%
$V_1 + V_2$	14%
$V_1 + V_2 + V_3$	17%

more attacks than pinprick. In about 50% of trigeminal neuralgia sufferers, attacks can be triggered by non-noxious stimuli touching small areas around the face, nose, and lips. These "trigger zones" can be as small as 1 to 2 mm in diameter. The pain intensity is independent of the trigger zone size. In most patients, the pain will start within the trigger zone, but in 5% to 9% of patients, the pain occurs outside of it. Most individuals have a refractory period (a time after the stimulation of a trigger zone), during which restimulation will not elicit an attack of trigeminal neuralgia. The length of the refractory period is proportional to the duration and severity of the prior painful attack.

A patient experiencing a trigeminal neuralgia attack typically freezes in place with the hands slowly rising to the area of pain on the face but not touching it. He or she then grimaces or quirks the face with a tic-like motion (tic douloureux) and then either remains in this position or cries out in pain.

DIAGNOSIS AND TESTING

In 1988, the International Headache Society (IHS) established diagnostic criteria for idiopathic trigeminal neuralgia (Table 23–2) (Headache Classification Committee of the International Headache Society, 1988). Trigeminal neuralgia is diagnosed by its clinical presentation and an examination that is normal except for the presence of trigger zones. Fifteen percent to 25% of individuals exhibit sensory loss on examination. This is hardly

Table 23–2 International Headache Society criteria for trigeminal neuralgia

1. Paroxysmal attacks of facial or frontal pain that lasts for a few seconds to less than 2 minutes
2. At least four of the following five characteristics are needed to make the diagnosis:
   a. Distribution along one or more divisions of the trigeminal nerve
   b. Sudden intense, sharp, superficial stabbing and burning pain quality
   c. Severe pain
   d. Evidence of trigger zones
   e. Asymptomatic between attacks

ever recognized by the patient. Most physicians feel that one must investigate for symptomatic or secondary trigeminal neuralgia if sensory loss is identified on examination. The most common underlying causes of trigeminal neuralgia include multiple sclerosis, basilar artery aneurysm, neoplasms (epidermoid, acoustic neuroma, meningioma, trigeminal neuroma), arterial or venous compression, syringobulbia, and brainstem infarction. Other authorities believe that sensory loss is not abnormal unless it is marked and progressive. Most who find sensory loss on examination will have the patient undergo neuroimaging, specifically a magnetic resonance imaging (MRI) study, to rule out an underlying pathologic process. An MRI can also visualize neurovascular contacts, while magnetic resonance angiography (MRA) can establish the true relationship between nerve and vessel. The probability that a surgical procedure, such as microvascular decompression, will be beneficial to the patient is enhanced if MRI/MRA discloses a vascular loop compressing the trigeminal nerve at the root entry zone. Majoie et al. (2000) assessed the diagnostic yield of MRI in patients who had symptoms and signs related to the trigeminal nerve. A normal examination and trigeminal neuralgia symptoms alone were highly correlated with a negative MRI study. Impaired sensation, subjective feelings of facial numbness, other positive neurologic signs and symptoms, progression of symptoms and signs, and symptoms that had been present for less than 1 year correlated with an abnormal MRI. Trigeminal evoked potentials may also may be a valuable diagnostic aid in the search for underlying compressive lesions of the trigeminal nerve. Sundaram et al. (1999) demonstrated abnormal trigeminal evoked potentials in all patients with trigeminal neuralgia resulting from known intracranial mass lesions, suggesting that trigeminal evoked potentials should be considered in the normal workup of patients who have trigeminal neuralgia and negative MRI. If the evoked potential responses are abnormal, then nerve compression is still the most likely cause of the patient's trigeminal neuralgia symptoms. Trigeminal evoked potentials may also be useful to predict recovery of nerve function after pain-relieving techniques, such as microvascular decompression. Leandri et al. (1998) examined ten trigeminal neuralgia patients who had MRI- and MRA-documented neurovascular contact. Immediate recovery of preprocedure abnormal trigeminal evoked potentials after decompression suggested recovery of nerve function and a good clinical outcome.

PATHOGENESIS

The true cause of trigeminal neuralgia is unknown. It is believed that both peripheral and central dysfunction play an important role. It has been suggested that chronic focal demyelination secondary to irritation of the trigeminal nerve at the root entry zone (usually caused by vascular compression) leads to increased firing rates in trigeminal primary afferents, as well as impairment of the efficacy of the inhibitory mechanisms in the trigeminal brain-stem complex, which normally controls this level of activity. This leads to a greater than normal excitability of the trigeminal brain-stem complex, which then responds to tactile stimuli as it typically would to noxious stimuli. Fromm (1991) suggested that in this setting there is increased paroxysmal firing of wide dynamic range (WDR) neurons, which are typically excited by noxious and non-noxious stimuli in the trigeminal nucleus caudalis, as well as hypersensitivity of low-threshold mechanoreceptors (LTMs) in the trigeminal nucleus oralis. The LTM neurons become hyperactive and start to fire at rates normally seen with noxious stimuli, resulting in paroxysmal trigeminal neuralgia. Hyperactivity of both LTM and WDR neurons may explain why both noxious and non-noxious stimuli trigger trigeminal neuralgia attacks. Raskin (1988) remarked that several features of trigeminal neuralgia suggest a centrally mediated process. These include the presence of refractory, continued volleys of pain after nerve stimulation and the central action of all medicines that are successful in treating trigeminal neuralgia.

TREATMENT

Both medical and surgical modalities may be used to treat trigeminal neuralgia. Patients are typically started with drug treatment. Drug therapy for trigeminal neuralgia dates back to the 1600s, when purgatives were used; but it was not until the 1940s, when phenytoin was first utilized for trigeminal neuralgia, that an effective therapy was available. Other important dates in the history of medical treatment for trigeminal neuralgia are 1962 (carbamazepine), 1976 (clonazepam), and 1980 (baclofen). New treatments are continually being tried for trigeminal neuralgia because most drugs have very low success rates with prevalent side effects. The drugs currently utilized for the treatment of trigeminal neuralgia will be discussed separately, with comments on mechanisms of action, pharmacokinetics, dosing strategies, and studies.

Carbamazepine

Carbamazepine is recognized as the best available drug for trigeminal neuralgia and is the first-line agent used by most physicians. Its proposed mechanism of action is decreasing the response of trigeminal mechanoreceptive neurons to peripheral stimulation. Carbamazepine has several important pharmacokinetic properties that make it unique. Since it causes its own induction of metabolism, a therapeutic level may not be maintained if the patient stays on the same dose. It is important to allow at least 20 days for autoinduction of metabolism to occur before looking at a maintenance dose. A serum concentration range of 24 to 43 μmol/l is targeted. The half-life of carbamazepine also changes over time. Initially, it is between 20 and 40 hours, but with chronic dosing it is between 11 and 27 hours. This unrecognized pharmacokinetic change may explain why the drug becomes less effective over time, especially if a constant dose is maintained. Counteracting these half-life changes by altering dose frequency could lead to less failure with chronic carbamazepine therapy.

To avoid neurotoxicity, carbamazepine

should be started at a low dose (100 mg one to two times a day). The dose can be increased by 100 to 200 mg every 3 days until pain relief is achieved. The usual maintenance dose is between 400 and 800 mg/day; most patients remain on less than 1,200 mg/day, although some need a dose of 1,500 mg/day or more. If the dose is below 800 mg/day, carbamazepine can be given twice daily; however, a dose that is above 800 mg/day must be given three to four times a day.

Adequately treated trigeminal neuralgia sufferers will not know if they are in an active pain phase or in remission. Pain-free patients should have their medications tapered to avoid unneeded treatment exposure and neurotoxicity. It is helpful for patients to maintain pain calendars to demonstrate changes in the pain pattern (intensity or frequency). When individuals have been pain-free for 4 to 6 weeks, carbamazepine may be tapered. This should be done slowly, by 100 mg every 3 to 7 days. If pain paroxysms return, the dose can be increased to the smallest pain-relieving level.

Drowsiness is a common initial side effect of carbamazepine; it usually abates after several days. Daytime drowsiness can be minimized by giving larger doses at bedtime. This schedule may have the added benefit of being more therapeutic to the patient as it provides higher morning drug serum concentrations, and most attacks of trigeminal neuralgia occur in the morning. Other side effects include dizziness, nausea, vomiting, nystagmus, ataxia, and diplopia. Carbamazepine may activate latent psychosis and cause agitation in the elderly. Hematologic side effects occur in 2% to 6% of patients and include leukopenia and aplastic anemia. A complete blood count is recommended every 2 weeks for the first 2 months of therapy. In addition, liver and renal function tests should be completed before starting the drug, 2 weeks into dosing, and then at 8- to 12-week intervals. Leukopenia, which resolves spontaneously in 10% of patients, may develop. If this occurs, discontinuation of the drug or blood count monitoring at 2-week intervals is mandatory. Maintaining the same carbamazepine dose for several days will usually alleviate minor central nervous system (CNS) side effects.

Carbamazepine is highly effective. It delivers pain relief in up to 80% of individuals, both initially and in the short term. Relief occurs within several hours to several days after starting the drug; 94% of patients experience pain relief within 48 hours (Zakrzewska, 1995a). Over time, however, fewer responders continue to have sustained relief. Taylor et al. (1981) followed patients for 16 years and found that although 69% had initial benefit, carbamazepine was effective in only 56% by the end of the study. About 5% to 19% of individuals are carbamazepine-intolerant.

Phenytoin

Phenytoin was the first effective drug for trigeminal neuralgia but is now a second- or third-line agent. Its proposed mechanism of action is depression of the response of spinal trigeminal neurons to maxillary nerve stimulation. Pharmacokinetically, phenytoin follows zero order of kinetics, so a small increase in dosage can lead to a rapid rise in plasma levels and a heightened risk of neurotoxicity.

The starting dose of phenytoin is 200 mg/day. The usual target dose is between 300 and 500 mg/day given in three divided doses. Phenytoin, in its parenteral form, can be utilized as acute therapy for trigeminal neuralgia in the emergency department. Phenytoin 250 mg IV given over 5 minutes can abort a trigeminal neuralgia attack immediately, and the pain relief may last from 4 hours to 3 days (Raskin, 1988). Studies utilizing fosphenytoin in the same manner have not been undertaken.

Side effects of phenytoin include gum hyperplasia, hirsutism, depression, and impaired memory. Coadministered carbamazepine can raise serum phenytoin concentrations, while phenytoin can decrease the half-life of carbamazepine.

In most individuals, pain improves within 24 to 48 hours. Initial effectiveness is up to 60% (Zakrzewska, 1995a). There are no good comparison data with other medicinal therapies in the literature. Phenytoin's effectiveness decreases over time, with less than 30% of patients responding after 2 years.

Baclofen

Baclofen is a γ-aminobutyric acid (GABA) analog that can be used alone or in combination with phenytoin or carbamazepine. Its proposed mechanism of action is suppression of the response of spinal trigeminal neurons to maxillary nerve stimulation. Oral baclofen has rapid gastrointestinal absorption, with peak serum concentrations occurring within 3 to 8 hours. Baclofen has a very short serum half-life, so a multiple daily dosing regime is required to maintain serum concentrations. Baclofen is excreted via the kidneys.

As monotherapy, baclofen is started at 5 to 10 mg three times a day. The dose can be increased by 5 to 10 mg every other day until pain is relieved. The normal maintenance dose is between 50 and 60 mg/day in four to six divided doses. The typical maximum tolerated dose is 80 mg/day. Because of baclofen's short half-life, additional doses should be interspersed between previous doses. When a patient is pain-free, baclofen can be tapered gradually; hallucinations, anxiety, and seizures may develop if it is tapered too quickly. Baclofen should be tapered by no more than 5 to 10 mg/week.

When baclofen is combined with other medication, the dosage of each drug needed for pain relief is often lower than what was needed as monotherapy. If baclofen is added to carbamazepine, the carbamazepine dose should be reduced to 600 mg/day and baclofen added at its normal dosing schedule (5 to 10 mg three times a day, with 5 to 10 mg increasing increments every other day). If baclofen is added to phenytoin, the phenytoin dose should be reduced to 300 mg/day and baclofen started at its normal dosing schedule.

The most common side effects of baclofen include drowsiness, dizziness, and gastrointestinal discomfort. About 10% of patients cannot tolerate the drug.

Newer Agents

Clonazepam was studied by Court and Case (1976), who found it to be effective in 65% of individuals with trigeminal neuralgia. Six-teen of these patients did not respond to carbamazepine, and of these, eight did well on clonazepam. Even though a number of patients had good pain relief on clonazepam on a 6 to 8 mg dose, 85% had ataxia or dizziness. Clonazepam should be started at an initial dose of 0.5 mg three times a day and increased by 0.5 mg every 3 to 5 days until pain relief is obtained. The normal therapeutic dosing range is between 1.5 and 8 mg/day. Side effects include drowsiness, fatigue, and dizziness, which can be decreased by dividing the dosing schedule.

Valproic acid was studied by Peiris et al. (1980), in an open-label study using 600 to 1,200 mg/day. Thirteen of 20 patients had a good response (six became pain-free and three had a greater than 50% reduction in pain). Four responders required combination therapy to achieve pain relief. The initial dose of valproic acid is 250 to 500 mg/day, increasing by 125 to 250 mg/week up to 1,500 mg/day or higher if tolerated. Valproic acid is given two to three times a day. One problem is that it may take weeks to see a response. Valproic acid in the form of divalproex sodium may be better tolerated.

Lamotrigine, a sodium channel modulator, is a new oral agent for trigeminal neuralgia. Zakrzewska et al. (1997) studied 14 patients using lamotrigine as an add-on therapy to carbamazepine or phenytoin. Eleven of 13 patients had better efficacy on lamotrigine than on placebo. Pain relief usually began within 24 hours of finding a therapeutic dose. The normal pain-relieving dose was 400 mg/day. This was a very short trial, lasting for only 2 weeks, so the long-term efficacy of lamotrigine could not be ascertained. Lunardi et al. (1997) utilized lamotrigine as monotherapy for trigeminal neuralgia with a 3- to 8-month follow-up. Eleven of 15 patients had an excellent response on only 150 to 250 mg/day. Eight patients became pain-free on lamotrigine. Lamotrigine should be started at 25 mg/day and the dose increased by 25 mg every third to seventh day up to 400 mg/day. Individuals respond between 150 to 400 mg/day. Lamotrigine has several benefits compared to carbamazepine and phenytoin. It has a better side effect profile, and there is no autoinduction of metabolism, so dosing is stable over time. If used in combination with carbamazepine or phenytoin, it does not alter their metabolism. Lamotrigine's major side effect is a drug rash that can evolve into Stevens-Johnson syndrome. The rash normally starts early in therapy. If a rash appears, the drug should be stopped immediately.

Pimozide is a dopamine receptor antagonist. In a double-blind, crossover trial, it was more effective than carbamazepine for trigeminal neuralgia. The overall dose is between 4 and 12 mg/day. Pimozide's major drawback is its poor side effect profile, which includes mental retardation, hand tremor, memory impairment, and parkinsonism, which affects up to 83% of patients (Lechin et al., 1989).

Gabapentin is anecdotally effective for trigeminal neuralgia. There are two isolated case reports in the literature (Sist et al., 1997). One of these individuals required 2,400 mg/day for pain relief, and the other needed 900 mg/day. The onset of pain relief came within 1 week of achieving a therapeutic drug level. Gabapentin was also shown to be successful for treating multiple sclerosis–induced trigeminal neuralgia (Khan, 1998). Seven patients who had been refractory to treatment were treated with gabapentin. Six patients had complete pain relief, while the seventh had partial pain relief. Pain relief began 3 to 4 days after beginning therapy and was complete within 2 weeks. Gabapentin maintained its effect through 1 year of follow-up (Khan, 1998). Gabapentin is started at 300 mg/day and increased by 300 mg every other day until pain relief is achieved. There is probably no top dose of gabapentin, but most limit the dose to 4,000 to 5,000 mg/day. Compared to carbamazepine and phenytoin, gabapentin has minimal side effects and is better tolerated by older patients.

Oxcarbazepine, a keto derivative of carbamazepine, has recently obtained FDA approval for the treatment of epilepsy. It is probably equal or superior to carbamazepine in the treatment of trigeminal neuralgia. Oxcarbazepine has very rapid oral absorption, with maximum blood concentrations occurring within 1 hour of dosing. Farago (1987)

treated 13 patients with oxcarbazepine for a mean of 11 months. Treatment resulted in pain reduction or complete pain relief in all patients. In six patients, pain relief occurred within 24 hours, and all patients had pain relief by 72 hours. The effective oxcarbazepine dose was 10 to 20 mg/kg of body weight. Zakrzewska and Patsalos (1989) used oxcarbazepine to treat six patients who were refractory to carbamazepine; all had some pain relief within 24 hours of the initial dose. In an open-label trial, 13 of 15 patients who were switched from carbamazepine to oxcarbazepine demonstrated pain reduction, while ten became pain-free on doses of 900 to 1,800 mg/day (Remillard, 1994). Oxcarbazepine should be started at a dose of 150 to 300 mg and increased every third day by 150 to 300 mg increments until there is pain relief (the total dose needed is usually <1,200 mg/day). Oxcarbazepine's side-effect profile appears to be better than that of carbamazepine, although the risk of hyponatremia is the same.

Topiramate, a novel antiepileptic, was successful at treating refractory trigeminal neuralgia in multiple sclerosis patients. In an open-label, consecutive case series, five patients became completely pain-free on topiramate. Four patients had pain relief with 200 mg, while a single patient needed 300 mg. All but one patient were able to discontinue their other trigeminal neuralgia medications. Patients remained pain-free on topiramate through 6 months of follow-up (Din et al., 2000).

Following is a list of rules for medical therapy in trigeminal neuralgia.

1. Do not overtreat. Look for remissions and taper the drug if the patient has been pain-free for 4 to 6 weeks, but be alert for recurrences. Pain diaries are useful to document pain-free intervals.
2. Chronic anticonvulsant therapy, especially in an older population, can cause cognitive impairment. Use the smallest pain-relieving dose possible.
3. Many trigeminal neuralgia patients become less responsive to medication with time. Try the drug to its fullest potential,

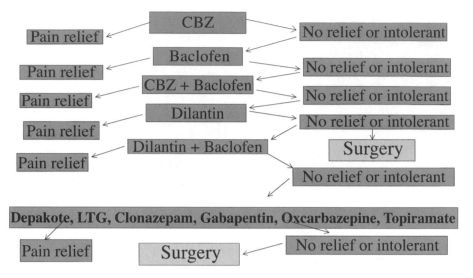

Figure 23–1 Algorithm for the treatment of trigeminal neuralgia.

recognize changes in pharmacokinetics (e.g., changing half-life of carbamazepine over time), and adjust doses accordingly.

4. Minimize medication side effects by carefully titrating doses throughout the day, avoiding peaks and troughs.

5. Aim for monotherapy, but polypharmacy is an acceptable and successful treatment scheme in trigeminal neuralgia.

6. Lamotrigine, gabapentin, topiramate, and oxcarbazepine may be more effective and better tolerated than carbamazepine and phenytoin.

Figure 23–1 is an algorithm for a drug-treatment scheme for trigeminal neuralgia. Most authorities start with carbamazepine and, if this fails, add baclofen. If carbamazepine and baclofen fail, consider phenytoin, alone or with baclofen. Clonazepam, depakote, gabapentin, topiramate, oxcarbazepine, and lamotrigine may be more useful than phenytoin and/or baclofen and should be tried closer to the top of the algorithm than previously considered. Table 23–3 provides a dosing schedule for medications that can be utilized for trigeminal neuralgia.

Nonmedical Therapy for Trigeminal Neuralgia

A recent trend in pain management has been nonmedicinal alternatives to medical therapy.

Acupuncture may have some benefit in trigeminal neuralgia. Shuhan et al. (1991) studied the role of acupuncture in 1,500 trigeminal neuralgia patients. The treatment course was 10 days (daily or every other day) and was repeated in 3 to 5 days if unsuccessful. Most patients required an average of 26 sessions to obtain relief. Five hundred and thirty-nine patients were followed from 1 to 6 years, and 99.2% of them were helped. About 44% had a recurrence of trigeminal neuralgia attacks, but the attacks were less severe than they were before therapy. Patients who had a shorter past history of trigeminal neuralgia had the best response. There was no correlation between success of acupuncture and pain distribution or the patient's age or gender. This was not a controlled trial.

Table 23–3 Drug therapy for trigeminal neuralgia

Medication	Dose range (mg/day)	Time to relief
Carbamazepine	400–800	24–48 hours
Phenytoin	300–500	24–48 hours
Baclofen	40–80	?
Clonazepam	1.5–8	?
Valproic acid	500–1,500	Weeks
Lamotrigine	150–400	24 hours
Pimozide	4–12	?
Gabapentin	900–2,400	1 week
Oxcarbazepine	900–1,800	24–72 hours
Topiramate	25–400	?

Surgical Treatment for Trigeminal Neuralgia

Candidates for surgical therapy for trigeminal neuralgia include patients who have failed medical therapy (which occurs about 30% of the time) or patients who initially responded but later became intolerant to medical therapy. About 50% of trigeminal neuralgia sufferers will require surgery (Table 23–4).

Extracranial Peripheral Denervation

Extracranial peripheral denervation previously was the most common surgical technique utilized for trigeminal neuralgia. The goal of this procedure is to interrupt signals from trigeminal peripheral afferents by temporarily or permanently destroying the afferent fibers via chemical, thermal, or traumatic measures. The location of the trigeminal neuralgia pain or trigger zones determines which nerve branch needs to be denervated. Peripheral denervation is performed at the supraorbital notch for ophthalmic division pain, the infraorbital notch for maxillary division pain, and the mental foramen for mandibular division pain. Lidocaine and bupivocaine are used for temporary denervation, while more permanent denervation is achieved with alcohol, freezing, and heating. Cutting or avulsing the nerve via neurectomy is also a surgical treatment option. Extracranial peripheral denervation has many advantages. There is good pain relief, with a 50% to 100% success rate. Only a small area of denervation is necessary, and there is no risk of corneal denervation or keratitis. It is an office procedure and requires only a brief postoperative recovery period. Finally, it enables the patient to appreciate what loss of sensation would mean if a more permanent procedure, such as radiofrequency thermocoagulation of the gasserian ganglion, were to be performed (Zakrzewska, 1995b). A major disadvantage of extracranial peripheral denervation is that it can be a very painful procedure if not performed under sedation, and elderly sufferers of trigeminal neuralgia are at increased risk of complications with anesthesia. Peripheral denervation provides only short-term pain relief. With lidocaine, pain returns in hours to days; with alcohol, it returns in 6 to 18 months; with freezing, it returns in 4 to 14 months; and with neurectomy, it returns in 20 to 30 months. Serious complications of peripheral denervation are rare but include skin necrosis and eye hemorrhage if denervation is completed in the ophthalmic division. Extracranial peripheral denervation is now recommended for the elderly patient with a short life expectancy or the patient who needs immediate pain relief and is medically unfit for a more invasive procedure. Extracranial peripheral denervation studies are plagued by methodologic issues, including the use of nonspecific diagnostic criteria, end points that are not defined, a length of follow-up that is not documented, and a lack of prospective observations.

Percutaneous Denervation of the Gasserian Ganglion and Retrogasserian Rootlets

Percutaneous denervation of the gasserian ganglion and retrogasserian rootlets involves partial destruction of the trigeminal nerve with either heat [radiofrequency (RF)], glycerol, or balloon compression. These techniques are presently the most commonly used surgical procedures for trigeminal neuralgia. Under radiographic control, a device is inserted into the cheek and directed through the foramen ovale into the area of the gasserian ganglion and rootlets, and the specific denervating agent is then used.

RADIOFREQUENCY THERMOCOAGULATION

Radiofrequency thermocoagulation is the most commonly used surgical treatment for

Table 23–4 Surgical procedures for trigeminal neuralgia

1. Peripheral techniques: These cause selective trauma to branches of the trigeminal nerve and try to prevent conduction of afferent painful stimuli.
2. Gasserian ganglion techniques: These are directed at the trigeminal root and try to cause selective damage to A delta and C fibers.
3. Posterior fossa surgery: This is done to restore functional anatomy by removing compressive lesions.

trigeminal neuralgia. More than 90% of patients experience relief from the initial procedure. The response is almost always immediate. Pain recurrence rates range from 4% to 65% (Zakrzewska, 1995d) and correlate with length of follow-up. The longest follow-up study of RF has been 13 years. Radiofrequency thermocoagulation has less denervation at the initial procedure and one of the lowest recurrence rates of all trigeminal neuralgia surgical procedures. Side effects of RF thermocoagulation include moderate dysesthesias in 5% to 25% of patients, severe dysesthesias in 2% to 10%, corneal sensory loss in 20%, and anesthesia dolorosa in 1% to 5% (Zakrzewska, 1995d). The minor side effects can be reduced by making the end point hypoalgesia rather than analgesia. Major side effects include intracranial hemorrhage, stroke, and infection. Weakness of the muscles of mastication occurs in about 53% of individuals (Onofrio, 1975), is usually temporary, and resolves in 3 to 6 months. Radiofrequency thermocoagulation has the advantage of being a highly specific procedure that is safe in the elderly and delivers immediate pain relief. It has a very low recurrence rate, with low mortality. Disadvantages include cost and the need for skilled hands. The procedure can cause corneal anesthesia if done in the ophthalmic division, and sensory loss can go beyond the area affected by the technique. Anesthesia dolorosa and keratitis may occur.

GLYCEROL TRIGEMINAL RHIZOTOMY

Glycerol trigeminal rhizotomy is an alternative to RF. Sterile glycerol acts as a mild denervating agent when injected into the gasserian ganglion. Glycerol rhizotomy is effective in up to 90% of individuals, and 50% experience pain relief within 24 hours. Others may not experience pain relief until 7 to 10 days after the procedure. Glycerol rhizotomy has a high recurrence rate; 28% of patients experience a recurrence within 1 year and 50% by 2 years (often within 6 to 12 months). Documented ranges of recurrence rates are 10% to 72% (Arias, 2000; Fujimaki et al., 1990). The procedure has very few side effects, but some form of sensory loss may occur in 26% to 71% of patients; this is less than

with RF lesions. Glycerol trigeminal rhizotomy is a highly specific technique that is safe in the elderly and requires no general anesthesia. It is less complicated than RF thermocoagulation. There is incomplete sensory loss and no mortality. Disadvantages include delayed pain relief, which can take up to 10 days. There are many initial failures since the procedure needs correct needle placement, and it has a fairly high recurrence rate. Glycerol trigeminal rhizotomy is particularly useful for the patient with ophthalmic division pain. Corneal anesthesia and keratitis occur less frequently with glycerol than with RF thermocoagulation.

PERCUTANEOUS BALLOON COMPRESSION

Percutaneous balloon compression is a technique used infrequently. Under general anesthesia, a Fogarty balloon catheter is inserted through the foramen ovale. The balloon is then inflated, causing compression of the gasserian ganglion. Initial success rates are high, between 80% and 90%. About 28% of patients, however, will have some recurrence, with a mean time of 6.5 months (Meglio and Cioni, 1989). Problems with the technique (compared with RF and glycerol denervation) include general anesthesia requirements and increased risk of intracranial hemorrhage with large trochar insertion; also, as this is not a selective procedure, the amount of sensory loss is not known until the procedure has been completed. Autonomic dysfunction from balloon inflation can induce bradycardia and hypotension. Thus, cardiac disease is a contraindication to percutaneous balloon compression.

MICROVASCULAR DECOMPRESSION

Microvascular decompression (MVD) is based on the theory that trigeminal neuralgia is due to a vascular loop compressing the trigeminal nerve at the root entry zone, leading to focal irritation, demyelination, and subsequent pain. As many as 96% of patients who undergo MVD for trigeminal neuralgia have documented vessel compression of the trigeminal nerve. Hamlyn and King (1992) found that 90% of patients who underwent vascular decompression had vessel compression compared to only 13% of age- and gender-matched nontrigeminal neuralgia cadaver patients. Most vascular loops leading to trigeminal nerve irritation are arterial and arise from the superior cerebellar artery. Venous compression occurs about 12% to 15% of the time.

Microvascular decompression was initially used by Dandy and perfected by Janetta. It requires a suboccipital retromastoid craniectomy. If a vascular compressive lesion is identified, the trigeminal nerve is decompressed by placing synthetic material between the nerve and the compressing vessel. Barker et al. (1996) completed a long-term outcome study of MVD on 1,185 patients over a 20-year period and showed that 80% had complete pain relief following the procedure, while 7.6% obtained partial relief. At 10 years, 70% continued to show excellent results, meaning that they had pain relief and no extra medications were needed, while 4% had partial relief. Of patients who did not have complete relief, 34% resumed chronic medication, 20% had an additional ablative procedure, and 22% had an ablative procedure plus needed chronic medication. Recurrence rates were minimal, only 1% to 6%, and most occurred within the first 2 years. The belief is that if there is no pain relapse within 2 years of MVD, patients will probably remain pain-free. The advantages of MVD include a long-lasting response, preservation of nerve function, no risk of anesthesia dolorosa, and a low recurrence rate. Factors increasing recurrence rates after MVD include female gender, symptoms present for longer than 8 years, venous compression, lack of immediate postoperative pain relief, less significant vascular contact with the trigeminal nerve, and a history of dull background pain between attacks (Zakrzewska, 1995c). Disadvantages include possible mortality and the risks of damaging cranial nerves other than the trigeminal nerve, especially the trochlear nerve. Complications from MVD include death in 0% to 1% of patients (cerebellar hemorrhage and infarction) (Zakrzewska, 1995c), intracranial hemorrhage or stroke in 1% to 2%, hearing loss in up to 21% (permanent in 3% to 8%) (van Loveren et al., 1982; Kolluri and Heros, 1984; Piatt and Wilkins, 1984; Bederson and Wilson, 1989), and sensory loss in 5% to 31%

(Szapiro and Sindou, 1985). In most institutions, MVD is carried out if RF thermocoagulation has failed, but others utilize MVD as a first-line therapy for medically refractory trigeminal neuralgia.

What is the role of repeat exploration if the initial MVD procedure has failed to alleviate pain or if pain has recurred? Speculated causes of MVD failure include incomplete vascular decompression with the initial procedure, recurrence of vascular compression, slippage of the synthetic implant, or scarring of the implant leading to nerve compression. Kureshi and Wilkins (1998) performed repeat exploration in 31 patients, 23 of whom had trigeminal neuralgia and 8 hemifacial spasm. On repeat exploration, they noted that the initial implant was in good position (nondisplaced) in 100% of patients. A new compressive element (artery, scarred implant, bony ridge) was noted in 30% of patients. Postsurgical complication after repeat exploration occurred in 30% of patients, typically involving hearing loss or facial weakness. The authors concluded that repeat exploration in failed MVD is unwarranted because of the lack of finding any significant compressive lesions on repeat exploration and the relatively high complication rate of the procedure. Instead of repeat exploratory surgery, the patient could be sent for another form of ablative procedure (i.e., RF rhizotomy) or tried again on medications. Jannetta and Bissonette (1985) looked at 51 patients with mild MVD and found persistent arterial or venous compression in 44 and scarred implants in 5 patients on repeat exploration. Bederson and Wilson (1989) found no abnormality on repeat exploration in 90% of 20 studied patients, while Cho et al. (1994) found that 23% of 53 patients had arterial loop compression on repeat exploration, 13% had venous compression, and 13% had implant compression. There is no consensus on the role of repeat exploration in failed MVD.

Gamma Knife Radiosurgery

Gamma knife radiosurgery, a form of stereotactic radiosurgery, is one of the newest therapeutic techniques for trigeminal neuralgia. The procedure entails the use of a stereotactic head frame, stereotactic imaging of the tri-geminal nerve root entry zone, and radiation of the trigeminal nerve, usually 2 to 4 mm anterior to the brain stem. The normal radiation dose is 70 to 80 Gy. The brain stem normally receives <20% of the total radiation dosage. Young et al. (1997) examined 51 patients after gamma knife radiosurgery; 49 had idiopathic trigeminal neuralgia and two had multiple sclerosis–induced trigeminal neuralgia. All patients were medical nonresponders, and 22 were surgical nonresponders. Thirty-eight of 51 patients (74.5%) were completely pain-free after gamma knife radiosurgery. A 50% to 90% decrease in facial pain was seen in another 13.7% of patients, while 11.1% failed the procedure. Follow-up was for 6 to 36 months, with mean follow-up being 16.3 months. Most patients (80.4%) remained pain-free or continued with marked pain reduction. Time to initial pain relief could be quite long, anywhere from 1 to 120 days, with a mean of 14 days. Kondziolka et al. (1996) reported on a five-center study of gamma knife radiosurgery for trigeminal neuralgia. Fifty percent of individuals became pain-free, and pain was reduced by 50% to 90% in another 34% of patients. Ten percent failed to respond. Overall, 84% of patients felt they had an excellent to good response. Mean follow-up time was 9.2 months. A problem with this study was that different techniques were used in different institutions, which suggests possible inconsistencies in the results. In addition, there was a very short follow-up period. The advantages of gamma knife radiosurgery in trigeminal neuralgia include a very short procedure time (only 2.5 to 3 hours), the need for only local anesthesia, and efficacy that is almost equal to more invasive procedures. There appears to be a low complication rate: only 6% of the patients in the Kondziolka et al. (1996) study had complications, and only one patient in the Young et al. (1997) study had complications. A disadvantage of gamma knife radiosurgery is that onset to pain relief may be slow. Most trigeminal neuralgia patients cannot wait months for pain relief as the syndrome can be excruciating and disabling. Also, there has been no long-term follow-up of gamma knife radio-surgery in trigeminal neuralgia. Finally, no one knows what the true delayed radiation complications of gamma knife radiosurgery are (especially in young patients). The proposed mechanism of action of gamma knife radiosurgery for trigeminal neuralgia is inactivating pathologic ephaptic transmission without damaging normal axonal conduction. Gamma knife radiosurgery costs three times more than percutaneous denervation and about 40% less than MVD.

GLOSSOPHARYNGEAL NEURALGIA

Glossopharyngeal neuralgia is an uncommon facial pain syndrome that was first described by Weisenburg (1910). Its incidence is between 0.2% and 1.3% of trigeminal neuralgia (White and Sweet, 1969a). Symptoms typically begin after the sixth decade (Rushton et al. 1981). Since the pain is felt in the sensory distribution of the glossopharyngeal and vagus nerves, some authors use the term "vagoglossopharyngeal neuralgia" for this disorder. Like trigeminal neuralgia, it may go into remission (Rushton et al., 1981). Glossopharyngeal nueralgia and trigeminal neuralgia occur in a combined form in 10% of patients.

Glossopharyngeal neuralgia is characterized by paroxysmal pain in the throat, tonsillar fossa, tongue, and ear. The onset is abrupt, and it may persist for several seconds to 1 minute. Attacks of pain are invariably triggered not by chewing but by swallowing, paricularly cold liquids, and, on occasion, by yawning or sneezing. As many as 2% of patients lose consciousness during pain paroxysms, probably due to bradycardia. The physical examination is normal, yet occasionally a trigger zone within the preauricular or postauricular area, the neck, or the external auditory canal is identified. Application of a local anesthetic to the oropharynx has both therapeutic and diagnostic implications (Rushton et al., 1981).

The evaluation of a patient with glossopharyngeal neuralgia should include an MRI scan with contrast. Secondary glossopharyngeal neuralgia may be due to an oropharyngeal malignancy, a peritonsillar infection, or vascular compression wherein a loop of a posterior fossa vessel compresses the nerve.

Glossopharyngeal neuralgia is treated with an anticonvulsant medication, such as carbamazepine, phenytoin, or baclofen. Patients who are refractory to medical therapy can be treated surgically with intracranial sectioning of the glossopharyngeal nerve and the upper rootlets of the vagus nerve. Microvascular decompression of the 9th cranial nerve is also effective (Kondo, 1998).

ATYPICAL FACIAL PAIN

Atypical facial pain includes those types of facial pain that do not represent "typical" or classifiable pain syndromes. The term was introduced by Frazier and Russell (1924), largely to distinguish trigeminal neuralgia from the myriad of other causes of facial pain. Fay (1932) was the first to postulate that nondescript facial pain not only may be due to an underlying vascular mechanism but could represent a referred pain syndrome in some patients.

The term "atypical facial pain" has been questioned over the years by several experienced clinicians. Rushton et al. (1959) wrote "Danger exists in considering atypical facial pain an entity since this would imply a common cause, and its use would assume that a definite diagnosis has been made." We agree with Raskin (1988) that a preferable term is "facial pain of unknown cause." If "typical" atypical facial pain exists, it should be considered only after facial pain secondary to anatomic and pathophysiologic disturbances have been excluded. An abnormal neurologic examination is not compatible with the diagnosis of atypical facial pain. A complete general and neurologic examination and sometimes consultations with colleagues in otorhinolaryngology, dentistry, and occasionally ophthalmology may by necessary. Appropriate imaging studies may be necessary to exclude nasopharyngeal and sinus neoplasms, structural abnormalities at the skull base, and dental conditions, such as maxillary and/or cryptic mandibular microabscesses. The possibility of squamous cell and basal cell carcinoma of the face should also be considered. The evaluation may also necessitate a chest roentgenogram or chest CT if referred pain from lung cancer is suggested by the history (smoker, weight loss) or examination (digital clubbing) (Capobianco, 1995), As our knowledge of this most troublesome disorder advances, other causes of pain will most certainly be identified.

Patients in whom "typical" atypical facial pain is eventually diagnosed possess the following features, which distinguish this pain disorder from the major facial neuralgias (Solomon and Lipton, 1988, 1990; Campbell, 1988). The pain is steady, generally unilateral (on occasion may become bilateral), and poorly localized yet typically involving the eye, nose, cheek, temple, or jaw. The pain may spread over the area supplied by the cervical roots. The pain is usually described as deep and aching yet is not infrequently characterized graphically as tearing, ripping, crushing, or pulling. Absent are the paroxysms of short duration (1 to 30 seconds) followed by freedom from pain seen in trigeminal neuralgia. Although the patient reports intense pain, quite often the patient does not appear to be in outward distress. The pain is generally present all day every day and often worsens over time. Absent are the trigger zones characteristic of the neuralgias. Attacks are not precipitated by cold air, cold water in the mouth, swallowing, talking, chewing, shaving, or washing the face. The typical patient is a woman in her thirties or forties, who is often depressed. The depression does not imply a causal relationship but may reflect the effect of unresolved pain. The pain is not significantly reduced or eliminated by division of the 5th or 9th cranial nerve. Surgical procedures are often performed in vain and only serve to aggravate the underlying problem. Some patients may suffer from a form of migraine involving the face, so-called facial migraine. This diagnosis should be considered if the facial pain is intermittent, throbbing, and associated with nausea, photophobia, and/or phonophobia. A careful search for triggering factors, such as menses, alcohol ingestion, exertion, or changes in the sleep–wake cycle, may provide a useful clue as to a migrainous mechanism. In such situations, a trial with antimigraine medications, both acute and preventive, may prove helpful. Cluster headache, the so-called lower-half form, should also be considered, particularly if the pain is of short duration and associated with ipsilateral autonomic accompaniments (Campbell, 1988).

Many patients with chronic, long-standing atypical facial pain require a multifaceted treatment approach. These patients often have undergone numerous surgical (dental, nasal, or sinus) procedures to no avail. Treatment can include pain-relieving or analgesic medications, antimigraine as well as antineuralgic medications, and nonpharmacologic treatment treatment strategies, including biofeedback and relaxation techniques.

REFERENCES

Arias, M.J. (2000). Percutaneous retrogasserian glycerol rhizotomies for trigeminal neuralgia. A prospective study of 100 cases. *Neurosurgery* 65:32–36.

Barker, G.G., P.J. Jannetta, D.J. Bissonette et al. (1996). The long-term outcome of microvascular decompression for trigeminal neuralgia. *N. Engl. J. Med.* 334:1077–1083.

Bederson, J.B. and C.B. Wilson (1989). Evaluation of microvascular decompression and partial sensory rhizotomy in 252 cases of trigeminal neuralgia. *J. Neurosurg.* 71:359–367.

Brewis, M., D.C. Poskanzer, C. Rolland et al. (1966). Neurological disease in an English city. *Acta Neurol. Scand.* 42:1–89.

Campbell, J.K. (1988). Facial pain due to migraine and cluster headache. *Semin. Neurol.* 8:255–347.

Capobianco, D.J. (1995). Facial pain as a symptom of nonmetastatic lung cancer. *Headache* 35: 581–585.

Cho, D.Y., G.S. Chang, Y.C. Wang et al. (1994). Repeat operations in failed microvascular decompression for trigeminal neuralgia. *Neurosurgery* 35:665–670.

Court, J.E. and C.S. Kase (1976). Treatment of tic douloureaux with a new anticonvulsant (clonazepam). *J. Neurol. Neurosurg. Psychiatry* 39: 297–299.

Din, M.U., M. Zvartan-Hind, A. Gilari et al. (2000). Topiramate relieved refractory trigeminal neuralgia in multiple sclerosis patients [Abstract]. *Neurology* 54:A60.

Duff, J.M., R.J. Spinner, N.M. Lindor et al. (1999). Familial trigeminal neuralgia and contralateral hemifacial spasm. *Neurology* 53:216–218.

Farago, F. (1987). Trigeminal neuralgia: Its treatment with two new carbamazepine analogues. *Eur. Neurol.* 26:73–83.

Fay, T. (1932). Atypical facial neuralgia, a syndrome of vascular pain. *Ann. Otol. Laryngol. 41*: 1030–1062.

Frazier, C.H. and E.C. Russell (1924). Neuralgia of the face. An analysis of 754 cases with relation to pain and other sensory phenomena before and after operation. *Arch. Neurol. Psychiatry 11*:557–563.

Fromm, G.H. (1991). Pathophysiology of trigeminal neuralgia. In *Trigeminal Neuralgia: Current Concepts Regarding Pathogenesis and Treatment* (G.H. Fromm and B.J. Sessle, eds.), pp. 105–130. Butterworth-Heinemann, Boston.

Fujimaki, T., T. Fukushima, and S. Miyazaki (1990). Percutaneous retrogasserian glycerol injection in the management of trigeminal neuralgia: Long-term follow-up results. *J. Neurosurg.* 73:212–216.

Hamlyn, P.J. and T.T. King (1992). Neurovascular compression in trigeminal neuralgia: A clinical and anatomical study. *J. Neurosurg.* 76:948–954.

Harris, W. (1926). Chronic paroxysmal trigeminal neuralgia. In *Neuritis and Neuralgia* (W. Harris, ed.), pp. 150–222. Oxford University Press, Oxford.

Headache Classification Committee of the International Headache Society (1988). Classification and diagnostic criteria for headache disorders, cranial neuralgia, and facial pain. *Cephalalgia* 8: 1–96.

Jannetta, P.J. and D.J. Bissonette (1985). Management of the failed patient with trigeminal neuralgia. *Clin. Neurosurg.* 32:334–347.

Jassim, S.A. (1994). Patient's assessment of outcome after radiofrequency thermocoagulation for management of trigeminal neuralgia. University of London, London. Dissertation.

Katusic, S., C.M. Beard, E. Bergstralh (1990). Incidence and clinical features of trigeminal neuralgia. *Ann. Neurol.* 27:89–95.

Khan, O.A. (1998). Gabapentin relieves trigeminal neuralgia in multiple sclerosis patients. *Neurology* 51:611–614.

Kolluri, S. and R.C. Heros (1984). Microvascular decompression for trigeminal neuralgia. A five year follow-up study. *Surg. Neurol.* 22:235–240.

Kondo, A. (1998). Follow-up results of using microvascular decompression for treatment of glossopharyngeal neuralgia. *J. Neurosurg.* 88: 221–225.

Kondziolka, D., L.D. Lunsford, J.C. Flickinger et al. (1996). Stereotactic radiosurgery for trigeminal neuralgia: A multiinstitutional study using the gamma unit. *J. Neurosurg.* 84:940–945.

Kureshi, S.A. and R.H. Wilkins (1998). Posterior fossa exploration for persistent or recurrent trigeminal neuralgia or hemifacial spasm: Surgical findings and therapeutic implications. *Neurosurgery* 43:1111–1116.

Kurland, L.T. (1958). Descriptive epidemiology of selected neurologic and myopathic disorders with particular reference to a survey in Rochester, Minnesota. *J. Chron. Dis.* 8:378–418.

Leandri, M., P. Eldridge, and J. Miles (1998). Recovery of nerve conduction following microvascular decompression for trigeminal neuralgia. *Neurology* 51:1641–1646.

Lechin, F., B. van der Dijs, M.E. Lechin et al. (1989). Pimozide therapy for trigeminal neuralgia. *Arch. Neurol.* 46:960–963.

Lunardi, G., M. Leandri, C. Albano et al. (1997). Clinical effectiveness of lamotrigine and plasma levels in essential and symptomatic trigeminal neuralgia. *Neurology* 48:1714–1717.

Majoie, C.B., F.J. Hulsmans, J.A. Castelijns et al. (2000). Symptoms and signs related to the trigeminal nerve: Diagnostic yield of MR imaging. *Radiology* 209:557–562.

Meglio, M. and B. Cioni (1989). Percutaneous procedures for trigeminal neuralgia: Microcompression versus radiofrequency thermocoagulation (personal experience). *Pain* 38:9–16.

Onofrio, B.M. (1975). Radiofrequency percutaneous gasserian ganglion lesions. Results in 140 patients with trigeminal pain. *J. Neurosurg.* 42:132–139.

Peiris, J.B., G.L. Perera, S.V. Devendra et al. (1980). Sodium valproate in trigeminal neuralgia. *Med. J. Aust.* 2:278.

Penman, J. (1968). Trigeminal neuralgia. In *Handbook of Clinical Neurology* (P.J. Vinken and G.W. Bruyn, eds.), pp. 296–322. Elsevier, Amsterdam.

Piatt, J.H. and R.H. Wilkins (1984). Treatment of tic douloureaux and hemifacial spasm by posterior fossa exploration: Therapeutic implications and various neurovascular relationships. *Neurosurgery* 14:462–471.

Pollack, I.F., P.J. Jannetta, and D.J. Bissonette (1988). Bilateral trigeminal neuralgia: A 14-year experience with microvascular decompression. *J. Neurosurg.* 68:559–565.

Raskin, N.H. (1988). Facial pain. In *Headache* (N.H. Raskin, ed.), pp. 333–374. Churchill Livingstone, New York.

Remillard, G. (1994). oxcarbazepine and intractable trigeminal neuralgia. *Epilepsia* 35:28–29.

Rothman, K.J. and R.R. Monson (1973). Epidemiology of trigeminal neuralgia. *J. Chron. Dis.* 26:1–12.

Rushton, G., J.A. Gibilisco, and N.P. Goldstein (1959). Atypical facial pain. *JAMA* 171:545–548.

Rushton, J.G. and H.N. MacDonald (1957). Trigeminal neuralgia. Special considerations of nonsurgical treatment. *JAMA* 165:437–440.

Rushton, J.G., J.C. Stevens, and R.H. Miller (1981). Glossopharyngeal (vagoglossopharyngeal) neuralgia. *Arch. Neurol.* 38:201–205.

Shuhan, G., X. Benren, and Z. Yuhuan (1991). Treatment of primary trigeminal neuralgia with acupuncture in 1500 cases. *J. Tradit. Chin. Med.* 11:3–6.

Sist, T., V. Filadora, M. Miner et al. (1997). Gabapentin for idiopathic trigeminal neuralgia: Report of two cases. *Neurology* 48:1467.

Solomon, S. and R.B. Lipton (1988). Atypical facial pain: A review. *Semin. Neurol.* 8:332–338.

Solomon, S. and R.B. Lipton (1990). Facial pain. *Neurol. Clin. November* 8:913–928.

Sundaram, P.K., A.S. Hegde, B.A. Chandramouli et al. (1999). Trigeminal evoked potentials in patients with symptomatic trigeminal neuralgia due to intracranial mass lesions. *Neurology* 47:94–97.

Szapiro, J. and M. Sindou (1985). Prognostic factors in microvascular decompression for trigeminal neuralgia. *Neurosurgery* 17:920–929.

Taylor, J.C., S. Brauer, and L.E. Espir (1981). Long-term treatment of trigeminal neuralgia with carbamazepine. *Postgrad. Med. J.* 5:16–18.

van Loveren, H., J.M. Tew, J.T. Keller et al. (1982). A 10 year experience in the treatment of trigeminal neuralgia: Comparison of percutaneous stereotoxic rhizotomy and posterior fossa exploration. *J. Neurosurg.* 57:757–765.

Weisenburg, T.H. (1910). Cerebello-pontine tumor diagnosed for six years as tic douloureux. The symptoms of irritation of the 9th and 12th cranial nerves. *JAMA* 54:1600–1604.

White, J.C. and W.H. Sweet (1969a). *Pain and the Neurosurgeon: A 40-Year Experience.* Charles C. Thomas, Springfield, IL.

White, J.C. and W.H. Sweet (1969b). Periodic migrainous neuralgia. In *Pain and the Neurosurgeon. A 40-year Experience* (J.C. White and W.H. Sweet, eds.), pp. 123–256. Charles C. Thomas, Springfield, IL.

Yoshimasu, F., L.T. Kurland, and L.R. Elveback (1972). Tic douloureaux in Rochester, Minnesota 1945–1969. *Neurology* 22:952–956.

Young, R.F., S.S. Vermeulen, P. Grimm et al. (1997). Gamma knife radiosurgery for treatment of trigeminal neuralgia: Idiopathic and tumor-related. *Neurology* 48:608–614.

Zakrzewska, J.M. (1995a). Medical management. In *Trigeminal neuralgia* (J.M. Zakrzewska, ed.), pp. 80–107. W.B. Saunders, London.

Zakrzewska, J.M. (1995b). Peripheral surgery. In *Trigeminal Neuralgia* (J.M. Zakrzewska, ed.), pp. 108–123. W.B. Saunders, London.

Zakrzewska, J.M. (1995c). Posterior fossa surgery. In *Trigeminal Neuralgia* (J.M. Zakrzewska, ed.), pp. 157–168. W.B. Saunders, London.

Zakrzewska, J.M. (1995d). Surgery at the level of the gasserian ganglion. In *Trigeminal Neuralgia* (J.M. Zakrzewska, ed.), pp. 125–156. W.B. Saunders, London.

Zakrzewska, J.M. (1995e). History. In *Trigeminal Neuralgia* (J.M. Zakrzewska, ed.), pp. 1–3. W.B. Saunders, London.

Zakrzewska, J.M., Z. Chaudhry, T.J. Nurmikko et al. (1997). Lamotrigine (Lamictal) in refractory trigeminal neuralgia: Results from a double-blind, placebo-controlled, crossover trial. *Pain* 73:223–230.

Zakrzewska, J.M. and P.N. Patsalos (1989). Oxcarbazepine—a new drug in the management of intractable trigeminal neuralgia. *J. Neurol. Neurosurg. Psychiatry* 52:472–476.

24

Giant Cell Arteritis and Polymyalgia Rheumatica

RICHARD J. CASELLI
GENE G. HUNDER

Headache is the most common presenting symptom of giant cell (temporal) arteritis (GCA) in elderly patients (Caselli et al., 1988a; Hollenhorst et al., 1960). Headache is a prominent symptom in approximately 70% of patients and the initial symptom in a third (Caselli et al., 1988a). The headache itself may be clinically nonspecific, but it generally represents a new symptom in patients who do not have a history of prior headaches or a new headache subtype in patients with pre-existing chronic headaches. It is characteristically throbbing, continuous, and focally worst in the temporal or, less often, occipital region. Many patients have clinically evident swollen, erythematous, and painful superficial temporal arteries (Fig. 24–1). An elevated erythrocyte sedimentation rate (ESR) or C-reactive protein (CRP) can provide a timely diagnosis and guide early therapeutic intervention, and the diagnosis can be subsequently confirmed with a temporal artery biopsy. Corticosteroid therapy generally produces symptomatic relief within days. Despite commensurate normalization of the ESR and CRP, active vasculitis probably continues for at least several weeks. Also, GCA can involve the aortic arch and its branches, resulting in a wide variety of vascular complications; therefore, prompt diagnosis and treatment are imperative.

PATHOLOGICAL CONSIDERATIONS

Histopathology

Patients with GCA have damage to the blood vessel wall, which is primarily the result of cellular immune mechanisms. Activated $CD4^+$ T-helper cells respond to an antigen (presumably elastin), the precise identity of which remains uncertain, that is presented by macrophages (Banks et al., 1983; Weyand et al., 1994; Shiiki et al., 1989; Wawryk et al., 1991). The inflammatory response often appears to be centered about the internal elastic lamina (Wilkinson and Russell, 1972) and results in the formation of multinucleated giant cells that represent the histological hallmark of GCA (Fig. 24–2). The multinucleated giant cells frequently contain elastic fiber fragments (Banks et al., 1983), suggesting that the specific antigen inciting the inflammatory response may be elastin (Hunder et al., 1993; Hellman, 1993).

Vascular Topography

The superficial temporal artery (STA) is involved in almost all patients, i.e., the term "temporal arteritis." However, GCA is more a disease of the aortic arch (Cardell and Han-

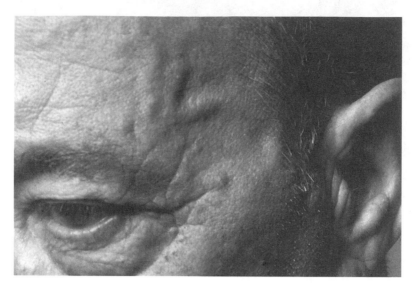

Figure 24–1 Seventy-year-old man with giant cell arteritis. A portion of the anterior branch of the left temporal artery is visibly swollen. It was tender and thickened to palpation.

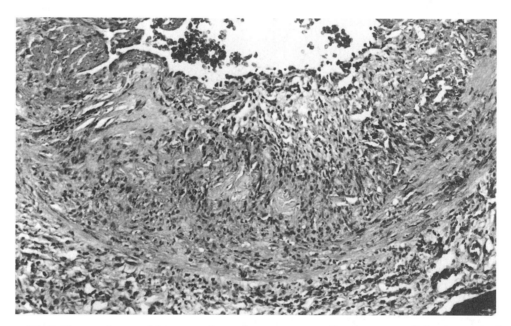

Figure 24–2 Temporal artery biopsy specimen showing active inflammation in all three vascular layers (intima, media, adventitia). The lumen is partially shown, at the top of the figure, and is narrowed. In most temporal artery biopsy specimens with giant cell arteritis, the media, especially the inner media in the region of the internal elastic lamina, is involved to the greatest extent and the intimal and adventitial layers are involved to a lesser degree than in this patient. (Hematoxylin and eosin stain, original ×200.)

ley, 1951; Heptinstall et al., 1954; Klein et al., 1975; Östberg, 1972; Evans et al., 1995) and its branches (Fig. 24–3), even though the aortic arch involvement is less than the STA involvement. Aortic arch–derived vessels that are occasionally involved include the coronary arteries (Cardell and Hanley, 1951; Östberg, 1972); the subclavian, axillary, and proximal brachial arteries (Heptinstall et al., 1954; Klein et al., 1975; Östberg, 1972; Andrews, 1966; Howard et al., 1984; Pollock et al., 1973); and cervicocephalic arteries, including

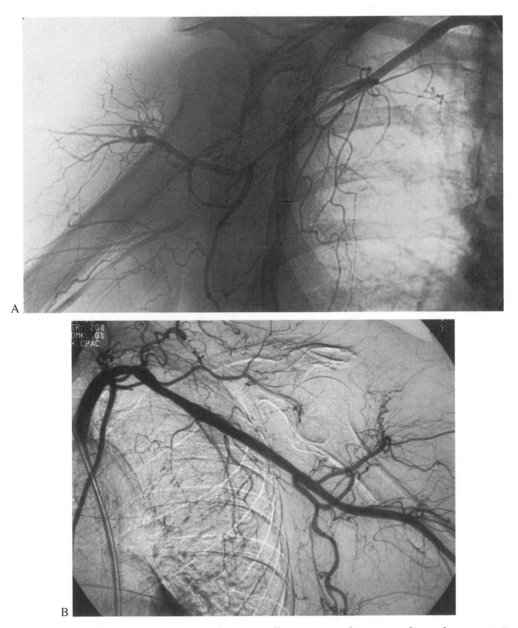

Figure 24–3 Angiogram in a patient with giant cell arteritis and aortic arch syndrome. *A*: Right subclavian artery and distal vessels. The distal axillary artery tapers progressively and becomes occluded at the axillary–brachial artery junction. The proximal brachial artery fills again via the abundant collateral vessels. *B*: Left subclavian artery shows a focal, smooth-walled, tapered area typical of vasculitis. There are prominent collateral vessels seen distally (shown), which resulted from a more distal severe brachial artery stenosis (not shown).

the carotid and vertebral arteries (Wilkinson and Russell, 1972; Cardell and Hanley, 1951; Heptinstall et al., 1954; Klein et al., 1975; Östberg, 1972; Evans et al., 1995; Andrews, 1966; Hamrin et al., 1965; Howard et al., 1984; Pollock et al., 1973; Bruk, 1967; Cooke et al., 1946; Crompton, 1959; Graham et al., 1981; Mowat and Hazelman, 1974; Russell, 1959; Whitfield et al., 1963). In fatal cases of GCA, autopsy studies have shown that the vertebral arteries are involved as frequently as the STAs (Wilkinson and Russell, 1972; Heptinstall et al., 1954; Crompton, 1959). Vertebral arteritis is extracranial, but it may extend intracranially up to 5 mm beyond dural penetration following the internal elastic lamina (Wilkinson and Russell, 1972). Because intracranial arteries lack an internal elastic lamina, GCA does not cause a widespread intracranial cerebral vasculitis and basilar artery involvement is rare (Heptinstall et al., 1954; Gibb et al., 1985). Intraorbital branches, especially the posterior ciliary and ophthalmic arteries, are commonly affected (Wilkinson and Russell, 1972; Crompton, 1959; Barricks et al., 1977; Wagener and Hollenhorst, 1958). Less often, the descending aorta (Klein et al., 1975; Östberg, 1972; Evans et al., 1994b, 1995), mesenteric (Klein et al., 1975), renal (Klein et al., 1975), iliac, and femoral (Cardell and Hanley, 1951; Heptinstall et al., 1954; Klein et al., 1975; Östberg, 1972; Caselli et al., 1988b) arteries are affected. Pulmonary arterial involvement also has been described (Heptinstall et al., 1954; Klein et al., 1975).

CRANIOFACIAL PAIN SYNDROMES IN THE GIANT CELL ARTERITIS PATIENT

Headache

The headache of GCA may have no pathognomonic features, but some qualities can be diagnostically suggestive. The most important feature is that the headache is either a new finding in a patient without a history of headaches or a new headache type in a patient with a history of chronic headaches. The headache quality is usually described as throbbing, generalized, and continuous. The temples are often focally painful and generally hurt to touch. Patients occasionally describe tender red cords in their temples (Fig. 24–1) or scalp tenderness when combing their hair. Rarely, the headache is predominantly occipital. One-third of patients lack these clinical signs of temporal or occipital artery inflammation. Approximately 5% of patients experience visual scintillations, suggestive of a migraine aura (Caselli et al., 1988a; Campbell and Caselli, 1991), though not specifically in a fixed temporal relationship with the headache. It is not known what significance these scintillations may have, but they should be viewed as a possible sign of retinal or optic nerve ischemia due to the vasculitis rather than a benign migrainous aura. A very rare cause of headache in the GCA patient is intracerebral hemorrhage (Hollenhorst et al., 1960), but its infrequency suggests that it is probably unrelated to vasculitis.

Other Craniofacial Pain Syndromes

Occipitonuchal pain may result from vasculitic involvement of the occipital arteries, or it may be part of the more generalized proximal limb, spine, and truncal pain that characterizes polymyalgia rheumatica (PMR), which occurs in approximately 50% of GCA patients and is the initial symptom in 25% of GCA patients (Caselli et al., 1988a). Ischemia of jaw and tongue muscles can cause jaw and tongue claudication. Jaw claudication occurs in approximately 40% of patients and is the initial symptom in roughly 4% (Caselli et al., 1988a). Tongue claudication occurs in approximately 4% of patients and is rarely the initial symptom (Caselli et al., 1988a). Rare cranial neuropathic syndromes, which may be a source of discomfort to patients, include transient hemianesthesia of the tongue (Caselli et al., 1988a), lingual paralysis (Kinmont and McCallum, 1964), and facial pain due to facial artery vasculitis (Das and Laskin, 1966), which might be mistaken for trigeminal neuralgia. Approximately 15% of patients with GCA have carotidynia (Caselli et al., 1988a). Presumably, this reflects carotid vasculitis, but angiographic studies of such patients who lack other signs and symptoms of carotid artery disease are lacking.

NEUROLOGICAL DISEASE IN THE SETTING OF ACTIVE GIANT CELL ARTERITIS

The following complications may accompany the headache of GCA and are important features of the disease that the headache may portend.

Central Nervous System Complications

Optic Neuropathy

Optic neuropathy is one of the most feared complications of GCA. Amaurosis fugax occurs in 10% to 12% of patients with GCA (Caselli et al., 1988a; Huston et al., 1978), and permanent loss of vision due to anterior ischemic optic neuropathy (AION) occurs in 8% (Caselli et al., 1988a) to 23% (Koorey, 1984). Prior to the advent and widespread use of corticosteroid therapy, however, most series reported that patients with transient loss of vision went on to develop permanent, bilateral loss of vision due to AION (Hollenhorst et al., 1960; Mowat and Hazelman, 1974; Russell, 1959; Wagener and Hollenhorst, 1958). Following monocular onset, the second eye became affected within days (Wagener and Hollenhorst, 1958). Prompt diagnosis and effective corticosteroid therapy has drastically reduced the number of patients with permanent loss of vision due to GCA (Hall et al., 1983). Most often, AION results from vasculitis of the posterior ciliary artery and, occasionally, from vasculitis or occlusion of the central retinal artery (Hollenhorst et al., 1960; Wagener and Hollenhorst, 1958). During acute AION, ophthalmoscopy shows sludging of blood in retinal arterioles, which can be orthostatically sensitive (Hollenhorst, 1967). Diagnostically important funduscopic signs of optic nerve swelling may lag behind visual loss and the acute ophthalmoscopic finding of papillary and retinal ischemia by roughly 36 hours (Wagener and Hol-

lenhorst, 1958). Occasionally, however, optic neuropathy is entirely retrobulbar without acute funduscopic changes (Wagener and Hollenhorst, 1958). In acute AION, the optic disk becomes pale with blurred margins due to papilledema (Wagener and Hollenhorst, 1958). As AION evolves, the absolute amount of disk elevation tends to be modest (less than 3 diopters in most cases), with infrequent areas of disk hemorrhage (Barricks et al., 1977). Optic disk edema resolves within 10 days or so and is replaced within 2 to 4 weeks by optic atrophy, even in retrobulbar cases (Wagener and Hollenhorst, 1958). Residual visual field defects are usually altitudinal (Wagener and Hollenhorst, 1958). In patients with central retinal artery occlusion, there may be pallor and edema of the entire retina and optic disk together with a macular cherry red spot (Hollenhorst et al., 1960).

Ocular Motility Disorders

Diplopia occurs in roughly 2% (Caselli et al., 1988a) to 14% (Hollenhorst et al., 1960; Huston et al., 1978) of patients with GCA. It may be static (in cases of oculomotor nerve infarction) or fluctuate daily (similar to myasthenia gravis) (Hollenhorst et al., 1960; Russell, 1959; Hollenhorst, 1967). Any level of the oculomotor apparatus can be involved, including the extraocular muscles, nerves (Dimant et al., 1980), and brain stem (Monteiro et al., 1984); but the extraocular muscle is the most common site (Russell, 1959; Barricks et al., 1977). Ptosis and miosis may occur together (Horner's syndrome) or separately, as well as in conjunction with other oculomotor disturbances (Dimant et al., 1980; Monteiro et al., 1984).

Cerebrovascular Disease

Clinically auscultable bruits reflect the topographic distribution of GCA. Carotid bruits occur in 10% to 20% of GCA patients and are often bilateral (Caselli et al., 1988a; Hamrin et al., 1965). Sixty percent of patients with bilateral carotid bruits also have upper limb bruits or claudication or both (Caselli et al., 1988a). Approximately 40% of GCA patients who have carotid bruits sustain some type of ischemic eye or brain complication (amaurosis fugax, transient ischemic attack, permanent visual loss, or stroke), although permanent deficits (permanent visual loss and stroke) do not occur more often than in GCA patients without carotid bruits (Caselli et al., 1988a). The known propensity of GCA to affect carotid and vertebral arteries should be considered in GCA patients with transient ischemic attacks (TIAs) and cerebral infarction (Caselli et al., 1988a; Caselli, 1990), even though atherosclerosis, hypertension, and cardiac disease remain the most important causes of cerebral infarction in elderly patients with or without GCA (Huston et al., 1978). Approximately 4% of GCA patients experience a TIA or stroke at some point during their illness (Caselli et al., 1988a). A relatively greater proportion of TIAs and cerebral infarctions occurs in the vertebrobasilar territory than the carotid territory in GCA patients compared to the general population (Caselli et al., 1988a). Unfortunately, there are few clinical features that reliably distinguish a vasculitic from an atheromatous cause, although in rare instances atheroembolic material has been observed funduscopically or angiographically in the setting of active GCA (Caselli et al., 1988a; Hollenhorst, 1967). Lacunar infarction syndromes due to hypertensive small vessel disease would not specifically be expected to result from a cervicocephalic arteritis, but it may be difficult to reliably distinguish a small from a large vessel stroke syndrome acutely or without neuroimaging.

Neuro-otological Disorders

One of several vasculitides that can lead to acute auditory nerve infarction is GCA, but it is a rare occurrence (Hollenhorst et al., 1960; Caselli et al., 1988a). Acute unilateral hearing loss is the most suggestive symptom, but we have seen GCA patients with vertigo that resolved with corticosteroid therapy (Caselli et al., 1988a).

Encephalopathy

The differential diagnosis of encephalopathy in the GCA patient is extensive and can relate to the disease itself, complications of treatment, or unrelated factors. Acute encephalopathy may be caused by GCA itself as a result of cerebral infarction (Wilkinson and Russell, 1972; Heptinstall et al., 1954; Cooke et al., 1946; Russell, 1959; Gibb et al., 1985; Caselli, 1990; Tomer et al., 1992). Cognitive changes may result from thalamic, mesial temporal, and mesencephalic involvement in some cases; and magnetic resonance imaging (MRI) or computed tomography (CT) should be performed. Acute encephalopathy is a poor prognostic sign, and many such patients progress to coma and death (Wilkinson and Russell, 1972; Heptinstall et al., 1954; Cooke et al., 1946; Russell, 1959; Gibb et al., 1985). With steroid therapy, some patients may stabilize and, over time, experience some recovery (Caselli, 1990; Tomer et al., 1992). One comatose patient had triphasic waves on the electroencephalogram, and steroid treatment led to complete recovery (Tomer et al., 1992). Recurrent episodes of acute encephalopathy with progressive cognitive impairment can lead to a more chronic multi-infarct dementia due to cervicocephalic arterial involvement by GCA (Caselli, 1990). In our experience, encephalopathy and dementia due to GCA are uncommon (Caselli et al., 1988a; Caselli, 1990), although earlier literature suggested that they were frequent (Paulley and Hughes, 1960; Vereker, 1952). Corticosteroid therapy itself may cause encephalopathy primarily (steroid psychosis) or secondarily. There are numerous potential steroid-related complications, such as metabolic abnormalities and systemic and central nervous system infections (which occur more commonly in immunocompromised hosts). Finally, diseases that are prevalent in the elderly and unrelated to GCA can cause encephalopathy and dementia, such as degenerative and vascular dementias, chronic subdural hematoma, and sedating medications.

Seizures

Although there is no evidence that GCA directly causes seizures, seizures may complicate the clinical course of any patient who has sustained a cortical infarction, whether or not the underlying mechanism was related to GCA. Seizures may also complicate the clinical course of patients with encephalopathy related primarily or secondarily to steroids, so there are various reasons that seizures may occur in the patient with GCA.

Myelopathy

On rare occasions, GCA may cause acute cervical myelopathy (Caselli et al., 1988a; Gibb et al., 1985; Brennan and Sandyk, 1982; Cloake, 1951). The vasculitis presumably extends to the anterior spinal artery from the vertebral arteries (Gibb et al., 1985). Myelopathic involvement may presage a fatal outcome (Gibb et al., 1985), although prompt treatment with corticosteroids may permit neurological stabilization (Caselli et al., 1988a) and improvement (Brennan and Sandyk, 1982).

Peripheral Nervous System Complications

Mononeuropathies

Occasionally, GCA affects large peripheral arteries and their branches (Klein et al., 1975), which can include the nutrient arteries of peripheral nerves (Caselli et al., 1988a) and result in mononeuropathies or mononeuritis multiplex (Russell, 1959; Caselli et al., 1988b; Dux et al., 1981; Feigal et al., 1985; Fryer and Singer, 1971; Massey and Weed, 1978; Meneely and Bigelow, 1953; Sànchez et al., 1983; Shapiro et al., 1983; Warrell et al., 1968). The incidence of acute ischemic mononeuropathies in GCA patients is difficult to estimate but is probably around 2% (Caselli et al., 1988b). Prognosis for neurological recovery with corticosteroid treatment is good provided that vascular compromise does not lead to loss of the affected limb (Caselli et al., 1988b). Essentially all named peripheral nerves can be involved as ischemic mononeuropathies. Among the spinal nerves, the fifth cervical nerve has been reported by several authors (Caselli et al., 1988b; Fryer and Singer, 1971; Sànchez et al., 1983; Shapiro et al., 1983) to be susceptible to GCA. Patients with GCA also can develop mononeuropathies that occur at common compression sites and are unrelated to vasculitis. For example, approximately 5% have carpal tunnel syndrome (Caselli et al., 1988b). In some cases, median nerve compression might be related to PMR-induced wrist synovitis.

Peripheral Neuropathy

Mild abnormalities of nerve conduction studies and electromyography (EMG) are common in elderly patients. Although such findings may suggest a peripheral neuropathy, the relationship of such neuropathies to GCA is uncertain. In other patients, however, antecedent ischemic mononeuropathies may accrue and eventually resemble a "diffuse," severe, peripheral neuropathy (Caselli et al., 1988b; Feigal et al., 1985; Warrell et al., 1968). However, this is much less likely to be caused by GCA than by other vasculitides.

Myopathy

Giant cell arteritis does not cause an inflammatory myopathy, although there are rare examples of localized inflammation in muscle (Andrews, 1966). Polymyalgia rheumatica may falsely lead to the clinical suspicion of a myopathy, and steroid therapy commonly causes a mild, non-inflammatory myopathy ("steroid myopathy"). In typical cases of PMR without vasculitic involvement of the peripheral nervous system, EMG results are normal (Caselli et al., 1988b).

LABORATORY EVALUATION

Blood Tests

When a patient's diagnosis is suspected to be GCA, an ESR should be performed immediately and the results obtained that same day so that steroid therapy may be instituted promptly. Though nonspecific, the combination of headache and an elevated ESR in an elderly patient is highly suspicious for GCA. The ESR is elevated in approximately 97% of patients with GCA who are not taking corticosteroids. The mean value is 85 [standard deviation (SD) 32] mm in 1 hour (Westergren method) (Campbell and Caselli, 1991). Other acute-phase reactant proteins are also increased. Increasingly, CRP is used to monitor disease activity; it is more sensitive than ESR in some patients. Other common laboratory abnormalities include a normochromic microcytic anemia (mean hemoglobin value 11.7 g/dl, SD 1.6) and thrombocytosis (mean platelet count $427 \times 10^3/\mu l$, SD 116×10^3) (31). Mild elevations of serum transaminases and alkaline phosphatase occur in 15% of patients, and elevations of plasma α_2 globulins occurs in 72% (Campbell and Caselli, 1991).

Temporal Artery Biopsy

The ESR or CRP are essential tests for early diagnosis and help to guide therapy in the acute setting, but GCA is a chronic disease that requires long-term steroid use. Greater diagnostic specificity than that provided solely by these tests is therefore important. Confirmation by temporal artery biopsy (TAB) should be considered in every patient in whom GCA is suspected. Glucocorticoids can be started before the TAB if necessary, but if this is done, TAB should be performed as soon as possible (preferably within a few days) to avoid steroid-induced histological suppression or alteration of vasculitis in the TAB specimen that would make diagnostic accuracy more problematic. However, patients may continue to have histological evidence of GCA on TAB as long as 6 weeks after the institution of steroids, even if there has been clinical resolution of symptoms (Achkar et al., 1994; Evans et al., 1994b). We recommend a 5 cm specimen from the most symptomatic side, and we obtain bilateral specimens if frozen sections are negative (Caselli and Hunder, 1993). If the TAB segment is long (4 to 6 cm) and multiple histological sections are taken, 86% of cases will be correctly diagnosed by unilateral biopsy (Hall and Hunder, 1984). Histological features include intimal proliferation with luminal stenosis, disruption of the internal elastic lamina by a mononuclear cell infiltrate, invasion and necrosis of the media progressing to panar-

teritic involvement by mononuclear cells, giant cell formation with granulomata within the mononuclear cell infiltrate, and variably, intraluminal thrombosis (Fig. 24–2). Involvement of the affected artery is often patchy (skip lesions) (Hall et al., 1983; Hall and Hunder, 1984).

Aortic Arch and Cerebral Angiography

Aortic arch and cerebral angiography are not routine diagnostic tests for GCA, but some patients with GCA undergo them for stroke-related symptoms. In such patients, the vertebral and external carotid arteries (including the superficial temporal artery) may show vasculitic changes of alternating stenotic segments (Caselli et al., 1988a) or occlusion (Caselli, 1990) (Fig. 24–2). Angiography of the STA, however, is less reliable than TAB for establishing a diagnosis. Internal carotid arteries may be occluded (Caselli et al., 1988a; Howard et al., 1984; Caselli, 1990; Cull, 1979), but they rarely have a characteristic vasculitic pattern. Subclavian, axillary, and proximal brachial arterial involvement produces a characteristic angiographic pattern of vasculitis that consists of long, smooth stenotic segments alternating with nonstenotic segments and tapered occlusions (Heptinstall et al., 1954; Klein et al., 1975; Östberg, 1972; Evans et al., 1995; Andrews, 1966; Hamrin et al., 1965; Howard et al., 1984; Pollock et al., 1973) (Fig. 24–3).

TREATMENT AND PROGNOSIS

Oral corticosteroids remain the mainstay of treatment. Most patients will require prednisone for 1 to 2 years, with initial doses of 40 to 60 mg daily. If a patient presents with an acute neurological syndrome or rapidly worsening neurological status, whether it be visual loss, mononeuritis multiplex, or acute encephalopathy, treatment may begin with an intravenous pulse over several days (1,000 mg methylprednisolone/day) or a very high oral dose of steroids (up to 120 mg prednisone), though there is no controlled study that has compared the efficacy and safety of this more aggressive regimen to conventional therapy. The starting dose is then tapered over a few weeks so that by the end of the first month of therapy most patients are taking about 40 mg of prednisone daily. Subsequent reductions by 2.5 to 5 mg amounts may be made every 1 to 3 weeks as tolerated. A patient with GCA who has a relapse may require only a modest increment in dose to control the flare in symptoms.

Following the initiation of steroid treatment, the headache usually resolves within days. The ESR may drop within days and become normal in a week or two. Neurological deficits can improve, but irreversible end-organ infarction may preclude clinically significant gains in some patients. Occasionally, a mild headache may persist for 2 to 4 weeks without any other clinical or laboratory signs of disease activity. Mild jaw claudication may persist up to several weeks before resolving completely. Neurovascular complications may occur during the initial tapering of corticosteroid dosage, typically around 1 month after beginning treatment (Caselli et al., 1988a), emphasizing the utility of ESR monitoring and the importance of small steroid decrements.

Chronic steroid therapy is fraught with complications. These include diabetes mellitus, vertebral compression fractures, steroid myopathy, steroid psychosis, and immunosuppression-related infections. Alternate therapeutic strategies would therefore be of potentially great utility for many patients. None have yet been shown to be reliably effective and safe, however. Some studies have suggested that much lower doses and more rapid tapering schedules are sufficient. One such study advocated initiating treatment with 20 mg of prednisolone daily and tapering it to 10 mg daily within 3 months (Lundberg and Hedfors, 1990). Although many patients may respond to this regimen with symptomatic improvement of headache, PMR, and reduction of ESR, a substantial number of patients will experience symptomatic worsening of symptoms (Lundberg and Hedfors, 1990). Headache and PMR, though they are the most common symptoms of GCA, are not the reason these patients are treated with high-

dose steroids. Higher doses are required to prevent irreversible ischemic ophthalmological and neurological complications. Trials of other immunosuppressant drugs, including azathioprine (De Silva and Hazleman, 1986), methotrexate (Krall et al., 1989), cyclophosphamide (De Vita et al., 1992), and dapsone (Demaziere, 1989), have been undertaken for their steroid-sparing effects. Steroid dosages have been successfully lowered in some patients on each of these drugs, but inconsistently. Toxicity can be a significant problem, particularly with dapsone and cyclophosphamide. Azathioprine has no acute effect, and its steroid-sparing effects may not be evident for 1 year (De Vita et al., 1992). Limited experience suggests that cyclophosphamide may be the most consistently effective immunosuppressant other than corticosteroids (Caselli and Hunder, 1993; De Vita et al., 1992; Demaziere, 1989) and may permit more rapid steroid tapering when instituted following a relapse. However, it is also the most toxic agent.

In summary, GCA is an important neurological disease that must be familiar to all medical practitioners who work with elderly patients. Although it commonly presents with headache, it is not a disease confined to the province of a headache subspecialist.

REFERENCES

Achkar, A.A., J.T. Lie, G.G. Hunder et al. (1994). How does previous corticosteroid treatment affect the biopsy findings in giant cell (temporal) arteritis? *Ann. Intern. Med.* 120:987–992.

Andrews, J.M. (1966). Giant-cell ("temporal") arteritis. A disease with variable clinical manifestations. *Neurology* 16:963–971.

Banks, P.M., M.D. Cohen, M.W. Ginsburg et al. (1983). Immunohistologic and cytochemical studies of temporal arteritis. *Arthritis Rheum.* 26:1201–1207.

Barricks, M.E., D.B. Traviesa, J.S. Glaser et al. (1977). Ophthalmoplegia in cranial arteritis. *Brain* 100:209–221.

Brennan, M.J.W. and R. Sandyk. (1982). Reversible quadriplegia in a patient with giant-cell arteritis. *S. Afr. Med. J.* 62:81–82.

Bruk, M.I. (1967). Articular and vascular manifestations of polymyalgia rheumatica. *Ann. Rheum. Dis.* 26:103–116.

Campbell, J.K. and R.J. Caselli. (1991). Headache and other craniofacial pain. In *Neurology in Clinical Practice: Principles of Diagnosis and Management* (W.G. Bradley, R.B. Daroff, G.M. Fenichel et al., eds.), pp. 1507–1561, Butterworth-Heinemann, Boston.

Cardell, B.S. and T. Hanley. (1951). A fatal case of giant-cell or temporal arteritis. *J. Pathol. Bacteriol.* 63:587–597.

Caselli, R.J. (1990). Giant cell (temporal) arteritis: A treatable cause of multi-infarct dementia. *Neurology* 40:753–755.

Caselli, R.J., J.R. Daube, G.G. Hunder et al. (1988a). Peripheral neuropathic syndromes in giant cell (temporal) arteritis. *Neurology* 38:685–689.

Caselli, R.J. and G.G. Hunder. (1993). Giant cell (temporal) arteritis and cerebral vasculitis. In *Current Therapy in Neurologic Disease*, 4th ed. (R.T. Johnson and J.W. Griffin, eds.), pp. 196–201, B.C. Decker, St. Louis.

Caselli, R.J., G.G. Hunder, and J.P. Whisnant. (1988b). Neurologic disease in giant cell (temporal) arteritis. *Neurology* 38:352–359.

Cloake, P.C.P. (1951). Temporal arteritis. *Proc. R. Soc. Med.* 44:847–852.

Cooke, W.T., P.C.P. Cloake, A.D.T. Govan et al. (1946). Temporal arteritis: A generalized vascular disease. *Q. J. Med.* 15:47–75.

Crompton, M.R. (1959). The visual changes in temporal (giant-cell) arteritis: Report of a case with autopsy findings. *Brain* 82:377–390.

Cull, R.E. (1979). Internal carotid artery occlusion caused by giant cell arteritis. *J. Neurol. Neurosurg. Psychiatry* 42:1066–1067.

Das, A.K. and D.M. Laskin. (1966). Temporal arteritis of the facial artery. *J. Oral Surg.* 24:226–232.

Demaziere, A. (1989). Dapsone in the long term treatment of temporal arteritis [letter]. *Am. J. Med.* 87:3.

De Silva, M. and B.L. Hazleman. (1986). Azathioprine in giant cell arteritis/polymyalgia rheumatica: A double-blind study. *Ann. Rheum. Dis.* 45:136–138.

De Vita, S., A. Tavoni, G. Jeraitano et al. (1992). Treatment of giant cell arteritis with cyclophosphamide pulses [letter]. *J. Intern. Med.* 232:373–375.

Dimant, J., D. Grob, and N.G. Brunner. (1980). Ophthalmoplegia, ptosis, and miosis in temporal arteritis. *Neurology* 30:1054–1058.

Dux, S., S. Pithk, and J.B. Rosenfeld. (1981). Popliteal neuritis complicating temporal arteritis. *Harefuah* 101:291.

Evans, J.M., K.P. Batts, and G.G. Hunder. (1994a). Persistent giant cell arteritis despite corticosteroid treatment. *Mayo Clin. Proc.* 69:1060–1061.

Evans, J.M., C.A. Bowles, J. Bjornsson et al. (1994b). Thoracic aneurysm and rupture in gi-ant cell arteritis. *Arthritis Rheum.* 37:1539–1544.

Evans, J.M., M.O. O'Fallon, and G.G. Hunder. (1995). Increased incidence of aortic aneurysm and dissection in giant cell (temporal) arteritis. A population based study. *Ann. Intern. Med.* 122:502–507.

Feigal, D.W., D.L. Robbins, and J.C. Leek. (1985). Giant cell arteritis associated with mononeuritis multiplex and complement-activating 19S IgM rheumatoid factor. *Am. J. Med.* 79:495–500.

Fryer, D.G. and R.S. Singer. (1971). Giant-cell arteritis with cervical radiculopathy. *Bull. Mason Clin.* 25:143–151.

Gibb, W.R.G., P.A. Urry, and A.J. Lees. (1985). Giant cell arteritis with spinal cord infarction and basilar artery thrombosis. *J. Neurol. Neurosurg. Psychiatry* 48:945–948.

Graham, E., A. Holland, A. Avery et al. (1981). Prognosis in giant-cell arteritis. *BMJ* 282:269–271.

Hall, S. and G.G. Hunder. (1984). Is temporal artery biopsy prudent? *Mayo Clin. Proc.* 59:793–796.

Hall, S., S. Persellin, J.T. Lie et al. (1983). The therapeutic impact of temporal artery biopsy. *Lancet* 2:1217–1220.

Hamrin, B., N. Jonsson, and T. Landberg. (1965). Involvement of large vessels in polymyalgia arteritica. *Lancet* 1:1193–1196.

Hellman, DB. (1993). Immunopathogenesis, diagnosis, and treatment of giant cell arteritis, temporal arteritis, polymyalgia rheumatica, and Takayasu's arteritis. *Curr. Opin. Rheumatol.* 5:25–32.

Heptinstall, R.H., K.A. Porter, and H. Barkley. (1954). Giant-cell (temporal) arteritis. *J. Pathol. Bacteriol.* 67:507–519.

Hollenhorst, R.W. (1967). Effect of posture of retinal ischemia from temporal arteritis. *Arch. Ophthalmol.* 78:569–577.

Hollenhorst, R.W., J.R. Brown, H.P. Wagener et al. (1960). Neurologic aspects of temporal arteritis. *Neurology* 10:490–498.

Howard, G.F. III, S.U. Ho, K.S. Kim et al. (1984). Bilateral carotid artery occlusion resulting from giant cell arteritis. *Ann. Neurol.* 15:204–207.

Hunder, G.G., J.T. Lie, J.J. Goronzy et al. (1993). Pathogenesis of giant cell arteritis. *Arthritis Rheum.* 36:757–761.

Huston, K.A., G.G. Hunder, J.T. Lie et al. (1978). Temporal arteritis. A 25-year epidemiologic, clinical, and pathologic study. *Ann. Intern. Med.* 88:162–167.

Kinmont, P.D.C. and D.I. McCallum. (1964). Skin manifestations of giant-cell arteritis. *Br. J. Dermatol.* 76:299–308.

Klein, R.G., G.G. Hunder, A.W. Stanson et al. (1975). Large artery involvement in giant cell (temporal) arteritis. *Ann. Intern. Med. 83*:806–812.

Koorey, D.J. (1984). Cranial arteritis. A twenty-year review of cases. *Aust. N. Z. J. Med. 14*:143–147.

Krall, P.L., D.J. Mazenec, and W.S. Wilke. (1989). Methotrexate for corticosteroid-resistant polymyalgia rheumatica and giant cell arteritis. *Cleve. Clin. Med. J. 56*:253–257.

Lundberg, I. and E. Hedfors. (1990). Restricted dose and duration of corticosteroid treatment in patients with polymyalgia rheumatica and temporal arteritis. *J. Rheumatol. 17*:1340–1345.

Massey, E.W. and T. Weed. (1978). Sciatic neuropathy with giant-cell arteritis [letter]. *N. Engl. J. Med. 298*:917.

Meneely, J.K., Jr. and N.H. Bigelow. (1953). Temporal arteritis. A critical evaluation of this disorder and a report of three cases. *Am. J. Med. 14*:46–51.

Monteiro, M.L.R., J.R. Coppeto, and P. Greco. (1984). Giant cell arteritis of the posterior cerebral circulation presenting with ataxia and ophthalmoplegia. *Arch. Ophthalmol. 102*:407–409.

Mowat, A.G. and B.L. Hazleman. (1974). Polymyalgia rheumatica—a clinical study with particular reference to arterial disease. *J. Rheumatol. 1*:190–202.

Östberg, G. (1972). Morphological changes in the large arteries in polymyalgia arteritica. *Acta Med. Scand. Suppl. 533*:135–164.

Paulley, J.W. and J.P. Hughes. (1960). Giant-cell arteritis, or arteritis of the aged. *BMJ 2*:1562–1567.

Pollock, M., J.B. Blennerhassett, and A.M. Clarke. (1973). Giant cell arteritis and the subclavian steal syndrome. *Neurology 23*:653–657.

Russell, R.W.R. (1959). Giant-cell arteritis. A review of 35 cases. *Q. J. Med. 28*:471–489.

Sànchez, M.C., J.L.C. Arenilla, D.A. Gutierrez et al. (1983). Cervical radiculopathy: A rare symptom of giant cell arteritis. *Arthritis Rheum. 26*:207–209.

Shapiro, L., T.A. Medsger, Jr., and J.J. Nicholas. (1983). Brachial plexitis mimicking C5 radiculopathy—a presentation of giant cell arteritis [letter]. *J. Rheumatol. 10*:670–671.

Shiiki, H., T. Shimokama, and T. Watanabe. (1989). Temporal arteritis: Cell composition and the possible pathogenetic role of cell mediated immunity. *Hum. Pathol. 20*:1057–1064.

Tomer, Y., M.Y. Neufeld, and Y. Shoenfeld. (1992). Coma with triphasic wave pattern in EEG as a complications of temporal arteritis. *Neurology 42*:439–441.

Vereker, R. (1952). The psychiatric aspects of temporal arteritis. *J. Ment. Sci. 98*:280–286.

Wagener, H.P. and R.W. Hollenhorst. (1958). The ocular lesions of temporal arteritis. *Am. J. Ophthalmol. 45*:617–630.

Warrell, D.A., S. Godfrey, and E.G.J. Olsen. (1968). Giant-cell arteritis with peripheral neuropathy. *Lancet 1*:1010–1013.

Wawryk, S.O., H. Ayberk, A.W. Boyd et al. (1991). Analysis of adhesion molecules in the immunopathogenesis of giant cell arteritis. *J. Clin. Pathol. 44*:497–501.

Weyand, C.M., K.C. Hicok, G.G. Hunder et al. (1994). Tissue cytokine patterns in patients with polymyalgia rheumatica and giant cell arteritis. *Ann. Intern. Med. 121*:484–491.

Whitfield, A.G.W., M. Bateman, and W.T. Cooke. (1963). Temporal arteritis. *Br. J. Ophthalmol. 47*:555–566.

Wilkinson, I.M.S. and R.W.R. Russell. (1972). Arteries of the head and neck in giant cell arteritis: A pathological study to show the pattern of arterial involvement. *Arch. Neurol. 27*:378–391.

IV

Special Topics

25

Headaches in Children and Adolescents

A. DAVID ROTHNER
PAUL WINNER

Headache is a frequent symptom in children and adolescents. An acute headache often accompanies a systemic infection. An acute or subacute headache may accompany an organic disorder. A chronic headache may be secondary to migraine or stress. A headache disorder affects the lifestyle of the child and his or her family. It results in significant disability, including time lost from school and parental absence from work. The majority of children and adolescents with headache never consult a physician, however (Sillanpaa et al., 1991).

Although historical references to headaches date back over 5,000 years, children's headaches have largely been ignored. It was not until 1873 that William Henry Day, a British pediatrician, devoted a chapter in his pediatric textbook to headaches in children (Day, 1873). The modern era of the study of headaches in children and adolescents began in 1962, when Bille performed a study of 9,000 schoolchildren (Bille, 1962). To date, the literature regarding headaches in children consists of only five textbooks (Friedman and Harms, 1967; Barlow, 1984; Hockaday, 1988; McGrath, 2001; Winner and Rothner, 2001); however, several journals are devoted to headaches in children and are useful resources (Rothner, 1995a; Smith, 1995; Hamalainen, 1997).

This chapter discusses the epidemiology, clinical features, management, and prognosis of headaches in children and adolescents. The genetics, anatomy, pathology, and pathophysiology of pain and migraine are briefly reviewed.

EPIDEMIOLOGY

Epidemiologic studies of headaches in children and adolescents can be divided into studies of (1) migraine headaches, (2) tension-type headaches, and (3) all types of headache combined. These studies can be further divided into those that look at individual populations and those that look at individuals who attend specialized headache clinics. Only a few studies have looked at cluster headaches in children and adolescents.

Before 1988, when the International Headache Society (IHS) published its criteria for headache classification and diagnosis (Headache Classification Committee of the IHS (1988), epidemiologic studies lacked standardized definitions. Because of this, estimates of the prevalence and incidence of primary headache disorders varied greatly not only in children and adolescents but also in adults. Epidemiologic studies of headache in children are complicated by the inability of young children to describe their pain or remember other features associated with their headaches. Headaches vary considerably from attack to attack, which complicates data gathering.

Incidence refers to the rate of onset of new cases of a particular disease in a defined population. *Prevalence* refers to the frequency with which a specific disorder is seen in the population at a given time. Most studies do not look at incidence or prevalence in children who are under 7 years of age.

By the age of 3, 3% to 8% of children have experienced a headache (Sillanpaa, 1976, 1994; Zuckerman et al., 1987). By age 5, 19.5% have had a headache, and by age 7, 37% to 51.5% have had a headache (Bille, 1962; Sillanpaa, 1983; Sillanpaa et al., 1991). Headache prevalence ranges from 57% to 82% in 7- to 15-year-olds (Bille, 1962; Sillanpaa, 1983; Sillanpaa et al., 1991). Headache prevalence increases from ages 3 to 11 in both boys and girls; however, prevalence is higher in 3- to 5-year-old boys than it is in 3- to 5-year-old girls (Mortimer et al., 1992). Cross-sectional studies have shown that overall headache prevalence increases from preschool-aged to school-aged children and then to adolescents. In boys, headache prevalence is stable from 7 to 14 years of age and declines thereafter, whereas girls show an increase in headache prevalence from 7 to 22 years of age (Sillanpaa, 1983, 1994).

Migraine prevalence in the pediatric age group has been well studied. At the age of 7 years, prevalence ranges from 1.2% to 3.2% (Bille, 1962; Mortimer et al., 1992; Sillanpaa, 1976). Between 7 and 15 years of age, prevalence ranges from 4% to 11% (Bille, 1962; Mortimer et al., 1992; Sillanpaa, 1976, 1994). In 1992, a study of 1,083 children between 3 and 11 years of age was performed within a single U.K. general practice; it utilized a structured interview, and 98.1% of patients participated (Mortimer et al., 1992). Three sets of diagnostic criteria were used. The results showed that migraine prevalence was higher in boys than girls at 3 to 5 years of age and at 5 to 7 years of age. Prevalence was equal in boys and girls aged 7 to 11 years and

was higher in girls after age 11. Stewart et al. (1992) conducted telephone interviews with more than 10,000 individuals between the ages of 12 and 29 years. Based on 392 males and 1,018 females with migraine, they estimated age- and sex-specific incidence rates for migraine with and without aura. The incidence of migraine was lower in males than females. The incidence of migraine with aura in males was 6.6/1,000 person-years and peaked at 5 to 6 years of age. The peak incidence of migraine without aura in males was 10/1,000 person-years and peaked at 10 to 11 years of age. New cases of migraine were uncommon in men in their twenties. The incidence of migraine with aura in females was 14.1/1,000 person-years and peaked at 12 to 13 years of age; the incidence of migraine without aura was 18.9/1,000 person-years and peaked at 14 to 17 years of age.

Data concerning the incidence and prevalence of tension-type headaches in children and adolescents are not readily available and vary greatly from study to study. Bille (1962) suggested that by age 15 frequent, nonmigrainous headaches are three times more prevalent in children than are migraine headaches. Abu-Arefeh and Russell (1994) studied 2,165 Aberdeen schoolchildren between 5 and 15 years of age and estimated the prevalence of tension-type headache at 0.9%. Schwartz et al. (1998) looked at the epidemiology of tension-type headaches in 13,345 subjects from the community who were between the ages of 18 and 65. In the youngest age group, the prevalence of episodic tension-type headache was 34.5% in men and 40.8% in women. The frequency of tension-type headache between the ages of 18 and 29 was 1.7/month in men and 2.5/month in women. The overall prevalence peaked in the 30- to 39-year age group and declined thereafter. Further studies that look specifically at the incidence and prevalence of episodic and chronic tension-type headaches in children and adolescents are needed. The incidence and prevalence of mixed or comorbid headaches have not been reviewed (Gladstein et al., 1993, 1997). The concept of transformed migraine has not been established in children or adolescents.

The incidence and prevalence of cluster headaches in individuals under the age of 20 has not been well studied. The typical age at onset of cluster headaches is in the late twenties, but one series found that 10% of patients were between 10 and 19 years of age (Pearce, 1980). Onset under the age of 10 has been reported, but this is quite unusual (Ekbom et al., 1978; Maytal et al., 1992).

CLASSIFICATION

Prior to the publication of IHS Headache Classification System in 1988, several classifications were used for headaches in children (Headache Classification Committee of the International Headache Society, 1988). These dealt mainly with migraine and included the criteria established by Vahlquist (1955), Deubner (1977), Congdon and Forsythe (1979), and Prensky and Sommer (1979). Several studies have compared the diagnosis of migraine in children utilizing these various criteria to test the agreement between the various classifications (Gherpelli et al., 1998; Maytal et al., 1997; Mortimer et al., 1992; Seshia et al., 1994). Still others have looked at the IHS criteria and were concerned as to their lack of specificity in children and adolescents. Others have proposed revisions to the IHS criteria for children and adolescents with migraine (Winner et al., 1997; Hamalainen et al., 1995; Seshia and Wolstein, 1995; Seshia, 1996; Gallai et al., 1995; Wober-Bingol et al., 1996; Metsahonkala and Sillanpaa, 1994; Winner et al., 1995; Gherpelli et al., 1998; Maytal et al., 1997). The major suggestions were to shorten the duration of the migraine attack to 1 hour and to remove hemicrania as a criterion since many children have headaches that are either bitemporal or bifrontal. An additional suggestion was to require either photophobia or phonophobia instead of both. Revised IHS criteria may be useful for classifying pediatric migraine in the future.

To date, no studies have addressed tension-type headaches in children or whether or not the current IHS criteria are appropriate for children and adolescents (Gladstein et al., 1993, 1997). A common problem in adolescents is comorbid migraine and tension-type headaches. Little is known about the frequency of this disorder in the childhood and adolescent age groups (Gladstein et al., 1997).

Clinically, it is helpful to classify headache using the temporal pattern plotted against the severity (Rothner, 1995b). Five patterns can be identified: acute, acute recurrent (migraine), chronic progressive (organic), chronic nonprogressive (tension-type), and mixed (migraine and tension-type) (Figs. 25–1, 25–2).

An acute headache is a single event with no history of a previous similar event. Acute headaches are often associated with febrile illnesses. If the acute headache is associated with neurologic symptoms or signs, an organic process should be suspected. The differential diagnosis of an acute headache involves a wide variety of disorders that can be seen in the pediatrician's office or in the emergency room (Kandt and Levine, 1987; Burton et al., 1997) (Table 25–1).

Acute recurrent headaches are usually migrainous (Rothner, 1986). These headaches are painful but not life-threatening. If migraine headaches are associated with neurologic symptoms or signs, other potentially life-threatening etiologies must be considered.

Chronic progressive headaches worsen in frequency and severity. As time progresses, they are often accompanied by symptoms of increased intracranial pressure or abnormal neurologic signs and progressive neurologic disease. An organic process is most likely (Cohen, 1995) (Table 25–2).

Chronic nonprogressive headaches, also known as tension-type headaches, occur frequently, daily, or constantly (Gladstein and Holden, 1996; Jensen and Rothner, 1995; Solomon et al., 1992). The episodic variety occurs less than 10 to 15 days a month, and the chronic variety occurs more than 15 days a month. They are not associated with symptoms of increased intracranial pressure or progressive neurologic disease. Examinations are normal, and laboratory studies, including imaging studies, are negative. Psychologic factors are important.

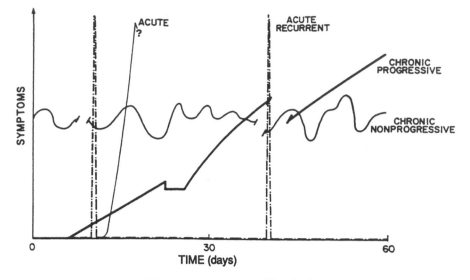

Figure 25–1 Types of headache.

The mixed or comorbid headache syndrome is a combination of acute recurrent headache (migraine) superimposed on a pattern of daily or episodic chronic, nonprogressive headache (tension-type) (Gladstein et al. 1997; Rothner, 1995b). These headaches are not life-threatening, although the pain may be disabling. Both genetic and psychologic factors are important.

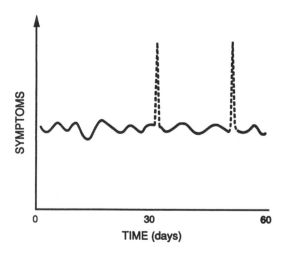

Figure 25–2 Temporal pattern of mixed headaches, which are characterized by a continuous daily headache with intermittent migrainous headache.

PATHOPHYSIOLOGY

Headaches caused by inflammation, irritation, displacement, traction, dilation, or invasion of pain-sensitive structures are the same in children as in adults. Perception of pain, however, is modified by psychologic factors, ethnic factors, age, and previous experience with pain (Schechter, 1984). Pain should not be taken as an absolute indicator of disease severity. Younger children with chronic pain may exhibit developmental regression and be-

Table 25–1 Acute headache

Generalized	Localized
Systemic infection	Sinusitis
Central nervous system	Otitis
infection	Ocular abnormality
Toxins: lead, CO	Dental disease
Postseizure	Trauma
Electrolyte imbalance	Occipital neuralgia
Hypertension	Temporomandibular joint
Hypoglycemia	dysfunction
Post-lumbar puncture	
Trauma	
Embolic	
Vascular thrombosis	
Hemorrhage	
Collagen disease	
Exertional	
Shunt malfunction	

Table 25–2 Chronic progressive headache

Tumor
Pseudotumor
Brain abscess
Subdural hematoma
Hydrocephalus

havioral difficulty. Chronic pain affects eating, sleeping, playing, and school functioning. Emotional and personality considerations assume even greater importance in the older child and adolescent. Headache may be a cause of school failure and absenteeism and is often provoked by problems with peers, family, or school. Depression and anxiety frequently coexist (Martin and Smith, 1995). Current concepts regarding the pathogenesis of migraine are based on biochemical studies and technologies that measure cerebral blood flow, as well as biochemical markers. These studies have been combined to produce the neurovascular hypothesis, which considers migraine an inherited sensitivity of the trigeminal vascular system (Moskowitz, 1991). The pathophysiology of migraine is similar in children and adults. Studies looking at the pathophysiology of this disorder in children have been performed less frequently than studies in adults (Puca and de Tommaso, 1999).

EVALUATION

The evaluation of the child or adolescent with headache is the key to appropriate treatment (Rothner, 1995b). A properly obtained history will differentiate the various headache types and their etiologies. A private interview with adolescents is helpful.

The history should begin with details of early childhood development, school function, previous medical problems, previous medications for both headache and other disorders, and drug and alcohol use. Patient and parent should be queried regarding anxiety, tension, and nervousness. Symptoms of depression should be explored. The family his-

tory should detail any members with a history of headaches or psychologic/psychiatric disorders. A second set of questions deals with the headache itself. A suggested format is found in Table 25–3. A third set of questions deals with symptoms of increased intracranial pressure or progressive neurologic disease, including ataxia, lethargy, seizures, visual disturbances, focal weakness, personality change, and loss of intellectual abilities.

Potentially ominous headache etiologies should be explored if (1) headache severity has increased dramatically, (2) the headache awakens the child from sleep, or (3) there has been a change in an established headache pattern. Patients with migraine or tension-type headaches have no symptoms of increased intracranial pressure or progressive neurologic disease.

Following the history, a general physical examination should be performed. Any abnormality of blood pressure or temperature should be noted. The skin must be closely examined for neurocutaneous abnormalities such as are seen in neurofibromatosis. The skull and neck should be both palpated and auscultated. The sinuses and jaws should be

Table 25–3 Headache database

1. Do you have one type or two types of headache?
2. How did the headache begin?
3. How long has the headache been present?
4. Are the headaches static, intermittent, or progressive?
5. How often does the headache occur?
6. Do the headaches occur at any special time or under special circumstances?
7. Are the headaches related to specific foods, medications, or activities?
8. Are there warning symptoms?
9. Where is the pain located?
10. What is the quality of the pain?
11. Are there associated symptoms?
12. How long does the headache last?
13. What do you do during the headache?
14. What makes the headache better?
15. What makes the headache worse?
16. Do symptoms continue in between the headaches?
17. Are you being treated for any other problem?
18. Do you take any medication for any reason regularly or intermittently?
19. Does anyone else in your family have headaches?
20. What do you think is causing your headache?

examined for inflammation, tenderness, or temporomandibular joint dysfunction. Most patients with migraine or tension-type headaches have a completely normal physical examination, especially between attacks.

When performing the neurologic examination, one should look carefully for signs of trauma or nuchal rigidity. Head circumference, optic fundi, eye movements, strength, reflexes, and coordination should be recorded. Any abnormality in the neurologic examination requires further investigation as children and adolescents with migraine and tension-type headaches have normal neurologic examinations between attacks.

LABORATORY TESTS

The choice of laboratory tests is based on the differential diagnosis. "Routine" laboratory tests are not helpful when patients have migraine or tension-type headaches. If, however, the patient is critically ill or the history suggests increased intracranial pressure or progressive neurologic disease, further testing is necessary.

Under certain circumstances, blood tests may be helpful. If the patient has had a stroke-like illness, coagulation factors, lactate and pyruvate levels, lipid analysis and platelet count may be indicated. If a rash is found and an infectious process is suspected, viral studies and/or Lyme titers may be of value. Nine percent of children with migraine have benign focal epileptiform discharges without any evidence of epilepsy (Kinast et al., 1982); therefore, the electroencephalogram (EEG) is of limited value in the routine evaluation of migraine and tension-type headaches (Kinast et al., 1982; Gronseth and Greenberg, 1995). However, if a patient has had abnormal movements or alteration or loss of consciousness, EEG may be diagnostic. Evoked potentials and brain electrical activity monitoring (BEAM) have not proven to be of value.

The diagnosis of structural central nervous system (CNS) disorders has been revolutionized by computed tomography (CT) and magnetic resonance imaging (MRI). Both are safe, rapid, and accurate methods of evaluating the intracranial contents. They are useful in diagnosing congenital malformations, cranial infections, trauma, neoplasms, degenerative disorders, and neurocutaneous and vascular abnormalities. In acute situations, they may be life-saving. Although MRI incurs greater cost, takes longer, and may require sedation, it can demonstrate lesions not visible on CT, including sinus pathology, white matter changes, and disorders of the craniospinal junction. Most patients with migraine or tension-type headaches, no symptoms of progressive neurologic disease or increased intracranial pressure, and a normal neurologic examination do not require imaging. Numerous studies have demonstrated that imaging in these patients is normal or shows unrelated abnormalities (Dooley et al., 1990; Maytal et al., 1995).

Psychologic interviews and projective tests are useful in individuals with chronic, recurring, or disabling headaches who are unresponsive to initial treatment (McGrath, 1990; Cooper et al., 1987; Jensen and Rothner, 1995). When academic problems coexist, psycho-educational testing may be indicated. Personality tests, such as the Minnesota Multiphasic Personality Inventory for Adolescents and the Parent Inventory for Children, are helpful. Headache patients frequently exhibit a variety of behavioral symptoms. Psychologic factors and learned behavioral patterns may maintain the symptoms. Experience and research support the value of headache diaries, structured interviews, self-report measures, and objective psychologic testing. The evaluation should assess the pain, the patient, and the patient's environment. Close attention should be paid to the interaction between the parent and the child. Many parents consciously or unconsciously "enable" the continuation of the child's pain syndrome. The family should view the psychiatrist or psychologist as part of a team working to resolve the patient's difficulties. Emphasize that the pain is genuine and that the goal of assessment is to investigate factors that may be causing, worsening, or maintaining the pain. An additional goal is helping the patient and family to deal with the pain.

SPECIFIC HEADACHE SYNDROMES

Acute Generalized Headache

Kandt and Levine (1987) studied 37 children who were seen in a pediatric office for generalized headache. Thirty percent of the children had infections, such as pharyngitis and otitis. Infectious disorders were present in 22 of the 37. They found that patients with a family history of migraine were more likely to have headache, and sleep disorders were more common in headache patients. If an acute headache is associated with neurologic symptoms or signs, an organic disorder must be suspected and further evaluation undertaken.

Five to seventeen percent of children who present to emergency rooms with headache have a serious, life-threatening disorder (Rothner, 1995c). Burton et al. (1997) reported on 696 patients with headache who were seen in a pediatric emergency room. These patients represented 1.3% of the total emergency room visits. Twenty-four percent of patients were 2 to 5 years of age, 57.6% were 6 to 12 years of age, and 18.1% were 13 to 18 years of age. Thirty-nine percent had viral illnesses, 16% had sinusitis, 15.6% had migraine, 6.6% had post-traumatic headaches, 4.9% had streptococcal pharyngitis, and 4.5% had tension-type headaches. Serious conditions included 5.2% of patients with viral meningitis and one case each of shunt malfunction, hydrocephalus, lymphoma, and trauma. Lewis and Qureshi (2000) stated that the most common cause of headache seen in a pediatric emergency room (57%) was an upper respiratory tract infection. Migraine without aura was seen in 18% of patients, and cause was undetermined in 7%. They noted, however, that 17.5% had serious neurologic problems, including 9% with viral meningitis, 2.6% with brain tumors, 2% with shunt malfunctions, 1.3% with intracranial hemorrhage, 1.3% with postictal headache, and 1.3% with headache secondary to trauma. They emphasized that all children with *"serious"* problems exhibited neurologic symptoms or clear-cut abnormalities on examination. Evaluation of a child with headache in the emergency room

is directed toward ruling out organic disease and life-threatening illness and then relieving the pain (American College of Emergency Physicians, 1996). The history is truncated if the patient has altered sensorium, is in severe pain, or is seriously ill. An organic disorder should be suspected if the headache is accompanied by neurologic symptoms or abnormalities on the neurologic examination. Patients with life-threatening headache may require extensive laboratory testing, including neuroimaging and lumbar puncture.

The treatment of acute headache, in the practitioner's office or in the emergency room, depends on its etiology (Table 25–1). The diagnosis should be established prior to treatment. Treatment of pain and associated symptoms should not include medications that alter mental status, change clinical signs, or compound the primary disorder. Only after the diagnosis has been established and the patient stabilized should narcotics, analgesics, or sedatives be considered. At the conclusion of the emergency intervention, the patient should be given an appointment for ongoing treatment.

Migraine

Acute Recurrent Headache

Migraine is an acute recurrent headache characterized by episodic, periodic, and paroxysmal attacks of pain separated by pain-free intervals. They *do not* occur daily. The Headache Classification Committee of the IHS (1988) has suggested criteria for the diagnosis of migraine (see Chapter 9). Several revisions have been suggested that apply specifically to children. Migraine attacks are often precipitated by trigger phenomena, but adequate documentation of the role of triggers in the pathogenesis of migraine is not available (Peatfield et al., 1984). Provocative factors include anxiety, stress, fatigue, excessive sleep, lack of sleep, minor head injury, exercise, menses, travel, illness, diet, odors, medications, and hunger. Specific foods that contain vasoactive substances have been implicated, including preserved meats such as bacon, salami, and ham due to the presence of nitrites;

aged cheese and red wine due to the presence of tyramine; Asian food due to monosodium glutamate; and chocolate due to phenylethylamine.

Whether a true migraine personality exists is not known (Cunningham et al., 1987). Some research has suggested that migraine attacks are precipitated by emotional reactions. Some authors have stated that patients with migraine are shy, withdrawn, obese, stubborn, and inflexible. Others describe children with migraine as fearful, sensitive, and easily frustrated. More recent studies, however, have not demonstrated a specific migraine personality that differs from the general population.

Migraine is a familial disorder, although disagreement exists regarding the mode of inheritance (Gardner and Hoffman, 1998). If one looks at the families of children with migraine, 50% to 90% of relatives also have migraine. Whether migraine is inherited as an autosomal dominant disorder with variable penetrance or is a complex, multifactored hereditary disorder has not been determined. Familial hemiplegic migraine has been associated with mutations in chromosomes 9 and 1 (Joutel et al., 1993; Ducros et al., 1997).

Some authors have correlated pediatric migraine with an increased incidence of car sickness, sleep disturbance, syncope, mitral valve prolapse, and Tourette's syndrome (Barabas et al., 1983a,b, 1984; Raskin and Knittle, 1976; Litman and Friedman, 1978). These relationships require further study.

It should be emphasized that pediatric and adult migraines differ. Approximately 15% to 30% of children have migraine with aura and 60% true hemicrania during repeated headaches (Winner et al., 2000b). Children appear to have fewer attacks per month in their younger years. Their attacks tend to be shorter in duration. They tend to be relieved by sleep and seem less severe and more easily controlled. As children mature into adolescents, the prevalence of migraine with aura appears to increase slightly, as does the prevalence of hemicrania. The number of attacks per month and the number of morning attacks increase as well. The duration of the attack increases, and the attacks become

more difficult to treat. In later adolescence, migraine headaches may be superimposed on daily or almost-daily tension-type headaches. This is called mixed or comorbid headache syndrome. More data concerning this entity are needed.

Migraine with Aura

Migraine with aura is less prevalent in children and adolescents than migraine without aura. When it is present, the aura is visual or somatic and may include brightly colored lights, moving lights, distorted images, scotomata, visual field defects, or fortification spectra. In addition, distortions of somatic perception, such as the "Alice in Wonderland" syndrome, may occur (Lippman, 1952; Golden, 1979). Somatic disturbances, such as dysphasia, dysesthesia, hemiplegia, and speech disturbances, are less frequent. The aura usually lasts 20 minutes and may be followed by a unilateral headache contralateral to the aura or a bilateral headache, which is usually described as severe and throbbing. This headache is frequently associated with pallor, anorexia, abdominal pain, photophobia, phonophobia, and nausea and vomiting. Patients with this disorder retire to their rooms. Their headaches are frequently relieved by sleep.

Migraine without Aura

Migraine without aura is the most prevalent form of migraine in children and adolescents (Winner et al., 2000b). Although no visual aura is present, many children experience a prodrome or autonomic aura prior to the headache. This phenomenon may be accompanied by personality change, pallor, irritability, and lethargy. The autonomic aura may last from minutes to hours and is followed by the headache, which is usually throbbing, severe, and bifrontal or bitemporal. It is usually associated with abdominal pain, anorexia, and nausea and vomiting. These children are bothered by light and/or sound and attempt to sleep. Many awake feeling refreshed. There is a wide variation in the frequency, severity, and duration of migraine among children. It is shorter in children than in adults and usually occurs twice a month. Migraine without aura is not usually associated with neurologic symptoms or signs.

Migraine headaches associated with transient neurologic disturbances have been called *complex* or *complicated* migraine by some authors (Barlow, 1984; Hockaday, 1988). The neurologic deficits are presumed to be secondary to neuronal dysfunction, and the syndromes are described by their vascular territories or neurologic deficits. Most resolve spontaneously and leave no sequelae. When patients have headaches associated with neurologic symptoms and/or signs, it is important to differentiate "complex" migraine from serious underlying intracranial conditions. The incidence of complex migraine is not known. Different authors describe different methods of evaluating these patients, but MRI and magnetic resonance angiography (MRA) have been suggested to rule out significant vascular pathology (Prager and Mikulis, 1991). Electroencephalography may be necessary if alteration or loss of consciousness has taken place. In most instances, invasive angiography is not necessary. Data concerning treatment of these conditions are anecdotal.

Hemiplegic Migraine

Hemiplegic migraine is the association of recurrent hemiparesis and headache (Bradshaw and Parsons, 1965; Terwindt et al., 1996; Glista et al., 1975). Hemiparesis may precede, accompany, or follow the headache, which usually resolves before the hemiparesis. The headache is contralateral to the hemiparesis. Neuronal dysfunction accompanied by vasoconstriction, producing ischemia in the distribution of the middle cerebral artery, is thought to cause the hemiparesis. The patient may also have a visual field defect or aphasia. If attacks alternate from side to side, unilateral structural abnormalities are less likely. The differential diagnosis of headache in association with unilateral neurologic deficits includes thromboembolism, arteriovenous malformation, moyamoya disease, mitochondrial disorder, and tumor. Cardiac disease, oral contraceptive use, smoking, or

hypercoagulable states may play a contributory role. If a headache is associated with meningismus, a CT scan followed by a lumbar puncture may be indicated to rule out hemorrhage. Cerebrospinal fluid pleocytosis has been reported during some hemiplegic migraine attacks. Some attacks may be precipitated by minor head trauma. In some children, the attacks are familial (Joutel et al., 1993; Ducros et al., 1997; Gardner and Hoffman, 1998), and have been linked to mutation on chromosomes 1 and 19.

Ophthalmoplegic Migraine

Ophthalmoplegic migraine is rare (Ostergaard et al., 1996; Vijayan, 1980). It is the association of a complete or incomplete third nerve palsy and ipsilateral headache. The headache may precede, accompany, or follow the neurologic abnormality. The pain is retroorbital and severe. Neurologic examination reveals a dilated, poorly reactive pupil. The eye is deviated laterally because of the unopposed action of the sixth nerve. Ptosis and diplopia may also be present. The ophthalmoplegia persists for a variable period of time after the headache has disappeared. Permanent sequelae may occur. The third nerve dysfunction may be secondary to edema of the internal carotid artery within the cavernous sinus or edema of the distal basilar artery. The third nerve may enhance when an MRI with contrast is done during or shortly after the attack. An MRA is also needed. The differential diagnoses of patients with a painful third nerve palsy include an aneurysm at the junction of the internal carotid artery and the posterior communicating artery as well as Tolosa-Hunt syndrome. Corticosteroids may decrease the duration of the ophthalmoplegia.

Basilar Artery Migraine

Basilar artery migraine was first described by Bickerstaff (1961). It is identified by recurrent attacks of occipital headache and neurologic symptoms referable to the cortex, cerebellum, and brain stem. The syndrome affects adolescents more frequently than adults. Occipital involvement may cause visual symptoms, including visual field cuts or blindness. Bilateral sensory symptoms, dizziness, vertigo, ataxia, dysesthesia, dysarthria, (rarely) quadriparesis, and loss of consciousness may also occur. These symptoms may precede the occipital headache. Nausea and vomiting frequently follow. The symptoms usually clear completely (Golden and French, 1975). The differential diagnoses include temporal lobe epilepsy, vascular disease, demyelinating disease, and occipital neuralgia. Electroencephalography between or during attacks may reveal occipital spike discharges. The condition must be differentiated from occipital epilepsy (Andermann and Zifkin, 1998).

Confusional Migraine

Confusional migraine is a disorder that simulates a toxic encephalopathy (Gascon and Barlow, 1970; Ehyai and Fenichel, 1978). Headache is followed by confusion and a communicative disorder, which may be an expressive or receptive aphasia. Drug abuse is frequently suspected. The neurologic examination shows "confusion" and may or may not show focal features. Evaluation should include toxicology screening, EEG, imaging studies, and possibly lumbar puncture to rule out encephalitis. The EEG may show slowing over the dominant hemisphere. The disorder, which may be the first manifestation of migraine or appear in individuals who have had previous migraine attacks or previous episodes of confusion and usually clears in 6 to 12 hours. Data concerning the efficacy of preventive measures in these syndromes are not available.

Migraine Variants

The IHS includes only two clinical entities as migraine variants: benign paroxysmal vertigo and alternating hemiplegia of childhood. Most pediatric neurologists would include paroxysmal torticollis, cyclic vomiting, retinal migraine, and possibly "Alice in Wonderland syndrome" in this category. Most would exclude alternating hemiplegia (Rho and Chugani, 1994).

BENIGN PAROXYSMAL VERTIGO

Benign paroxysmal vertigo is not uncommon in children, although incidence figures are lacking (Fenichel, 1967; Dunn and Snyder, 1976). It more commonly affects younger children, who develop sudden unsteadiness and grab on to whatever is near them for stability. Consciousness is not lost. Nystagmus may be present. Vomiting may or may not occur. The spells last only minutes, and afterward the child is normal and will resume play or want to sleep. The spells usually occur in clusters over days to weeks and then subside. Laboratory evaluation is probably unnecessary in clear-cut cases. In less clear-cut cases, EEG and MRI scanning should be performed.

This disorder evolves into common migraine in later childhood and adolescence. Although antihistamine therapy has been suggested, no definitive therapeutic studies have been performed.

PAROXYSMAL TORTICOLLIS

Paroxysmal torticollis may be a variant of basilar migraine (Snyder, 1969; Chutorian, 1974). It is characterized by attacks of head tilt, vomiting, and ataxia that last from hours to days. It usually occurs in younger children. There is often a family history of migraine. This syndrome may evolve into more typical migraine in later years. In clear-cut cases, no evaluation is necessary; however, in problematic cases, EEG and MRI may be necessary. No studies have shown that specific medications are effective at preventing recurrence.

CYCLIC VOMITING

Cyclic vomiting is a symptom complex that occurs in infants, children, and, less commonly, adolescents and adults. It is characterized by repeated episodes of severe vomiting and dehydration (Simon and Russell, 1986; Fleisher and Matar, 1993). Between events, these children are healthy. Headache is not usually part of this syndrome. It is necessary to rule out intermittent bowel obstruction and metabolic disease prior to arriving at the diagnosis of cyclic vomiting. According to several authors, migraine prophylaxis can be effective at decreasing the frequency and severity of attacks (Andersen, 1997). General treatment measures include hydration, antiemetics, and sedation.

"ALICE IN WONDERLAND" SYNDROME

"Alice in Wonderland" syndrome consists of bizarre visual illusions and spatial distortions that precede migraine headaches (Hupp et al., 1989; Golden, 1979). Children may describe micropsia, macropsia, metamorphopsia, or teleopsia before the headache begins. This type of visual abnormality has also been reported in infectious mononucleosis, complex partial seizures, and drug ingestion.

RETINAL MIGRAINE

Retinal migraine is also called ocular or ophthalmic migraine (Shevell, 1996). It is uncommon in children and adolescents. Patients report sudden, momentary monocular blackouts or grayouts or blinding visual disturbances that may or may not be followed by a headache. Examination of the fundus during an attack may disclose retinal vein and artery constriction and retinal pallor. Some patients suffer visual sequelae, presumably due to retinal infarction. Evaluation for hypocoagulable states, embolic sources, and other vascular abnormalities should be carried out.

ALTERNATING HEMIPLEGIA OF CHILDHOOD

Alternating hemiplegia consists of attacks of hemiparesis, monoparesis, or quadriparesis, accompanied by decreased tone and occasionally involuntary movements (Rho and Chugani, 1994). Children are normal at the onset of symptoms. Symptoms are often reversed by sleep. Over time, more attacks occur, and children demonstrate developmental problems. This may be a mitochondrial disorder. Children with alternating hemiplegia may be helped by flunarazine.

Treatment

Once a diagnosis of migraine has been made, a treatment plan should be formulated. No treatment is indicated if attacks are infrequent and easily relieved by sleep. For some patients, episodic symptomatic or abortive

therapy will suffice. For others, a combination of symptomatic therapy, abortive therapy, and preventive therapy will be needed. Unfortunately, the use of medication to treat migraine in children is not well substantiated by appropriate studies. The use of a headache calendar is valuable for determining the frequency and severity of headaches before, during, and after treatment. It may demonstrate patterns of headache not previously suspected. Symptomatic treatment is used to encourage sleep and suppress pain, nausea, and vomiting. Abortive treatment is used to end attacks after they have begun by interfering with the migraine cascade. Preventive treatment is used to decrease the frequency and severity of future attacks. Nonpharmacologic treatments, including biofeedback, counseling, and stress reduction, have also been suggested as both abortive and preventive treatment (Wasiewski and Rothner, 1999).

Symptomatic Treatment

The mainstay of the pharmacologic management of childhood migraine is intermittent oral analgesics (Table 25–4). Overuse of these medications (more than two or three times weekly) can lead to both increased headache and rebound headache. Acetaminophen, ibuprofen, naproxen sodium, and ketorolac used early in the course of the headache at appropriate doses are frequently effective (Bruni et al., 1991; Graf and Riback, 1995; Hamalainen et al., 1997). Two medications in combination, such as acetaminophen and ibuprofen, may be helpful. Combination medications, which may include barbiturates or narcotics, play a secondary role if the initial agents fail (Solomon, 1995; Wasiewski and Rothner, 1999). Narcotics should be avoided during the initial stages of treatment as they may not only exacerbate the nausea and vomiting but lead to tolerance, addiction, and abuse.

Antiemetics may be useful since anorexia, abdominal pain, and vomiting occur in 90% of patients (Jones et al., 1989; Tek et al., 1990). Gastric stasis and nausea and vomiting may preclude the use of oral analgesics. An-

Table 25–4 Migraine symptomatic treatment

Medication	Dosage	Comment
Analgesics		
Acetaminophen[a]	10–15 mg/kg Q 4–6 h	Available as suppository
Ibuprofen[a]	4–10 mg/kg Q 6–8 h	No suppository available
Acetaminophen + codeine[b]	0.5–1 mg/kg Q 6–8 h	No suppository available
Fioricet	1 tablet Q 6 h	Number of tablets should be limited
Antiemetics		
Trimethobenzamide	15–20 mg/kg divided Q 6 h	100 or 200 mg suppository
Perchlorperazine[b]	0.4 mg/kg divided Q 6–8 h	2.5, 5, or 25 mg suppository, extrapyramidal reactions

[a]May be used together.
[b]Use with caution.

tiemetics alone may provide substantial relief and are surprisingly effective at eliminating all symptoms, including headache. These agents may be administered orally, rectally, or by injection. Dystonic reactions may occur and should be anticipated.

Abortive Treatment

Abortive agents that are commonly utilized include ergot preparations, nonsteroidal anti-inflammatory drugs (NSAIDs), a combination drug (Midrin), and the triptans (Silberstein and Young, 1995; Yuill et al., 1972) (Table 25–5). Medications can be administered orally, intranasally, parenterally, or rectally.

Ergotamine tartrate is a useful agent, but the risk of nausea and ergot rebound withdrawal headaches limits its value in patients in the pediatric and adolescent age groups. One should generally limit ergot use to no more than twice weekly. Adverse effects include nausea, vomiting, and vasoconstriction. An intranasal formulation of dihydroergota-

mine (DHE) has been approved for adult use. Dihydroergotamine (DHE-45), which needs dosage adjustment depending on age, can be used intramuscularly, subcutaneously, or intravenously with a concomitant antiemetic. Children between the ages of 6 and 9 years should receive 0.1 mg/dose, those between the ages of 9 and 12 should receive 0.5 mg/dose, and those between the ages of 12 and 16 should receive 0.75 mg/dose. It may be helpful to bring the child to the office on a day when he or she does not have a migraine and to give the child a test dose of DHE to make sure it does not cause significant nausea. If nausea occurs, the dose can be lowered. In general, problems can be avoided by lowering the dose, diluting the DHE with 30 to 60 cc of saline, and administering the solution intravenously over a period of one-half to one hour (Linder, 1994). In addition, 20 to 30 minutes prior to the administration of DHE, metoclopramide can be given to prevent nausea or vomiting. In addition to preventing nausea, metoclopramide has antido-

Table 25–5 Migraine abortive medication

Medication	Dosage	Comment
Midrin/duradrin[a]	2 caps at onset	>50 kg–max 5 caps
	1 additional cap/h ×3	<50 kg–max 3 caps
Ergot[a]	2 mg sublingual, may repeat once in 1 h	>50 kg
Sumatriptan[a]	SQ 0.06–0.1 mg/kg	See Protocol (Linder, 1994)
	Oral 25 mg	<50 kg
	Oral 50 mg	>50 kg
	Nasal 5 mg	<50 kg
	Nasal 20 mg	>50 kg
Naratriptan[a]	2.5 mg	>50 kg
Zomitriptan[a]	2.5–5.0 mg	>50 kg
Dihydroergotamine nasal spray[a]	As directed	>50 kg

[a]Not approved for children <18 years

paminergic effects, which can be helpful in treating migraine. Some children are sensitive to antiemetics, such as metoclopramide, and may develop extrapyramidal side effects, which can be readily reversed with 1 mg/kg diphenhydramine. Extrapyramidal side effects may also be seen with oral metoclopramide; if so, they usually occur between the fifth and eighth doses and are readily reversible with diphenhydramine. Phenergan, which is easily administered and has a rapid onset of efficacy, may be substituted for metoclopramide.

Nonsteroidal anti-inflammatory drugs, including naproxen, flurbiprofen, and meclofenamate, are useful for the acute treatment of migraine (Pradalier et al., 1988; Lewis et al., 1994). The maximal allowable dosage should be utilized at the onset of the attack.

Isometheptene mucate, a sympathomimetic agent that includes acetaminophen and a mild sedative, is useful for adolescents with migraine (Yuill et al., 1972). It is generally better tolerated than the ergots.

The triptan drugs are currently being studied in children and adolescents. These agents have no known analgesic activity. They are well absorbed orally, intranasally, and parenterally. A double-blind, placebo-controlled trial of sumatriptan was conducted at 35 sites with 302 adolescents (Winner et al., 2000a). Tablets of 25, 50, and 100 mg were tested. All tested doses of sumatriptan were statistically significantly superior to placebo at 180 and 240 minutes, with 74% pain relief at 4 hours. Recurrence rates varied from 18% to 28% with all three doses. No significant adverse events were noted in this study.

Sumatriptan nasal spray was studied in a randomized, double-blind, placebo-controlled study of adolescents whose ages ranged from 12 to 17 years. A single attack was treated. In this study, 5, 10, and 20 mg doses were studied. At 1 hour post-dose, headache relief was noted in 56% of patients using 10 mg compared with 41% of the placebo group. All three doses were superior to placebo with respect to the cumulative percentage of patients who attained headache relief within 2 hours. When reviewing the pain-free data, the 20 mg dose of sumatriptan nasal spray

helped 36% of patients. There was no difference with regard to headache recurrence among the treatment groups compared with the placebo group. The most common adverse event was taste disturbance. If this side effect is removed from the calculation, the overall incidence of adverse events for the nasal treatment group is similar to the placebo group. No serious adverse event was reported. Sumatriptan 20 mg nasal spray provided rapid relief and was well tolerated in the adolescent migraine population (Rothner et al., 2000).

A 5 mg tablet formulation of rizatriptan was evaluated in patients aged 12 to 17 years in a double-blind, placebo-controlled, parallel-group, single-attack study (Winner et al., 2000c). Sixty-six percent of the adolescents had pain relief at 2 hours with this dosage. Headache-free status at 2 hours was 32%. There were no serious adverse events. The most common adverse events were fatigue, dizziness, somnolence, dry mouth, and nausea. Forty-four percent of adolescent patients on 5 mg of rizatriptan reported no functional disability at 2 hours. Further studies of rizatriptan, zolmitriptan, and naratriptan are being conducted in the pediatric and adolescent populations. Adverse effects associated with the triptans include tingling, dizziness, warm/hot sensations, and injection site reactions. Headache recurrence is less of a problem in adolescents than in adults.

Prophylactic Treatment

Preventive therapy should be considered when individuals have frequent and or prolonged attacks that interfere with their ability to function (Table 25–6). Many medications have been used for migraine prophylaxis, including methysergide, β blockers, calcium channel blockers, NSAIDs, tricyclic antidepressants, and cyproheptadine (Curran et al., 1967; Diamond and Medina, 1976; Olesen, 1986; Peatfield et al., 1986; Couch et al., 1976; Lavenstein, 1991). The anticonvulsant sodium valproate has also been successfully utilized in the prophylaxis of migraine (Hering and Kuritzky, 1992).

Table 25–6 Migraine prophylactic treatment

Drug	Daily dosage	Comment
Cyproheptadine	0.25 mg/kg 1/3 A.M.-2/3 HS	Sedation appetite stimulation
Propranolol	0.6–1.5 mg/kg, divided 3 doses	Cardiac, vivid dreams depression
Amitriptyline	0.1–2 mg/kg HS	Cardiac, sedation
Verapamil	4–8 mg/kg, divided 3 doses	Cardiac, constipation
Depakote	10–30 mg/kg, divided 2 or 3 doses	Hepatic or pancreatic dysfunction, anorexia or weight gain.

Methysergide is rarely used today because of the risk of serious complications, such as pleural and peritoneal fibrosis.

Cyproheptadine is used for migraine prophylaxis in children. However, its use for this purpose has not been supported by medical research, and the drug does not have an approved indication for headache. A nightly dose of 4 to 12 mg is used. Common side effects include fatigue and weight gain (Lavenstein, 1991).

Nonsteroidal anti-inflammatory drugs are widely prescribed as analgesics and antipyretics (Pradalier et al., 1988). They are valuable in acute and preventive migraine treatment. Those reported to have prophylactic activity in migraine include aspirin, naproxen, flurbiprofen, ketoprofen, flufenamic acid, and fenoprofen. Adverse effects are relatively common. Gastrointestinal effects include dyspepsia, heartburn, nausea, vomiting, diarrhea, constipation, abdominal pain, and bleeding. Renal effects include decreased glomerular filtration rate and water retention. Both indomethacin and fenoprofen appear to be more nephrotoxic than other NSAIDs.

The β blockers are first-line drugs for migraine prophylaxis (Diamond and Medina, 1976; Ludvigsson, 1974). They also may have anxiolytic effects. The β blockers that are effective in migraine prophylaxis include propranolol and timolol. The β blockers are generally well tolerated, but they are contraindicated in patients with bronchospastic disease, diabetes, and Wolff-Parkinson-White syndrome. Side effects include depression, fatigue, sleep disorders, and decreased athletic endurance. Studies utilizing β blockers in children have had conflicting results. One of three studies found them to be effec-

tive, whereas two found no difference from placebo (Ludvigsson, 1974; Forsythe et al., 1984; Olness et al., 1987).

Calcium entry blockers, including verapamil, diltiazem, flunarazine, nimodipine, and nicardipine, have been useful in the prophylaxis of migraine. Data regarding their efficacy vary. They are not convincingly effective in children. The most common adverse effects are daytime sedation, weight gain, depression, and constipation.

Flunarazine, a drug not available in the United States, has been found to be effective and well-tolerated in two European childhood studies of migraine prophylaxis (Pothmann, 1987; Sorge et al., 1988).

Valproate, an anticonvulsant, has been evaluated for efficacy in migraine in adults (Hering and Kuritzky, 1992). Treatment with valproate significantly reduced the number and severity of migraine attacks. To date, it has not been well studied in childhood or adolescent migraine. No correlation was found between valproate levels and the frequency, severity, or duration of migraine attacks. In the adult population, no serious side effects were reported. Hepatic toxicity may occur in younger children; however, this is rare. Reported common side effects include weight gain, tremor, hair loss, and nausea. There is concern regarding valproate's possible relationship to polycystic ovaries.

Antidepressant medications are effective in migraine prophylaxis (Gomersall and Stuart, 1973; Moreland et al., 1979), and tricyclic antidepressants are more effective than the newer selective serotonin reuptake inhibitors (SSRIs) (Hershey et al., 2000). The selection of a specific antidepressant should be based primarily on whether or not the patient has a sleep disturbance. Patients who initiate and maintain sleep easily are better able to tolerate nonsedating drugs. Patients who have difficulty initiating and maintaining sleep respond better to sedating drugs. Nonsedating antidepressants include protriptyline and desipramine. Sedating antidepressants include amitriptyline, nortriptyline, and imipramine. Patients frequently are intolerant of the anticholinergic side effects, such as dry mouth, blurred vision, urinary retention, and constipation, of antidepressants. These medications should be initiated at low dosages and increased slowly. Cardiac conduction problems can occur with all tricyclic antidepressants and may cause prolongation of the P–R, QRS, and Q–T intervals. Selective SSRIs have not been well studied in migraine in children.

Nonpharmacologic Therapy

Nonpharmacologic preventive measures that may reduce headache frequency include patient/parent education, sleep hygiene, diet, and exercise. Sleep hygiene can have a significant effect on childhood headaches. A balanced diet, avoiding skipping meals and foods that precipitate migraine, can be useful. Food triggers may affect 5% to 15% of patients. Regular exercise, although not well studied, may be beneficial in reducing headache frequency. Studies involving biofeedback have proven it to be as effective as β blockers (McGrath and Reid, 1995). If stress is a significant contributing feature, counseling, relaxation therapy, and cognitive training have been helpful (Larson and Melin, 1988).

Prognosis

The short-term prognosis for migraine in children is favorable, with greater than 50% of patients reporting improvement within 6 months of medical intervention, regardless of the treatment method used (Hockaday, 1978; Bille, 1981). The long-term prognosis suggests that two-thirds of children go into remission for 2 or more years through adolescence and early adulthood. About 60% of migraineurs who had adolescent-onset mi-

graines, however, reported ongoing migraine after 30 years of age. Congden and Forsythe (1979) reported that 37 of 108 children (34%) had headache remission. Sillanpaa (1994) suggested that the remission rate for those whose onset was before 8 years of age was 22%, and boys were more likely to remit than girls. The remission rate for those whose onset was between 8 and 14 years of age was 25%, and girls were more likely to remit than boys, by a ratio of 3:2. The prognosis of childhood migraine is better in boys than in girls but is, at best, variable.

CHRONIC PROGRESSIVE HEADACHES

Chronic progressive headache implies a pathologic process within the cranium (Cohen, 1995) (Table 25–2). Increased intracranial pressure may be present. The symptoms and signs are progressive and worsen over time. Prominent in this group of disorders are hydrocephalus, brain tumor, pseudotumor cerebri, brain abscess, intracranial hemorrhage, and chronic subdural hematoma. Toxic processes, endocrine disturbances, congenital anomalies, degenerative disorders, and metabolic conditions may cause progressive headache; but this is rare. When the child's symptoms are progressive, rapid intervention to appropriately diagnose and treat the condition is mandatory. When increased intracranial pressure is present, associated symptoms may include progressive nausea, vomiting, focal weakness, ataxia, personality change, lethargy, visual disturbances, intellectual deterioration, and seizures. The general physical examination and the neurologic examination may rarely be normal or may demonstrate papilledema, a sixth nerve palsy, or other focal neurologic signs. When neurologic signs are present, their localization may lead to a specific diagnosis. If a cranial or intracranial process is suspected, MRI scanning may be diagnostic. Lumbar puncture should be considered as an initial diagnostic test only when acute bacterial meningitis is suspected. In other situations, it should be preceded by an imaging study to exclude a mass lesion.

Hydrocephalus is a condition in which increased ventricular volume with or without increased pressure is secondary to an obstruction or decreased cerebrospinal fluid (CSF) absorption (Abbott et al., 1991; Cohen, 1995). It may be secondary to a congenital anomaly, such as aqueductal stenosis, or it may develop following bacterial meningitis or intracranial hemorrhage. Symptoms and signs are those of nonlocalized increased intracranial pressure. When the disorder is chronic, macrocephaly may be present. The MRI is diagnostic, and a diversion procedure, such as a third ventriculostomy or a shunting procedure, is the treatment of choice.

Brain tumors are the second most frequent type of neoplasm in children and adolescents (Gilles, 1991; Honig and Charney, 1982). Headaches usually are progressive in frequency and severity, but temporary plateaus can occur. The pain is secondary to traction on pain-sensitive structures or obstruction of CSF flow with resultant hydrocephalus. The headache is not always localizing. Supratentorial tumors may cause frontal headaches, posterior fossa tumors may cause occipital headache, and hemispheric tumors may cause unilateral pain. Normal activity, such as changing position, defecating, coughing, or exertion, may exacerbate the pain. Although the quality of the pain and its severity are not diagnostic, it frequently is more severe in the morning and associated with and relieved by vomiting. Approximately 70% of children with brain tumors have headache as their presenting symptom. It may awaken them at night. The MRI is usually diagnostic. Various treatment modalities, including surgery, radiation, and chemotherapy, singly or in combination, are utilized.

Pseudotumor cerebri is increased intracranial pressure without evidence of an infection, mass lesion, or hydrocephalus (Corbett, 1983; Baker et al., 1989). Patients usually have headache and papilledema, as well as an associated sixth nerve palsy and diplopia. Visual field testing may reveal an enlarged blind spot. Pseudotumor without papilledema has been reported (Marcelis and Silberstein, 1991). Tinnitus may be present. The MRI reveals normal to small ventricles. Lumbar puncture demonstrates normal chemistries but elevated pressure. The disorder has been associated with a variety of conditions, including obesity, menstrual irregularity, chronic otitis, and various medications. Treatment consists of careful observation, removal of offending agents, diuretic or steroid administration, and repeated lumbar punctures, with removal of sufficient CSF to return the pressure to normal. If vision is threatened, lumbar peritoneal shunt or surgical decompression of the optic nerve may be indicated.

Brain abscess is rare but may occur in patients with cyanotic congenital heart disease, chronic infections, or immunosuppression secondary to chemotherapy or human immunodeficiency virus infection (Tekkok and Erbengi, 1992). There may be single or multiple abscesses. Symptoms include fever, headache, focal weakness, and seizures. Abnormal neurologic signs include papilledema and focal neurologic deficits. The MRI is usually diagnostic. Antibiotics and surgical drainage are the treatments of choice.

Both intracranial hemorrhage and subdural hematoma may be secondary to head trauma (accidental or secondary to child abuse), blood dyscrasia, or vascular abnormality, including malformations and aneurysms (Roach and Riela, 1995; Dhellemmes et al., 1985). Symptoms include headache, vomiting, lethargy, and focal neurologic symptoms. The examination may reveal macrocephaly, papilledema, retinal hemorrhages, and focal neurologic abnormalities. The CT scan demonstrates blood and MRI with MRA usually demonstrates the abnormality. Therapies include corticosteroids, surgical drainage, or a shunting procedure.

CHRONIC NONPROGRESSIVE HEADACHES

Chronic nonprogressive headaches are common in adolescents (Solomon et al., 1992; Gladstein et al., 1997). Bille (1962) stated that they are three times more common than migraine by age 15. Their etiology is unknown. Many believe that these headaches are associated with emotional stress and no identifiable organic substrate. This category also includes stress-related headaches, headaches caused by conversion reaction, headaches that are depressive equivalents, and headaches related to malingering. This group does not include migraine headaches that are precipitated by stress. The disorder may occur alone or in association with migraine. It may occur episodically, less than 15 times a month, or chronically, more than 15 times a month. These headaches seem to be less common in children under 10 to 12 years of age and more frequent in adolescents (Akhtar et al., 1998). They affect females more frequently than males. The frequent nonmigrainous headaches described by Bille (1962) are tension-type headaches and occur in 16% of adolescents by 15 years of age.

The clinical features of chronic nonprogressive headaches in adolescents have not been well defined (Gladstein and Holden, 1996). The IHS criteria have not been reexplored with special attention to children or adolescents. The symptoms are similar to those noted in adults. Headaches are frequently described as frontal and pressure- or band-like. Associated tenderness in the occipital and cervical regions may be present. There is no aura. Patients who have both disorders describe the pain as less severe than migraine. Although some patients have mild nausea, they usually do not vomit. The pain may be present for the entire day or a portion of the day, or may come and go throughout the day. Many adolescents with this disorder continue their usual activities. Few seem bothered by light or noise. Patients frequently describe the headaches in a nonspecific manner and may also describe mild blurred vision, fatigue, and dizziness. Many take medications in excess. Others stop taking medications entirely, feeling they are not helpful.

Details concerning school absence, headaches in other family members, alcohol and drug abuse, divorce, parental absence from the home, or the death of a close relative or friend may be important. Some patients have a previous history of recurrent abdominal pain or limb pain for which no cause was found. Some have a history of chronic behavioral difficulties. A noncephalic illness or trauma may precede the chronic headaches. When asked, many adolescents identify aggravating factors, such as fatigue due to erratic sleep patterns and stressful situations at home and at school. The headache also seems to aggravate fatigue, impair concentration, and cause irritability and anxiety. It rarely awakens the patient from sleep. Weather and food do not play important roles. In many patients, physical activity and exercise exacerbate the headache. A subset of patients have excessive school absences combined with high achievement.

General physical and neurologic examinations are normal. Laboratory testing is generally not needed, but patients frequently have had tests done prior to consultation or request them. Routine blood counts, sedimentation rates, and metabolic profiles have been nonrevealing. Scanning by CT or MRI in these patients shows no abnormality or unrelated minor abnormalities. A psychologic evaluation or counseling may enable patients to recognize their "stress." Many parents inadvertently perpetuate their children's chronic headaches by providing secondary gain in the form of attention and relief from stress.

If an adolescent has had daily or constant headaches for longer than 8 weeks, no symptoms of increased pressure or progressive neurologic disease, a normal general physical examination, and a normal neurologic examination, an organic etiology is unlikely and a psychologic interview and testing may lead to the appropriate diagnosis and treatment.

Patients with chronic headache frequently show a variety of psychologic and behavioral symptoms. The psychologic factors and learned behavioral patterns often maintain the patient's symptoms. The methodologies used to evaluate such patients differ, but direct and indirect measures, including a headache diary, structured self-report measures, and objective psychologic testing, are useful. The evaluation should assess the pain itself, including antecedents, precipitants, and responses; the effects on the patient, including global psychologic and social functioning; and the patient's environment, including family, school, and social factors.

Depression, overt and covert, as well as anxiety have been studied in patients with chronic nonprogressive headaches (Larson, 1988; Andrasik et al., 1988). Controlled studies of depression indicate significantly more depressive symptoms in these patients when compared with headache-free controls. In addition, significantly more anxiety is reported. Other concerns include stress, but what is considered stressful by one individual may seem trivial to another. Precipitants in children and adolescents with chronic headache include genetic predisposition, achievement motivation and fear of failure, somatic preoccupation, and major negative life changes or life events, including divorce, moving, or the death of a close friend or relative.

Acute episodic tension-type headache in a child or teenager does not present a serious management problem unless it becomes chronic or daily and results in altered function. The occasional use of over-the-counter analgesics, including acetaminophen and ibuprofen, either separately or combined; resting in a dark room; applying an ice pack; and avoiding stressful situations are usually sufficient. Daily or frequent use of aspirin, acetaminophen, NSAIDs, caffeine-containing compounds, barbiturate-containing compounds, and narcotic analgesics should be avoided as they may cause physical side effects and actually perpetuate the headache (Symons, 1998). Discontinuation of these compounds is necessary in order to achieve a successful outcome.

Many forms of psychologic intervention are useful, including relaxation training, stress management training, and behavioral contingency management (Richter et al., 1986; Labbe and Williamson, 1984). The treatment may range from self-taught relaxation to intensive multidisciplinary family intervention programs. Biofeedback and relaxation training have been used with success. Parents should be taught to reinforce normal behaviors.

Daily tricyclic antidepressant medications combined with the above psychologic interventions may be useful, even if overt depression is not present (Couch et al., 1976; Hershey et al., 2000). The efficacy of these medications at improving chronic nonprogressive headaches in adults without depression has been studied. Tricyclic antidepres-

sants are more beneficial than SSRIs. If more serious underlying psychopathology is suspected, a psychiatric consultation may be needed. Patients may also benefit from physical therapy, daily exercise, sleep regulation, and an improved diet.

The outcome of these therapies and the long-term prognosis in these patients have not been well studied. Since the pathogenesis of this disorder is not well understood but stress, anxiety, and depression seem to participate, the combination of psychologic and medical interventions used in a conservative fashion seems reasonable. Patients must return to school and discontinue excessive analgesics.

OTHER HEADACHES

Pediatric and adolescent patients may have the mixed headache syndrome, which is migraine superimposed on chronic nonprogressive headaches (Gladstein and Holden, 1996; Rothner, 1995b). The combination is not uncommon and requires a combined psychologic and pharmacologic approach (Rothner, 1995c).

Cluster headaches are rare in children and uncommon in adolescents (Ekbom et al., 1978; Maytal et al., 1992). They consist of severe unilateral pain that lasts 30 to 45 minutes, is located behind or around the eye, and may be associated with ptosis, miosis, nasal congestion, rhinorrhea, and injection of the conjunctiva. Attacks occur several times a day and frequently awaken the patient. Episodes occur for several weeks or months and then disappear for months to years. Treatment includes steroids, methysergide, ergotamine, oxygen, lithium, and triptans (Maytal et al., 1992).

Temporomandibular joint dysfunction may present with unilateral pain just below the ear (Belfer and Kaban, 1982; Pillemer et al., 1987) that is aggravated by chewing. Patients may describe jaw clicking or locking. The incidence of this disorder in children and adolescents is not known. It may be seen in patients with arthritis or after injury to the jaw. On examination, these patients have tenderness over the jaw and limitation of mouth opening. In most patients, however, the disorder is associated with muscle spasms, fatigue, stress, malocclusion, bruxism, teeth clenching, and excessive gum chewing. A combination of muscle relaxants, anti-inflammatory drugs, and counseling may be beneficial. Major dental surgery and costly therapeutic programs are usually unnecessary.

Occipital neuralgia is a syndrome that includes pain in the posterior part of the head, starting at the upper neck or base of the skull (Dugan et al., 1962; Hammond and Danta, 1978). It may be unilateral or bilateral. The pain may be brought on by movement, especially hyperextension of the head. It may be seen in athletes or individuals involved in flexion/extension automobile accidents. Physical examination is normal or may show cervical tenderness, limitation of motion, and decreased sensation over the C2 dermatome. An MRI that focuses on the cervicocranial junction can help rule out a congenital anomaly or other pathologic process. Treatment modalities vary but may include a soft cervical collar, analgesics, muscle relaxants, local injections, and physical therapy. Only rarely is surgery needed. The prognosis is quite good.

Four syndromes that are infrequently seen in pediatric and adolescent medicine are specifically responsive to indomethacin (Mathew, 1981). These include exertional headaches precipitated by sports; cyclic migraine, in which the patient exhibits cycles of migraine headache daily for several weeks followed by 3 to 4 months without headache; chronic paroxysmal hemicrania, which is characterized by multiple, unilateral, daily bouts of pain that last 5 to 30 minutes; and hemicrania continua, which occurs predominantly in females and is characterized by severe, steady, unilateral, nonparoxysmal hemicrania localized to the frontal part of the head and not associated with nausea and vomiting. Indomethacin can be dramatically helpful in these patients, but its use must be carefully monitored.

REFERENCES

Abbott, R., F.J. Epstein, and J.H. Wisoff (1991). Chronic headaches associated with a function-ing shunt: Usefulness of pressure monitoring. *Neurosurgery* 28:72.

Abu-Arefeh, I. and G. Russell (1994). Prevalence of headache and migraine in school children. *BMJ* 309:765–769.

Akhtar, N.D., L.K. Mannik, K.M. O'Neil et al. (1998). Distribution of headache syndromes among children of various ages. *Neurology* 50: A–83 (abstr).

American College of Emergency Physicians (1996). Clinical policy for the initial approach to adolescents and adults presenting to the emergency department with a chief complaint of headache. *Ann. Emerg. Med.* 27:821–844.

Andermann, F. and B. Zifkin (1998). The benign occipital epilepsies of childhood: An overview of the idiopathic syndromes and of the relationship to migraine. *Epilepsia* 40:1320–1323.

Andersen, J.M., K.S. Sugerman, J.R. Lockhart et al. (1997). Effective prophylactic therapy for cyclic vomiting syndrome in children using amitriptyline or cyproheptadine. *Pediatrics* 100: 997–981.

Andrasik, F., E. Kabela, S. Quinn et al. (1988). Psychological functioning of children who have recurrent migraine. *Pain* 34:43–57.

Baker, R.S., R.J. Baumann, and J.R. Buncic (1989). Idiopathic intracranial hypertension (pseudotumor cerebri) in pediatric patients. *Pediatr. Neurol.* 5:5–11.

Barabas, G., M. Ferrari, and W.S. Matthews (1983a). Childhood migraine and somnambulism. *Neurology* 33:948.

Barabas, G., W.S. Matthew, and M. Ferrari (1983b). Childhood migraine and motion sickness. *Pediatrics* 72:188.

Barabas, G., W.S. Matthews, and M. Ferrari (1984). Tourette's syndrome and migraine. *Arch. Neurol.* 41:871–872.

Barlow, C.F. (1984). *Headaches and Migraine in Childhood.* Oxford-Blackwell Scientific Publishers, Philadelphia.

Belfer, M.L. and L.B. Kaban (1982). Temporomandibular joint dysfunction. *Pediatrics* 69: 564–567.

Bickerstaff, E.R. (1961). Basilar artery migraine. *Lancet* 1:15–17.

Bille, B. (1981). Migraine in children and its prognosis. *Cephalalgia* 1:71–75.

Bille, B.S. (1962). Migraine in school children. *Acta Paediatr. Scand.* 51 (Suppl. 136): 1–151.

Bodensteiner, J.B. (2001). Pediatric Headaches. (A.D. Rothner, ed). *Semin. Pediatr. Neurol.* 8.

Bradshaw, P. and M. Parsons (1965). Hemiplegic migraine: A clinical study. *QJM* 34:65–85.

Bruni, O., F. Cortesi, V. Guidetti et al. (1991). Acetylsalicylic vs. acetaminophen in childhood and adolescence acute migraine. In *Juvenile Headache* (V. Gallai and V. Guidetti, eds.), pp. 421–424. Excerpta Med.-Elsevier, Amsterdam.

Burton, L.J., B. Quinn, J.L. Pratt-Cheney et al. (1997). Headache etiology in a pediatric emergency department. *Pediatr. Emerg. Care* 13:1–4.

Chutorian, A.M. (1974). Benign paroxysmal torticollis, tortipelvis and retrocollis in infancy [abstract]. *Neurology* 24:366–367.

Cohen, B.H. (1995). Headaches as a symptom of neurological disease. *Semin. Pediatr. Neurol.* 2: 144–150.

Congdon, P.J. and W.I. Forsythe (1979). Migraine in childhood: A study of 300 children. *Dev. Med. Child Neurol.* 21:209–216.

Cooper, P.J., H.N. Bawden, P.R. Camfield et al. (1987). Anxiety and life events in childhood migraine. *Pediatrics* 79:999–1004.

Corbett, J.J. (1983). Problems in the diagnosis and treatment of pseudotumor cerebri. *Can. J. Neurol. Sci.* 10:221–229.

Couch, J.R., D.K. Ziegler, and R.S. Hassanein (1976). Amitriptyline in the prophylaxis of migraine. *Neurology* 26:121–127.

Cunningham, S.J., P.J. McGrath, H.B. Ferguson et al. (1987). Personality and behavioral characteristics in pediatric migraine. *Headache* 27: 16–20.

Curran, D.A., H. Hinterberger, and J.W. Lance (1967). Methysergide. *Headache* 1:74–122.

Day, W.H. (1873). *Essays on Diseases of Children.* J & A Churchill, London.

Deubner, D.C. (1977). An epidemiologic study of migraine and headache in 10–20 year olds. *Headache* 17:173–180.

Dhellemmes, P., J.P. Lejeune, J.L. Christiaens et al. (1985). Traumatic extradural hematoma in infancy and childhood. *J. Neurosurg.* 62:861–864.

Diamond, S. and J.L. Medina (1976). Double-blind study of propranolol for migraine prophylaxis. *Headache* 16:24–27.

Dooley, J.M., P.R. Camfield, M. O'Neill et al. (1990). The value of CT scans for children with headaches. *Can. J. Neurol. Sci.* 17:309–310.

Ducros, A., A. Joutel, V. Biousse et al. (1997). Mapping of a second locus for familial hemiplegic migraine to 1q21-q23 and evidence of further heterogeneity. *Ann. Neurol.* 42:885–890.

Dugan, M.C., S. Locke, and J.R. Gallagher (1962). Occipital neuralgia in adolescents and young adults. *N. Engl. J. Med.* 267:1166–1172.

Dunn, D.W. and C.H. Snyder (1976). Benign paroxysmal vertigo of childhood. *Am. J. Dis. Child.* 130:1099–1100.

Ehyai, A. and G.M. Fenichel (1978). The natural history of acute confusional migraine. *Arch. Neurol.* 35:368–369.

Ekbom, K., B. Ahlborg, and R. Schele (1978). Prevalence of migraine and cluster headache in Swedish men of 18. *Headache* 18:9–19.

Fenichel, G.M. (1967). Migraine as a cause of benign paroxysmal vertigo of childhood. *J. Pediatr.* 71:114–115.

Fleisher, D.R. and M. Matar (1993). The cyclic vomiting syndrome: A report of 71 cases and literature review. *J. Pediatr. Gastroenterol. Nutr.* 17:361–369.

Forsythe, W.I., D. Gillies, and M.A. Sills (1984). Propranolol (Inderal) in the treatment of childhood migraine. *Dev. Med. Child Neurol.* 26: 737–741.

Friedman, A.P. and E. Harms (1967). *Headaches in Children.* Thomas, Springfield, IL.

Gallai, V., P. Sarchielli, F. Carboni et al. (1995). Applicability of the 1988 IHS criteria to headache patients under the age of 18 years attending 21 Italian headache clinics. *Headache* 35: 146–153.

Gardner, K. and E.P. Hoffman (1998). Current status of genetic discoveries in migraine: Familial hemiplegic migraine and beyond. *Curr. Opin. Neurol.* 11:211–216.

Gascon, G. and C.F. Barlow (1970). Juvenile migraine presenting as an acute confusional state. *Pediatrics* 45:628–635.

Gherpelli, J.L.D., L.M. Nagae Poetscher, A.M.M.H. Souza et al. (1998). Migraine in childhood and adolescence. A critical study of the diagnostic criteria and of the influence of age on critical findings. *Cephalalgia* 18:333–341.

Gilles, F.H. (1991). The epidemiology of headache among children with brain tumor. *J. Neurooncol.* 10:31–46.

Gladstein, J. and E.W. Holden (1996). Chronic daily headaches in children and adolescents: A two-year prospective study. *Headache* 36:349–351.

Gladstein, J., E.W. Holden, L. Peralta et al. (1993). Diagnoses and symptom patterns in children presenting to a pediatric headache clinic. *Headache* 33:497–500.

Gladstein, J., E.W. Holden, P. Winner et al. (1997). Chronic daily headache in children and adolescents: Current status and recommendations for the future. *Headache* 37:626–629.

Glista, C.G., J.F. Mellinger, and E.D. Rooke (1975). Familial hemiplegic migraine. *Mayo Clin. Proc.* 50:307–311.

Golden, G.S. (1979). The Alice in Wonderland syndrome in juvenile migraine. *Pediatrics* 63: 517–519.

Golden, G.S. and J.H. French (1975). Basilar artery migraine in young children. *Pediatrics* 56: 722–726.

Gomersall, J.D. and A. Stuart (1973). Amitriptyline in migraine prophylaxis. *J. Neurol. Neurosurg. Psychiatry* 36:684–690.

Graf, W.D. and P.S. Riback (1995). Pharmacologic treatment of recurrent pediatric headache. *Pediatr. Ann.* 24:477–484.

Gronseth, G.S. and M.K. Greenberg (1995). The utility of the electroencephalogram in the evaluation of patients presenting with headache: A review of the literature. *Neurology* 45:1263–1267.

Hamalainen M.L. (1997). Optimal drug treatment of recurrent headaches and migraine in children—a clinical and pharmacological study (thesis). Department of Clinical Pharmacology, University of Helsinki, Helsinki, Finland.

Hamalainen, M.L., K. Hoppu, and P.R. Santavuori (1995). Effect of age on the fulfillment of the IHS criteria for migraine in children at a headache clinic. *Cephalalgia* 15:404–409.

Hamalainen, M.L., K. Hoppu, E. Valkeila et al. (1997). Ibuprofen or acetaminophen for the acute treatment of migraine in children: A double-blind, randomized, placebo-controlled, crossover study. *Neurology* 48:103–107.

Hammond, S.R. and G. Danta (1978). Occipital neuralgia. *Clin. Exp. Neurol.* 15:258–270.

Headache Classification Committee of the International Headache Society (1988). Proposed classification and diagnostic criteria for headache disorders, cranial neuralgias, and facial pain. *Cephalgia* 8:1–96.

Hering, R. and A. Kuritzky (1992). Sodium valproate in the prophylactic treatment of migraine: A double-blind study versus placebo. *Cephalalgia* 12:81–84.

Hershey, A.D., S.W. Powers, A.L. Bentti et al. (2000). Effectiveness of amitriptyline in the prophylactic management of childhood headaches. *Headache* 40:539–54.

Hockaday, J.M. (1978). Late outcome of childhood onset migraine and factors affecting outcome, with particular reference to early and late EEG findings. In *Current Concepts in Migraine Research* (R. Greene, ed.), pp. 41–48. Raven Press, New York.

Hockaday, J.M. (ed.) (1988). *Migraine in Childhood*. Butterworths, London.

Honig, P.J. and E.B. Charney (1982). Children with brain tumor headaches. *Am. J. Dis. Child.* 136:121.

Hupp, S.L., L.B. Kline, and J.J. Corbett (1989). Visual disturbances of migraine. *Surv. Ophthalmol.* 33:221–236.

Jensen, V. and A.D. Rothner (1995). Chronic nonprogressive headaches in children and adolescents. *Semin. Pediatr. Neurol.* 2:151–158.

Jones, J., D. Sklar, J. Dougherty et al. (1989). Randomized double-blind trial of intravenous prochlorperazine for the treatment of acute headache. *JAMA* 261:1174–1176.

Joutel, A., M.G. Bousser, V. Biousse et al. (1993). A gene for familial hemiplegic migraine maps to chromosome 19. *Nat. Genet.* 5:40–45.

Kandt, R. and R. Levine (1987). Headache and acute illness in children. *J. Child. Neurol.* 2:22–27.

Kinast, M., H. Lueders, A.D. Rothner et al. (1982). Benign focal epileptiform discharges in childhood migraine (BFEDC). *Neurology* 32:1309.

Labbe, E.E. and D.A. Williamson (1984). Treatment of childhood migraine using autogenic feedback training. *J. Consult. Clin. Psychol.* 52:968–976.

Larson, B. (1988). The role of psychological, health behavior and medical factors in adolescent headache. *Dev. Med. Child Neurol.* 30:616–625.

Larson, B. and L. Melin (1988). The psychological treatment of recurrent headache in adolescents: Short-term outcome and its prediction. *Headache* 28:187–195.

Lavenstein, B.A. (1991). Comparative study of cyproheptadine, amitriptyline, and propranolol in the treatment of preadolescent migraine. *Cephalalgia* 11(Suppl. 11):122–123.

Lewis, D.W., M.T. Middlebrook, L. Hehallick et al. (1994). Naproxen for migraine prophylaxis. *Ann. Neurol.* 36:542–543.

Lewis, D.W. and F. Qureshi (2000). Acute headache in children and adolescents presenting to the emergency department. *Headache* 40:200–203.

Linder, S.L. (1994). Treatment of childhood headache with dihydroergotamine mesylate. *Headache* 34:578–580.

Lippman, C.W. (1952). Certain hallucinations peculiar to migraine. *J. Nerv. Ment. Dis.* 116:346–351.

Lipton, R.B. (1997). Classification and epidemiology of headaches in children. *Current Opinion Neurol.* 10:231–236.

Litman, G.I. and H.M. Friedman (1978). Migraine and the mitral valve prolapse syndrome. *Am. Heart J.* 96:610–614.

Ludvigsson, J. (1974). Propranolol used in prophylaxis of migraine in children. *Acta Neurol. Scand.* 50:109–115.

Marcelis, J. and S.D. Silberstein (1991). Idiopathic intracranial hypertension without papilledema. *Arch. Neurol.* 48:392–399.

Martin, S.E. and M.S. Smith (1995). Psychosocial factors in recurrent pediatric headache. *Pediatr. Ann.* 24:469–474.

Mathew, N.T. (1981). Indomethacin-responsive headache syndromes. *Headache* 21:147–150.

Maytal, J., R.S. Bienkowski, M. Patel et al.(1995). The value of brain imaging in children with headaches. *Pediatrics* 96:413–416.

Maytal, J., R.B. Lipton, S. Solomon et al. (1992). Childhood onset cluster headaches. *Headache* 32:275–279.

Maytal, J., M. Young, A. Shechter et al. (1997). Pediatric migraine and the International Headache Society (IHS) criteria. *Neurology* 48:602–607.

McGrath, P.A. (1990). *Pain in Children: Nature, Assessment, and Treatment*. Guilford, New York.

McGrath, P.A. (2001). *The Child with Headache: Diagnosis and Treatment.* IASP Press, Seattle.

McGrath, P.J. and G.J. Reid (1995). Behavioral treatment of pediatric headache. *Pediatr. Ann.* 24:486–491.

Metsahonkala, L. and M. Sillanpaa (1994). Migraine in children—an evaluation of the IHS criteria. *Cephalalgia* 14:285–290.

Moreland, T.J., O.V. Storli, and T.E. Mogstad (1979). Doxepin in the prophylactic treatment of mixed vascular and tension headache. *Headache* 19:382–383.

Mortimer, J., J. Kay, and A. Jaron (1992). Epidemiology of headache and childhood migraine in an urban general practice using ad hoc, Vahlquist and IHS criteria. *Dev. Med. Child. Neurol.* 34:1095–1101.

Moskowitz, M. (1991). The visceral organ brain: Implications for the pathophysiology of vascular head pain. *Neurology* 41:182–186.

Olesen, J. (1986). Role of calcium entry blockers in the prophylaxis of migraine. *Eur. Neurol.* 25(Suppl. 1):72–79.

Olness, K., J.T. MacDonald, and D.L. Uden (1987). Comparison of self-hypnosis and propranolol in the treatment of juvenile classic migraine. *Pediatrics* 79:593–597.

Ostergaard, J.R., H.U. Moller, and T. Christensen (1996). Recurrent ophthalmoplegia in childhood: Diagnostic and etiologic considerations. *Cephalalgia* 16:276–277.

Pearce, J.M.S. (1980). Chronic migrainous neuralgia, a variant of cluster headache. *Brain* 103:149–159.

Peatfield, R.C., J.R. Fozard, and F.C. Rose (1986). Drug treatment of migraine. In: *Handbook of Clinical Neurology*, Vol. 48 (F.C. Rose, ed.), pp. 173–216. Elsevier, Amsterdam.

Peatfield, R.C., V. Glover, J.T. Littlewood et al. (1984). The prevalence of diet-induced migraine. *Cephalgia* 4:179–183.

Pillemer, F.G., B.J. Masek, and L.B. Kaban (1987). Temporomandibular joint dysfunction and facial pain in children: An approach to diagnosis and treatment. *Pediatrics* 80:565–570.

Pothmann, R. (1987). Migraneprophylaxe mit flunarizin und azetylsalizylsaure. Eine dobbelblindstudie. *Monatsschr. Kinderheilkd.* 135:646–649.

Pradalier, A. (1988). Treatment review: Non-steroid anti-inflammatory drugs in treatment of long-term prevention of migraine attacks. *Headache* 28:550–557.

Prager, J.M. and D.J. Mikulis (1991). The radiology of headache. *Med. Clin. North Am.* 75:525–544.

Prensky, A.L. and D. Sommer (1979). Diagnosis and treatment of migraine in children. *Neurology* 29:506–510.

Puca, F. and M. de Tommaso (1999). Clinical neu-

rophysiology in childhood headache. *Cephalalgia* 19:137–146.

Raskin, N.H. and S.C. Knittle (1976). Ice cream headache and orthostatic symptoms in patients with migraine. *Headache* 16:222–225.

Rho, J.M. and H.T. Chugani (1998). Alternating hemiplegia of childhood: insights into its pathophysiology. *J. Child Neurol.* 13:39–45.

Richter, I., P.J. McGrath, P.J. Humphreys et al. (1986). Cognitive and relaxation treatment of pediatric migraine. *Pain* 25:195–203.

Roach, E.S. and A.R. Riela (1995). Intracranial hemorrhage. *Pediatr. Cerebrovasc. Disord.* 5:69–83.

Rothner, A.D. (1986). The migraine syndrome in children and adolescents. *Pediatr. Neurol.* 2:121–126.

Rothner, A.D. (ed.) (1995a). Headache in children and adolescents. *Semin. Pediatr. Neurol.* 2:101–107.

Rothner, A.D. (1995b). The evaluation of headaches in children and adolescents. *Semin. Pediatr. Neurol.* 2:109–118.

Rothner, A.D. (1995c). Miscellaneous headache syndromes in children and adolescents. *Semin. Pediatr. Neurol.* 2:159–164.

Rothner, A.D., P. Winner, R. Nett et al. (2000). One-year tolerability and efficacy of sumatriptan nasal spray in adolescents with migraine: results of a multicenter, open-label study. *Clin. Ther.* 22:1533–1546.

Schechter, N.L. (1984). Recurrent pains in children: An overview and approach. *Pediatr. Clin. North Am.* 31:949–968.

Schwartz, B.S., W.F. Stewart, D. Simon et al. (1998). Epidemiology of tension-type headache. *JAMA* 279:381–383.

Seshia, S.S. (1996). Specificity of IHS criteria in childhood headache. *Headache* 36:295–299.

Seshia, S.S. and J.R. Wolstein (1994). International Headache Society classification and diagnostic criteria in children: A proposal for revision. *Dev. Med. Child Neurol.* 37:879–882.

Seshia, S.S., J.R. Wolstein, C. Adams et al. (1994). International Headache Society criteria and childhood headache. *Dev. Med. Child Neurol.* 36:419–428.

Shevell, M.I. (1996). Acephalgic migraines of childhood. *Pediatr. Neurol.* 14:211–215.

Silberstein, S.D. and W.B. Young (1995). Safety and efficacy of ergotamine tartrate and dihydroergotamine in the treatment of migraine and status migrainous. *Neurology* 45:577–584.

Sillanpaa, M. (1976). Prevalence of migraine and other headache in Finnish children starting school. *Headache* 15:288–290.

Sillanpaa, M. (1983). Changes in the prevalence of migraine and other headaches during the first seven school years. *Headache* 23:15–19.

Sillanpaa, M. (1994). Headache in children. In *Headache Classification and Epidemiology* (J.

Olesen, ed.), pp. 273–281. Raven Press, New York.

Sillanpaa, M., P. Piekkala, and P. Kero (1991). Prevalence of headache at preschool age in an unselected child population. *Cephalalgia* 11: 239–242.

Simon, D.N.K. and G. Russell (1986). Abdominal migraine: A childhood syndrome defined. *Cephalalgia* 6:223–228.

Smith, M.S. (ed.) (1995). Headaches. *Pediatr. Ann.* 24:446–491.

Snyder, C.H. (1969). Paroxysmal torticollis in infancy. A possible form of labyrinthitis. *Am. J. Dis. Child.* 117:458–460.

Solomon, G.D. (1995). The pharmacology of medications used in treating headache. *Semin. Pediatr. Neurol.* 2:165–177.

Solomon, S., R.B. Lipton, and L.C. Newman (1992). Clinical features of chronic daily headache. *Headache* 32:325–329.

Sorge, F., R. DeSimone, E. Marano et al. (1988). Flunarazine in prophylaxis of childhood migraine. A double-blind, placebo-controlled, crossover study. *Cephalalgia* 8:1–6.

Stewart, W.F., R.B. Lipton, D.D. Celentano et al. (1992). Prevalence of migraine headache in the United States. *JAMA* 267:64–69.

Symons, D.N.K. (1998). Twelve cases of analgesic headache. *Arch. Dis. Child.* 78:555–556.

Tek, D.S., D.S. McClellan, J.S. Olshaker et al. (1990). A prospective, double-blind study of metoclopramide hydrochloride for the control of migraine in the emergency department. *Ann. Emerg. Med.* 19:1083–1087.

Tekkok, I.H. and A. Erbengi (1992). Management of brain abscess in children. Review of 130 cases over a period of 21 years. *Childs Nerv. Syst.* 8: 411–416.

Terwindt, G., J. Haan, R.A. Ophoff et al. (1996). Familial hemiplegic migraine: Clinical comparison of families linked and unlinked to chromosome 19. *Cephalalgia* 16:153–155.

Vahlquist, B. (1955). Migraine in children. *Int. Arch. Allergy* 7:348–355.

Vijayan, N. (1980). Ophthalmoplegic migraine: Ischemic or compressive neuropathy? *Headache* 20:300–304.

Wasiewski, W.W. and A.D. Rothner (1999). Pediatric migraine headache: Diagnosis, evaluation, and management. *Neurologist* 5:122–134.

Winner, P., A.D. Rothner, J. Saper et al. (2000a). A randomized, double-blind, placebo-controlled study of sumatriptan nasal spray in the treatment of acute migraine in adolescents. *Pediatrics* 106:989–992.

Winner, P., et al. (2000b). Demographic and migraine characteristics of adolescent patients: the Glaxo Wellcome adolescent clinical trials database. *Headache* 40:438 (abstr).

Winner, P, et al. (2000c). Clinical profile of rizatriptan 5 mg in adolescent migraines. *Headache*, 437.

Winner, P., W. Martinez, L. Mate et al. (1995). Classification of pediatric migraine: Proposed revisions to the IHS criteria. *Headache* 35:407–410.

Winner, P. and A.D. Rothner (2001). *Headache in Children and Adolescents*. BC Decker, London.

Winner, P., W. Wasiewski, J. Gladstein et al. (1997). Multicenter prospective evaluation of proposed pediatric migraine revisions to the IHS criteria. *Headache* 37:545–548.

Wober-Bingol, C., C. Wober, and C. Wagner-Ennsgraber (1996). IHS criteria for migraine and tension-type headache in children and adolescents. *Headache* 36:231–238.

Yuill G.M. (1972). A double-blind crossover trial of isometheptene mucate compound and ergotamine in migraine. *Br. J. Clin. Pract.* 26:76–79.

Zuckerman, B., J. Stevenson, and V. Bailey (1987). Stomachaches and headaches in a community sample of preschool children. *Pediatrics* 79: 677–682.

26

Behavioral Management
of Headache

KENNETH A. HOLROYD
DONALD B. PENZIEN
GAY L. LIPCHIK

Harold G. Wolff is often honored at the same time his work is ignored. He is justifiably honored for his groundbreaking formulation of pathophysiological mechanisms in migraine and tension headache and for experimental studies that established the study of benign headache as a legitimate scientific enterprise. At the same time, the thesis of over two decades of Wolff's work, that to truly understand psychophysiological disorders such as headache we need to understand how psychosocial and physiological variables interact during stress to induce symptom episodes, is ignored (Simmons and Wolff, 1954; Wolff, 1948, 1953; Wolff and Wolff, 1948). Toward this end, Wolff developed innovative methods of observing psychological and physiological responses as people coped with naturalistic stressors or with cleverly designed laboratory stressors. He also vigorously pursued efforts to integrate knowledge from the social and medical sciences that would be necessary to this understanding. Simmons and Wolff (1954) state the thesis concisely: "it is the joint province of both social and physical (medical) scientists to work on the central linkage, namely, how specified stresses work to evoke particular (psychophysiological) protective reaction patterns." This focus on *psy-chophysiology*, the interaction of psychological and physiological variables in generating headaches and on the integration of relevant knowledge from the social and medical sciences, would place him in the mainstream of behavioral medicine today.

Wolff's approach to clinical work is also often forgotten in today's busy practice environment, where 10-minute clinic visits may focus primarily on identifying the best medication to prescribe. His systematic clinical observations and research describe how thoughts, behaviors, and bodily reactions evolve in response to stress to induce headache episodes. The contemporary behavior therapist would recognize Wolff's (1953) observation of how migraines often occur

at the peak or the sequel of actively functioning protective reaction patterns which have been operating for days, weeks, or longer. These involve all the bodily adjustments that accompany great efforts in work, cumulative tension, over-alertness, perfectionism, operating according to schedules, delayed actions, and the relentless pursuit of approval.

Prior to the development of behavior therapy, few methods were available to Wolff to help patients control the "bodily adjustments" induced by "great efforts in work," "cumulative tension," hyperarousal or "overalertness," "perfectionism," the "relentless pursuit of approval," unceasing schedules of activity, etc. Teaching patients to prevent or manage these "bodily adjustments" is the primary goal of the behavioral and cognitive-behavioral interventions we discuss in this chapter.

OVERVIEW OF BEHAVIORAL INTERVENTIONS

The most commonly used behavioral interventions for headache can be grouped into three categories: (1) relaxation training, (2) biofeedback training, and (3) cognitive-behavior (stress-management) therapy. Although these treatments attempt to influence both the frequency and the severity of headaches, they emphasize the prevention of headache episodes. Behavioral treatments may also reduce psychological symptoms, affective distress, or somatic complaints. For some, these latter benefits may be appreciated as much as, or more than, reduced headache activity.

Behavior therapies may be a treatment option for headache sufferers who have at least one of the following characteristics: (1) a preference for nonpharmacological interventions; (2) poor tolerance of pharmacological treatment; (3) medical contraindications to pharmacological treatments; (4) inadequate response to pharmacological treatment; (5) pregnancy, planned pregnancy, or nursing; (6) a history of excessive use of analgesic or other acute medications; and (7) life stress, deficient coping skills, or comorbid psychological disorder that aggravates headache problems or disability. The long-term goals of behavior therapy include reduced frequency and severity of headaches, reduced headache-related disability and affective distress, reduced reliance on poorly tolerated or unwanted pharmacotherapies, and enhanced personal control of headaches.

Relaxation Training

The therapeutic value of relaxation training has been recognized for over 100 years (Call,

1898; Stebbins, 1893). The three most widely used types of relaxation training are (1) *progressive muscle relaxation*, i.e., alternately tensing and relaxing selected muscle groups throughout the body (Bernstein and Borkovec, 1973; Jacobson, 1934); (2) *autogenic training*, i.e., the use of self-instructions of warmth and heaviness to promote a state of deep relaxation (Schultz and Luthe, 1959); and (3) *meditation*, the use of a silently repeated word or sound to promote mental calm and relaxation (Benson, 1975). Relaxation skills are typically used as preventive therapy. Relaxation skills enable headache sufferers to exert control over headache-related physiological responses and to lower sympathetic arousal. Relaxation may also provide an activity break, as well as help patients gain a sense of mastery or self-control over their symptoms. Relaxation training may involve ten or more treatment sessions, but fewer sessions are needed for uncomplicated headache problems. Patients are instructed to practice relaxation techniques for 20 to 30 minutes a day and to integrate relaxation into their daily activities as they master brief relaxation techniques.

Biofeedback Training

Biofeedback refers to any procedure that provides information about physiological processes (usually through the use of electronic instrumentation) in the form of an observable display (an audio tone or visual display). The patient uses the "feedback" he or she receives about a physiological function to self-regulate the response being monitored (Schwartz, 1995) (Fig. 26–1).

The two types of biofeedback training most often used in the treatment of recurrent headache disorders are thermal (hand-warming) feedback, which is feedback of skin temperature from a finger, and electromyographic (EMG) feedback, which is feedback of electrical activity from muscles of the scalp, neck, and sometimes the upper body (Fig. 26–1). Biofeedback training is commonly administered in conjunction with relaxation training and may require a dozen or more treatment sessions. As with relaxation

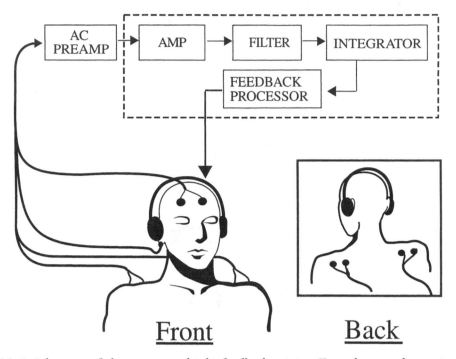

Figure 26–1 Schematic of electromyographic biofeedback training. Frontal area and trapezius muscles are being monitored with ground on the ear lobe.

training, patients are instructed to practice the self-regulation skills they are learning for about 20 to 30 minutes a day and to integrate these skills into their daily lives.

Cognitive-Behavior (Stress-Management) Therapy

The rationale for using cognitive-behavior therapy or stress-management training in headache management derives from the observation that the way individuals cope with everyday stresses can precipitate, exacerbate, or maintain headaches and increase headache-related disability and distress (Holroyd and Andrasik, 1982; Holroyd et al., 1982). Cognitive-behavior therapy focuses on the cognitive and affective components of headache, and it is typically administered in conjunction with relaxation training. Cognitive-behavioral interventions alert patients to the role their thoughts play in generating stress responses and to relationships between stress, coping efforts, and headaches. Patients are taught to employ more effective strategies for coping with headache-related stresses and

headaches themselves. Cognitive-behavior therapy commonly requires from three to 12 or more treatment sessions. Greater psychotherapeutic skill is required to administer cognitive-behavior therapy than to administer relaxation training or biofeedback training.

EFFICACY OF BEHAVIORAL TREATMENTS

Migraine

In February 1999, the U.S. Agency for Health Care Policy and Research (AHCPR, now the Agency for Healthcare Research and Quality) released a series of technical reports that systematically reviewed controlled trials of medical, behavioral, and physical treatments for migraine that were published between 1966 and 1996. The evidence report of most relevance here reviewed randomized, controlled trials and other prospective, comparative clinical trials of behavioral and physical treatments for migraine (Duke University

Center for Clinical Health Policy Research, 1999). Overall, 355 behavioral and physical treatment articles were identified, of which 70 controlled trials of behavioral treatments for migraine were reviewed and 39 trials were included in the evidence report. The behavioral treatments included were relaxation training, biofeedback training, cognitive-behavioral (or stress-management) therapy, hypnosis, and various combinations of these interventions.

Measures of *headache index* (a composite score of headache frequency, severity, and/or duration) and headache frequency were used to calculate an effect-size score, a standardized difference in headache index. A larger effect size reflects a larger improvement. Because fewer than half the available trials provided sufficient information for the calculation of an effect size, this analysis could

have been conducted with an unrepresentative sample of studies. Therefore, the meta-analysis was repeated using average percentage improvement in migraine from pre- to post-treatment rather than effect-size data as the former could be calculated for a larger number of studies (Fig. 26–2).

Effect-size and percent improvement data from the AHCPR evidence report are presented for the four behavioral treatments that were found to be more effective than wait-list control (Fig. 26–2). These four treatments yielded 35% to 55% reduction in migraine activity. Insufficient evidence was available to judge the effectiveness of other psychological interventions, including hypnosis and cephalic vasomotor biofeedback. These findings are consistent with results from earlier, more inclusive meta-analyses (Blanchard amd Andrasik, 1982; Blanchard et

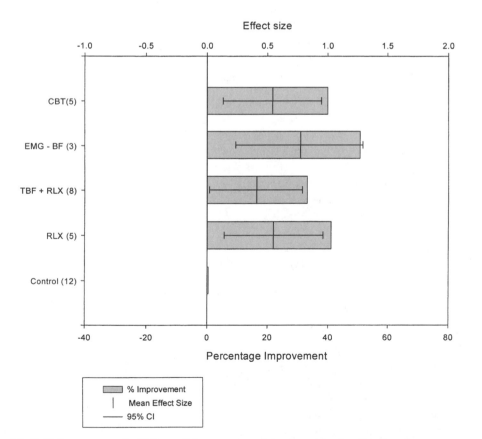

Figure 26–2 Effect size with 95% confidence interval (top axis) and percent reduction in migraine (bottom axis). *CBT*, Cognitive behavior therapy; *EMG-BF*, electromyographic biofeedback training; *TBF + RLX*, thermal biofeedback training plus relaxation training; *RLX*, relaxation training; *Control*, headache monitoring control.

al., 1980; Haddock et al., 1997; Penzien et al., 1985). Drawing on the AHCPR evidence report, the U.S. Headache Consortium on Management of Migraine in Primary Care Settings (American Academy of Family Physicians, American Academy of Neurology, American Headache Society, American College of Emergency Physicians, American College of Physicians, American Osteopathic Association and National Headache Foundation) developed clinical guidelines for the management of migraine, which conclude: "Relaxation training, thermal biofeedback combined with relaxation training, EMG biofeedback, and cognitive-behavioral therapy may be considered as treatment options for the prevention of migraine" (Campbell et al., 2000; Silberstein and Rosenberg, 2000).

Tension-type Headache

Although the AHCPR evidence report on the treatment of tension-type headache has not yet been released, effect-size and percent improvement data from preliminary analyses are presented in Fig. 26–3 for the four behavioral treatments that were more effective than wait-list control and for the best validated preventive drug therapy (D. McCrory, personal communication; McCrory et al., 1996). Each of these four behavioral treatments yielded a 40% to 50% reduction in tension-type headache activity when results were averaged across trials. These findings also are consistent with earlier, more inclusive meta-analyses using different statistical techniques (Blanchard and Andrasik, 1982; Blanchard et al., 1980; Bogaards and ter Kuile, 1994; Haddock et al., 1997; Holroyd and Penzien, 1986) (Fig. 26–3).

Maintenance of Improvements

It is relatively well established that improvements in migraine and tension-type headache achieved with psychological treatments tend to be maintained, at least for the 3- to 9-month follow-up periods that have most frequently been evaluated. For example, improvements reported at such short-term follow-up evaluations have been larger than improvements observed at post-treatment

evaluations in 65 patient samples included in two meta-analytic reviews (Holroyd and Penzien, 1986; Penzien et al., 1985). Long-term (greater than 1 year) follow-up results also have been positive but are less definitive because a significant proportion of patients are typically lost to follow-up over longer periods. However, at least 45% reductions in headache activity have been reported in 14 of 15 studies that used daily headache recordings to assess improvement 1 to 3 years following psychological treatment and in three studies that assessed improvement 5 to 7 years following treatment (Blanchard, 1987, 1992; Gauthier and Carrier, 1991; Holroyd and French, 1995).

In sum, there is considerable empirical evidence that relaxation training, EMG and thermal biofeedback training, and cognitive-behavior therapy yield clinically significant reductions in headache activity. Even in the most conservative of meta-analytic reviews, these treatments average about a 40% improvement in migraine or tension-type headache activity.

CLINICAL ISSUES IN ADMINISTERING BEHAVIORAL TREATMENTS

A number of problems can interfere with the acquisition of self-regulation skills or with the effective use of these skills to manage headaches. Fortunately, most of these problems can be prevented or effectively managed. This section provides basic information about the nuts and bolts of behavioral treatment, emphasizing the prevention of commonly encountered problems and responses to problems that inevitably arise. Additional clinical tips can be found in Arena and Blanchard (1996), Blanchard and Andrasik (1985), Duckro et al. (1995), Holroyd et al. (1988, 1998), Martin (1993), Penzien and Holroyd (1994), and Schwartz (1995).

Treatment Rationale

Patients may view their headaches as outside their control ("Headaches just happen") or as the result of a personal deficiency ("It must

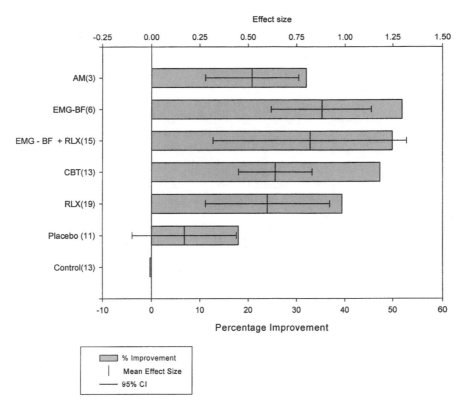

Figure 26–3 Effect size with 95% confidence interval (top axis) and percent reduction in tension-type headache activity (bottom axis). *AM*, amitriptyline HCl; *EMG-BF*, electromyographic biofeedback training; *EMG-BF + RLX*, electromyographic biofeedback training plus relaxation training; *CBT*, cognitive-behavior therapy; *RLX*, relaxation training; *Placebo*, pseudotherapy or false biofeedback training; *Control*, headache monitoring control.

be my fault I have headaches"). Either belief can undermine the patient's motivation to actively manage headache problems and lead to an attitude of helplessness. Conceptualizing headaches within a psychobiological model (Bakal, 1982) that emphasizes the joint influence of environmental, biological, and psychological factors, with no one factor regarded as the sole cause of a headache episode, can help patients appreciate the relevance of psychological/behavioral interventions. With this model, relaxation or biofeedback training is introduced as a method for learning to regulate physiological responses that lead to headaches. Stress-management (cognitive-behavioral) interventions are introduced to manage stresses that induce physiological responses which may trigger, aggravate, or maintain headache episodes.

Homework Assignments

Homework is central to the success of behavioral interventions. Therefore, it is important to emphasize the importance of activities that will occur outside of therapy. One type of homework assignment involves collecting information that will be needed in subsequent treatment sessions. For example, patients may monitor their physical reactions, thoughts, and emotional responses to headache-related stresses. This information is then used to teach the individual how to effectively use headache-management skills. A second type of homework is designed to encourage patients to experiment with using skills learned during relaxation, biofeedback, or stress-management training so that problems encountered in using these skills to manage headaches can be addressed.

Treatment begins with homework assignments that are easy to complete. This often
helps overcome patients' initial resistance to
homework and provides success experiences
that increase patients' self-confidence in their
ability to complete difficult homework assignments later. For example, relaxation skills are
introduced in a graded fashion, beginning
with the detailed tensing and relaxing of 16
or more muscle groups and proceeding in
graduated steps to brief relaxation techniques
that can be used throughout the day. Self-
regulation skills also are practiced in quiet,
headache-free periods before being used to
control physiological responses throughout
the day or to abort an anticipated headache
episode. Audiotapes and treatment manuals
can repeat and extend what is learned in
treatment sessions and present homework
assignments.

Patients frequently encounter problems
that interfere with completion of homework
assignments. Perhaps the most common
problem is lack of time. We suggest working
with the patient to establish priorities and encourage the therapist to approach problems
as normal difficulties that can be overcome.
For example, if a patient reports that inter-
ruptions interfere with the completion of
homework assignments, we suggest problem-
solving with the patient to identify a time that
can be set aside and kept relatively free from
distractions. If a patient frequently forgets to
practice homework tasks, develop environmental and subjective cues to assist the patient in remembering and initiating homework assignments.

Therapist Attitude and Patient Self-efficacy

Patients' confidence in their ability to manage
their headaches can be more important than
their abilities to regulate specific physiological
responses (Blanchard et al., 1993; Holroyd
and Martin, 2000; Holroyd et al., 1984).
Therefore, it is important for the therapist to
attend to the patients' perceptions of their
performance as well as to their actual performance during skill training. Most patients require encouragement. We recommend that

the therapist review the patient's performance with optimism, initially magnifying
small successes and approaching problems as
normal and manageable phases of treatment.

Acquiring Headache Management Skills

Patients may experience a variety of difficulties in acquiring headache-management skills.
The obstacles that therapists most frequently
encounter in relaxation and biofeedback
training arise in three principal areas: (1) the
patients' attitudes and beliefs regarding treatment, (2) environmental events and experiences that interfere with learning skills, and
(3) maintenance or generalization from the
clinic to the home environment. Similar obstacles are commonly encountered in stress-
management training: understanding of the
therapy rationale, monitoring headache-
related stresses, identifying a target problem,
and acquisition and application of stress- and
headache-coping skills. Tables 26–1, 26–2,
and 26–3 outline a number of these commonly encountered problems and offer strategies that may be useful in responding to
them.

REFRACTORY HEADACHE PROBLEMS

This section addresses the use of behavioral
treatments for patients who are likely to be
unresponsive to first-line behavioral and drug
therapies. Information about the efficacy of
behavioral interventions and clinical issues
that arise when using behavioral interventions
with difficult-to-treat headache problems is
discussed.

Excessive Medication Use

Headaches resulting from chronic, excessive
medication use (analgesics, ergotamines, etc.)
are notably refractory to both pharmacological (Kudrow, 1982; Mathew et al., 1990) and
nonpharmacological (Michultka et al., 1989)
therapies. One retrospective review of patient
records (Michultka et al., 1989) found that
less than one-third of "high medication con-

Table 26–1 Relaxation training: problems and solutions

Problems	Solutions
Patient's attitude	
Patient is self-critical or hesitant during training.	Identify self-critical thoughts and help patient to challenge them. Offer reassurance.
Patient is overly concerned about performance.	Suggest that trying hard is counterproductive; instruct in alternative attitude of passive volition.
Patient is hesitant to relinqush control.	Discuss fears about loss of control; explain that the novelty of sensations of relaxation may be triggering anxiety.
Learning the Skill	
Patient falls asleep when practicing relaxation.	Do not schedule relaxation practice just after meals or before bedtime. Practice seated rather than lying down.
Patient's concentration is disturbed by thoughts or feelings.	Use imagery techniques (e.g., placing interfering thoughts in an imaginary trunk or closet) or autogenic phrases (e.g., peaceful, calm) to focus attention. Do not fight thoughts, but let them pass through the mind.
Certain muscles are difficult to relax.	Repeat tensing–relaxing sequence with specific muscles; use muscle-stretching exercises prior to relaxation practice.
Maintenance and generalization	
Patient reports no carry-over effect after relaxation.	Introduce brief cue-controlled relaxation techniques to use periodically throughout the day. Identify thoughts or situations that evoke arousal.
Patient has difficulty detecting difference between sensations of tension and relaxation.	Use partial tensing of muscles (discrimination training) to help patient identify subtle cues of relaxation.

Adapted with permission from Holroyd, K.A., D.D. Penzien, and J.E. Holm (1988). Clinical issues in the treatment of recurrent headache disorders. In *Innovations in Clinical Practice: A Source Book* (P.A. Keller and L.G. Ritt, eds.). Professional Resource Exchange, Sarasota, FL.

sumption" patients achieved clinically significant reductions in headache activity (50% or greater reduction in headache activity) following behavioral treatment, while more than half of patients with the same primary headache diagnosis using lower levels of medication showed this level of improvement. High medication consumption in this study was defined by a score of 40 or greater, the equivalent of approximately six aspirin or three Fiorinal a day, on a commonly used weighted medication index developed by Coyne et al. (1976).

Several clinical series (Baumgartner et al., 1989; Blanchard et al., 1992; Diener et al., 1989; Mathew et al., 1990; Rapoport et al., 1984) have documented the benefits of analgesic and abortive medication withdrawal combined with pharmacological and behavioral therapy. Baumgartner et al. (1989) reported on a 17-month follow-up evaluation that demonstrated that medication withdrawal accompanied by prophylactic pharmacotherapy and relaxation training produced significant reductions in headache activity in 61% of patients who had been us-

ing high levels (35 to 40 doses/week) of medication. Uncontrolled case series suggest that medication withdrawal combined with behavioral therapy or behavior therapy and prophylactic pharmacotherapy can be effective in managing headaches aggravated by high levels of medication use. However, the benefits of behavior therapy or prophylactic medication in facilitating medication withdrawal have not been evaluated in controlled trials.

It is important to help patients understand rebound headaches and to provide clear guidelines for using problem medications. In addition, the behavioral factors that can influence analgesic consumption need to be assessed. For example, some patients take analgesics in anticipation of a headache even though they are unable to accurately predict the headache onset. Often, it is anxiety and fear of a headache rather than a valid signal for the onset of a headache that cues the individual to take medication. For other patients, it is the mood-altering effects of barbiturate- or caffeine-containing medications that reinforce their excessive medication use. Behavioral interventions can be used to

Table 26–2 Biofeedback training: problems and solutions

Problem	Solution
Patient's attitudes and beliefs	
Patient is intimidated by equipment or biofeedback task.	Begin with easy to master responses (e.g., forearm flexor or frontal EMG).
Patient perceives the biofeedback task as an achievement challenge.	Allow patient to practice without therapist. Encourage attitude of playful experimentation.
Learning the skill	
Patient is unable to alter feedback signal or believes changes in signal are unrelated to actions.	Alternate direction of feedback (e.g., increase rather than decrease EMG or temperature). Reduce signal threshold to make task easier. Alter feedback signal. Have patient experiment with a variety of mental strategies (e.g., imagery, focus on sensations, etc.).
The physiological parameter changes in the wrong direction.	Patient may perceive task as a performance challenge. In thermal biofeedback, consider using short training periods (15 minutes or less) because autoregulatory mechanisms may oppose vasodilatation after 15–20 minutes.
Lack of variability in physiological parameter makes learning difficult.	Investigate possible interfering effects of medications (e.g., ergotamine, sumatriptan). Alternate direction of feedback.
Maintenance and generalization	
Patient shows inconsistency in control of physiological response from session to session.	Emphasize home practice. Examine use of medications or other interfering agents (e.g., caffeine, nicotine) prior to session.
Patient has difficulty recognizing subjective cues and continues to rely on feedback signal to indicate control of physiological response.	Gradually fade feedback during training session. Have patient record subjective cues during day to heighten awareness of cues. Rehearse recognizing and controlling physiological response in imagination.
Patient controls response during session but reports being unable to control response in natural environment.	If daily life stress disrupts patient's performance, consider stress management. Encourage patient initially to attempt to control response in "easy" situations with few distractions or pressures.

Adapted with permission from Holroyd, K.A., D.D. Penzien, and J.E. Holm (1988). Clinical issues in the treatment of recurrent headache disorders. In *Innovations in Clinical Practice: A Source Book* (P.A. Keller and L.G. Ritt, eds.). Professional Resource Exchange, Sarasota, FL.

help patients distinguish valid signs of headache onset from anxiety or fear of headaches and to teach skills for managing anxiety. Patients may require a high level of support when they reduce or eliminate analgesic use, especially during the period of increased headache severity that follows.

Chronic Daily Headache

Chronic daily headache is a heterogeneous group of conditions that are associated with near-daily headaches, including those with primarily migrainous features ("chronic migraine" or "transformed migraine") and headaches with primarily tension-type features (e.g., chronic tension-type headache) (see Chapter 12). There is considerable disagreement about how to conceptualize chronic daily headaches. However these headache disorders are conceptualized, there is general

agreement that chronic daily headaches tend to be refractory to standard monotherapy with either drug or nondrug therapies and, thus, create special problems for treatment. Unfortunately, in the absence of agreed-upon diagnostic criteria, trials with this population have not been conducted.

Near-daily headaches (frequent episodes of severe headaches) may respond poorly to relaxation and biofeedback therapies, even when excessive medication use is not an aggravating factor. For example, Blanchard and colleagues (1989) found that patients who recorded near-daily (one or fewer headache-free days during a 4-week baseline), at times intensely painful headaches were less likely to benefit from relaxation or EMG biofeedback than were patients with more episodic headaches (two or more headache-free days a week). While 13% of the former patients showed at least a 50% reduction in headache

Table 26–3 Stress-Management therapy: problems and solutions

Problems	Solutions
Treatment rationale	
Patient does not see behavior as influencing stress responses or headaches.	Use personal examples to illustrate how cognitions influence stress responses. Review rationale using concrete examples.
Monitoring stress and identifying a target problem	
Patient presents a large number of stressful situations.	Be alert to common themes that cut across multiple problems. List problems from largest to smallest. Choose manageable problem as an initial focus. Structure session to maintain focus on selected problem.
Headaches are not clearly stress-related, or patient is unable to identify stress-related thoughts.	Review headache records and analyze situations associated with headache. First, use physical cues and stressful events or times associated with headaches to recognize onset of episode, then identify concrete thoughts present prior to onset. Use events that occur in therapy to identify automatic thoughts occurring in the "here and now."
Headache always present.	Identify factors associated with exacerbation rather than onset of headache. Consider focusing on potential aggravating factors (e.g., chronic stress, depression).
Patient's and therapist's preferred target problems differ.	Openly discuss difference of opinion; defer to patient if preference is strongly held.
Coping skills training and application	
Patient does not attempt, or attempts but "fails" homework assignment.	Examine patient's thoughts about homework assignment for clues to maladaptive thoughts/beliefs. Frame assignment as opportunity to learn. Break assignment into easier tasks.
Patient believes external pressures prevent change (e.g., inflexibility in job situation).	Be alert to thoughts or beliefs that prevent patient from seeing alternatives. Experiment with small change (e.g., muscle stretching during bathroom break). Examine persons who the patient identifies as effective copers for models of feasible change. Brainstorm without requiring that alternatives generated be perceived as feasible.
Maladaptive thoughts seem self-evidently true to patient.	Offer a variety of alternative explanations of same "facts." Reverse roles with patient.
Friction or difficulties in therapeutic alliance.	Openly discuss conflict. Be alert to possibility that difficulty provides information about coping. Admit errors.

Adapted with permission from Holroyd, K.A., D.D. Penzien, and J.E. Holm (1988). Clinical issues in the treatment of recurrent headache disorders. In *Innovations in Clinical Practice: A Source Book* (P.A. Keller and L.G. Ritt, eds.). Professional Resource Exchange, Sarasota, FL.

activity, more than 50% of the latter patients showed this level of improvement. Because only about 10% of the patients with near-daily headaches in this study met criteria for excessive medication use, near-daily headaches for the most part could not be assumed to be a product of medication overuse.

Results from the Treatment of Chronic Tension-type Headache (TCTH) trial described below (see Combining Behavioral and Drug Therapy) suggest that cognitive-behavior therapy yields moderate reductions in chronic tension-type headaches. However, the full benefits of cognitive-behavior therapy were not observed for a number of months in this study, possibly because patients must apply headache management skills for several months before they impact near-daily headaches. Patients in this study with co-morbid migraine headaches (maximum of one migraine day a month) were equally responsive to cognitive-behavior therapy as patients with chronic tension-type headache only. However, patients with chronic daily headaches characterized by frequent severe or migraine-like headaches may be more difficult to treat. Controlled studies of behavioral therapies with chronic daily headache are needed but probably must await agreed-upon diagnostic criteria for distinguishing the different forms of chronic daily headache.

When excessive medication use appears to be aggravating headaches, patients need to reduce medication use as described above. Clinicians commonly assume that patients with chronic daily headache require aggressive multimodal therapy, e.g., conjoint prophylactic medications and multiple behavioral interventions; however, no controlled trials of multimodal treatment are available. Typically, behavioral interventions for near-daily headaches focus on pain management, reduction of pain-related disability, and prevention of mild pain progressing to disabling pain because these patients rarely experience a headache-free period and, thus, rarely have an opportunity to use headache-management skills to prevent headaches. Unremitting pain frequently contributes to sleep disturbances, family problems, psychological distress, and functional impairment, which in turn may serve to maintain or exacerbate headaches. These problems, when present, need to be addressed with the patient. For example, the prolonged presence of a headache may exert a psychological toll on the patient, such that over time the patient feels "sick and tired of being sick and tired." The negative thoughts ("I can't handle this," "My day is ruined," "I'll never get over these headaches") and emotions (anxiety, fear, and depression) elicited by the continual head pain can add to the burden of headaches or become headache triggers themselves. The link between psychological distress and headaches can be addressed with the patient through cognitive therapy. Relaxation training can be employed to assist with sleep problems and to prevent mild headaches from progressing to more intense headaches.

Comorbid Psychiatric Disorders

Epidemiological findings reveal an association between both anxiety and mood disorders and migraine, while clinical studies find similarly elevated rates of anxiety and mood disorders in chronic tension-type headache (Breslau and Davis, 1993; Breslau et al., 1994;

Goncalves and Monteiro, 1993; Guidetti et al., 1998; Holroyd et al., 2000b; Merikangas et al., 1990, 1993; Puca et al., 1999). Of course, psychiatric disorders occur in only a small proportion of recurrent headache sufferers in the general population (Penzien et al., 1993). It is widely believed that patients with comorbid psychiatric disorders are less likely to respond to first-line pharmacological and/or behavioral therapies than are patients without a comorbid diagnosis, although controlled studies evaluating this possibility have not been conducted.

For the patient with a comorbid mood or anxiety disorder, the addition of short-term cognitive-behavioral therapy may be particularly useful. Cognitive-behavioral interventions for depression (Beck et al., 1979; Dobson, 1989; Robinson et al., 1990) fit well with cognitive-behavioral interventions for recurrent headache disorders, so evaluation of a treatment that integrates these interventions for the headache sufferer who is clinically depressed makes sense. Similarly, there are several empirically validated cognitive-behavioral interventions for the treatment of anxiety disorders (Barlow, 1988; Borkovec and Whisman, 1996; Gould et al., 1997) that could easily be adapted to a behavioral headache-management protocol. Adapting existing behavioral treatment protocols to the needs of patients with comorbid psychological disorders may yield positive treatment outcomes for this subpopulation, just as adapting behavioral protocols to the needs of older adults has resulted in significantly improved outcomes for older headache patients. Unfortunately, there are no controlled trials for either behavioral therapy or combined pharmacological and behavioral therapies for the treatment of comorbid psychological and headache disorders. Such studies are needed.

A psychological disorder may complicate treatment in a number of ways. Depression can be a consequence of living with chronic, disabling headaches and may respond as headaches improve. On the other hand, preexisting depression or anxiety may precipitate or exacerbate headache episodes so that neither headaches nor affective distress improves until the comorbid psychopathology is treated. Occasionally, headaches are a manifestation of a primary psychological disorder (e.g., a somatization disorder may be present when headache is one of a long list of presenting physical complaints). In addition, comorbid personality disorders can complicate headache treatment because of the difficult interpersonal style of the patient (e.g., borderline patients may be inappropriately manipulative, histrionic patients may greatly exaggerate physical complaints, passive/dependent patients may excessively rely on health-care providers, narcissistic patients may be demanding).

Combined psychological and pharmacological treatment should be considered for patients who experience comorbid psychological and headache disorders (Holroyd et al., 1998). Brief, focused attention to the specific psychological problems that precipitate or exacerbate headache episodes, interfere with treatment compliance, or interfere with the use of self-regulatory skills is usually sufficient. Biofeedback training may provide a nonthreatening way to introduce the patient to the process of psychological treatment and, thus, to encourage the patient to acknowledge psychological difficulties and accept treatment for psychological disorders.

ALTERNATE TREATMENT FORMATS

A variety of different formats for the delivery of behavioral treatments have been explored, with the goal of reducing treatment cost and increasing availability. Minimal-contact or home-based treatment reduces the number of clinic visits required for behavioral treatment, while group treatment reduces the therapist time per patient that is required at each clinic visit. Preliminary efforts have also been made to use the mass media or the internet to teach behavioral headache-management skills in a self-help treatment format without formal therapist contact.

Limited-Contact and Group Treatment

In a minimal-contact or "home-based" treatment format, headache-management skills are introduced and problems patients encounter in acquiring or using these skills are addressed in a few clinic visits; however, written materials and audiotapes also are used to enable patients to acquire headache-management skills at home that typically would be taught in clinic sessions. As a result, only three or four (monthly) clinic sessions and two or three brief phone calls (where problems that arise in the use of home study materials are addressed) may be required to complete limited-contact behavioral treatment. This contrasts with the 8 to 16 (often weekly) clinic sessions sometimes required for completely therapist-administered, "clinic-based" treatment.

Studies that have directly compared the effectiveness of the same behavioral intervention in therapist-administered and minimal-contact treatment formats have reported that they yield similar outcomes (Haddock et al., 1997; Nash and Holroyd, 1992; Rowan and Andrasik, 1996). A meta-analytic review of results from 13 studies found no clear differences in dropout rate, reduction in headache activity, or proportion of patients showing clinically significant improvements with home-based and clinic-based treatments for adults (Haddock et al., 1997).

For many adults, a limited-contact treatment format provides a cost-effective method of providing behavioral treatment. Some proportion of patients will, of course, continue to require more therapist-intensive treatment. Individuals who excessively use analgesic medication, who are clinically depressed, or who suffer from near-daily headache problems may require more intensive treatment. Other patients simply do not persist in efforts to learn or apply self-regulation skills without regular contact with a health professional.

Behavioral treatments are often administered in small groups (rather than individually), and this is as true for the treatment of recurrent headache disorders as for other problems. Although the effectiveness of the same behavioral intervention administered individually and in a group has not been directly compared in the treatment of recurrent headache disorders, there is no indication that these two treatment formats differ in effectiveness. A recent meta-analysis of ten studies where behavioral treatments were administered in a group treatment format reported a 53% reduction in headache activity (Penzien et al., 1992), a level of improvement similar to that reported when the same behavioral interventions are individually administered. Where patient flow is adequate, group rather than individual administration of treatment allows the cost of treatment to be reduced and health professionals' time to be efficiently used.

Self-Help Treatment

Behavioral treatments could be made available to a wider range of individuals, including the significant number of individuals who do not currently seek medical treatment, if patients were able to learn behavioral headache-management skills at home without the face-to-face assistance of a health professional. The availability of behavioral treatment in a self-help treatment format also would facilitate the incorporation of behavioral interventions into public health efforts to manage headaches. However, efforts to eliminate therapist contact and create a completely self-help treatment format have been rare and suffered from extremely high dropout rates (Kohlenberg, 1981). The primary problem may be that self-help treatments lack mechanisms to provide corrective feedback when users encounter problems in learning or to maintain the motivation of the user during the months that may be required to learn to effectively use headache-management skills.

A novel public health effort in the Netherlands attempted to remedy the limitations of self-help treatment by providing accompanying instruction via television and radio: television programs were used to demonstrate headache-management skills and radio programs to help participants solve the problems encountered in applying these skills (de Bruin-Kofman et al., 1997). Relaxation, cognitive, and pain-management skills were covered in home-study materials (a workbook and three audio cassettes) that were purchased by approximately 15,000 viewers; each of these headache-management skills was

then demonstrated in the course of ten TV programs. In addition, ten radio programs spaced throughout the training period provided the opportunity for participants to submit questions and listen to discussions of representative problems encountered by participants. Unfortunately, methodological limitations of the program-evaluation component of this study, including the assessment of outcome in only a subsample (n = 271) of participants, limit the conclusions that can be drawn about the effectiveness of this pioneering self-help program. However, the 164 participants who completed the evaluation did record a 50% average reduction in headache frequency, as well as a reduction of about 4.5 days of lost work time over the previous 4 months. This study at least raises the possibility that the mass media can be used to improve the results obtained with self-help materials and offers one model for a population-based public health intervention.

Diagnosis, evaluation, and delivery of treatment materials were all conducted over the internet in a recent study of applied relaxation therapy (Strom et al., 2000). Unfortunately, over half of the individuals enrolled dropped out, leaving 45 participants who completed either applied relaxation training or assessment-only control conditions. Moreover, patients who completed the applied relaxation condition showed only modest reductions in headache activity (33% reduction in headache index) and differed from controls only on a subset of outcome measures. These results are similar to those obtained with self-help workbooks alone, possibly because applied relaxation training in this study consisted primarily of workbook material sent via e-mail. Additional studies that make greater use of the capacity of the internet to individualize treatment and to provide social support and assistance (e.g., via chat groups) thus appear warranted. Legal and liability issues also need to be resolved before investigators in the United States are likely to offer diagnostic and treatment procedures to the general population. However, for patients who are already receiving treatment at a "bricks-and-mortar" clinic, the internet initially might be used to make available additional educational and behavioral interventions, as well as to monitor and collect outcome data.

The effectiveness of limited-contact treatment formats for administering behavioral interventions is relatively well established. In contrast, the effectiveness of self-help behavior therapy has yet to be established. Because little is known about the individuals who can benefit from self-help interventions, there is a risk that ineffective self-help treatments will lead some users to delay seeking more effective or urgently needed treatment. On the other hand, the availability of even modestly effective self-help materials would allow behavioral interventions to be more easily incorporated into the diverse treatment settings where headache disorders are treated, as well as into public health efforts to reduce the disability associated with recurrent headache disorders.

THERAPEUTIC MECHANISMS

Tension-type Headache

Efforts to understand how psychological treatments produce reductions in tension headache activity have focused primarily on EMG biofeedback training. The initial development of EMG biofeedback training was guided by the assumption that feedback of pericranial muscle activity enables the individual to acquire control of muscle activity associated with tension-type headaches and, thereby, to reduce tension type headaches (Fig. 26–4a). Unfortunately, studies that have examined relationships between the self-regulation of pericranial EMG activity and improvement following EMG biofeedback training have provided little support for this model (Andrasik and Holroyd, 1980; Holroyd et al., 1984; Martin and Mathews, 1978; Rokicki et al., 1997). Especially problematic is the finding that, at least under some conditions, feedback for increasing or for maintaining constant pericranial muscle activity can be as effective at controlling tension type headaches as feedback for reducing pericranial muscle activity (Andrasik and Holroyd, 1980; Holroyd et al., 1984).

The second model postulates that reductions in tension type headache activity are consequences of cognitive and behavioral changes induced by biofeedback training (Fig. 26–4b). Studies finding that changes in self-efficacy, and not EMG changes induced by biofeedback training, predict improvement following training (Holroyd et al., 1984; Rokicki et al., 1997) provide some initial support for this model. Improvements in tension-type headache activity following biofeedback training have also been hypothesized to result because biofeedback training remedies deficits in central pain modulation that underlie chronic tension-type headache (Fig. 26–4b'). However, initial attempts to test this possibility by examining the effects of EMG biofeedback training on electrophysiological measures thought to index the integrity of relevant supraspinal pain-modulation systems have yielded conflicting results (Rokicki et al., 1997; Schoenen, 1989). Unfortunately, our ability to assess, or even to identify, relevant supraspinal pain-modulation systems involved in tension-type headache is limited (Bendtsen et al., 1996; Lipchik, et al., 1996, 1997, 2000). Negative findings may thus reflect our inability to accurately identify or assess the operation of relevant supraspinal pain-modulation systems rather than the failure of biofeedback training to affect these mechanisms.

Recent work on the pathophysiology of tension-type headache appears to implicate the sensitization of trigeminal pain transmission pathways, at least in chronic tension-type headache (Bendtsen et al., 1997). Although direct measures of this trigeminal sensitization are not available, future studies of change mechanisms in EMG biofeedback training might examine the effects of biofeedback training on measures of pericranial muscle tenderness, pain threshold, and pain tolerance that are likely to be indirectly influenced by trigeminal sensitization (Ashina et al., 1999).

Migraine

Efforts to examine how behavioral treatments produce improvements in migraine have fo-

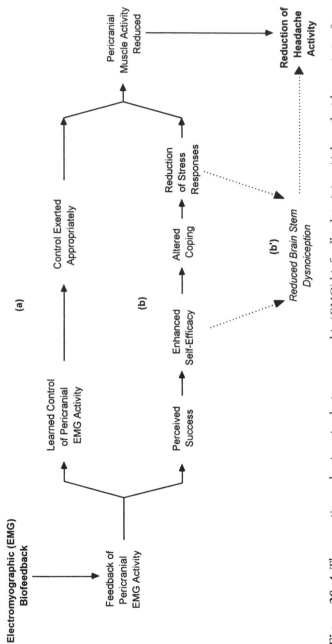

Figure 26–4 Therapeutic mechanisms in electromyographic (*EMG*) biofeedback training. (Adapted with permission from Holroyd, K.A., D.B. Penzien, K.G. Hursey et al. (1984). Change mechanisms in EMG biofeedback training: Cognitive changes underlying improvements in tension headache. *J. Consult. Clin. Psychol.* 52:1039–1053.)

cused primarily on thermal (hand-warming) biofeedback training. Several studies have found that biofeedback training for either hand warming or hand cooling is associated with improvements in migraine (Blanchard et al., 1997; Gauthier et al., 1981; Kewman and Roberts, 1980; Largen et al., 1981), calling into question the role of hand warming as a therapeutic mechanism. However, efforts to test the hypothesis that the improvements in migraine observed with thermal biofeedback training are mediated by the same changes in self-efficacy that have been implicated as therapeutic mechanisms in EMG biofeedback training (Holroyd et al., 1984) have failed to support this hypothesis (Blanchard et al., 1994; French et al., 1997). Although changes in cerebral blood flow associated with volitional hand warming have long been hypothesized to underlie the effectiveness of thermal biofeedback training, efforts to examine cerebrovascular change mechanisms during biofeedback training using radioactive xenon-inhalation techniques or transcranial Doppler assessments of cerebral blood flow velocity have yielded no clear findings (Mathew et al., 1980; McGrady et al., 1994; Wauquier et al., 1995).

Olness and colleagues (1999) examined the intriguing hypothesis that relaxation training improves migraines by preventing stress-induced mast cell activation. Mast cell activation is of interest because it releases vasoactive and nociceptive substances (e.g., nitric oxide, histamine, serotonin) that may play a role in activating the trigeminovascular system. Olness et al. (1999) reported that young migraine sufferers (ages 5 to 12 years) who benefited from three relaxation training sessions (≤ 1 migraine month following treatment) showed greater reductions in an index of mast cell activation (assessed via urinary tryptase levels) than untreated controls. Although the authors reported no statistical analyses, our analysis of the authors' data indicates that urinary tryptase levels decreased more frequently (9 of 10) in relaxation responders than in untreated controls (4 of 14; $p < 0.05$) at the 24-week evaluation, but this difference was not significant at the 12-week evaluation. Although the small number of

subjects and the large intersubject variability in urinary tryptase levels render this finding preliminary, this hypothesis deserves further attention.

Efforts to understand change mechanisms in the behavioral treatment of migraine have yielded few clear results. No study has convincingly demonstrated that hand warming is a necessary component of thermal biofeedback training, though this possibility has not been excluded either. Efforts to identify cognitive change mechanisms in thermal biofeedback training also have been inconclusive. It may be that the focus on craniovascular mechanisms has been misguided. Studies reporting that psychophysiological measures of neuronal excitability, such as contingent negative variation, are normalized with successful (drug) therapy (Schoenen et al., 1986) and that the products of neuronal activation are altered by relaxation training (Olness et al., 1999) may provide a more promising model for future research.

BEHAVIOR THERAPY, HORMONES, AND HEADACHES

There has been a tendency to assume that headaches associated with hormonal changes or aggravated by hormonal preparations are less responsive than other headaches to either behavioral therapy or drug therapy (Holroyd and Lipchik, 2000).

Menstruation-Related Migraine

Only a few studies have evaluated the effectiveness of behavioral treatments specifically for menstrual migraine, and these studies have yielded conflicting results (Table 26–4). Three studies have examined the effects of relaxation/biofeedback therapy specifically on menstrual migraine, with two studies (Gauthier et al., 1991; Szekely et al., 1986) reporting positive results and one (study 2 in Kim and Blanchard, 1992) reporting negative results. Two additional studies have examined the effectiveness of relaxation/biofeedback therapies on overall headache activity in women who experienced menstrual mi-

Table 26–4 Response of menstrual migraines to behavioral treatment

Authors	Definition of MM[a]	Results	Comments
Gauthier et al. (1991) (n = 39)	−3 to +3 days from start of menstruation	MM = NMM 49% of patients have >50% reduction in MM	Not clear subjects on oral contraceptives were excluded
Kim and Blanchard (1992) (study 1 n = 98)	Self-identification	MM = NMM 42% of MM patients have >50% reduction in headaches	MM and NMM not distinguished in diary recordings
Kim and Blanchard (1992) (study 2 n = 15)	Self-identification and verification by diary	MM = NMM 27% of patients have >50% reduction in MM	Reductions in neither MM nor NMN significant
Szekeley et al. (1986) (n = 8)	−7 to +7 days from start of menstruation	MM = NMM 50% of patients have >50% reduction in MM	Cluster and tension headache included; improvements not significant
Solbach et al. (1984) (n = 136)	−3 to +3 days from start of menstruation	Direct comparison not reported,[b] approx. 13% reduction in headaches in MM sufferers[c]	MM and NMM not distinguished in diary recordings

[a]MM, menstrual migraine; NMM = non-menstrual migraine.

[b]Indirect comparison suggested MM < NMM.

[c]Reduction in frequency from pretreatment to final 12-week block.

graines, with one reporting positive results (study 1 in Kim and Blanchard, 1992) and one negative results (Solbach et al., 1984). The inability to unambiguously identify menstrually related migraine, and thus the use of slightly different definitions of menstrual migraine in different studies, makes it difficult to compare results across studies.

One study nonetheless provides reasonable evidence that menstrually related migraines need not be refractory to behavioral therapy. Gauthier and colleagues (1991) compared improvements in headaches associated with menstruation (occurring within 3 days of the beginning of a menstrual period) and in headaches occurring at other times in women who received either thermal or cephalic vasomotor biofeedback training. Similar improvements were observed in menstrual and nonmenstrual headaches, with about half of women showing clinically significant (≥50%) improvement in each type of headache. Improvements in menstrual and nonmenstrual headaches also were equally likely to be maintained at a 6-month follow-up.

Pregnancy

Behavioral interventions are attractive for managing headaches during pregnancy be-

cause, unlike drugs, behavioral interventions would not be expected to pose risks to the developing baby. Moreover, behavioral interventions may reduce the nausea and vomiting that are sometimes associated with pregnancy. However, migraines may remit during the second or third trimester, making it difficult to evaluate the effectiveness of headache therapies during pregnancy. Uncontrolled studies thus provide limited information about the effectiveness of therapy during pregnancy.

Marcus et al. (1995) suggested that behavior therapy may prove to be a promising treatment during pregnancy. In this study, 31 pregnant women were randomized to either a 2-month (eight-session) treatment that included education, relaxation/thermal biofeedback training, and physical therapy exercises or to a pseudotherapy control treatment that included much of the same educational material plus biofeedback training to decrease (rather than increase) finger temperature. For most women, the treatment program was initiated during the second trimester (18th week of pregnancy on average) and, thus, completed before delivery. Women who received the active treatment showed substantially larger reductions in headache activity (81% vs. 33% reduction) and were more likely to show clinically significant improvements (73% vs. 29%) following treatment than women in the control condition. Moreover, improvements were maintained throughout the perinatal period and at 3- and 6-month follow-up evaluations (Scharff et al., 1996). These initial findings should encourage greater experimentation with the use of behavioral intervention to manage headaches during pregnancy.

COMBINING BEHAVIORAL AND DRUG THERAPY

Migraine

The comparative effectiveness and combined effects of behavioral and drug therapies have rarely been directly assessed (Holroyd, 1993). Consequently, the effectiveness of these two treatment modalities can best be examined via a meta-analysis of the separate drug therapy and behavior therapy literatures. In a meta-analysis of these two literatures, Holroyd et al. (1991b) found that virtually identical improvements in migraine have been reported with propranolol HCl (25 clinical trials) and relaxation/thermal biofeedback training (35 clinical trials): each yielded a 55% reduction in migraine activity in the typical patient, while the average patient treated with pill placebo showed only a 12% reduction in migraine activity. Less information is available concerning the effectiveness of prophylactic agents other than propranolol; however, in direct comparisons, other agents have generally proven to be no more effective than propranolol in the average patient (Holroyd et al., 1991b). Prophylactic drug and behavioral therapies may thus be equally viable for uncomplicated migraine.

Two of three studies that have evaluated the combination of propranolol and relaxation/thermal biofeedback training found this combination treatment to be highly effective at managing recurrent migraines, yielding more than a 70% headache reduction on average (Holroyd et al., 1992; Mathew, 1981). In fact, combined therapy proved to be significantly more effective than relaxation/bio-

feedback training alone in both studies, but in the Mathew (1981) study the combined treatment was no more effective than propranolol alone. Additional clinical trials are needed to provide information about the distinct benefits of psychological and preventive drug therapies for both moderate- and high-severity migraine (Holroyd, in press). For example, for frequent disabling (high-severity) migraines, a trial might ask if preventive drug therapy, psychological treatment or combined therapy best add to benefits achieved with new abortive (triptan) therapies. For less frequent and disabling (moderate-severity) migraine, a trial might ask if drug therapy or brief home-based psychological treatment is more cost-effective in the long-term management of migraines.

In developing an algorithm for combining preventive drug and behavioral therapies in clinical practice, we have argued that if migraines are frequent or severe or psychological problems complicate treatment, conjoint behavior and drug therapy should be considered (Holroyd et al., 1998). If migraines are less frequent and not complicated by psychological problems, behavioral and drug therapies may be equally viable for many patients. In the latter case, patient preference, treatment costs, and the presence of medication contraindications (e.g., possibility of pregnancy, breast-feeding) might influence the choice of treatment modality. Larger-scale studies examining the separate and combined effects of behavioral and prophylactic drug therapies, particularly in patients also using triptan therapies, are needed.

Tension-type Headache

The comparative effectiveness of preventive drug and behavioral therapies in the management of tension-type headache has been examined in four studies: two studies of EMG biofeedback training and two studies of cognitive-behavior therapy. In the first study (Bruhn et al., 1979), chronic tension-type headache sufferers (n = 28) were randomized to 16 EMG biofeedback training sessions or to an individualized medical management program that included drug therapy (antide-

pressant medication, analgesics, muscle relaxants, sedatives), physical therapy, or combined drug/physical therapy depending on
the clinician's assessment of the patient's
needs. Biofeedback training, but not medical
management, yielded significant reductions in
headache activity, with 54% of patients in the
biofeedback-training group but only 10% of
patients in the medical-management group
showing at least a 50% reduction in headache activity. Improvements with biofeedback
training also were maintained at a 6-month
follow-up. The authors suggest that in this severely disabled population "Drug therapy and
physical therapy reinforce a tendency to dependent behavior . . . but biofeedback edu-
cates the patient to control his own well
being."

A second study (Reich and Gottesman,
1993) (n = 50) examined the benefits of
adding amitriptyline (dose adjustment to 75
mg/day) to EMG biofeedback training from
multiple muscle sites (suboccipital, cervical,
trapezius, sterncleidomastoid, and masseter)
over 30 training sessions. Diagnoses are not
reported, but patients appear to have had frequent and, in many cases, chronic tension-
type headaches. Amitriptyline initially enhanced the effectiveness of biofeedback
training; however, beginning at month 8 and
continuing through the 24-month observation
period, the combined treatment showed no
advantage over biofeedback training alone. In
fact, at the 20- and 24-month observation
periods, patients who received biofeedback
training alone recorded significantly fewer
hours of headache activity than patients who
received combined amitriptyline/biofeedback
training. The relatively poor results obtained
with combined treatment at these two follow-
up assessments probably reflects the fact that
patients were weaned from amitriptyline at
month 16.

The recently completed TCTH trial (Holroyd et al., 2000a) extends findings from an
earlier study that found brief cognitive-
behavior therapy at least as effective as amitriptyline at reducing frequent tension-type
headache activity (Holroyd et al., 1991a). The
TCTH trial evaluated the separate and combined effects of cognitive-behavior therapy

(three-session minimal-contact treatment format) and tricyclic antidepressant medication
(amitriptyline to 100 mg/day or, if not tolerated, nortriptyline to 75 mg/day) in 203
patients with chronic (mean 26 headache
days/month) tension-type headache. Both
antidepressant medication and cognitive-
behavior therapy reduced headache activity, analgesic medication consumption, and
headache-related disability at the 6-month
evaluation, with improvements in headache
activity and analgesic medication use occurring more rapidly with antidepressant medication than with cognitive-behavior therapy
(Fig. 26–5). However, patients who received
the combined treatment were significantly
more likely (64% of patients) than patients
who received antidepressant medication
(38% of patients) or cognitive-behavior therapy (35% of patients) alone to show clinically
significant (≥50%) reductions in headache
activity. This suggests that antidepressant
medication and brief cognitive-behavior therapy are each capable of producing moderate
improvements in near-daily tension-type
headache activity, although antidepressant
medication may produce more rapid improvements. Combining these two treatments
may increase the probability that patients will
show clinically significant reductions in headache activity.

SPECIAL POPULATIONS

Children and Adolescents

Migraine

Headaches occur in close to 70% of children,
with epidemiological surveys suggesting that
1% to 3% of 7-year-olds and 4% to 11% of
7- to 11-year-olds suffer from migraine (Lipton and Stewart, 1997; Sillanpaa, 1983). The
female-to-male sex ratio increases from about
age 12 to age 42 and probably approaches
2:1 by late adolescence. In a seminal 40-year
follow-up of children 7 to 15 years of age who
experienced at least one disabling migraine a
month, Bille (1997) found that over half of
the children continued to experience mi-

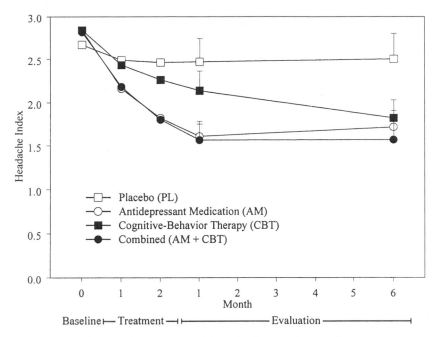

Figure 26–5 Mean headache index scores with standard error for the four treatment groups. Headache index is calculated as a mean of four daily (0–10 scale) pain ratings. One month baseline, two month treatment/dose adjustment period and 6-month evaluation period.

graines as adults. About half also had children with headache problems that appeared to be migraines. Successful control of headaches in children and adolescents may thus have the potential to prevent the development of chronic headache problems in adulthood.

Information about the effectiveness of behavioral interventions with children and adolescents is more limited than for adults. Nonetheless, published studies raise the possibility that behavioral treatments are even more effective with children and adolescents than they are with adults. Summarizing results from five early studies where thermal biofeedback training was administered in conjunction with relaxation (autogenic) training, Blanchard (1992) concluded that about 70% of children showed clinically significant improvements (50% or greater reduction in migraine activity) with this treatment, better results than are typically found with adults. Table 26–5 summarizes results from more recent studies, where it can be seen that empirical support continues to accumulate for the effectiveness of relaxation training, thermal biofeedback training, and cognitive-

behavior therapy. Hermann et al. (1995a) also have summarized much of this literature in a meta-analytic review. Positive results have been reported with home- and school-based interventions as well as phone-based self-administered behavioral treatment. Data are too limited to determine if the addition of a parent intervention to patient-focused behavioral treatment improves treatment outcomes. Also, the lack of pseudotherapy or placebo-controlled studies is a limitation of this literature because it is likely that children are more responsive than adults to placebo.

The comparative effectiveness of preventive drug and behavioral therapies in the management of migraine in children and adolescents has been addressed in only two studies. In the first study (Olness et al., 1987), combined relaxation and self-hypnosis training (five treatment sessions) yielded significantly better results than propranolol (3 mg/kg daily) in 33 children between the ages of 6 and 12 years with migraine with aura. In fact, while combined relaxation/self-hypnosis produced better results than placebo, results achieved with propranolol and placebo did

Table 26-5 Pediatric treatment studies

Clinic and home-based studies

Study	Helm-Hylkema et al. (1990)	Allen and McKeen (1991)	McGrath et al. (1992)	Labbe (1995)	Hermann et al. (1997)	Allen and Shriver (1998)	Mehta (1992)
Sample size	20	15	87	30	32	27	18
Age range (years)	10–19	7–12	11–18	7–18	8–16	7–18	N/A
Mean age (years)	N/A	N/A	N/A	12	11.8 ± 2.1	N/A	10.7
Sex ratio (M/F)	4/16	N/R	24/63	17/13	19/13	11/16	11/7
HA type	Migraine	Migraine	Migraine	Migraine	Migraine	Migraine	Recurrent HA
Type of study	Comparative group outcome	Multiple baseline	Controlled group outcome	Controlled group outcome	Single group outcome	Comparative group outcome	Single group outcome
Treatment condition	1. CBT/RLX + TBF winter (8 sessions) 2. CBT/RLX + TBF summer (8 sessions)	TBF (home-based) + PI (3, 6, 9 weeks baseline)	1. CBT/RLX self-administered (8 weeks) 2. CBT/RLX clinic (8 weeks) 3. UC	1. TBF + RLX (10 sessions, 7 weeks) 2. RLX (10 sessions, 7 weeks) 3. WLC	TBF (home-based) 4 sessions, 8 weeks	1. TBF 2. TBF + pain behavior management	RLX, Cog, PI (10–14 sessions)
Outcome measure Result (% improvement at end of TX)	HA diary 1. 56.4% 2. 13.7% HA frequency	HA diary 47% HA index	HA diary 1. 50.3% 2. 47.8% 3. 5.8% HA index 1 = 2 > 3	HA diary 1. 83.3% 2. 81.1% 3. 24.4% HA index 1 = 2	HA diary 59.6% HA index	HA diary 1. 21.4% 2. 63.4% HA frequency 1 < 2	HA diary 86.9% HA frequency
% Sample improved	NS ($p < 0.08$) N/A	87% (13/15)	1. 66.7% (16/24) 2. 43.5% (10/23) 3. 24% (6/25)	1. 100% (10/10) 2. 90% (9/10) 3. 60% (6/10)	68.8% (22/32)	1. 46.2% (6/13) 2. 71.4% (10/14)	33% (6/18)
% Improved	N/A	≥70%	50%	≥50%	≥50%	≥50%	50%–80%
Follow-up (months)	9–12	8	12	6	N/A	12	3
% Change (end of TX to FU)	N/A	Maintained Improvement	1. 36.1% 2. 19.3% 3. N/A	1. 90.9% 2. 71.4% 3. 9.7%	N/A	1. 51.5% 2. 40%	38%

Study	Bussone et al. (1998)	Grazzi et al. (1990)	Womack et al. (1988)	Barry and Baeyer (1997)	Griffiths and Martin (1996)	Kroner-Herwig et al. (1998)	Sartory et al. (1998)
Sample size	30	10	119	29	42	50	30
Age range (years)	11–15	12–15	4–20	7–12	10–12	8–14	8–16
Mean age (years)	N/A	N/A	12.5 ± 3.3	9	11	11	11.3
Sex ratio (M/F)	15/15	5/5	60/59	10/19	21/21	20/30	17/13
HA type	Tension	Tension	Tension or migraine	Tension or migraine	Tension or migraine	Tension or tension + migraine	Migraine or tension + migraine
Type of study	Comparative group outcome	Single group outcome	Single group outcome	Controlled group outcome	Controlled group outcome	Controlled group outcome	Comparative group outcome
Treatment condition	1. EMG-BF/RLX (10 sessions, 5 weeks) 2. Self-RLX (10 sessions, 5 weeks)	EMG-BF (12 sessions, 6 weeks)	EMG-BF and/or TBF + RLX (8 weekly sessions)	1. CBT/RLX + PI (2 sessions, 2 weeks) 2. UC	1. CBT/RLX clinic (8 sessions) 2. CBT/RLX home-based (3 sessions) 3. WLC	1. RLX + PI 2. RLX 3. EMG-BF + PI 4. EMG-BF 5. UC	1. RLX + CBT (10 sessions) 2. Cephalic vasomotor feedback + CBT (10 sessions)
Outcome measure	HA diary	HA diary	HA diary	HA diary	HA diary	HA diary	HA diary
Result (% improvement at end of TX)	1. 54.2% 2. 56.5% HA index	88.6% HA index	N/A	1. 6.8% 2. 41.8% HA freq.	1. 87% 2. 65.4% 3. 13.3% HA index	1. 46.5% 2. 16.6% 3. 45.5% 4. 71.8% 5. 24.1% HA frequency (1+2+3+4/4 > 5)	1. 33% 2. 42% HA frequency
% Sample improved	1 = 2 N/A	90% (9/10)	44.5% (53/119)	1 < 2 1. 16.7% (2/12) 2. 11.8% (2/17)	1 = 2 > 3 1. 80% (12/15) 2. 62% (9/15) 3. 25% (3/12)	1. 70% (7/10) 2. 40% (4/10) 3. 60% (6/10) 4. 80% (8/10) 5. 40% (4/10)	1 = 2 1. 80% (12/15) 2. 53.3% (8/15)
% Improved	N/A	≥50%	≥50%	≥50%	≥50%	≥50%	≥50%
Follow-up	12 months	12 months	≥6 months	N/A	9 weeks	6 months	8 months
% Change (end of TX to FU)	1. 86% 2. 60%	61.8%	N/A	N/A	1. 66.7% 2. 44.4% 3. N/A	1. 0% 2. 42.9% 3. 41.7% 4. 81.8% 5. N/A	1. -39% 2. -31%

(Table continued on following page)

Table 26–5 Pediatric treatment studies (*Continued*)

School-based treatment studies

Study	Osterhaus et al. (1993)	Larsson and Carlsson (1996)	Larsson, et al. (1990)	Larsson and Melin (1986)
Sample size	41	26	48	31
Age range (years)	12–19	10–15	16–18	16–18
Mean age (yars)	14.8	N/A	N/A	N/A
Sex ratio (M/F)	10/31	1/25	5/43	1/30
HA type	Migraine	Tension	Tension or tension + migraine	Tension or tension + migraine
Type of study	Controlled group outcome	Controlled group outcome	Controlled group outcome	Controlled group outcome
Treatment condition	1. CBT/RLX + TBF (8 sessions) 2. WLC	1. RLX (10 sessions, 5 weeks) 2. UC	1. Self-RLX (5 weeks) 2. WLC	1. RLX (9 sessions, 5 weeks) 2. INF[a] (9 sessions, 5 weeks) 3. UC
Outcome measure	HA diary	HA diary	HA diary	HA diary
Result (% improvement at end of TX)	1. 44.1% 2. 3.4% HA index	1. 34% 2. 15% HA frequency	1. 16.3% 2. −2.0% HA index	1. 40% 2. 10% 3. −6% HA frequency
% Sample improved	1 > 2 1. 45% (14/32) 2. 11% (1/9)	1 > 2 1. 69% (9/13) 2. 8% (1/13)	NS (p = 0.08) 1. 19.4% (6/31) 2. 0% (0/17)	1 > 3 1. 81.8% (9/11) 2. 7.7% (1/13) 3. 0% (0/7)
% Improved	≥50%	≥50%	≥50%	≥50%
Follow-up (months)	7	6	N/A	6
% Change (end of TX to FU)	1. 17.9% 2. N/A	1. 6.5% 2. −19.6%	N/A	1. 33.3% 2. 6.7% 3. 88%

CBT, cognitive behavioral therapy; RLX, relaxation therapy; TBF, thermal biofeedback; PI, parent involvement; UC, unrelated control group; WLC, wait listed control group; EMG-BF, electromyographic biofeedback; Self-RLX, self-relaxation without instruction or assistance; INF, information contact group; TX, treatment; FU, follow-up

This table, when combined with the similar table summarizing early studies in Blanchard (1992), provides a reasonable summary of studies evaluating behavioral treatments for headache in children and adolescents.

not differ. Similar findings were reported by Satory et al. (1998), who compared the efficacy of metoprolol (50 or 100 mg/day depending on body weight) and two behavioral treatments in 43 children with migraine aged 8 to 16 years. Behavioral treatments combined stress management with either relaxation training or cephalic vasomotor biofeedback and were administered in ten sessions over 6 weeks. Combined relaxation/stress-management training yielded the best outcomes, producing clinically significant (>50%) reductions in 80% of patients, while metoprolol yielded the poorest results, yielding clinically significant improvement in only 42% of patients.

Evidence for the effectiveness of behavior therapy appears to be stronger than for drug therapy for migraine (Forsythe et al., 1984; Olness et al., 1987). Larger studies of behavioral therapies in primary-care or pediatric settings are needed, including studies that evaluate nurse- or paraprofessional-administered home-based and self-administered treatments that could be practically integrated into busy medical practice settings. Ideally, such studies would include a pseudotherapy or placebo control and a usual care or drug therapy comparison group, as well as provide information about the relative effectiveness of treatments in pre- and post-pubertal females.

Tension-type Headache

Good data on the prevalence of tension-type headache in children are lacking, although Bille (1962) found that approximately 15% of children and adolescents aged 7 to 15 experienced nonmigrainous headaches by age 15, the large proportion of which were probably tension-type headaches.

Although behavioral interventions have rarely been evaluated in young children with tension-type headache, there are some encouraging data with adolescents. For example, in a reanalysis of data from three early studies, Larsson and Melin (1988) concluded that therapist-administered relaxation training produced larger improvements (63% reduction in headache activity) in adolescents (aged 16 to 18) with episodic tension-type headaches than a pseudotherapy control treatment. Recent studies are summarized in Table 26–5, where it can be seen that EMG biofeedback training has yielded quite positive results with tension-type headache (Bussone et al., 1998; Grazzi et al., 1990). School-based, nurse-administered relaxation training (Larsson and Carlsson, 1996), but not self-administered relaxation training (Larsson et al., 1990), also has shown promise.

More information is needed about the effectiveness of behavioral interventions for both episodic and chronic tension-type headache and about the relative effectiveness of drug and behavioral interventions with tension-type headache.

Older Adults

The prevalence of headaches tends to decrease with age (Lipton et al., 1994). Nonetheless, it has been estimated that recurrent headaches are a significant problem for approximately 17% of individuals over the age of 65 (Cook et al., 1989). Pharmacological treatment of headaches in the older adult can be problematic because of side effects and the likelihood that patients are already using multiple medications for other problems. Thus, behavioral interventions are attractive for older adults.

For behavioral intervention to be effective with older adults, the standard procedures for administering them must be modified. Retrospective analyses of clinical outcomes with behavioral therapy (Blanchard et al., 1985a,b; Diamond and Montrose, 1984) and a meta-analytic review of results from 37 studies evaluating behavioral treatments (Holroyd and Penzien, 1986) suggested that adults over 50 years of age with tension-type headaches were likely to be unresponsive to behavioral interventions. Fortunately, subsequent prospective studies where treatment procedures were tailored for older adults have reported positive results, particularly with combined cognitive-behavior therapy and relaxation training (e.g., Arena et al., 1991; Mosley et al., 1995; Nicholson and Blanchard, 1993). These findings suggest that relatively straightforward adjustments in treatment procedures effectively eliminate the adverse effect of age on treatment outcome that was observed in earlier studies.

Mosley et al. (1995) found cognitive-behavior therapy plus relaxation training to be more effective than relaxation training alone in patients from 60 to 78 years of age (mean 68 years), illustrating these latter findings. Sixty-four percent of patients (from 60 to 78 years old) who received 12 sessions of cognitive-behavior therapy achieved clinically significant improvements ($\geq$50% reduction in headache activity) in tension-type headache activity. To facilitate learning of headache-management skills, supplementary audiotapes and written materials designed to assist patients in practicing and learning skills were provided, and weekly phone contacts following each session were used to answer questions and identify problems. Detailed verbal and written explanations of treatment procedures, frequent reviews of the material covered, and additional time to practice elementary skills before more advanced skills were introduced also were provided.

MEASURING HEADACHE IMPACT

It is widely recognized that pain measures provide only limited information about the impact that a pain disorder has on a person's life. Attention has thus been devoted to the development of measures to capture the psychosocial impact of recurrent headache disorders (Dahlof, 1993; Holroyd et al., 1999; Solomon, 1997). Characteristics of measures that have been used in recent studies are summarized in Table 26–6. These measures vary in their specificity (for migraine, for headache in general, or for medical conditions in general), in the dimensions they assess (primarily disability but other impact dimensions as well), in the time frame they address (a single migraine episode or a month or longer period of time), and in the availability of supportive psychometric data. Increasing attention is likely to be paid to the ability of treatments to ameliorate the psychosocial impact of headaches as well as to reduce pain and associated symptoms in fu-

ture clinical trials evaluating drug and behavioral therapies.

FUTURE DIRECTIONS

Impact of Triptans

Triptans are playing an increasingly important role in migraine management (Adelman et al., 1998). The high cost of the triptans means that methods are needed to help patients use these medications in an optimal fashion. Strategies for recognizing the early onset of migraines; deciding when to use analgesic, abortive, or rescue medications; timing intake of the selected medication; and evaluating the effects of different medications for moderate and severe migraines already have been incorporated into some behavioral migraine-management programs. In fact, the same interventions that help patients identify the best times to use behavioral migraine-management skills can be used to teach patients to effectively time their intake of analgesic and abortive medications. Such adherence interventions are likely to be an integral part of behavioral interventions in the future, and the impact of behavioral treatment on triptan use should be evaluated in future studies.

Integration of Behavioral Therapy into Primary-Care Settings

Behavior therapy is more likely to be available in subspecialty headache clinics than in primary-practice settings. Patients referred for behavioral therapy also are likely to have long-standing or complicated headache problems or comorbid psychopathology that prompts referral. However, behavioral interventions may be more effective at preventing the evolution of severe or complicated headache problems than at treating these problems once they are well established. Patients in primary-practice settings may therefore be more likely to benefit from behavioral interventions than patients seen in subspecialty headache clinics.

Table 26–6 Quality of life and disability measures used to assess the impact of headache

Measure	Description	Internal consistency[a]	Test–retest reliability[b]	Convergent validity[c]	Content validity[d]	Discriminative validity[e]	Sensitivity examples[f]
Headache-specific measures							
MQoLQ Migraine Quality of Life Questionnaire (Santanello et al., 1995; Hartmaier et al., 1995)	Measures 24 h QoL changes associated with acute migraine attack. Consists of five domains: Work, Social, Energy/Vitality, Feelings/Concerns, Symptoms.	°°	? / °°	Migraine diary	Items based on general health-related QoL literature, clinical migraine experts, and patients	°° Migraine with nausea/vomiting vs. no nausea/vomiting; Migraine-free period vs. 24 h post-migraine	°°°° Rizatriptan vs. placebo (Ahrens et al., 1999; Santanello et al., 1997)
MSQoL Migraine-Specific Quality of Life Measure (Wagner et al., 1996b)	Measures general QoL among people with migraines.	°°	°	° Migraine severity PGWB SF-36	Developed using needs-based model (Hunt et al., 1986), based on ethnographic interviews with migraine patients and literature reviews	?	?
MSQoL Quality of Life Questionnaire (Jhingran et al., 1997; Martin et al., 2000)	Measures general QoL among people with migraines. Consists of three dimensions: Role Function-Restriction, Role Function-Preventative, Emotional Function	°°	?	° Disease severity	Items included only if meaningful to both patients and clinicians	?	°° Improves with sumatriptan (Jhingran et al., 1996)
QLH-Y Quality of Life Headache in Youth (Langeveld et al., 1996, 1997)	Measures QoL for adolescents between ages 12 and 18 who experience chronic HA or migraines. Consists of five subdomains: Psychological Functioning, Functional Status, Physical Status, Social Functioning, Satisfaction with Life in General.	°°	°°	°° Diary QLH-Y Parent ratings of child QLH-Y	Derived from existing measurements of psychological functioning, social functioning, and satisfaction with life and health	°° HA vs. HA-free Captured changes in HA status	?

(Table continued on following page)

Table 26–6 Quality of life and disability measures used to assess the impact of headache (*Continued*)

Measure	Description	Internal consistency[a]	Test–retest reliability[b]	Convergent validity[c]	Content validity[d]	Discriminative validity[e]	Sensitivity examples[f]
HDI Headache Disability Inventory (Jacobson et al. 1994, 1995)	Measures functional and emotional impact of HA on everyday life.	°°	°°° Long and short term	°° Migraine severity	Derived from patient perceptions of HA-related disability, based on existing scales for hearing and dizziness disability	?	°° CBT vs. placebo and amitriptyline vs. placebo (Holroyd et al., 2000a)
MWPLQ Migraine Work and Productivity Loss Questionnaire (Davies et al., 1999)	Measures impact of migraine and migraine therapy on paid work. Consists of seven domains: Time Management, Work Quality, Work Quantity, Bodily Effort, Interpersonal Demands, Mental Effort, and Environmental Factors.	°°	?	°° Migraine diary SF-36	?	?	°° Rizatriptan vs. usual care
HImQ Headache Impact Questionnaire or MIDAS Migraine Disability Assessment (Stewart et al., 1998, 1999b; Lipton et al. 1998)	Measures pain and activity limitations due to HA. Focused on disability. Most recent version consists of five easy to quantify items.	°°°	°°°	°°° Migraine diary Physician's judgment of disability	Items based on previous population-based and managed care-based studies of migraine. Reviewed by international group of HA clinicians and researchers.	°° Severe vs. less severe HA as determined by physicians	?
QoLQ Quality of Life Questionnaire (Cavallini et al., 1995)	Measures impact of HA on QoL during and between attacks for both episodic and chronic HA. Consists of six major concepts: Physical Functioning, Role Functioning, Social Functioning, Mental Health, Symptoms, and Health Perception.	?	?	?	Based on international guidelines, including functional state, physical symptoms, psychological conditions, social interactions	°° Episodic HA vs. chronic daily HA	?

Instrument					
RIIP Recurrent Illness Impairment Profile (Headache Version) (Wittrock et al., 1991) Measures functional impairment associated with episodic or recurrent illnesses. Consists of two subscales: General Functional Impairment and Employment-Specific Functional Impairment.	°°	°° Migraine severity	? ?	° Tension HA vs. migraine vs. tension HA and migraine	?

General measures used with headache

Instrument					
SSAP Subjective Symptom Assessment Profile (Dahlof and Dimenas, 1995) General measure of subjective symptoms. Consists of six dimensions: Emotional Distress, Gastrointestinal Symptoms, Peripheral Vascular Symptoms, Cardiac Symptoms, Sex Life, and Dizziness. A subset of questions is considered migraine-specific.	°°	? ?	? Developed as a general measure of QoL (Dimenas et al., 1990)	°° Migraine vs. HA-free	° Some improvement on three dimensions after stepped care drug treatment (Dahlof, 1995)
MSEP Minor Symptom Evaluation Profile (Dahlof and Dimenas, 1995; Dahlof, 1993) General measure of subjective central nervous system–related symptoms that impact well-being. Consists of three dimensions: Contentment, Vitality, and Sleep.	°°	°° NHP PGWB	°° Developed as a general assessment of CNS-related symptoms and QoL (Dahlof et al., 1989)	° Migraine vs. HA-free	°°° Improves with sumatriptan (Dahlof et al., 1992) Improves with diclofenac-K (Dahlof and Bjorkman, 1993)
PGWB Psychological General Well-Being (Wagner, 1996b; Dahlof and Dimenas, 1995) General measure of changes in well-being. Consists of six dimensions: Anxiety, Depressed Mood, Positive Well-being, Self-control, General Health, and Vitality.	°°	? ?	? Developed as a general measure of QoL (Dupuy, 1984)	°° Migraine vs. HA-free	?

(Table continued on following page)

Table 26–6 Quality of life and disability measures used to assess the impact of headache (*Continued*)

Measure	Description	Internal consistency[a]	Test–retest reliability[b]	Convergent validity[c]	Content validity[d]	Discriminative validity[e]	Sensitivity examples[f]
MOS SF-20 Medical Outcomes Study Short Form Health Survey (20) (Solomon et al., 1993; Skobierands et al., 1993)	General measure of disease impact. Consists of six health components: Physical Functioning, Role Functioning, Social Functioning, Mental Health, Health Perceptions, and Pain.	°°	?	— Poor in one study (Holroyd et al., 2000)	Developed as a brief version of the MOS for general assessment of QoL (Stewart et al., 1988)	°°° HA vs. HA-free with other chronic diseases Tension vs. HA-free	— Poor in one 6-month study of outpatients (Skobierands et al., 1993)
MOS SF-36 Medical Outcomes Study Short Form Health Survey (36) (Osterhaus et al., 1994; Essink-Bot et al., 1995; Durham et al., 1998; Monzon and Lainez, 1998)	General measure of disease impact. Consists of nine components: Physical Functioning, Role Functioning-Physical, Role Functioning-Emotional, Social Functioning, Bodily Pain, Mental Health, Vitality, General Health, and Change in Health	°°°	°°	°° SF-20 NHP	Developed as a brief version of the MOS for general assessment of QoL (Ware and Sherbourne, 1992)	°°°° Migraine vs. HA-free Migraine vs. severe-HA Migraine vs. chronic daily HA	°°° Improves with sumatriptan (Jhingran et al., 1996; Litaker et al., 1997) improves with guided imagery (Mannix et al., 1999)
NHP Nottingham Health Profile (Jenkinson, 1990; Erdman et al., 1993; Essink-Bot et al., 1997, 1995; Passchier et al., 1996)	General measure of health-related QoL. Consists of six areas of health: Energy, Pain, Emotional Reactions, Sleep, Social Isolation, and Physical Mobility.	°	?	°° SF-36	Developed as a general measure of perceived health (Hunt et al. 1986)	°° HA vs. HA-free subjects	?

[a]*Internal consistency*, the degree to which items within a scale measure the same construct, determined by inter-item correlations, usually Chronbach's alpha.

[b]*Test–retest reliability*, the degree to which an individual's scores on a scale are stable over time, determined by correlating individuals' scores from two different testing times.

[c]*Convergent validity*, the degree to which a scale coherently relates to other measures of the same construct, determined here by positive correlations with other related measures.

[d]*Content validity*, the degree to which scale items are relevant to and representative of the targeted construct, determined here by considering how the scale is constructed and items are chosen.

[e]*Discriminative validity*, the degree to which a scale is able to differentiate individuals in groups that vary on the targeted construct, determined by significantly different scores according to diagnosis.

[f]*Sensitivity*, the degree to which a scale is able to capture changes in the targeted construct due to treatment, determined here by score changes after some treatment.

Key to Ratings System: ?, no evidence found; —, negative evidence; °, low support from one source; °°, moderate to high support from one source; °°°, moderate to high support from multiple sources; °°°°, moderate to high support from multiple, independent sources.

Key to abbreviations: QoL, quality of life; HA, headache; CBT, cognitive behavior therapy.

If behavioral therapy is to be successfully integrated into the primary-practice setting, a brief, easy-to-use assessment device will be needed, to allow the primary-care practitioner to identify patients who are likely to benefit from behavioral therapy; the format (self-administered, home-based, or clinic-based delivery) and the provider (physician, physician assistant, nurse, technician, consulting psychologist) of behavioral treatment need to be identified; and behavioral interventions need to be simplified for use in this setting. One promising approach is an entirely home-based treatment program administered via instructional materials and supervised over the phone by paraprofessionals (P. McGrath, personal communication; McGrath et al., 1992). Such a program might require only that the primary-care practitioner provide a patient with a pamphlet that describes the program and a phone number to contact to begin treatment. A second approach that has shown promise with chronic disorders such as depression and diabetes makes use of nurses or other health professionals to teach disease-management skills (Von Korff et al., 1997; Wagner et al., 1996a). Ideally, individual programs for the management of prevalent psychological (e.g., anxiety and mood disorders) and pain (e.g., back pain, migraine) disorders would be organized in a similar fashion so that the physician would need to learn only one system in order to administer programs for multiple disorders.

Information Technology

Developments in computer and information technologies offer new ways to bring behavioral principles to bear on the management of recurrent headache disorders. For example, computer information systems that typically serve only medical record keeping and scheduling functions might also support effective headache management. A computer system might flag patients likely to benefit from special attention, including patients who are depressed, who use problematic levels of analgesic or abortive medication, or who have made emergency room visits for headache problems. A computer system also might be designed to encourage clinicians to use empirically based treatments by displaying relevant clinical guidelines when a patient's record is called up or updated. Automated telephone assessment and other communication technologies also make it possible to cost-effectively assess clinical outcomes even if patients do not return for follow-up visits. Systematic feedback of clinical outcomes then allows headache-management problems and patterns to be identified and corrected.

The availability and low cost of hand-held computers also have led investigators to consider computerizing the headache diary (Hermann et al., 1995b; Holroyd and Chen, 2000; Honkoop et al., 1999). Potential advantages of the hand-held computer include the ability to monitor the time of each diary entry, to efficiently collect large amounts of data without unduly burdening the patient, to transmit data directly to the investigator over a wireless network or via modem, and the possibility of two-way communication between the patient and either a host website or a health professional. Hand-held computer technology has the potential both to enhance the quality and the quantity of data that can be collected and, by providing two-way electronic communication between the patient and healthcare professional, to change the way educational and behavioral interventions are administered. Although this new technology is likely to initially be used to improve the quality of data collected in research, it is likely to be employed for the administration of educational and behavioral interventions as well in the next decade.

REFERENCES

Adelman, J.L., A. Brod, R.L. Von Seggem et al. (1998). Migraine preventive medications: A reappraisal. *Cephalalgia* 18:605–611.

Ahrens, S.P., M.V. Farmer, D.L. Williams et al. (1999). Efficacy and safety of rizatriptan wafer for the acute treatment of migraine. *Cephalalgia* 19:525–530.

Allen, K. and M. Shriver (1998). Role of parent-mediated pain behavior management strategies in biofeedback treatment of childhood migraines. *Behav. Ther.* 29:477–490.

Allen, K.M. and L.R. McKeen (1991). Home-based multicomponent treatment of pediatric migraine. *Headache* 31:467–472.

Andrasik, F. and K.A. Holroyd (1980). A test of specific and nonspecific effects in the biofeedback treatment of tension headache. *J. Consult. Clin. Psychol.* 48:575–586.

Arena, J.G. and E.B. Blanchard (1996). Biofeedback and relaxation therapy for chronic pain disorders. In *Psychological Approaches to Pain Management: A Practitioner's Handbook* (R.J. Gatchel and D.C. Turk, eds.). Guilford Press, New York. 179–230.

Arena, J.G., S.L. Hannah, G.M. Bruno et al. (1991). Electromyographic biofeedback training for tension headache in the elderly: A prospective study. *Biofeedback Self-Regulation* 35:187–195.

Ashina, M., L.H. Lassen, L. Bendtsen et al. (1999). Effect of inhibition of nitric oxide synthase on chronic tension-type headache: A randomized crossover trial. *Lancet* 353:287–289.

Bakal, D.A. (1982). *The Psychobiology of Chronic Headache*. Springer, New York.

Barlow, D.H. (1988). *Anxiety and Its Disorders*. Guilford Press, New York.

Barry, J. and C. Baeyer (1997). Brief cognitive-behavioral group treatment for children's headache. *Clin. J. Pain* 13:215–220.

Baumgartner, C., P. Wesseley, C. Bingolet al. (1989). Long-term prognosis of analgesic withdrawal in patients with drug-induced headaches. *Headache* 29:510–514.

Beck, A.T., A.J. Rush, B.F. Shaw et al. (1979). *Cognitive Therapy of Depression*. Guilford Press, New York.

Bendtsen, L., R. Jensen, J. Brennum et al. (1996). Exteroceptive suppression of temporal muscle activity is normal in chronic tension-type headache and not related to actual headache state. *Cephalalgia* 16:251–256.

Bendtsen, L., J. Norregard, R. Jensen et al. (1997). Evidence of qualitatively altered nociception in patients with fibromyalgia. *Arthritis Rheum.* 40:98–102.

Benson, H. (1975). *The Relaxation Response*. William Morrow, New York.

Bernstein, D.A. and T.D. Borkovec (1973). *Progressive Relaxation Training: A Manual for the Helping Professions*. Research Press, Champaign, IL.

Bille, B. (1962). Migraine in school children. *Acta Paediatr. Scand.* 51:1–151.

Bille, B. (1997). A 40-year follow-up of school children with migraine. *Cephalalgia* 17:488–491.

Blanchard, E.B. (1987). Long-term effects of behavioral treatment of chronic headache. *Behav. Ther.* 23:375–385.

Blanchard, E.B. (1992). Psychological treatment of benign headache disorders. *J. Consult. Clin. Psychol.* 60:537–551.

Blanchard, E.B. and F. Andrasik (1982). Psychological assessment and treatment of headache: Recent developments and emerging issues. *J. Consult. Clin. Psychol.* 50:859–879.

Blanchard, E.B. and F. Andrasik (1985). *Management of Chronic Headaches: A Psychological Approach*. Pergamon Press, Elmsford, NY.

Blanchard, E.B., F. Andrasik, T.A. Ahles et al. (1980). Migraine and tension headache: A meta-analytic review. *Behav. Ther.* 11:613–631.

Blanchard, E.B., F. Andrasik, K.A. Appelbaum et al. (1985a). The efficacy and cost-effectiveness of minimal-therapist-contact, non-drug treatments of chronic migraine and tension headache. *Headache* 25:214–220.

Blanchard, E.B., F. Andrasik, D.D. Evans et al. (1985b). Biofeedback and relaxation treatments for headache in the elderly: A caution and a challenge. *Biofeedback Self-Regulation* 10:69–73.

Blanchard, E.B., K.A. Appelbaum, C.L. Radnitz et al. (1989). The refractory headache patient: I. Chronic, daily, high-intensity headache. *Behav. Res. Ther.* 27:403–410.

Blanchard, E.B., M. Kim, C. Hermann et al. (1994). The role of perception of success in the thermal biofeedback treatment of vascular headache. *Headache Q.* 5:231–236.

Blanchard, E.B., M. Kim, C.U. Hermann et al. (1993). Preliminary results of the effects on headache relief of perception of success among tension headache patients receiving relaxation. *Headache Q.* 4:249–253.

Blanchard, E.B., M.L. Peters, C. Herman et al. (1997). Direction of temperature control in the thermal biofeedback treatment of vascular headache. *Appl. Psychophysiol. Biofeedback* 22:227–246.

Blanchard, E.B., A.E. Taylor, and M.P. Dentinger (1992). Preliminary results from the self-regulatory treatment of high-medication-consumption headache. *Biofeedback Self-Regulation* 17:179–202.

Bogaards, M.C. and M.M. ter Kuile (1994). Treatment of recurrent tension headache: A meta-analytic review. *Clin. J. Pain* 10:174–190.

Borkovec, T.D. and M.A. Whisman (1996). Psychosocial treatments for generalized anxiety disorder. In *Long-Term Treatment of Anxiety Disorders* (M. Mavissakalian and R. Prien, eds.). American Psychiatric Association, Washington, D.C.

Breslau, N. and G.C. Davis (1993). Migraine, physical health and psychiatric disorder: A prospective epidemiologic study in young adults. *J. Psychiatr. Res.* 27:211–221.

Breslau, N., K. Merikangas, and C.L. Bowden (1994). Comorbidity of migraine and major affective disorders. *Neurology* 44 Suppl. 7):S17–S22.

Bruhn, P., J. Olesen, and B. Melgaard (1979). Controlled trial of EMG feedback in muscle contraction headache. *Ann. Neurol.* 6:34–36.

Bussone, G., L. Grazzi, D. D'Amico, et al. (1998). Biofeedback-assisted relaxation training for young adolescents with tension-type headache: A controlled study. *Cephalalgia* 18:463–467.

Call, A.P. (1898). *Power Through Repose*. Little Brown, Boston.

Campbell, J.K., D.B. Penzien, and E.M. Wall (2000). Evidence-based guidelines for migraine headache: Behavioral and physical treatments. US Headache Consortium. Available from http://www.aan.com.

Cavallini, A., K.G. Micieli, G. Bussone et al. (1995). Headache and quality of life. *Headache* 35:29–35.

Cook, N.R., D.A. Evans, H. Funkenstein et al. (1989). Correlates of headache in a population-based cohort of elderly. *Arch. Neurol.* 46:1338–1344.

Coyne, L., J. Sargent, J. Segerson, et al. (1976). Relative potency scale for analgesic drugs: Use of psychophysical procedures with clinical judgments. *Headache* 16:70–71.

Dahlof, C. (1993). Assessment of health-related quality of life in migraine. *Cephalalgia* 13:233–237.

Dahlof, C. and R. Bjorkman (1993). Diclofenac-K (50 and 100 mg) and placebo in the acute treatment of migraine. *Cephalalgia* 13:117–123.

Dahlof, C. and E. Dimenas (1995). Migraine patients experience poorer subjective well-being/quality of life between attacks. *Cephalalgia* 15:31–36.

Dahlof, C., E. Dimenas, and B. Olofsson (1989). Documentation of an instrument for assessment of subjective CNS-related symptoms during cardiovascular pharmacotherapy. *Cardiovasc. Drugs Ther.* 3:919–927.

Dahlof, C., C. Edwards, and A. Toth (1992). Sumatriptan injection is superior to placebo in the acute treatment of migraine—with regard to both efficacy and general well-being. *Cephalalgia* 12:214–220.

Dahlof, C.G.H. (1995). Health-related quality of life under six months' treatment of migraine—an open clinic-based longitudinal study. *Cephalalgia* 15:414–422.

Davies, G.M., N. Santanello, W. Gerth et al. (1999). Validation of a migraine work and productivity loss questionnaire for use in migraine studies. *Cephalalgia* 19:497–502.

de Bruin-Kofman, A.T., H. van de Wiel, N.H. Groenman et al. (1997). Effects of a mass media behavioral treatment for chronic headache: A pilot study. *Headache* 37:415–420.

Diamond, S. and D. Montrose (1984). The value of biofeedback in the treatment of chronic headache: A four-year retrospective study. *Headache* 24:5–18.

Diener, H.C., J. Dichgans, E. Scholz et al. (1989). Analgesic-induced chronic headache: Long-term results of withdrawal therapy. *J. Neurol.* 236:9–14.

Dimenas, E., C. Dahlof, B. Olofsson et al. (1990). An instrument for quantifying subjective symptoms among untreated and treated hypertensives: Development and documentation. *J. Clin. Res. Pharmacoepidemiol.* 4:205–217.

Dobson, K.S. (1989). A meta-analysis of the efficacy of coginitive therapy for depression. *J. Consult. Clin. Psychol.* 57:414–419.

Duckro, P.N., W.D. Richardson, and J.E. Marshall (1995). *Taking Control of Your Headaches*. Guilford Press, New York.

Duke University Center for Clinical Health Policy Research (1999). *Behavioral and Physical Treatments for Migraine Headache* (PB127946). Agency for Health Care Policy and Research, Durham, NC.

Dupuy, H.J. (1984). The Psychological General Well-Being (PGWB). In *Assessment of Quality of Life in Clinical Trials of Cardiovascular Therapies* (N.K. Wenger, N.T. Mattson, C.D. Furberg et al., eds.). LeJacq, New York.

Durham, C.F., K.R. Alden, J. Dalton et al. (1998). Quality of life and productivity in nurses reporting migraine. *Headache* 38:427–435.

Erdman, R.A., J. Passchier, M. Kooijman et al. (1993). The Dutch version of the Nottingham Health Profile: Investigations of psychometric aspects. *Psychol. Rep.* 72:1027–1035.

Essink-Bot, M., P.F.M. Krabbe, G.J. Bonsel et al. (1997). An empirical comparison of four generic health status measures. *Med. Care* 35:522–537.

Essink-Bot, M., L. van Royen, P. Krabbe et al. (1995). The impact of migraine on health status. *Headache* 35:200–206.

Forsythe, W., D. Gillies, and M. Sills (1984). Propranolol (Inderal) in the treatment of childhood migraine. *Dev. Med. Child Neurol.* 26:737–741.

French, D.J., J.G. Gauthier, C. Roberge et al. (1997). Self-efficacy in the thermal biofeedback treatment of migraine sufferers. *Behav. Ther.* 28:109–125.

Gauthier, J., R. Bois, D. Allaire et al. (1981). Evaluation of skin temperature biofeedback training at two different sites for migraine. *J. Behav. Med.* 4:407–419.

Gauthier, J.G. and S. Carrier (1991). Long-term effects of biofeedback on migraine headache: A prospective follow-up study. *Headache* 31:605–612.

Gauthier, J.G., A. Fournier, and C. Roberge (1991). The differential effects of biofeedback in the treatment of menstrual and non-menstrual migraine. *Headache* 31:82–90.

Goncalves, J.A. and P. Monteiro (1993). Psychiatric analysis of patients with tension-type headache. In *Tension-Type Headache: Classification,*

Mechanisms, and Treatment (J. Olesen and J. Schoenen, eds.). Raven Press, New York.

Gould, R.A., M.W. Otto, M.H. Pollack et al. (1997). Cognitive behavioral and pharmacological treatment of generalized anxiety disorder: A preliminary meta-analysis. *Behav. Ther.* 28:285–305.

Grazzi, I., F. Leone, F. Frediani et al. (1990). A therapeutic alternative for tension headache in children: Treatment and 1-year follow-up results. *Biofeedback Self-Regulation* 15:1–6.

Griffiths, J. and P. Martin (1996). Clinical- versus home-based treatment formats for children with chronic headache. *Br. J. Health Psychol.* 1:151–166.

Guidetti, V., F. Galli, P. Fabrizi et al. (1998). Headache and psychiatric comorbidity: Clinical aspects and outcome in an 8 year follow-up study. *Cephalalgia* 18:455–462.

Haddock, C.K., A.B. Rowan, F. Andrasik et al. (1997). Home-based behavioral treatments for chronic benign headache: A meta-analysis of controlled trials. *Cephalalgia* 17:113–118.

Hartmaier, S.L., N.C. Santanello, R.S. Epstein et al. (1995). Development of a brief 24-hour migraine-specific quality of life questionnaire. *Headache* 35:320–329.

Helm-Hylkema, H., J. Orlebeke, L. Enting et al. (1990). Effects of behavior therapy on migraine and plasma β-endorphin in young migraine patients. *Psychoneuroendocrinology* 15:39–45.

Hermann, C., E.B. Blanchard, and H. Flor (1997). Biofeedback treatment for pediatric migraine: Prediction of treatment outcome. *J. Consult. Clin. Psychol.* 65:611–616.

Hermann, C., M. Kim, and E.B. Blanchard (1995a). Behavioral and pharmacological intervention studies of pediatric migraine: An exploratory meta-analysis. *Pain* 60:239–256.

Hermann, C., M.L. Peters, and E.B. Blanchard (1995b). Use of hand-held computers for symptom-monitoring: The case of chronic headache. *Mind Body Med.* 1:59–69.

Holroyd, K. (1993). Integrating pharmacologic and non-pharmacologic treatments. In *Headache Diagnosis and Interdisciplinary Treatment* (C.D. Tolison and R.S. Kunkel, eds.). Williams and Wilkins, Baltimore.

Holroyd, K., M. Stensland, G. Lipchik et al. (2000b). Psychosocial correlates and impact of chronic tension-type headaches. *Headache* 40:3–16.

Holroyd, K.A. (in press). Assessment and psychological treatment of recurrent headache disorders. *J. Consult. Clin. Psychol.*

Holroyd, K.A. and F. Andrasik (1982). A cognitive-behavioral approach to recurrent tension and migraine headache. In *Advances in Cognitive-Behavioral Research and Therapy* (P.E. Kendall, ed.). Academic Press, New York.

Holroyd, K.A., M. Appel, and F. Andrasik (1982). A cognitive-behavioral approach to the treatment of psychophysiological disorders. In *Stress Prevention and Management: A Cognitive-Behavioral Approach* (D. Meichenbaum and M. Jaremko, eds.), pp. 219–257. Plenum Press, New York.

Holroyd, K.A. and Y. Chen (2000). A hand-held computer headache diary program: Monitoring headaches, medication use, and disability in real time. Presented at the American Headache Society Convention, Montreal, Canada. June 23–25.

Holroyd, K.A., G.E. Cordingley, J.L. France et al. (1992). Combining propranolol and biofeedback for treatment of migraine. *Headache* 32:254–255.

Holroyd, K.A. and D. French (1995). Recent advances in the assessment and treatment of recurrent headaches. In *Handbook of Health and Rehabilitation Psychology* (A.J. Goreczny, ed.). Plenum Press, New York.

Holroyd, K.A. and G.L. Lipchik (2000). Sex differences in recurrent headache disorders. In *Sex, Gender and Pain: From the Bench Top to the Clinic* (R.B. Fillingim, ed.), pp. 251–279. IASP Press, Seattle.

Holroyd, K.A., G.L. Lipchik, and D.B. Penzien (1998). Psychological management of recurrent headache disorders: Empirical basis for clinical practice. In *Best Practice: Developing and Promoting Empirically Supported Interventions* (K.S. Dobson and K.D. Craig, eds.), pp. 193–212. Sage: Newbury Park, CA.

Holroyd, K.A., P. Malinoski, M.K. Davis et al. (1999). The three dimensions of headache impact: Pain, disability and affective distress. *Pain* 83:571–578.

Holroyd, K.A. and P.R. Martin (2000). Psychological treatments for tension-type headache. In *The Headaches* (J. Olesen, P. Tfelt-Hansen, and K.M.A. Welch, eds.), 2nd ed., pp. 643–649. Lippincott–Williams and Wilkins, Philadelphia.

Holroyd, K.A., Nash, J.M., J.D. Pingel et al. (1991a). A comparison of pharmacological (amitriptyline HCl) and nonpharmacological (cognitive-behavioral) therapies for chronic tension headaches. *J. Consult. Clin. Psychol.* 59:387–393.

Holroyd, K.A., F.J. O'Donnell, G.L. Lipchik et al. Management of chronic tension-type headache with (tricyclic) antidepressant medication, stress-management therapy, and their combination: a randomized controlled trial. *Cephalalgia* 20:294–295.

Holroyd, K.A. and D.B. Penzien (1986). Client variables in the behavioral treatment of recurrent tension headache: A meta-analytic review. *J. Behav. Med.* 9:515–536.

Holroyd, K.A., D.B. Penzien, and G. Cordingley (1991b). Propranolol in the management of recurrent migraine: A meta-analytic review. *Headache* 31:333–340.

Holroyd, K.A., D.D. Penzien, and J.E. Holm (1988). Clinical issues in the treatment of recurrent headache disorders. In *Innovations in Clinical Practice: A Source Book* (P.A. Keller and L.G. Ritt, eds.). Professional Resource Exchange, Sarasota, FL.

Holroyd, K.A., D.B. Penzien, K.G. Hursey et al. (1984). Change mechanisms in EMG biofeedback training: Cognitive changes underlying improvements in tension headache. *J. Consult. Clin. Psychol.* 52:1039–1053.

Honkoop, P.C., M.J. Sorbi, G.L.R. Godaeri et al. (1999). High-density assessment of the IHS classification criteria for migraine without aura: A prospective study. *Cephalalgia* 19:201–206.

Hunt, S., J. McEwen, and S.P. McKenna (1986). *Measuring Health Status*. Croom Helm: London.

Jacobson, E. (1934). *Progressive Relaxation*. University of Chicago Press: Chicago.

Jacobson, G.P., N.M. Ramadan, S.K. Aggarwal et al. (1994). The Henry Ford Hospital Headache Disability Inventory (HDI). *Neurology* 44:837–842.

Jacobson, G.P., N.M. Ramadan, L. Norris et al. (1995). Headache Disability Inventory (HDI): Short-term test–retest reliability and spouse perceptions. *Headache* 35:534–539.

Jenkinson, C. (1990). Health status and mood state in a migraine sample. *Int. J. Soc. Psychiatry* 36:42–48.

Jhingran, P., R.K. Cady, J. Rubino et al. (1996). Improvements in health-related quality of life with sumatriptan treatment for migraine. *J. Fam. Pract.* 42:36–42.

Jhingran, P., J.T. Osterhaus, D.W. Miller et al. (1997). Development and validation of the migraine-specific quality of life questionnaire. *Headache* 38:295–302.

Kewman, D. and A.H. Roberts (1980). Skin temperature biofeedback and migraine headache: A double-blind study. *Biofeedback Self-Regulation* 5:327–345.

Kim, M. and E.B. Blanchard (1992). Two studies of the non-pharmacological treatment of menstrually-related migraine headaches. *Headache* 32:197–202.

Kohlenberg, R.J. (1981). Self-help treatment of migraine headache: A controlled outcome study. *Headache* 21:196–200.

Kroner-Herwig, B., U. Mohn, and R. Pothmann (1998). Comparison of biofeedback and relaxation in the treatment of pediatric headache and the influence of parent involvement on outcome. *Appl. Psychophysiol. Biofeedback* 23:143–157.

Kudrow, L. (1982). Paradoxical effects of frequent analgesic use. In *Advances in Neurology: Headache: Physiopathological and Clinical Concepts* (M. Critchley, A.P. Friedman, S. Gorini et al., eds.). Raven Press, New York.

Labbe, E. (1995). Treatment of childhood migraine with autogenic training and skin temperature biofeedback: A component analysis. *Headache* 35:10–13.

Langeveld, J.H., H. Koot, and J. Passchier (1997). Headache intensity and quality of life in adolescents. How are changes in headache intensity in adolescents related to changes in experienced quality of life? *Headache* 37:37–42.

Langeveld, J.H., H.M. Koot, and M.C. Loonen (1996). A quality of life instrument for adolescents with chronic headache. *Cephalalgia* 16:183–196.

Largen, J.W., R.J. Mathew, K. Dobbins et al. (1981). Specific and non-specific effects of skin temperature control and migraine management. *Headache* 21:36–44.

Larsson, B. and J. Carlsson (1996). A school-based, nurse-administered relaxation training for children with chronic tension-type headache. *J. Pediatr. Psychol.* 21:603–614.

Larsson, B. and L. Melin (1988). The psychological treatment of recurrent headache in adolescents—short-term outcome and its prediction. *Headache* 28:187–195.

Larsson, B., L. Melin, and A. Döberl (1990). Recurrent tension headache in adolescents treated with self-help relaxation training and muscle relaxant drug. *Headache* 30:665–671.

Larsson, B.M. and L. Melin (1986). Chronic headaches in adolescents: treatment in a school setting with relaxation training as compared with information-contact and self-registration. *Pain* 25:325–336.

Lipchik, G.L., K.A. Holroyd, C.R. France et al. (1996). Central and peripheral mechanisms in chronic tension-type headache. *Pain* 64:467–475.

Lipchik, G.L., K.A. Holroyd, F.O. O'Donnell et al. (in press). Exteroceptive suppression periods and pericranial muscle tenderness in chronic tension-type headache: Effects of psychopathology, chronicity, and disability. *Cephalalgia*.

Lipchik, G.L., K.H. Holroyd, F. Talbot et al. (1997). Pericranial muscle tenderness and exteroceptive suppression of temporalis muscle activity: A blind study of chronic tension-type headache. *Headache* 37:368–376.

Lipton, R.B., S.D. Silberstein, and W.F. Stewart (1994). An update on the epidemiology of migraine. *Headache* 34:319–328.

Lipton, R.B. and W.F. Stewart (1997). Epidemiology and comorbidity of migraine. In *Headache* (P.J. Goadsby and S.D. Silberstein, eds.). Butterworth-Heinemann, Boston.

Lipton, R.B., W.F. Stewart, J. Sawyer et al. (1998). Attributes necessary for a new instrument assessing the burden of migraine: Clinical utility of the Migraine Disability Assessment (MIDAS) questionnaire. Presented at the American Association for the Study of Headache Convention, San Francisco, CA. June 26–28.

Litaker, D.G., G.D. Solomon, and J.R. Genzen (1997). Using pretreatment quality of life perceptions to predict response to sumatriptan in migraineurs. *Headache* 37:630–634.

Mannix, L.K., R.S. Chandurkar, L.A. Tusek et al. (1999). Effect of guided imagery on quality of life for patients with chronic tension-type headache. *Headache* 39:326–334.

Marcus, D.A., L. Scharff, and D.C. Turk (1995). Nonpharmacological management of headache during pregnancy. *Psychosom. Med.* 57:527–535.

Martin, B.C., D.S. Pathak, M.L. Sharfman et al. (2000). Validity and reliability of the Migraine-Specific Quality of Life Questionnaire (MSQ version 2.1). *Headache* 40:204–215.

Martin, P.R. (1993). *Psychological Management of Chronic Headaches.* Guilford Press, New York.

Martin, P.R. and A.M. Mathews (1978). Tension headaches: Psychophysiological investigation and treatment. *J. Psychosom. Res.* 22:389–399.

Mathew, N.T. (1981). Prophylaxis of migraine and mixed headache: A randomized controlled study. *Headache* 21:105–109.

Mathew, N.T., R. Kurman, and F. Perez (1990). Drug induced refractory headache—clinical features and management. *Headache* 30:634–638.

Mathew, R.J., J.W. Largen, K. Dobbins et al. (1980). Biofeedback control of skin temperature and cerebral blood flow in migraine. *Headache* 20:12–28.

McCrory, D.C., D.B. Penzien, J.C. Rains et al. (1996). Efficacy of behavioral treatments for migraine and tension-type headache: Meta-analysis of controlled trials. *Headache* 36:172.

McGrady, A., A. Wauquier, A. McNeil et al. (1994). Effect of biofeedback-assisted relaxation on migraine headache and changes in cerebral blood flow velocity in the middle cerebral artery. *Headache* 34:424–428.

McGrath, P.J., P. Humphreys, D. Keene et al. (1992). The efficacy and efficiency of a self-administered treatment for adolescent migraine. *Pain* 49:321–324.

Mehta, M. (1992). Biobehavioral intervention in recurrent headaches in children. *Headache Q.* 3:426–430.

Merikangas, K.R., J. Angst, and H. Isler (1990). Migraine and psychopathology: Results of the Zurich cohort study of young adults. *Arch. Gen. Psychiatry* 47:894–852.

Merikangas, K.R., J.R. Merikangas, and J. Angst (1993). Headache syndromes and psychiatric disorders: Association and family transmission. *J. Psychom. Res.* 27:197–210.

Michultka, D.M., E.B. Blanchard, K.A. Appelbaum et al. (1989). The refractory headache patient: II. High medication consumption (analgesic rebound) headache. *Behav. Res. Ther.* 27:411–420.

Monzon, M.J. and M.J. Lainez (1998). Quality of life in migraine and chronic daily headache patients. *Cephalalgia* 18:638–643.

Mosley, T.H., C.A. Grotheus, and W.M. Meeks (1995). Treatment of tension headache in the elderly: A controlled evaluation of relaxation training and relaxation combined with cognitive-behavior therapy. *J. Clin. Geropsychol.* 1:175–188.

Nash, J. and K. Holroyd (1992). Home-based behavioral treatment for recurrent headache: A cost-effective alternative. *Am. Pain Soc. Bull.* 2:1–6.

Nicholson, N.L. and E.B. Blanchard (1993). A controlled evaluation of behavioral treatment of chronic headache in the elderly. *Behav. Ther.* 24:67–76.

Olness, K., H. Hall, J. Rozneicki et al. (1999). Mast cell activation in children with migraine before and after training in self-regulation. *Headache* 39:101–107.

Olness, K., J.T. MacDonald, and D.L. Uden (1987). Comparison of self-hypnosis and propranolol in the treatment of juvenile migraine. *Pediatrics* 79:593–597.

Osterhaus, J.T., R.J. Townsend, B. Gandek et al. (1994). Measuring the functional status and well-being of patients with migraine headache. *Headache* 34:337–343.

Osterhaus, S.O.L., J. Passchier, H. van der Helm-Hylkema et al. (1993). Effects of behavioral psychophysiological treatment on schoolchildren with migraine in a nonclinical setting: Predictors and process variables. *J. Pediatr. Psychol.* 18:697–715.

Passchier, J., M. de Boo, J.A. Quaak et al. (1996). Headache-related quality of life of chronic headache patients is predicted by the emotional component of their pain. *Headache* 36:556–560.

Penzien, D.B. and K.A. Holroyd (1994). Psychosocial interventions in the management of recurrent headache disorders 2: Description of treatment techniques. *Behav. Med.* 20:64–73.

Penzien, D.B., K.A. Holroyd, J.E. Holm et al. (1985). Behavioral management of migraine: Results from five dozen group outcome studies. *Headache* 25:162.

Penzien, D.B., J.C. Rains, and K.A. Holroyd (1992). A review of alternative behavioral treatments for headache. *Mississippi Psychologist* 17:8–9.

Penzien, D.B., J.C. Rains, and K.A. Holroyd (1993). Psychological assessment of the recurrent headache sufferer. In *Headache: Diagnosis and Treatment* (C.D. Tollison and R.S. Kunkel, eds.). Williams and Wilkins, Baltimore.

Puca, F., S. Genco, and M.P. Prudenzano (1999). Psychiatric comorbidity and psychosocial stress in patients with tension-type headache from headache centers in Italy. *Cephalalgia* 19:159–164.

Rapoport, A.M., F.D. Sheftell, S.M. Baskin et al. (1984). *Analgesic Rebound Headache*. New England Center for Headache, Stamford, CT.

Reich, B.A. and M. Gottesman (1993). Biofeedback and psychotherapy in the treatment of muscle contraction/tension-type headache. In *Headache Diagnosis and Interdisciplinary Treatment* (C.D. Tollison and R.S. Kunkel, eds.). Urban and Schwartzenberg, New York.

Robinson, L.A., J.S. Berman, and R.A. Neimeyer (1990). Psychotherapy for the treatment of depression: A comprehensive review of controlled outcome research. *Psychol. Bull.* 108:30–49.

Rokicki, L.A., K.A. Holroyd, C.R. France et al. (1997). Change mechanisms associated with combined relaxation/EMG biofeedback training for chronic tension headache. *Appl. Psychophysiol. Biofeedback* 22:21–41.

Rowan, A.B. and F. Andrasik (1996). Efficacy and cost-effectiveness of minimal therapist contact treatments of chronic headache: A review. *Behav. Ther.* 27:207–234.

Santanello, N., A. Polis, S. Hartmaier et al. (1997). Improvement in migraine-specific quality of life in a clinical trial of rizatriptan. *Cephalalgia* 17:867–872.

Santanello, N.C., S.L. Hartmaier, R.S. Epstein et al. (1995). Validation of a new quality of life questionnaire for acute migraine headache. *Headache* 35:330–337.

Sartory, G.M., B. Muller, J. Metsch et al. (1998). A comparison of psychological and pharmacological treatment of pediatric migraine. *Behav. Res. Ther.* 36:1155–1170.

Scharff, L., D.A. Marcus, and D.C. Turk (1996). Maintenance of effects in the nonmedical treatment of headaches during pregnancy. *Headache* 36:285–290.

Schoenen, J. (1989). Exteroceptive silent periods of temporalis muscle in headache. In *EMG of Jaw Reflexes in Man* (D. van Steenberghe and A. DeLaat, eds.). Leuven University Press, Leuven.

Schoenen, J., A. Maertens de Noordhout, and M. Timsit-Berthier (1986). Contingent negative variation and efficacy of beta-blocking agents in migraine. *Cephalalgia* 6:229–233.

Schultz, J. and W. Luthe (1959). *Autogenic Training: A Psychophysiologic Approach in Psychotherapy*, Vol. 1. Grune and Stratton, New York.

Schwartz, M.S. (1995). *Biofeedback: A Practitioner's Guide*. Guilford Press, New York.

Silberstein, S.D., and J. Rosenberg (2000). Multispecialty consensus on diagnosis and treatment of headache. *Neurology* 54:1553–1554.

Sillanpaa, M. (1983). Prevalence of headache in puberty. *Headache* 23:10–14.

Simmons, L.W., and H.G. Wolff (1954). *Social Science in Medicine*. Russell Sage Foundation, New York.

Skobierands, F.G., G.D. Solomon, and L.A. Gragg (1993). Quality of life changes in headache patients following six months of outpatient treatment: Use of the Medical Outcomes Study Instrument 37. *Headache* 33:283.

Solbach, P., J. Sargent, and L. Coyne (1984). Menstrual migraine headache: Results of a controlled, experimental outcome study of nondrug treatments. *Headache* 24:75–78.

Solomon, G.D. (1997). Evolution of the measurement of quality of life in migraine. *Neurology* 48 (Suppl. 3):S10–S15.

Solomon, G.D., F.G. Slobieranda, and L. Gregg (1993). Quality of life and well-being of headache patients: Measurement by the Medical Outcomes Study Instrument. *Headache* 33:351–358.

Stebbins, G. (1893). *Dynamic Breathing and Harmonic Gymnastics: A Complete System of Psychical, Aesthetic and Physical Culture*. Edgar S. Werber, New York.

Stewart, A.L., R.D. Hays, and J.E. Ware (1988). The MOS short-form General Health Survey: Reliability and validity in a patient population. *Med. Care* 26:724–735.

Stewart, W.F., R.B. Lipton, K. Kolodner et al. (1999a). Reliability of the migraine disability assessment score in a population-based sample of headache sufferers. *Cephalalgia* 19:107–114.

Stewart, W.F., R.B. Lipton, D. Simon et al. (1998). Reliability of an illness severity measure for headache in a population sample of migraine sufferers. *Cephalalgia* 18:44–51.

Stewart, W.F., R.B. Lipton, D. Simon et al. (1999b). Validity of an illness severity measure in a population sample of migraine sufferers. *Pain* 79:291–301.

Strom, L., R. Peterson, and G. Andersson (2000). A controlled trial of self-help treatment of recurrent headache conducted via the internet. *J. Consult. Clin. Psychol.* 68:722–727.

Szekely, B., D. Botwin, B.H. Eidelman et al. (1986). Nonpharmacological treatment of menstrual headache: Relaxation-biofeedback behavior therapy and person-centered insight therapy. *Headache* 26:86–92.

Von Korff, M., J. Gruman, J. Schaefer et al. (1997). Collaborative management of chronic illness. *Ann. Intern. Med.* 127:1097–1102.

Wagner, E.H., B.T. Austin, and M. von Korff (1996a). Improving outcomes in chronic illness. *Managed Care Q.* 4:12–25.

Wagner, T.H., D.L. Patrick, B.S. Galer et al. (1996b). A new instrument to assess the long-term quality of life effects from migraine: Development and psychometric testing of the MSQOL. *Headache* 36:484–492.

Ware, J.E. and C.D. Sherbourne (1992). The MOS 36-item Short-Form Health Survey (SF-36). I. Conceptual frameworks and item selection. *Med. Care 30*:473–483.

Wauquier, A., A. McGrady, L. Aloe et al. (1995). Changes in cerebral blood flow velocity associated with biofeedback-assisted relaxation treatment of migraine headaches are specific for the middle cerebral artery. *Headache 35*:358–362.

Wittrock, D.A., D.B. Penzien, J.H. Moseley et al. (1991). The recurrent illness impairment pro-file: Preliminary results using the headache version. *Headache Q.* 2:138–139.

Wolff, H.G. (1948). *Headache and Other Head Pain*. Oxford University Press, New York.

Wolff, H.G. (1953). *Stress and Disease*. Charles C Thomas, Springfield, IL.

Wolff, H.G. and S. Wolff (1948). *Pain*. Charles C Thomas, Springfield, IL.

Womack, W., M. Smith, and A. Chen (1988). Behavioral management of childhood headache: A pilot study and case history report. *Pain 32*:279–283.

27

Communicating with the Patient

VALERIE SOUTH
FRED SHEFTELL

Listen to the patient, he is telling you the diagnosis
Osler, 1904

Let us not begin with the assumption that doctors are to be accused of an inability to listen. Nor should we that think patients with headache ramble. We must, however, open our eyes to a serious threat to headache care: in the absence of true communication between those who suffer and those who treat, all that has been learned about headache disorders and their treatment is vulnerable.

Evidence suggests that improved communication between doctors and patients will result in improvement in diagnosis, treatment, and satisfaction. This chapter discusses barriers to effective communication while providing practical advice to those in the practice of medicine and those who receive medical care. We examine both provider and patient behaviors and their ability to influence outcomes.

BACKGROUND

Why Improve Communication?

Many headache patients are unhappy with their medical care. Most patients who seek help from a doctor never return for follow-up. A large-scale Canadian study (Edmeads et al., 1993) showed that only 32% of the 76% of those headache sufferers who sought medical attention returned for ongoing care. Slightly more than one-half of patients who did not return stated that they were unhappy with their doctors or had had problems with their medications. They gave the following reasons for their dissatisfaction with the physician: the doctor did not take me seriously, the doctor did not spend enough time with me, the doctor was not knowledgeable, the doctor's explanations were unclear.

Another study showed that patients' dissatisfaction with doctors' communicative ability far outweighed their dissatisfaction with doctors' technical abilities (Ben-Sira, 1976). In this study, patients gave the following reasons for their dissatisfaction: the doctor did not listen to me (Baron, 1985), the doctor used jargon, the doctor talked down to me.

Doctors are also dissatisfied. Physicians crave the gratification of helping people with their fears and not just their diseases. The barrier to providing optimal care most often cited by doctors is insufficient time (Daley, 1993).

Where Are Things Going Wrong?

Doctors feel that there is not enough time in the typical appointment to effectively communicate all the information patients need to have. The trend toward consulting with alternative practitioners may be partly caused by patient dissatisfaction with the time medical doctors can spend in the average patient appointment (MacGregor, 1997). Many medical doctors yearn for the past, when doctors were able to spend 5 or 6 hours with headache patients during their first interview (Sheftell, 1996). Of course, this was before extensive waiting lists, managed care, health-maintenance organizations, capitation, and departmental budget freezes; time spent talking to patients was highly valued, unlike today, when doctors who spend time talking with their patients often feel looked down upon by more technical peers (Daley, 1993). (Indeed, a glance at a current appointment schedule is all one needs to confirm this suspicion.) In the "old days," patients had not morphed into consumers either. Often, they did not question diagnoses or ask about side effects of medications, and they almost always complied with treatment regimes. Those days of passive patients and despotic doctors have given way to informed participatory partners, patients who take an active role in their health management and disease prevention and doctors who have come to expect and anticipate that most of their patients want to be well informed. However, these new roles have caused significant changes, and these changes have not necessarily been managed effectively. If one tries to treat active, informed, educated, empowered patients as passive partners in a fraction of the time previously allotted, frustration will arise at both ends of the stethoscope.

Effective Listening

Patients are talking more, and they think their doctors are not listening. Although physicians may be listening, if they fail to make that apparent through gestures or eye contact, it will be perceived that they are not (Buckman, 1992). The average time that a patient is allowed to talk before being interrupted by the physician is 18 seconds (Beckman and Frankel, 1984). Less than one-quarter of patients ever finish their initial address to the doctor. Many doctors who treat headache patients tell us that their patients are not very good at

telling a succinct story and that if they want to get through the appointment in the time allotted, it is necessary to interrupt. However, when patients were allowed to tell their stories without interruption, they usually spoke for no longer than 150 seconds. Physicians who interrupted saved, on average, only 132 seconds (Buckman, 1992). Furthermore, by interrupting, they sacrificed increased perceived competence of the doctor, enhanced compliance with the treatment plan, and improved overall satisfaction with the doctor.

More effective communication (beginning with more effective listening) will not solve all of the woes brought on by managed care and too-short appointments, but it will enhance the practice of medicine and it does not take as long as most people believe.

Are All Patients Treated Equally?

Just as we do not think of "the acute headache in room three," we cannot think of all patients en masse. The principle of Osler (1904), that it is more helpful to approach the person who has the disease than the disease the person has, is essential when treating headache patients. Patients' medical disorders must be viewed in the context of their life experiences, lifestyles, expectations, attitudes, and behaviors. Physicians need to adapt their approach to be understood, relevant, and practical. Despite this, few providers determine critical information about their patients' literacy levels, cultural preferences, or value systems.

Patients who are upwardly mobile, fully insured, computer-literate web surfers born and raised in the culture are treated differently from patients who may have financial difficulties, be in poorer health, or not speak the language. The doctors who treat these groups differently may be doing so without realizing it or understanding the full implication of their actions. Studies have shown that the information communicated by the doctor to the patient varies with the patient's age, income, health status, cultural background, and sociodemographic characteristics. Patients whose cultural, ethnic, and socioeconomic backgrounds differ from their physicians' are less likely to receive information from the provider.

Those at risk for ineffective communication include patients of lower socioeconomic status, as measured by occupation, insurance coverage, or income (Epstein et al., 1985; Ventures and Gordon, 1990). This is relevant to large numbers of people with migraine as a study (Stewart et al., 1992) in at least one country (United States) showed a strong association between higher prevalence of migraine and low household income.

Older patients, especially women (Root, 1987; Weisman, 1987), are at risk. Patients with poorer reported health status are also at risk, a fact that is significant because these individuals report substantially diminished functioning and well-being compared with the U.S. general population with no reported chronic conditions (Osterhaus et al., 1994).

Are All Doctors Viewed as Equal?

Academic knowledge and clinical competence are not the only factors that patients prize. Just as important is the physician's ability to impart this knowledge. Member organizations of the World Headache Alliance rated the number one desire of headache patients to be "to spend *time* with a knowledgeable doctor." Effectively relaying accurate information to the patient is just as important as getting the diagnosis right. Packard (1979) surveyed 100 outpatients and 50 doctors to determine what patients want from a medical consultation. While the doctors believed that the patients' foremost desire was pain relief, the patients stated that their most urgent desire was an explanation for their pain.

The tone of the consultation is very important. Perceived lack of warmth in the physician is a serious barrier to effective care (Korsch et al., 1968). While some remaining die-hard proponents of the old school may dismiss focusing on communication as overly emotional, we are not suggesting abandoning dress shoes in favor of sandals. However, it is important that doctors infuse their personality into their practice. Graham (1987) wrote "Any style will be effective providing it clearly demonstrates to the patient that the physician

is interested in him and his life as a person, as well as in the details of the medical complaint."

Dynamics of Doctor–Patient Relationships

The need to develop a personal style and effective approach to patients has been thought of as more of an art form than a science. Roter and Hall (1992) clarified this through their definition of the four prototypes of the physician–patient relationship (listed below), based on issues of control.

Paternalism

Physician control is high and patient control is low. The physician takes total charge of decision-making, which is ultimately "in the patient's best interests." The patient's role is to cooperate and obey. The stereotype is "Doctor knows best, dear."

Consumerism

Physician control is low and patient control is high. The physician accommodates the demands of the patient. The stereotype is "I just read something about drug A and my friend is taking drug B. I'd like those, please."

Default

Physician control is low and patient control is low. Stagnation and paralysis result since neither party takes responsibility for decisions.

Mutuality

Physician control is high and patient control is high. Both take an active role in decision-making. Mutuality is the authors' preference and recommendation. Mutuality embodies an alliance or partnership and implies an active role by the patient.

An external locus of control, characterized by the patient remaining passive and looking to the physician alone, leads to a poorer prognosis. These patients may say "You're the doctor—fix me!" and will often be searching for a magic bullet to take away the disease. This behavior can negatively influence the course of the illness as well as the treatment outcome. Examples include asthmatic patients who continue to smoke, patients with hyperlipidemia who do not follow diet or exercise regimes, or diabetics who drink alcohol to excess. An effective consultation can lead to recognizing behavioral issues that may affect outlook on, participation in, and outcome of therapy.

ACTION

Armed with the awareness that has been gleaned by using the preceding information, it is now time to enter the consultation suite and put it all together with some practical advice.

The patient–physician dichotomy begins with the patient holding all of the raw information required by the doctor but knowing very little about how the pieces fit together to create the full picture (Daley, 1993). Patients often struggle when translating symptoms into words. If the doctor is not a good coach, the entire game may fall apart. The onus is on both the physician and the patient to focus on communication and pave the way to effective care.

Practice Points for Doctors to Consider

Develop Communicative Potential

Communicating effectively is as important as conducting physical examinations. Expend your personal resources accordingly. Use patient-centered skills, such as giving information and counseling, vs. physician-centered behaviors, such as asking questions and giving directions (Roter et al., 1987). Developing your patient-centered skills is a science.

Set the Stage

Take the time to increase your comfort and the comfort of your patient (Buckman, 1992). Introduce yourself, shake hands, sit down. Avoid talking over a desk, yet establish yourself a culturally appropriate distance away from your patients so they do not feel either distanced from or smothered by you. Minimize distractions and move clutter out of the way.

Go for the "relaxed yet engaged" look. Patients will quickly pick up on boredom, distraction, or impatience.

Communicate to the patient that you take the problem seriously. Many headache patients have encountered doctors who have projected a less than serious attitude to their problems (Edmeads et al., 1993).

Touch the patient's head during the examination. Physical contact will establish in the patient's mind that you have thoroughly examined the affected part.

Assess Impact and Disability

Pain is a subjective experience that is often difficult to communicate. Migraine is more than just pain. Benign headache has a huge impact on all areas of life for those who suffer, and effectively communicating the associated disability can result in greater understanding by the physician. The use of such instruments as the Migraine Disability Assessment Questionnaire (MIDAS) and the Headache Impact Test (HIT) allows both patient and doctor to assess disability. Describing pain intensity, location, and characteristics does not have the same impact as stating "Doctor, these headaches are causing me to miss 3 or 4 days of work each month" or "My headaches don't allow me to care for my family several days a month."

Determine the Patient's Expectations

Ensure that realistic expectations are stated in the consultation. Establish the fact that headache control, not cure, is the goal. Disappointment will be inevitable if the patient thinks of the doctor as savior. Avoid speaking at great length without eliciting the patient's ideas or expectations.

Let the Patient Speak

Allow the patient to tell his or her entire story, including emotions and feelings

(Korsch et al., 1968). This will increase your patient's perception of your competence (Hall et al., 1981) and enhance compliance (Stewart, 1982).

Watch for Buried Questions

Often, the patient will not present the chief complaint first. This is usually not intentional, but the doctor might focus on the first complaint that the patient presents and spend the appointment on an issue that is not the patient's biggest concern.

If patients are afraid of the answer, they may be ambivalent about asking the question. These patients often ask the dreaded question in a soft voice while you are talking (Buckman, 1992). Should this occur, finish your sentence, and then say something like "I'm sorry, you were about to say something."

Patients who are uncomfortable or afraid to discuss their headache may bring the subject up as they are exiting the room. Avoid thinking "Well, it could not be that important or they would have brought it up long before this." Bring the patient back, either immediately or for another appointment.

Explain the Diagnosis

Although having a name for one's problem is therapeutic, the name alone will mean little to the average patient. Sharing how you formulated your conclusion will provide reassurance that you have "got it right." Failing to give an explanation of the diagnosis or to shine light on the cause of the illness is a barrier to effective consultation. A clear explanation of the disorder is more important to most patients than pain relief.

Explain the Tests

As important as outlining what to expect if a test is ordered is explaining why tests might not be ordered. The concept of tests being ordered only to rule out sinister causes of headache rather than to confirm a benign finding is not necessarily implicit.

Use Appropriate Language

In his book *The Doctor*, Edward E. Rosenbaum writes: "All my life I have listened to practitioners saying one thing and patients hearing another." Doctors use different language from patients (Bourhis et al., 1989). Nurses often become "communication brokers" as their tendency is to use language that is partway between that used by doctors and that used by patients. However, they may not be available to debrief the patient. Be clear, and avoid using medical jargon.

Speak to the Future

Do not shy away from the potential seriousness of the diagnosis, the prognosis, or how long the problem/symptoms will continue. Patients believe that this information is routinely kept from them. People believe that doctors withhold information to "protect them" in some way (Lipkin, 1979; Katz, 1984; Bell,1986).

Discuss the Treatment Plan

Formulating the treatment plan together with the patient will enhance accordance and result in compliant participation in the treatment regimen. Explain why you believe the plan you have outlined is the best one available, and be clear about any alternatives that may exist.

A second, third, or even fourth appointment may be needed to complete the initial phases of developing the treatment plan and explaining it effectively. Patients can assimilate only two or three important pieces of information per visit. They need time to process the information provided (Daley, 1993).

Take Time to Thoroughly Discuss Medication

If you do not prescribe medication, be sure the patient knows why. If you reduce a patient's medication, as may be the case in analgesic-overuse headache syndromes, be sure to provide thorough education and many reinforcing resources. When you prescribe medication, be sure that the patient knows its name, when to take it, its potential side effects, and how long it will take to work. Remember that the patient is more than just "the headache," and be aware of other medications he or she may be taking. Discuss potential interactions with alcohol as well as other drugs.

Discuss Lifestyle and Be Aware of Behavioral Issues

Headache diaries help identify suspected triggers and document medication use, menstrual periods, and other related events.

Behavioral issues are not a popular topic to discuss with headache patients. For years, the belief that headache disorders were caused by an unstable constitution or psychiatric illness stigmatized people with headache. Although we have come a long way since then and benign headache disorders such as migraine have firmly established their neurobiological roots, behavioral issues must be examined in the same light one would examine them in any other medical disorder.

When looking for behavioral components, start by asking the patient to describe a typical day. Behaviors with potential for negative impact on health include type A behaviors, a generalized high-intensity approach to life, self-sacrificing behaviors, negative cognitive styles, overly high self-expectations, behaviors that contribute to difficulties in work or personal relationships, passivity, and lack of initiative.

Give suggestions and directions regarding necessary lifestyle and behavior changes, and consider a referral to a behavioral colleague when issues are identified.

Provide Ongoing Education

Reinforce the office experience with as many "take-aways" and leads as possible. Information is available in many formats, from written publications to videos to World Wide Web sites. Quality patient-targeted information is available from more than 40 headache organizations worldwide (the World Headache Alliance website is http://www.w-h-a.org).

Several pharmaceutical manufacturers have published materials for patients.

Patients often have more information than you have provided, but there is a tendency to withhold it for fear that you might not appreciate it. Tell your patients that you not only welcome their questions but encourage them to seek out information from other sources.

Communicate Follow-Up Plans Effectively

Be sure the patient knows the follow-up plan, whether this is with you or another doctor. Patients need to know with whom to communicate if problems arise.

The Patient's Part

Although most of this chapter is directed to physicians, it is important to provide some information for patients since they need to be active participants in their care. Following are some useful tips for patients:

1. Prepare for your visit. Spend some time organizing your thoughts, and think about how to relate your symptoms and treatment to date. Bring notes if you need to. Take notes during the visit if this helps you.
2. Make the best use of everyone's time. You probably will not have all of the time you would like, and your doctor will not have all of the time he or she would like either. Try to focus on what motivated you to make this appointment, and present this complaint first. Do not wait until you are ready to leave before you present what is really bothering you.
3. Tell your story truthfully and do not minimize or exaggerate your symptoms.
4. Do not be eager to agree with any leading questions your doctor may ask. In an effort to speed up the process, the doctor may present you with a constellation of symptoms. You may feel that if you do not say you have all of them, an important diagnosis will be missed. This is not the case. It is important to present the symptoms of

your headache exactly as they are so that the doctor can make an accurate diagnosis.

5. Be assertive about getting medical attention if you believe your symptoms warrant it. If you call the office, explain your concerns and your need for an immediate appointment. Some offices make provision for urgent appointments. In emergency situations, head to an emergency department.

6. If you have "done your part" but are unhappy with the dynamic between you and your doctor, consider changing doctors (Baldwin and McInerney, 1996). People are often more inclined to change their mechanic than to change their doctor. Some say "Well, when something serious is wrong with me, I'll find a better doctor." Ask yourself if you can be sure that this doctor about whom you are not confident will know when something is seriously wrong.

SUMMARY

More has been learned about the pathogenesis and treatment of headache disorders in the last 10 years than at any other time in history. We are also better able to impart this knowledge to those who need treatment. When we are able to assign the same importance to both areas, the millions of people who suffer from headache will be assured a brighter future.

REFERENCES

Baldwin, F.D. and S. McInerney (1996). Doctor–patient relationships. In *Infomedicine: A Consumer's Guide to the Latest Medical Research*, pp. 43–59. New York, Little Brown and Co.

Baron, R.J. (1985). An introduction to medical phenomenology: I can't hear you when I'm listening. *Ann. Intern. Med.* 103:606–611.

Beckman, H.B. and R.M. Frankel (1984). The effect of physician behavior on the collection of data. *Ann. Intern. Med.* 101:692–696.

Bell, J.N. (1986). How much should your doctor tell you? *Today's Health July*:18–24.

Ben-Sira, Z. (1976). The function of the professional's affective behavior in client satisfaction. *J. Health Soc. Behav.* 17:3–11.

Bourhis, R.Y., S. Roth, and G. MacQueen (1989). Communication in the hospital setting: A survey of medical and everyday language use amongst patients, nurses and doctors. *Soc. Sci. Med.* 28:339–346.

Buckman, R. (1992). Basic communication skills. In *How to Break Bad News: A Guide for Health Care Professionals*, pp. 40–64. University of Toronto Press, Toronto.

Daley, J. (1993). Overcoming the barrier of words. In *Through the Patient's Eyes: Understanding and Promoting Patient-Centered Care* (M. Gerteis, S. Edgman-Levitan, J. Daley et al., eds.), pp. 72–95. Jossey-Bass, San Francisco.

Edmeads, J., H. Findlay, P. Tugwell et al. (1993). Impact of migraine and tension-type headache on life-style, consulting behavior, and medication use: A Canadian population survey. *Can. J. Neurol. Sci.* 20:131–137.

Epstein, A.M., W.C. Taylor, and G.R. Seage (1985). Effects of patients' socioeconomic status and physicians' training on practice on patient–doctor communication. *Am. J. Med.* 78:101–106.

Graham, J.R. (1987). The headache patient and the doctor. In *Psychiatric Aspects of Headache* (C.S. Adler, S.M. Adler, and R.C. Packard, eds.), pp. 34–40. Williams and Wilkins, Baltimore.

Hall, J.A., D.L. Roter, C.S. Rand et al. (1981). Communication of affect between patient and physician. *J. Health Soc. Behav.* 22:18–30.

Katz, J. (1984). *The Silent World of Doctor and Patient*. Free Press, New York.

Korsch, B.M., E.K. Gozzi, and V. Francis (1968). Gaps in doctor–patient communication. *Pediatrics* 42:855–870.

Lipkin, M. (1979). On lying to patients. *Newsweek June 4*:13.

MacGregor, E.A. (1997). The doctor and the migraine patient: Improving compliance. *Neurology* 48(Suppl. 3):S16–S20.

Osler, W. (1904). The master-word in medicine. In *Aequanimitas, with Other Addresses to Medical Students, Nurses and Practitioners of Medicine*. Blakiston, Philadelphia.

Osterhaus, J.T., R.J. Townsend, B. Gandek et al. (1994). Measuring the functional status and well being of patients with migraine headache. *Headache* 34:337–343.

Packard, R.C. (1979). What does the headache patient want? *Headache* 19:370–374.

Root, M.J. (1987). Communication barriers between older women and physicians. *Public Health Rep. July–August 101*(Suppl.):152–155.

Rosenbaum, E.E. (1988). *The Doctor*. Ballantine Books, New York.

Roter, D.L. and J.A. Hall. (1992). Models of the doctor–patient relationship. In *Doctors Talking with Patients/Patients Talking with Doctors: Im-*

proving Communication in Medical Visits, pp. 21–37. Auburn House, Westport, CT.

Roter, D.L., J.A. Hall, and N.R. Katz (1987). Relations between physicians' behaviors and analogue patients' satisfaction, recall and impressions. *Med. Care* 25:437–451.

Sheftell, F. (1996). The approach to the patient with headache. In *Office Practice of Neurology* (M.A. Samuels and S. Feske, eds.), pp. 1086–1096. Churchill Livingstone, New York.

Stewart, M.A. (1982). Factors affecting patient's compliance with doctor's advice. *Can. Fam. Physician* 28:1519–1526.

Stewart, W.F., R.B. Lipton, D.D. Celentano et al. (1992). Prevalence of migraine headache in the United States. Relation to age, income, race and other sociodemographic factors. *JAMA* 267:64–69.

Ventures, W. and P. Gordon (1990). Communication strategies in caring for the underserved. *J. Health Care Poor Underserved* 1:305–314.

Weisman, C.S. (1987). Communication between women and their health care providers: Research questions and unanswered questions. *Public Health Rep. July–August 101*(Suppl.): 147–151.

Index